BIOCHEMISTRY

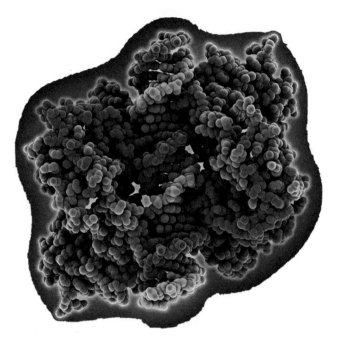

Cover Theme: *The tumour suppressor p53 (light pink, pink) complexed with DNA (blue, cyan). p53 prevents the proliferation of cells with damaged DNA and works to prevent cancer.*

BIOCHEMISTRY

As per the Competency-Based Medical Education Curriculum (NMC)

Sixth Edition

Pankaja Naik PhD
Professor
Department of Biochemistry
SMBT Institute of Medical Sciences and Research Center
Nashik, Maharashtra, India

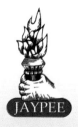

JAYPEE BROTHERS MEDICAL PUBLISHERS
The Health Sciences Publisher
New Delhi | London

Jaypee Brothers Medical Publishers (P) Ltd.

Headquarters

Jaypee Brothers Medical Publishers (P) Ltd
EMCA House
23/23-B, Ansari Road, Daryaganj
New Delhi - 110 002, India
Landline: +91-11-23272143, +91-11-23272703
+91-11-23282021, +91-11-23245672
Email: jaypee@jaypeebrothers.com

Corporate Office

Jaypee Brothers Medical Publishers (P) Ltd
4838/24, Ansari Road, Daryaganj
New Delhi 110 002, India
Phone: +91-11-43574357
Fax: +91-11-43574314
Email: jaypee@jaypeebrothers.com

Overseas Office

J.P. Medical Ltd
83 Victoria Street, London
SW1H 0HW (UK)
Phone: +44 20 3170 8910
Fax: +44 (0)20 3008 6180
Email: info@jpmedpub.com

Website: www.jaypeebrothers.com
Website: www.jaypeedigital.com

Inquiries for bulk sales may be solicited at: jaypee@jaypeebrothers.com

Biochemistry

First Edition: 2005
Second Edition: 2007
Third Edition: 2010
Fourth Edition: 2016
Fifth Edition: 2019
   Revised and Reprint: 2021

Sixth Edition: **2023**

ISBN: 978-93-5465-860-0

Printed at: Sterling Graphics Pvt. Ltd. India.

Dedicated to

My Students

_____

_____

_____

Preface to the Sixth Edition

It gives me immense pleasure to share with you an updated and highly improvised sixth edition of *"Biochemistry"*. In keeping with the previous competency-based medical education (CBME) content, I have revised the chapters and reorganized the content into thirty chapters to meet the needs of the student as per competency-based curriculum. In this edition many outdated topics have been removed.

To immediately draw students into the topic for study, each chapter opens with the competency and specific learning objectives as per the guidelines provided by National Medical Council of India (NMC) and various universities. I have thoroughly revised the learning objectives for every chapter and updated the text to ensure that all competencies and objectives are clearly addressed in a logical order.

Chapter overviews, illustrations, tables, figures, boxes, headings and subheadings make the content easier and more interesting to read. Revised self-assessment questions in the form of structured long essay questions (SLEQs), short essay questions (SEQs), short answer questions (SAQs), case vignette-based questions (CVBQs) and multiple choice questions (MCQs), have been provided at the end of each chapter to give an idea of the type of questions that are put across in the examination.

This is an attempt to make the book more acceptable for undergraduate medical students by presenting *"Biochemistry"*, sixth edition. I strongly feel that my students are my teachers and their suggestions and healthy criticism will be the great help in the future for the further improvement of this book. Their feedback gave me the opportunity to know the learner's needs in order to customize the knowledge that is reflected in this edition. I would like you to send me your feedback at *pankajanaik@gmail.com*.

Pankaja Naik

Acknowledgments

I express my profound gratitude to Honorable Shri Balasaheb Thorat (Former Minister of Revenue of Maharashtra and Trustee), and Honorable Dr Sudhirji Tambe (MLA and Trustee), SMBT Sevabhavi Trust, Nashik, Maharashtra, India, for their keen interest in all the academic activities of the faculty members. I find myself short of words to express my humble gratitude to Dr Harshal Tambe, the Dynamic Managing Trustee, SMBT Sevabhavi Trust, Nashik, Maharashtra, India, for his continuous support and encouragement. This edition would not have been possible without his relentless support and encouragement.

I wholeheartedly acknowledge the interest, and enthusiasm of Dr (Brig.) Vasant Pawar, Former Director, SMBT Sevabhavi Trust, Nashik, Maharashtra, India. He has always been supportive and a well-wisher in all my endeavors.

I extend my heartfelt thanks and sincere regards to Dr Pramod Ingle, Professor and Head, Department of Biochemistry, LTM Medical College and Lokmanya Tilak Municipal General Hospital, Sion, Mumbai, for giving his valued views for better presentation of this edition.

I am very grateful to Dr Manju Koshy, Professor and Head, Department of Biochemistry, SUT Academy of Medical Sciences, Thiruvananthapuram, Kerala; Dr Shashank Tyagi, Professor and Head, Department of Biochemistry, Government Medical College, Shivpuri, Madhya Pradesh; Dr Prashant Hisalkar, Professor and Head, Department of Biochemistry, Government Medical College, Dungarpur, Rajasthan; Dr Purnima Deysarkar, Professor and Head, Department of Biochemistry, Mahatma Gandhi Memorial Medical College, Indore, Madhya Pradesh; Dr Anupama Patne, Professor, All India Institute of Medical Sciences, Udaipur, Rajasthan, Dr Arti Karnik, Professor and Head, Department of Biochemistry, ACPM Medical College, Dhule, Maharashtra; Dr Sanjay Gaikwad, Professor and Head, Department of Biochemistry, Government Medical College, Jalgaon, Maharashtra; Dr Shamali Jungare, Associate Professor, Department of Biochemistry, Government Medical College, Jalgaon; for their professional support and providing balanced feedback in their friendly and cheerful style.

I am very grateful to the colleagues of my department, Ms Asmita Patil, Assistant Professor, Ms Shilpa Dhotre, Assistant Professor, Ms Anuja Mary Sabu, Assistant Professor, and Mr Ashok Katta, Assistant Professor for their valuable suggestions to the book.

I am grateful to all my colleagues and students from various institutes and universities across the world as reviewers. Their suggestions and thoughtful comments immensely helped me in maintaining excellence of the sixth edition.

My special thanks to Shri Jitendar P Vij (Group Chairman), Mr Ankit Vij (Group President) and Mr MS Mani (Group President) M/s Jaypee Brothers Medical Publishers (P) Ltd, New Delhi, India, for their vision and belief in this project and to make the book popular both at the national and international levels. I sincerely thank Dr Madhu Chaudhary (Director–Educational Publishing), Jaypee Brothers, Medical Publishers (P) Ltd, New Delhi, India, who inspired me all the time to take up the task and go ahead. I wish to thank Mr Chandrashekhar S Gawade (Zonal Manager–Mumbai) for his unfailing personal support the preparation of sixth edition of *"Biochemistry"*.

I am also thankful to Ms Pooja Bhandari (Production Head), Ms Sunita Katla (Executive Assistant to Group Chairman and Publishing Manager), Ms Samina Khan (Executive Assistant to Director–Educational Publishing), Dr Aditya Tayal (Team Leader–UG Publishing), Mr Rajesh Sharma (Production Coordinator), Ms Seema Dogra (Cover Visualizer), Ms Geeta Barik (Proofreader), Mr Akshay Thakur (Typesetter) and Gopal Kirola (Graphic Designer) of M/s Jaypee Brothers, Medical Publishers (P) Ltd New Delhi, India, for the efforts they put forth for the upcoming edition for medical students. Thanks for their careful attention, dedication in accomplishing this task on time. It was really nice to work with them.

I would like to acknowledge the hard work and dedication of Jaypee Brothers, Medical Publishers (P) Ltd New Delhi, India marketing department for supporting this book through its many editions.

Finally I want to thank my husband and my son for supporting me to complete the task successfully.

Contents

Competency Table

Competency number	Competency	Core (Y/N)	Chapter Number	Page Number
BI1.1	Describe the molecular and functional organization of a cell and its subcellular components.	Y	1	1–20
BI2.1	Explain fundamental concepts of enzyme, isoenzyme, alloenzyme, coenzyme and cofactors. Enumerate the main classes of IUBMB nomenclature.	Y	5	89–118
BI2.3	Describe and explain the basic principles of enzyme activity.	Y	5	89–118
BI2.4	Describe and discuss enzyme inhibitors as poisons and drugs and as therapeutic enzymes.	Y	5	89–118
BI2.5	Describe and discuss the clinical utility of various serum enzymes as markers of pathological conditions.	Y	5	89–118
BI2.6	Discuss use of enzymes in laboratory investigations (Enzyme-based assays)	Y	5	89–118
BI2.7	Interpret laboratory results of enzyme activities and describe the clinical utility of various enzymes as markers of pathological conditions.	Y	5	89–118
BI3.1	Discuss and differentiate monosaccharides, disaccharides and polysaccharides giving examples of main carbohydrates as energy fuel, structural element and storage in the human body.	Y	2	21–37
BI3.2	Describe the processes involved in digestion and assimilation of carbohydrates and storage.	Y	10	194–245
BI3.3	Describe and discuss the digestion and assimilation of carbohydrates from food.	Y	10	194–245
BI3.4	Define and differentiate the pathways of carbohydrate metabolism, (glycolysis, gluconeogenesis, glycogen metabolism, HMP shunt).	Y	10	194–245
BI3.5	Describe and discuss the regulation, functions and integration of carbohydrate along with associated diseases/disorders.	Y	10	194–245
BI3.6	Describe and discuss the concept of TCA cycle as a amphibolic pathway and its regulation.	Y	10	194–245
BI3.7	Describe the common poisons that inhibit crucial enzymes of carbohydrate metabolism (e.g., fluoride, arsenate).	Y	10	194–245
BI3.8	Discuss and interpret laboratory results of analytes associated with metabolism of carbohydrates.	Y	10	194–245
BI3.9	Discuss the mechanism and significance of blood glucose regulation in health and disease.	Y	10	194–245
BI3.10	Interpret the results of blood glucose levels and other laboratory investigations related to disorders of carbohydrate metabolism.	Y	10	194–245
BI4.1	Describe and discuss main classes of lipids (Essential/non-essential fatty acids, cholesterol and hormonal steroids, triglycerides, major phospholipids and sphingolipids) relevant to human system and their major functions.	Y	3	38–57
BI4.2	Describe the processes involved in digestion and absorption of dietary lipids and also the key features of their metabolism.	Y	11	246–292
BI4.3	Explain the regulation of lipoprotein metabolism and associated disorders.	Y	11	246–292
BI4.4	Describe the structure and functions of lipoproteins, their functions, interrelations and relations with atherosclerosis.	Y	11	246–292
BI4.5	Interpret laboratory results of analytes associated with metabolism of lipids.	Y	11	246–292
BI4.6	Describe the therapeutic uses of prostaglandins and inhibitors of eicosanoid synthesis.	Y	11	246–292

Competency number	Competency	Core (Y/N)	Chapter Number	Page Number
BI4.7	Interpret laboratory results of analytes associated with metabolism of lipids.	Y	11	246–292
BI5.1	Describe and discuss structural organization of proteins.	Y	4	58–88
BI5.2	Describe and discuss functions of proteins and structure-function relationships in relevant areas, e.g., hemoglobin and selected hemoglobinopathies.	Y	4	58–88
BI5.3	Describe the digestion and absorption of dietary proteins.	Y	12	293–332
BI5.4	Describe common disorders associated with protein metabolism.	Y	12	293–332
BI5.5	Interpret laboratory results of analytes associated with metabolism of proteins.	Y	12	293–332
BI6.1	Discuss the metabolic processes that take place in specific organs in the body in the fed and fasting states.	Y	13	333–345
BI6.2	Describe and discuss the metabolic processes in which nucleotides are involved.	Y	18	397–409
BI6.3	Describe the common disorders associated with nucleotide metabolism.	Y	18	397–409
BI6.4	Discuss the laboratory results of analytes associated with gout and Lesch Nyhan syndrome.	Y	18	397–409
BI6.5	Describe the biochemical role of vitamins in the body and explain the manifestations of their deficiency.	Y	9	160–193
BI6.6	Describe the biochemical processes involved in generation of energy in cells.	Y	8	147–159
BI6.7	Describe the processes involved in maintenance of normal pH, water and electrolyte balance of body fluids and the derangements associated with these.	Y	16 17	374–382, 383–396
BI6.8	Discuss and interpret results of Arterial Blood Gas (ABG) analysis in various disorders.	Y	17	383–396
BI6.9	Describe the functions of various minerals in the body, their metabolism and homeostasis.	Y	15	357–373
BI6.10	Enumerate and describe the disorders associated with mineral metabolism.	Y	15	357–373
BI6.11	Describe the functions of haem in the body and describe the processes involved in its metabolism and describe porphyrin metabolism.	Y	7 14	134–146 346–356
BI6.12	Describe the major types of haemoglobin and its derivatives found in the body and their physiological/pathological relevance.	Y	7	134–146
BI6.13	Describe the functions of the kidney, liver, thyroid and adrenal glands.	Y	25	498–524
BI6.14	Describe the tests that are commonly done in clinical practice to assess the functions of these organs (kidney, liver, thyroid and adrenal glands).	Y	25	498–524
BI6.15	Describe the abnormalities of kidney, liver, thyroid and adrenal glands.	Y	25	498–524
BI7.1	Describe the structure and functions of DNA and RNA and outline the cell cycle.	Y	6	119–133
BI7.2	Describe the processes involved in replication and repair of DNA and the transcription and translation mechanisms.	Y	19 20 21	410–425 426–438 439–452
BI7.3	Describe gene mutations and basic mechanism of regulation of gene expression.	Y	22	453–464
BI7.4	Describe applications of molecular technologies like recombinant DNA technology, PCR in the diagnosis and treatment of diseases with genetic basis.	Y	23	465–476
BI7.5	Describe the role of xenobiotics in disease.	Y	29	566–572
BI7.6	Describe the antioxidant defence systems in the body.	Y	30	573–580
BI7.7	Describe the role of oxidative stress in the pathogenesis of conditions such as cancer, complications of diabetes mellitus and atherosclerosis.	Y	30	573–580
BI8.1	Discuss the importance of various dietary components and explain importance of dietary fiber.	Y	24	477–497
BI8.2	Describe the types and causes of protein energy malnutrition and its effects.	Y	24	477–497
BI8.3	Provide dietary advice for optimal health in childhood and adult, in disease conditions like diabetes mellitus, coronary artery disease and in pregnancy.	Y	24	477–497
BI8.4	Describe the causes (including dietary habits), effects and health risks associated with being overweight/obesity.	Y	24	477–497
BI8.5	Summarize the nutritional importance of commonly used items of food including fruits and vegetables (macromolecules and its importance).	Y	24	477–497
BI9.1	List the functions and components of the extracellular matrix (ECM).	Y	26	525–532

Competency number	Competency	Core (Y/N)	Chapter Number	Page Number
BI9.2	Discuss the involvement of ECM components in health and disease.	Y	26	525–532
BI9.3	Describe protein targeting and sorting along with its associated disorders.	N	21	439–452
BI10.1	Describe the cancer initiation, promotion oncogenes and oncogene activation. Also focus on p53 and apoptosis.	Y	28	555–565
BI10.2	Describe various biochemical tumor markers and the biochemical basis of cancer therapy.	Y	28	555–565
BI10.3	Describe the cellular and humoral components of the immune system and describe the types and structure of antibody.	Y	27	533–554
BI10.4	Describe and discuss innate and adaptive immune responses, self/non-self recognition and the central role of T-helper cells in immune responses.	Y	27	533–554
BI10.5	Describe antigens and concepts involved in vaccine development.	Y	27	533–554
BI11.17	Explain the basis and rationale of biochemical tests done in the following conditions: • Myocardial infarction • Renal failure, gout • Proteinuria • Nephrotic syndrome • Edema • Jaundice • Liver diseases, pancreatitis, disorders of acid- base balance, thyroid disorders.	Y	25	498–524
BI11.23	Calculate energy content of different food Items, identify food items with high and low glycemic index and explain the importance of these in the diet.	Y	24	477–497
BI11.24	Enumerate advantages and/or disadvantages of use of unsaturated, saturated and trans fats in food.	Y	3	38–57

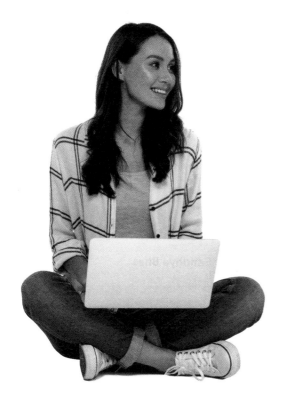

YOUR GUIDE AT EVERY STEP

Expert Knowledge Anytime, Anywhere

SCAN QR CODE FOR MORE DETAILS

WHY CHOOSE US

Video Lectures

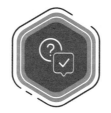

Self-Assessment Questions

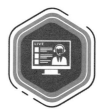

Top Faculty

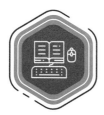

New CBME Curriculum

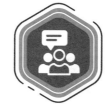

Clinical Case Based Approach

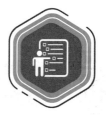

NEET Preparation

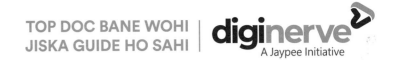
Video Lectures | Notes | Self-Assessment

UnderGrad Courses Available

Community Medicine
for UnderGrads — by Dr. Bratati Banerjee

Forensic Medicine & Toxicology
for UnderGrads — by Dr. Gautam Biswas

Medicine
for UnderGrads — by Dr. Archith Boloor

Microbiology
for UnderGrads — by Dr. Apurba S Sastry, Dr. Sandhya Bhat & Dr. Deepashree R

OBGYN
for UnderGrads — by Dr. K. Srinivas

Ophthalmology
for UnderGrads — by Dr. Parul Ichhpujani & Dr. Talvir Sidhu

Orthopaedics
for UnderGrads — by Dr. Vivek Pandey

Pathology
for UnderGrads — by Prof. Harsh Mohan, Prof. Ramadas Nayak & Dr. Debasis Gochhait

Pediatrics
for UnderGrads — by Dr. Santosh Soans & Dr. Soundarya M

Pharmacology
for UnderGrads — by Dr. Sandeep Kaushal & Dr. Nirmal George

Surgery
for UnderGrads — by Dr. Sriram Bhat M (SRB)

Cell, its Organelles and Transport Across Cell Membranes

Competency	Learning Objectives
BI 1.1: Describe the molecular and functional organization of a cell and its subcellular components.	1. Describe cell types and subcellular components. 2. Describe structure and functions of plasma membrane. 3. Describe structure and functions of subcellular organelles. 4. Describe structure and functions of cytoskeleton. 5. Describe cell fractionation and marker enzymes for different organelles. 6. Describe transport mechanisms across cell membrane.

◼ OVERVIEW

Biochemistry is the study of life on molecular level. Life is based on morphological units known as **cell**. Cells are often called the **"building blocks of life"**. Cells are the structural and functional units of all living organisms. Organisms can be classified as **unicellular** (consisting of a single cell such as bacteria) or **multicellular** (including plants and animals). Most unicellular organisms are classed as microorganisms.

In humans each cell type has unique structure; human cell types have certain architectural features in common, such as the **plasma membrane**, membrane around the nucleus and **organelles**, and a **cytoskeleton**. In this chapter, we review structure and function of organelles.

◼ CELL TYPES AND SUBCELLULAR COMPONENTS

Cells are of two types: **eukaryotic**, which contain a nucleus, and **prokaryotic**, which do not. Prokaryotes are **single-celled** organisms, while eukaryotes can be either **single-celled** or **multicellular**.

Prokaryotic Cells (Greek: pro: before, karyon: nucleus)

Prokaryotes include **bacteria** and **archaea**. Prokaryotic cells are simpler and smaller than eukaryotic cells, and **lack a nucleus**, and other membrane-bound organelles. The **DNA** of a prokaryotic cell consists of a single **circular**

chromosome. The nuclear region in the cytoplasm is called the **nucleoid**.

Archaea and **Bacteria** can be distinguished on genetic and biochemical grounds.

i. **Archaea** lives in extreme environments: salt lakes hot springs, highly acidic bogs, and the ocean depths. Archaea may be the most primitive of the groups.

ii. **Bacteria** live in soils, surface waters, and the tissues of other living or decaying organisms.

Components of Prokaryotic Cell

Cell envelope: It generally consisting of a plasma membrane covered by a **cell wall** which, for some bacteria, may be further covered by a third layer called a **capsule**. The envelope gives **rigidity** to the cell and separates the interior of the cell from its environment, serving as a protective filter. Some eukaryotic cells (plant cells and fungal cells) also have a cell wall.

- **Cytoplasm:** It contains the **genome (DNA)** and **ribosomes**. The DNA is condensed in a **nucleoid**. The nucleoid is not separated from the cytoplasm by a membrane. Prokaryotes can carry **extrachromosomal DNA** elements called **plasmids**, which are usually **circular**. Plasmids encode additional genes, such as **antibiotic resistance genes**.

- **Flagella and pili:** Flagella and pili project from the cell's surface. These are structures (not present in all prokaryotes) made of proteins that facilitate movement and communication between cells **(Figure 1.1)**.

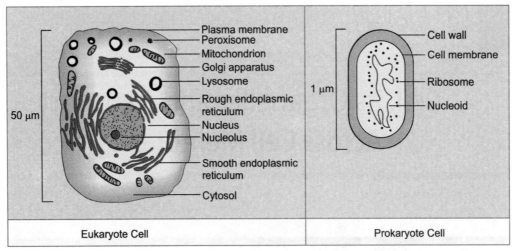

Figure 1.1: Cell structure of eukaryotic and prokaryotic cell.

Eukaryotic Cells (eu: good, karyon: nucleus)

Eukaryote include single cell organism such as yeast, fungi and multicellular plants and animals. Their cell volume is 1,000 to 10,000 times larger than most prokaryotic cells. The main distinguishing feature of eukaryotes as compared to prokaryotes is:

- Eukaryotes have a defined nucleus with a well-defined membrane that contains the bulk of the cell's DNA.
- They also have intracellular organelles surrounded by membrane. These intracellular membrane systems establish distinct cellular compartments. By compart-mentalization, different chemical reactions that require different environments can occur simultaneously.

There are other differences in chemical composition and biochemical activities between eukaryotes and prokaryotes. As an example:

- Prokaryotes do not contain **histones**, a highly conserved class of protein in all eukaryotes that complex with DNA.
- There are also differences in enzyme content and in **ribosomes**, involved in biosynthesis of proteins.

Table 1.1 and **Figure 1.1** describe some of the major structural features of the prokaryote and eukaryote cells

What are Viruses?

- ❖ **Viruses** are not living organism in the sense that cells are. Viruses are not classified as cells and therefore are neither unicellular nor multicellular organisms. They are incapable of replicate themselves outside their host cells and have virtually no biochemical activities of their own.
- ❖ Viruses are supramolecular complexes of nucleic acid, either DNA or RNA encapsulated in a protein coat, and in some instances, surrounded by a membrane envelope.
- ❖ Viruses are not alive; they are not even cellular. Instead, they are packaged bits of genetic material that can parasitize in order to reproduce.
- ❖ The protein coat serves to protect the nucleic acid and allow it to gain entry to the cells that are its specific hosts.

Contd...

Contd...

- ❖ Viruses infecting bacteria are called **bacteriophages** ("bacteria eaters"): different viruses infect animal cells and plants cells.
- ❖ Often they cause disintegration, or lysis of the cells they have infected. It is these cytolytic properties that are the basis of viral disease. In certain circumstances, the viral nucleic acid may integrate into the host chromosome and transform cells into a cancerous state.

Components of Eukaryotic Cell

All eukaryotic cells possess characteristic structure and organelles. A cell has three major components.

1. **Plasma membrane (cell membrane).**

TABLE 1.1: Structural features of eukaryotes and prokaryotes.

Organelle	Eukaryotes	Prokaryotes
Nucleus	Present	No define nucleus. DNA present but not separated from rest cell
Plasma membrane	Present	Present
Mitochondria	Present	Absent. Enzymes for oxidation reactions located on plasma membrane
Endoplasmic reticulum	Present	Absent
Ribosomes	Present 50S and 30S	Present 60S and 40S
DNA	Linear with histone	Circular
Chromosomes	More than one chromosome	Single chromosome
Cytoplasm	Contains various membrane bound organelles, such as mitochondria, lysosomes, peroxisomes and Golgi apparatus	Undifferentiated

2. **Cytoplasm with its organelles**.
   - Endoplasmic reticulum
   - Golgi apparatus
   - Mitochondria
   - Lysosomes
   - Peroxisomes
3. **Nucleus**

Table 1.2 shows major biochemical functions of subcellular organelles of the eukaryotic cell.

STRUCTURE AND FUNCTIONS OF CELL MEMBRANE

The cell membrane also called the **plasma membrane**, which envelops the cell. In animals, the plasma membrane is the outer boundary of the cell, while in plants and prokaryotes it is usually covered by a **cell wall**. This membrane serves to separate and protect a cell from its surrounding environment.

Structure of Cell Membrane

Most membranes composed primarily of **lipids** and **proteins**. The relative proportions of protein and lipid vary with the type of membrane, reflecting the diversity of biological roles. Plasma membrane consists of a **double layer of phospholipids**. Hence, the layer is called a **lipid bilayer (Figure 1.2)**. The hydrophobic portions of the phospholipid molecules, are repelled by water but are mutually attracted

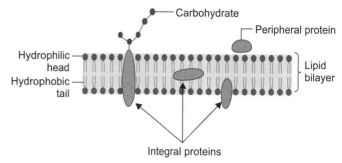

Figure 1.2: The basic organization of biological membrane.

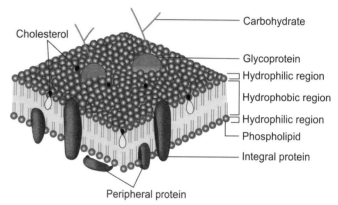

Figure 1.3: The fluid mosaic model of cell membrane.

to one another, and have natural tendency to attach to one another in the middle of the membrane, as shown in **Figure 1.2**.

The cell membrane is sometimes referred to as a **fluid mosaic membrane (Figure 1.3)** because it consists of a variety (mosaic) of proteins and lipids. The lipids present in the membrane are in fluid form that allows the flexibility of the membrane without disturbing the structural integrity. The fluidity of the membrane is mainly dependent on the lipid composition of the membrane. The membrane proteins are loosely attached and float in fluid phospholipid bilayer. Most of the interactions among its components are noncovalent, leaving individual lipid and protein molecules free to move laterally in the plane of the membrane. The approximate composition of cell membrane is:

- Protein: 55%
- Phospholipids: 25%
- Cholesterol: 13%
- Other lipids: 4%
- Carbohydrate: 3%

The different types of membrane include cell membrane, nuclear membrane, membrane of the endoplasmic reticulum, and membrane of the mitochondria, lysosomes and Golgi apparatus.

Membrane Lipids

Membrane Phospholipids

The basic **lipid bilayer** is composed of **phospholipid** molecules which are **amphipathic** (partly **hydrophobic**

TABLE 1.2: Biochemical functions of subcellular organelles of the eukaryotic cell.	
Subcellular organelles	*Function*
Plasma membrane	Transport of molecules in and out of cell, receptors for hormones and neurotransmitters
Lysosome	Intracellular digestion of macromolecules and hydrolysis of nucleic acid, protein, glycosaminoglycans, glycolipids, sphingolipids
Golgi apparatus	Post-translational modification and sorting of proteins and export of proteins
Rough endoplasmic reticulum	Biosynthesis of protein and secretion
Nucleus	Storage of DNA, replication and repair of DNA, transcription and post-transcriptional processing
Peroxisomes	Metabolism of hydrogen peroxide and oxidation of long chain fatty acids
Nucleolus	Synthesis of rRNA and formation of ribosomes
Mitochondrion	ATP synthesis, site for tricarboxylic acid cycle, fatty acid oxidation, oxidative phosphorylation, part of urea cycle and part of heme synthesis
Smooth endoplasmic reticulum	Biosynthesis of steroid hormones and phospholipids, metabolism of foreign compounds (cytochrome P450 detoxification)
Cytosol	Site for glycolysis, pentose phosphate pathway, part of gluconeogenesis, urea cycle and heme synthesis, purine and pyrimidine nucleotide synthesis

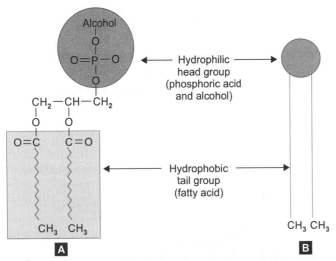

Figures 1.4A and B: Structure of phospholipid: (A) Common glycerophospholipid; (B) Diagrammatic representation of phospholipid.

and partly **hydrophilic**). One end of each phospholipid molecule (head group) is soluble in water; (hydrophilic). The other end (tail group) is soluble only in fats; (hydrophobic). The phosphate end of the phospholipid is hydrophilic and the free fatty acid portion is hydrophobic **(Figures 1.4A and B)**.

The phospholipid molecules spontaneously organize themselves in a **bilayer (Figure 1.2)**; with the hydrophobic tails facing the interior of the bilayer forming a hydrophobic region held together by intermolecular forces between the tails. The hydrophilic heads form a hydrophilic region on either side of the bilayer that can interact with both the water-based cytoplasm and the exterior of the cell. The principle phospholipids in the membrane are:

- **Glycerophospholipids:** Phosphatidylcholine, phosphatidylethanolamine, and phosphatidylserine
- **Sphinogophospholipid:** Sphingomyelin.

The lipid composition varies among different cell types, with **phosphatidylcholine** being the major plasma membrane phospholipid in most cell types. Each cell type and the organelles of each cell type have a characteristic set of membrane lipids. Plasma membrane for example, is enriched in **cholesterol** and contains no detectable **cardiolipin**; mitochondrial membrane is very low in cholesterol and sphingolipids but that contain cardiolipin.

Membrane Cholesterol

The cholesterol molecules in the membrane are also lipid in nature. Cholesterol, which is incorporated between the phospholipids, maintains **membrane fluidity**. The fluidity of a membrane depends on composition of lipids and the degree of unsaturation. The major determinant is its **cholesterol-phospholipid ratio**. In eukaryotes, the ratio is about 1:1. Higher cholesterol content reduces the fluidity of the membrane.

The changes in membrane fluidity may affect proteins that span the membrane (integral proteins), such as ion channels and receptors for neurotransmitters involved conducting the nerve impulse.

Functions of the Lipid Bilayer

- Cell membrane produces a **permeability barrier** between the interstitial fluid and the cytoplasm.
- The permeability of substance depends on whether it is lipid-soluble or water-soluble. Lipid-soluble substances such as oxygen, carbon dioxide, and alcohol can pass easily through the cell membrane, whereas water-soluble substances, such as ions, glucose and urea cannot pass easily.

Factors that influence bilayer fluidity

❖ **The length of the fatty acid tail:** Longer the phospholipid tails, the more interactions between the tails are possible and the less fluid the membrane will be.

❖ **Temperature:** As temperature increases, so does phospholipid bilayer fluidity. At lower temperatures, phospholipids in the bilayer do not have as much kinetic energy and they cluster together more closely, increasing intermolecular interactions and decreasing membrane fluidity. At high temperatures, the opposite process occurs, phospholipids have enough kinetic energy to overcome the intermolecular forces holding the membrane together, which increases membrane fluidity.

❖ **Cholesterol content of the bilayer:** Cholesterol has a somewhat more complicated relationship with membrane fluidity. It is a buffer that helps keep membrane fluidity from getting too high or too low at high and low temperatures. At low temperatures, phospholipids tend to cluster together, but steroids in the phospholipid bilayer fill in between the phospholipids, disrupting their intermolecular interactions and increasing fluidity. At high temperatures, the phospholipids are further apart. In this case, cholesterol in the membrane has the opposite effect and pulls phospholipids together, increasing intermolecular forces and decreasing fluidity.

❖ **The degree of saturation of fatty acids tails:** Phospholipid tails can be saturated or unsaturated. The terms saturated and unsaturated refer to whether or not double bonds are present between the carbons in the fatty acid tails. Saturated tails have no double bonds and as a result have straight, unkinked tails. Unsaturated tails have double bonds, and as a result, have crooked, kinked tails.

Membrane Proteins

The protein composition of membrane from different sources varies even more widely than their lipid composition, reflecting functional specialization. Two types of membrane proteins differ in their association with the membrane. Most of the membrane proteins are **glycoproteins**.

- **Integral membrane proteins:** Integral proteins that are protruding all the way through the membrane. They are very firmly associated with the lipid bilayer.

- **Peripheral membrane proteins:** Peripheral proteins that are attached only to one surface of the membrane and do not penetrate all the way through. Peripheral protein molecules are often attached to the integral proteins. They are associated with the membrane **through electrostatic interactions** and **hydrogen bonding** with the hydrophilic domains of integral proteins and with polar head groups of membrane lipids.

Functions of Membrane Proteins

- Integral membrane proteins function primarily as **channels (pores)** through which water molecules and water-soluble substances, especially ions, can diffuse between extracellular and intracellular fluids. These protein channels have also selective properties that allow preferential diffusion of some substance over others.
- Other integral proteins act as **carrier proteins** transporting substances that otherwise could not penetrate the lipid bilayer.
- These proteins even transport substances in the direction opposite to their electrochemical gradients for diffusion, which is called **"active transport"**.
- They can also serve as **receptors** for hormones and neurotransmitter.
- Integral proteins spanning the cell membrane provide a means of conveying information about the environment to the cell interior.
- Peripheral proteins function almost entirely as enzymes or as controllers of transport of substances through the cell membrane **"pores"**.
- One of the main roles of peripheral proteins is to direct and maintain both the intracellular cytoskeleton and components of the extracellular matrix.

Clinical Conditions Associated with Membrane Transport Protein

Multiple drug resistance
- ❖ In human **multiple drug transporter (MDR1) protein** (an integral membrane protein), called **P-glycoprotein** is responsible for resistance to some antitumor drugs.
- ❖ Over production of MDR1 is associated with treatment failure in cancers. When tumor cells are exposed to chemotherapeutic drugs such as **Adriamycin**, **Doxorubicin** and **Vinblastine**, MDR1 transporter protein pumps these drugs out of the cell before the drug can exert its effect and thus prevents its therapeutic effect.
- ❖ Highly selective **inhibitors** of multidrug transporters, which enhance the effectiveness of antitumor drugs that are otherwise pumped out of the tumor cells, are the objects of current drug discovery and design.

Cystic fibrosis
- ❖ Cystic fibrosis is caused by defects in a membrane bound protein called **cystic fibrosis transmembrane conductance regulator (CFTR) protein** which functions as a channel for chloride ions.
- ❖ The defect in CFTR is due to mutation. In mutation, there is deletion of **phenylalanine residue** at position **508** of the CFTR, which causes improper protein folding. Most of this protein is then degraded and its normal function is lost.

Membrane Carbohydrates

Membrane carbohydrates occur in combination with proteins or lipids in the form of **glycoproteins** or **glycolipids**. Some of the proteins and lipids on the external surface of the membrane contain short chains of **carbohydrate (oligosaccharides)** that extent into the aqueous medium. As well as many other carbohydrate compounds called **proteoglycans** are loosely attached to the outer surface of the cell. Thus the entire outside surface of the cell often has a loose carbohydrate coat called the **glycocalyx**. Carbohydrate constitutes 2–10% of the weight of cell membrane.

Functions of Membrane Carbohydrates

- Many of the carbohydrates have a negative electrical charge, which gives most cells an overall negative surface charge that repels other negative objects and restricts the uptake of hydrophobic compounds.
- The glycocalyx of some cell attaches to the glycocalyx of other cells, thus attaching cells to one another.
- Many of the carbohydrate act as **hormone receptor** such as insulin
- Some carbohydrate moieties involved into immune reactions.

> As the individual lipid and proteins of the plasma membrane are not covalently linked, the entire structure is flexible, allowing changes in the shape and size of the cell. The two sides of mammalian plasma membranes have different chemical composition and functions.

Functions of Plasma Membrane

- The plasma membrane maintains the physical integrity of the cell by preventing the contents of the cell from leaking into the outside fluid environment and at the same time facilitating the entry of nutrients, inorganic ions and most other charged or polar compounds from the outside.
- The functions of the plasma membrane are coordinated by specialized adhesion receptors called **integrins**. Integrins are integral transmembrane proteins. Integrins represent important cell receptors that regulate fundamental cellular process; such as attachment, movement, growth and differentiation.

> Because integrins play vital roles in the functions of the plasma membranes, they are also involved in many disease processes. They involved in the **initiation** and **progression of neoplasia, tumor, metastasis, immune dysfunction viral infection** and **osteoporosis**.

STRUCTURE AND FUNCTIONS OF SUBCELLULAR ORGANELLES

Cytoplasm is the internal volume bounded by the plasma membrane. The clear fluid portion of the cytoplasm in which the organelles are suspended is called **cytosol**. This contains mainly dissolved **proteins**, **electrolytes** and **glucose**. Five important organelles that are suspended in the cytosol are:

1. Endoplasmic reticulum
2. Golgi apparatus
3. Mitochondria
4. Lysosomes
5. Peroxisomes

Endoplasmic Reticulum (ER)

The endoplasmic reticulum is the interconnected, folded network of tubular structures in the cytoplasm. A portion of the endoplasmic reticulum has **ribosomes** bound to it, which give it a rough appearance in contrast with smooth endoplasmic reticulum which is devoid of ribosomes (**Figures 1.5A and B**). Endoplasmic reticulum and Golgi apparatus are involved in formation of other cellular organelles such as **lysosomes** and **peroxisomes**.

> ❖ The ribosomes which are not attached to the endoplasmic reticulum are **"free"** in the cell usually attached to the **cytoskeleton**. These ribosomes synthesize proteins used intracellularly and remain within the cell, either within the cytoplasm or directed to organelles bounded by a double membrane, such as the nucleus and mitochondria.
> ❖ During cell fractionation, the endoplasmic reticulum network is disrupted and membrane reseals to form small vesicles called **microsomes**; which can be isolated by differential centrifugation. Microsomes as such, do not occur in cell.

Functions of Rough Endoplasmic Reticulum

- The **rough endoplasmic reticulum** is the site for **synthesis of proteins** that are destined to be exported from the cell. Virtually all integral membrane proteins of the cell, except those located in the membranes of mitochondria are formed by ribosomes bound to the endoplasmic reticulum.
- The endoplasmic reticulum also has mechanisms for maintaining the quality of the proteins synthesized. The endoplasmic reticulum has three different sensor molecules that monitor the amounts of improperly folded proteins that accumulate.

Functions of Smooth Endoplasmic Reticulum

- **Smooth endoplasmic reticulum** is involved in **lipid synthesis** and contains enzymes termed **cytochromes**

P_{450} that catalyze hydroxylation of a variety of endogenous and exogenous compounds.

- These enzymes are important in **biosynthesis of steroid hormones** and removal of **toxic substances**

> ❖ Protein misfolding and aggregation are associated with **neurological diseases**.
> ❖ **Parkinson's disease, Alzheimer's disease, Huntington disease,** and **transmissible spongiform encephalopathy** (prion disease), are associated with improperly folded proteins due to mutation.
> ❖ All of these diseases result in the deposition of protein aggregates, called **amyloid** proteins. These diseases are consequently referred to as **amyloidosis**.
> ❖ Accumulation of nonfunctional proteins in ER contributes to a situation referred to as **Endoplasmic Reticulum Stress**, which is associated with **diabetes** and **cancer** as well as **neurodegenerative diseases**.

Golgi Apparatus

The Golgi (named for its discoverer **Camillo Golgi**) apparatus is a flat, membranous sac. The Golgi apparatus is also referred to as **Golgi complex**. In Golgi apparatus proteins are processed, modified and prepared for export from the cell. It works in association with endoplasmic reticulum, where proteins for certain destinations are synthesized (**Figure 1.6**).

As shown in **Figure 1.6**, small transport vesicles (ER vesicles) continually pinch of from the ER and shortly thereafter fuse with the Golgi apparatus. In this way, substances entrapped in the ER vesicles are transported from the ER to Golgi apparatus. The transported substances are then processed in the Golgi apparatus to form **lysosomes**, **peroxisomes**, secretory vesicles and other cytoplasmic components.

Functions of Golgi Apparatus

The Golgi apparatus participates in **post-translational modification** of proteins: such as complex branched chain oligosaccharide addition, sulfation and phosphorylation.

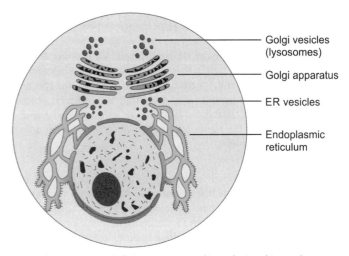

Figure 1.6: A Golgi apparatus and its relationship to the endoplasmic reticulum and nucleus.

Golgi vesicles (lysosomes)
Golgi apparatus
ER vesicles
Endoplasmic reticulum

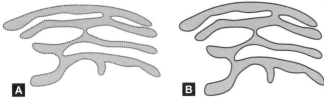

Figures 1.5A and B: Structure of endoplasmic reticulum. (A) Rough or granular endoplasmic reticulum; (B) Smooth or a granular endoplasmic reticulum.

Proteins which are synthesized in the endoplasmic reticulum passed through layers of the Golgi apparatus where enzymes in Golgi membranes catalyze transfer of carbohydrate units to proteins to form **glycoproteins** or to lipids to make **glycolipids**, a process that is important in determining the proteins eventual destination. The modified proteins are then sorted, packaged and transported to destination inside or outside the cell. Golgi apparatus plays the role of **post office mail sorting room**, the mail in this case being newly synthesized proteins.

Mitochondrion (Power House of Cell)

Mitochondria are organelles in **eukaryotic cells** that supply **energy** for all cellular metabolic activities. The number of mitochondria in cells varies as do their energy needs. Muscle cells of the **heart** contain the **largest number of mitochondria**. Mitochondria are called **Power plant** of the cell, since they generate most of the cell's energy in the form of **ATP**. **Erythrocytes** are an exception which derive their ATP from glycolysis due to **lack of mitochondria**. Each mitochondrion is bounded by **two membranes**.

- The relatively **porous** smooth **outer membrane** is permeable to most molecules.
- The **inner membrane**, which is **impermeable to ions** and a variety of organic molecules. The inner membrane projects inwards into folds that are called **cristae** (**Figure 1.7**).
- Together, both membranes create two separate compartments: the **intermembrane space** (between the outer and the inner membranes) and the **matrix** which is bounded by the inner membrane. The matrix side and the cytoplasmic side also called the **N** and **P** sides respectively, because the membrane potential is **negative** on the matrix side and **positive** on the cytoplasmic side.
- The outer and inner membranes both contain mechanism for translocation of specific proteins. There is variety of transmembrane system in the inner membrane for translocation of various metabolites.
- The outer membrane is permeable to most small molecules and ions because it contains many **mitochondrial porin** (pore forming protein) also known as **voltage-dependent anion channel (VDAC)** that permit access to most molecules. In contrast inner membrane is

impermeable to nearly all ions and polar molecules. Many transporters shuttles metabolites such as ATP, pyruvate, and citrate across the inner mitochondrial membrane.

> Mitochondrial DNA is usually described as being circular, but the recent research suggests that the mitochondrial DNA of many organisms may be linear.

Functions of Mitochondria

- The intermembrane space contains several **enzymes** involved in **nucleotide metabolism**.
- Whereas, the gel-like matrix (mitosol) consists of high concentration of enzymes required for the metabolic pathways of **oxidation of pyruvate** produced by glycolysis, fatty acids, and amino acids and some reactions in **biosynthesis of urea** and **heme**. The mitochondrial matrix is the site of most of the reactions of the **citric acid cycle** and **fatty acid oxidation**.
- Oxidative phosphorylation takes place in the inner mitochondrial membrane. Components of **electron transport** system and **oxidative phosphorylation** that are responsible for the synthesis of **ATP** are embedded in inner membrane. Also present are a series of proteins that are responsible for the transport of specific molecules and ions.
- Mitochondria also have a requisite machinery to catalyze **protein synthesis**. Mitochondria contain their own DNA, (mtDNA), which in human encodes 13 respiratory chain proteins, as well as small and large ribosomal RNAs and enough tRNAs to translate all codons
- In recent years, mitochondria have also been recognized as key regulators of apoptosis. Mitochondria have a key role in aging; cytochrome c, a component of the mitochondrial electron transport chain, is an initiator of **apoptosis**.

Genetic Diseases of Mitochondria

There are several hundred genetic diseases of mitochondrial function. Mutations in mtDNA are responsible for a number of diseases called **mitochondriopathies** that can be inherited. Mutations in mitochondrial DNA are transmitted from an affected mother to all her children but not from an affected father.

> It is worth noting that inheritance of mtDNA defects is through a maternal lineage, as mitochondria are present in large numbers in the ovum that forms the zygote. Male mitochondria are not present in the head of the sperm that fertilizes the ovum.

Many mitochondrial diseases involve **skeletal muscle** and **central nervous** systems. In some patients, exercise intolerance and muscle fatigue are due to mutations in mtDNA. Mitochondrial DNA damage may occur due to free radicals (superoxides) formed in the mitochondria.

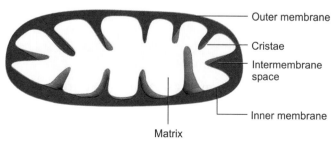

Outer membrane
Cristae
Intermembrane space
Inner membrane
Matrix

Figure 1.7: Structure of mitochondria.

- The first disease to be identified as due to a mutation of mitochondrial DNA was **Leber's Hereditary Optic Neuropathy, (LHON)** which leads to sudden blindness in early adulthood caused by degeneration of the optic nerve. Mutation in patients with this disease is a **single base substitution** that replaces an **arginine** residue in one of the subunits of **NADH-Q reductase** with **histidine**. Mutation impairs electron flow through the respiratory chain and reduces ATP synthesis. They lead to blindness because the optic nerve has a high energy demand and depends almost entirely on oxidative phosphorylation for its ATP supply.
- It has been suggested that a single mutation for a mitochondrial tRNA leads to **hypertension, high blood cholesterol** and **decreased level of plasma Mg^{2+}**.
- Mutation in mitochondrial rRNA results in antibiotic (such as streptomycin, paromomycin, and gentamycin) induced deafness.
- Organs that are highly dependent on oxidative phosphorylation, such as the nervous system and the heart, are most vulnerable to mutations in mtDNA.

Lysosomes

Lysosomes are organelles formed from Golgi apparatus and dispersed throughout the cytoplasm. The lysosomes are membrane bounded sacs containing **hydrolytic enzymes**. Lysosomes contain as many as forty different hydrolytic enzymes. The hydrolytic enzymes found in lysosomes include **proteases, nucleases, glycosidases, lipases, phosphatases and sulfatases**. All these enzymes function at acidic pH, so pH of lysosome matrix is maintain at about 5.

Among all organelles of the cytoplasm, the lysosomes have the thickest covering membrane to prevent the enclosed hydrolytic enzymes from coming in contact with other substances in the cell and therefore prevent their digestive actions. Disruption of the lysosomal membrane within cells leads to cellular digestion. Various pathological conditions such as **arthritis, allergic responses, several muscular diseases**, and drug-induced tissue destruction have been attributed to release of lysosomal enzymes.

Functions of Lysosomes

- Lysosomes are involved in digestion of intra- and extra-cellular substances that must be removed. Substances destined to be degraded are identified and taken up by lysosomes through endocytosis. Products of lysosomal digestion are released from lysosomes and are reutilized by the cell. Indigestible material called residual bodies are removed from the cell by exocytosis.
- During development, lysosomes play an important role in the formation of specialized tissues such as fingers and toes. For example, lysosomes digest the webbed tissues that join fingers and toes in the embryo.

Lysosomal Storage Disease

Genetic defects in lysosomal enzymes, or in proteins such as the **mannose-6-phosphate receptors** required for targeting the enzyme to the lysosome, lead to an abnormal accumulation of undigested material that may be converted to residual bodies particularly in neuronal cells. Genetic diseases such as the **Tay-Sachs disease** (an accumulation of partially digested gangliosides in lysosomes), and Pompe's disease (an accumulation of glycogen particles in lysosomes) are caused by the absence or deficiency of specific lysosomal enzymes. Such diseases, in which a lysosomal function is compromised, are known as **lysosomal storage disease**.

The lysosomal enzymes are synthesized at the rough ER and become glycosylated in the ER and Golgi apparatus. In the Golgi apparatus they finally acquire a mannose-6-phosphate residue on some of their oligosaccharides. Mannose-6-phosphate is a molecular tag that acts like a postal address to route the enzymes to the lysosomes. A partial list of lysosomal enzymes is given in **Table 1.3**. The enzyme content of lysosomes varies in different tissues and depends on specific tissue functions.

> In a number of lysosomal storage disease, individual lysosomal enzymes are missing, leading to accumulation of the substrate of the missing enzymes. The lysosomes become enlarged with undigested material, thereby interfering with normal cells function. One such case is **I-cell disease** also called **mucolipidosis II**, in which lysosomes contain dense **inclusion bodies** (**hence I cell**) of undigested glycosaminoglycan and glycolipids. These inclusions are due to missing of enzymes responsible for degradation of glycosaminoglycan from affected lysosomes. However, abnormally high levels of these enzymes are present in blood and urine.
>
> In **I cell disease** mannose residue of enzyme lacks phosphate. Mannose-6-phosphate directs enzymes from the Golgi complex to lysosomes where they normally function. Due to improper glycosylation of enzyme, they are exported (mistargeted) instead of being sequestered in lysosomes. I cell disease is characterized by sever **psychomotor retardation** and **skeletal deformities**.

Peroxisomes

Peroxisomes (organelles having ability to produce or utilize hydrogen peroxide) are similar to lysosome in that they are membranous sacs containing enzymes. The enzyme content of cellular peroxisome varies according to the need of the tissue. Liver peroxisomes contain three important detoxification enzymes; **catalase, peroxidase** and **D-amino acid oxidase**.

Functions of Peroxisomes

- Peroxisomes contain enzymes that are used for **detoxification** rather than for hydrolysis.
- Peroxisomes also participate in degradation of very long chain fatty acids and synthesis of **glycerolipids, plasmalogens** and **isoprenoids**.

TABLE 1.3: Lysosomal enzymes.

Type of enzymes	Specific substrate
Polysaccharide hydrolyzing Enzymes	
α-glucosidase	Glycogen
α-fucosidase	Membrane fucose
β-galactosidase	Galactosides
α-mannosidase	Mannosides
β-glucuronidase	Glucuronides
Hyaluronidase	Hyaluronic acid and chondroitin sulfates
Lysozyme	Bacterial cell wall
Protein hydrolyzing enzymes	
Cathepsins	Proteins
Collagenase	Collagen
Elastase	Elastin
Peptidases	Peptides
Nucleic acid hydrolyzing enzymes	
Ribonuclease	RNA
Deoxyribonucleases	DNA
Lipid hydrolyzing enzymes	
Lipases	Triacylglycerol and cholesterol esters
Esterase	Fatty acid esters
Phospholipase	Phospholipids
Phosphatases	
Phosphatase	Phosphomonoesters
Phosphodiesterase	Phosphodiester
Sulfatase	
Chondroitin sulfatase	Heparan sulfate
Arylsulfatase B	Dermatan sulfate

- In peroxisomes, a number of molecules which are not metabolized elsewhere are oxidized by enzymes by using molecular oxygen directly and produce hydrogen peroxide (H_2O_2). Hydrogen peroxide is destroyed further by catalase and peroxidases. By having both peroxide producing and peroxide utilizing enzymes in one compartment, cells protect themselves from the toxicity of hydrogen peroxide

Peroxisomal Diseases

Several diseases are associated with peroxisomes. Peroxisomal diseases are caused by mutations that affect either the synthesis of functional peroxisomal enzymes or their incorporation into peroxisomes. Defects in peroxisome lead to disorders such as:

Adrenoleukodystrophy: Mutation in the ATP-binding cassette (ABC) transport membrane protein of a fatty acid in the peroxisomal membrane

Zellweger's syndrome: Defective formation of peroxisomes, characterized by accumulation of long chain, **saturated**, **unbranched fatty acids** in liver and CNS, server neurological symptoms and early death.

Refsum's disease: Deficiency of **phytanoyl-CoA hydroxy-lase** required for α-oxidation of branched chain fatty acid; characterized by **peripheral neuropathy**, **ataxia** and **retinitis pigmentosa**.

Nucleus

Nucleus is the control center of the cell; it contains the DNA organized into chromosomes which carry genetic information. The nucleus is surrounded by a double membrane called **nuclear envelope**. The outer membrane is fused with the endoplasmic reticulum at multiple sites. **Nuclear pores** (multiprotein complexes) occur at points where the outer and inner membranes are connected **(Figure 1.8)**. Nuclear pores permits controlled movement of particles and large molecules between the nuclear matrix and the cytoplasm.

It is now considered that the nuclear envelope plays important roles other than just as a barrier between the nuclear matrix and the cytoplasm. The space enclosed by the nuclear envelope is called **nucleoplasm;** within this the **nucleolus** is present. Nucleolus is an organized structure of DNA, RNA and protein. Nucleolus is a major site of **RNA synthesis** and the site of assembly of ribosome.

The remaining nuclear DNA is dispersed throughout the nucleoplasm in the form of chromatin fibers). Chromatins are complexes of DNA with specific proteins such as histones. In the nucleus, these chromatin fibers are associated with nuclear **lamina**, a fibrous network made of **three proteins**, **A**, **B**, and **C**; lying beneath the inner nuclear membranes. At mitosis chromatin is condensed into discrete structures called **chromosomes**. The organization of the nuclear envelope, nucleolus, and chromatin is shown in **Figure 1.8**.

Functions of Nucleus

- DNA, the repository of genetic information is located in the nucleus as a DNA-protein complex, chromatin, which is organized into chromosomes. The nucleus contains the proteins and enzymes of replication of DNA and for repair of DNA that has been damaged.

- The major functional role of the nucleus is that of **replication**, synthesis of new DNA and **transcription**, synthesis of rRNA, tRNA and mRNA. All of the RNA molecules operate functionally outside the nucleus and seem to leave via the nuclear pores.

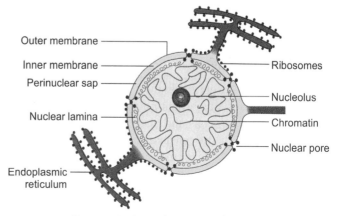

Figure 1.8: General structure of nucleus.

- The processing of RNA for assembly of ribosomes, required for protein synthesis in the cytosol, occurs in the nucleolus.

Hutchinson Gilford Progeria Syndrome (HG-PS)

Hutchinson-Gilford progeria syndrome is a genetic condition characterized by the intense, rapid appearance of aging beginning in childhood. Affected children typically look normal at birth and in early infancy, but then grow more slowly than other children and do not gain weight at the expected rate (failure to thrive).

They develop a characteristic facial appearance including prominent eyes, a thin nose, and loss of hair, wrinkled skin, atherosclerosis, and cardiovascular problems. This condition does not affect intellectual development or the development of motor skills such as sitting, standing, and walking. The aging process in these individuals is 6 to 8 times the normal rate of aging. These serious complications can worsen over time and are life-threatening for affected individuals

Progeria was first described in 1886 by Jonathan Hutchinson. It was also described independently in 1897 by Hastings Gilford. The condition was later named Hutchinson–Gilford progeria syndrome. The word progeria comes from the Greek words "pro", meaning "before" or "premature", and "gēras", meaning "old age".

Mutations in the *LMNA* gene cause Hutchinson-Gilford progeria syndrome. The *LMNA* gene provides instructions for making a protein called **lamin A**. This protein plays an important role in determining the shape of the nucleus within cells. It is an essential scaffolding (supporting) component of the nuclear envelope, which is the membrane that surrounds the nucleus. Mutations that cause Hutchinson-Gilford progeria syndrome result in the production of an abnormal version of the **lamin A protein**. The altered protein makes the nuclear envelope unstable and progressively damages the nucleus, making cells more likely to die prematurely. Researchers are working to determine how these changes lead to the characteristic features of Hutchinson-Gilford progeria syndrome.

CYTOSKELETON

The cytoplasm of most eukaryotic cells contains network of several types of proteins filaments that interact extensively with each other and with the component of the plasma membrane forming three-dimensional meshwork. Such an extensive intracellular meshwork of protein has been called **cytoskeleton**. Cytoskeleton is not a rigid permanent framework of the cell but is a dynamic, changing structure.

Functions of Cytoskeleton

- The cytoskeleton gives cells their characteristic shape and form, provides attachment points for organelles, fixing their location in cells and also makes communication between parts of the cell possible.
- It is also responsible for the separation of chromosomes during cell division.
- The internal movement of the cell organelles as well as cell locomotion and muscle fiber contraction could not take place without the cytoskeleton. It acts as **track** on

which cells can move organelles, chromosomes and other things.

Structure of Cytoskeleton

The cytoskeleton is an organized network of three protein filaments; **Microfilaments**, **microtubules** and **intermediate filaments**, differing in width, composition and specific function.

- **Microfilaments** consist of long thin strands of protein **actin**, which is also a main component of muscle. Actin filament form a meshwork just underlying the plasma membrane of many cells and are referred to **stress fiber** or **cell cortex** which is labile. They disappear as cell motility increases or upon **malignant transformation** of cells by chemical or oncogenic viruses.
- **Microtubules** are long, thin tubes composed of the protein **tubulin**. They rapidly assemble into tubular structures and disassemble depending on the needs of cells. Microtubules comprise the spindle fibers that separate chromosomes prior to cell division. Centrioles are composed of microtubules and function as the organizing center for the formation of spindle fibers.
- **Intermediate filaments** are so-called as their diameter is intermediate between that of microfilaments and of microtubules. These are formed from fibrous protein which cannot be easily disassembled as either the microtubules or the microfilaments can, except **lamin**. Protein structure of intermediate filaments varies with different tissue type. There are major seven classes of intermediate filaments as indicated in **Table 1.4**.

CELL FRACTIONATION AND MARKER ENZYMES FOR DIFFERENT ORGANELLES

Investigation of the biochemical properties of organelles requires subcellular fractionation in which the cell is first mechanically homogenized using isotonic 0.25 M sucrose solution to break cells and disperse their contents in an aqueous buffer to maintain the pH at its optimum value for organelle stability. Sucrose solution is used because it is not metabolized in most tissues and it has an osmotic pressure similar to that in organelles, thus balancing diffusion of water

TABLE 1.4: Types of cytoskeleton and their proteins.

Cytoskeleton protein	Types of protein present
Microfilaments	Actin filament
Microtubules	Tubulin
Intermediate filament	1. Keratin 2. Vimentin 3. Desmin 4. Glial fibrillary acidic protein (GFAP) 5. Peripherin 6. Neurofilament 7. Lamins

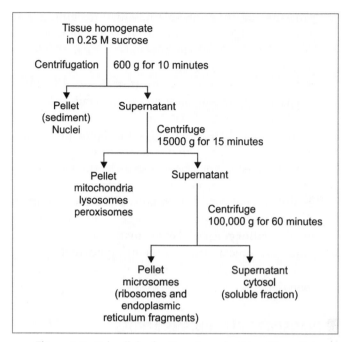

Figure 1.9: Subcellular fractionation of cell by differential centrifugation.

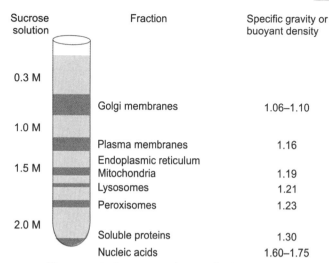

Figure 1.10: Separation of organelles by isopycnic centrifugation technique.

into and out of the organelles, which would swell and burst in a solution of lower osmolarity.

- By gently homogenization in an isotonic sucrose solution, the cell membrane is ruptured keeping most of the internal organelles intact. However, large fragile structures such as the endoplasmic reticulum, is broken into pieces that spontaneously form vesicles called **microsomes**.

- Then homogenate is centrifuged at different speeds. Large particles sediment more rapidly than small particles and soluble material does not sediment. In differential centrifugation, the homogenate is subjected to a series of centrifugation steps of increasing time and gravitational force **(Figure 1.9)**.

- The subcellular organelles, e.g., nuclei and mitochondria, which differ in size and specific gravity and thus sediment at different rates in a centrifugal field and can then, be isolated from homogenate by differential centrifugation. The dense nuclei are sediment first, followed by the mitochondria, and finally the microsomal fraction at the highest forces. After, all the particulate matter has been removed; the soluble remnant is the **cytosol**.

- Organelles of similar sedimentation coefficient obviously cannot be separated by differential centrifugation. For example, mitochondria isolated in his way are contaminated with lysosome and peroxisomes. These may be separated by **isopycnic centrifugation technique**.

Isopycnic Centrifugation Technique

In this technique, a density gradient is set up in a centrifuge tube; i.e., the density of the solution in the tube increases from the top to the bottom. Sucrose is often used as a medium.

Colloidal materials such as **Percoll**, which form density gradients with a low osmotic pressure, are often preferred.

Particles are sediment to an equilibrium position at which their density equals that of the medium at that point in the tube **(Figure 1.9)**. Different organelles are thus separated **according to their density, their size and shape being immaterial**.

After centrifugation to equilibrium, the gradient is fractionated and the separated organelles recovered as shown in **Figure 1.10**. Macromolecules, such as large proteins, nucleic acids and nucleoprotein complexes can also be separated by density gradient centrifugation technique.

Marker Enzymes for Different Organelles

The purity of isolated subcellular fraction is assessed by the analysis of **marker enzymes**. Marker enzymes are the enzymes that are located exclusively in a particular fraction, and thus become characteristic of that fraction.

Analysis of marker enzymes confirms the identity of the isolated fraction and indicates the degree of contamination with other organelles. For example, isolated **mitochondria** have a high specific activity of **cytochrome oxidase** but low **catalase** and **acid phosphatase**, the catalase and acid phosphatase activities being due to contamination with peroxisomes and lysosomes respectively. Some typical subcellular markers are given in **Table 1.5**.

▮ MEMBRANE TRANSPORT

Fundamental Properties of Biological Membranes

Cell membranes are highly fluid, dynamic structures consisting of **lipid bilayer** and associated proteins. Cell membranes form closed compartments around the cytoplasm to define cell boundaries. The cell membrane has **selective permeability**. The lipid bilayer of biological membranes is basically impermeable to ions and polar molecules.

TABLE 1.5: Marker enzymes of subcellular fractions.

Fraction	Enzymes
Plasma membrane	5'-nucleotidase, Na^+-K^+-ATPase
Nucleus	• DNA polymerase • RNA polymerase
Endoplasmic reticulum	Glucose-6-phosphatase
Golgi bodies	Galactosyltransferase
Lysosomes	• Acid phosphatase • β-glucuronidase
Mitochondria	• Succinate dehydrogenase • Cytochrome-c oxidase
Peroxisomes	Catalase
Cytosol	• Lactate dehydrogenase • Glucose-6-phosphate dehydrogenase

TABLE 1.6: Chemical composition of extracellular and intracellular fluid.

Substance	Extracellular fluid	Intracellular fluid
Na^+	140 mEq/L	10 mEq/L
K^+	4 mEq/L	140 mEq/L
Ca^{++}	2.4 mEq/L	0.0001 mEq/L
Mg^{++}	1.2 mEq/L	58 mEq/L
Cl^-	103 mEq/L	4 mEq/L
HCO_3^-	28 mEq/L	10 mEq/L
PO_4^{3-}	2 mEq/L	60 mEq/L
SO_4^{--}	1 mEq/L	2 mEq/L
Glucose	90 mg/dL	0–20 mg/dL
Amino acids	30 mg/dL	200 mg/dL
Cholesterol Phospholipids Natural fat	0.5 g/dL	2–95 g/dL
PO_2	35 mm Hg	20 mm Hg
PCO_2	46 mm Hg	50 mm Hg
pH	7.4	7.0
Protein	2 g/dL (5 mEq/L)	16 g/dL (40 mEq/L)

The lipid bilayer is not miscible with either the extracellular fluid (ECP) or the intracellular fluid (ICF). Therefore, it constitutes a barrier against movement of water molecules and water-soluble substances between extracellular and intracellular fluid compartments, thereby maintaining differences in composition between inside and outside of the cell (**Table 1.6**).

The membrane is sometimes referred to as a **fluid mosaic** (*see* **Figure 1.3**). Since, it consists of a mosaic (variety) proteins and lipid molecules that can move laterally in the plane of the membrane. The membrane mosaic is **fluid** because most of the interactions among its components are noncovalent, leaving individual lipid and protein molecules free to move laterally in the plane of the membrane.

- Selective membrane permeability is conferred by specific **transporters** and **ion channels**. Most of the membrane proteins can function as transport proteins. These proteins are highly selective for the types of molecules or ions that are allowed to cross the membrane. Different proteins function differently:
  - **Channel proteins:** Some proteins have watery spaces all the way through the molecule and allow free movements of water as well as selected ions or molecules; these are called channel proteins.
  - **Carrier proteins:** Others called carrier proteins bind with molecules or ions that are to be transported.
- The cells also transport certain **macromolecules** such as proteins, polysaccharides, and polynucleotides across the plasma membrane by independent mechanisms namely **endocytosis** and **exocytosis**.
- There are special areas of membrane structure—gap junction, through which adjacent cells may exchange material.

TRANSPORT MECHANISMS ACROSS CELL MEMBRANE

Transport mechanism through cell membrane can be broadly divided into three types (**Figure 1.11**):
1. Passive transport
2. Active transport
3. Vesicular transport

Passive Transport

- In passive transports, the substances pass through the membrane from both sides. The direction of transport of molecule is always from a **region of** higher concentration to lower concentration. It does not require energy in the form of ATP.
- There are three types of passive transport as follows:
  1. Simple diffusion
  2. Facilitated diffusion
  3. Osmosis

Simple Diffusion

Diffusion is a process of **passive transport** in which molecules move from the area of higher concentration to the area of lower concentration. The energy that causes diffusion is derived by the kinetic energy generated due to random motion of molecules.

- The examples of substances that pass through cell membranes by simple diffusion are transport of O_2, CO_2, urea, ammonia and ions.
- Across a membrane, diffusion of a molecule exists on both sides of the membrane. The net movement of molecule ceases when the concentration of molecule on both sides becomes equal and a diffusional equilibrium is achieved. Simple diffusion can occur through the cell membrane by two pathways (**Figure 1.12**):

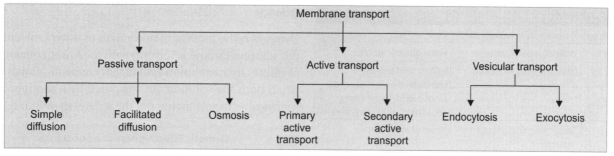

Figure 1.11: Types of membrane transport mechanism.

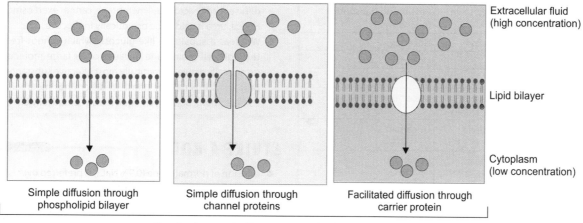

Passive transport—No energy required

Figure 1.12: Transport across the cell membrane by diffusion.

1. Through the interstices of lipid bilayer if the diffusing substance is lipid soluble and
2. Through watery (aqueous) channels formed by transmembrane proteins.

Simple Diffusion of Lipid-soluble Molecules through the Lipid Bilayer

Simple diffusion of lipid-soluble molecules occurs rapidly through the interstices of the lipid bilayer **(Figure 1.12)**. For example, **oxygen, nitrogen, carbon dioxide** and **alcohols** are lipid soluble, so all these can dissolve directly in lipid bilayer and diffuse through the cell membrane. The rate of diffusion of each of these substances through the membrane is directly proportional to its lipid solubility.

Simple Diffusion of Water and Other Lipid Insoluble Molecules through Protein Channels

Even though water is highly insoluble in the membrane lipids, it readily passes through **protein channels** that penetrate all the way through the membrane **(Figure 1.12)**. Other lipid insoluble molecules can pass through the **protein pore** in the same way as water molecules if they are water-soluble and small enough like ions, glucose and urea.

- **Protein pores** and **channels** are tubular pathways all the way from the extracellular to the intracellular fluid. Therefore substances can move by simple diffusion directly along these pores and channels from one side of the membrane to the other.

- **Pores** are composed of **integral cell membrane proteins** that form open tubes through the membrane and are always open. However, the diameter of a pore and its electrical charges provide selectivity that permits only certain molecules to pass through. These protein pores are called **aquaporins** or **water channels**. They permit rapid passage of water through cell membranes but exclude other molecules. The pore is too narrow to permit passage of any hydrated ions. At least 13 different types of aquaporins have been found in various cells of the human body.

- **Protein channels** are highly selective for transport of one or more **specific ions or molecules**; as they have characteristic diameter, shape, and the nature of the electrical charges and chemical bonds along its inside surfaces. A polypeptide subunit forms a **gate** at one end of the channel that opens in response to a specific stimulus.

Gating of protein channels provides a means of controlling ion permeability of the channels. The opening and closing of gates are controlled by the **electrical potential** across the cell membrane, e.g., Na^+ and Ca^+ channels and by the binding of a chemical substance ligand) either an ion or a specific molecule with the protein; this causes a conformational change in

TABLE 1.7: Glucose transporters in humans.

Transporter	Tissues where expressed	Role
GLUT 1	Ubiquitous (All tissues)	Basal glucose uptake
GLUT 2	Liver, pancreatic B cells, intestine	In liver and kidney, removal of excess glucose from blood, in pancreas regulation of insulin release
GLUT 3	Brain (neuronal), testis (sperm)	Basal glucose uptake
GLUT 4	Muscle, fat cell, heart	Activity increased by insulin
GLUT 5	Intestine, testis, kidney	Primarily fructose transport
GLUT 6	Spleen, leukocytes, brain	Possibly no transporter function
GLUT 7	Small intestine, colon	Uncertain
GLUT 8	Testis	Uncertain
GLUT 9	Liver, kidney	Uncertain
GLUT 10	Heart, lung, brain, liver, muscle, pancreas, kidney	Uncertain
GLUT 11	Heart, skeletal muscle, kidney	Uncertain
GLUT 12	Skeletal muscle, heart, prostatic gland, small intestine	Uncertain

the protein molecule that opens or closes the gate, e.g., acetylcholine channel. Acetylcholine opens the gate of this channel.

Facilitated Diffusion

This is also called **carrier-mediated diffusion**, as the process of diffusion is facilitated by a **carrier protein** in the membrane. There are many types of carrier proteins in membranes, each type having binding sites that are specific for a particular substance. Among the most important substances that cross cell membranes by facilitated diffusion are **glucose** and most of the **amino acids**. In case of glucose there are 12 glucose transporter molecules have been discovered in various tissues **(Table 1.7)**. Like simple diffusion, facilitated diffusion is also a downhill transport and does not require energy **(Figure 1.12)**.

- Facilitated diffusion is more rapid than simple diffusion. These diffusion processes are not coupled to the movement of other ions, they are known as **uniport transport** process.
- Sometimes, facilitated diffusion is regulated by hormones. For example, transport of glucose by GLUT-4 into muscle and adipose tissue is insulin dependent.
- In facilitated diffusion, the number of **carrier proteins** available determines the rate of diffusion. In simple diffusion, the rate of diffusion is proportional to the **concentration of the substance**.

In diabetes mellitus, glucose uptake by muscle and fat cells is impaired because the carrier GLUT-4 for facilitated diffusion of glucose requires insulin.

Osmosis

Osmosis is the process of movement of water (solvent) from the solution (Solute + Solvent) with the lower concentration of solutes to the solution with higher concentration of solute, when both the solution are separated by a semipermeable (permeable to solvent but not the solute) membrane.

Osmotic Effectiveness of a Substance

- ❖ A substance to exert osmotic pressure should be detained to one side of the membrane. Therefore, a substance like urea which can diffuse readily across cell membrane, cannot exert osmotic effects. Hence, urea is said to be osmotically ineffective.
- ❖ Whereas a substance like glucose, which cannot freely diffuse through cell membrane because of its large molecular size, is osmotically active. Osmotically most effective substance is plasma protein as it is neither transferred from nor metabolized in the compartment. Sodium chloride is also osmotically effective.

STRIKE A NOTE

- ❖ Infusion of normal saline (0.9% NaCl) is preferred over isotonic 5% glucose solution in blood volume depletion
- ❖ 5% glucose solution is isotonic, initially, when infused intravenously but later on becomes hypotonic because glucose is transferred into the cell and metabolized. However as glucose is rapidly metabolized, the net effect of infusion is like the infusion of a hypotonic solution. Whereas 0.9 % NaCl (the normal saline) is the satisfactory replacement in blood volume depletion.
- ❖ In diabetes, increased plasma osmolality due to very high plasma glucose concentration causes shrinkage of cells. Especially, dehydration of brain cell leads to coma

Active Transport

By passive transport processes, the composition of intracellular fluid tends to equalize with that of composition of extracellular fluid. However, this should never happen practically, as it threatens cell volume and intracellular solute concentrations that are not compatible with life. Therefore, nature maintains inequality of fluid composition of intracellular and extracellular compartments by providing special transport mechanisms to the cell membrane that oppose these equilibrating transport processes. These transport processes are called **active transport mechanisms (Figure 1.13)**.

When a cell membrane transports molecules or ions uphill (towards high concentration) against a concentration gradient or uphill against an electrical or pressure gradient, the process is called **active transport**. There are two common characteristics of active transport mechanisms

- **Uphill transport:** The transport occurs against the electrochemical gradient of the substance transported.
- **Utilizes energy:** Energy utilized for the active transport is derived from the breakdown of ATP.

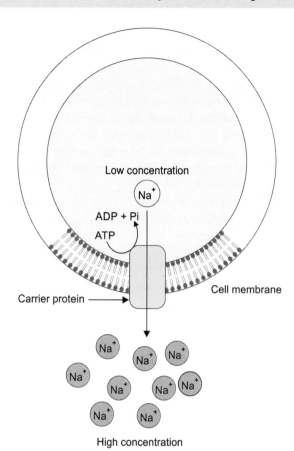

Figure 1.13: Active transport of sodium and potassium.

There are two types of active transport according to the source of energy used to cause transport.

1. Primary active transport
2. Secondary active transport

Primary Active Transport

Primary active transport is the transport mechanism that directly utilizes energy derived from hydrolysis of **ATP to ADP**. The mechanism is operated by **ion pumps**.

- In this process, the solute is transported against its electrochemical gradients, which requires energy in the form of ATP.
- As the ion pumps hydrolyze ATP, these are also called **ATPases**.
- The examples of primary active transports are:
  - **Na+-K+ ATPase** or **Na+-K+ pump**
  - **Calcium ATPase**
  - **H+-K+ ATPase**
  - **H+- ATPase**.
- Active transport depends on **carrier proteins**. These carrier proteins are capable of transporting substance against the concentration gradient hence energy is required. There are four major classes of active transporters.
  1. **P-type:** P signifies **phosphorylation**. P-type transporters are phosphorylated and dephosphorylated

during transport. Na+-K+ ATPase and Ca2+ ATPase are the examples of P-type ATPase.

2. **F-type transporters:** F-signifies energy coupling factor type. The most important example of this class is the **mitochondrial ATP synthase** present in mitochondria.
3. **V-type transporter:** V signifies vacuolar, V-type transporters pump protons into lysosomes, endosomes, Golgi vesicles and secretory vesicles.
4. **ABC transporters:** ABC transporters transport a variety of compounds out of the cells those includes ions, steroids, cholesterol, peptides, bile acids, drugs and xenobiotics. The most important example of this class is:
   - **CFTR protein:** Cystic fibrosis transmembrane conductance regulator (CFTR) protein is responsible for regulating the proper flow of **chloride and sodium** in and out of the cell membranes in the lungs and other organs. This protein functions as a channel across the membrane of cells that produce **mucus**, **sweat**, **saliva**, **tears**, and **digestive enzymes**. **Cystic fibrosis** occurs when the cystic fibrosis transmembrane conductance regulator (CFTR) protein is either not made correctly, or not made at all.
   - **MDR-1 protein** (multidrug resistance-1 protein). **P-glycoprotein 1** (permeability glycoprotein, **Pgp**) also known as **multidrug resistance protein 1 (MDR1)**. This transporter pumps a variety of drugs including many anticancer agents out of the cells.
   - **BRCP** (breast cancer resistance protein): BCRP physiologically functions as a part of a **self-defense mechanism** for the organism; it enhances elimination of toxic **xenobiotic** substances and harmful agents in the **gut** and **biliary tract**, as well as through the **blood-brain**, **placental**, and possibly **blood-testis barriers**. It was so named because it was initially cloned from a multidrug-resistant breast cancer cell line where it was found to confer resistance to chemotherapeutic agents in cancer cells.

STRIKE A NOTE

- ❖ ABC transporter pumps cytotoxic drugs from cancer cells out of the cells. This decreases effective concentration of drugs in the cells needed for killing cancer cells. Hence cancer cells become resistant to anticancer chemotherapy.
- ❖ Cardiac glycosides like **ouabain**, or **digitals** are used for the treatment of congestive heart failure to increase the contraction of heart muscle.
- ❖ These glycosides inhibit Na+-K+ pump by binding to the external surface of the carrier protein and interfering with the hydrolysis of the ATP. This result in less Na+ being pumped out of the cardiac cell and leads to an increase of the intracellular concentration of Na+ and prevents K+ influx (coming in).

Contd...

Contd...

> ❖ The intracellular accumulation of Na^+ decreases Na^+ gradient from outside to inside which results in slower extrusion of Ca^{++} by the Na^+-Ca^{++} exchanger and raise calcium ion concentration in cardiac muscle provides the extra calcium needed to increase the muscle contraction force.

Secondary Active Transport

Many cells have aided by other carrier mechanisms that transfer one solute against its concentration by using energy generated by gradient of other solute that was originally pumped by primary active transport **(Figure 1.14)**. Since the transport depends on primary active transport of sodium by the Na^+-K^+ pump, it is known as a **secondary active transport**.

- Typical example of secondary active transport is reabsorption of glucose from intestine and kidney tubules across intestinal and renal epithelial cell.
- When sodium ions are transported out of the cells by primary active transport (Na^+-K^+ pump) large concentration gradient of sodium ions develops across the cell membranes, (high concentration outside the cell and low concentration inside). This gradient generates energy, as the excess sodium outside the cell membrane is always attempting to diffuse to the interior. This diffusion energy of sodium can pull glucose along with the sodium through cell membrane from luminal fluid into the cell.

Vesicular Transport

- Vesicular transport is special for **macromolecules**. Macromolecules cannot be transported by diffusion or active transport process. Therefore they are transferred across the cell membrane mainly by vesicular transport. Amino acids, sugars, waste products of metabolism, cellular secretions, hormones, neurotransmitters and organisms are transported by this mechanism.
- Transport process occurs by either fusion of vesicle or formation of vesicle is called vesicular transport.
- The process by which cells **take up** large molecules is called **endocytosis** and the process by which cells **release** large molecules **from the cells to the outside** is called **exocytosis**.
- Fusion of vesicle with the cell membrane occurs in **exocytosis** and formation of vesicle from cell membrane occurs in **endocytosis**.
- In vesicular transport, formation and transport of vesicles are facilitated by some vesicular transport proteins. These proteins are **calthrin**, **coating proteins**, **dynamin** and **docking proteins**.

Endocytosis

Endocytosis is the process of transport in which a substance is taken into the cell by means of vesicle formation. It is the only process by which most macromolecules, such as most proteins, polysaccharides and polynucleotides can enter cells.

Endocytosis occurs by two mechanisms: **Constitutive** and **Clathrin-mediated**.

Constitutive Endocytosis

Endocytosis by **constitutive pathway** occurs in almost all cells. It is called "constitutive", as the process occurs continually and does not require any specific stimulus. The molecule or substance makes contact with the cell membrane that invaginates to form an **endocytic vesicle**. The non-cytoplasmic side of the membrane then fuses and the vesicle is pinched-off into the cytosol **(Figure 1.15)**.

Clathrin-mediated Endocytosis

- **Clathrin-mediated** endocytosis occurs at the specific site of the cell membrane. Clathrin is fibrillar protein located in the cell membrane beneath the receptor protein. Clathrin-mediated endocytosis internalizes various organisms, growth factors and lipoproteins **(Figure 1.16)**.
- These molecules first attach to specific receptors on the surface of the membrane.
- The receptors are generally concentrated in small pits on the outer surface of the cell membrane. These receptors are coated on the cytoplasmic side with a fibrillar protein called **clathrin** and contractile filaments of **actin** and **myosin**.
- Once the macromolecules (which are to be absorbed) have bound with the receptors, the entire pit invaginates inward, and the fibrillar protein by surrounding the invaginating pit causes it to close over the attached

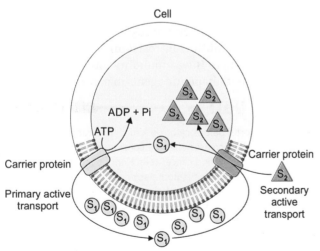

Figure 1.14: Diagrammatic representation of secondary active transport. Gradient of ion has been established by primary active transport movement of solute (S_1, often Na^+) down its electrochemical gradient provides the energy to drive cotransport of a second solute (S_2) against its electrochemical gradient.

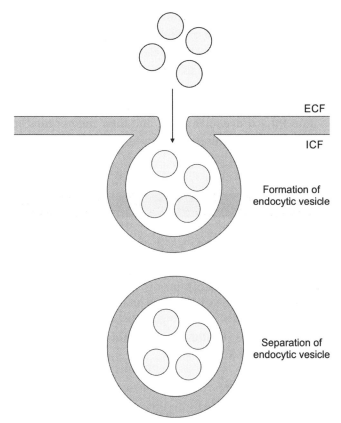

Figure 1.15: Constitutive endocytosis.
(ECF: extracellular fluid; ICF: intracellular fluid)

macromolecule along with a small amount of extracellular fluid.

- Then immediately, the invaginated portion of the membrane breaks away from the surface of the cell forming **endocyte vesicle** inside the cytoplasm of the cell.

STRIKE A NOTE

- ❖ A disadvantages consequence of receptors mediated endocytosis is that virus which cause diseases such as hepatitis (affecting liver cells), poliomyelitis (affecting motor neurons) and AIDS (affecting T-cells) initiate their infections cycles by entering cells via this mechanism.
- ❖ Receptor mediated endocytosis plays a key role in cholesterol metabolism.

Digestion of Endocyte Vesicles

- Immediately after a endocytotic vesicle appears inside a cell, one or more lysosomes become attached to the vesicle and empty their acid hydrolases to the inside of the vesicles.
- The macromolecules present in vesicle are digested to yield amino acids, simple sugars or nucleotides that can diffuse through the membrane of the vesicle into the cytoplasm and reused by the cell.
- What is left of the digestive vesicle, called the residual body, represent indigestible substances. In most instances, this is finally excreted through the cell

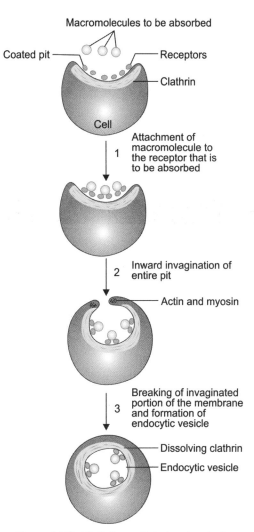

Figure 1.16: Clathrin-mediated endocytosis.

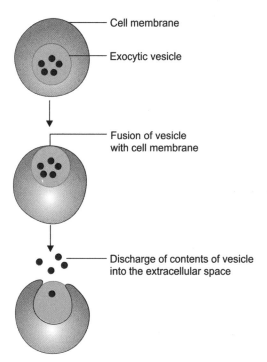

Figure 1.17: Process of exocytosis.

membrane by a process called **exocytosis**, which is opposite of endocytosis **(Figure 1.17)**.

Exocytosis

Exocytosis is the release of macromolecules from cells to the exterior, which is reverse of endocytosis. By exocytosis, hormones, neurotransmitters, digestive enzymes and undigested foreign particles are released from cells.

- The undigestible substances produced within the cytoplasm may be enclosed in membranes to form vesicles called **exocytic vesicles**.
- These cytoplasmic exocytic vesicles fuse with the internal surface of the plasma membrane.
- The vesicle then ruptures releasing their contents into the extracellular space and their membranes are retrieved (left behind) and reused **(Figure 1.17)**.

ASSESSMENT QUESTIONS

■ SHORT ESSAY QUESTIONS (SEQs)

1. Draw the structure of eukaryotic cell and write functions of the subcellular organelles.
2. Give structure and function of any two subcellular organelles.
3. With the help of diagram, describe the fluid mosaic model of cell membranes.
4. Enumerate transport processes across cell membrane with diagrams.
5. Write mechanism and importance of endocytosis, and exocytosis.

■ SHORT ANSWER QUESTIONS (SAQs)

1. Write types and functions of membrane proteins.
2. What are marker enzymes? Name the marker enzymes for lysosomes and mitochondria.
3. What are the functions of lysosomes?
4. What are the functions of peroxisomes?
5. What are the functions of membrane carbohydrates?
6. Write difference between passive and active transport.
7. Infusion of normal saline (0.9% NaCl) is preferred over isotonic 5% glucose solution; justify.
8. What are aquaporins? Write importance of aquaporins.
9. What are ABC transporters? Write most important example of ABC transporters

■ MULTIPLE CHOICE QUESTIONS (MCQs)

1. **The following is the metabolic function of ER:**
   a. RNA processing
   b. Fatty acid oxidation
   c. Synthesis of plasma protein
   d. ATP-synthesis
2. **In biologic membranes, integral proteins and lipids interact mainly by:**
   a. Covalent bond
   b. Both hydrophobic and covalent bond
   c. Hydrogen and electrostatic bond
   d. None of the above

3. **Plasma membrane is:**
   a. Composed entirely of lipids
   b. Mainly made up of proteins
   c. Mainly made up of lipid and protein
   d. Composed of only carbohydrates and lipids
4. **Select the subcellular component involved in the formation of ATP:**
   a. Nucleus   b. Plasma membrane
   c. Mitochondria   d. Golgi apparatus
5. **Mitochondrial DNA is:**
   a. Maternal inherited
   b. Paternal inherited
   c. Maternal and paternal inherited
   d. None of the above
6. **All of the following statements about the nucleus are true, *except*:**
   a. Outer nuclear membrane is connected to ER
   b. It is the site of storage of genetic material
   c. Nucleolus is surrounded by a bilayer membrane
   d. Outer and inner membranes of nucleus are connected at nuclear pores
7. **Golgi apparatus is produced from which organelle?**
   a. Endoplasmic reticulum
   b. Plasma membrane
   c. Mitochondria
   d. Ribosomes
8. **Peroxisomes arise from:**
   a. Golgi membrane
   b. Lysosomes
   c. Mitochondria
   d. Pre-existing peroxisomes and budding off from the smooth ER
9. **Na$^+$ - K$^+$ ATPase is the marker enzyme of:**
   a. Nucleus   b. Plasma membrane
   c. Golgi bodies   d. Cytosol
10. **The rough endoplasmic reticulum in the cells is because of the presence of:**
    a. Mitochondria associated with ER
    b. Ribosomes on the surface of ER
    c. Ca granules on the surface of ER
    d. Sulphur granules on the surface of ER

11. **In human which cell lacks nucleus:**
    a. Lymphocyte
    b. Monocytes
    c. RBC
    d. Neutrophils

12. **Microtubules are made up of by which protein?**
    a. Tubulin
    b. Myosin
    c. Actin
    d. None of these

13. **No membrane surrounds in this organelle:**
    a. Lysosome
    b. Nucleolus
    c. Golgi body
    d. Nucleus

14. **The cytoskeleton includes all of the following, *except*:**
    a. Microtubules
    b. Intermediate filaments
    c. Myosin filaments
    d. Actin filaments

15. **Ribosomes are found:**
    a. Only in the nucleus
    b. In the cytoplasm
    c. Attached to the rough endoplasmic reticulum
    d. Both b and c

16. **The Golgi apparatus is involved in:**
    a. Packaging proteins into vesicles
    b. Altering or modifying proteins
    c. Producing lysosomes
    d. All of the above

17. **Which of the following are involved with the movement or transport of materials or organelles throughout the cell?**
    a. Rough endoplasmic reticulum
    b. Cytoskeleton
    c. Smooth endoplasmic reticulum
    d. All of the choices are true

18. **Lysosomes are produced by the:**
    a. Nucleus
    b. Mitochondria
    c. Golgi apparatus
    d. Ribosomes

19. **Major site of RNA synthesis is:**
    a. Nucleoplasm
    b. Nucleolus
    c. Nucleus
    d. All

20. **Mitochondria is an organelle of which process, *except*:**
    a. Glycolysis
    b. Krebs' cycle
    c. Biosynthesis of urea
    d. Fatty acid oxidation

21. **Give name of organelle, which is surrounded by a double layered wall.**
    a. Lysosome
    b. Plasma membrane
    c. Golgi apparatus
    d. Nucleus

22. **Assertion: A cell membrane shows fluid behavior.**

    Reason: A membrane is a mosaic or composite of diverse lipids and proteins.
    a. Both Assertion and Reason are true and the Reason is the correct explanation of the Assertion.
    b. Both Assertion and Reason are true but the Reason is not the correct explanation of the Assertion.
    c. Assertion is true statement but Reason is false.
    d. Both Assertion and Reason are false statements

23. **Assertion: Eukaryotic cells have the ability to adopt a variety of shapes and carry out directed movements.**
    Reason: There are three principal types of protein filaments; actin filament, microtubules and intermediate filaments, which constitute the cytoskeleton.
    a. Both assertion and reason are true and the reason is the correct explanation of the assertion.
    b. Both assertion and reason are true but the reason is not the correct explanation of the assertion.
    c. Assertion is true statement but reason is false.
    d. Both assertion and reason are false

24. **Gases such as oxygen and carbon dioxide cross the plasma membrane by:**
    a. Secondary active transport
    b. Passive diffusion through the lipid bilayer
    c. Specific gas transport proteins
    d. Primary active transport

25. **A substance can only be accumulated against its electro-chemical gradient by:**
    a. Facilitated diffusion
    b. Passage through ion channels
    c. Diffusion through a uniport
    d. Active transport

26. **Which of the following is an example of primary active transport?**
    a. Cl^-- HCO_3^- exchange
    b. Na^+ - H^+ exchange
    c. Na^+-Ca^{2+} exchange
    d. Na^+, K^+ ATPase

27. **The sodium pump:**
    a. Exchanges extracellular Na^+ for intracellular K^+
    b. Is important for maintaining a constant cell volume
    c. Can only be inhibited by metabolic poisons
    d. Is an ion channel

28. **Which of the following statements regarding exocytosis is correct?**
    a. Is always employed by cells for secretion
    b. Is used to deliver material into the extracellular space
    c. Takes up large molecules from the extracellular space
    d. Allows the retrieval of elements of the plasma membrane

29. **Endocytosis is used by cells to:**
    a. Ingest bacteria and cell debris
    b. Retrieve elements of the plasma membrane after exocytosis
    c. Secrete large molecules into the extracellular space
    d. None of the above

30. **The sodium-potassium pump transports:**
    a. More Na^+ out than K^+ in
    b. K^+ out and Na^+ in on a one-for-one basis
    c. Na^+ out and K^+ in on a one-for-one basis
    d. K^+ and Na^+ in the same direction

31. **Exocytosis is a process by which cells:**
    a. Pass substances out of the cell in vesicles
    b. Pass substances out of the cell through the membrane by osmosis
    c. Release substances directly into the extracellular fluid through a pore
    d. Release substances directly into the extracellular fluid through a pit

32. Cystic fibrosis results from defective ion channels for:
    a. Na^+
    b. Cl^-
    c. Ca^{++}
    d. H^+

33. Substances transported by facilitated diffusion:
    a. Move passively through specific channels from an area of greater concentration to one of lower concentration
    b Must have movements coupled to those of other substances
    c. May flow to a region of higher concentration by the expenditure of energy
    d. Are restricted to only one direction through the membrane

34. The methods of membrane transport that don't require protein channels or carriers are:
    a. Exocytosis
    b. Diffusion
    c. Phagocytosis
    d. All of the above

35. In erythrocyte glucose transport is an example of:
    a. Simple diffusion
    b. Active transport
    c. Facilitated diffusion
    d. Ion driven active transport

36. Which of the following is correct for active transport processes?
    a. Transport molecules or ions against concentration gradient.
    b. Transport molecules or ions against electrical gradient
    c. Are often referred to as pumps.
    d. All of the above

37. Facilitated diffusion transport molecules:
    a. Against concentration gradient
    b. With the concentration gradient
    c. Always use energy
    d. Does not require carrier protein

38. The exocytosis requires which ion:
    a. Ca^{2+} b. Na^+
    c. K^+ d. Fe^+

■ ANSWERS FOR MCQs

1. c	2. c	3. c	4. c	5. a
6. c	7. a	8. d	9. b	10. b
11. c	12. a	13. c	14. c	15. d
16. d	17. d	18. c	19. b	20. a
21. d	22. a	23. a	24. b	25. d
26. d	27. b	28. b	29. a	30. a
31. a	32. b	33. a	34. d	35. c
36. d	37. b	38. a		

Chemistry of Carbohydrates

Competency	Learning Objectives
BI 3.1: Discuss and differentiate monosaccharides, di-saccharides and polysaccharides giving examples of main carbohydrates as energy fuel, structural element and storage in the human body.	1. Give definition, functions and classification of carbohydrates with examples. 2. Discuss monosaccharides: Structure and isomerism. 3. Describe biologically important monosaccharide derivatives. 4. Describe the formation of glycosides and its therapeutic importance. 5. Describe the formation of glycosides and its therapeutic importance. 6. Discuss disaccharides with examples and importance. 7. Discuss polysaccharides with examples and importance. 8. Describe glycoproteins and their functions. 9. Describe concept of glycation and glycosylation.

■ OVERVIEW

The carbohydrates are widely distributed both in animal and plant tissues. Chemically, they contain the elements **carbon**, **hydrogen** and **oxygen**. The empirical formula of many simple carbohydrates is $[CH_2O]_n$. Hence, the name **carbohydrate**, i.e., hydrated carbon. They are also called **saccharides**. In Greek, **saccharon** means sugar. Although many common carbohydrates confirm the empirical formula $[CH_2O]_n$, others like deoxyribose, rhamnohexos do not. Some carbohydrates also contain **nitrogen**, **phosphorus** or **sulfur**.

This chapter introduces the major classes of carbohydrates with examples and their structural and functional roles.

■ DEFINITION, FUNCTIONS AND CLASSIFICATION OF CARBOHYDRATES

Definition

Carbohydrates may be defined chemically as **aldehyde** or **ketone** derivatives of polyhydroxy (more than one hydroxy group) alcohols or as compounds that yield these derivatives on hydrolysis.

Classification of Carbohydrates

Carbohydrates are classified into three groups:
1. Monosaccharides
2. Oligosaccharides
3. Polysaccharides.

Monosaccharides (Greek: Mono = one)

Monosaccharides are the simplest carbohydrates. Monosaccharides are colorless, crystalline solids that are freely soluble in water but insoluble in nonpolar solvents. Most have a sweet test. Monosaccharides are also called **simple sugars**. The term sugar is applied to carbohydrates that are soluble in water and sweet to test. They consist of a single polyhydroxy aldehyde or ketone unit, and thus cannot be hydrolyzed into a simpler form. They may be subdivided into different groups as follows:
- Depending upon the **number of carbon atoms** they possess, e.g.,
  - Trioses
  - Tetroses

- Pentoses
- Hexoses
- Heptoses.

● Depending upon the functional **aldehyde (CHO)** or **ketone (C=O)** group present:

- Aldoses
- Ketoses.

Classification of monosaccharides based on the number of carbon and the type of functional group present with examples is given in **Table 2.1**. **The most abundant monosaccharide in nature is six carbon sugar D-glucose**. Biologically important monosaccharides are listed in **Table 2.2**.

Oligosaccharides (Greek: Oligo = few)

Oligosaccharides consist of a short chain of monosaccharide units (2–10 units), joined together by a characteristic bond called **glycosidic bond** which, on hydrolysis gives two to ten molecules of simple sugar (monosaccharide) units. Oligosaccharides are subdivided into different groups based on the number of monosaccharide units present **(Table 2.3)**.

● The disaccharides which have two monosaccharide units are the most abundant in nature.

● Raffinoses, stachyose, Verbascose are indigestible oligosaccharides present in large amounts in legumes, especially beans.

● In cells, most oligosaccharides consisting of three or more units, do not occur as free entities but are joined to non-sugar molecules (lipids or proteins) in **glycoconjugates (glycolipids** and **glycoproteins)**.

Polysaccharides (Greek: Poly = many) or Glycans

Polysaccharides are polymers consisting of hundreds or thousands of monosaccharide units. They are also called **glycans** or **complex carbohydrates**. They may be either **linear**, (e.g., cellulose) or **branched**, (e.g., glycogen) in structure. Polysaccharides have **high molecular weight** and are only **sparingly soluble in water in the cold**. They form colloidal solutions when heated with water. They are **not sweetish** and do not exhibit any of the properties of aldehyde or ketone group. Polysaccharides are of two types **(Figure 2.1)**:

1. Homopolysaccharide (homoglycans)
2. Heteropolysaccharide (heteroglycans).

Homopolysaccharides (Homoglycans)

A polysaccharide made up of several units of one and the same type of monosaccharide unit only is called homopolysaccharide. The most common homoglycans are:

● Starch
● Dextrins
● Glycogen

TABLE 2.1: Classification of monosaccharide and their examples.

No. of carbon	Type of sugar	Aldoses	Ketoses
3	Trioses	Glyceraldehyde	Dihydroxyacetone
4	Tetroses	Erythrose	Erythrulose
5	Pentoses	Ribose, xylose	Ribulose, xylulose
6	Hexoses	Glucose, galactose and mannose	Fructose
7	Heptoses	Glucoheptose	Sedoheptulose

TABLE 2.2: Biologically important monosaccharides.

Type of monosaccharide	Example	Importance
Trioses	Glyceraldehyde and Dihydroxyacetone	• Intermediates in the glycolysis • Precursor of glycerol which is required for the formation of lipid like triacylglycerol, and phospholipid
Tetroses	D-Erythrose	Intermediate product of carbohydrate metabolism (Hexose monophosphate pathway)
Pentoses	D-Ribose D-Ribulose D-Xylulose L-Xylulose	• Structural element of nucleic acid RNA and coenzymes, e.g., ATP, NAD, NADP and flavoproteins • Intermediate product of pentose phosphate pathway • Intermediate product of pentose phosphate pathway • Constituent of proteoglycans and glycoproteins • Intermediate in uronic acid pathway. Excreted in urine in essential pentosuria
Hexoses	D-Glucose D-Fructose D-Galactose D-Mannose	• The main sugar of the body which is carried by blood and utilized by the tissue for energy purposes. Excreted in urine in diabetes mellitus • Can be converted to glucose in the liver and so used in the body for energy purpose • Can be converted to glucose in the liver and metabolized • Synthesized in mammary gland to make the lactose of milk • A constituent of glycolipids, proteoglycans and glycoproteins • A constituent of glycoprotein, glycolipids and blood group substances
Heptoses	Sedoheptulose	An intermediate in the pentose phosphate pathway

TABLE 2.3: Classification of oligosaccharides and their examples.

Type of oligosaccharide	Number of monosaccharide	Example	Type of monosaccharide present
Disaccharide	Two	Maltose	Glucose + Glucose
		Lactose	Glucose + Galactose
		Sucrose	Glucose + Fructose
		Isomaltose	Glucose + Glucose
Trisaccharide	Three	Raffinose	Glucose + Galactose + Fructose
Tetrasaccharide	Four	Stachyose	2 molecules of galactose + Glucose + Fructose
Pentasaccharide	Five	Verbascose	3 molecules of galactose + Glucose + Fructose

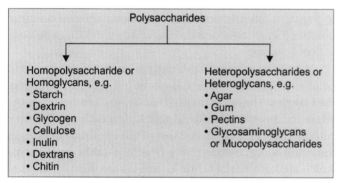

Figure 2.1: Classification of polysaccharide.

- Dextrans
- Inulin and
- Dietary fiber cellulose.

Some homopolysaccharides serve as a storage form of monosaccharides used as fuel, e.g., starch and glycogen, while others serve as structural elements in plants, e.g., cellulose.

Heteropolysaccharides (Heteroglycans)

They contain two or more different types of monosaccharide units or their derivatives. Plants heteropolysaccharides are **agar**, **gum**, **pectins**, etc. Heteropolysaccharide present in human beings is glycosaminoglycans (mucopolysaccharides), e.g.,

- Heparin
- Chondroitin sulfate
- Hyaluronic acid
- Dermatan sulfate
- Keratan sulfate
- Blood group polysaccharides.

Functions of Carbohydrates

- Certain carbohydrates like sugar and starch are a **dietary staple** in most parts of the world.
- Glucose is the major **metabolic fuel** of living beings.

- Homopolysaccharides, like glycogen serve as **storage forms** of carbohydrate in animals.
- Glucose is the precursor for the synthesis of:
  - **Glycogen** (storage form of carbohydrate)
  - **Ribose** and **deoxyribose** (constituents of nucleic acids RNA and DNA)
  - **Galactose** (constituent of lactose of milk)
  - **Glycolipids**, **glycoproteins** and **proteoglycans**.
- Proteoglycans (heteropolysaccharides) serve as structural component and provide **protection**, **shape** and **support** to cells, tissues and organs.
- Nondigestible carbohydrates like cellulose, agar, gum and pectin serve as **dietary fibers**.
- The oligosaccharides attached to plasma membrane (the glycocalyx) are central players in cell-cell recognition and adhesion, cell migration during development, blood clotting, the immune response, wound healing and other cellular processes.
- Derivative of glucose, e.g., **glucuronic acid** is also involved in detoxification reactions.

■ MONOSACCHARIDE: STRUCTURE AND ISOMERISM

Structure of Glucose

The structure of glucose can be represented in a **straight chain form** or **cyclic ring (Haworth projection) form**. The common monosaccharaides have cyclic structures. For simplicity the structure of aldoses and ketoses are represented as straight chain molecules **(Figure 2.2)**. In fact in aqueous solution sugars that contain four or more carbons are not open chains. Rather the open chain forms of these sugars cyclize into rings.

In solution, the aldehyde (CHO) or ketone (C=O) group of monosaccharide form a covalent bond with the oxygen of a hydroxyl (OH) group of the same molecule, to form derivatives called **hemiacetal** or **hemiketal**, respectively.

- The **C-1 aldehyde** in the open chain form of glucose reacts with the **C-5 hydroxyl group** of the same molecule. The resulting cyclic six membered ring is called **glucopyranose** because of its similarity to **pyran ring**.
- Similarly, the **C-2 keto** group in the open chain form of a fructose reacts with C-5 hydroxyl group to form a five membered ring is called a **fructofuranose** because of its similarity to **furan ring**.
- In case of glucose the six membered **glucopyranose** is much more stable however in case of fructose the more common and stable form is **fructofuranose**.
- During cyclization the carbonyl carbon becomes a new **chiral** (asymmetric) center. This carbonic carbon is called an **anomeric** carbon atom. Asymmetric anomeric carbon produces two possible stereoisomers designated α and β **(Figure 2.2)**.

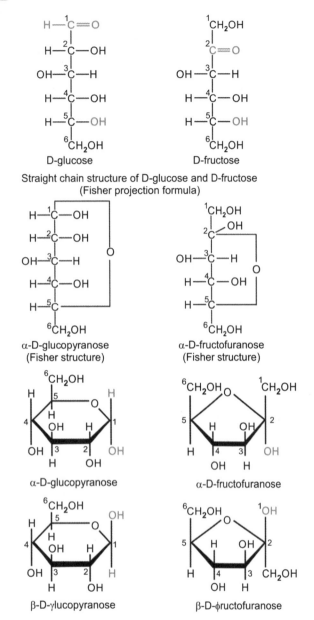

Figure 2.2: Structure of D-glucose and D-fructose.

Isomerism

All monosaccharides except **dihydroxyacetone** contain one or more asymmetric (chiral) carbon atoms exhibits **isomerism**. The compounds possessing identical molecular formula but different structures are referred to as **isomers**. The phenomenon of existence of isomers is called **isomerism**.

Isomerism in sugars is biologically significant because the enzymes that act on sugars are strictly stereospecific.

The compounds possessing identical molecular formula but different structures are referred to as **isomers**. The five types of isomerism exhibited by sugar are as follows:

1. Ketose-aldose isomerism
2. D and L isomerism

3. Optical isomerism
4. Epimerism
5. Anomerism.

Ketose-Aldose Isomerism

Glucose and fructose are isomers of each other having the same chemical (molecular) formula $C_6H_{12}O_6$, but they differ in structural formula with respect to their functional groups. There is a **keto** group in position two of fructose and an **aldehyde** group in position one of glucose (**Figure 2.3**). This type of isomerism is known as **ketose-aldose isomerism**.

D and L Isomerism

D and L isomerism depends on the orientation of the H and OH groups around the asymmetric carbon atom adjacent to the terminal primary alcohol carbon, e.g., carbon atom number 5 in glucose determines whether the sugar belongs to D or L isomer.

When OH group on this carbon atom is on the right, it belongs to **D-series**, when it is on the left; it is the member of the **L-series**. The structures of D and L-glucose based on the reference monosaccharide, D and L glyceraldehyde, a three carbon sugar (**Figure 2.4**). Most of the monosaccharides in the living beings belong to the D-series (unlike amino acids which are L isomers). D and L isomers are mirror images of each other. These two forms are called **enantiomers**.

Optical Isomerism

The presence of **asymmetric carbon** atoms exhibits **optical activity** on the compound. Optical activity is the capacity of a substance to rotate the plane polarized light passing through it.

When a beam of plane polarized light is passed through a solution of carbohydrates it rotates the light either to the right and is said to be **dextrorotatory (+)** or to the left and is said to be, **levorotatory (–)**.

The direction of rotation of polarized light is independent of the D and L isomerism. of the sugar, so it may be designated D (–), D (+), L (–), or L (+). For example, the naturally occurring form of fructose is the D (–) isomer.

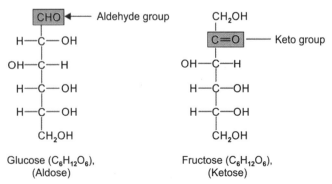

Figure 2.3: Aldose-ketose isomerism.

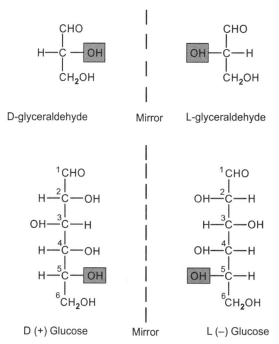

Figure 2.4: D and L isomers (enantiomeric pairs) of glyceraldehyde and glucose.

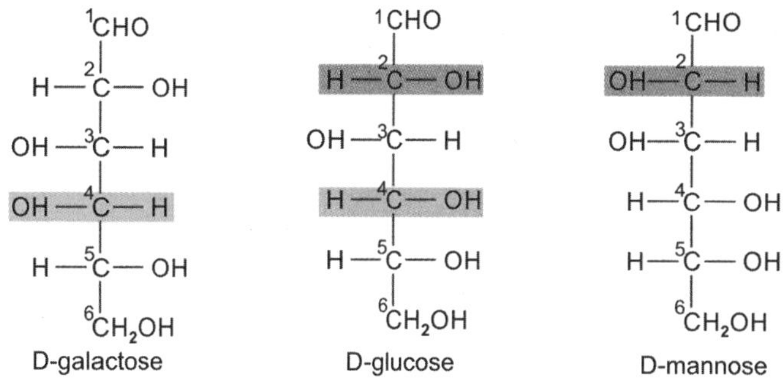

Figure 2.5: Epimers of glucose.

In solution, glucose is dextrorotatory that is why glucose solutions sometimes known as **dextrose**.

> Confusingly, dextrorotatory (+) was at one time called *d*-, and levorotatory (–) *l*-. This nomenclature is obsolete, but may sometimes be found; it is unrelated to D- and L-isomerism.

When equal amount of dextrorotatory (+) and levorotatory (–) isomers are present, the resulting mixture has no net rotation of plane polarised light and has no optical activity. Since the activity of each isomer cancel one another, such a mixture is said to be a **racemic mixture**.

Epimerism

When two monosaccharides differ from each other in their configuration around a single **asymmetric carbon** (other than anomeric carbon) atom, they are referred to as **epimers** of each other.

For example, galactose and mannose are two epimers of glucose **(Figure 2.5)**. They differ from glucose in the configuration of groups (H and OH) around C-4 and C-2 respectively. Galactose and mannose are not epimers of each other as they differ in configuration at two asymmetric carbon atoms around C-2 and C-4. Biologically, the most important epimers of glucose are mannose and galactose.

Anomerism

α and β Anomerism

The predominant form of glucose and fructose in a solution are not an open chain. Rather, the open chain form of this sugar in solution cyclize into rings. An additional asymmetric center is created when glucose cyclizes. Carbon-1

of glucose in the open chain form becomes an asymmetric carbon in the ring form **(Figure 2.6)** producing two possible stereoisomerisms, designated α and β.

The designation α means that the hydroxyl group attached to C-1 is below the plane of the ring, β means that it is above the plane of the ring. Isomeric forms of monosaccharides that differ only in their configuration about the carbonyl carbon atom are called anomers and carbonyl carbon is called anomeric carbon. The C-1 carbon of glucose is the anomeric carbon atom and so, α and β forms are **anomers**.

BIOLOGICALLY IMPORTANT MONOSACCHARIDE DERIVATIVES

Monosaccharide may undergo various reactions to form **carbohydrate derivatives**. In addition to simple hexoses such as glucose, galactose and mannose, there are a number of sugar derivatives in which a hydroxyl group in the parent compound is replaced with another substituent, or a carbon atom is oxidized to a carboxyl group. Several of these are important metabolic and structural components of living organism. Some important sugar derivatives of monosaccharide are:

- Sugar phosphates
- Amino sugars
- Deoxy sugars
- Sugar acids
- Sugar alcohols.

After modification, a transformed molecule of sugar is not considered as sugar anymore because its function and characteristics has changed. Abbreviations for common monosaccharide derivatives are given in **Table 2.4**.

Sugar Phosphates

Phosphorylated derivatives of certain monosaccharides are frequently formed during metabolic reactions. The first step in the breakdown of glucose is its conversion into **glucose-6-phosphate**. Glucose 6 Phosphate **(Figure 2.7)** plays an important role in glycolysis. The addition of the phosphate group gives the sugar a negative charge which prevents sugars from crossing lipid membranes. It can

α-D-glucose

D-glucose
(open chain formula)

β-D-glucose

α-D-glucose

β-D-glucose

Above
the plane

Below
the plane

Figure 2.6: Binding of OH group of C-5 to the CHO group of C-1 generated a new asymmetric carbon atom at C-1.

TABLE 2.4: Abbreviations for common monosaccharide derivatives.	
Monosaccharide derivative	*Abbreviations*
Glucuronic acid	GlcA
Glucosamine	GlcN
Galactosamine	GalN
N-Acetylgalactosamine	GalNAc
N-acetylglucosamine	GlcNAc
Iduronic acid	IdoA
Muramic acid	Mur
N-Acetylmuramic acid	Mur2Ac
N-Acetylneuraminic acid (a sialic acid)	Neu5Ac

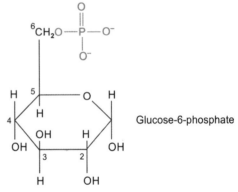

Glucose-6-phosphate

Figure 2.7: Phosphoric acid ester of glucose.

be converted into glycogen and stored in the liver and muscles.

Several important phosphorylated derivatives of sugars are components of **nucleotides**. Phosphorylation also activates sugars for subsequent chemical transformation.

> Phosphorylation of sugar within cell is essential to prevent diffusion of the sugar out of the cell. Phosphorylation makes sugars anionic; the negative charge prevents these sugars from spontaneously leaving the cell by crossing lipid-bilayer membranes. Most cells do not have plasma membrane transporters for phosphorylated sugars, thus phosphorylation trap the sugar inside the cell.

Amino Sugars

In amino sugar a hydroxyl group (most commonly on carbon 2) of a sugar is replaced by an amino group. Examples of amino sugars include (**Figure 2.8**):

- Glucosamine
- Galactosamine
- Mannosamine
- N-Acetylglucosamine
- N-acetylneuraminic acid (sialic acid).

The most common amino sugar of animal cells is **D-glucosamine**, **D-galactosamine** and **D-mannosamine** in which the hydroxyl at C-2 of the parent compound is replaced with an **amino group**.

- In **N-acetylglucosamine** amino group of amino sugar is commonly condensed with **acetic acid**. These amino sugars are found in **glycoproteins** and **proteoglycans** (**glycosaminoglycans**) in which hydroxyl groups can also be sulphated.

- Several antibiotics such as **erythromycin**, **carbomycin** contain amino sugar.

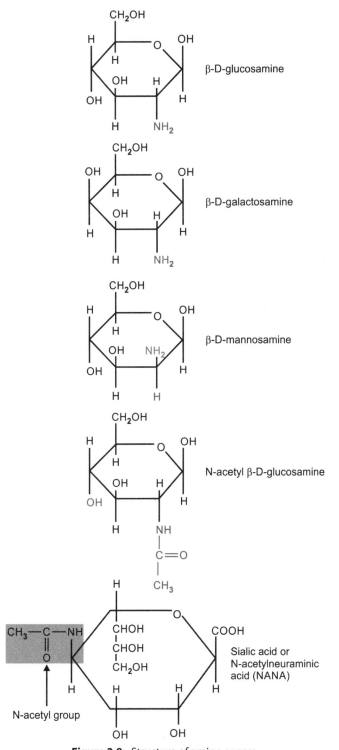

Figure 2.8: Structure of amino sugars.

- **N-acetylneuraminic acid** (often referred to as **sialic acid**) is a nine carbon sugar derived from **D-mannosamine** and **pyruvic acid**. Sialic acids are acetylated derivatives of neuraminic acid in which amino ($-NH_2$) or hydroxyl (OH) group is acetylated **(Figure 2.8)**.
- Sialic acid occurs in many glycoproteins and glycolipids of animal cell surfaces, providing **sites of recognition** by other cells.

Deoxy Sugars

Monosaccharide in which one of the OH group is substituted by **hydrogen group** is known as **deoxy sugars**. Two important deoxy sugars found in cells are **L-fucose** and **Deoxyribose (Figure 2.9)**.

- **Deoxyribose:** Deoxyribose is the most commonly known deoxy sugar. Deoxyribose found in **nucleic acid DNA**. It is present in the backbone of DNA double helices. In the DNA backbone, deoxyribose sugars are bound to phosphate groups via phosphodiester linkages, and are each covalently attached to one of the four DNA nitrogenous bases. They therefore play very important roles in the flexibility of the DNA backbone.
- **L-fucose:** The substitution of hydrogen for the hydroxyl group at C-6 of L-galactose produces L-fucose. L-fucose is found in **complex oligosaccharide** components of **glycoproteins** (such as ABO blood group antigens), and **glycolipids**.

Sugar Acids

- Oxidation of aldehyde group of glucose to the carboxyl group produces **gluconic acid (Figure 2.10)**. Gluconic acid is used in medicine as a harmless counter ion while administering positively charged drugs such as **quinine** or ions such as **Ca^{2+}**. Other aldoses yield other aldonic acids.
- Oxidation of the terminal CH_2OH group (C_6) of glucose, galactose or mannose forms the corresponding **uronic acid; glucuronic acid (Figure 2.10), galacturonic** or **mannuronic acid**. Two uronic acids important

Figure 2.9: Structure of deoxy sugars.

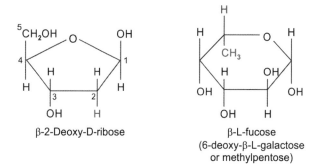

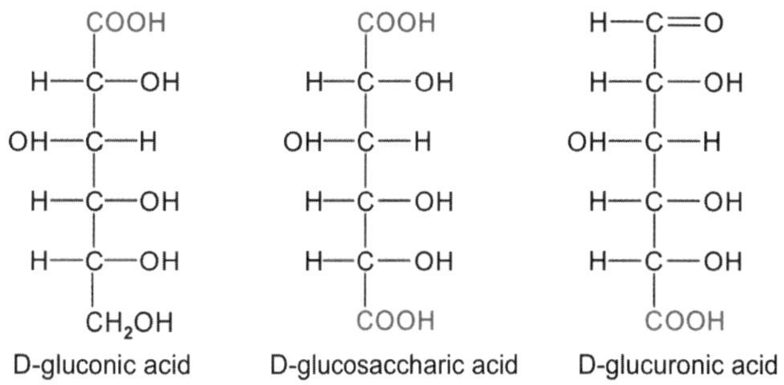

Figure 2.10: Sugar acids produced by oxidation of glucose.

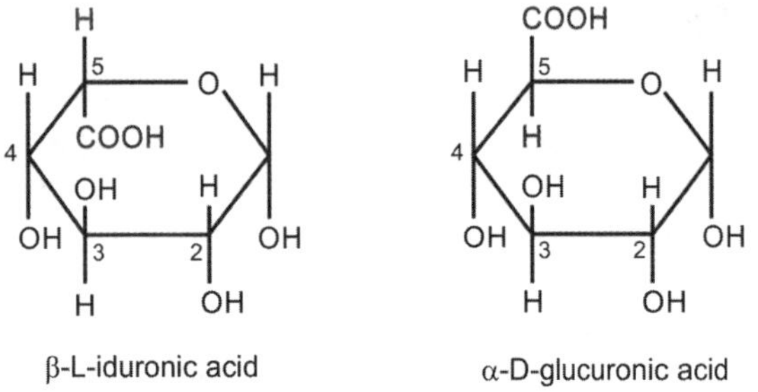

Figure 2.11: Structure of uronic acids.

D-glucose —Reduction→ D-sorbitol

D-mannose —Reduction→ D-mannitol

D-fructose —Reduction→ D-mannitol + D-sorbitol

D-galactose —Reduction→ Dulcitol

Figure 2.12: Reduction of sugar to form alcohol.

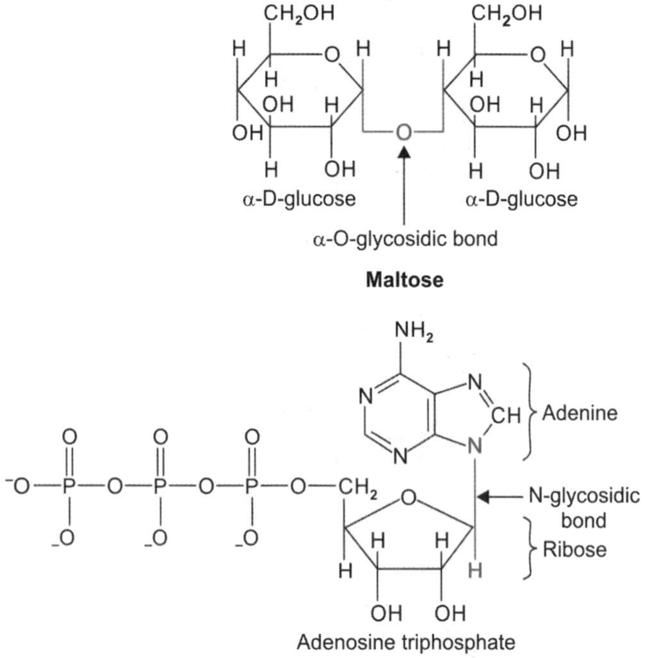

Figure 2.13: The O- and -N type of glycoside bonds.

in animals are **D-glucuronic acid** and its epimer, **L-iduronic acid (Figure 2.11)**. Both D-glucuronic acid and L-iduronic acid are abundant in connective tissue.

- In liver glucuronic acid is combined with molecules such as steroids, certain drugs and bilirubin and make them water soluble. This process helps to remove waste products from the body.
- Oxidation of both aldehyde and terminal primary alcohol groups to carboxyl groups, form **saccharic acid (Figure 2.10)**. For example, glucose to **glucosaccharic acid**, mannose to **mannaric acid** and galactose to **mucic acid**. Mucic acid test is used for the identification of galactose (mucic acid forms insoluble crystals).

Sugar Alcohols

Both aldoses and ketoses may be reduced by enzymes or non-enzymatically to the corresponding polyhydroxy alcohols. The alcohols formed from glucose, mannose, and galactose are **sorbitol**, **mannitol** and **dulcitol (Figure 2.12)**.

- Mannitol, the sugar alcohol derived from mannose, is frequently used medically as an osmotic diuretic to reduce cerebral edema.
- Sorbitol, the sugar alcohol derived from glucose, often accumulates in the lenses of diabetics and produces cataracts.

GLYCOSIDE AND ITS IMPORTANCE

Glycosides are formed when **hydroxyl (OH) group of anomeric carbon** (a carbon carrying the **ketone** or **aldehyde** functional group) of monosaccharides condense with **a hydroxyl (OH)** or **amine (–NH) group of a second compound** that may or may not be another carbohydrate with elimination of water molecule.

- If a second group is a hydroxyl (OH) group, it is called **O-glycosidic bond**. For example, the glycosidic bond of disaccharide like lactose, maltose sucrose is of O-glycosidic bond **(Figure 2.13)**.
- If a second group is an amine (–NH), it is called **N-glycosidic bond**. For example, the bond formed between a hydroxyl (OH) group of ribose sugar and **–NH of nitrogenous base adenine** to form nucleotides such as ATP **(Figure 2.13)**.
- Glycosides are named for the sugar that provides the anomeric hydroxyl group. Thus, if glucose provides anomeric hydroxyl group the resultant molecule is a **glucoside**; if it galactose resultant molecule is **galactoside** and so on.
- The non-carbohydrate moiety of a glycoside is known as the **aglycone**. The aglycone may be methanol, glycerol, sterol, phenol or a base such as adenine.

Therapeutic Importance of Glycosides

- Glycosides are important in medicine because of their action on the heart. **Cardiac glycosides** such as, **ouabain** and **digoxin** increase heart muscle contraction and are used for treatment of **congestive heart failure**. They act by inhibiting the **Na^+/K^+ ATPase** that blocks the active transport of Na^+.
- Other glycosides are found in many antibiotics such as **streptomycin**. **Anthracyline glycosides** (daunorubicin and doxorubicin) are used to treat **leukemia** and wide range of **cancer**.

DISACCHARIDES: EXAMPLES AND IMPORTANCE

Disaccharides consist of **two monosaccharide** units joined by an **O-glycosidic bond**; they are crystalline, water soluble and sweet to test. Disaccharides may be reducing or non-reducing on the basis of the presence or absence of free reducing group (aldehyde or ketone). Sucrose, lactose and maltose are the most physiologically important disaccharides **(Table 2.3)**.

Maltose

Maltose contains two glucose residues, joined by glycosidic linkage between C-1 (the anomeric carbon) of one glucose residue and C-4 of the other, leaving one free anomeric carbon of the second glucose residue, which can act as a reducing agent. Thus, maltose is a reducing disaccharide.

In maltose sugar-sugar linkage is through oxygen atom. The numerical description like (1→4) **of glycosidic bond** represents the number of carbon atoms that connect the two sugars as shown in **Figure 2.14**. The sugar contributing anomeric carbon is written first.

- Maltose is a sweet carbohydrate, but compared to other common sweet carbohydrates, such as sucrose (table sugar) and fructose, it is a lot less sweet. Due to its lack of sweetness, it isn't often added to products as a sweetener.
- Maltose is produced as an intermediate product in the digestion of starch by the action of the enzyme

α-amylase. The amylase can either break the starch into individual glucose units or into the disaccharide **maltose** which in turn hydrolysed to two molecules of glucose by **maltase** and then be used as **energy**.

Isomaltose

Isomaltose is a disaccharide similar to maltose, but with **α-1→6** linkage instead of the α-1→4 linkage. Isomaltose is a reducing sugar. It consists of two glucose molecules linked by an **(α-1→6) glycosidic bond (Figure 2.14)**.

Isomaltose is derived from the digestion of starch. It is hydrolyzed to glucose in the intestinal tract by an enzyme called **isomaltase** and then be used as **energy**.

Lactose (Milk Sugar)

Lactose is present in milk. Lactose contains one unit of **β-D-galactose** and one unit of **β-D-glucose** that are linked by β **(1→4) glycosidic** linkage **(Figure 2.14)**. The anomeric carbon of the bond comes from β-D-galactose making lactose a β-D-glycosidic. The anomeric carbon of the glucose unit is available for oxidation and thus lactose is a reducing disaccharide.

- In the intestine, lactose is hydrolysed to **glucose** and **galactose** by an enzyme **lactase** in human. Glucose and galactose are used by our body for energy and various functions.

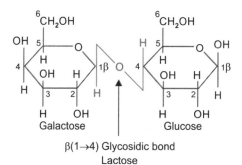

Figure 2.14: Structure of nutritionally important disaccharides.

TABLE 2.5: Clinically important carbohydrates.

Name of sugar	Clinical significance
L-Xylulose	Found in urine in essential pentosuria (hereditary disease)
D-Glucose	Found in urine (glycosuria) in diabetes mellitus (hyperglycemia)
D-Fructose	Accumulation of fructose occur in hereditary fructose intolerance and leads to hypoglycemia
D-Galactose	Failure to metabolize galactose leads to galactosemia and cataract
D-Lactose	In lactose intolerance, due to deficiency of **lactase** enzyme, malabsorption of lactose leads to diarrhea and flatulence
Sucrose	In sucrase deficiency, malabsorption leads to diarrhea and flatulence
Glycogen	In glycogen storage disease (hereditary disorder) accumulation of glycogen occur that leads to hypoglycemia

- Lactose has clinical significance **(Table 2.5)**. Lactose maldigestion is due to the normal reduction of the activity of **lactase**. Lactose intolerance is the inability to digest lactose that results in intestinal discomfort such as **bloating**, **diarrhea**, and **gas**.

STRIKE A NOTE

- **Lactose:** Reducing disaccharide made up of galactose and glucose.
- **Lactulose:** Reducing disaccharide made up of galactose and fructose. Synthetic osmotic laxative.
- **Lactase:** Enzyme which hydrolyse lactose to galactose and glucose.
- **Lactate:** End product of anaerobic glycolysis.

Sucrose (Common Table Sugar)

Sucrose is a disaccharide of **glucose** and **fructose**. It is formed by plant but not by human beings. Sucrose is an intermediate product of photosynthesis. Commonly used **table sugar** is nothing but sucrose. In contrast to maltose and lactose, sucrose contains no free anomeric carbon atom. The anomeric carbon of both monosaccharide units is involved in the glycosidic bond **(Figure 2.14)**. Sucrose is therefore a non-reducing sugar. Sucrose is hydrolysed to **fructose** and **glucose** by an enzyme **sucrase** is also called **invertase**. The **fructose** and **glucose** are metabolized to release **energy**.

Sucrose has clinical significance **(Table 2.5)**. **Sucrose intolerance** or genetic sucrase-isomaltase deficiency is the condition in which **sucrase-isomaltase**, an enzyme needed for proper metabolism of sucrose and starch is not produced or the enzyme produced is either partially functional or non-functional in the small intestine. A deficiency or absence of sucrase-isomaltase function is likely to cause chronic **intestinal discomfort** such as **bloating**, **diarrhea**, and **gas** whenever a person eats food containing sucrose or starch.

- In food industry, hydrolysed sucrose is called **invert sugar**, and the enzyme that hydrolyzes it is called **invertase**.
- The specific rotation of the sucrose (dextrorotatory) before hydrolysis is positive (+66.4°), but after hydrolysis it becomes **negative**.
- Hydrolysis of sucrose yields a mixture of **dextrorotatory D-glucose** (specific rotation = +52.7°) and **levorotatory D-fructose** (specific rotation = –92°).
- **Hydrolytic mixture** is called **"invert sugar"** because fructose is strongly levorotatory changes (inverts) the weaker dextrorotatory action of sucrose.

POLYSACCHARIDES (GLYCANS): EXAMPLES AND IMPORTANCE

Carbohydrates composed of ten or more monosaccharide units or their derivatives (such as amino sugars and uronic acids) are generally classified as polysaccharides. Polysaccharides are colloidal in size. Monosaccharide units are joined together by **glycosidic linkages**. Another term for polysaccharides is a **glycans**.

Polysaccharides play vital roles in **energy storage** and in maintaining the **structural integrity** of an organism. Polysaccharides are subclassified in to two groups **(Figure 2.1)**:

1. **Homopolysaccharides (Homoglycans):** When a polysaccharide is made up of several units of one and the same type of monosaccharide unit only, it is called homopolysaccharide.
2. **Heteropolysaccharides (Heteroglycans):** They contain two or more different types of monosaccharide units or their derivatives.

Homopolysaccharides or Homoglycans

The most important storage polysaccharides are **starch** in plant cell and **glycogen** in animal cells.

Starch

Starch is the most important storage polysaccharides in **plants**. Starch is a homopolymer of glucose called a **glucosan** or **glycan**. It is the most important dietary carbohydrate in cereals, potatoes, legume and other vegetables. Starch contains two types of glucose polymer, **amylose** (13% to 20%) and **amylopectin** (80% to 87%).

- **Amylose** consists of long, unbranched chains of **D-glucose** residues connected by α-$1\rightarrow4$ linkages **(Figure 2.15)**. Such chains vary in molecular weight from a few thousand to more than a million.
- **Amylopectin** also has a high molecular weight (up to 200 million) but unlike amylose is highly branched. The branch points in amylopectin are connected by α-$1\rightarrow6$ bonds and occur at an interval of 24 to 30 residues of glucose. Thus amylopectin is a branched

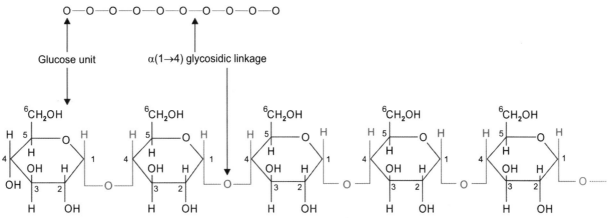

Figure 2.15: Amylose (unbranched polymer of glucose) type of structure, glucose units joined by α-(1→4) linkages.

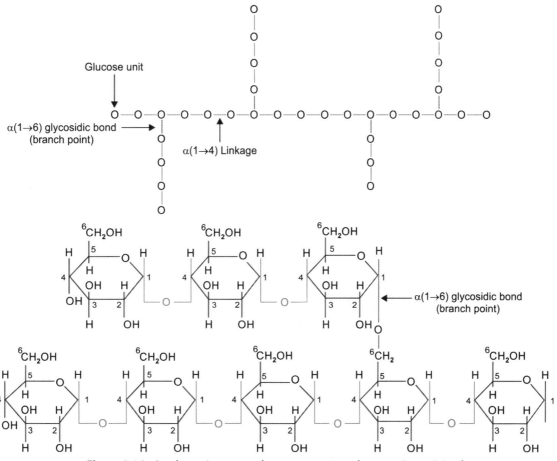

Figure 2.16: Amylopectin type or glycogen structure, glucose units are joined by α-(1→4) and α-(1→6) glycosidic linkages.

polymer having both α-(1→4) and α-(1→6) linkages **(Figure 2.16)**.

Dextrin

Partial hydrolysis of starch by acids or α-amylase (enzyme) produces substances known as dextrins. These also occur in honey. All dextrins have few free aldehyde groups and can show mild reducing property. They are not fermented by yeast.

Glycogen (Animal Starch)

Glycogen is the major **storage form of carbohydrate (glucose)** in animals, found mostly in **liver** and **muscle**. It is often called **animal starch**. Glycogen is especially abundant in liver where it may constitute as much as 7% of the wet weight. The structure of glycogen is similar to that of amylopectin, except that it is more highly branched, having α-(1→6) linkages at an intervals of about 8 to 10 glucose units **(Figure 2.17)**.

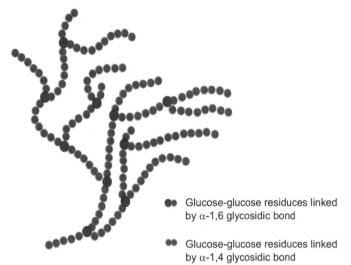

● ● Glucose-glucose residuces linked
        by α-1,6 glycosidic bond

● ● Glucose-glucose residues linked
        by α-1,4 glycosidic bond

Figure 2.17: Diagrammatic representation of glycogen molecule.

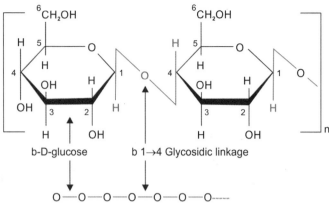

Figure 2.18: Structure of cellulose.

Function

- The function of muscle glycogen is to act as a readily available source of glucose for energy within muscle itself.
- Liver glycogen is a storage form of glucose and concerned with maintenance of the blood glucose.

Why Glucose is Stored in the form of Glycogen?

❖ The stored glycogen is insoluble and contributes little to the **osmolarity** of the **cytosol**. Storage of glucose in a large polymer like **glycogen is not osmotically active**.

❖ However, free glucose molecules cannot be stored because **glucose is osmotically active**, which would be threateningly elevate osmolarity; leading to osmotic imbalance of the cell, causing entry of water in to the cell that might rupture the cell.

Cellulose

Cellulose is the chief constituent of cell wall of plants. It is an **unbranched polymer** of glucose and consists of long straight chains which are linked by β-(1→4) glycosidic linkages and not α-(1→4) as in starch and glycogen **(Figure 2.18)**.

- Since humans lack an enzyme **cellulase** that can hydro-lyze the β-(1→4) glycosidic linkages of polysaccharides, **cellulose cannot be digested** and **absorbed** and does not serve as a souse of energy and has no food value unlike starch. It is however, a significant component of the diet since it acts as a **dietary fiber**.
- The ruminant can utilize cellulose because they have in their digestive tract microorganisms whose enzymes hydrolyse cellulose and ferment the products to short chain fatty acids as a major energy source.

Inulin

Inulin is a polymer of **D-fructose** (Fructosans) linked together by β-(1→2) **glycosidic linkage**. It is readily soluble in water. It occurs in the tubers of some plants, e.g., chicory, bulb of onion and garlic. Inulin is not hydrolyzed by α-amylase due to β configuration of glycosidic bond and so is not utilized as food. Inulin has **clinical importance**; it is used to determine the glomerular **filtration rates (kidney function test)**.

Dextran

Dextrans are bacterial and yeast polysaccharides made up of (α-1→6) linked poly D-glucose; all have (α-1→3) branches, and some also have (α-1→2) or (α-1→4) branches.

Clinical Importance of Dextran

High molecular weight dextran has importance in medicine because of its use as **plasma substitute** or expander. Dextran solution is used in transfusion to increase the volume of plasma in the treatment of various conditions such as hemorrhage and shock.

It works by restoring blood plasma lost through severe bleeding. Severe blood loss can decrease oxygen levels and can lead to organ failure, brain damage, coma, and possibly death. Plasma is needed to circulate red blood cells that deliver oxygen throughout the body.

- Dextran is used to treat **hypovolemia** (decreased volume of circulating blood plasma), that can result from surgery, trauma or injury, severe burns, or other causes of bleeding.
- Dextran should not be used in severe kidney disease, severe congestive heart failure, or uncontrolled bleeding.
- Synthetic dextrans for example **Sephadex** used for fractionation of proteins by chromatography.
- Dental plaque, formed by bacteria growing on the surface of teeth is rich in dextrans, which are adhesive and allow the bacteria to stick to teeth and to each other. Dextrans also provide a source of glucose for the bacterial metabolism.

Heteroglycans

Agar

Agar is vegetable mucilage obtained from seaweeds. Cell walls of certain marine red algae contain agar. Agar is a mixture of sulphated heteropolysaccharides made up of **D-galactose** and **L-galactose** derivatives. Agar swells strongly in hot water, which upon cooling sets to a gel.

● Agar is a **nondigestible** and is at times given to provide bulk to the feces in the treatment of constipation.

● Agarose is the agar. The gel forming property of agarose makes it useful in the biochemistry laboratory. Agarose gels are used as inert supports for the **electrophoretic separation** of **nucleic acid**s.

● Agar is also used to media for the growth of bacterial colonies.

● Another commercial use of agar is for the **capsules** in which some vitamins and drugs are packaged. The dried agar material dissolves readily in the stomach and is metabolically inert.

Gum and Pectin

Gum and pectin are known as **non-cellulose fiber**. These fibers bind a number of small organic compounds including carcinogens, cholesterol and bile acids, thereby **reducing plasma cholesterol**. Pectin and gum **slow the rate of gastric emptying** and retard the rate of digestion and absorption of many nutrients. This effect is beneficial to diabetics because it can **reduce the rise in blood glucose** following a carbohydrate rich meal.

Glycosaminoglycans Or Mucopolysaccharides

Glycosaminoglycans (GAGs) are **heteropolysaccharides** of the extracellular matrix. They are not found in plants. Glycosaminoglycans were first isolated from mucin which led to the original name as **mucopolysaccharide**. One component is always an amino sugar hence the name **glycos-aminoglycans**.

Structure of GAG

The glycosaminoglycans are linear, **unbranched** polymers composed of **repeating disaccharide** units.

● One of the two monosaccharides in repeating disaccharide of glycosaminoglycans is always **amino sugar** (hence the name glycosaminoglycans), either

N-acetylglucosamine or N-acetylgalactosamine (Figure 2.8).

● The other component of the repeating disaccharide in most cases an **uronic acid**, usually **D-glucuronic acid (GlcUA)** or **L-iduronic (IDUA) acid (Figure 2.11)**. L-iduronic is a **5′-epimer** of glucuronic acid.

● Some glycosaminoglycans contain **esterified sulfate** groups. The **sulfate groups** and the **carboxylic groups** of the uronic acid residues give glycosaminoglycans a very high **negative charge**. The negatively charged carboxyl and sulfate groups on the proteoglycan bind positively charged ions and form hydrogen bonds with water molecules, thereby producing **gel like matrix**. The **sulfated glycosaminoglycans** are attached to extracellular proteins to form **proteoglycans**. Proteoglycans consist of up to **95% carbohydrate** by weight.

● The polymer of GAG is attached covalently to extra-cellular proteins called **core protein** (except hyaluronic acid) to form **proteoglycan monomer**. Linking of GAG chain to core protein occurs by a core **trisaccharide linker (Gal-Gal-Xyl)**. A resulting structure resembles a **bottle brush (Figure 2.19)**.

● The proteoglycan monomer associate with a molecule of **hyaluronic acid** to form **proteoglycan aggregates (Figure 2.20)**. The association is not covalent, but occurs primarily through ionic interaction between core protein and the hyaluronic acid. The association is stabilized by additional small protein called **link proteins**. With the exception of hyaluronic acid, all the GAGs contain sulfate group.

Occurrence of GAGs

GAGs in the form of proteoglycans are found in the:
● Synovial fluid of joints
● Vitreous humor of the eye

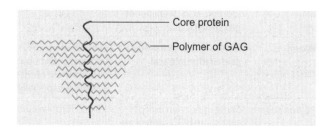

Figure 2.19: Bottle brush structure of proteoglycan monomer.

- Arterial walls
- Bones
- Cartilage.

Types of GAGs

The major glycosaminoglycans are:
- Hyaluronan/hyaluronic acid.
- Chondroitin sulfate

- Keratan sulfate I and II
- Dermatan sulfate
- Heparin
- Heparan sulfate

The different types of glycosaminoglycans differ from each other in a number of following properties:
- Amino sugar composition
- Uronic acid composition
- Linkages between these components
- Chain length of the disaccharides
- The presence or absence of sulfate groups and their positions of attachment to the constituent sugars
- The nature of core proteins to which they are attached
- The nature of the linkage to core protein
- Their tissue and subcellular distribution
- Their biologic functions.

The structure, distribution and functions of each of the glycosaminoglycans will now be briefly discussed. The structural repeating disaccharide unit, location and functions of the glycosaminoglycans are summarized in **Table 2.6**.

Functions of GAGs

- They act as structural component. They are major components of the extracellular matrix or ground substance.
- The negatively charged carboxyl and sulfate groups on the proteoglycan bind positively charged ions and from hydrogen bonds with water molecules, thereby producing gel like matrix. The gel provides a flexible mechanical support for the ECM and functions as a **cushion** and **lubricant** against mechanical shocks.
- Because the long negative charged glycosaminoglycan chains repel each other, the proteoglycans occupy a very

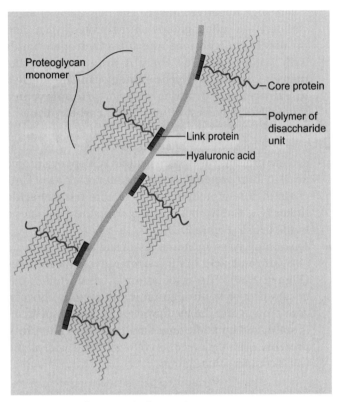

Figure 2.20: Proteoglycan aggregate.

TABLE 2.6: Structure, distribution and functions of glycosaminoglycans (GAGs).			
GAG	**Repeating disaccharide unit**	**Location**	**Function**
Hyaluronic acid	N-acetyl glucosamine-glucuronic acid	Synovial fluid of joints, vitreous humor of the eye, loose connective tissue and umbilical cord	Serve as lubricant and shock absorber, facilitate cell migration in embryogenesis, morphogenesis, wound healing
Chondroitin sulfate	N-acetyl-galactosamine-glucuronic acid	At sites of calcification in bone and cartilage, certain neurons	Provide an endoskeletal structure helping to maintain their shape. Have role in compressibility of cartilage in weight bearing
Keratan sulfate	N-acetyl-glucosamine-galactose (no uronic acid)	Cornea, loose connective tissue, cartilage	Transparency of cornea
Dermatan sulfate	N-acetyl-galactosamine-L-iduronic acid (5-epimer of glucuronic acid)	Skin, blood vessels and heart valves	Transparency of cornea and maintain the overall shape of the eye
Heparin	Glucosamine-glucuronic acid or Iduronic acid	Unlike other GAGs that are extracellular compounds heparin is an intracellular component of mast cells, that line arteries, especially in liver, lung and skin	Serves as an anticoagulant (binds antithrombin III) causes release of lipoprotein lipase from capillary walls
Heparan sulfate	Same as heparin except that some glucosamine are acetylated	Skin, fibroblast and aortic wall	Are component of plasma membrane where they may act as receptor and may also participate in the mediation of cell growth, cell-cell communication

large space and act as **"molecular sieves"** determining which substances enter and leave cells

- They also give **resilience** (elasticity) to substances such as cartilage, permitting compression and re-expansion. When a solution of glycosaminoglycans is compressed, the water is squeezed out and glycosaminoglycans are forced to occupy a smaller volume. After releasing compression the glycosaminoglycans spring back to their original hydrated volume.
- Facilitate cell migration, e.g., hyaluronan.
- Play role in corneal transparency, e.g., keratan sulfate I and dermatan sulfate.
- Have structural role in sclera, e.g., dermatan sulfate.
- Act as anticoagulant, e.g., heparin.
- They are components of plasma membranes, where they may act as **receptors** and participate in **cell adhesion** and **cell-cell communications**, e.g., heparin sulfate.
- Determine charge selectiveness of renal glomerulus, e.g., heparin sulfate.
- They are components of synaptic and other vesicles, e.g., heparin sulfate.

STRIKE A NOTE

- ❖ Site of synthesis of GAG is ER and Golgi apparatus.
- ❖ Glycosaminoglycan with no Uronic acid is keratan sulfate.
- ❖ Glycosaminoglycan with not sulfate group is hyaluronan.
- ❖ GAG that helps in cell communication is Hyaluronan.
- ❖ GAG found in bacteria is hyaluronan.
- ❖ Glycosaminoglycan not covalently linked to protein is hyaluronan.
- ❖ **Hyaluronidase**, an enzyme secreted by some pathogenic bacteria, can hydrolyze the glycosidic linkages of hyaluronan, rendering tissues more susceptible to bacterial invasion. A similar enzyme in sperm hydrolyzes an outer glycosaminoglycan coat around the ovum, allowing sperm penetration.
- ❖ Glycosaminoglycans are generally extracellular, only intracellular glycosaminoglycan is heparin.
- ❖ The **sulfate** and **carboxylic groups** of the uronic acid residues give glycosaminoglycans a very high **negative charge**.
- ❖ Mucin clot test (Rope test) is to detect hyaluronan in the synovial fluid.
- ❖ GAG that gives corneal transparency is keratan Sulphate I and Dermatan Sulphate.
- ❖ GAG that have role in compressibility of cartilage in weight bearing are Hyaluronan and chondroitin sulphate.
- ❖ Osteoarthritis, the most common form of arthritis, results when water is lost from proteoglycan with aging. Other forms of arthritis result from the proteolytic degradation of aggrecan and collagen in the cartilage.
- ❖ The **mucopolysaccharidoses** are genetic hereditary disorders (1:30,000 birth) characterized by excessive accumulation of glycosaminoglycans in various tissues causing symptoms such as skeletal and extracellular matrix deformities and mental retardation.

■ GLYCOPROTEINS

Glycoproteins are proteins to which oligosaccharides are covalently attached to their polypeptide chain. Glyco-proteins contain much shorter carbohydrate chain than proteoglycans. These oligosaccharide chains are often branched instead of linear and do not contain repeating disaccharides and may or may not be negatively charged (as proteoglycans).

- Almost all plasma proteins in humans with the notable exception of **albumin** are glycoproteins.
- The proportion of carbohydrate in glycoprotein varies considerably. It ranges from 1% to more than 85% of its weight and may be simple or very complex in the structure. For example **immunoglobulin IgG** contains less than 4% of its mass as carbohydrates whereas human **gastric glycoprotein (mucin)** contains more than 80% carbohydrates and **glycophorin** a membrane constituent of human erythrocytes contain as much as 85%.
- The oligosaccharide components of glycoprotein are composed primarily of eight types of sugars, **xylose, Fucose, galactose, glucose, mannose, N-acetyl galactosamine, N-acetyl glucosamine**, and **N-acetylneuraminic acid**.
- The oligosaccharide may be attached to the protein through O-glycosidic link or N-glycosidic link. In O-glycosidic link sugar chain is attached to a hydroxyl group of either serine or threonine of side chain. In N-glycosidic link the sugar chain is attached to the amide group of aspargine side chain.

Functions of Glycoproteins

- Almost all the plasma proteins of humans are glycoproteins, except **albumin**.
- Many integral membrane proteins are glycoproteins.
- Membrane bound glycoproteins participate in:
  - Cell surface recognition (by other cells, hormones and viruses)
  - Cell surface antigenicity (such as blood group antigens).
- Most proteins that are secreted, such as **antibodies, hormones** and **coagulation factors** are glycoproteins.
- Glycoproteins serve as **lubricant** and **protective agent**, e.g., glycoproteins are components of extracellular matrix and mucin of the gastrointestinal and urogenital tracts where they act as protective agent and biological lubricants.
- It also serves as transport molecules, such as **transferrin** and **ceruloplasmin**.
- The biological function of the carbohydrate chains of the glycoproteins are as follows:
  - Regulate the lifespan of proteins. For example, loss of sialic acid residues from the end of oligosaccharide chains of erythrocytes results in the removal of red blood cells from the circulation.
  - Serve as recognition signals to facilitate cell-cell interaction (e.g., Sperm-oocyte) and targeting of proteins.

■ Stabilization of protein against denaturation and facilitate its solubility.

GLYCATION AND GLYCOSYLATION

Glycation and glycosylation are two mechanisms which add carbohydrates to the proteins. Glycosylation is an enzymatic process and produces a mature protein, which is functional while glycation is a non-enzymatic process and has serious pathological consequences.

● **Glycation:** Glycation is the nonenzymatic covalent attachment of free sugars to the proteins. Glycations occur mainly in the bloodstream. Glycation affects both function and stability of proteins and has serious pathological consequences. For example glycated hemoglobin. The increased level of which occur in diabetes mellitus.

● **Glycosylation:** It is posttranslational modification of proteins in which a defined carbohydrate is added to a predetermined region of a protein. It is a enzymatic attachment of sugar to protein. It is an essential biochemical process. The endoplasmic reticulum and Golgi apparatus play a major role in glycosylation reactions involved in the biosynthesis of glycoproteins.

ASSESSMENT QUESTIONS

STRUCTURED LONG ESSAY QUESTION (SLEQs)

1. Describe carbohydrates under following headings:
   i. Definition
   ii. Classification with examples
   iii. Functions
2. Describe glycosaminoglycans under following headings:
   i. Structure
   ii. Types
   iii. Functions
3. Describe biologically important sugar derivatives of monosaccharide under following headings:
   i. Types
   ii. Importance

SHORT ESSAY QUESTIONS (SEQs)

1. What is glycogen? Write its importance.
2. What is glycosaminoglycan? Give different types and their function.
3. What is glycoproteins? Write its importance.

SHORT ANSWER QUESTIONS (SAQs)

1. Write functions of carbohydrates.
2. Name different types of glycosaminoglycans.
3. Give diagrammatic representation of proteoglycan aggregate.
4. What are difference between glycoproteins and proteoglycan? Give example of each.
5. Name any two biologically important sugar derivatives with their functions.
6. What is glycoside? Name any two therapeutic important glycosides.
7. Give clinically important monosaccharide with its clinical significance.
8. Write difference between glycation and glycosylation.
9. Write dietary importance of cellulose.

MULTIPLE CHOICE QUESTIONS (MCQs)

1. **All the following are composed exclusively of glucose, *except*:**
   a. Glycogen   b. Starch
   c. Lactose   d. Maltose
2. **The carbohydrate of the blood group substances is:**
   a. Sucrose   b. Fucose
   c. Arabinose   d. Maltose
3. **Which of the following carbohydrate is dietary fiber?**
   a. Cellulose   b. Starch
   c. Glycogen   d. Inulin
4. **Glycosaminoglycans are:**
   a. Disaccharide   b. Homoglycans
   c. Heteroglycans   d. None of the above
5. **Which of the following glycosaminoglycans is unsulfated?**
   a. Chondroitin sulfate   b. Heparin
   c. Hyaluronic acid   d. Keratan sulfate
6. **Which of the following GAGs does not contain uronic acid?**
   a. Hyaluronic acid   b. Keratan sulfate
   c. Heparin   d. Heparan sulfate
7. **Which of the following is not hydrolyzed by α-amylase?**
   a. Starch   b. Glycogen
   c. Cellulose   d. Dextrin
8. **A polysaccharide which is called animal starch is:**
   a. Glycogen   b. Starch
   c. Inulin   d. Dextrin
9. **The homopolysaccharide used for intravenous infusion as plasma substitute is:**
   a. Agar   b. Inulin
   c. Dextrans   d. Starch
10. **The polysaccharide used in assessing the glomerular filtration rate (GFR) is:**
    a. Glycogen   b. Agar
    c. Inulin   d. Hyaluronic acid

11. The constituent unit of inulin is:
    a. Glucose
    b. Fructose
    c. Mannose
    d. Galactose

12. Cellulose is:
    a. Non-starch polysaccharide
    b. Glycoprotein
    c. Oligosaccharide
    d. Heteropolysaccharides

13. Keratan sulfate is found in abundance in:
    a. Heart muscle
    b. Liver
    c. Adrenal cortex
    d. Cornea

14. Glucose on oxidation gives which of the following, *except*:
    a. Mucic acid
    b. Glucosaccharic acid
    c. Gluconic acid
    d. Glucuronic acid

15. What monosaccharides make up a sucrose (table sugar) molecule?
    a. Galactose and fructose
    b. Galactose and maltose
    c. Lactose and fructose
    d. Glucose and fructose

16. Glucose is a building block for, *except*:
    a. Cellulose
    b. Glycogen
    c. Inulin
    d. Starch

17. The sugar found in milk is:
    a. Galactose
    b. Glucose
    c. Fructose
    d. Lactose

18. An L-isomer of monosaccharide formed in human body is:
    a. L-Fructose
    b. L-Erythrose
    c. L-Erythrulose
    d. L-Xylulose

19. N–Acetylglucosamine is present in:
    a. Keratan sulfate
    b. Chondroitin sulfate
    c. Heparin
    d. All of these

20. Amylose is a constituent of:
    a. Cellulose
    b. Starch
    c. Glycogen
    d. All of the above

21. Synovial fluid contains which of the following GAGs:
    a. Heparin
    b. Hyaluronic acid
    c. Chondroitin sulfate
    d. Keratin sulfate

22. In humans carbohydrates are stored as:
    a. Glucose
    b. Glycogen
    c. Starch
    d. Cellulose

23. Which of the following carbohydrate is intracellular?
    a. Heparin
    b. Hyaluronic acid
    c. Chondroitin sulfate
    d. None of the above

24. Following glycosaminoglycans are extracellular, *except*:
    a. Heparin
    b. Hyaluronic acid
    c. Chondroitin sulfate
    d. Keratin sulfate

25. Which of the following proteoglycan exclusively consists of serine and glycine in their protein?
    a. Heparin
    b. Keratin sulfate
    c. Chondroitin sulfate
    d. Dermatan sulfate

26. Hyaluronic acid is present in:
    a. Vitreous humor
    b. Mast cell
    c. Cornea
    d. Dermis

27. Heparin is:
    a. Polysaccharide
    b. Proteoglycan
    c. Carbohydrate
    d. All of the above

28. Sucrose is hydrolyzed to fructose and glucose by an enzyme which called _____.
    a. Hydrolase
    b. Phosphorylase
    c. Ligase
    d. Invertase

29. Which of the following is the sugar alcohol?
    a. Sorbitol
    b. Mannitol
    c. Dulcitol
    d. All of these

30. Glycosidic bond in lactose is:
    a. β-(1$\rightarrow$2)
    b. β-(1$\rightarrow$4)
    c. α-(1$\rightarrow$4)
    d. α-(1$\rightarrow$2)

31. L-Iduronic acid is epimer of:
    a. D-Glucuronic acid
    b. Galactose
    c. Mannose
    d. Glucose

ANSWERS FOR MCQs

1. c	2. b	3. a	4. c	5. c
6. b	7. c	8. a	9. c	10. c
11. b	12. a	13. d	14. a	15. d
16. c	17. d	18. d	19. a	20. b
21. b	22. b	23. a	24. a	25. a
26. a	27. d	28. d	29. d	30. b
31. a				

Chemistry of Lipids

Competency	Learning Objectives
BI 4.1: Describe and discuss main classes of lipids (Essential/non-essential fatty acids, cholesterol and hormonal steroids, triglycerides, major phospholipids, and sphingolipids) relevant to human system and their major functions. **BI 11.24:** Enumerate advantages and/or disadvantages of use of unsaturated, saturated and trans fats in food.	1. Give definition, functions, and classification of lipids with examples. 2. Give definition, functions, and classification of fatty acids with examples. 3. Describe essential fatty acids, its importance and deficiency manifestations. 4. Describe advantages of unsaturated fatty acids and disadvantages of saturated and trans fats in food. 5. Describe composition and importance of triglycerides. 6. Describe composition, types, and clinical importance of phospholipids. 7. Describe structure, types, and clinical importance of sphingolipids. 8. Describe structure, types, and functions of lipoproteins. 9. Describe structure and biological importance of cholesterol.

■ OVERVIEW

Lipids are naturally occurring water insoluble substances. Due to predominance of hydrocarbon chains in their structure, lipids have hydrophobic nature. They perform outstanding range of functions in living organisms. Some lipids are vital energy reserves others are the primary structural components of biological membranes. Still other lipids act as hormones, antioxidants, pigments or vital growth factors, and vitamins. This chapter describes the structures, properties and functions of the major lipid classes found in living organism.

■ LIPIDS: DEFINITION, CLASSIFICATION, AND FUNCTIONS

Definition of Lipids

Lipids may be defined as organic substances insoluble in water but soluble in organic solvents like chloroform, ether, and benzene; they are esters of fatty acids with alcohol or are substances capable of forming such esters and are utilizable by the living organism.

Classification of Lipids

There are many different methods of classifying lipids. The most commonly used classification of lipids is modified from Bloor as follows:

- Simple lipid
- Complex or compound lipid
- Derived lipids.

Simple Lipid

These are esters of fatty acids with various alcohols. Depending on the type of alcohols, these are subclassified as **(Figure 3.1)**:

- Neutral fats or triacylglycerol or triglycerides
- Waxes.

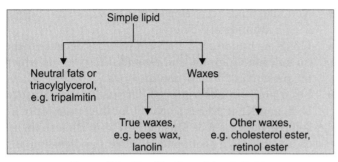

Figure 3.1: Classification of simple lipids.

Neutral fats or Triacylglycerol or Triglycerides

These are esters of fatty acids with alcohol **glycerol**, for example, **tripalmitin**. Because they are **uncharged**, they are termed **neutral fat**. The fats we eat are mostly triglycerides. A fat in **liquid state** is called **oil**, e.g., vegetable oils like groundnut oil, mustered oil, corn oil, etc.

Waxes

- These are esters of fatty acids with higher molecular weight **monohydric long chain alcohols**. These compounds have no importance as far as human metabolism is concerned. But they are widespread in nature. They are protective coatings on the leaves, stem and fruits of plants, and the skin and fur of animals. These are widely used in pharmaceutical, cosmetic, and other industries in the manufacture of lotions, ointments, and polishes For example:
  - **Lanolin** (from lamb's wool)
  - **Bees-wax**
  - **Spermaceti oil** (from whales).
- Waxes also contain long chain alcohols, aldehydes, and steroid alcohols, for example, **cholesterol ester**, **vitamin A ester** (retinol) and **Vitamin D ester** (cholecalciferol).

Complex or Compound Lipid

These are esters of fatty acids, with alcohol containing additional (prosthetic) groups. These are subclassified according to the type of prosthetic group present in the lipid as follows:
- Phospholipids
- Sphingolipids
- Lipoproteins.

Phospholipids

Lipids containing, in addition to fatty acids and an alcohol, a **phosphoric acid** residue are called phospholipid. They frequently have nitrogen containing bases and other substituents. Phospholipids may be classified on the basis of the type of alcohol present in them as **(Figure 3.2)**:
- Glycerophospholipids
- Sphingophospholipids.

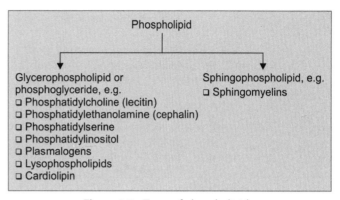

Figure 3.2: Types of phospholipids.

Glycerophospholipids

The alcohol present is **glycerol**. Glycerophospholipids are the membrane lipids. Examples of glycerophospholipids are:
- Phosphatidyl choline (lecithin)
- Phosphatidylethanolamine (cephalin)
- Phosphatidylserine
- Phosphatidylinositol
- Lysophospholipid
- Plasmalogens
- Cardiolipins.

Sphingophospholipids

The alcohol present in sphinogophospholipid is **sphingosine**. An example of sphinogophospholipid is **sphingomyelin**. Sphingomyelins are the only phosphorus containing sphingolipids. Sphingomyelins are most abundant in nervous tissue.

Sphingolipids

Sphingolipids are composed of one molecule of the long-chain **amino alcohol sphingosine**, one molecule of **fatty acid**, and a **polar head group** (like glucose, di-, tri-, or tetrasaccharide, complex oligosaccharide, phosphocholine) that is joined by a **glycosidic** linkage in some cases and a **phosphodiester** in others. There are two types of sphingolipids, deferring in their head groups **(Figure 3.3)**:
1. Sphinogophospholipid
2. Glycolipids/Glycosphingolipids.

- Sphinogophospholipid contains **phosphocholine** or **phosphoethanolamine** as their polar head group and

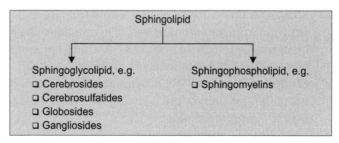

Figure 3.3: Types of sphingolipids.

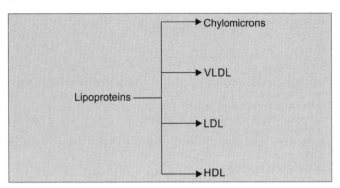

Figure 3.4: Types of lipoproteins.

therefore classified as **phospholipids,** e.g., **sphingomyelins**.

- **Glycosphingolipids** have head groups with one or more **sugars**. They do not contain phosphate, e.g., cerebrosides, globosides and gangliosides. **Gangliosides**, the most complex sphingolipids, have oligosaccharides as their polar head groups and one or more residues of **N-acetylneuraminic acid (NANA)** which is often called **sialic acid**.

Lipoproteins

Lipoproteins are formed by combination of **lipid** with a prosthetic group **protein**, e.g., serum lipoproteins like **(Figure 3.4):**

- Chylomicrons
- Very low density lipoprotein (VLDL)
- Low density lipoprotein (LDL)
- High density lipoprotein (HDL).

Derived Lipids

Derived lipids include the products obtained after the hydrolysis of simple and compound lipids. For example, e.g., Fatty acids, glycerol, steroids, other alcohols, fatty aldehydes, hydrocarbons, ketone bodies, lipid soluble vitamins and micronutrients and hormones.

Functions of Lipids

The biological functions of the lipids are as diverse as their chemistry.

- **Storage form of energy:** The fats and oils are the principle stored forms of energy in living organisms.
- **Structural lipids:** Phospholipids and sterols are major structural components of biological membranes. These lipids play a passive role in the cell by forming impermeable barriers that separate cellular components.
- **Cholesterol,** a sterol, is a **precursor of many steroid hormones**, **vitamin D**, and is also an important component of plasma membrane.
- Lipid acts as a **thermal insulator** in the subcutaneous tissues and around certain organs.

- Nonpolar lipids act as **electrical insulators** in the myelin sheath around nerve fibers.
- Lipids are important dietary constituents because of the **fat soluble vitamins**, and **essential fatty acids** which are present in the fat of natural foods.
- Lipid helps in absorption of fat soluble vitamins (A, D, E, and K). It acts as a solvent for the transport of fat soluble vitamins. Bile salts derived from cholesterol act as a emulsifying agent and facilitate the digestion and absorption of lipids.
- Lipids, for example:
  - Arachidonic acid functions as precursor of prostaglandins and leukotrienes.
  - Phosphatidylcholine functions as surfactant in the alveolar membrane.
  - Inositol triphosphate and diacylglycerol participates as a second messenger in hormone action.

FATTY ACIDS: DEFINITION, FUNCTIONS, AND CLASSIFICATION

Definition of Fatty Acids

Fatty acids are long **hydrocarbon chains** ($-CH_2-CH_2-CH_2-$....) of various lengths (ranging from 4 to 36 carbons long) with a **carboxyl group (–COOH)** at one end, and a **methyl group (–CH$_3$)** at the other end. Fatty acids represented by a chemical formula R-COOH, where R—stands for hydrocarbon chain. In some fatty acids, this hydrocarbon chain is unbranched and fully saturated (contains no double bond); in others, the chain contains one or more double bonds **(Table 3.1)**.

- The fatty acids are **amphipathic** in nature, that is each has **hydrophilic (COOH)** and **hydrophobic (hydrocarbon chain)** groups in the structure.
- The hydrocarbon chain is almost invariable unbranched in animal fatty acids.

TABLE 3.1: Some naturally occurring fatty acids and their carbon numbers.

Fatty acid	*Number of carbons*
Saturated fatty acids	
Lauric acid	12
Myristic acid	14
Palmitic acid	16
Stearic acid	18
Arachidic acid	20
Lignoceric acid	24
Unsaturated fatty acids	
Palmitoleic acid (ω-7)	16
Oleic acid (ω-9)	18
Linoleic acid (ω-6)	18
Linolenic acid (ω-3)	18
Arachidonic acid (ω-6)	20

- Fatty acids in biological systems usually contain even number atoms, typically between 14 and 24 **(Table 3.1)**. The 16- and 18-carbon fatty acids are most common.
- The configuration of the double bonds in most unsaturated fatty acids is cis.
- Fatty acids occur mainly as **esters of glycerol** in neutral fats and oil.

Importance of Fatty Acids

Fatty acids have three major physiological functions:

1. Fatty acids serve as a major fuel for most cells and they are precursors of all other classes of lipids.
2. They serve as building blocks of **phospholipids** and **glycolipids**. These amphipathic molecules are important components of biological membranes.
3. Fatty acid derivatives serve as **hormones**, e.g., **prostaglandins** and intracellular messenger like **phosphatidylinositol**.

Numbering of Fatty Acids and Representation of Double Bonds

- Fatty acid carbon atoms are numbered from the **carboxyl carbon (carbon no. 1)**. The carbon atoms adjacent to the carboxyl carbons 2, 3, and 4 are also known as α, β, and γ respectively. The terminal **methyl carbon** is called the ω (omega; the last letter in the Greek alphabet) or **n-carbon (Figure 3.5)**.
- The symbol Δ (delta) is used for indicating the number and position of the double bonds. Two systems are used to designate the position of double bond; **C-system** and **ω-system**.

C-system

In C-system the **carboxyl carbon** is assigned the **number 1** (C-1), and the carbon next to it is C-2. The positions of any double bonds is represented by the symbol Δ (delta), are specified relative to C-1 followed by a superscript number indicating the lower-numbered carbon in the double bond. By this system, oleic acid a C-18 fatty acid with one double bond between C-9 and C-10 is represented as $18:1:\Delta^9$ **(Figure 3.6)**.

ω-system

This method is widely used by **nutritionists**. In this system, the **carbon atom of the methyl group** in a fatty acid is called the ω carbon and is given the **number 1 (C-1)**. In ω-system the oleic acid is denoted as $18:1:\omega\text{-}9$ **(Figure 3.6)** to indicate that, it has 18 carbon atoms and one double bond.

$\omega\text{-}9$ represents the double bond position, which is found between 9th and 10th carbon atoms, the first carbon atom being that of the methyl (omega carbon) group. Likewise:

- In **ω-6 unsaturated fatty acids**, the first double bond occurs between the 6th and 7th carbon atoms, e.g., **linoleic acid**
- In **ω-3** the first double bond occurs between the 3rd and 4th carbon atoms, e.g., **linolenic acid**.

Classification of Fatty Acids

Fatty acids are classified into four major classes **(Figure 3.7)**.

1. Straight chain fatty acid
2. Branched chain fatty acid
3. Substituted fatty acids
4. Cyclic fatty acid

Straight Chain Fatty Acids

Fatty acids, in which the carbons are arranged linearly, are subclassified into two classes:

1. Saturated fatty acids
2. Unsaturated fatty acids.

Saturated Fatty Acids

There is no double bond in the hydrocarbon chain of these fatty acids and are in extended conformation and so can be packed together into a compact structure. Saturated fatty acids are subclassified into:

- **Even carbon acids** carry even number of carbons, e.g., palmitic acid and stearic acid
- **Odd carbon acids** carry odd number of carbons, e.g., propionic acid.

Unsaturated Fatty Acids

They contain double bonds in their hydrocarbon chains. They are in cis configuration. This configuration produces a rigid bend in the aliphatic chain and compact packing is prevented, consequently the unsaturated fatty acids are loosely packed and are therefore more easily disturbed by heat. This accounts the low melting point of unsaturated fatty acids and is usually liquid at room temperature. These are subclassified according to the number of double bonds present in the structure:

- **Monoenoic** or **monounsaturated fatty acids** carry a single double bond in molecule, e.g., oleic acid.
- **Polyenoic** or **polyunsaturated fatty acids (PUFAs)** contain two or more double bonds. PUFAs with a double bond between: C-3 and C-4 are called omega-3 (**ω-3**) **fatty acids** and C-6 and C-7 are **omega-6 (ω-6) fatty acids**. The first carbon atom is that of the methyl group.

$$\underset{\omega}{\overset{16}{CH_3}} - \overset{15}{CH_2} - \overset{14}{CH_2} - \overset{13}{CH_2} - \overset{12}{CH_2} - \overset{11}{CH_2} - \overset{10}{CH_2} - \overset{9}{CH_2} - \overset{8}{CH_2} - \overset{7}{CH_2} - \overset{6}{CH_2} - \overset{5}{CH_2} - \overset{4}{CH_2} - \underset{\beta}{\overset{3}{CH_2}} - \underset{\alpha}{\overset{2}{CH_2}} - \overset{1}{COOH}$$

Palmitic acid

Figure 3.5: Numbering of fatty acid carbon.

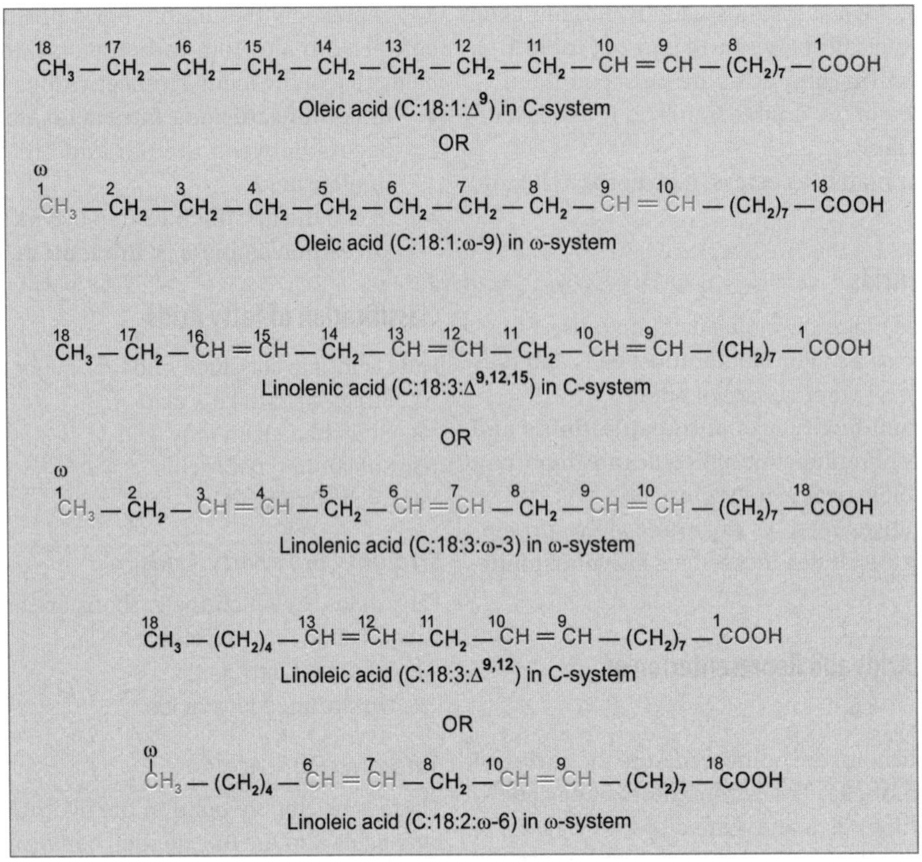

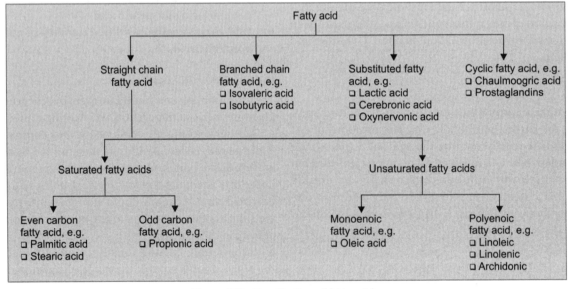

Figure 3.6: Representation of double bonds of unsaturated fatty acids.

Figure 3.7: Classification of fatty acids.

Naturally occurring polyunsaturated fatty acids belong to ω-6 and ω-3 series are (**Table 3.2**):

- Linoleic acid (18:2: ω-6) having two double bonds.
- Linolenic acid (18:3: ω-3) having three double bonds.
- Arachidonic acid (20:4: ω-6) having four double bonds.

The family of **polyunsaturated fatty acids (PUFAs)** with a double bond between the third and fourth carbon from the methyl end of the chain are of special impotence in human nutrition. Because the physiological role of PUFAs is related more to the position of the first double bond near the methyl end of the chain than to that near the carboxyl end.

TABLE 3.2: Omega classification of fatty acids with examples.

Series	Examples
ω-3	• α Linolenic acid • Timnodonic acid (Eicosapentaenoic acid) • Cervonic acid (Docosahexaenoic acid) (DHA)
ω-6	• Linoleic acid • γ Linolenic acid (GLA) • Arachidonic acid
ω-9	• Oleic acid • Elaidic acid

Branched Chain Fatty Acids

These are less abundant than straight chain acids in animal and plant, e.g., **isovaleric acid** and **isobutyric acid**.

Substituted Fatty Acids

In substituted fatty acids one or more hydrogen atoms have been replaced by another group, e.g., lactic acid of blood, cerebronic acid, and oxynervonic acids of brain glycolipids, ricinoleic acid of castor oil.

Cyclic Fatty Acids

Fatty acids bearing cyclic groups are present in some bacteria and seed lipids, e.g., chaulmoogric acid of chaulmoogra seed.

ESSENTIAL FATTY ACIDS: IMPORTANCE AND DEFICIENCY MANIFESTATIONS

Humans can biosynthesize many saturated and monounsaturated fatty acids. However, humans cannot synthesize the two main types of polyunsaturated fatty acids, **Linoleic (ω-6)** and **Linolenic (ω-3)** acids. But plants can synthesize both.

- Humans lack the enzymes to introduce double bonds at carbon atoms beyond C_9 in the fatty acid chain. Hence, humans cannot synthesize linoleic acid ($18:2:\Delta^{9,12}$) and linolenic acid ($18:2:\Delta^{9,12,15}$) having double bonds beyond C_9. Because they are necessary precursors for the synthesis of other products, **linoleic acid** and **linolenic acid** are **essential fatty acids** for mammals. They must be obtained from the dietary plant material.
- Ingested dietary **linoleic acid** may be converted to other polyunsaturated acids, particularly **arachidonic acid**.
- Similarly, **linolenic acid** is converted to two important derivatives, **eicosapentaenoic acid (EPA)** and **Docosahexaenoic acid (DHA)**.

Functions of Essential Fatty Acids (EFA)

- **Linoleic acid** is an essential precursor for synthesis of **arachidonic acid** ($20:4:\Delta^{5,8,11,14}$) from which **eicosanoids** having important regulatory functions are produced which includes:
  - Prostaglandins
  - Thromboxane
  - Prostacyclin
  - Leukotrienes.
- **Linolenic acid** is the precursors for the synthesis of a variety of other unsaturated fatty acids. Human can synthesize two other ω-3 polyunsaturated acids, important in cellular function:
  - Eicosapentaenoic acid (EPA)
  - Docosahexaenoic acid (DHA).

EPA and DHA are important for proper fetal development, including neuronal, retinal, and immune function. EPA and DHA may affect many aspects of cardiovascular function including inflammation, peripheral artery disease, major coronary events, and anticoagulation. EPA and DHA have been linked to promising results in prevention, weight management, and cognitive function in those with very mild Alzheimer's disease.

EPA and DHA have been associated with fetal development (neuronal, retinal), immune function cardiovascular function, cognitive function, and prevent Alzheimer's disease.

- **Maintenance of structural integrity:** EFAs are constituent of **structural lipids** of the cell and are concerned with the structural integrity of the mitochondrial membrane. Their deficiency decreases efficiency of biological oxidation. Arachidonic acid is present in membranes and accounts for 5 to 15% of the fatty acids in phospholipids.
- **Development of retina and brain:** Docosahexaenoic acid (DHA: ω-3) is present in high concentration in retina, cerebral cortex, testes, and sperm. DHA is particularly needed for development of the brain and retina during the neonatal period and is supplied via the placenta and milk. Therefore, a small daily intake of EFA is now recommended. This may be especially important when the nervous system is developing.
- **Skin protector:** It covalently binds another fatty acid attached to cerebrosides in the skin forming an unusual lipid (**acylglucosylceramide**) that helps to make the skin impermeable to water. This formation of linoleic acid may help to explain the red **scaly dermatitis** and other skin problems associated with a dietary deficiency of essential free fatty acids.
- **Antiatherogenic effect:** Essential fatty acids have antiatherogenic effect. Ingestion of polyunsaturated fatty acids increases esterification and excretion of cholesterol, thereby lowering serum cholesterol level.

Deficiency Manifestations

A disease state known as **essential fatty acid deficiency** occurs if EFAs are excluded from the diet for long periods. The syndrome in the humans is characterized by **dermatitis** and **poor wound healing**. These problems clear up when the patients are fed diet containing EFA.

ADVANTAGES OF UNSATURATED FATTY ACIDS AND DISADVANTAGES OF SATURATED AND TRANS FATS IN FOOD

Unsaturated fatty acids having **double bonds** can occur in two isomeric forms: *Cis* and *Trans*. In **cis isomer**, similar or identical groups are on the **same side** of a double bond and when such groups are on opposite sides of a double bond, the molecule is said to be a *trans* isomer **(Figure 3.8)**.

- In nearly all naturally occurring unsaturated fatty acids, the double bonds are in the *cis* **configuration**.
- *Trans* fatty acids, are produced by fermentation in the rumen of dairy animals and are obtained from dairy products and meat. As well as *trans* fatty acids, are produced during the **catalytic hydrogenation** of vegetable oils to make **margarine**. The purpose of hydrogenation is to change the physical properties of oils into solid products, which are easier to manipulate. Examples of food products that may contain trans fats include cookies, crackers, doughnuts, and fried foods.

Advantages of Use of Unsaturated Fatty Acids in the Diet

Unsaturated fats are considered the **'healthy fats'** and they are important to include as part of a healthy diet. These fats help reduce the risk of high **blood cholesterol** levels and have other health benefits when they replace saturated fats in the diet.

Unsaturated fats are liquid at room temperature, unlike saturated fats that are solid at room temperature. Healthy unsaturated fats come in two main forms, polyunsaturated and monounsaturated. These differ in their chemical structure and they have slightly different health benefits as a result.

- Unsaturated fats in the diet help in reducing the weight.
- They help to reduce the risk of cardiovascular diseases by decreasing LDL cholesterol and blood pressure.
- They help to reduce the risk of cancers like prostate cancer in males and breast cancer in females.
- They increase the sensitivity of tissues to insulin in those with or without high blood sugar there by reducing the incidence of diabetes mellitus.
- They help in reducing inflammation by reducing the expression of inflammatory genes.

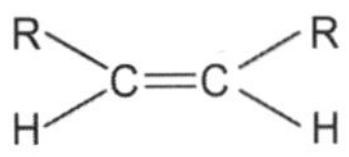

Cis isomer
Both R groups are on the same side of carbon-carbon double bond

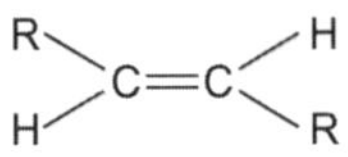

Trans isomer
R groups are on different side of the carbon-carbon double bond

Figure 3.8: *Cis* and *trans* forms of unsaturated fatty acids.

Advantages of Use of Omega-3 Polyunsaturated Acids in the Diet

- Decrease the risk of cardiovascular disease.
- Lower the production of thromboxane and tendency of the platelet aggregation.
- They are anti-inflammatory. They promote the synthesis of less inflammatory prostaglandins and leukotrienes.
- Decreases serum triglycerides.
- An imbalance in omega-6 and omega-3 polyunsaturated acids in the diet is associated with an increased risk of cardiovascular disease. The optimal dietary ratio of omega-6 to omega-3 PUFAs is in between 1:1 and 4:1. The mediterrnean diet which has been associated with lowered cardiovascular risk is richer in omega-3 PUFAs obtained in fish oils. The fish oils are especially rich in EPA and DHA. Fish oil supplements are often prescribed for individuals with a history of cardiovascular disease and in hyperlipoproteinemia with hypertriglyceridemia.
- Important in infant development, as discussed above.

> Dietary sources of unsaturated fats include:
> - Olives and olive oil
> - Peanut butter and peanut oil
> - Vegetable oils, such as sunflower, corn, or canola
> - Fatty fish, such as salmon and mackerel
> - Nuts and seeds, such as almonds, peanuts, cashews, and sesame seeds

Disadvantages of Use of Saturated Fats in Food

A saturated fat on the other hand is a type of fat in which the fatty acid chains have all single bonds. Food sources rich in saturated fat include meat and dairy products, such as:

- Cheese
- Butter
- Ice-cream
- High-fat cuts of meat
- Coconut oil
- Palm oil
  - Consumption of more saturated fats in diet increases the risk of cardiovascular diseases by increasing the level of LDL cholesterol and buildup of cholesterol in arteries.
  - Many high-fat foods such as pizza, baked goods, and fried foods have a lot of saturated fat. Eating too much fat can add extra calories to diet and leads to gain weight.
  - Consumption of high amounts of saturated fats increases the insulin resistance thereby aggravating the risk of diabetes mellitus.

Disadvantages of Use of *Trans* Fats in Food

Trans fatty acids present in high amounts in processed foods, fast foods and bakery items, and fried foods.

- There is now strong evidence that dietary intake of trans fatty acids "(trans fats)" leads to a higher incidence of cardiovascular disease.
- Dietary trans fatty acids raise the level of **triacylglycerol** and **LDL bad cholesterol** and lower the level of **good cholesterol HDL**.
- Trans fatty acids compete with essential fatty acids, hence aggravate essential fatty acid deficiency.
- Consumption of trans fatty acids for long terms may raise the **risk factor for cardiovascular diseases** like **atherosclerosis** and **coronary artery disease**, and **diabetes mellitus**.
- It also increases the body's inflammatory response.

STRIKE A NOTE

- ❖ When lipid rich foods are exposed too long to the oxygen in air, they may spoil and become **rancid**. The unpleasant test and smell associated with rancidity result from the oxidative cleavage of double bonds in unsaturated fatty acids, which produces aldehydes and carboxylic acids of shorter chain length and therefore higher volatility; these compounds pass readily through the air to our nose.
- ❖ To improve the self-life of vegetable oils used in cooking and to increase their stability at high temperatures used in deep frying, commercial vegetable oils are prepared by partial hydrogenation. This process converts many of the *cis* double bonds in the fatty acids to single bonds and increases the melting temperature of the oils so that they are solid at room temperature (margarine is produced from vegetable oil in this way).
- ❖ Partial hydrogenation has another, undesirable effect: Some *cis* double bonds are converted to trans double bonds. There is now strong evidence that dietary intake of *trans* fatty acids "(*trans* fats)" leads to a higher incidence of cardiovascular disease.
- ❖ Dietary *trans* fatty acids raise the level of triacylglycerol and of LDL bad cholesterol and lower the level of good cholesterol HDL.
- ❖ Many natural vegetable fats and oils may contain antioxidants like vitamin E which prevent onset of rancidity. Therefore, vegetable fats can be preserved for a longer time than animal fats. Overheating and repeated heating of oil leads to formation of peroxides. Therefore, overheating or repeated heating of oil is an unhealthy practice.

▊ TRIGLYCERIDE: COMPOSITION AND IMPORTANCE

Triacylglycerols are the **simplest lipids**, also referred to as **triglycerides, fats**, or **neutral fats**.

- These are **esters of fatty acids** with **glycerol**. Triacylglycerol is the major storage and **transport** forms of fatty acids.
- These are composed of three fatty acids, which are esterified with a single glycerol through their carboxyl groups, resulting in a loss of negative charge and formation of **neutral fat (Figure 3.9)**. As the polar hydroxyl groups of glycerol and polar carboxyl groups of the fatty acids are bound in ester linkages, triacylglycerols are **nonpolar**, **hydrophobic**, and **neutral** (in charges) molecules, essentially **insoluble in water**.

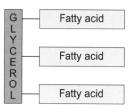

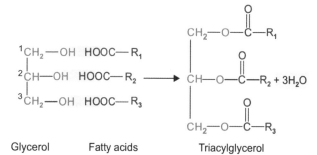

Figure 3.9: Triacylglycerol.

The fatty acid moiety in lipid ester is known as an **acyl group**.

- Three general types of glycerides occur. **Monoacylglycerides**, **diacylglycerides**, and **triacylglycerides**, consist respectively of one, two, or three molecules of fatty acid esterified to a molecule of glycerol.
- Triacylglycerols containing the same kind of fatty acid in all three positions are called **simple triacylglycerols** and are named after the fatty acid they contain, e.g., **simple triacylglycerols** of palmitic acid is called **tripalmitin**.
- **Mixed triacylglycerols** contain two or more different fatty acids. The stereospecific numbering (SN) of the glycerol carbon atom is shown in **Figure 3.9**.
  - The fatty acid on carbon 1 of the glycerol is usually saturated.
  - That on carbon 2 is usually unsaturated, and
  - That on carbon 3 can be either.
- The presence of the unsaturated fatty acid(s) decreases the melting temperature of the lipid and remains in liquid form (oil). Most triacylglycerol molecules contain fatty acids of varying lengths may be unsaturated or saturated or a combination. Depending on their fatty acid composition triacylglycerol is referred to as **fats** or **oils**.
  - Fats which are solid at room temperature contain large proportion of saturated fatty acids.
  - Oil is quid at room temperature because of their relatively high unsaturated fatty acid content.

Lipids have lower specific gravities than water, which explains why mixtures of oil and water have two phases: oil with the lower specific gravity, floats on the aqueous phase.

Occurrence

Many foods contain triacylglycerol. Most natural fats, such as those in vegetable oils, dairy products and animal fat are complex mixtures of simple and mixed triacylglycerol. These contain a variety of fatty acids differing in chain length and degree of saturation. Vegetable oils such as corn and olive oil are composed largely of triacylglycerol with unsaturated fatty acids, and thus are liquids at room temperature.

Triacylglycerols containing only saturated fatty acids, such as **tristearin**, the major component of **beef fat**, are white greasy solids at room temperature.

Importance of Triacylglycerols

Triacylglycerols are highly concentrated stores of metabolic energy. Triacylglycerols have two significant advantages over other forms of metabolic fuel, polysaccharides such as glycogen.

- The carbon atoms of fatty acids are more reduced than those of sugars and oxidation of triacylglycerides yields twice the energy as the oxidation of carbohydrates. Furthermore, triacylglycerol are hydrophobic and therefore unhydrated, so they are stored in a nearly anhydrous form, they no need to carry the extra weight of water of hydration that is associated with stored glycogen (2 g per gram of glycogen). Consequently, a gram of nearly anhydrous fat stores more than six times as much energy as a gram of hydrated glycogen.
- The glycogen stores provide enough energy to sustain physiological function for about 24 hours; whereas the triacylglycerol stores allow survival for several weeks.
- Obese persons may have 15 or 20 kg of triacylglycerol deposited in their adipocytes, sufficient to supply energy needs for months. In contrast, the human body can store less than a day's energy supply in the form of glycogen.
- Carbohydrates (glucose and glycogen) do offer certain advantages as quick sources of metabolic energy, one of which is their ready solubility in water.

PHOSPHOLIPIDS: COMPOSITION, TYPES, AND CLINICAL IMPORTANCE

Phospholipids are the major lipid constituents of **cell membranes**. They comprise about 40% of the lipids in the erythrocyte membrane and over 75% of the lipids in the inner mitochondrial membrane. A phospholipid molecule is constructed from four components:

1. Fatty acid (one or more)
2. Glycerol or sphingosine (a backbone to which fatty acids are attached)
3. Phosphate and
4. Nitrogenous base/alcohol (attached to the phosphate).

Like fatty acids, phospholipids are **amphipathic** in nature, fatty acid components provide hydrophobic region (nonpolar tail), whereas the reminder of the molecule has hydrophilic properties (polar head) **(Figure 3.10)**.

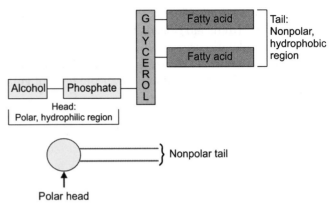

Figure 3.10: Schematic structure of amphipathic phospholipid.

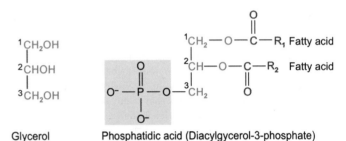

Figure 3.11: Structure of glycerol and phosphatidic acid.

Types of Phospholipid

There are two types of phospholipids **(Figure 3.2)**
1. Glycerophospholipid or phosphoglyceride
2. Sphingophospholipid.

Glycerophospholipids or Phosphoglycerides

Phospholipids derived from **glycerol** are called glycerophospholipids or phosphoglycerides. In glycerophospholipids, the hydroxyl groups at C-1 and C-2 of glycerol are esterified with carboxyl groups of the two fatty acids. The C-3 hydroxyl group of the glycerol is esterified with **phosphoric acid**. The resulting compound called, **phosphatidic acid (diacylglycerol 3-phosphate) (Figure 3.11)**.

Phosphatidic acid is the simplest phosphoglyceride. Only small amounts of phosphatidic acid are present in membranes. However, phosphatidic acid is a key intermediate in the biosynthesis of the other **glycerophospholipids**. The major glycerophospholipids are derived from phosphatidic acid by the formation of an ester bond between the phosphate group of phosphatidic acid and hydroxyl group of one of the several alcohols. The common alcohol moieties of glycerophospholipids are the **choline, ethanolamine, amino acid serine, inositol,** and **glycerol (Figure 3.12)**. Different types of glycerophospholipids are discussed below.

Phosphatidylcholine (Lecithin)

The most common phospholipid in mammals is phosphatidylcholine; comprising approximately 50% of the membrane

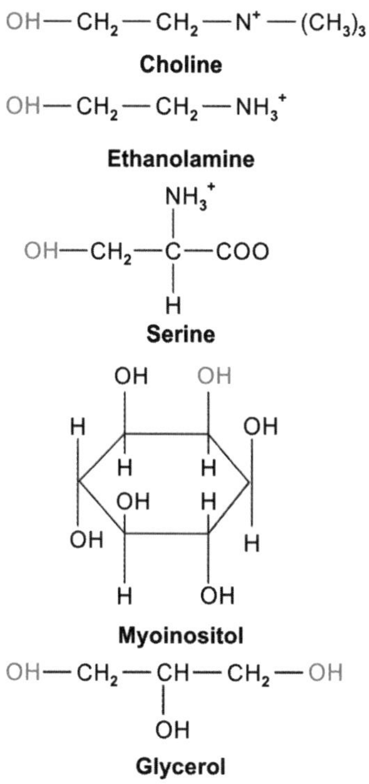

OH—CH$_2$—CH$_2$—N$^+$—(CH$_3$)$_3$

Choline

OH—CH$_2$—CH$_2$—NH$_3$$^+$

Ethanolamine

OH—CH$_2$—C—COO

NH$_3$$^+$ / H

Serine

Myoinositol

OH—CH$_2$—CH—CH$_2$—OH

OH

Glycerol

Figure 3.12: The common alcohol moieties or nitrogen bases of glycerophospholipids.

mass. These are phosphoglycerols containing **choline** (**Figure 3.13**), commonly called **lecithin**.

- These are most abundant phospholipids of the **cell membrane** having both structural and metabolic functions and represent a large proportion of the body's store of choline. Choline is a store of labile methyl groups.
- Dipalmitoyl phosphatidylcholine is an important phosphatidylcholine found in lungs, secreted by **pulmonary type II epithelial cell**. Normal lung function depends on a constant supply of **dipalmitoyl lecithin**. It is a major component of **lungs surfactant**.

Respiratory Distress Syndrome (RDS)

Respiratory distress syndrome (RDS) is a breathing disorder that affects newborns due to a failure in biosynthesis of **dipalmitoyl phosphatidylcholine**. RDS rarely occurs in full-term infants. The disorder is more common in premature infants. In fact, nearly all infants born before 28 weeks of pregnancy develop RDS.

- RDS is more common in premature infants because their lungs are not able to make enough surfactant. Surfactant is a liquid that composed of **dipalmitoyl phosphatidylcholine**. Surfactant coats the inside of the lungs. It helps keep them open so breathing can occur after birth.
- Phosphatidylcholine, in combination with specific proteins and other phospholipids, (such as phosphatidyl glycerol and phosphatidylinositol) is found in the extracellular fluid and surrounds the alveoli of the lungs, where it decreases the surface tension of the fluid to prevent lung collapse (atelectasis) during breathing.

- Premature infants may suffer from respiratory distress syndrome because their immature lungs do not synthesize enough **dipalmitoyl lecithin**.
- Without enough surfactant, the lungs tend to collapse, when the infant exhales (breathes out) and the infant suffer from breathing problems. The lack of oxygen can damage the baby's brain and other organs if proper treatment is not given.
- Some full-term infants develop RDS because they have faulty genes that affect the formation of surfactant.

The maturity of the fetal lung can be assessed from the **lecithin/sphingomyelin (L/S) ratio in amniotic fluid**. A ratio of 2 or above is evidence of pulmonary maturity. Lung maturation can be accelerated by giving the mother **glucocorticoids** shortly before delivery. Administration of natural or synthetic surfactant is also used in the prevention and treatment of respiratory distress syndrome.

Signs and Symptoms of RDS

Most infants who develop RDS show signs of breathing problems. They include:

- Rapid, shallow breathing
- Sharp pulling in of the chest below and between the ribs with each breath
- Murmuring sounds
- Widening of the nostrils
- The infant also may have pauses in breathing that last for a few seconds. This condition is called **apnea**.

STRIKE A NOTE

- ❖ Excess choline is associated in the development of heart disease.
- ❖ Gut bacteria convert excess choline into trimethylamine (TMA), a gas that smells like rotten fish, and the liver converts TMA into trimethylamine-N-oxidase (TMAO).
- ❖ TMAO stimulates cholesterol uptake by macrophages, a process that can result in atherosclerosis.
- ❖ Foods rich in phosphatidylcholine, such as red meats and dairy products, may also result in TMAO production

Phosphatidylethanolamine (Cephalin)

They differ from lecithin in having nitrogenous base **ethanolamine** in place of choline (**Figure 3.13**). **Thromboplastin** (coagulation factor III), which is needed to initiate the clotting process, is composed mainly of cephalin.

Phosphatidylserine

Phosphatidylserine makes up 10% of the phospholipids in mammals. It contains the amino acid **serine** rather than ethanolamine and is found in most tissues (**Figure 3.13**).

- Phosphatidylserine is a component of the cell membrane which plays a key role in **cell cycle signaling**; specifically it plays an important role in **apoptosis (programmed cell death)**.
- Phosphatidylserine is normally located in the inner leaflet of the plasma membrane bilayer but is moved to

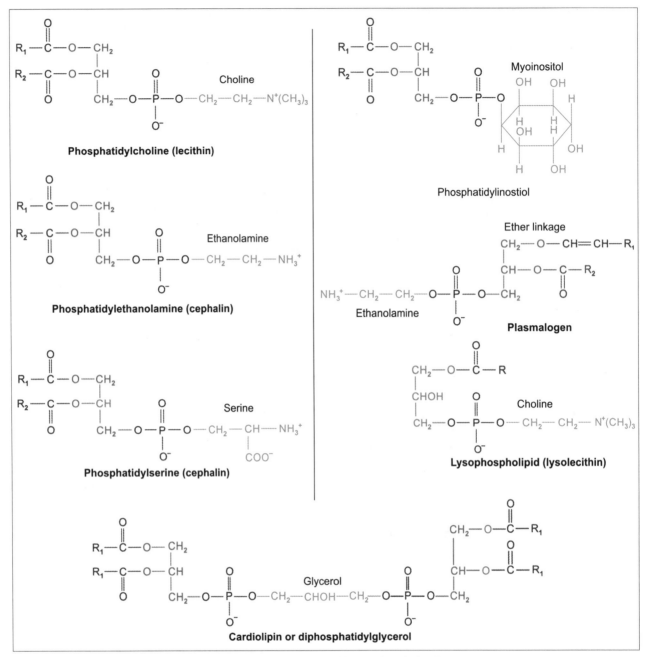

Figure 3.13: Structure of different phospholipids.

the outer leaflet in **apoptosis**. There, it serves to attract phagocytes to consume the cell remnants after apoptosis is complete.

> Phosphatidylserine is translocated from one side of the membrane to the other by an ATP-binding cassette translocase.

Phosphatidylinositol

In phosphatidylinositol, inositol is present as the stereoisomer **myoinositol (Figure 3.13)**.

- Phosphatidylinositol is a precursor of **second messenger**.
- On stimulation by hormones like **oxytocin** and **vasopressin** it is cleaved into **diacylglycerol** and **inositol**

triphosphate **(IP$_3$)**, both of which act as internal signals or **second messengers**.

Inositol or myo-inositol is a sugar alcohol with half the sweetness of sucrose (table sugar). It is made naturally in humans from glucose. A human kidney makes about two grams per day. Other tissues synthesize it too, and the highest concentration is in the brain, where it plays an important role by making other neurotransmitters and growth factors and participates in osmoregulation.

Plasmalogens

Structurally, the plasmalogens resemble phosphatidylethanolamine but possess an **ether link** on C-1 of glycerol instead of the ester link **(Figure 3.13)**. In some instances, choline, serine, or inositol may be substituted for ethanolamine.

- These are found in brain and in cardiac muscle.
- These constitute as much as 10 to 30% of the phospholipids of brain and heart.
- **Platelet activating factor (PAF)** is a plasmalogen and involved in platelet aggregation and degranulation.
- Plasmalogens may have protective effect against reactive oxygen species.

Lysophospholipids

Lysophospholipids are intermediates formed in the metabolism of phosphoglycerols.

- These are phosphoglycerols containing only one acyl radical, for example, lysophosphatidylcholine (lysolecithin) **(Figure 3.13)**.
- Lysophosphatidylcholine important in the metabolism and interconversion of phospholipids.
- It is also found in oxidized lipoproteins.

Cardiolipin (Diphosphatidyl Glycerol)

Cardiolipin is composed of two molecules of **phosphatidic acid** and a molecule of **glycerol** in which two molecules of phosphatidic acid esterified through their phosphate groups to a molecule of glycerol **(Figure 3.13)**.

- Cardiolipin is found only in mitochondrial membrane and is required for the mitochondrial function.
- Decreased cardiolipin levels cause mitochondrial dysfunction in aging and pathological conditions including heart failure, hypothyroidism, and Barth syndrome (cardioskeletal myopathy).
- This is only human phosphoglyceride that is **antigenic** and is recognized by antibodies raised against **Treponema pallidum**, the bacterium that causes **syphilis**.

Sphingophospholipids

Phospholipid derived from alcohol **sphingosine** instead of glycerol is called sphinogophospholipid **(Figure 3.14)**. **Sphingomyelin** is the only phospholipid in membranes that is not derived from glycerol. Instead, the alcohol in sphingomyelin is **sphingosine**, an amino alcohol that contains a long, unsaturated hydrocarbon chain. Carbons C-1, C-2, and C-3 of sphingosine molecule are structurally similar to the three carbons of glycerol in glycerophospholipids.

- When a fatty acid is attached to $-NH_2$ group on C-2 of sphingosine the resulting compound is called, **ceramide** (sphingosine-fatty acid complex) **(Figure 3.15)**, which is structurally similar to a diacylglycerol. In all sphingolipids, the amino group of ceramide is **acylated**. In addition, primary hydroxyl group of sphingosine is esterified to **phosphorylcholine**.
- Sphingomyelin are present in the **plasma membranes** of cells. Sphingomyelins are especially predominant in

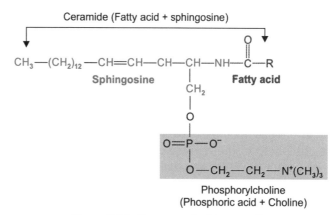

Figure 3.14: Structure of sphingomyelin.

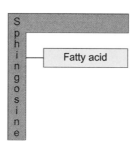

Figure 3.15: Schematic structure of ceramide.

myelin sheath that surrounds and **insulates the axons** of some neurons, thus the name "Sphingomyelin". They play a role in **cell signaling** and in **apoptosis** (process of programmed **cell death** of abnormal, unneeded cells)

- Sphingomyelin of the myelin sheath that surrounds nerve fibers contains predominantly longer chain fatty acids such as **lignoceric** and **nervonic acids**, whereas a grey matter of the brain has sphingomyelin that contains primarily **stearic acid**.

Importance of Phospholipids

- Phospholipids are the major lipid constituents of cellular membranes. They comprise about 40% of the lipids in the erythrocyte membrane and over 75% of the lipids in the inner mitochondrial membrane.
- They regulate **permeability of membranes** as well as activation of some membrane bound enzymes.
- Phospholipids are of importance in **insulating the nerve impulse** (like the plastic or rubber covering around an electric wire) from the surrounding structures, e.g., sphingomyelins act as an electrical insulator in the myelin sheath around nerve fibers.
- Phospholipids act as a lipotropic factor. **Lipotropic factor** is the component that prevents **fatty liver**, i.e., accumulation of fat in the liver. Lecithin represents a storage form of lipotropic factor choline and labile methyl group.
- These are good **emulsifying agents** that help in transport, intestinal absorption and metabolic interactions of lipids.

- Thromboplastin (coagulation factor III), which is needed to initiate the clotting process, is composed mainly of cephalin.
- Phospholipid (lecithin) acts as **lung surfactant**, which prevents alveolar collapse (atelectasis).
- Phospholipids, to some extent, are an **anticholesterol agent**, as lecithin plays an important role in the esterification of free cholesterol to cholesterol ester and thus help in the **reverse cholesterol transport (***see* **Chapter 11; Lipid Metabolism)** and in the removal of cholesterol from the body.
- Phosphatidylinositol is a precursor of second messenger for the activity of certain hormones.
- In mitochondria cardiolipin is necessary for optimum functions of the electrons transport process.
- Plasmalogens (platelet activating factor) involved in platelet aggregation and degranulation.
- Sphingomyelin play a role in cell signaling and in apoptosis.

STRIKE A NOTE

- ❖ Sphingosine is biosynthesized by condensation of palmitoyl-CoA and serine.
- ❖ Ceramide is a precursor for sphingolipids (sphingomyelin, cerebroside, and gangliosides).
- ❖ Ceramide serve as second messengers in the regulations of cell growth, differentiation, and death.
- ❖ Ceramide itself induces programmed cell death or apoptosis in some cell type.
- ❖ Cancer cells prevent ceramide-induced cell death
- ❖ It appears that cancer cells destroy the apoptotic signal by converting it into a pro-mitotic signal.
- ❖ Ceramidase removes the fatty acid from ceramide, generating sphingosine.
- ❖ Sphingosine is then converted into sphingosine1-phosphate by sphingosine kinase, which stimulates cell division.
- ❖ Thus, cancer cells convert a potentially lethal signal molecule into one that promotes tumor growth. Efforts are underway to develop inhibitors of ceramidase for use of chemotherapeutic agents.

SPHINGOLIPIDS: STRUCTURE, TYPES, AND FUNCTIONS

Sphingolipids are composed of one molecule of the long-chain **amino alcohol sphingosine**, one molecule of **fatty acid**, and a **polar head group** (like glucose, di-, tri-, or tetrasaccharide, complex oligosaccharide, phosphocholine) that is joined by a **glycosidic** linkage in some cases and a **phosphodiester** in others. There are two types of sphingolipids, deferring in their head groups **(Figure 3.3)**:
1. Sphingogophospholipid
2. Sphingoglycolipids/Glycosphingolipids (Glycolipids)

Sphinogophospholipid

Sphingophospholipids contain **phosphocholine** or **phosphoethanolamine** as their polar head group and therefore

classified as **phospholipids,** e.g., **sphingomyelins** (for details refer phospholipids).

Glycolipids/Glycosphingolipids

Glycolipids (ceramide + carbohydrate), as their name implies, are sugar containing lipids. Glycolipids like sphingomyelins are derived from **sphingosine**. The amino group of sphingosine is esterified by a fatty acid, as in sphingomyelin. They do not contain phosphate; rather, one or more sugar units are attached to the hydroxyl group of sphingosine. Glycolipids are widely distributed in every tissue of the body, particularly in nervous tissue such as brain. Four classes of glycolipids have been distinguished:
1. Cerebrosides
2. Sulfatides
3. Globosides
4. Gangliosides.

Cerebrosides (Ceramide + Monosaccharides)

Cerebroside **(Figure 3.16)** is the simplest glycolipid in which there is only one sugar residue, either **glucose** or **galactose** linked to ceramide and named as **glucocerebroside** and **galactocerebroside** respectively.

Galactocerebroside is found in high concentration in nerve tissue membrane and glucocerebroside is the predominant glycolipid of extraneural (non-neural) tissues, where it functions as an intermediate in the synthesis of more complex glycolipids, e.g., **gangliosides**.

Sulfatides (Ceramide + Monosaccharide + Sulfate)

Sulfatides are cerebrosides in which the monosaccharide contains a sulfate ester **(Figure 3.16)**. The most common sulfatide is **sulfogalactoceramide** which is found in high amounts in myelin.

Globosides (Ceramide + Oligosaccharide)

Globosides contains two or more sugar molecules, most often **galactose**, and **glucose** or **N-acetyl galactosamine**, attached to ceramide **(Figure 3.16)**. These glycolipids are important constituents of the RBC-membrane and are the determinants of the **A**, **B**, and **O blood group** system.

> Cerebrosides and globosides are sometimes called **neutral glycolipids**, as they have no charge at pH 7.

Gangliosides (Cerebroside + Oligosaccharides + N-acetylneuraminic Acid)

Gangliosides are complex glycolipids, derived from glucocerebroside. Ganglioside contains **oligosaccharides** as their polar head groups and one or more molecules of **sialic acid**, which is usually **N-acetylneuraminic acid (NANA)** attached to ceramide. Deprotonated sialic acid gives

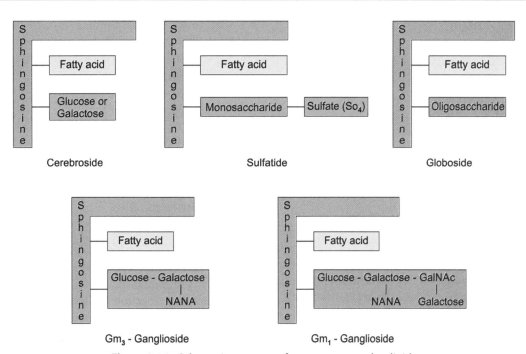

Figure 3.16: Schematic structure of some common glycolipids.

gangliosides the negative charge at pH 7 that distinguishes them from globosides.

- Several types of gangliosides such as **GM₁**, **GM₂**, **GM₃**, etc., have been isolated from brain and other tissues. G represents Ganglioside; M represents mono which indicates presence of one sialic acid residue and subscript number assigned on the basis of chromatographic migration of ganglioside.
- The simplest ganglioside found in tissues is GM₃. GM₁ is a more complex ganglioside derived from GM₃ **(Figure 3.16)**.
- Gangliosides are involved in special roles in cell **membrane receptors** for certain polypeptide hormones, for a number of drugs and viruses.
- GM₁ is a compound which is known to be the **receptor** in human intestine for **cholera toxin**. In cholera, cholera toxin produced by the intestinal bacterium *Vibrio cholera* enters cells after attaching to specific gangliosides on the intestinal epithelial cell surface. GM1 is a compound which is known to be the receptor in human intestine for cholera toxin.

Importance of Sphingolipids

- Glycolipids are an important constituent of the nervous tissue, such as, brain and outer leaflet of cell membrane.
- Gangliosides are an important constituent of specific receptors for certain polypeptide hormones, a number of drugs and viruses.
- They are found in the specific sites on the nerve endings to which neurotransmitter molecules become bound during the chemical transmission of an impulse from one nerve cell to the next.

- Glycolipids are antigenic and act as blood group antigens. The carbohydrate moieties of certain glycolipids define the human blood groups and therefore, determine the type of blood group.

Disorders of Sphingolipids

Sphingolipids are a class of lipids containing a backbone sphingosine instead of glycerol. This includes **sphingomyelin**, **cerebroside**, and **gangliosides**. There are several disorders of sphingolipid metabolism, known as **sphingolipidoses**. Some of these are:

1. **Niemann–Pick disease** is caused by a rare genetic defect in the lysosomal enzyme **sphingomyelinase**, which cleaves phosphocholine from sphingomyelin. Sphingomyelin accumulates in the brain, spleen, and liver. The disease becomes evident in infants and causes **mental retardation** and **early death**.
2. **Gaucher disease**, in which **glucocerebroside** accumulates in brain, liver, spleen, and bone marrow due to inherited deficiency of lysosomal enzyme of β-**glucosidase**. This disorder is associated with mental retardation and enlargement of liver and spleen.
3. In **Tay–Sachs diseases**, ganglioside **GM₂** accumulates in the brain and spleen due to lack of the lysosomal enzyme **hexosaminidase A**. The symptoms of Tay-Sachs disease are progressive developmental retardation, paralysis, blindness and death by age of 3 or 4 years.
4. **Guillain-Barre syndrome** is a serious autoimmune disorder, in which the body makes antibodies against its own gangliosides. The resulting inflammation damages the peripheral nervous system, leading to temporary or sometimes permanent paralysis.

LIPOPROTEINS: COMPOSITION, TYPES, AND IMPORTANCE

Lipids (triacylglycerol, cholesterol, cholesterol esters, and phospholipids) are essentially insoluble in water. To facilitate their transport, they are carried in the blood plasma as **lipoproteins**. Lipoproteins are macromolecular complexes of specific carrier proteins called **apolipoproteins** and various combinations of phospholipids, cholesterol, cholesterol esters, and triacylglycerols.

Apolipoproteins (apo means detached or separated) combine with lipids to form several types of lipoprotein particles. These lipoprotein particles consist of hydrophobic lipids such as **triacylglycerols** and **cholesterol esters** in the central, which is surrounded by a single surface layer of **amphipathic phospholipids** and **free cholesterol** molecules and hydrophilic **apoproteins** at the surface **(Figure 3.17)**.

Types of Lipoproteins

Different combinations of lipids and proteins produce different types of lipoprotein particles of different densities **(Table 3.3)**. The main four types of lipoprotein are:

1. Chylomicrons
2. Very low density lipoproteins (VLDL)
3. Low density lipoprotein (LDL)
4. High density lipoprotein (HDL)

The site of synthesis of four main lipoproteins and their functions are summarized in **Table 3.4**.

- The density of these lipoproteins is inversely proportional to triacylglycerol content.
- As the density increases, the diameter of the particle decreases as shown in **Figure 3.18**.

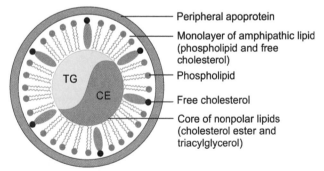

Peripheral apoprotein

Monolayer of amphipathic lipid (phospholipid and free cholesterol)

Phospholipid

Free cholesterol

Core of nonpolar lipids (cholesterol ester and triacylglycerol)

Figure 3.17: Structure of lipoprotein.
(TG: triacylglycerol; CE: cholesterol ester)

- **Chylomicrons** containing about **2% protein** and **98% triacylglycerol** have the **lowest density**.
- While **HDL** contains **55% of protein** and **45% of lipid** have the **highest density**.
- **Triacylglycerol** is the predominant lipid in **chylomicrons** and **VLDL**.
- **Cholesterol** is the predominant lipid in **LDL**.
- **Phospholipid** is the predominant lipid in **HDL**.

Percentage of three major lipid classes, i.e., triacylglycerols, cholesterol, and phospholipids present in lipoproteins are shown in **Table 3.3**. These lipoproteins can be separated by **ultracentrifugation**.

Apolipoproteins

At least 10 distinct **apolipoproteins** are found in the lipoproteins of human plasma **(Table 3.5)**, distinguishable by their size, their reactions with specific antibodies and their characteristic distribution in the lipoprotein classes. These protein components act as **signals**, targeting lipoproteins to specific tissues or **activating enzymes** that act on the lipoproteins.

Association between ApoE Alleles and Alzheimer Disease

- ❖ In human, there are three common alleles, ApoE-3, ApoE-4, and ApoE-2 of the gene encoding apolipoprotein E.
- ❖ It has been observed that the ApoE-4 allele is common in humans with Alzheimer disease.
- ❖ Individuals who inherit ApoE-4 have an increased risk of late onset Alzheimer disease.
- ❖ The molecular basis for the association between Apo-E and Alzheimer disease is not yet known.
- ❖ It is also not clear how ApoE-4 might affect the growth of the amyloid fibers, the causative agent of the disease.

Importance of Lipoprotein

Each class of lipoprotein has a specific function, determined by its point of synthesis, lipid composition, and apolipoprotein content.

1. Chylomicrons carry dietary triacylglycerol, cholesterol, and other lipids from the intestine through blood to peripheral tissue.
2. Very low density lipoprotein transfer triacylglycerol and cholesterol in excess of the liver's own needs through blood to peripheral tissue.

		Composition (Weight %)				
Lipoprotein	Density (g/mL)	Protein	Phospholipids	Free cholesterol	Cholesteryl esters	Triglyceride
Chylomicrons	<1.006	2	9	1	3	85
VLDL	0.95–1.006	10	18	7	12	50
LDL	1.006–1.063	23	20	8	37	10
HDL	1.063–1.210	55	24	2	15	4

TABLE 3.3: Characteristics of major classes of human plasma lipoproteins.

TABLE 3.4: The four main lipoproteins and their site of synthesis and function.

Lipoprotein	Site of synthesis	Functions
Chylomicrons	Intestine	Transport of dietary lipids from intestine to peripheral tissues
VLDL	Liver	Transport endogenous triacylglycerol from liver to peripheral tissues
LDL	Plasma VLDL	Transport cholesterol from liver to peripheral tissues
HDL	Liver and intestine	• Transport free cholesterol from peripheral tissues to the liver where it can be catabolized (Reverse cholesterol transport) • Reservoir of apo C-II and apo E required for the metabolism of chylomicrons and VLDL

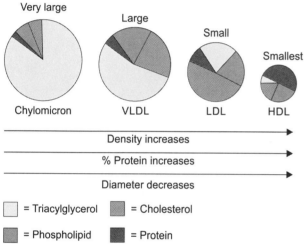

Figure 3.18: Lipoprotein with increasing densities and their composition.

TABLE 3.5: Apolipoproteins of the human plasma lipoproteins.

Apolipoproteins	Lipoprotein association	Function
ApoA I	HDL	Activates LCAT
ApoA II	HDL	Inhibits LCAT
ApoA IV	Chylomicrons, HDL	Activates LCAT; cholesterol transport/clearance
ApoB 48	Chylomicrons	Cholesterol transport/clearance
ApoB 100	VLDL, LDL	Binds to LDL receptor
ApoC I	VLDL, HDL	Not known
ApoC II	Chylomicrons, VLDL, HDL	Activates lipoprotein lipase
ApoC III	Chylomicrons, VLDL, HDL	Inhibits lipoprotein lipase
Apo D	HDL	Not known
Apo E	Chylomicrons, VLDL, HDL	Triggers clearance of VLDL and chylomicron remnants

3. Low-density lipoprotein is the major carrier of cholesterol in blood. The role of LDL is to transport cholesterol to peripheral tissues and regulate de novo cholesterol synthesis at these sites.
4. High-density lipoprotein picks up cholesterol released into the plasma from dying cells and from membranes undergoing turnover and delivers the cholesterol to the liver for excretion.

Abnormal Form of Lipoproteins

Lipoprotein (a) and **lipoprotein-x** are the variant of LDL and associated with clinical conditions.

❖ Lipoprotein-a (LPa) occurs in very small amounts in normal human plasma. LPa is similar to LDL in lipid composition. Apolipoprotein-a is bound to **apo B100** by a **disulfide linkage**. It may interfere with the action of **plasminogen**, impairing the process of **clot resolution** (fibrinolysis). Apo (a) contains structural units similar to those present in **plasminogen** and so LPa competes with plasminogen for binding with tissue plasminogen receptors and impairs the function of plasminogen and subsequent impairs **thrombolysis**. Several studies have shown that an excess plasma level (more than 0.30 g/L) of LPa is a risk factor and an independent predictor of **coronary heart disease**.

❖ **Lipoprotein-x (LP-x)** is an abnormal lipoprotein found in patients with obstructive **liver disease of LCAT** (Lecithin: cholesterol acyl transferase) **deficiency**. The composition of LP-x differs from that of LDL, and consists of almost **entirely free cholesterol** and **phospholipids**. LP-x from patients with obstructive disease has been reported to lack of ApoA-I a powerful activator of LCAT.

■ CHOLESTEROL: STRUCTURE AND IMPORTANCE

Cholesterol is the major **sterol** in animal tissues. It is the precursor of other important steroids. Cholesterol is widely distributed in all the cells of the body, but particularly in nervous tissue. It occurs in animal fats, but not in the plant fats.

All steroids have a similar cyclic nucleus resembling **phenanthrene** (ring A, B, and C) to which a **cyclopentane ring** (D) is attached **(Figure 3.19)**.

● **Cholesterol** consists of **steroid nucleus**, having **19-carbon** atoms **(Figure 3.20)**.

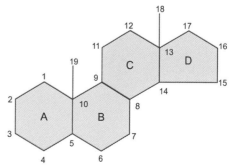

Figure 3.19: The steroid nucleus, phenanthrene (ring A, B, and C), to which cyclopentane D ring is attached.

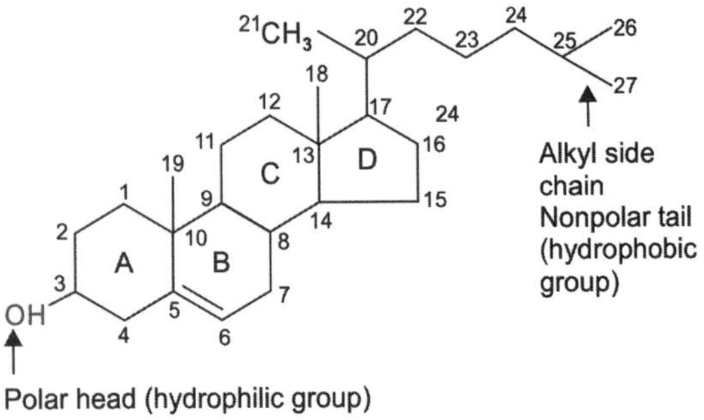

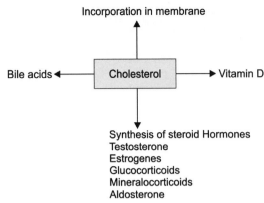

Figure 3.20: The structure of cholesterol.

- **Methyl** side chains are shown as single bonds at position C_{10} and C_{13}.
- Cholesterol, a **27-carbon** compound, has **8-carbon alkyl side chain** attached to the D ring at C_{17} and a **hydroxyl group** attached to C_3 of the A ring, with one **double bond** between carbon atoms **5** and **6 (Figure 3.20)**.
- Cholesterol is **amphipathic**, with a **polar** head the hydroxyl group at C_3 and a **nonpolar**, the steroid nucleus and alkyl hydrocarbon side chain at C_{17}.
- Most of the cholesterol in the body exists as a **cholesterol ester**, with a fatty acid attached to the hydroxyl group at C_3.
- Plants do not contain cholesterol. They have other steroid that is known as **phytosterols**. The most abundant of phytosterols are **(Figure 3.21)**:
  - **β-sitosterol** in which the chain attached to C_{17} contains 10 rather than 8 carbon atoms.
  - **Ergosterol,** the sterol of yeast contains a methyl group at C_{24}, double bond in the side chain and two double bonds in the B-ring. Unlike plant and animal, bacteria (with rare exception) do not contain sterols.

Functions of the Cholesterol

It is a major structural constituent of the **cell membranes** and **plasma lipoproteins**.

Figure 3.22: Metabolic importance of cholesterol.

Cholesterol serves as the precursor for a variety of biologically important products **(Figure 3.22)** which are given below:

1. The **steroid hormones** synthesized from **cholesterol** help to control metabolism, inflammation, immune functions, salt and water balance, development of sexual characteristics, and the ability to withstand illness and injury. The **steroid hormones** synthesized from **cholesterol** are of two types:
   - **Corticosteroids:** Made in the adrenal cortex, (hence cortico) for example, **glucocorticoids** and **mineralocorticoids**.
   - **Sex hormones:** Made in the gonads or placenta for example, **androgens** (male sex hormones), **estrogens** and **progesterone** (female sex hormones)
2. Cholesterol also serves as the precursor for **bile acids** and **vitamin D**
   - Bile acids, derived from cholesterol, act as a detergent in the intestine, emulsifying dietary fats to make them readily accessible to digestive enzyme lipase.
   - Vitamin D is a hormone essential in calcium and phosphate metabolism.

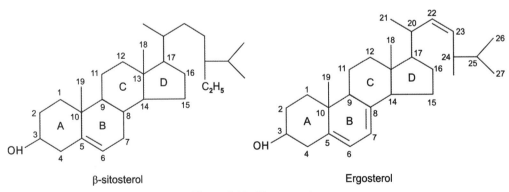

β-sitosterol

Ergosterol

Figure 3.21: Phytosterols.

ASSESSMENT QUESTIONS

■ STRUCTURED LONG ESSAY QUESTIONS (SLEQs)

1. Describe lipids under following headings:
   i. Definition
   ii. Classification with examples
   iii. Functions
2. Describe phospholipids. Under following headings:
   i. Definition
   ii. Types with examples
   iii. Functions
3. Describe sphingolipids under following headings:
   i. Definition
   ii. Types with examples
   iii. Functions
4. Describe fatty acids under following headings:
   i. Definition
   ii. Classification with examples
   iii. Functions

■ SHORT ESSAY QUESTIONS (SEQs)

1. What is cholesterol write its importance in the body.
2. What is PUFA? Give examples and functions of PUFA.
3. Write functions of phospholipids.
4. Write structure, types and functions of lipoproteins.
5. Write types and functions of glycolipids.
6. What is surfactant? Which phospholipid acts as surfactant? Explain its importance in the body in health and disease.
7. Name amphipathic lipids and its importance.

■ SHORT ANSWER QUESTIONS (SAQs)

1. What is pulmonary surfactant and its clinical importance?
2. What is cardiolipin? Write its importance.
3. What is lecithin? Write its importance.
4. Write importance phosphatidyl inositol.
5. What are essential fatty acids? Name the essential fatty acids.
6. What is a ceramide and write type of lipids formed from a ceramide?
7. Do LDL and HDL carry out the same function? Justify the answer.
8. Write various types of lipoproteins and their associated major apolipoproteins?
9. What is triacylglycerol? Write its importance.
10. Disadvantage of use of trans fatty acids in food.
11. Advantages of use of unsaturated fatty acids.

■ MULTIPLE CHOICE QUESTIONS (MCQs)

1. **The precursor for vitamin D is:**
   a. Cholesterol
   b. Arachidonic acid
   c. Triacylglycerol
   d. Phospholipids

2. **Which of the following lipids is deficient in infants with respiratory distress syndrome?**
   a. Sphingomyelins
   b. Cardiolipins
   c. Leukotrienes
   d. Dipalmitoyl phosphatidylcholine

3. **The highest quantity of lipid and lowest concentration of protein are found in:**
   a. Chylomicrons
   b. Very low-density lipoproteins
   c. Low-density lipoproteins
   d. High-density lipoproteins

4. **Methylated form of phosphatidyl ethanolamine is known as:**
   a. Phosphatidylinositol
   b. Phosphatidylserine
   c. Phosphatidylcholine
   d. Lysophosphatidylcholine

5. **Which ring of the cholesterol molecule contains a double bond?**
   a. A-ring
   b. B-ring
   c. C-ring
   d. D-ring

6. **All of the following statements are true for phosphoglycerides, *except*:**
   a. They are major storage of metabolic energy
   b. They are found in cell membrane
   c. They are amphipathic
   d. They are derived from glycerol

7. **All of the following are sphingolipids, *except*:**
   a. Sphingomyelin
   b. Cerebroside
   c. Phosphatidylinositol
   d. Ganglioside

8. **The lipoprotein particles that have the highest concentration of triacylglycerol are:**
   a. VLDL
   b. HDL
   c. LDL
   d. Chylomicrons

9. **All of the following statements about prostaglandins are true, *except*:**
   a. They are derived from arachidonic acids
   b. They are potent biologic effectors
   c. They were first observed to cause uterine contraction
   d. They are synthesized only in prostate gland

10. **Glycerol is the backbone of:**
    a. Glycerophospholipid
    b. Sphingophospholipid
    c. Glycolipids
    d. Cholesterol esters

11. **All of the following statements about lipids are true, *except*:**
    a. They are esters of fatty acids
    b. They have poor solubility in water
    c. They are a source of energy
    d. They are polyhydroxy aldehydes

12. Which of the following statements about cholesterol is true?
    a. It is saturated
    b. It contains 27-carbon atom
    c. It is a major sterol of plants
    d. It contains four hexane rings fused together

13. Which of the following phospholipids has an antigenic activity?
    a. Lecithin
    b. Cardiolipin
    c. Sphingomyelin
    d. Cephalin

14. Which of the following glycolipids is known to be the receptor in human intestine for cholera toxin?
    a. GM1
    b. GM3
    c. Globoside
    d. Cerebroside

15. Which of the following is the major storage and transport form of fatty acids?
    a. Cholesterol
    b. Triacylglycerol
    c. Albumin
    d. Phospholipid

16. Triglycerides are:
    a. Esters of higher fatty acids with acetyl alcohol
    b. Esters of fatty with cholesterol
    c. Esters of stearic acid with retinol
    d. Esters of fatty acids with glycerol

17. Which of the following is a phospholipid?
    a. Cerebroside
    b. Lecithin
    c. Gangliosides
    d. Kerasin

18. Which of the following is saturated fatty acid?
    a. Palmitic acid
    b. Oleic acid
    c. Linoleic acid
    d. Linolenic acid

19. Arachidonic acid is formed from:
    a. Stearic acid
    b. Palmitic acid
    c. Linoleic acid
    d. Oleic acid

20. Sphingomyelinase deficiency is seen in:
    a. Niemann-Pick disease
    b. Gaucher's disease
    c. Tay-Sachs disease
    d. Guillain-Barre syndrome

21. Ganglioside is composed of all *except*:
    a. Oligosaccharide
    b. Phosphate
    c. Ceramide
    d. Sialic acid

22. Which of the following comprise an important part of lung surfactant?
    a. Lecithin
    b. Cephalin
    c. Cholesterol
    d. Plasmalogens

23. Tay-Sachs is an inherited disorder due to deficiency of:
    a. Lecihtinase
    b. Hexosaminidase A
    c. Sphingomyelinase
    d. Phospholipase B

24. Cerebrosides and Gangliosides have the following similarities, *except*.
    a. Both are compound lipids
    b. Both contain sphingosine
    c. Both are found in brain and nervous tissues
    d. Both are degraded by the enzyme glucocerebrosidase

25. Thromboxanes:
    a. Inhibit platelet aggregation
    b. Produces vasodilation
    c. Enhances platelet aggregation
    d. Relaxes smooth muscles

26. In addition to alcohol and fatty acids, some of the lipids may contain:
    a. Phosphoric acid
    b. Nitrogen base
    c. Carbohydrates
    d. All of the above

27. A membrane phospholipid that does not contain glycerol is:
    a. Lecithin
    b. Sphingomyelin
    c. Cardiolipin
    d. Ceramide

28. Which are the examples of phospholipids, *except*:
    a. Lecithin
    b. Cephalin
    c. Sphingosine
    d. Sphingomyelins

29. Glycolipids contain a special alcohol called:
    a. Sphingosine
    b. Cholesterol
    c. Sorbitol
    d. Glycerol

30. Chaulmoogra acid is an example of:
    a. Substituted fatty acids
    b. Cyclic fatty acids
    c. Branched chain FA
    d. Unbranched fatty acids

31. From which EFA, prostaglandins and leukotrienes are synthesized in the body.
    a. Linoleic acid
    b. Linolenic acid
    c. Arachidonic acids
    d. All of the above

32. Docosahexaenoic acid is formed from dietary:
    a. Linoleic acid
    b. Linolenic acid
    c. Arachidonic acid
    d. Palmitic acid

33. Which are the examples of glycerophospholipid?
    a. Cephalin
    b. Lecithin
    c. Phosphatidyl serine
    d. All of the above

34. Which of the following does not contain 'Glycerol'?
    a. Cephalin
    b. Lecithin
    c. Plasmalogen
    d. Sphingomyelins

35. Apolipoprotein A is found in:
    a. HDL
    b. LDL
    c. Chylomicron
    d. VLDL

36. Ganglioside type GM-3 contains:
    a. Ceramide
    b. Oligosaccharide
    c. Neuraminic acid
    d. All of the above

37. If choline moiety is replaced by ethanolamine, the net product is:
    a. Cerebroside
    b. Sphingomyelin
    c. Cephalin
    d. Plasminogen

38. Eicosanoids include the:
    a. Prostaglandins
    b. Leukotrienes
    c. Thromboxane
    d. All of the above

39. The lipid that mainly functions as fuel reserve in animals is:
    a. Triglycerides
    b. Cholesterol
    c. Phospholipid
    d. Lipoprotein

40. The phospholipid that produces second messenger in hormonal action is:
    a. Phosphatidyl lecithin
    b. Plasmalogen
    c. Phosphatidyl Inositol
    d. Phosphatidyl ethanolamine

41. Which of the following is the cardio protective fatty acid?
    a. Palmitic acid
    b. Stearic acid
    c. Oleic acid
    d. Omega 3 fatty acid

42. Which of the following is an inhibitor of platelet aggregation?
    a. Leukotriene-A_4
    b. Prostacyclin
    c. Thromboxane-A_2
    d. Prostaglandin H_2

43. Which of the following is correct with regards to function of phospholipid?
    a. Synthesis of steroid hormones
    b. Storage form of lipid
    c. Surfactant
    d. Transport form of fatty acids

44. Glycosphingolipids are made up of, *except*:
    a. Oligosaccharide
    b. Glycerol
    c. Sphingosine
    d. Fatty acids

45. The following fatty acid does not belong to ω-6 series:
    a. Linoleic acid
    b. Arachidonic acid
    c. Linolenic acid
    d. Oleic acid

▮ ANSWERS FOR MCQs

1. a	2. d	3. a	4. c	5. b
6. a	7. c	8. d	9. d	10. a
11. d	12. b	13. b	14. a	15. b
16. d	17. b	18. a	19. c	20. a
21. b	22. a	23. b	24. d	25. c
26. d	27. b	28. c	29. a	30. b
31. c	32. b	33. d	34. d	35. a
36. d	37. c	38. d	39. a	40. c
41. d	42. b	43. c	44. b	45. a,c,d

4 CHAPTER

Chemistry of Amino Acids and Proteins

Competency	Learning Objectives
BI 5.1: Describe and discuss structural organization of proteins. **BI 5.2:** Describe and discuss functions of proteins and structure-function relationships in relevant areas, e.g., hemoglobin and selected hemoglobinopathies.	1. Describe amino acids: Definition, general nature, classification with examples and their importance. 2. Describe nonstandard amino acids. 3. Describe properties of amino acids. 4. Describe biologically important peptides. 5. Describe proteins: Definition, classification with examples and functions. 6. Describe and discuss structural organization of proteins at different levels with examples and its biological importance. 7. Describe denaturation of protein. 8. Describe structure-function relationship of hemoglobin and myoglobin and importance of proteins structure-function relationships in hemoglobinopathies. 9. Describe plasma proteins with functions and clinical significance. 10. Describe acute phase response and acute phase proteins.

OVERVIEW

Proteins are the most abundant class of organic compounds in human body, which mediate virtually every process that takes place in cell. Proteins are polymers of **amino acids**. Biochemical functions of proteins include catalysis, transport, contraction, protection, structure, and metabolic regulation.

Polymerization of amino acids yields a **polypeptide**. The properties of proteins depend on the characteristic sequence of amino acids that defines both its three-dimensional structure and its biological function. The sequence of amino acids in a protein is dictated by the DNA and the uniqueness of each living organism is due to its quality of specific proteins. Here we consider the fundamental structure, properties and functions of amino acids, peptides and proteins.

AMINO ACID: DEFINITION, GENERAL NATURE, AND CLASSIFICATION

Definition

Amino acids are the building blocks, of proteins joined by a specific type of covalent linkage known as **peptide bonds**. Each amino acid unit within the polypeptide is referred to as a **residue**.

There are 22 amino acids that are found in proteins and of these, only 20 are specified by the universal genetic code. These 20 amino acids of proteins are often referred to as the **standard** or **primary** or **normal amino acids**.

Nature of Amino Acids

All the 20 amino acids found in proteins **(Table 4.1)** have a **carboxyl (–COOH)** and **amino group (–NH$_2$) groups**

TABLE 4.1: The 20, L-α-amino acids (standard amino acids) found in proteins.

Name	Symbol	Structural formula
Aliphatic side chain		
Glycine	Gly (G)	H—CH—COO$^-$ │ NH$_3^+$
Alanine	Ala (A)	CH$_3$—CH$_3$—COO$^-$ │ NH$_3^+$
Valine	Val (V)	CH$_3$ \CH—CH—COO$^-$ CH$_3$/ │ NH$_3^+$
Leucine	Leu (L)	H$_3$C \CH—CH$_2$—CH—COO$^-$ H$_3$C/ │ NH$_3^+$
Isoleucine	Ile (I)	CH$_3$ \CH$_2$ \CH—CH—COO$^-$ CH$_3$/ │ NH$_3^+$
Hydroxylic (OH) group containing side chains		
Serine	Ser (S)	CH$_2$—CH—COO$^-$ │ │ OH NH$_3^+$
Threonine	Thr (T)	CH$_3$—CH—CH—COO$^-$ │ │ OH NH$_3^+$
Tyrosine	Tyr (Y)	See aromatic group containing side chain amino acids
Sulfur containing side chains		
Cysteine	Cys (C)	CH$_2$—CH—COO$^-$ │ │ SH NH$_3^+$
Methionine	Met (M)	CH$_2$—CH$_2$—CH—COO$^-$ │ │ S—CH$_3$ NH$_3^+$
Side chains containing acidic groups (–COOH) and their amides		
Aspartic acid	Asp (D)	COO$^-$—CH$_2$—CH—COO$^-$ │ NH$_3^+$
Asparagine	Asn (N)	H$_2$N—C—CH$_2$—CH—COO$^-$ ‖ │ O NH$_3^+$
Glutamic acid	Glu (E)	-OCC—CH$_2$—CH$_2$—CH—COO$^-$ │ NH$_3^+$
Glutamine	Gln (Q)	NH$_2$—C—CH$_2$—CH$_2$—CH—COO$^-$ ‖ │ O NH$_3^+$
Basic groups containing side chains		
Arginine	Arg (R)	H—N—CH$_2$---CH$_2$—CH—COO$^-$ │ │ C=NH$_3^+$ NH$_3^+$ │ NH$_2$

Contd...

Contd...

Name	Symbol	Structural formula
Lysine	Lys (K)	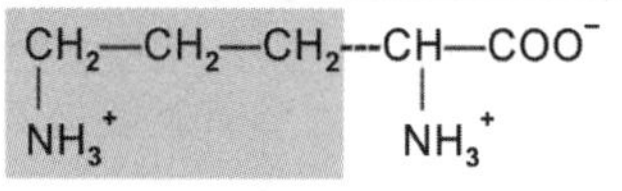 CH_2—CH_2—CH_2---CH—COO^- with NH_3^+ and NH_3^+
Histidine	His (H)	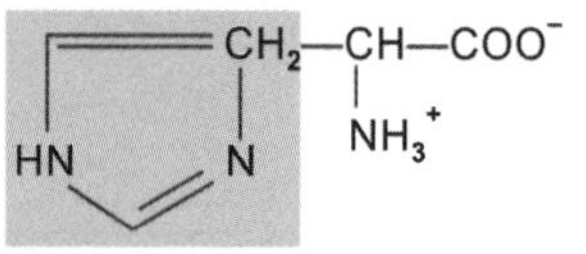 imidazole ring–CH_2—CH—COO^- with NH_3^+; HN, N
Aromatic group containing side chains		
Histidine	His (H)	See above
Phenylalanine	Phe (F)	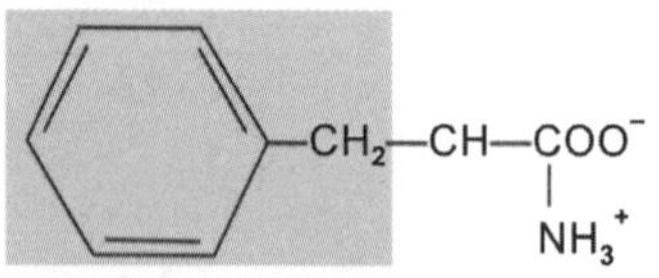 benzene ring—CH_2—CH—COO^- with NH_3^+
Tyrosine	Tyr (Y)	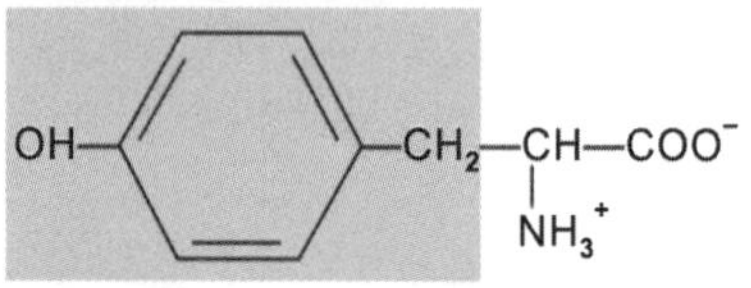 OH–benzene ring—CH_2—CH—COO^- with NH_3^+
Tryptophan	Trp (W)	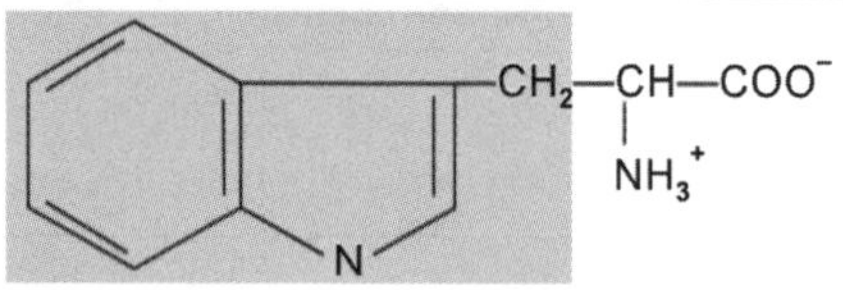 indole ring—CH_2—CH—COO^- with NH_3^+; N
Imino acids		
Proline	Pro (P)	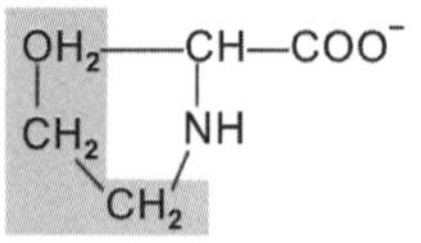 OH_2—CH—COO^-; CH_2, NH; CH_2

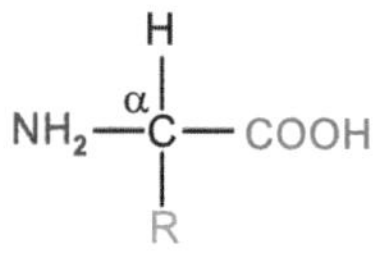

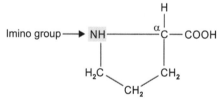

Figure 4.1: General structure of α-amino acid found in protein.

Figure 4.2: Structure of proline.

bound to the same carbon atom called the **α-carbon (Figure 4.1)**.

- Amino acids differ from each other in their side chains or R groups, attached to the α-carbon, which vary in structure, size, and electric charges and therefore influence the solubility of amino acid in water.
- When R group contains additional carbons in a chain, they are designated β, γ, δ, ε, etc., proceeding out from the α-carbon.
- The standard amino acids have been assigned three letters abbreviations and one letter symbol. The abbreviations for amino acids are the first three letters of their names, except for **asparagine (Asn)**, **glutamine (Gln)**, **isoleucine (Ile)**, and **tryptophan (Trp)**.
- The symbols for many amino acids are the first letters of their names (e.g., **G** for glycine and **L** for leucine);

the other symbols have been agreed on by convention **(Table 4.1)**.

- One of the 20 amino acids, **proline** is an **imino (–NH) acid** not an amino (–NH_2) acid as are other 19 **(Figure 4.2)**. The side chains of proline and its α-amino group form a ring structure and thus proline differs from other amino acids in that it contains an **imino** group, rather than amino group.

Classification of Amino Acids

There are five ways of classifying amino acids depending on the:

1. Chemical nature of the amino acid in the solution.
2. Structure of the side chain of the amino acids.

3. Nature or polarity of the side chain of the amino acids.
4. Nutritional requirement of amino acids.
5. Metabolic fate of amino acids.

Classification based on Chemical Nature of the Amino Acid in Solution

According to this type of classification amino acids are classified as:
1. Neutral amino acids
2. Acidic amino acids
3. Basic amino acids

- **Neutral amino acids:** The amino acids which are neutral in solution are monoamino monocarboxylic acids (i.e., having one amino group and one carboxylic group), e.g.,

  - Glycine
  - Alanine
  - Valine
  - Leucine
  - Isoleucine
  - Serine
  - Threonine
  - Cysteine
  - Methionine
  - Proline
  - Phenylalanine
  - Tyrosine
  - Tryptophan
  - Asparagine
  - Glutamine

- **Acidic amino acids:** These are acidic in solution and are monoamino dicarboxylic acids, e.g.,
  - Aspartic acid
  - Glutamic acid
- **Basic amino acids:** These are basic in solution and are diamino monocarboxylic acids, e.g.,
  - Lysine
  - Arginine
  - Histidine.

Classification based on Chemical Structure of Side Chain of the Amino Acid

According to this type of classification, amino acids are classified as:
1. Aliphatic amino acids
2. Hydroxy amino acids
3. Sulfur containing amino acids
4. Dicarboxylic acid and their amides
5. Diamino acids
6. Aromatic amino acids
7. Imino acids

- **Aliphatic amino acids:** Amino acids having aliphatic side chain, e.g.,
  - Glycine
  - Alanine
  - Valine
  - Leucine
  - Isoleucine
- **Hydroxy amino acids:** Amino acids having hydroxy group in the side chain, e.g.,
  - Threonine
  - Serine
- **Sulfur containing amino acids:** Amino acids having sulfur in the side chain, e.g.,
  - Cysteine
  - Methionine
- **Dicarboxylic acid and their amides:** Amino acids having carboxylic group in their side chain, e.g.,
  - Glutamic acid
  - Glutamine (amide of glutamic acid containing terminal carboxamide in place of carboxylic group)
  - Aspartic acid
  - Asparagine (amide of aspartic acid containing terminal carboxamide in place of carboxylic group)
- **Diamino acids:** Amino acids having amino group ($-NH_2$) in the side chain, e.g.,
  - Lysine
  - Arginine
  - Histidine
- **Aromatic amino acids:** Amino acids containing aromatic ring in the side chain, e.g.,
  - Phenylalanine
  - Tyrosine
  - Tryptophan
- **Imino acids or heterocyclic amino acids:** This amino acid has a secondary amino, i.e., imino (–NH) group not a primary one NH_2, e.g.,
  - Proline.

Classification based on Nature or Polarity of Side Chain of Amino Acid

According to this type of classification amino acids are classified into two major classes (**Figure 4.3**). While describing protein structure, it is most useful to classify amino acids on the basis of polarity of side chain of amino acids. Few amino acids are somewhat difficult to characterize or do not fit perfectly in any one group, particularly **glycine**, **histidine**, and **cysteine**. Their assignments to particular groupings are the results of considered judgments rather than absolutes.

1. **Hydrophilic or polar amino acids:** The side chains of the hydrophilic amino acids contain polar groups that may be either **charged** or **uncharged**. The R groups of these amino acids interact favorably with water and are more soluble in water or more hydrophilic than those of nonpolar amino acids because they contain functional groups that form hydrogen bond.
   - *Charged hydrophilic amino acids:* The charged side chains are of two types:
     - **Negatively charge side chain:** The side chains of the acidic amino acids, e.g., aspartic acid (aspartate) and glutamic acid (glutamate) have carboxyl groups that are negatively charged within the physiologic pH range.
     - **Positively charge side chain:** The side chains of basic amino acids, lysine, arginine, and histidine have a positive charge at physiological pH.
   - *Uncharged hydrophilic amino acids:* Six amino acids are polar but uncharged. The uncharged side chains

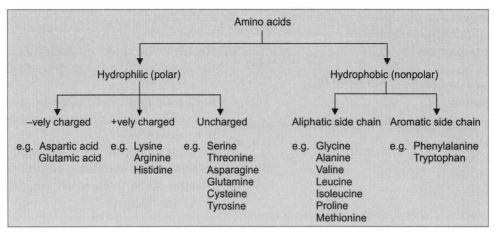

Figure 4.3: Classification of amino acid based on polarity.

of other amino acids have oxygen, sulfur or nitrogen atoms, enabling them to form hydrogen bonds with water. Although they are uncharged, these amino acids are hydrophilic, e.g.,

♦ Threonine and serine, and tyrosine with OH group in the hydrophobic side chain
♦ Asparagine and glutamine with amide group containing terminal carboxamide in place of carboxylic group
♦ Cysteine with thiol group (–SH) in the side chain.
♦ Methionine sulfur containing amino acid is hydrophobic because it contains aliphatic side chain that includes a thioester (–S–) not the thiol (–SH) group.

2. **Hydrophobic or nonpolar amino acids:** The side chains of hydrophobic amino acids interact poorly with water. They have either **aliphatic** or **aromatic** side chains.

■ Glycine (Although it is grouped with the nonpolar amino acids, it's very small side chain makes no real contribution to hydrophobic interaction.)
■ Alanine
■ Valine
■ Leucine
■ Isoleucine
■ Methionine has an aliphatic side chain that contains highly nonpolar thioester (–S–) group.
■ Proline has an aliphatic side chain with a distinctive cyclic structure
■ Hydrophobic amino acids with aromatic side chain are, phenylalanine and tryptophan.

Classification of Amino Acid based on Nutritional Requirement

Nutritionists divide amino acids into two groups:

1. **Essential amino acids:** Those amino acids which cannot be synthesized in the body. Hence these amino acids are to be supplied in the diet.
2. **Nonessential amino acids:** Amino acids which can be synthesized in the body. Hence not required in the diet.

TABLE 4.2: Essential and nonessential amino acids.	
Essential amino acids	*Nonessential amino acids*
Mnemonic: PVT. TIM. HALL	
• Phenylalanine	• Glycine
• Valine	• Serine
• Threonine	• Alanine
• Tryptophan	• Cysteine
• Isoleucine	• Proline
• Methionine	• Tyrosine
• Histidine	• Glutamic acid
• Arginine	• Aspartic acid
• Lysine	• Glutamine
• Leucine	• Asparagine

Table 4.2 shows essential and nonessential amino acids in humans.

Essential Amino Acids

● Ten amino acids essential for humans include:

■ Phenylalanine   ■ Methionine
■ Valine   ■ Histidine
■ Threonine   ■ Arginine
■ Tryptophan   ■ Lysine
■ Isoleucine   ■ Leucine

The mnemonics used for essential amino acids are **PVT. TIM. HALL** or **L. VITTHAL (MP) (Table 4.2).**

● Among the ten essential amino acids, **arginine** and **histidine** are known as **semiessential** amino acids since these amino acids are synthesized partially in human body but inadequate to support growth of children. Growing children require them in the diet, but not essential in adult.

● Enough **arginine** is synthesized by the urea cycle to meet the needs of an adult, but in growing children it is synthesized inadequately.

● Although **histidine** is considered essential, unlike the other essential it does not fulfil the criteria of inducing negative nitrogen balance promptly upon removal from the diet.

- Arginine and histidine become essential in diet during periods of rapid growth as in childhood and pregnancy.
- A deficiency of even one essential amino acid impairs protein synthesis and leads to a negative nitrogen balance, (nitrogen excretion exceeds nitrogen intake). In this state, more protein is degraded than is synthesized, and so more nitrogen is excreted than is ingested.

Nonessential Amino Acids

Some amino acids are **nutritionally nonessential** to human beings because they can be synthesized in human body and are not required in diet, e.g.,

- Glycine
- Proline
- Serine
- Glutamic acid
- Glutamine
- Alanine
- Tyrosine
- Cysteine
- Aspartic acid
- Asparagine

Classification of Amino Acid based on Metabolic Fate

On the basis of their catabolic end products, the twenty standard amino acids are divided in three groups (**Table 4.3**):
1. Glucogenic amino acids
2. Exclusive ketogenic amino acids
3. Both glucogenic and ketogenic

- **Glucogenic amino acids:** These amino acids serve as precursor of gluconeogenesis for glucose formation. The amino acids that are degraded to pyruvate, α-ketoglutarate, succinyl-CoA, fumarate, and/or oxaloacetate can be converted into glucose (by gluconeogenesis) are the glucogenic amino acids.
  - Thirteen out of the twenty standard amino acids are glucogenic amino acids.
  - These are; glycine, alanine, serine, aspartic acid, asparagine, glutamic acid, glutamine, proline, valine, methionine, cysteine, histidine, and arginine.
- **Ketogenic amino acids:** The amino acids that are degraded to acetyl-CoA are termed ketogenic amino acids because they can give rise ketone bodies (acetoacetate, acetone and β-hydroxybutyrate).
  - The seven amino acids—phenylalanine, tyrosine, tryptophan, threonine, isoleucine, leucine, and lysine are ketogenic amino acids.

- The amino acids degraded to pyruvate (alanine, cysteine, glycine, and serine) are also potentially ketogenic because pyruvate can be converted to acetyl-CoA.
  - **Leucine** and **lysine** are exclusively ketogenic amino acid.
- **Both glucogenic and ketogenic:** Those, which can be converted to both glucose and ketone bodies. Five amino acids, **phenylalanine**, **tyrosine**, **tryptophan threonine**, and **isoleucine** are both glucogenic and ketogenic.

Importance of Amino Acids

- **Formation of proteins:** Amino acids are joined to each other by peptide bonds to form proteins and peptides
- **Formation of glucose:** Glucogenic amino acids are converted to glucose in the body
- **Enzyme activity:** The thiol (–SH) group of cysteine has an important role in certain enzyme activity
- **Transport and storage form of ammonia:** Amino acid glutamine play an important role in transport and storage of amino nitrogen in the form of ammonia
- **As a buffer:** Both free amino acids and some amino acids present in protein can potentially act as buffer, e.g., histidine can serve as the best buffer at physiological pH
- **Detoxification reactions:** Glycine, cysteine and methionine are involved in the detoxification of toxic substances.
- **Formation of biologically important compounds:** In addition to being the building blocks of proteins and peptides, amino acids serve as precursors of many kinds of **biomolecules**, e.g., purines, pyrimidines, neurotransmitters, hormones, heme, and vitamins (**Table 4.4**) that have important and diverse biological roles.

TABLE 4.4: Biologically important compounds formed by amino acids.

Amino acid	Formation of biologically important compound
Tyrosine	Hormone, e.g., thyroxine, skin-pigment, melanin
Tyrosine and phenylalanine	Hormone, e.g., epinephrine, norepinephrine, and dihydroxyphenylalanine (DOPA)
Glutamic acid (neurotransmitter)	γ-Aminobutyric acid (GABA)
Tryptophan	Vitamin niacin
Glycine, arginine and methionine	Creatine
Glycine and cysteine	Bile salts
Glycine	Heme
Aspartic acid and glutamic acid	Pyrimidine bases
Glycine, aspartic acid, and glutamine	Purine bases
β-alanine	Coenzyme-A
Histidine	Histamine
Tryptophan	Serotonin

TABLE 4.3: Classification of amino acid based on metabolic fate.

Exclusive glucogenic	Exclusive ketogenic	Both ketogenic and glucogenic
• Glycine, Alanine, Serine • Cysteine, Aspartic acid • Asparagine, Glutamic acid • Glutamine, Proline, Histidine • Arginine, Methionine, Valine	• Leucine • Lysine	• Tryptophan • Phenylalanine • Tyrosine • Threonine • Isoleucine

21st and 22nd Amino Acid

There are actually 22 rather than 20 amino acids specified by the known genetic code. The two extra ones are **selenocysteine** and **pyrrolysine** each found in very few proteins but both offering intimation into the complexities of code evolution. **Selenocysteine** and **pyrrolysine** coded by **stop codon UGA** and **UAG** respectively. This process of converting stop codons **to** a coding codon is called **recoding**.

21st amino acid
Selenocysteine

Selenocysteine is the 21st amino acid occurs uncommonly in at least 25 human selenoproteins. It contains **selenium** rather than the **sulfur** of the cysteine **(Figure 4.4)**. Precursor amino acid for selenocysteine is **serine**. Serine provides the carbon skeleton of selenocysteine.

❖ It is encoded in a special way by **UGA codon**, which is normally a stop codon. A special unusual type of tRNA called **tRNA^Sec** recognizes selenoproteins-specific UGA codon and no other codons. Selenocysteine is incorporated in peptides during translation rather than produced through a post-translational modification.

❖ Selenocysteine is a constituent of several human proteins and enzymes. It is located in the active site of enzymes that participate in oxidation-reduction reactions. These include; **glutathione peroxidase**, **thioredoxin reductase** and **iodothyronine deiodinase** that converts thyroxine to triiodothyronine. Selenocysteine participate in the catalytic mechanism of these enzymes. The replacement of selenocysteine by cysteine impairs catalytic activity.

❖ Impairments in human selenoproteins leads to **tumorigenesis** and **atherosclerosis**, and are associated with selenium deficiency **cardiomyopathy (Keshan disease)**.

22nd amino acid
Pyrrolysine

Pyrrolysine (abbreviated as Pyl or O) is a naturally occurring, genetically coded amino acid used by some anaerobic methanogen archaea. These organisms produce methane as a required part of their metabolism.

❖ It is similar to **lysine**, but with an added **pyrroline ring** linked to the end of the lysine side chain.

❖ This amino acid is encoded by **UAG** (normally a stop codon)

❖ Pyrrolysine was discovered in 2002 at the active site of methyl-transferase enzyme from a methane-producing archaeon, *Methanosarcina barkeri*.

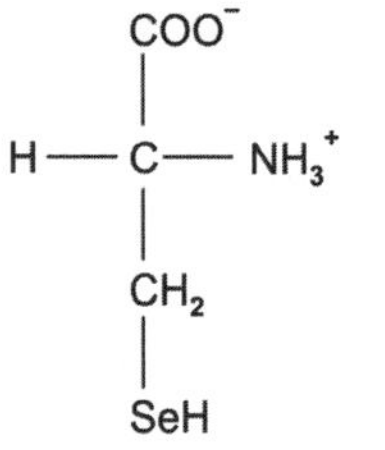

▮ NONSTANDARD AMINO ACIDS

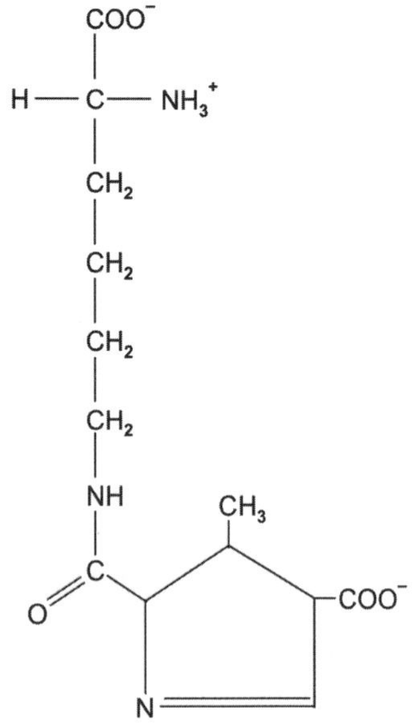

There are approximately 300 amino acids present in various animal, plant and microbial systems, but only **20 amino acids** are **standard** and **present in protein** because they are coded by genes. All of the proteins on the earth are made up of the same 20 amino acids.

Other amino acids are **modified** or **derived amino acids** and called **nonprotein amino acids**. Some amino acids are modified after a protein has been synthesized by **post-translational modifications**; others are amino acids present in living organisms but not as constituents of proteins. Derived amino acids do not have a genetic code.

Figure 4.4: Structure of 21st (selenocysteine) and 22nd (pyrrolysine) amino acids.

TABLE 4.5: Derived amino acids which occur in proteins.

Amino acid	Occurrence or significance
Cystine	Two cysteine molecules join to form cystine. Found in protein having disulfide bond, e.g., insulin, immunoglobulin
4-hydroxy proline	Found in collagen
5-hydroxy lysine	Found in collagen
Desmosine	Found in elastin
Gamma carboxy glutamate	Found in clotting factors, like prothrombin that bind calcium
Methyl lysine	Present in myosin

TABLE 4.6: Derived/nonslandered amino acids which do not occur in proteins.

Amino acid	Occurrence or significance
Glutamate-γ semialdehyde	Serine catabolite
β-Alanine	Formed from cytosine and uracil. It is present in pantothenic acid, acyl carrier protein and of coenzyme A
Homocysteine	Derived from methionine
γ-Aminobutyric acid	Brain tissue
β-Aminoisobutyric acid	End-product in pyrimidine metabolism; found in urine of patients with an inherited metabolic disease
Ornithine	Urea cycle intermediate
Citrulline	Urea cycle intermediate
Homoserine	Cysteine biosynthesis intermediate

Derived amino acids result from reaction at an **amino group**, **carboxy group**, **or side-chain** of amino acids. These are classified into:

1. Derived amino acids present in proteins **(Table 4.5)**
2. Derived amino acids not present in proteins **(Table 4.6)**.

PROPERTIES OF AMINO ACIDS

- All amino acids (except glycine) are optically active. **Glycine** is **optically inactive** because, glycine does not contain an asymmetric carbon atom.

- Amino acids are colorless because they do not absorb visible light. However, **tyrosine**, **phenylalanine**, and **tryptophan** absorb **ultraviolet light** in the range of **250–290 nm**. The ability of proteins to absorb ultraviolet light is predominantly due to the presence of the **tryptophan**, which absorbs maximum ultraviolet light.

- All of the 20 amino acids found in proteins are exclusively of the **L-configuration** except glycine. Because glycine is not optically active and, thus, it is neither D nor L. However, two free D-amino acids **D-serine** and **D-aspartic acid** have been found to be present in the human brain.

> Certain microorganisms secrete free D-amino acids, or peptides that may contain both D- and L- α-amino acids.
> ❖ Several of these bacterial peptides are of therapeutic value, including the **antibiotics bacitracin** and **gramicidin A**, and the antitumor agent **bleomycin.**
> ❖ Certain other microbial peptides are, however, toxic. For example amino acid present in the seeds of **legumes** of the genus *Lathyrus* can result in **Lathyrism**, a terrible irreversible disease in which individual lose control of their limbs.

Ionization of Amino Acids

All amino acids have at least one **carboxyl** and one **amino** functional group. Both of these groups are **ionizable**. Due to ionizing property of amino acids, amino acids exhibit:

- Acid-base behavior
- Amphoteric nature
- Zwitterion formation
- Buffering activity.

Acid-Base Behavior

Amino acids can act as **acids** and **bases**. The **carboxyl** and **amino** groups of amino acids, along with the **ionizable R** groups of some amino acids, function as weak bases and acids.

- The **carboxyl** (-COOH) group of an amino acid can donate proton (H⁺) and behave as an acid (proton donor), forming a negatively charged **anion**.

- **Amino** group (-NH₂) of an amino acid can accept the proton (H⁺) which behave as a base (proton acceptor), forming positively charged **cation (Figure 4.5)**.

- At physiological pH (around 7.4) the carboxyl group will be unprotonated and the amino group will be protonated. An amino acid with no ionizable R-group would be electrically neutral at this pH (as they have both positive and negative charges on the same amino acids). This type of molecule is termed a **zwitterion** (German word means "hybrid ion"). Such zwitterion can act as either an acid (proton donor) or base (proton acceptor).

Amphoteric Properties

- As amino acids are capable of acting as both an **acid** (i.e., proton donor) and a **base** (i.e., proton acceptor) these are regarded as ampholytes. Substances having a dual nature are called **amphoteric** (Greek word **ampho** means **both)** and are often called **ampholytes** (amphoteric electrolytes).

- Behavior of amino acids as acid or base and ionization state varies with pH.
  - At acidic pH, amino acid is **positively charged** because at acidic pH the amino group is ionized, protonated (-NH₃⁺) and the carboxyl group is not ionized (COOH).
  - As pH is raised, i.e., at alkaline pH amino acid is **negatively charged** as the carboxylic group is ionized to give up a proton (COO⁻) and amino group is remained in unionizsed (NH₂) form.

- Between these pH ranges, there is a certain pH at which both carboxyl and amino groups are ionizsed and that pH is called **isoelectric pH** or **isoelectric point (PI)**. At isoelectric pH though both carboxyl and amino groups are ionizsed, the molecule as a whole is electrically neutral, i.e., amino acid bears no net charge (zwitterion) and therefore does not move in an electric field. Isoelectric pH or isoelectric point (PI) is constant for every amino acid. The solubility of the amino acid is least at its isoelectric pH.

> ❖ In laboratory altering the charge on amino acids and their derivatives by varying the pH facilitates the physical separation of amino acids, peptides, and proteins.
> ❖ In the clinical laboratory, knowledge of the pI guides selection of conditions for electrophoretic separations as well as chromatographic separations.

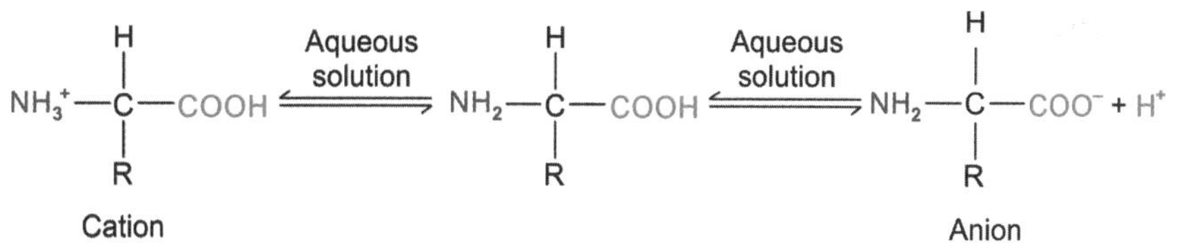

Figure 4.5: Ionization of amino acid.

Zwitterion Formation

- When an amino acid lacking ionizable R group, is dissolved in water at neutral pH, it exists in solution as the **dipolar ion**, or **zwitterion** (hybrid ion) which means that they have both positive and negative charges on the same amino acids and the overall molecule is **electrically neutral**. The (neutral) zwitterion is the usual form of amino acids exist in solution.
  - The α-**COOH** group is ionized to form a negatively charged anion (COO⁻) and
  - The α-**NH₂** group is protonated to form a positively charged cation (NH₃⁺)
- The molecular species, which contain an equal number of ionizable groups of opposite charge and as a result bear no net charge are called **zwitterions**. A zwitterion can act as either an acid (proton donor) or a base (proton acceptor) **(Figure 4.6)**.
- When the pH of the surrounding medium is lowered below the pI (isoelectric pH) value **(pH < pI)** of an amino acid its carboxyl group accepts a proton to form protonated (COOH) form. This form of amino acid carries net **positive charge**. Conversely when the pH of the surrounding medium is above the pI value **(pH > pI)** of an amino acid its NH₃⁺ group loses its proton and

becomes uncharged. This form of amino acid carries net **negative charge (Figure 4.7)**.

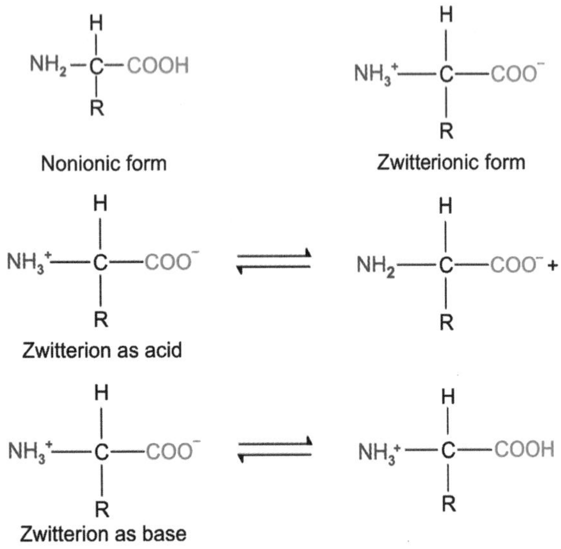

Buffering Action of Amino Acid

A buffer system consists of a weak acid (the proton donor) and its conjugate base (the proton acceptor). Amino acid can act as weak acid (the proton donor) or weak base (the proton acceptor). In addition, each of the acidic and basic amino acids contains an ionizable group in its side chain. Thus, both free amino acids and some amino acids present in proteins can potentially act as buffer. Maximum buffer capacity occurs at pH equal to the pKa. So amino acid which has pKa range near physiologic pH can act as effective buffer.

Among the 20 standard amino acids, **histidine** serves as the best buffer at physiological pH. The imidazole group (side chain) of histidine has a **pKa of 6.5–7.4**. Hence at physiological pH histidine has maximum buffering capacity.

Protein containing histidine residues therefore buffer effectively near physiological pH. All other amino acids have pKa value, too far away from pH 7 to be an effective physiological buffer. The acidic amino acids have pKa below histidine's pKa and the basic amino acids have pKa far above histidine's pKa and thus among all amino acids histidine is the best amino acid buffer under physiological conditions.

Structural and Functional Importance of α-R Groups of Amino Acid

- Each amino acid differs in terms of its R-group. Chemical properties of each amino acid depend on its R group.
- The nature of R-group of the amino acids dictates structure-function relationships of peptides and proteins.
- Since **glycine**, the smallest amino acid (smallest R-group) can be accommodated in places inaccessible to other amino acids, it often occurs where peptides bend sharply.
- The hydrophobic R groups of **alanine, valine, leucine,** and **isoleucine** and the aromatic R groups of **phenylalanine, tyrosine,** and **tryptophan** typically occur primarily in the interior of proteins shielded from direct contact with water.
- Conversely, the **hydrophilic amino acids basic (lysine, arginine and histidine) and acidic amino acids**

Figure 4.6: Nonionic and zwitterionic forms of amino acid. A zwitterion can act as either an acid (proton donor) or base (proton acceptor).

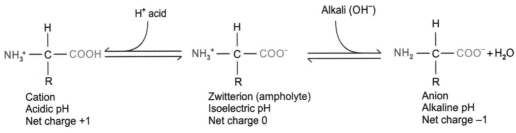

Figure 4.7: Ionic forms of amino acid in acidic, basic and isoelectric pH.

(aspartic acid, glutamic acid) are generally found on the exterior of proteins as well as in the active centers of enzymatically active proteins.

- **Histidine** plays unique roles in enzymatic catalysis. The imidazole ring of histidine allows it to act as either a proton donor or acceptor at physiological pH. Hence, it is frequently found in the reactive center of enzymes.
- Similarly the ability of histidine in hemoglobin to buffer the H^+ ions from carbonic acid ionization in red blood cells is very important. It is this property of hemoglobin that allows it to exchange O_2 and CO_2 at the tissues or lungs, respectively.
- The primary **hydroxyl group** of **serine** and **threonine** as well as the **thiol (–SH)** group of **cysteine** are involved in enzymatic catalysis. The hydroxyl groups of **serine**, **tyrosine**, and **threonine** frequently serve as the points of covalent attachment for phosphoryl groups that regulate protein function.

STRIKE A NOTE

- ❖ Amino acids not coded by genetic code are all the derived amino acids.
- ❖ Amino acids coded by stop codon are: Selenocysteine and pyrrolysine.
- ❖ Amino acid with no asymmetric carbon, no optically active carbon is glycine.
- ❖ All of the 20 standard amino acids except glycine are of the L-configuration. Glycine is neither D nor L. However
- ❖ Aromatic amino acids absorb UV light.
- ❖ Amino acids are colorless because they do not absorb visible light.
- ❖ Only two amino acids, leucine and lysine are exclusively ketogenic.
- ❖ At physiological pH imidazole group of histidine has the maximum buffering capacity.
- ❖ Most abundant amino acid in the protein present in the body is alanine.

BIOLOGICALLY IMPORTANT PEPTIDES

Peptide and Proteins

Although amino acids serve other functions in cells, their most important role is as **constituents of proteins**. Proteins are polymers of amino acids. In polymer amino acids are linked to each other by **peptide bonds**, in which the **carboxyl group** of one amino acid is joined to the **amino group** of the second, with the **loss of a molecule of water** to yield a simplest peptide, **dipeptide (Figure 4.8)**.

- The amino acids present in a peptides, called **amino acid residues** (the part left over after losing the water molecule).
- A chain made up of just a few amino acids linked together is called an **oligopeptide** (oligo: few) while a typical protein, which is made up of many amino acids is called a **polypeptide** (poly: many).

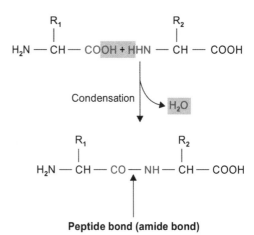

Peptide bond (amide bond)

Figure 4.8: Formation of peptide bond.

- Proteins are polypeptides with thousands of amino acids residues and of greatly different length.
- Although the term 'protein'; and 'polypeptide' are sometimes interchangeable, molecules referred to as **polypeptides** generally have molecular weights below 10,00, and those called **proteins,** have higher molecular weights.

In 1953, Frederick Sanger determined the amino acid sequence of **insulin**, a protein hormone. This work is a landmark in biochemistry because it showed for the first time that a protein has a precisely defined amino acid sequences consisting only L-amino acids linked by peptide bonds. Currently, the complete amino acid sequences of more than 2,000,000 peptides are known.

Isopeptide Bond/Atypical Peptide Bond/Pseudopeptide Bond

- ❖ Isopeptide bond is an amide bond between **side chain amines** or **carbonyl carbons** on the side chain rather than α-amine or α-carbonyl.
- ❖ In glutathione, for example, the γ-carboxyl group of glutamic acid is linked to the α-amino group of cysteine.
- ❖ Isopeptide bonds occur post-translationally, can be formed spontaneously or enzymatically
- ❖ As proteases cannot hydrolyse isopeptide bond, it makes the protein resistant to action of proteases.
- ❖ For example; glutathione, thyrotropin releasing hormone.

- There are many naturally occurring small polypeptides and oligopeptides, some of which have important biological activities and are called **biologically important peptides**. A number of **hormones** and **neurotransmitters** are peptides. Additionally, **several antibiotics** and **antitumor agents** are peptides. A few of them are listed below (**Table 4.7**).
1. **Glutathione:** Glutathione (GSH) is a **tripeptide** (γ-glutamyl–cysteinyl–glycine) containing **glutamate, cysteine** and **glycine**. Glutathione is found in all mammalian cells except **the neurons**. Glutathione is an **antioxidant**. Glutathione plays a key role in detoxification of H_2O_2 and organic peroxides.

TABLE 4.7: Biologically important peptides.

Peptide	Example
Tripeptide	• Glutathione • Thyrotropin releasing hormone (TRH)
Pentapeptide	Enkephalins
Octapeptide	Angiotensin II
Nonapeptide	• Oxytocin • Vasopressin [ADH] • Bradykinin
Decapeptide	Angiotensin-I

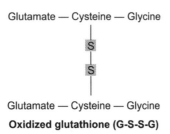

Glutamate — Cysteine — Glycine

SH

Reduced glutathione (GSH)

Glutamate — Cysteine — Glycine

S

S

Glutamate — Cysteine — Glycine

Oxidized glutathione (G-S-S-G)

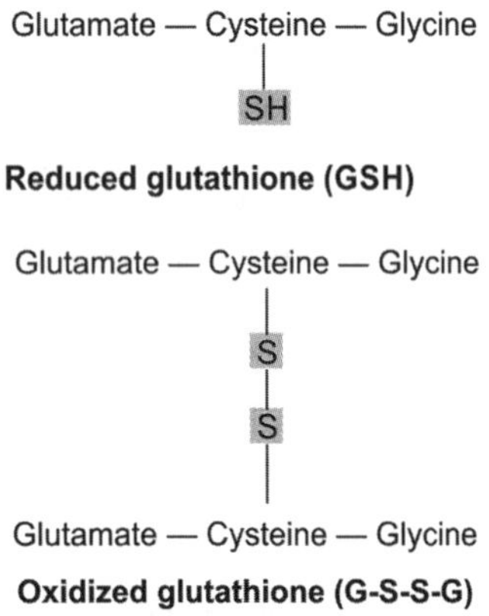

Figure 4.9: Reduced and oxidized glutathione.

Glutathione may exist as the **reduced (GSH)** or **oxidized (G-S-S-G)** form **(Figure 4.9)** and can thus play a role in some **oxidation–reduction reactions**. In oxidized form, two molecules of glutathione are linked by disulfide bond. The sulfhydryl (–SH–) is the functional group primarily responsible for the functions of glutathione.

♦ The reduced form of glutathione with a free sulfhydryl (–SH–) group serves as a **redox buffer** regulating the redox state of the cell by maintaining an appropriate equilibrium between its oxidized and reduced state (ratio of reduced to oxidized glutathione is 500:1).

♦ It helps in keeping the enzymes in an active state by preventing the oxidation of sulfhydryl (–SH–) group of enzyme to disulfide (–S-S–) group.

♦ Reduced glutathione is essential for maintaining the normal structure of red blood cells and for keeping hemoglobin in the ferrous state. Cells with lowered level of reduced glutathione are more susceptible to hemolysis.

♦ Glutathione plays a key role in detoxification by reducing H_2O_2 and organic peroxides, (lipid peroxides) the harmful byproduct of metabolism **(Figure 4.10)**.

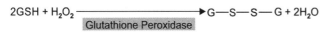

$$2GSH + H_2O_2 \xrightarrow{\text{Glutathione Peroxidase}} G—S—S—G + 2H_2O$$

Figure 4.10: Role of glutathione in detoxification of H_2O_2.

♦ Glutathione is involved in transport of amino acids across the cell membrane of the kidney and intestine via γ-**glutamyl cycle** or **Mester cycle)**.

2. **Thyrotropin releasing hormone:** Thyrotropin releasing hormone (TRH) is a hypothalamic hormone of three amino acid residues. It stimulates the release of hormone thyrotropin, from the anterior pituitary gland.

3. **Enkephalins:** Enkephalins a pentapeptide formed in the CNS that bind to receptors in certain cells of brain and induce analgesia (deadening of pain sensations). Enkephalins represent one of the body's own mechanisms for control of pain. The enkephalins receptors also bind morphine, heroin and other addicting drugs

4. **Angiotensin:** Angiotensin II is a vasoconstrictor and elevates the arterial pressure and also promotes the synthesis of a steroid hormone called aldosterone that promotes sodium retention.

> Liver synthesizes **angiotensinogen**, a protein that occurs in the blood. A circulating proteolytic enzyme, **renin**, catalyzes the hydrolysis of angiotensinogen to **angiotensin I**, which is converted to **angiotensin II** by an enzyme **angiotensin converting enzyme (ACE) (Figure 4.11)**. ACE inhibitors like **captopril** and **enalapril** are commonly used for the treatment of hypertension and congestive heart failure.

5. **Oxytocin:** This is a 9-amino acid residue hormone secreted by posterior pituitary and stimulates uterine contractions.

6. **Vasopressin:** This is a 9-amino acid residue hormone secreted by posterior pituitary and it increases blood pressure and has an antidiuretic action.

7. **Bradykinin:** It contains, 9-amino acid residue. It is a powerful vasodilator and causes contraction of smooth muscle. It is formed in the blood under a certain condition and is mainly responsible for causing intense peripheral and visceral pain by stimulating the pain receptors.

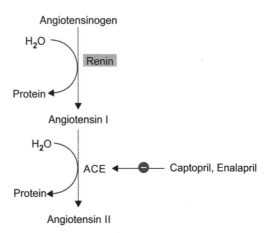

Figure 4.11: Conversion of angiotensinogen to angiotensin II.

Aspartame: It is a commercially synthesized dipeptide **L-aspartyl phenylalanyl methyl ester**. This compound is an artificial sweetener and is intensely sweet. So it is used in food stuffs as low calorie sweetener under the name *aspartame* or *nutra sweet*. Its drawback is that its content of phenylalanine makes it unsuitable for consumption by phenylketonurics.

PROTEIN: DEFINITION, CLASSIFICATION, AND FUNCTIONS

Definition

Proteins are macromolecules composed of one or more polypeptide chains, each with a characteristic sequence of amino acids linked by peptide bonds.

Classification

Proteins have been classified in several ways. They are most conveniently classified on the basis of their:
- Function
- Molecular shape
- Composition
- Nutritional quality.

Classification of Proteins based on Functions

Of all the molecules encountered in living organisms, proteins have the most diverse function. In a functional classification, they are grouped according to their biological role. Some functions that proteins serve and examples of specific functional proteins are as follows:

Catalytic Proteins or Enzymes

Catalytic proteins called the **enzymes** accelerate thousands of biochemical reactions in such process as digestion, and metabolism, e.g.,
- Glucokinase
- Dehydrogenases
- Transaminases
- Hydrolytic enzymes, pepsin, trypsin, etc.

Transport Proteins

Transport proteins in blood plasma bind and carry specific molecules or ions from one organ to another, e.g.,
- Hemoglobin of erythrocytes binds oxygen and carries it to the peripheral tissues.
- Apolipoproteins carry lipids from the liver to other organs.
- Other kinds of transport proteins are present in the plasma membrane and intracellular membranes. These bind glucose, amino acids or other substances and transport them across the membrane.
- Transferrin and ceruloplasmin are serum proteins that transport **iron** and **copper**, respectively.

Storage Proteins

Many proteins serve as storage form of essential components, e.g.,
- Apoferritin stores iron in the form of ferritin
- Myoglobin stores oxygen in muscles.

Contractile Proteins

Some proteins have the ability to contract and function in the contractile system of skeletal muscle, e.g.,
- Actin
- Myosin.

Structural Proteins

Many proteins serve as supporting filaments or sheet to give biological structure, strength or protection, e.g.,
- Collagen, a fibrous protein of tendon
- Cartilage, elastin of ligaments
- Keratin of hair and nails.

Defense Proteins

Many proteins defend against invasion of foreign substances, such as viruses, bacteria and cells from other organism. Examples of defense proteins are:
- Immunoglobulins or antibodies
- Fibrinogen and thrombin are blood clotting proteins that prevent loss of blood when the vascular system is injured.

Regulatory Proteins

Some proteins regulate cellular or physiological activity, e.g.,
- Cellular **receptors** that recognize hormones and neurotransmitters are proteins.
- Insulin and glucagon are peptide hormones that regulate blood glucose levels. Growth hormone stimulates cell growth and division.
- Growth factors, such as platelet-derived growth factor (PDGF) and epidermal growth factor (EGF) are polypeptides that control cell division and differentiation.

Stress Response Protein

A capacity of living organisms to survive a variety of abiotic stress is mediated by certain proteins, e.g.,
- **Cytochrome P$_{450}$** an enzyme that converts a variety of toxic substances into less toxic derivatives.
- **Metallothionein**, a cysteine-rich intracellular protein found in all mammalian cells that binds to and sequesters toxic metals, such as cadmium, mercury, and silver.
- **Heat shock proteins (HSPs):** Heat shock proteins are a family of proteins that are produced by cells in response to exposure to stressful conditions. They were first described in relation to **heat shock** but are now known to also be expressed during other stresses including

exposure to cold, UV light, and during wound healing or tissue remodeling. If proteins are severely damaged, HSPs promote their degradation.

Classification based on Molecular Shape of the Proteins

In this type of classification, proteins are classified as follows:

Fibrous Proteins

Fibrous proteins are also called **scleroproteins**. They are insoluble, high molecular weight fibers. The fibers are long and thin. These have axial ratio (length/breadth), greater than 10 **(Figure 4.12)**. Examples of fibrous proteins are:
- Collagen found in cartilage and tendons
- Elastin found in elastic tissue such as tendon and arteries
- Keratin of hair, skin, and nail.

Keratins, those in mammals are called α-*keratins*, being almost entirely α-helical in structure in contrast to β-*keratins* which are made up of β-sheets and occurs in feathers.

Globular Proteins

They are also called **spheroproteins**, on account of their spherical or ovoid shape. In globular proteins, the polypeptide chain is compactly folded and coiled and have axial ratio (length/breadth) of less than 10 **(Figure 4.12)**. These are soluble proteins of relatively low molecular weight. This group includes mainly:
- Albumin
- Globulin
- Many enzymes
- Histones
- Protamine
- Actin, troponin, etc.

Classification of Proteins based on Composition of Protein

According to the joint committee of the **American Society of Biological Chemists and American Physiological** Society, proteins are classified into three main groups as follows:
1. Simple proteins
2. Conjugated proteins
3. Derived proteins.

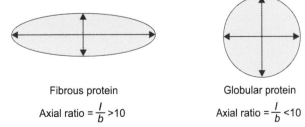

Figure 4.12: Diagrammatic representation of fibrous and globular proteins (*l* = length, *b* = breadth).

Simple Proteins

Many proteins containing only amino acid residues and no other chemical constituents; these are considered simple proteins. For example:
- **Albumins:** The albumins are **soluble in water, coagulated by heat**. It is deficient in glycine, e.g., egg albumin, lactalbumin of milk.
- **Globulins:** The globulins are insoluble in water, but they are **soluble in dilute neutral salt solution and are heat coagulable**, e.g., ovoglobulin of egg yolk, serum globulin, legumin of peas.
- **Glutelins:** The glutelins are **soluble in dilute acids and alkalies,** but they are **insoluble in neutral solvents**. They are plant proteins, e.g., glutelin of wheat and oryzenin of rice.
- **Prolamins or alcohol soluble proteins:** The prolamins are soluble in **70–80% alcohol**, but they are **insoluble in water**, **neutral solvent** or **absolute alcohol**. The prolamins are rich in proline but are **deficient in lysine**. They are plant proteins, e.g., zein of corn, gliadin of wheat.
- **Histones:** The histones are **soluble in water, but are not coagulated by heat**. Histones are basic proteins as they are rich in basic amino acids. The histones, being basic, usually occur in tissues in salt combinations with acidic substances, such as nucleic acids (RNA and DNA).
- **Protamines:** They are strongly basic and rich in basic amino acid arginine. The protamines are **soluble in water but are not heat coagulable**. Like histones they occur in tissues with nucleic acids.
- **Scleroprotein:** Scleroprotein also called **albuminoid** is insoluble in water, and in dilute solutions of salt, acids and bases. The most important scleroproteins are **collagen**, **keratin** and **fibroin**. All scleroproteins have a fibrillar structure. In natural state, scleroproteins (except elastin) are not hydrolyzed by proteolytic enzymes and therefore have no nutritive value.

Conjugated Proteins

Some proteins contain permanently associated chemical components in addition to amino acid; these are called conjugated proteins. The nonamino part of a conjugated protein is referred to as the **prosthetic** (additional) group. Conjugated proteins are classified on the basis of the chemical nature of their prosthetic groups as follows **(Table 4.8)**:
- **Nucleoproteins:** The nucleoproteins are composed of simple basic proteins (histones or protamines) with **nucleic acids (RNA and DNA) as the prosthetic groups**.
- **Glycoproteins:** These consist of simple protein and **carbohydrate** as a prosthetic group, e.g., mucin of saliva, immunoglobulins, and hormones like TSH, FSH, and LH.

TABLE 4.8: Conjugated proteins.

Class	Prosthetic group	Example
Nucleoproteins	Nucleic acid	Histones or protamines
Glycoproteins	Carbohydrates	• Immunoglobulins • Mucin of saliva • TSH, FSH, and LH
Chromoproteins: • Hemoproteins • Flavoproteins	Color prosthetic group • Heme (iron porphyrin) • Flavin nucleotides	• Hemoglobin, Cytochromes, Catalase, peroxidase • Succinate dehydrogenase
Phosphoproteins	Phosphate Groups	Casein of milk Vitellin of egg yolk
Lipoproteins	Lipid	Chylomicrons, LDL, HDL, VLDL
Metaloproteins	Metallic elements • Iron • Zinc • Calcium • Molybdenum • Copper	 • Ferritin • Carbonic anhydrase, Alcohol dehydrogenase, DNA polymerase, carboxypeptidase • Calmodulin • Dinitrogenase • Ceruloplasmin, Plastocyanin

- **Chromoproteins:** Chromoproteins are composed of simple proteins with a **colored prosthetic group**, e.g.,
  - Hemoproteins (heme as a prosthetic group), e.g., hemoglobin, cytochromes, catalase, peroxidase
  - Flavoproteins (flavin nucleotide as a prosthetic group), e.g., succinate dehydrogenase.
- **Phosphoproteins:** The phosphoproteins are formed by a combination of protein with **phosphate group** as a prosthetic group, e.g., casein of milk and vitellin of egg yolk.
- **Lipoproteins:** The lipoproteins are formed by a combination of protein with a prosthetic group **lipid**, e.g., serum lipoproteins like:
  - Chylomicrons
  - Very low-density lipoprotein (VLDL)
  - Low-density lipoprotein (LDL)
  - High-density lipoprotein (HDL).
- **Metalloproteins:** The prosthetic group is **metallic elements** such as: iron, zinc, calcium, molybdenum, copper, etc. For example:
  - Ferritin is an iron-containing protein
  - Carbonic anhydrase, alcohol dehydrogenase, carboxy-peptidase and DNA polymerase are zinc-containing proteins
  - Calmodulin is calcium-containing protein
  - Dinitrogenase is molybdenum-containing protein
  - Ceruloplasmin-plastocyanin is a copper-containing protein.

Derived Proteins

This class of proteins as the name implies, includes those substances formed from simple and conjugated proteins. Derived proteins are subdivided into **primary-derived** proteins (denatured protein) and **secondary-derived** proteins.

- **Primary-derived proteins (denatured proteins):** These protein derivatives are formed by agents, such as heat, acids, alkalies, etc. which cause only slight changes in the protein molecule and its properties without hydrolytic cleavage of peptide bond **(Figure 4.13)**. These are:
  - **Proteans:** These are the earliest product of protein hydrolysis by action of dilute acids or enzymes, e.g., myosan from myosin and fibrin from fibrinogen.
  - **Metaproteins:** The metaproteins are formed by further action of acids and alkalies on proteans, e.g., acid and alkali albuminates.
- **Secondary-derived proteins:** These substances are formed in the progressive hydrolytic cleavage of the peptide bonds of metaproteins (coagulated proteins) into progressive smaller molecules, e.g., **(Figure 4.13)**.
  - Proteoses
  - Peptones
  - Peptides

Classification of Proteins based on Nutritional Value

Proteins present in different foods vary in their nutritional quality because of the differences in their amino acid composition. **The quality of protein depends on the pattern of essential amino acids it supplies.** The best quality protein is the one which provides essential amino acid pattern very close to the pattern of the tissue proteins.

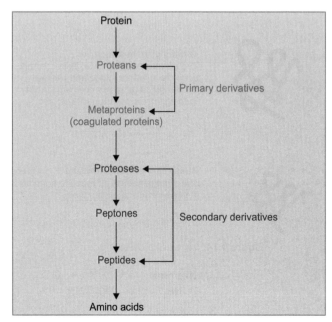

Figure 4.13: Successive stages of the complete hydrolytic decomposition of a native protein molecule into amino acids.

According to the nutritional quality, proteins are classified as follows:

- **Complete protein or first class proteins:** Complete protein or first class proteins are nutritionally rich. They contain all the **essential amino acid** in the required proportion, e.g., egg proteins, casein of milk.
- **Incomplete proteins:** They lack one essential amino acid. For example, pluses are deficient in methionine and cereals are deficient in lysine.
- **Poor proteins:** They lack many essential amino acids. For example, zein from corn lacks tryptophan and lysine.

STRUCTURAL ORGANIZATION OF PROTEINS

Proteins are linear polymers of **amino acids**. Protein structure is the **three-dimensional conformation** of the

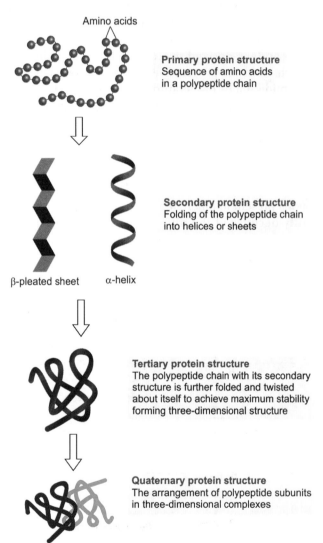

Figure 4.14: Levels of protein structure.

polypeptide. This conformation, in turn, will determine the function of the protein. The structure of proteins is described at four levels: **primary**, **secondary**, **tertiary**, and **quaternary** level **(Figure 4.14)**.

- Proteins that consist of a single polypeptide chain are generally considered at three levels of organization, **primary**, **secondary**, and **tertiary structure**.
- For protein that contains two or more polypeptide chains there is a **quaternary** level of structure.

Primary Structure of Protein

The unique **sequence**, or **order**, of **amino acids** in a polypeptide chain is known as the protein's **primary structure**.

- In the primary structure a series of amino acids joined by **peptide bonds** or an **amide bond (Figure 4.8)** in which α-**carboxyl group** of one amino acid is covalently joined to the α-**amino group** of the second, with the loss of a molecule of water. Peptide bonds are made during the process of **protein biosynthesis (translation)**.
- Each protein has a characteristic and unique **amino acid sequence**. Each amino acid unit in a polypeptide chain is called a **residue** or **moiety**. The term residue reflects, the part left over after losing the water molecule; a hydrogen atom from its amino group and the hydroxyl group from its carboxylic group.
- The end of the polypeptide that has a **free amino group** is called the **N-terminus** while the end with the free **carboxyl** is termed the **C-terminus (Figure 4.15)**.

Importance of Primary Structure

- The function of a protein depends on its amino acid sequence. The sequence and number of amino acids of protein is determined by the DNA of the gene. Primary structure determines the 3-D conformation of the protein. This conformation, in turn, determines the function of the protein.
- A change in the gene's DNA sequence may lead to a change in the amino acid sequence of the protein. Even changing just one amino acid in a protein's sequence can affect the protein's overall structure and function. For example, a single amino acid change is associated with sickle cell anemia, an inherited disease that affects red blood cells.
- Knowledge of the sequence of amino acids provides important information about:
  - Protein structure and function

$$\text{NH}_3^+ - \overset{1}{\text{C}}\text{H} - \text{CO} - \text{NH} - \overset{2}{\text{C}}\text{H} - \text{CO} - \text{NH} - \overset{3}{\text{C}}\text{H} - \text{CO} - \text{NH} - \overset{4}{\text{C}}\text{H} - \text{COO}^-$$

N-terminal .... C-terminal

$R_1 \qquad R_2 \qquad R_3 \qquad R_4$

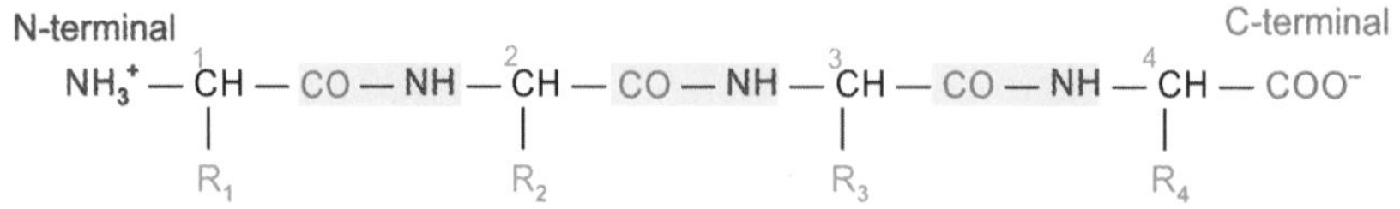

Figure 4.15: Backbone of a polypeptide chain showing N-terminal, C-terminal and variable side (R).

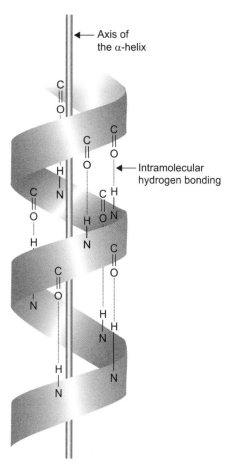

← Axis of
the α-helix

← Intramolecular
hydrogen bonding

Figure 4.16: Schematic diagram of α-helical structure of protein. Each oxygen of a C=O group of a peptide bond forms a hydrogen bond with the hydrogen atom attached to the nitrogen in a peptide bond.

- Cellular location, chemical modification, and half-life of a protein.
- As well as the history of evolution of life on earth.

STRIKE A NOTE

❖ The spatial (three-dimensional) arrangement of amino acids in a protein is called its **conformation**.

❖ Proteins in any of their folded, functional conformations are called **native proteins**.

❖ The function of a protein depends on its amino acid sequence. The primary structure of a protein determines how it folds up into its unique three-dimensional structure, and this in turn determines the function of the proteins.

❖ Post-translational modification such as disulfide bond formation, phosphorylation and glycosylation are usually also considered a part of the primary structure, and cannot be read from the gene.

Secondary Structure of Protein

The folding of primary polypeptide chains into regular or ordered structures is called **secondary structure**. Folding of a polypeptide chain occurs due to **hydrogen bonds** between atoms (CO and NH of peptide bond) of the **backbone** (polypeptide chain apart from the R groups is called backbone). Hydrogen bonds are formed between the **carbonyl oxygen (CO)** of one amino acid and the **amino hydrogen (NH)** of another amino acid of the backbone. Thus, secondary structure does not involve R group atoms. There are few types of secondary structure that are particularly stable and occur widely in proteins.

In 1951 Linus Pauling and Robert Corey proposed two common structures called **α-helix** and **β-pleated sheet**. Subsequently, other structures such as **β-turn** and **loop** were identified. Although the β-turn and omega loop are not common/regular structures, these are well defined and contribute with α-helices and β-sheets to form the final protein structure.

α-Helix

It is called 'α' because it was the first structure elucidated by Pauling and Corey. The α-helix has a coiled structure **(Figure 4.16)**.

- In α-**helix**, the carbonyl (C=O) oxygen of one amino acid is bonded to the hydrogen of amino (N-H) group of an amino acid that is four down the chain. For example, the CO group of amino acid 1 would form a hydrogen bond to the N=H of amino acid 5 **(Figure 4.17)**.
- This pattern of bonding pulls the polypeptide chain into a helical structure with each turn of the helix containing 3.6 amino acids and rise along the helical axis is 5.4 Å. Thus, distance along the axis between adjacent amino acids is **1.5 Å**.
- These hydrogen bonds have essentially optimal **nitrogen to oxygen (N=O)** distance of **2.8 Å**.
- The R groups of the amino acids stick outward from the helix.
- Essentially all α helices found in proteins are **right handed**.

Examples of Proteins Containing α-helical Structures

The α-helical **content of proteins ranges widely, from none to almost 100%. For example:**

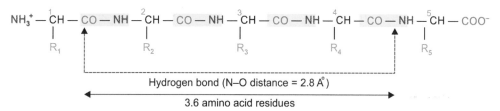

Figure 4.17: Formation of hydrogen bond in α-helix. In α-helix, the CO group of residue 1 forms hydrogen bond with the NH group of residue 4.

- About 75% of residues in **ferritin** (a protein that stores iron) are in α-helices
- About 25% of all **soluble proteins** are composed of α-helices.
- Many proteins that span biological membranes also contain α-helices
- Whereas in others their contribution may be small, e.g., chymotrypsin and cytochrome or absent, in collagen and elastin.

β-Pleated Sheet Structure

Pauling and Corey discovered a second type of structure which they named **β-conformation** (β because it was the second structure they elucidated). In the β-conformation, the backbone of the polypeptide chain (called β strand) is stable into a **zigzag** structure rather than helical structure (**Figure 4.18**). The zigzag structure of the individual polypeptide segments gives rise to a **"pleated"** appearance (like the pleats in a curtain) of the overall sheet and these structures are therefore often called **"β-pleated sheet"**.

- In a **β-pleated sheet**, two or more segments of a polypeptide chain line up (arranged) side by side, forming a **sheet-like** structure held together by **hydrogen bonds**.
- However, in contrast to **intrachain** hydrogen bond in α-helix, in a **β-pleated sheet interchain** hydrogen bonds are formed between two adjacent polypeptide chains (**Figure 4.19**).
- The strands of a β-pleated sheet can run in the same direction with respect to N-terminal and C-terminals (**parallel**) or opposite direction (**antiparallel**) (**Figure 4.19**).
- The distance between adjacent amino acids along β strand is approximately 3.5 Å, in contrast with a distance of 1.5 Å along α-helix.

Examples of Proteins Containing β-sheets Structures

Many proteins contain both α helices and β-pleated sheets, though some contain just one type of secondary structure. For example, **fatty acid binding proteins, transthyretin** are made almost entirely from **β-sheets**. Like α-helix, β-sheets are found in both **fibrous** and **globular** proteins. For example,

- Antiparallel β-sheet conformation is less common in human proteins. The best example in nature is **silk fibrion**.
- Parallel β-sheet occur in flavodoxin
- Both parallel and antiparallel β-sheet occur in carbonic anhydrase.

The β-pleated sheet occurs as a principal secondary structure in proteins found in people with **amyloidosis**. The proteins that accumulate are called amyloid fibrils rich in β-sheets. These are misfolded proteins derived from immunoglobulins. Amyloid fibrils are insoluble and their accumulation in tissues and organs disrupt normal physiological process. The amyloid deposit is produced in certain chronic inflammatory diseases, in some cancers and in the brain disorders, like **Alzheimer disease**.

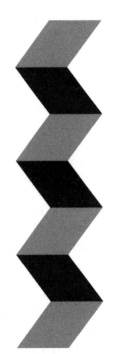

Figure 4.18: Schematic diagram of β-pleated sheet structure of protein.

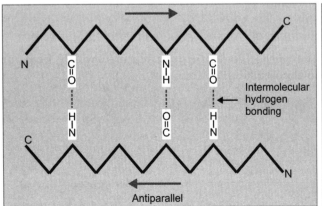

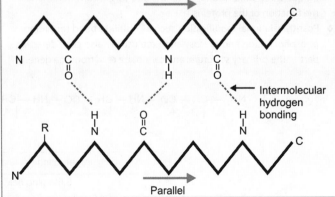

Figure 4.19: Parallel and antiparallel β-pleated sheet structure.

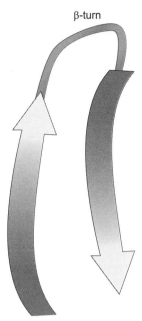

Figure 4.20: Two antiparallel beta strands connected by a bend, i.e., β-turn.

Turns

Turns (sometimes called reverse turns) are a type of **secondary structure**. As the name suggests, it causes a turn in the structure of a **polypeptide chain**.

- Turns refer to short segments of amino acids that join two units of a secondary structure in a protein; such as two adjacent strands of an antiparallel β-sheet **(Figure 4.20)**.
- Most proteins have a compact, globular shape due to reversals in the direction of their polypeptide chains. Turns give rise to **tertiary structure**; causing interruptions in the secondary structures (α-**helices** and β-**strands**).
- There are at least five types (α, β, γ, δ, and π) of turns. Of these, the β-turns are the most common form.
- β-turn involves four amino acyl residues. First amino acyl residue is hydrogen bonded to the fourth resulting in a tight 180° turn. **Proline** and **glycine** often are present in β-turn which provides flexibility and facilitates the turn. β-**turn is a space saving method of turning a corner**. Thus, turns make polypeptide chains to a compact molecule.

Random Coils

- Not all portions of proteins are necessarily ordered. Some sections of a protein assume no regular, distinct structure and are sometimes said to lack **secondary structure**, though they may have **hydrogen bonds**.
- Protein may contain **"disordered"** regions, often at the extreme amino or carboxyl terminal. Such segments are described as **random coils**.

Contd...

Contd...

- Random coils provide flexibility to their structure. This structural flexibility enables such regions to act as ligand-controlled switches that affect protein structure and function.
- In many instances, these disordered regions assume an ordered conformation upon binding of a ligand.

Super Secondary Structure/Motif

- Super secondary structures are intermediate between secondary and tertiary structures. These are simply a combination of secondary structures which is modified into a more complex structure. These combinations are called **motif** or **super secondary structure**.
- Super secondary structures, or motifs, are characteristic combinations of a secondary structures. These structures result from packing specific adjacent secondary structure motifs, such as:
  - Helix-turn-helix (α-helix separated from another α-helix by a turn)
  - β-barrel (a more complex modified structure of β-sheet)
  - Leucine zipper (DNA binding motif with leucine at every seventh position)
  - Zinc finger (DNA binding motif which require Zinc for its activity
- Both leucine zipper and zinc finger motifs are found in **transcription factors** that interact with DNA. Helix-turn-helix is found in DNA binding motif.

Domain

Three-dimensional confirmations with all secondary structural types; helices, sheets, bends and loops assemble to form **domain**. Domain is a section of protein structure sufficient to perform a particular chemical and physical function such as binding of substrate.

STRIKE A NOTE

- Most abundant amino acid in α-helix is methionine followed by glutamate.
- Amino acid least present in α-helix is proline.
- Glycine does not favor α-helix
- Amino acids with branches at β-carbon atom valine, threonine and isoleucine, tends to destabilize α-helix.
- Serine and asparagine tend to disrupt α helices.
- Proline tends to disrupt both α-helices and β-strand.
- Most abundant amino acid in β-sheet is valine.
- Amino acid least present in β-sheet is proline.
- Most abundant amino acid in turns is proline followed by glycine
- Glycine readily fits into all structures, but its conformational flexibility renders it well suited to β-turns.

Tertiary Structure of Protein

The overall **three-dimensional folded compact** and **biologically active conformation** of a protein is referred to

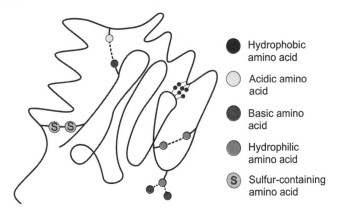

Figure 4.21: Schematic tertiary structure of protein.

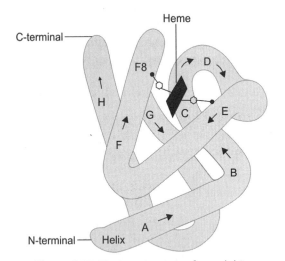

Figure 4.22: Tertiary structure of myoglobin.

as its **tertiary structure**. This structure reflects the overall shape of the molecule.

- The polypeptide chain with its secondary structure is further folded and twisted about itself in such a way as to achieve maximum stability forming three-dimensional structures **(Figure 4.21)**. An example of proteins having tertiary structures is myoglobin **(Figure 4.22)**.

- Amino acids residues which are very distant from one another in the sequence can be brought very near due to the folding.

- A tertiary structure is stabilized by interactions among amino acids which may be far apart from each other in the primary sequence, and are in different types of secondary structure but which are close to each other in the folded three-dimensional structure.

- The tertiary structure is primarily due to interactions between the **R groups** of the amino acids. The non-covalent interactions stabilize the three-dimensional structure of a protein.

- Bonds involved in tertiary structure include:
  1. **Hydrogen bonds:** Between polar R groups
  2. **Hydrophobic interactions:** Force formed due to interaction between nonpolar hydrophobic R groups of amino acid residues.

3. **Van der Waals forces:** Van der waals forces are extremely weak and act only on extremely short distances include both an attractive and a repulsive component (between both polar and nonpolar side chain of amino acid residues).

4. **Ionic (electrostatic) bonds or salt bridges:** R groups with like charges repel one another, while those with opposite charges can form an ionic bond.

5. **Dipole-dipole interactions:** Forces occur between polar molecules.

6. **Disulfide bond (covalent bond** that can contribute to tertiary structure): A covalent bond formed between the **sulfhydryl groups (–SH)** of side chain of **cysteine** residues in the same or different peptide chains. Disulfide bonds are common in structural protein like keratin and extracellular enzyme, e.g., ribonuclease but are rare in intracellular globular protein. These disulfide bonds help to stabilize against denaturation and confer additional stability.

Quaternary Structure of Protein

Many proteins are made up of a single polypeptide chain and are called **monomeric** proteins and have only three levels of structure. They do not exhibit a quaternary structure. However, some proteins are made up of **multiple polypeptide chains (polymeric)** and have a quaternary structure.

- The arrangement of these polypeptide subunits in three-dimensional complexes is called the quaternary structure of the protein.

- Adult **hemoglobin** is a good example of a protein with quaternary structure, being composed four polypeptide chains, (two identical α-chains and two identical β-chains **(Figure 4.23)**. Another example is **DNA polymerase**, an enzyme that synthesizes new strands of DNA and is composed of ten subunits.

- The subunits of polymeric protein are held together by the same types of noncovalent interactions that contribute to tertiary structure, e.g.:

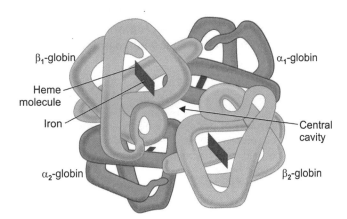

Figure 4.23: Quaternary structure of polymeric protein hemoglobin.

Legend (Figure 4.21):
- Hydrophobic amino acid
- Acidic amino acid
- Basic amino acid
- Hydrophilic amino acid
- Sulfur-containing amino acid

- Hydrophobic interactions
- Hydrogen bond
- Ionic bonds
- Disulfide bonds.

Bonds Responsible for Protein Structure

Protein structure is stabilized by two types of bonds:
 1. Covalent bond, e.g.,
    ➢ Peptide bonds
    ➢ Disulfide bond.
 2. Noncovalent bond, e.g.,
    ➢ Hydrogen bond
    ➢ Hydrophobic bond or interaction
    ➢ Electrostatic or ionic bond or salt bond or salt bridge
    ➢ Van der Waals interactions.

DENATURATION OF PROTEIN

Denaturation of a protein is a nonspecific alteration in **secondary**, **tertiary**, and **quaternary** structures of protein molecule when treated with denaturing agent.

- The **secondary**, **tertiary**, and **quaternary** structures of protein are stabilized by **Hydrogen bonds**, **ionic bonds** and **hydrophobic bonds** to maintain its three-dimensional conformation (native state).
- This conformation can be disturbed and disorganized by the rupture of ionic bond, hydrogen bonds, and hydrophobic bond without breakage of any peptide linkage. Everything lost in denaturation except the primary structure (i.e., peptide bond)
- This conformation can be disrupted by a number of external factors including **temperature**, **pH**, and **removal of water**, **presence of hydrophobic substances**, and **presence of metal ions**. The loss of secondary, tertiary or quaternary structure due to exposure to a stress factor is called **denaturation**.
- Denaturation results in unfolding of the protein into a random or misfolded shape **(Figure 4.24)**. Cooked meat or boiled egg, milk paneer, etc. are the examples of denatured proteins.
- Denaturation of proteins leads to:
  - Unfolding of natural coils of native protein
  - Decrease in solubility and increase in perceptibility
  - Loss of biological activities (e.g., enzyme activity) and antigenic properties
  - Increased digestibility.

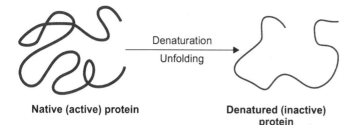

Native (active) protein　　　　**Denatured (inactive) protein**

Figure 4.24: Denaturation of protein.

Denaturing Agents

- **Physical agents:** Heat, ultraviolet rays and ionizing radiations can denature proteins.
- **Chemical agents:** Acids, alkalis and certain acid solutions of heavy metals, e.g., mercury, lead, detergents; organic solvents like alcohol, acetone, etc. urea solution, guanidine solution denature proteins.
- **Mechanical means:** Vigorous shaking or grinding leads to denaturation of the protein.

Significance of Denaturation

- Digestibility of native protein is increased on denaturation by gastric HCl or by heat on cooking. Denaturation causes unfolding of native polypeptide coil so that hidden peptide bonds are exposed to the action of proteolytic enzyme in the gut. It also increases reactivity of certain groups.
- Denaturation property of a protein is used in blood analysis to eliminate the proteins of the blood (deproteinization of blood).

Coagulation

Denaturation may, in rare cases be reversible, in which case the protein refolds into its original native structure, when the denaturing agent is removed. However, most proteins, once denatured, remain permanently disordered and called **irreversible denaturation** or **coagulation**, e.g., coagulated egg white of boiled egg.

STRUCTURE-FUNCTION RELATIONSHIP OF PROTEINS

Proteins are made by linking together various amino acids. Each protein has a characteristic and unique amino acid sequence. The unique sequence or order of amino acids is known as the protein's **primary structure**. Primary structure dictates the 3-D conformation of protein. This conformation, in turn, will determine the function of the protein. Even change in sequence by amino acid, changes the protein structure and function.

Structure-Function Relationship of Hemoglobin and Myoglobin

Hemoglobin and **myoglobin** illustrate both protein structure function relationships. A comparison of myoglobin and hemoglobin explains some key aspects of protein structure and function. Both myoglobin and hemoglobin have similarity in binding oxygen. However hemoglobin is remarkably efficient oxygen carrier, able to use as much as 90% of its potential oxygen-carrying capacity effectively. Under similar conditions, myoglobin would be able to use only 7% of its potential capacity. What accounts for this dramatic difference?

- Particularly, hemoglobin's multiple subunits (polymeric) with quaternary structure **(Figure 4.23)** compared to myoglobin's single subunit (monomeric) **(Figure 4.22)** with **no quaternary structure** give rise to these differences.
- Myoglobin exists as a **single polypeptide**, whereas hemoglobin comprises **four polypeptide** chains. The four chains in hemoglobin bind oxygen **cooperatively**, meaning that the binding of oxygen to a site in one chain increases the probability that the remaining chains will bind oxygen (*see* **Figure 7.8**). The cooperative loading or unloading of oxygen from hemoglobin is an exclusive property of **polymeric** protein.
- Furthermore, the oxygen binding properties of hemoglobin are modulated by the binding of **hydrogen ions** and **carbondioxide** in a manner that enhances oxygen carrying capacity. In this regard, hemoglobin acts as an **allosteric protein**, with an ability to change shapes, or undergo allosteric conformational changes.
- Both **cooperative** and the **response to modulators** are made possible by variations in the **quaternary structure of hemoglobin**.
- However, **myoglobin**, a **monomeric protein** does not exhibit cooperative binding effect. That is why myoglobin unsuitable as an O_2 transport protein, but well suited for O_2 storage.

Importance of Protein Structure-Function Relationships in Hemoglobinopathies

Hemoglobinopathies are a group of disorders due to alterations in hemoglobin structure. Mutations that alter amino acid sequence of a globin chain of hemoglobin can affect the function of hemoglobin which leads to disease condition

- The sequence of amino acids in protein is determined by the DNA of the gene. A change in the gene's DNA sequence may lead to a change in the amino acid sequence of the protein. Even changing just one amino acid in a protein's sequence can affect the protein's overall structure and function.
- Altered amino acid sequence alters the physiologic properties and functions of hemoglobin and form variant hemoglobin For example:
  - Sickle hemoglobin (HbS)
  - Hemoglobin C (HbC) and
  - Hemoglobin M (HbM)
- These variant hemoglobins lead to **sickle cell disease**, **HbC disease** or **Cooley's hemoglobin** and **HbM diseases** or **methemoglobin**
  Sickle cell disease: In sickle Hb, the **glutamic acid** that is normally the sixth amino acid of the β chain of hemoglobin is replaced by a **valine**

```
 1    2    3    4    5    6    7    8
Val—His—leu—Thr—Pro—Glu—Glu—Lys—(β-chain
                                   of HbA)

Val—His—leu—Thr—Pro—Val—Glu—Lys—(β-chain
                                   of HbS)
```

- When HbS deoxygenated, it becomes **insoluble and** forms polymers of **deoxy-HbS**. Normal hemoglobin (HbA) remains soluble on deoxygenation. **Polymerization of deoxy-HbS forms insoluble long tubular fibre** and deform the red blood cells.
- The altered properties of HbS result from a single amino acid substitution, a **nonpolar, hydrophobic, Valine (Val) instead** of a **polar, hydrophilic Glutamic acid (Glu)** residue at position 6 in the two β-chains.

- **HbM diseases or methemoglobinemia:** HbM disease is due to mutation in **histidine** residue (either α- or β-chains) to which heme is attached, is replaced by **tyrosine**. Tyrosine stabilizes iron in the ferric (Fe^{3+}) form instead of ferrous (Fe^{2+}) form which cannot bind oxygen.
- **HbC disease or Cooley's hemoglobin:** In HbC, the **glutamic acid** at position six in β-chain is replaced by **lysine** residue due to mutation. This disease is characterized by accumulation of crystals of HbC which leads to a mild **hemolytic anemia**.

■ PLASMA PROTEINS AND THEIR FUNCTIONS

The plasma proteins are:
- Albumin
- Globulin
  - α_1-globulin
  - α_2-globulin
  - β-globulin
  - γ-globulin
- Fibrinogen.

What is plasma and serum?

- ❖ **Plasma** is obtained by centrifuging blood that has been treated with an anticoagulant to prevent clotting.
- ❖ The **serum** is different from plasma in its protein content. The serum contains only the **albumin** and **globulin**.
- ❖ The plasma contains the **albumin** and **globulin** and **fibrinogen**.
- ❖ The fibrinogen is absent in serum because, it is converted into fibrin during the coagulation of the blood.
- ❖ Thus **serum = plasma – fibrinogen**.

The normal reference range of plasma proteins are:
- Total protein   6–8 g%
- Serum albumin   3.5–6 g%
- Serum globulin   2–3.5 g%
- Fibrinogen   200–400 mg%
- A/G ratio   1.2:1–1.6:1

TABLE 4.9: Major classes of plasma proteins, their functions and diagnostic importance.

Classes	Examples	Principal functions	Diagnostic importance
Prealbumin	• Thyroxine binding prealbumin (TBPA) • Retinal binding prealbumin (RBPA)	• Transport of hormone thyroxine • Transport of vitamin A	Liver disease, thyrotoxicosis malnutrition
Albumin		Exert colloidal osmotic pressure and transport function	Malnutrition, liver, kidney and GI disease, malignancy
α_1-Gloublin	• Retinal binding protein (RBP) • α1-fetoprotein (AFP) • α1-protease inhibitor (API) or α1-antitrypsin (AAT) • α1-acid glycoprotein (AAG) • Prothrombin	• Transport of vitamin A • Unknown • Antiprotease, natural inhibitor of proteolytic enzyme elastase • Tissue repair • Blood clotting	— • Neural tube defects, also as a tumor marker • API-deficiency in lung disorders • Inflammatory disease of GIT and malignant neoplasm • Coagulation screen, also as a liver function test
α_2-Globulins	• Ceruloplasmin • Haptoglobin • Thyroxine binding protein (TBG) • α2-Macroglobulin (AMG)	• Transport of copper • Conservation of iron by binding free hemoglobin • Transport thyroxine hormone • Natural antiprotease, inhibits thrombin, trypsin and pepsin	• Wilson's disease • Hemolytic disorders • Thyroid disease • Myeloma, peptic ulcer nephrotic syndrome, cirrhosis, collagen disease
β-Globulins	• Hemopexin • Transferrin • C-reactive protein (CRP) • β2-microglobulin (BMG)	• Binds heme and prevents loss of iron • Transport of iron • Body's defense mechanism • Body's defense mechanism	• Hemolytic disorders • Iron deficiency • Nonspecific test that may be used instead of ESR • Monitoring myeloma, renal failure
γ-Globulins	• Immunoglobulins • IgG, IgA, IgM, IgD, and IgE	Body's defende mechanisms	Liver disease, infections, autoimmune disease and paraproteinemia
Fibrinogen		Blood coagulation	

Synthesis of Plasma Proteins

All the **albumin** and **fibrinogen** are essentially synthesized by the **liver** only. Similarly 50 to 80% of the globulin is formed in the liver. The remainder of the globulins is formed almost entirely in the **lymphoid tissues**. They are **gamma globulins** that form the **antibodies** used in the immune system. In severe liver disease there is thus lowered concentration of plasma albumin but globulin fraction may not show substantial fall, as immunoglobulins are not synthesized by the liver. **The A/G ratio therefore can be altered in the liver disease**. A brief summary of different plasma proteins and their functions is given in **Table 4.9**.

Separation of Plasma Proteins

Electrophoresis is the most commonly employed analytical technique for the separation of plasma/serum proteins. Serum proteins separated on cellulose acetate membrane by electrophoresis generally have five bands namely, **albumin**, α_1-**globulin**, α_2-**globulin**, β-**globulin**, γ-**globulin**. These five bands appear as five peaks on the densitometer graph **(Figures 4.25A and B)**.

- Serum protein electrophoretic patterns provide useful **diagnostic information**.
- Different electrophoretic patterns of serum associated with various disorders, compared with normal serum are shown in **Figures 4.26A to E**.

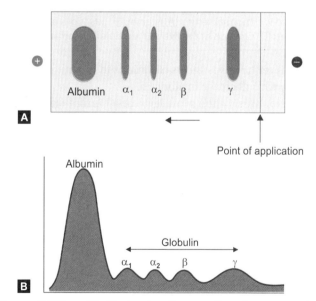

Figures 4.25A and B: Electrophoretic separation of serum proteins: (A) Electrophoretogram of normal serum on cellulose acetate strip; (B) Densitometry scanning from cellulose acetate strip converts bands to characteristic peaks of albumin, α_1-globulin, α_2-globulin, β-globulin, and γ-globulin.

- Changes in serum protein fractions associated with various conditions are given below:
  - Infective hepatitis shows slight decrease in albumin and significant increased γ-globulins.

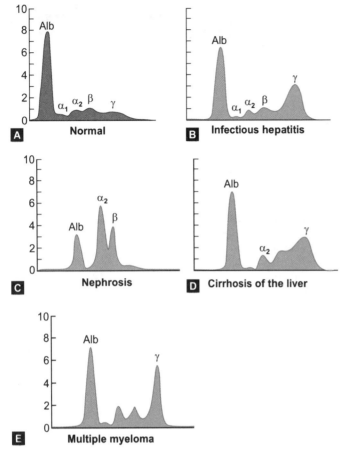

Figures 4.26A to E: Different electrophoretic patterns of serum compared with normal serum. (A) Normal; (B) Infectious hepatitis; (C) Nephrosis; (D) Cirrhosis of the liver; (E) Multiple myeloma.

- Liver cirrhosis shows elevations in β- and γ-globulins with a decrease in albumin.
- Nephrosis shows low level of albumin, significantly elevated α_2-globulin and elevated β-globulin.
- Multiple myeloma shows marked increase in γ-globulin.

Major Classes of Plasma Proteins

Prealbumin

Prealbumin, a minor band can be seen running ahead of albumin when separation of protein is good. Prealbumin is synthesized in liver. Following are the examples of prealbumin:

- **Thyroxine Binding Prealbumin (TBPA):** It is minor transport protein for thyroxine hormone. TBPA also binds retinol binding protein. About one-third of the TBPA of human serum circulates as the **TBPA-RBP complex** and is known as **transthyretin**.
- **Retinol Binding Prealbumin (RBPA):** It transports vitamin A (retinol)
  Low levels of prealbumin occur in:
  - Hepatitis
  - Early cirrhosis

- Thyrotoxicosis (syndrome due to excessive amounts of thyroid hormone)
- Deficiency of zinc (Zn is required for RBPA synthesis).

Albumin

Albumin is a major protein in plasma accounting for approximately 50% of plasma protein mass.

- Albumin is a **globular protein** consisting of single polypeptide chain with a molecular weight of about **69000** in the human. It comprises some **585 amino acid** residues.
- It has **no carbohydrate** side chains, but is highly soluble in water due to its high net negative charge at physiological pH.
- Albumin is synthesized by the hepatic parenchymal cells. Albumin is exclusively synthesized by the liver for this reason; serum albumin levels are determined to assess liver function (synthesis decreased in liver diseases). The liver synthesizes approximately 12 g of albumin per day. The synthetic rate of albumin is controlled by colloidal osmotic pressure (COP) and protein intake.

Functions of Albumins

- Albumin's primary function is the maintenance of colloidal **osmotic pressure** in both vascular and extravascular spaces. Because of its relatively low molecular mass and high concentration, albumin makes the biggest contribution (75 to 85%) of the oncotic pressure of human plasma. Thus, albumin plays a predominant role in maintaining blood volume and body fluid distribution. Very low plasma albumin concentration develops edema **(Figures 4.26A to E)**.
- A second important function of albumin is to bind to and thereby facilitate the transport of many metabolites which are poorly soluble in water such as:
  - Fatty acids
  - Bilirubin
  - Calcium
  - Certain steroid hormones
  - Copper
  - Some of the plasma tryptophan
  - A variety of drugs (those which are poorly soluble) like sulfonamides, penicillin G, dicumarol, aspirin, digoxin is all carried by albumin.
- **Buffering function:** Among the plasma proteins, albumin has maximum buffering capacity due to its high concentration in blood.

Clinical Significance

Serum albumin measurements are used to assess the various clinical conditions, e.g., **hypoalbuminemia**, **hyperalbuminemia**, and **analbuminemia**.

Hypoalbuminemia

Decreased levels of plasma albumin are seen in various disorders, some of which are discussed in the following text. Hypoalbuminemia may be due to physiological or pathological causes **(Table 4.10)**. There are 5 main reasons to the occurrence of low plasma albumin level which are:

1. **Reduced synthesis:** This may be due to:
   - Severe and prolonged protein energy malnutrition
   - Intestinal malabsorptive diseases and

TABLE 4.10: Causes of hypoalbuminemia.	
Physiological	• Pregnancy • Physical exercise

Pathological	• Impaired synthesis, e.g.,
	  ➢ Malnutrition
	  ➢ Malabsorption
	  ➢ Chronic liver disease
	• Increased catabolism, e.g., in
	  ➢ Injury, e.g., major surgery or trauma
	  ➢ Infection
	  ➢ Fever and
	  ➢ Malignant disease
	• Abnormal distribution
	  ➢ Severe burns
	  ➢ Tissue injury
	  ➢ Activation of the innate immune system
	• Abnormal or excessive losses, e.g., in:
	  ➢ Nephrotic syndrome
	  ➢ Gastrointestinal tract diseases
	  ➢ Burns or certain skin diseases
	  ➢ Hemorrhage
	  ➢ Inflammation
	• Overhydration due to hemodilution

- Liver diseases (as liver is the site of synthesis of albumin).

2. **Abnormal distribution:** This is due to increased capillary permeability in the **acute phase response** which permits plasma to leak into the extravascular compartment, when there is sequestration of proteins, e.g.:
   - Severe burns
   - Tissue injury
   - Activation of the innate immune system.

3. **Increased catabolism:** Increased catabolism occurs as a result of:
   - Injury, e.g., major surgery or trauma
   - Infection
   - Fever
   - Malignant disease.

4. **Abnormal or excessive losses:** The liver can normally replace albumin losses of up to 5 g/day. Greater losses may occur in:
   - Nephrotic syndrome
   - Gastrointestinal tract disease
   - Burns or certain skin diseases
   - Hemorrhage
   - Inflammation.

In nephrotic syndrome, large amounts of protein are lost in the urine and hypoalbuminemia and edema develop **(Figure 4.27)**. Inflammatory disease of the intestinal tract is associated with increased gastrointestinal loss of albumin. Acute or chronic inflammations are the most

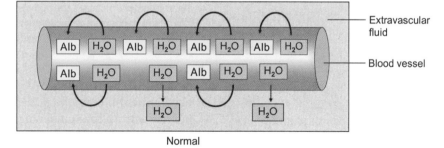

Normal

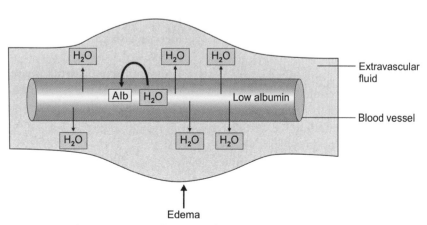

Edema

Figure 4.27: Development of edema in hypoalbuminemia.

(Alb: albumin)

common cause of hypoalbuminemia resulting from hemodilution, loss of protein into the extravascular space.

5. **Overhydration:** Hypoalbuminemia can be induced by overhydration due to hemodilution.

Hyperalbuminemia

Increased levels of plasma albumin are present only in acute dehydration and have no clinical significance.

Analbuminemia

Analbuminemia is a rare hereditary abnormality. Certain human suffer from genetic mutations that impair their ability to synthesize **albumin**. Individual whose plasma is completely devoid of albumin are said to exhibit analbuminemia.

Although albumin is normally the major determinant of oncotic pressure, person suffering from analbuminemia, show only moderate edema due to compensatory increase in plasma globulin concentration.

Globulins

Globulins are bigger in size than albumin. Globulins constitute several fractions. These are:

1. α_1-globulin
2. α_2-globulin
3. β-globulin
4. γ-globulin

α_1-Globulins

Following are the examples of α_1-globulin:

1. Retinol binding protein (RBP)
2. α_1-fetoprotein (AFP)
3. α_1-protease inhibitor (API) OR also known as α_1 antitrypsin (AAT)
4. α_1-acid glycoprotein (AAG)
5. Prothrombin.

- **Retinol Binding Protein (RBP):** Retinol (vitamin A) is transported in plasma bound to RBP. Most retinol RBP in the plasma is reversibly complexes with **transthyretin** (thyroxine binding protein).
- **α_1-fetoprotein (AFP):** This is present in the tissues and plasma of the fetus. Plasma concentration of AFP falls very rapidly after birth, but minute amount (up to 15 mg/L) is present in plasma of adults. The function of α_1-fetoprotein is unclear, but it may play an **immunoregulatory** role during pregnancy.
  - Alpha fetoprotein is a low molecular weight glycoprotein synthesized mainly in the fetal yolk sac and liver.
  - Its production is almost completely repressed in the normal adult. It can diffuse slowly through capillary membranes and appears in the fetal urine, and hence in the amniotic fluid, and in maternal plasma.

- The reason for high concentrations in fetal neural tube defects in amniotic fluid and maternal plasma is not clear, but the protein may leak from the exposed (open) neural tube vessels.

Measurements of AFP
❖ In the pregnancy, by measuring the concentration of amniotic fluid and plasma AFP, diagnosis of **open neural tube defects** (increased AFP) and **Down's syndrome** (decreased AFP) before birth is possible.
❖ Open neural tube defects are a group of congenital abnormalities caused by; failure of the neural tube (the embryological structure from which the brain and spinal cord develop). Down's syndrome is a form of mental subnormality due to a chromosome defect.
❖ Plasma AFP is greatly increased in hepatoma (cancer of liver) and used as a tumor marker.

- **α_1-Protease inhibitor (API) or also known as α_1 antitrypsin (AAT):** API is one of the plasma proteins, that inhibits activity of **proteases** particularly **elastase**, which degrades elastin, a protein that gives elasticity to the lungs. In a normal individual, the activity of elastase is regulated by API. A genetic deficiency in API can lead to **emphysema** (lung disorder). Excessive cigarette smoking also leads to emphysema. As cigarette smoke inhibits the activity of API.

Cigarette Smoke and Emphysema
❖ Cigarette smoke inhibits the activity of API by oxidizing a specific methionine residue in API. Thus API can no longer inhibit elastase activity.
❖ Cigarette smoke increases the number of neutrophils in the lung and neutrophils increases the amount of elastase.
❖ Elastase then causes the tissue breakdown and loss of elasticity in the lungs leads to emphysema.

- **α_1-acid Glycoprotein (AAG):** AAG also known as **orosomucoid**, contains a high percentage of carbohydrate with a large number of **sialic acid** residues, AAG is synthesized by liver parenchymal cells. AAG is the major constituent of the seromucoid fraction of plasma. Its true physiological function is unknown. AAG levels increases in GI inflammatory disease and malignant neoplasm.
- **Prothrombin:** It is synthesized by liver with the help of vitamin K and involved in **blood clotting**. Liver damage causes lengthening of prothrombin time.

α_2-Globulins

Following are the examples of α_2-globulin:

1. Ceruloplasmin (Ferroxidase)
2. Transcortin or corticosteroid binding globulin
3. Haptoglobin
4. Thyroxine binding globulin (TBG)
5. α_2-Macroglobulin (AMG).

- **Ceruloplasmin (ferroxidase):** This is a copper containing plasma protein synthesized by liver, is a ferroxidase required for the oxidation of Fe^{2+} to Fe^{3+}. Fe^{3+} is then bound to transferrin in blood. It is essential for the transport and utilization of iron.

  Ceruloplasmin is also the major transport protein for copper, an essential trace element. Plasma ceruloplasmin level is reduced in **Wilson's disease (see Chapter 15)** in patients with malnutrition and in the nephrotic syndrome.

- **Transcortin or corticosteroid binding globulin:** This binds cortisol. It is synthesized in liver and synthesis is increased by estrogen.

- **Haptoglobin (Hp):** Haptoglobin (Hp) is a plasma glycoprotein that binds extra-corpuscular hemoglobin (Hb) to form a noncovalent complex (Hb-Hp). Since the Hb-Hp complex is too large to pass through the glomerulus, this protects the kidney from the formation of harmful precipitates and prevents the loss of iron associated hemoglobin in the urine. Patients suffering from hemolytic anemias exhibit low levels of haptoglobin.

- **Thyroxine-binding globulin (TBG):** TBG is synthesized in liver. TBG has a electrophoretic mobility between α_1- and α_2-globulins. It transports thyroxine hormone (T_3 and T_4). Thyroxine is also carried by **thyroxine binding prealbumin (TBPA)**, which is also a globulin, and moves ahead of the albumin in electrophoresis. TBG binds T_3 and T_4 with 100 times more affinity than TBPA.

- **α_2-Macroglobulin (AMG):** This is major α_2-globulin, which is a natural inhibitor of **endopeptidase** such as trypsin, chymotrypsin, plasmin, thrombin, etc. Plasma AMG is decreased in myeloma, peptic ulcer and increased in nephrotic syndrome, cirrhosis, and collagen disorders.

β-globulin

Following are the examples of β-globulin:
1. Hemopexin
2. Transferrin
3. β_2-Microglobulins (BMG)
4. C-reactive protein (CRP).

- **Hemopexin:** Hemopexin is a β_1-globulin that binds **free heme**, but not the hemoglobin. Albumin will bind some metheme (ferric heme) to form methemoglobin, which then transfers the metheme to hemopexin. Like haptoglobin, hemopexin also plays an important role in the conservation of iron by preventing its loss in the urine.

- **Transferrin (Tf):** Transferrin is a β_1-globulin. In human, iron is transported through the plasma protein **transferrin,** a glycoprotein synthesized by the liver. It transports iron (two molecules of Fe^{3+} per molecule of transferrin) through blood to the sites where iron

TABLE 4.11: Acute phase reactants (proteins).

Positive acute phase reactants	Negative acute phase reactants
C-reactive protein (CRP)	Albumin
Antiprotease inhibitors (API) or α1-antitrypsin (AAT)	Prealbumin
Fibrinogen	Transferrin
Hepcidine	Retinal binding protein
Serum amyloid A	Antithrombin

is required. The concentration of Tf in plasma is approximately 300 mg/dL, sufficient to carry a total of 300 microgram of iron per decilitre of plasma.

- Increased serum levels of transferrin are seen in **iron deficiency anemia** and **pregnancy**.
- Low levels occur in chronic infections and in malnutrition.

> Glycosylation of transferrin is impaired in chronic alcoholism. The presence of carbohydrate-deficient transferrin (CDT), which can be measured by isoelectric focusing (IEF), is used as a biomarker of chronic alcoholism.

- **C-reactive protein (CRP):** C-reactive protein (CRP) is synthesized by the liver. CRP is involved in the body's response to foreign compounds. The level of CRP rises when there is an inflammation or an infection.
  - It is one of a group of proteins called **acute phase proteins (Table 4.11)**. The levels of acute phase **proteins** increase in response to certain inflammation.
  - Because CRP levels often go up before the symptoms of pain or fever, the CRP test is especially useful for tracking infections.
  - It is also useful in differentiating bacterial from viral infections because the **level of CRP is increased in bacterial infections only**.

> It was initially thought that CRP might be a pathogenic secretion since it was elevated in a variety of illnesses, including cancer. Later it is demonstrated that, it is a native protein synthesize by liver. CRP was so named because CRP is named because it reacts with Capsular–polysaccharides (C-polysaccharide) of the cell wall of pneumococci bacteria.

- **β_2-microglobulins:** This protein forms part of the **human leukocyte antigen (HLA) system**. It is derived from myeloid and lymphoid cells and is normally synthesized at the constant rate. Plasma levels are increased whenever; there is malignant lymphoid or myeloid proliferation and renal failure.

- **γ-globulins:** The immunoglobulins are **γ-globulins**, called **antibodies**. All antibodies are immunoglobulin but all immunoglobulins may not be antibodies. They constitute about 20% of all the plasma proteins. Immunoglobulins are produced by **plasma cells** and to some extent by **lymphocytes**. The primary function of antibodies is to protect against infectious agents or their products.

Structure, function and characteristics of different types of immunoglobulin are discussed later in **Chapter 27: Immune System**.

Fibrinogen (Blood Clotting Factor I)

It is a glycoprotein and constitutes about 4% of total plasma proteins. It is synthesized in liver and secreted in blood where it is involved in **blood coagulation**. During blood coagulation, fibrinogen is converted to fibrin which polymerizes to form fibrin clot. Plasma level of fibrinogen decreases in severe hepatic diseases.

Functions of Plasma Proteins

- **Maintenance of colloidal osmotic pressure (oncotic pressure):** The principal function of albumin is to provide colloidal osmotic pressure in the plasma, which, in turn, prevents loss of plasma from the capillaries and controls the distribution of water in the body **(Figure 4.27)**.
- **Maintenance of blood pressure:** The plasma proteins provide viscosity to the blood, which is important to maintain the blood pressure. Albumin provides more viscosity than other plasma proteins.
- **Maintenance of acid-base balance:** Proteins play a part in maintaining the blood pH. This is because of the buffering action of protein. Proteins are negatively charged at body pH and therefore, act as bases accepting H^+ ions.
- **Role in transport or binding mechanism:** Proteins, **albumin**, **α-globulin**, and **β-globulin** serve as carriers for various cations and some compounds that are relatively insoluble in water, e.g., Albumin transports bilirubin, free fatty acids, calcium ions, and metals like Cu^{2+}, Zn^{2+}, steroid hormones and a variety of drugs
  - Ceruloplasmin transports Cu^{2+}
  - Lipoproteins transport lipids
  - Transferrin transports iron
  - Transcortin transports cartisol
  - Hptoglobin binds extracorpuscular hemoglobin
  - Haemopexin binds heme
  - Retinol binding proteins transports vitamin A
  - Thyroxine binding protein transports thyroxine hormone
- **Role of protein in defense mechanism of body:** The **gamma globulin** plays an important role in the defense mechanism of the body. These molecules act as **antibodies** and are called **immunoglobulins**. The antibody reacts with antigens of disease causing micro-organisms. In addition to gamma globulin, $β_2$-**microglobulins** are also involved in defense mechanism.
- **Involvement in inflammatory responses:** Some proteins are involved in inflammatory (immediate defensive reaction) responses, e.g., **C-reactive protein**

(CRP) is involved in body's response to foreign compounds (acute phase response).

- **Enzymatic function of proteins:** The globulins perform a number of enzymatic functions in the plasma, e.g., blood coagulation factors.
- **Role in blood coagulation:** Fibrinogen is essential for the coagulation of blood. During coagulation of blood, the fibrinogen polymerizes into long fibrin thread, thereby forming blood clots that help to repair leaks in the circulating system.

ACUTE PHASE RESPONSE AND ACUTE PHASE PROTEINS (REACTANTS)

- The acute phase response is a nonspecific response to the stimulus of tissue following **trauma**, **infection**, **inflammation**, **burn**, etc.
- Acute phase reactants (APR) are **inflammation markers** that show significant changes in serum concentration during inflammation. These are produced in the liver during acute and chronic inflammatory states.
- Interleukin-6 (primary cytokine), tumor necrosis factor-alpha (TNF-α), and interferon-gamma (IFN-γ) are responsible to induce the production of acute-phase reactants.
- Acute phase reactants cause several adverse effects. These include:
  - Fever
  - Anemia of chronic disease
  - Anorexia
  - Somnolence (drowsiness)
  - Lethargy
  - Amyloidosis, and
  - Cachexia (fat and muscle loss, anorexia, weakness).

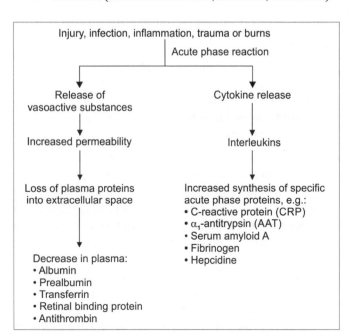

Figure 4.28: Mechanism of acute phase response.

- Acute phase reactants can be classified as **positive** or **negative**, depending on their serum concentrations during inflammation **(Table 4.11)**.
  - Positive acute phase reactants are upregulated, and their concentrations increase during inflammation. Positive acute phase reactants include procalcitonin (precursor protein of the hormone calcitonin), C-reactive protein, ferritin, fibrinogen, hepcidin, and serum amyloid A.
  - Negative acute phase reactants are downregulated, and their concentrations decrease during inflammation. Negative acute phase reactants include albumin, prealbumin, transferrin, retinol-binding protein, and antithrombin
- An increase or decrease in the concentration of several specific proteins occurs some hours after the injury. The mechanism of acute phase response mediated through formation of vasoactive substances and cytokines such as interleukins is shown in **Figure 4.28**.

ASSESSMENT QUESTIONS

STRUCTURED LONG ESSAY QUESTIONS (SLEQs)

1. Describe proteins under following headings:
   i. Definition
   ii. Classification by various ways with examples
   iii. Functions
2. Describe amino acids under following headings:
   i. Definition
   ii. Classification by various ways with examples
   iii. Functions
3. Describe structure of protein under following headings:
   i. Primary with diagram and examples
   ii. Secondary with diagram and examples
   iii. Tertiary with diagram and examples
   iv. Quaternary with diagram and examples
4. Describe plasma proteins under following headings:
   i. Types
   ii. Functions
   iii. Clinical significance

SHORT ESSAY QUESTIONS (SEQs)

1. Describe structure-function relationship of proteins with examples.
2. Give the importance of the 21st amino acid.
3. Give bonds responsible for the three-dimensional structure of proteins.
4. With help of diagram write secondary structure of protein.
5. Write functional classification of proteins with examples.
6. What is denaturation of protein? Write its importance.
7. Name biologically important peptides. Write structure and function of glutathione.
8. Give definition, name, and importance of essential amino acids.
9. Give importance of protein structure-function relationships in hemoglobinopathies.
10. What is acute phase reaction? Give different types of acute phase reactants.
11. Write functions of plasma proteins.

SHORT ANSWER QUESTIONS (SAQs)

1. Enumerate four biologically important compound derived from amino acids.
2. Among twenty amino acids why histidine has maximum buffering capacity?
3. Define peptide. Give important functions of two biologically important peptides.
4. Enumerate essential amino acids.
5. Enumerate the forces/bonds that stabilize structure of proteins?
6. What is meant by quaternary structure of a protein? Name a protein, abundantly found in blood that has a quaternary structure.
7. Define denaturation of proteins with example.
8. What are the functions of glutathione?
9. What is importance of primary structure of protein?
10. Give any two clinical conditions associated with changes in plasma protein fractions.

MULTIPLE CHOICE QUESTIONS (MCQs)

1. **All amino acids found in proteins are optically active, *except*:**
   a. Serine
   b. Glycine
   c. Threonine
   d. Tyrosine

2. **Which of the following amino acid is not occurring in proteins?**
   a. β-alanine
   b. α-aminobutyrate
   c. β-aminobutyrate
   d. All of the above

3. **The greatest buffering capacity at physiological pH would be provided by a protein, rich in which of the following amino acids:**
   a. Glycine
   b. Lysine
   c. Histidine
   d. Valine

4. **The three-dimensional shape of a protein is maintained mainly by:**
   a. Strong covalent interactions
   b. Multiple weak interactions
   c. Interaction with other proteins
   d. Interaction with prosthetic groups

5. Which of the following amino acid is exclusively ketogenic?
   a. Leucine
   b. Phenylalanine
   c. Threonine
   d. Isoleucine

6. In humans all of the following amino acids are essential, *except*:
   a. Valine
   b. Isoleucine
   c. Glycine
   d. Phenylalanine

7. During denaturation of protein the following bonds are disrupted, *except*:
   a. Hydrogen
   b. Hydrophobic
   c. Peptide
   d. Van der Waals forces

8. The imino acid present in protein is:
   a. Phenylalanine
   b. Valine
   c. Leucine
   d. Proline

9. Glycine is used for synthesis of the following, *except*:
   a. Heme
   b. Serotonin
   c. Purine
   d. Creatine

10. Which class of amino acids contains only nonessential amino acids?
    a. Aromatic
    b. Acidic
    c. Branched chain
    d. Basic

11. Which of the following is a nonprotein amino acid?
    a. Proline
    b. Histidine
    c. Ornithine
    d. Asparagine

12. Which of the following is a kind of secondary structure?
    α. α-helix
    b. β-bend
    c. Triple helix
    d. All of the above

13. Glutathione is found in all mammalian cells, *except*:
    a. RBC
    b. Neurons
    c. Skeletal muscle
    d. Argentaffin cells

14. Albumin is deficient in which of the following amino acid?
    a. Glycine
    b. Tryptophan
    c. Cystine
    d. Methionine

15. Which of the following acts as a redox buffer?
    a. Insulin
    b. Glucagon
    c. Glutathione
    d. Angiotensin

16. The important source of nitrogen for the body is:
    a. Carbohydrate
    b. Lipids
    c. Proteins
    d. All the above

17. Which of the following type of amino acids are present in biological proteins?
    a. L-α
    b. D-α
    c. L-β
    d. D-β

18. In which of the following amino acid imidazole ring is present?
    a. Histidine
    b. Alanine
    c. Tryptophan
    d. Valine

19. Glucogenic amino acids are that:
    a. Which contains glucose in its structure
    b. Acts as precursors for carbohydrates biosynthesis
    c. On biological oxidation it gives energy equal to glucose
    d. All of the above

20. The pH at which the molecule acts as zwitterion is called as:
    a. Isoelectric pH
    b. Isoelectric focusing
    c. Optimum pH
    d. Neutral pH

21. Amino acids can be identified by:
    a. Biuret test
    b. Ninhydrin test
    c. Molisch's test
    d. None of the above

22. The polypeptide responsible for uterine contraction is:
    a. Oxytocin
    b. Glutathione
    c. Vasopressin
    d. Angiotensin

23. The vasopressin is polypeptide which:
    a. Stimulate kidney to retain water
    b. Stimulate kidney to loss water
    c. Constrict the blood vessels
    d. All of the above

24. The polypeptide that protects RBC membrane is:
    a. Oxytocin
    b. Glutathione
    c. Vasopressin
    d. Angiotensin

25. Proteins are made up from how many standard amino acids:
    a. 15
    b. 18
    c. 20
    d. 100

26. Which of the following amino acids is hydroxy amino acid?
    a. Serine
    b. Isoleucine
    c. Leucine
    d. All of the above

27. Which of the following amino acid is considered as basic amino acid?
    a. Tryptophan
    b. Histidine
    c. Proline
    d. Hydroxyproline

28. Which of the following is sulfur-containing amino acid?
    a. Cysteine
    b. Cystine
    c. Methionine
    d. All of the above

29. Vitamin niacin is synthesized from:
    a. Tyrosine
    b. Tryptophan
    c. Cystine
    d. Glycine

30. Which of the following amino acid is involved in synthesis of creatine?
    a. Glycine
    b. Arginine
    c. Methionine
    d. All of the above

31. Glycine is used for the synthesis of:
    a. Heme
    b. Niacin
    c. Serotonin
    d. Thyroxine

32. Those amino acids can be synthesized by the body is called as:
    a. Essential amino acids
    b. Nonessential amino acids
    c. Semiessential amino acids
    d. None of the above

33. Proteins are linear chains of amino acids that are linked together by:
    a. Peptide bonds
    b. Hydrogen bonds
    c. Hydrophobic bond
    d. Glycosidic bonds

34. Which amino acids are involved in "detoxification" reaction?
    a. Glycine
    b. Cystine
    c. Methionine
    d. All of the above

35. Which of the following is fibrous protein?
    a. Collagen   b. Elastin
    c. Keratin   d. All of the above

36. Which of the following is true for α-helix structure of protein?
    a. There are 3.6 amino acids per turn
    b. It is called α because it was the first structure elucidated by Pauling and Corey
    c. The helix is stabilized by hydrogen bond
    d. All of the above

37. All of the following are glycoproteins, *except*:
    a. Collagen   b. Albumin
    c. IgG   d. Transferrin

38. Which one of the following list is correct?
    a. Serine and tryptophan both have hydroxyl groups in their side chains
    b. The most abundant amino acid in collagen is proline
    c. Glutamine and asparagine have amide groups on their side chains
    d. All amino acids found in proteins except proline, have a hydrogen atom attached to their α-carbon

39. Which one of the following statement is correct concerning denaturation or hydrolysis of proteins?
    a. Denaturation alters the primary structure of a protein and destroys its biological activity
    b. Proteins can be denatured by exposure to acids, alkalis or concentrated solutions of urea or by elevated temperatures
    c. Most proteins become more soluble when denatured
    d. Denaturation decreases digestibility

40. Select the correct statement concerning the varying levels of structure found in proteins.
    a. The secondary and tertiary structures of protein depend on its amino acid sequence
    b. The secondary structure of protein is the three-dimensional configuration
    c. The primary, secondary and tertiary structures of a protein are destroyed when the protein is denatured
    d. Protein secondary structures are stabilized by disulfide bonds

41. The sequence of amino acids in a polypeptide is called the:
    a. Primary structure
    b. Secondary structure
    c. Tertiary structure
    d. Quaternary structure

42. All of the following are hemoproteins, *except*:
    a. Myoglobin
    b. Cytochrome
    c. Catalase
    d. Albumin

43. All are true about glutathione, *except*:
    a. It is a tripeptide
    b. It converts hemoglobin to methemoglobin
    c. It conjugates xenobiotics
    d. It is cofactor of various enzymes

44. Guanidinium group is associated with:
    a. Tyrosine   b. Arginine
    c. Histidine   d. Lysine

45. Which of the following is aromatic amino acid with a hydroxyl R group?
    a. Tyrosine   b. Serine
    c. Threonine   d. Methionine

46. Replacing alanine by which amino acid will increase UV absorbance of protein at 280 nm wavelength:
    a. Leucine   b. Proline
    c. Arginine   d. Tryptophan

47. Which of the following special amino acid is not formed by post-translational modification?
    a. Triiodothyronine
    b. Hydroxyproline
    c. Hydroxylysine
    d. Selenocysteine

48. Which of the following have a positive charge in physiological pH?
    a. Arginine   b. Aspartic acid
    c. Isoleucine   d. Valine

49. Selenocysteine is coded by:
    a. UAG   C. UAA
    b. UGA   d. GUA

50. Polar amino acids is/are:
    a. Serine   b. Tryptophan
    c. Tyrosine   d. Valine
    e. Lysine

51. Nonpolar amino acid are:
    a. Alanine   b. Tryptophan
    c. Isoleucine   d. Lysine
    e. Tyrosine

52. Hydrophobic amino acids are:
    a. Methionine   b. Isoleucine
    c. Tyrosine   d. Alanine
    e. Asparagine

53. Basic amino acids is/are:
    a. Leucine   b. Arginine
    c. Lysine   d. Histidine

54. Which of the following amino acid is responsible for the absorption of UV light in proteins?
    a. Leucine
    b. Proline
    d. Tryptophan
    c. Arginine

55. Which among the following is the structure of myoglobin?
    a. Monomer
    b. Homodimer
    c. Heterodimer
    d. Tetramer

56. Denaturation is resisted by which of the following bond?
    a. Peptide bond   b. Hydrogen bond
    c. Disulphide bond   d. Electrostatic bond

57. Polypeptide formation in amino acid is by:
    a. Primary structure
    b. Secondary structure
    c. Tertiary structure
    d. Quaternary structure

58. In forming 3D structure following factors help:
    a. Peptide bond
    b. Amino acid sequence
    c. Interaction between polypeptide
    d. Chaperon
    e. Side chain

■ ANSWERS FOR MCQs

1. b	2. d	3. c	4. b	5. a
6. c	7. c	8. d	9. b	10. b
11. c	12. d	13. b	14. a	15. c
16. c	17. a	18. a	19. b	20. a
21. b	22. a	23. a	24. b	25. c
26. a	27. b	28. d	29. b	30. d
31. a	32. b	33. a	34. b	35. b
36. d	37. b	38. c	39. b	40. a
41. a	42. d	43. b	44. b	45. a
46. d	47. d	48. a	49. b	50. a,e
51. a,b,c,e	52. a,b,c,d		53. b,c,d	54. d
55. a	56. a	57. a	58. b,c,d,e	

Enzymes

Competency	Learning Objectives
BI 2.1: Explain fundamental concepts of enzyme, isoenzyme, alloenzyme, coenzyme and cofactors. Enumerate the main classes of International Union of Biochemistry and Molecular Biology (IUBMB) nomenclature. **BI 2.3:** Describe and explain the basic principles of enzyme activity. **BI 2.4:** Describe and discuss enzyme inhibitors as poisons, drugs and as therapeutic enzymes. **BI 2.5:** Describe and discuss the clinical utility of various serum enzymes as markers of pathological conditions. **BI 2.6:** Discuss use of enzymes in laboratory investigations (enzyme-based assays). **BI 2.7:** Interpret laboratory results of enzyme activities and describe the clinical utility of various enzymes as markers of pathological conditions.	1. Describe enzymes: Definition, general properties and IUBMB classification with examples. 2. Describe various cofactor and coenzyme. 3. Describe the basic principles of enzyme activity: Mechanism and enzyme specificity. 4. Describe enzyme kinetics: Factors affecting the enzyme activity. 5. Describe regulation of enzyme activity. 6. Describe enzyme inhibition: Types, examples, kinetics, clinical and therapeutic importance and enzyme inhibitors as poisons. 7. Describe isoenzymes: Definition, examples and diagnostic importance. 8. Describe alloenzyme with example. 9. Describe diagnostically important serum enzymes. 10. Describe serum enzyme assays (profile) in: myocardial infarction and liver diseases, and pancreatitis. 11. Describe use of enzymes in laboratory for investigations (enzyme-based assays). 12. Describe therapeutic uses of enzymes.

■ OVERVIEW

Enzymes (from Greek *enzymos*, "leavened" means an agent that modify a whole) are biological materials with catalytic properties, i.e., they increase the rate of chemical reactions in biological and *in vitro* (in the laboratory) systems, that otherwise proceed very slowly. Deficiencies in the quantity or catalytic activity of key enzymes can result from genetic defects, nutritional deficits or toxins. The study of enzymes and of the changes in the enzyme activity that occur in body fluids has become a valuable diagnostic tool for the elucidation of various diseases and for testing organ function.

■ ENZYMES: DEFINITION, GENERAL PROPERTIES AND IUBMB CLASSIFICATION WITH EXAMPLES

Definition, General Properties of Enzyme

Enzymes are specialized **proteins** that **catalyze biological reactions**. Enzymes have extraordinary catalytic power, often far greater than that of synthetic or inorganic catalysts. Virtually every reaction that occurs within a cell requires the action of an enzyme.

- They functions in aqueous solutions under very mild conditions of temperature and pH.

- The catalytic activity of enzyme depends on their native **protein conformation**.
- If an enzyme is denatured or dissociated into its subunits, catalytic activity is usually lost. Thus the primary, secondary, tertiary, and quaternary structures of protein enzymes are essential to their catalytic activity.

Ribozymes

- Ribozymes are catalytically active RNA molecules.
- Enzymes are **proteins** with the exception of a few classes of RNA molecule.
- In some cases, RNAs have a catalytic activity. These unusual catalytic RNAs are known as **ribozymes**.
- **Ribozymes** (ribosomal RNA) most frequently catalyze **cleavage** and **ligation** of specific phosphodiester bonds and peptide bond formation during protein synthesis on the ribosome.
- **Peptidyl transferase** is the activity of ribosomal RNA responsible for peptide bond formation during protein synthesis.

Zymogen or Proenzyme

A number of proteolytic enzymes found in the blood or in the digestive tract are present in an **inactive (precursor)** form, called **zymogen** or **proenzyme, (Table 5.1)** which must be cleaved to be activated.

Their synthesis in a zymogen or proenzyme (inactive) form prevents them from catalyzing reactions in the cell where they are synthesized. For example, chymotrypsin is secreted by the pancreas as **chymotrypsinogen**. It is activated in the digestive tract by the proteolytic enzyme **trypsin**, which cleaves off a small peptide from N-terminal region of chymotrypsinogen. The cleavage changes the conformation of the enzyme and creates a binding site for the substrate.

Precursor proteins or inactive enzyme names have the prefix *"pro"* like prothrombin, proelastase, etc. or suffix *"ogen"* like chymotrypsinogen, trypsinogen, pepsinogen, which are produced and stored as inactive proenzymes or zymogen form.

IUBMB Classification and Nomenclature of Enzymes

The enzyme nomenclature and classification scheme was described in 1961 by **Enzyme Commission** of the International Union of Biochemistry (IUB). According to this classification, each enzyme is characterized by a code number called **enzyme code number** or **'EC' number**. According to this system, enzymes are classified into **six classes**, based on the type of reaction catalyzed.

- However, it has become apparent that none of these could describe the important group of enzymes that catalyze the movement of ions or molecules across membranes or their separation within membranes. Several of these involve the hydrolysis of ATP and they were previously classified as ATPases (EC 3: Hydrolases), although the hydrolytic reaction is not their primary function.
- In August 2018, these enzymes have been classified under a new EC class, **EC-7 category** describing **Translocases**, by the Enzyme Commission, **International Union of Biochemistry and Molecular Biology (IUBMB)**.
- Each enzyme is assigned a four-digit EC number, the first three digits of which define the reaction catalyzed and the fourth of which is a unique identifier (serial number).

The seven classes as per **IUBMB** are as follows:
1. EC-1: Oxidoreductase
2. EC-2: Transferase
3. EC-3: Hydrolase
4. EC-4: Lyase
5. EC-5: Isomerase
6. EC-6: Ligase
7. EC-7: Translocases

Table 5.2 describes the seven classes of enzymes with examples recommended by IUBMB

EC-1: Oxidoreductase

The enzymes involved in oxidation and reduction reactions are called **oxidoreductase** and are classified into four groups as follows.
1. Dehydrogenases
2. Oxygenases (monooxygenase and dioxygenase)
3. Oxidases
4. Hydroperoxidases

- **Dehydrogenases:** They catalyze the removal of hydrogen from a substrate but are not able to use oxygen as a hydrogen acceptor. These enzymes, therefore, require specific **coenzymes** as acceptor of hydrogen atoms. The coenzymes of dehydrogenases may be either nicotinamide coenzymes (NAD^+ or $NADP^+$) or flavin coenzymes (FMN or FAD). For example:
  - Lactate dehydrogenase (LDH)
  - Succinate dehydrogenase (SDH)
  - Glucose-6-phosphate dehydrogenase (G-6PD)
- **Oxygenases:** They catalyze the direct transfer and incorporation of oxygen into a substrate molecule. The two types of oxygenases are:

TABLE 5.1: Zymogens (inactive enzymes) secreted by stomach and pancreas.

Site of synthesis	Zymogen	Active form of enzyme
Stomach	Pepsinogen	Pepsin
Pancreas	Chymotrypsinogen	Chymotrypsin
	Trypsinogen	Trypsin
	Procarboxypeptidase	Carboxypeptidase

TABLE 5.2: International IUBMB classification of enzymes.

Class	Type of reaction catalyzed	Examples
EC-1: Oxidoreductases	Oxidation-reduction reactions (transfer of electrons, hydride ions or H atoms)	• Lactate dehydrogenase (LDH) • Succinate dehydrogenase (SDH) • Glucose-6-phosphate dehydrogenase (G6PD) • Homogentisate oxidase • Tryptophan pyrrolase (Dioxygenase) • L-amino acid oxidase • Xanthine oxidase • Cytochrome oxidase • Phenylalanine hydroxylases • Tyrosine hydroxylase • Tryptophan hydroxylase
EC-2: Transferases	Group (like amino, carboxyl, methyl or phosphoryl, etc.) transfer reactions	• Aspartate transaminase (AST) • Alanine transaminase (ALT) • Ornithine carbamoyltransferase • Hexokinase • Creatine kinase
EC-3: Hydrolases	Hydrolysis reactions (enzymes of this class catalyze the cleavage of **C-O**, **C-N**, **C-C** and some other bonds with the addition of water)	• Lipase • α-amylase • Trypsin • Chymotrypsin • Lactase • Sucrase • Alkaline phosphatase • Pepsin
EC-4: Lyases	Cleavage of C-O, C-C and C-N or other bonds by means other than hydrolysis or oxidation, giving rise to compound with double bonds or catalyze the reverse reaction by the addition of group to a double bond. In cases where addition of groups to double bonds occur, then synthase (not synthetase of group EC-6), is used in the name	• Aldolase • Porphobilinogen synthase • Fumarase • Argininosuccinase • Carbonic anhydrase • Cysteine desulfurase • Decarboxylase
EC-5: Isomerases	Transfer of groups within molecules to yield isomeric forms	• Phosphoglucomutase • Triphosphate isomerase • Phosphohexose isomerase • Glucose epimerase • Retinal isomerase
EC-6: Ligases	Joining of two molecules by condensation reactions at the expense of ATP hydrolysis. They may form **C-O**, **C-S**, **C-N**, **C-C** or other bonds	• Glutamine synthetase • Pyruvate carboxylase • DNA ligases
EC-7: Translocases	Catalyze the movement of ions or molecules across membranes or their separation within membranes	• ADP/ATP translocases • Ornithine translocase • Carnitine-acylcarnitine translocase

1. **Dioxygenases** which catalyze the incorporation of both atoms of molecular oxygen into substrate. Examples are:
   ♦ Homogentisate oxidase
   ♦ Tryptophan pyrrolase (Dioxygenase)
2. **Mono-oxygenases**, this enzyme incorporate only **one atom** of molecular oxygen into the substrate in the form of **hydroxyl group**, while the other oxygen atom of O_2 is reduced to H_2O_2 by reducing equivalents donated by coenzymes. Examples are:
   ♦ Phenylalanine hydroxylases
   ♦ Tyrosine hydroxylase
   ♦ Tryptophan hydroxylase

Cytochrome P_{450} is mono-oxygenases (mixed function oxidase) important for the detoxification of many drugs and for the hydroxylation of steroids.

• **Oxidases:** They catalyze the removal of hydrogen from a substrate in the form of H_2O or H_2O_2 (hydrogen peroxide), using oxygen as a hydrogen acceptor, e.g., **cytochrome oxidase** (cytochrome aa_3), **L-amino acid oxidase, xanthine oxidase**, etc.

• **Hydroperoxidases:** They use hydrogen peroxide or organic peroxide as substrate. There are two types of hydroperoxidases, **peroxidases** and **catalases**.

Hydroperoxidases protect the body against harmful peroxides. Accumulation of peroxides can lead to generation of free radicals, which in turn disrupt membranes and cause diseases like cancer and atherosclerosis.

EC-2: Transferase

Those enzymes that catalyze the transfer of a functional group such as, **amino**, **carboxyl**, **methyl** or **phosphoryl,** etc. from one molecule to another are called transferases. These reactions can be illustrated as follows:

Some common enzymes in this category include:

- **Aminotransferase or transaminase:** Transfer of amino group from an amino acid to a keto acid
- **Kinase:** Transfer phosphate group usually from ATP to a substrate.
- **Transmethylase:** Transfer methyl group
- **Phosphorylase:** Transfer phosphate group from inorganic phosphate to a substrate.
- **Transketolase:** Transfer ketone group
- **Transaldolase:** Transfer aldehyde group.

EC-3: Hydrolase

Enzymes of this class catalyze the cleavage of **C-O, C-N, C-C** and some other covalent bonds with the addition of water. All digestive enzymes are hydrolases. These can be illustrated as follows:

- **Peptidases (trypsin, pepsin, chymotrypsin, elastase, carboxypeptidase):** Hydrolyze peptide bond of protein.
- **Amylase:** Hydrolyze glycosidic bond of carbohydrates
- **Exonucleases and endonucleases:** Hydrolyze phosphodiester bond of nucleic acid.
- **Esterase and lipases:** Hydrolyze ester bond of lipids.

EC-4: Lyase

Lyase catalyze the cleavage of **C-O, C-C** and **C-N** bonds by means other than hydrolysis or oxidation, giving rise to compound with double bonds or catalyze the reverse reaction by the addition of group to a double bond. In cases where reverse reaction is important, then synthase (not synthetase of group EC-6), is used in the name. This type of reaction is illustrated as follows:

Examples of lyses are:

- *Decarboxylase:* Cleave C-C bond and remove CO_2
- *Aconitase, enolase, fumarase, and aldolase:* Form double bond by removal or addition of groups.
- HMG-CoA lyase, argininosuccinate lyase
- Most synthase belong to lyases

EC-5: Isomerases

Isomerases catalyze intramolecular rearrangement (structural or geometric changes) in a molecule. They are called **epimerases**, **isomerases** or **mutases**, depending on the type of isomerism involved. The examples are as follows:

- All enzymes with isomerase in its name
- Racemases
- Mutase like phosphoglucomutase

EC-6: Ligases (Synthetases)

Ligases catalyze the joining of two molecules coupled with the hydrolysis of ATP. They may form **C-O, C-S, C-N, C-C**. The examples are as follows:

- Pyruvate carboxylase
- Acetyl-CoA carboxylase
- Propionyl-CoA carboxylase

EC-7: Translocases (A new EC Class)

Translocases catalyze the movement of ions or molecules across membranes or their separation within membranes. They were previously classified as **ATPases (EC 3: Hydrolases)**. The subclasses are designated based on types of ions or molecules translocated.

For example:

- **Carnitine-acylcarnitine translocase:** It is responsible for transporting both carnitine-fatty acid complexes and carnitine across the inner mitochondrial membrane (since fatty acids cannot cross the mitochondrial membranes without assistance.
- **Ornithine translocase:** It is responsible for transporting ornithine from cytosol into mitochondria in urea cycle.
- **ADP/ATP translocases:** Catalyzes the exchange of cytosolic adenosine diphosphate (ADP) and mitochondrial adenosine triphosphate (ATP) across the inner mitochondrial membrane. ATP produced from oxidative phosphorylation is transported from the mitochondrial matrix to the cytoplasm.

■ COFACTORS AND COENZYMES

Some enzymes require an additional chemical component for its catalytic activity. This additional group is called **cofactor** which may be either one or more **inorganic ions,** such as Fe^{2+}, Mg^{2+}, Mn^{2+} or Zn^{2++} **(Table 5.3)** or a complex **organic molecule** called a **coenzyme**.

- Coenzymes are thermostable, low molecular weight, non-protein organic substances.
- Coenzymes act as transient carriers of specific functional groups. Most are derived from **vitamins (Table 5.4)**.
- Some enzymes require both a coenzyme and one or more metal ions for activity.
- Cofactors are associated **reversibly** with enzymes.

TABLE 5.3: Inorganic ions that serve as cofactors for enzymes.

Ions	Enzymes
Cu^{2+}	Cytochrome oxidase, tyrosinase, amino acid oxidase
Fe^{2+} or Fe^{3+}	Cytochrome oxidase, catalase, and peroxidase
K^+	Pyruvate kinase, propionyl-CoA carboxylase, and acetyl-CoA thiolase
Mg^{2+}	Hexokinase, glucose-6-phosphatase, and pyruvate kinase
Mn^{2+}	Arginase, ribonucleotide reductase
Mo^+	Dinitrogenase, nitrate reductase
Ni^{2+}	Urease
Se	Glutathione peroxidase
Zn^{2+}	Carbonic anhydrase, alcohol dehydrogenase, and carboxypeptidase

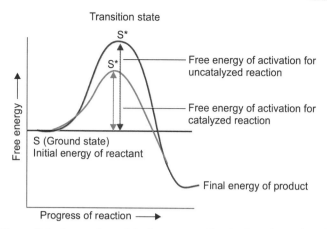

Figure 5.1: Comparison of the free energy of activation of a catalyzed and uncatalyzed reaction.

(S* = Transition state)

- An enzyme which is tightly bound to metal ion is called **metalloenzyme**.
- Enzymes which have metal as cofactor, i.e., loosely bound to them are termed **metal-activated enzyme**.
- An enzyme without its cofactor is referred to as an **apoenzyme** or **apoprotein**. A complete catalytically active enzyme is called **holoenzyme**. **Apoenzyme + Cofactor = Holoenzyme**.
- A coenzyme or metal ion that is very tightly or even covalently bound to the enzyme protein is called a **prosthetic** group.

Coenzymes Derived from Nonvitamin Precursors

- ❖ **Lipoate** which functions as a carrier of acyl groups and electrons
- ❖ **Coenzyme-Q** acts as hydrogen acceptor from flavoproteins (NADH-dehydrogenase and succinate dehydrogenase)
- ❖ **Tetrahydrobiopterine** serves as a source of hydrogen.

◼ MECHANISM AND ENZYME SPECIFICITY

Enzymes are highly effective catalysts. A chemical reaction of a substrate **S** to form product **P** goes through a transition state **S*** that has a higher free energy (energy in biological systems is described in terms of free energy, G) than does either

S or P. **Figure 5.1** shows the changes in energy during the conversion of a molecule of reactant 'S' to product P through the transition state S*.

- Enzymes accelerate reactions by facilitating the formation of the transition state. The star denotes the transition state. The transition state is a transitory molecular structure that is no longer the substrate but is not yet the product.
- The transition state is the least stable because it is the one with the highest free energy.
- The difference in the free energy between the transition state and the substrate is called **Gibbs free energy** of **activation** or simply the **activation energy**, symbolized by $\Delta G^* = Gs^* - Gs$.

In **Figure 5.1** the peak of free energy activation, represents the transition state, in which the high energy intermediates (S*) are formed during the conversion of a reactant to a product.

Enzymes function to lower the activation energy or in other words, enzymes facilitate the formation of the transition state. With an enzyme as a catalyst, the reaction may easily proceed at the normal physiological temperature. The rates of uncatalyzed chemical reactions are often slow because of activation energy.

TABLE 5.4: Some common coenzymes and their functions.

Vitamins	Coenzymes	Coenzyme for
Thiamine (vitamin B_1)	Thiamine pyrophosphate (TPP)	Oxidative decarboxylation and transketolase reaction
Riboflavin (vitamin B_2)	Flavin adenine dinucleotide and flavin mononucleotide (FAD and FMN)	Oxidation and reduction reactions
Niacin	Nicotinamide adenine dinucleotide (NAD) Nicotinamide adenine dinucleotide Phosphate (NADP)	Oxidation and reduction reactions
Pyridoxine (vitamin B_6)	Pyridoxal phosphate (PLP)	Transamination, deamination, and decarboxylation reactions of amino acids
Biotin	Biocytin	Carboxylation reactions
Folic acid	Tetrahydrofolate (THF)	Carrier of one carbon group
Pantothenic acid	Coenzyme A	Acyl carrier
Cyanocobalamin vitamin B_{12}	Methylcobalamin and deoxyadenosylcobalamin	Transfer of CH_3 group and isomerization

Mechanism of Enzyme Action

Formation of an **enzyme-substrate (ES)** complex is the first step in enzymatic catalysis. Substrate is bound through multiple **noncovalent interactions** at the **active site** of the enzyme forming an ES complex which is subsequently converted to product and free enzyme.

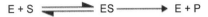

- The **active site** of an enzyme is the region that binds the substrate and which contains the specific amino acid residues, **binding residues** and **catalytic residues** and possesses three-dimensional structures.
- **Binding residues** recognize and bind the correct substrate to form ES complex.
- **Catalytic residues** create a chemical environment that enhances the reaction rate and ES complex is converted to an enzyme (E) and a product (P).

Two models for substrate binding to the active site of the enzyme have been proposed to explain the specificity that an enzyme has for its substrate:

1. Lock and key model or rigid template model of Emil Fischer
2. Induced fit model or hand-in-glove model of Daniel E Koshland.

Lock and Key Model or Rigid Template Model of Emil Fischer

This model is proposed by Emil Fischer in 1890.

- In this model, enzyme is preshaped and the active site has a rigid structure that is complementary to that of the substrate **(Figure 5.2)**.
- This model is called lock and key model, because in this model the substrate fits into the active site in much the same way that a key fits into a lock.
- This model has been useful in understanding how some enzymes can bind only a specific substrate but will not bind another compound with an almost identical structure. For example, most enzymes in carbohydrate metabolism can bind the D-isomer of hexoses but cannot bind the corresponding L-isomer, which differs only in the configuration around a single carbon atom.
- This model explains all mechanisms but do not explain the changes in the enzyme activity in the presence of allosteric modulators.

Induced Fit Model or Hand-in-glove Model of Daniel E Koshland

Fischer's model explained the specificity of enzyme-substrate interaction but, the implied rigidity of the enzymes active site failed to explain the dynamic changes that must take place during catalysis. A model that accounts for both of these aspects of enzyme catalysis is the **induced fit model of Daniel E Koshland (Figure 5.3)**.

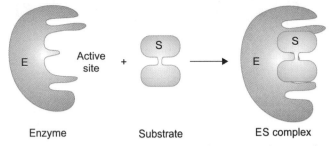

Figure 5.2: Representation of formation of an ES-complex according to the Fischer's lock and key model. The active site of the enzyme is complementary in shape to that of substrate.

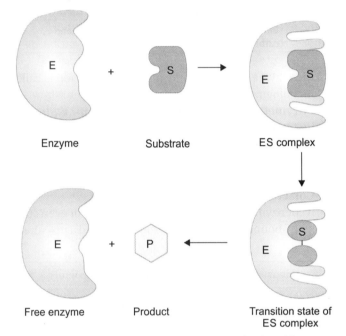

Figure 5.3: Schematic representation of induced fit model of Koshland.

- In the Fischer's model, the catalytic site is presumed to be preshaped to fit the substrate. However, Daniel E Koshland in 1958 postulated that the **enzymes are flexible and shapes of the active site can be modified by the binding of the substrate**.
- In the induced fit model, the substrate induces a conformational change in the enzyme, in the same manner in which placing a hand (substrate) into a glove (enzyme) induces changes in the glove's shape. Therefore, this model is also known as **hand-in-glove model**.
- Conformational change in enzyme aligns catalytic residues which participate in catalysis.
- The enzyme in turn induces reciprocal changes in its bound substrate that alters their orientation and configuration and strains the structure of the bound substrate. Such change helps to bring the ES-complex into its **transition state (Figure 5.3) with liberation of energy**.
- The intrinsic binding energy due to the substrate-enzyme interaction is made available for the transformation of

the substrate into product. This model is believed to describe more accurately the specificity of substrate binding than do lock and key model of E Fischer.

Specificity of Enzyme Action

Specificity refers to the ability of an enzyme to discriminate between two competing substrates. Enzymes are highly specific both in the type of reaction catalyzed and in their choice of substrates. Specificity makes it possible for a number of enzymes to coexist in the cell without interfering in each other's actions.

Types of Specificity

The following types of specificity have been recognized:
1. Substrate specificity
2. Reaction specificity
3. Stereospecificity

Substrate Specificity

There are following types of substrate specificity:
1. Absolute substrate specificity
2. Relative substrate specificity
3. Broad substrate specificity.

- **Absolute substrate specificity:** Certain enzymes will act on only one substrate and catalyze one reaction, e.g., glucokinase, lactase, urease, **(Figure 5.4)**.
- **Relative substrate specificity:** In this case, enzyme acts on more than one substrate. The relative substrate specificity is of two types:
  1. Group specificity
  2. Bond specificity.
  - In **group specificity**, an enzyme acts on more than one substrate containing a particular group, e.g., chymotrypsin acts on several proteins by hydrolyzing peptide bonds attached to aromatic amino acids. Trypsin hydrolyzes peptide linkages involving arginine or lysine.
  - In **bond specificity**, an enzyme acts on more than one substrate containing a particular kind of bond, e.g., salivary α-amylase cleaves α-(1→4) glycosidic bonds of carbohydrates, lipase hydrolyzes ester bonds of lipids.
- **Broad substrate specificity:** In this case, an enzyme acts on more than one structurally-related substrates, e.g., hexokinase catalyzes the phosphorylation of more

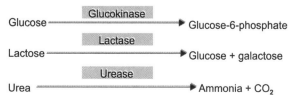

Figure 5.4: Absolute substrate specificity.

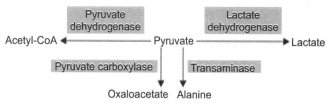

Figure 5.5: Example of reaction specificity.

than one kind of hexoses such as glucose, fructose and mannose.

Reaction Specificity

In this case, an enzyme is specific to a particular reaction but not to substrate (s) and catalyzes only one type of reaction. For example, pyruvate can undergo several reactions. Each reaction is catalyzed by a separate enzyme, which catalyzes only that reaction and none other as shown in **Figure 5.5**.

Stereospecificity

Many enzymes show specificity toward stereoisomers, i.e., they act on only one type of isomer of a given compound. For example:
- L-lactate dehydrogenase will act only on L-lactic acid and not D-lactic acid.
- Likewise, L-amino acid oxidase and D-amino acid oxidase are distinct enzymes which act only on L and D-amino acids respectively.
- D-glucose oxidase can similarly act only on D-glucose and not on L-glucose.
- Salivary α-amylase acts on the α-1,4 glycoside linkages and is inactive on β-1,4 glycoside linkages.

Isomerase and epimerase do not show stereospecificity.

ENZYME KINETICS: FACTORS AFFECTING THE VELOCITY OF ENZYME REACTION

Enzyme Kinetics

Kinetics means **velocity** or **rate**. The study of reaction rates and how they change in response to changes in experimental parameters is known as **enzyme kinetics**. This is the oldest approach for understanding enzyme mechanism, and one that remains most important today. Knowledge about the kinetics of an enzyme is useful to know:
- Detailed mechanism of action of enzyme
- Their role in metabolism
- Factors that affect its activity
- Mechanisms of inhibition
- Can do analysis, diagnosis, and treatment of the disease. Enzymes are target for drugs used in treatment, e.g., **allopurinol** is the drug for the treatment of **gout**, act through inhibiting enzyme **xanthine oxidase**

We study the effect of various variables or factors on the velocity or rate. The rate of enzyme reaction is greatly influenced by:

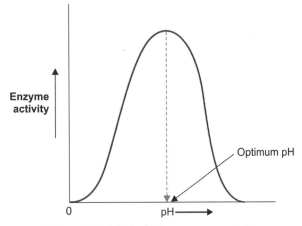

Figure 5.6: Effect of pH on enzyme activity.

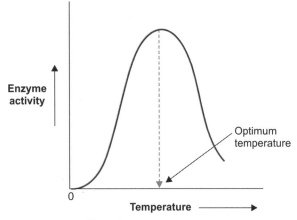

Figure 5.7: Effect of temperature on enzyme activity.

- pH, i.e., H^+ ion concentration
- Temperature
- Enzyme concentration
- Substrate concentration
- Inhibitors

Hydrogen Ion Concentration

Each enzyme has an **optimum pH**, a pH at which the enzyme has maximum activity. Below or above this pH, enzyme activity is decreased. The optimum pH differs from enzyme to enzyme, e.g., optimum pH for **pepsin is 1.2** and for **trypsin 8.0**.

A bell-shaped curve is obtained when enzyme activity is plotted against pH **(Figure 5.6)**. As enzymes are proteins, changes in pH can alter the following:

- Ionization state of the amino acid residues present in the active site of the enzyme. Enzyme activity is related to the ionic state of active site of the enzyme.
- The ionization state of the substrate. The active site of an enzyme may require particular ionic state of the substrate for optimum activity.
- Ionization of residues that is responsible for maintaining the enzyme protein conformation.
- It may dissociate the apoenzyme from the prosthetic group (coenzyme).
- Drastic change in pH denatures the enzyme protein.

All these affect the enzyme substrate complex formation and decrease the rate of enzyme reaction.

> As pH affects the enzyme activity, in enzyme studies buffers are used to keep enzyme at an optimum or at least a favorable H^+ ion concentration.

Temperature

Enzyme catalyzed reactions show an increase in rate with increasing temperature only within a relatively small and low temperature range. Each enzyme shows the highest activity at a particular temperature called **optimum temperature**.

The activity progressively declines both above and below this temperature **(Figure 5.7)**.

- Increase in velocity is due to the increase in the kinetic energy to pass over the energy barrier and form the product of the reaction. Further elevation of the temperature results in a decrease in reaction velocity as a result of temperature-induced denaturation of the enzyme protein.
- Low temperature also decreases enzyme activity and enzymes may be completely inactive at temperature of 0°C and below. **The inactivity at low temperature is reversible**. So, many enzymes in tissues or extracts may be preserved for months by storing at –20°C or –70°C. Most of the body enzymes have the optimum temperature close to 37–38°C and have progressively less activity as the temperature rises.
- The reaction velocity of most chemical reactions increase with temperature approximately doubles for each 10°C rise called temperature coefficient Q_{10}.

Enzyme Concentration

The velocity of a reaction is directly proportional to the amount of enzyme present as long as the amount of substrate is not limiting. The substrate must be present at a concentration sufficient to ensure that all of the enzyme molecules have substrate bound to their active site **(Figure 5.8)**.

Substrate Concentration

The key factor affecting the rate of a reaction catalyzed by an enzyme is the **concentration of substrate** [S]. The effect on V_0 (initial velocity) of varying substrate concentration [S], when enzyme concentration is held constant, is shown in **Figure 5.9**.

For a given quantity of enzyme, the velocity of the reaction increases as the concentration of the substrate is increased. At first, this relationship is almost linear, but later, the reaction curve becomes **hyperbolic** in shape.

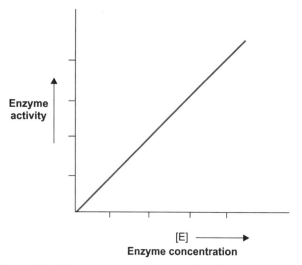

Figure 5.8: Effect of enzyme concentration of enzyme activity.

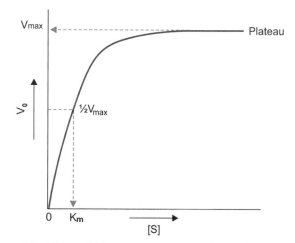

Figure 5.9: Effects of substrate concentration [S] on the initial velocity of an enzyme catalyzed reaction keeping enzyme concentration constant.

(V_0: Initial velocity, V_{max}: Maximum velocity, K_m: 1/2 V_{max}: Michaelis-Menten constant, [S]: Substrate concentration)

As we know that, enzyme first combines reversibly with its substrate to form an **enzyme-substrate complex (ES)**. The ES complex then breaks down to yield the **free enzyme** and the **product P**. At any given instant, in an enzyme catalyzed reaction, the enzyme exists in two forms, the free or uncombined form **E** and the combined form **ES**.

$$E + S \rightleftharpoons ES \longrightarrow E + P$$

- Initially at low substrate concentration [S], most of the enzyme will be in the uncombined or free form E. Here, the rate will be proportional to substrate concentration [S].
- The maximum velocity (V_{max}) of the catalyzed reaction is observed when virtually all of the enzymes are present as the ES complex and concentration of enzyme E is vanishingly small.
- Under these conditions, the enzyme is saturated with its substrate, and all the free enzymes will have been converted into ES form. So that any further increase in substrate concentration [S] has no effect on the rate. This condition exist when [S] sufficiently high that essentially all the free enzyme has been converted to the ES form.

- After the ES complex breaks down to yield the product P, the enzyme is free to catalyze the reaction of another molecule of substrate under saturating conditions. The saturation effect is responsible for the plateau observed in **Figure 5.9**. In general, the reaction is said to be in steady state when the rate of synthesis of ES is equal to its rate of degradation.

Michaelis-Menten Constant (K_m) and its Importance

- Leonor Michaelis and Maud Menten introduced a mathematical illustration to describe the action of enzymes with two constants, V_{max} and K_m.
- The **Michaelis constant (K_m)** is the concentration of the substrate when half of the active binding sites of an enzyme are occupied by the substrate. It can be defined as; the substrate concentration at which velocity (V_0) is half the maximal velocity $V_{max}/2$ **(Figure 5.9)**. The constant helps to show the affinity of the enzyme for their substrate.
- This value is given as the concentration of the substrate (mM) at half of V_{max}. The K_m value of an enzyme depends on the particularly on **substrate** and **environmental conditions** such as **pH**, **temperature** and **ionic strength**. The K_m can vary greatly from enzyme-to-enzyme and even for different substrates of the same enzyme **(Table 5.5)**.
- K_m provides an amount of the substrate concentration required for significant catalysis to occur. If the normal concentration of substrate is near K_m the enzyme will display significant activity.
- K_m does represent a measure of the affinity of the enzyme for its substrate in the ES complex.
  - An enzyme with a high K_m has a low affinity for the substrate, and a high concentration of the substrate is needed in order for the enzyme to become saturated.
  - Conversely, an enzyme with a low K_m has a high affinity for the substrate and a less amount of substrate is needed in order achieve V_{max}.

TABLE 5.5: K_m for some enzymes and substrates.		
Enzymes	*Substrates*	*K_m (mM)*
Hexokinase (brain)	ATP	0.4
	D-glucose	0.05
	D-fructose	1.5
Carbonic anhydrase	HCO_3^-	26
β-galactosidase	D-lactose	4.0
Threonine dehydratase	L-threonine	5.0
Chymotrypsin	Glycyltyrosinylglycine	108
	N-Benzoyltyrosinamide	2.5

Physiological Relevance of K_m

The physiological importance of K_m is illustrated by the sensitivity of some individuals to **alcohol**. Such persons exhibit facial flushing and tachycardia (increased heart rate) after intake of even small amount of alcohol. Normally in the liver ethanol (alcohol) is converted to acetaldehyde by an enzyme alcohol dehydrogenase.

- ❖ The cause of symptoms of alcoholic is due to the accumulation of acetaldehyde in the body. Acetaldehyde is then oxidized to acetate by liver enzyme acetaldehyde dehydrogenase. Most people have two forms of the acetaldehyde dehydrogenase.
  1. A low K_m mitochondrial form.
  2. A high K_m cytosolic form.
- ❖ In susceptible persons, the mitochondrial enzyme is less active due to the substitution of a single amino acid and acetaldehyde is converted to acetate only by cytosolic enzyme. Because this enzyme has a high K_m (less affinity for substrate) less acetaldehyde is converted into acetate and leads to accumulation of acetaldehyde in blood which accounts for the physiological effects of alcoholics.

Maximum Velocity (V_{max}) and its Importance

- The **maximal velocity (V_{max})** refers to the point at which the increase in concentration of the substrate does not increase the rate of a reaction catalyzed by an enzyme **(Figure 5.9)**. This occurs because the substrate molecules saturate the active sites of the enzyme and are not able to form more complexes with the enzyme. This value is given as a rate (mmol/s), which is the maximum velocity of the reaction when the enzyme is saturated.
- V_{max} or maximum velocity reveals the **turnover number** of an enzyme, which is the number of substrate molecules converted into products by an enzyme molecule in a unit time when the enzyme is fully saturated with substrate. The V_{max} of a reaction is an index of the catalytic efficiency of an enzyme.
- The V_{max} is useful in comparing the activity of one enzyme with that of another.
- Every enzyme has the characteristics V_{max} and K_m which are sensitive to changes in **pH**, **temperature** and **ionic strength**.

Lineweaver-Burk Plot or Double-reciprocal Plot

A graphical representation of 1/V on y-axis and 1/S on x-axis is called **Lineweaver-Burk plot** or **double-reciprocal plot**.

- **Figure 5.9** shows a simple graphical method for obtaining an approximate value for K_m and V_{max}. A more convenient procedure, using a **double-reciprocal plot** is presented by Lineweaver-Burk equation. This equation is obtained by taking the reciprocal of the Michaelis-Menten equation.

$$\frac{1}{V_0} = \frac{K_m}{V_{max}} \cdot \frac{1}{[S]} + \frac{1}{V_{max}}$$

- When $1/V_0$ is plotted against $1/[S]$, straight line obtained **(Figure 5.10)**, with: A slope equal to K_m/V_{max}.

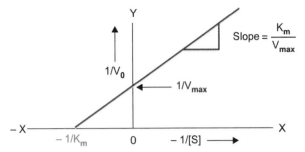

Figure 5.10: Lineweaver-Burk plot (double-reciprocal plot).

- The point, at which line intersects the y-axis, is numerically equal to $1/V_{max}$ and the point at which the line intersects the x-axis is numerically equal to $-1/K_m$.
- The values of K_m and V_{max} can be readily calculated from the values of these two intercepts. Also, this plot is useful to determine the mechanism of action of enzyme inhibitors.

■ REGULATION OF ENZYME ACTIVITY

In cell metabolism, groups of enzymes work together in sequential chains or systems to carry out a given metabolic process. In such enzyme systems, the reaction product of the first enzyme becomes the substrate of the next and so on **(Figure 5.11)**. The activity of enzymes must often be regulated so that they function at the proper time and place. This regulation is essential for coordination of the vast array of biochemical processes taking place at any instant in an organism.

In each enzyme system, there is at least one enzyme that regulates the rate of overall metabolic sequence as per the cells demand. Such regulatory enzymes not only have catalytic function, but are also capable of increasing or decreasing their catalytic activity in response to certain signals. Such enzymes, whose activity is modulated through various types of molecular signals, are called regulatory enzymes. In most multienzyme systems, the first enzyme of the sequence is the *regulatory enzyme*. Enzyme activity is regulated by short-term and long-term mechanism:

- **Short-term mechanisms are by:**
  - Allosteric or noncovalent control of enzymes
  - Reversible covalent modification of enzymes
  - Proteolytic cleavage of proenzymes/zymogens
- **Long-term mechanism is by:**
  - Induction and repression of enzyme synthesis (long term regulation)

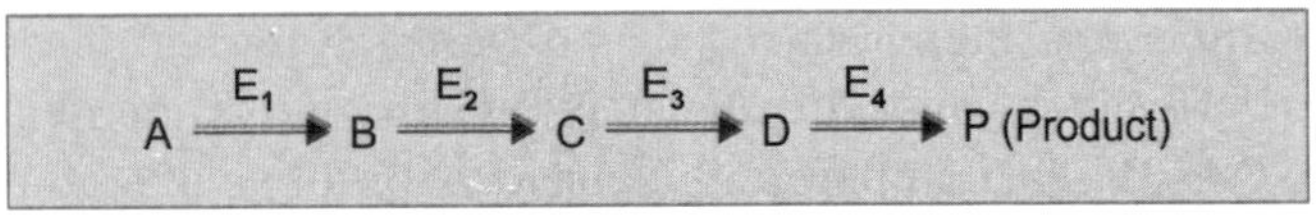

$$A \xrightarrow{E_1} B \xrightarrow{E_2} C \xrightarrow{E_3} D \xrightarrow{E_4} P \text{ (Product)}$$

Figure 5.11: Schematic representation of multienzyme system responsible for converting A to P via four sequential enzyme catalyzed steps.

Allosteric or Noncovalent Regulation of Enzymes

Allosteric Enzyme

The term allosteric derives from Greek word, allo = "other" and steros = "space" or site. **Allosteric enzymes are those having other site**. Like all enzymes, allosteric enzymes have catalytic sites which bind the substrate and transform it, but they also have one or more regulatory or allosteric sites for binding **regulatory metabolites** which is called **effector** or **modulator** or **modifier**.

Allosteric enzymes may be inhibited or stimulated by their effectors or modulators **(Figure 5.12)** and effectors that inhibit enzyme activity are termed **negative effectors** whereas those that increase enzyme activity are called *positive effectors.* **Some examples are given in Table 5.6**.

Just as the catalytic site of an enzyme is specific for its substrate, the allosteric site is specific for its modulators. Allosteric enzyme molecules are generally larger and more complex than those of simple enzymes. Most of them have two or more polypeptide chains or subunits.

Allosteric enzymes do not obey the Michaelis-Menten behavior. A **sigmoid saturation curve** results rather than the classical **hyperbolic** substrate saturation curve as shown by nonregulatory enzyme **(Figure 5.13)**.

Feedback Allosteric Regulation

In some multienzyme systems, the first enzyme of the sequence is the regulatory allosteric enzyme and has distinctive characteristics.

- It is inhibited by the end product of the multienzyme system whenever the end product of such metabolic reaction produced in excess of the cell's needs. The end product of the sequence acts as a **specific inhibitor** of the first or regulatory enzyme in the sequence.
- The whole enzyme system thus slows down to bring the rate of production of its end product back into balance with the cell's needs. This type of regulation is called **allosteric feedback regulation (Figure 5.14)**.

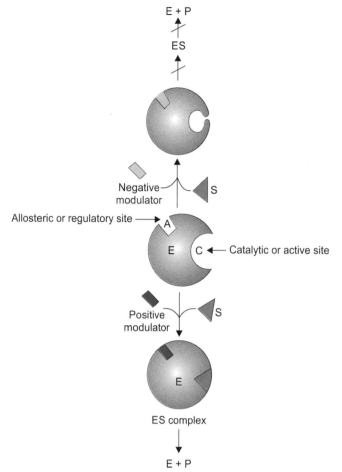

Figure 5.12: Mechanism for the inhibition and stimulation by modulator of allosteric enzyme.

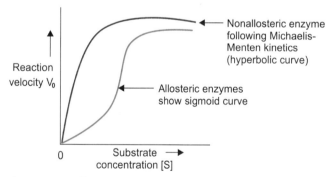

Figure 5.13: Effect of substrate concentration on reaction velocity for an allosteric enzyme.

TABLE 5.6: Allosteric enzymes and its modulators.			
Pathways	**Enzymes**	**Inhibitors**	**Activators**
Glycolysis	Phosphofructokinase-1 Pyruvate kinase	ATP and citrate ATP and acetyl-CoA	AMP –
Conversion of pyruvate to acetyl-CoA	Pyruvate dehydrogenase	ATP, NADH and acetyl-CoA	–
TCA cycle	Isocitrate dehydrogenase	ATP	ADP
Glycogenolysis	Glycogen phosphorylase	ATP	AMP
Gluconeogenesis	Fructose-1,6-bisphosphatase Pyruvate carboxylase	AMP –	ATP and citrate Acetyl-CoA
Fatty acid synthesis	Acetyl-CoA carboxylase	–	Citrate

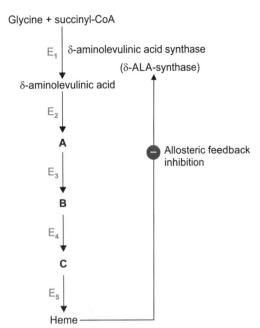

Figure 5.14: Feedback inhibition. First enzyme δ-ALA-synthase is an allosteric enzyme inhibited by its end product heme.

Reversible Covalent Modification

Covalent modification of enzymes is a means of regulating enzyme activity. The covalent attachment/removal of a molecule to an enzyme modifies its activity. Most modifications are reversible. Some of the common methods of covalent modifications are **(Table 5.7)**:

- Phosphorylation and dephosphorylation (most common covalent modification)
- Acetylation and deacetylation
- ADP ribosylation
- Ubiquitination.

Phosphorylation and Dephosphorylation

- **Phosphorylation and dephosphorylation** are the most common means of covalent modification. The enzymes catalyzing phosphorylation reactions are called **protein kinases**. ATP is the most common donor of phosphoryl group. Phosphoryl group of ATP is transferred to a specific amino acid of the enzyme,

commonly one of the three hydroxyl group containing amino acids; **serine**, **threonine** or **tyrosine**.
- **Protein phosphatase** reverses the effects of kinases by catalyzing the removal of phosphoryl groups attached to proteins.
- For example, phosphorylation of **glycogen phosphorylase** (an enzyme that degrades glycogen to glucose) increases activity whereas the removal of phosphate from glycogen phosphorylase inactivates the enzyme.

Acetylation and Deacetylation

- The attachment of acetyl groups and their removal are another common means. Histone (proteins), that are packaged with DNA into chromosomes are extensively acetylated and deacetylated *in vivo* on lysine residues. More heavily acetylated histones are associated with genes that are being actively transcribed.
- The acetyltransferase and deacylase enzymes are themselves regulated by phosphorylation. Thus, the covalent modification of an enzyme can be controlled by the covalent modification of the modifying enzyme.

ADP-ribosylation

Poly-ADP-ribosylation, also known as parylation, is the post-translational modification process by which polymers of ADP-ribose (adenosine diphosphate-ribose) are covalently attached to proteins by PAR (Poly-ADP-ribose) polymerase enzymes. The polymerase covalently attaches ADP-ribose polymer to histones and other DNA-associated proteins. Parylation regulates chromatin organization, DNA repair, transcription and replication and other processes.

Ubiquitination

The attachment of the small **protein ubiquitin** can signal that a protein is to be destroyed, the ultimate means of regulation. The protein **cyclin** must be ubiquitinated and destroyed before a cell can enter anaphase and proceed through the cell cycle.

Proteolytic Cleavage of Proenzymes/Zymogens

Many enzymes are activated by specific **proteolytic cleavage**. Some enzymes are inactive until the cleavage of one or few specific peptide bonds. Such an inactive form of enzyme is called a **zymogen** or **proenzyme**. Proteolytic cleavage does not require an energy source such as ATP. As well as proteolytic activation, in contrast with allosteric control and reversible covalent modification, takes place just **one in the life** of an enzyme molecule. Specific proteolysis is a common means of activating enzymes.

	Donor molecules	Examples of modified protein	Enzyme functions
TABLE 5.7: Covalent modifications of enzyme activity.			
Modifications			
Phosphorylation	ATP	Glycogen phosphorylase Glycogen synthase	Glycogen metabolism
Acetylation	Acetyl-CoA	Histones	DNA packing into chromosome
Ubiquitination	Ubiquitin	Cyclin	Control of cell cycle
ADP-ribosylation	NAD+	RNA polymerase	Transcription

- The digestive enzymes that hydrolyze proteins are synthesized as zymogens in the stomach and pancreas **(Table 5.1)**.
- Some protein hormones are synthesized as inactive precursors. For example, insulin is derived from **proinsulin** by proteolytic removal of a peptide.
- Blood clotting is mediated by a cascade of proteolytic activations.
- The fibrous protein collagen, the major constituent of skin and bone, is derived from **procollagen**.
- Programmed cell death, or **apoptosis**, is mediated by proteolytic enzymes called **caspases**, which are synthesized in precursors form as **precaspases**.

Induction and Repression of Enzyme Synthesis

The regulatory mechanism described above modifies the activity of existing enzyme molecules. However, cells can also regulate the amount of enzyme present, usually by altering the rate of enzyme synthesis.

The increased (induction) or decreased (repression) synthesis of the proteins (enzymes) leads to an alteration in the total amount of active sites rather than influencing the efficiency of existing enzyme molecules. Enzymes, subject to regulation of synthesis, are often those that are needed at only one stage of development or under selected physiologic conditions. For example, elevated levels of insulin, due to high blood glucose levels, cause an increase in the synthesis of key enzymes involved in glucose metabolism.

In contrast, enzymes that are in constant use are usually not regulated by altering the rate of enzyme synthesis. Alterations in enzyme levels due to induction or repression of protein synthesis are slow (hours to days) compared to allosteric changes in activity which occur in seconds to minutes.

ENZYME INHIBITION: TYPES, EXAMPLES, KINETICS, CLINICAL AND THERAPEUTIC IMPORTANCE AND ENZYME INHIBITORS AS POISONS

Enzyme inhibitors are molecules that interfere with catalysis, slowing or halting enzymatic reactions. There are varieties of naturally occurring and synthetic compounds, which have the ability to bind reversibly or irreversibly to specific enzymes and alter their activity.

- From the study of enzyme inhibitors valuable information can be obtained about
    - Substrate specificity of enzymes
    - The nature of the functional groups at the active site
    - The mechanism of the catalytic activity.
- Enzyme inhibitors also are very useful in elucidating metabolic pathways in cells.
- Moreover, enzyme inhibitors include **drugs**, **antibiotics**, **toxins** and **antimetabolites** as well as many **natural**

products of the enzyme reactions have therapeutic applications.

Most enzyme inhibitors act **reversibly**, but there are also **irreversible inhibitors** that permanently modify the target enzyme.

- Reversible inhibitors bind to enzymes through **noncovalent** bonds. Reversible inhibition implies that the activity of the enzyme is restored fully when the inhibitor physically is removed from the system.
- An irreversible in contrast with reversible inhibitor dissociates very slowly from its target enzyme because it has become tightly bound to the enzyme, either covalently or noncovalently.

Types of Enzyme Inhibition

Different types of enzyme inhibitions are:
1. Competitive or substrate analog inhibition
2. Noncompetitive inhibition
3. Uncompetitive inhibition
4. Suicide inhibition

Using **Lineweaver-Burk plot**, it is possible to distinguish three forms of reversible inhibition: competitive, noncompetitive and uncompetitive inhibition.

Competitive Inhibitor

The competitive inhibitors (I) often **resemble the substrate** and binds to the **active site** (substrate binding site) of the enzyme, the substrate is thereby prevented from binding to the same active site. Formation of an EI complex rather than ES complex occurs **(Figure 5.15)**.

A competitive inhibitor diminishes the rate of catalysis by reducing the proportion of ES complex. By increasing the substrate concentration competitive inhibition can be relieved and thus it is a **reversible type of inhibition**.

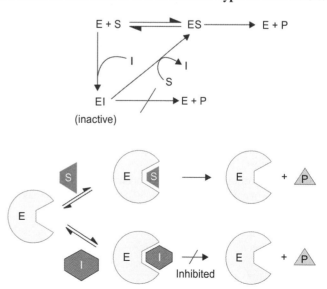

Figure 5.15: A competitive inhibitor binds at the active site and prevents the substrate from binding.

(E = Enzyme; S = Substrate; I = Competitive inhibitor; P = Product)

When substrate concentration [S] far exceeds [I], the substrate successfully competes with the inhibitor for the binding to the enzyme and reaction exhibits a **normal V$_{max}$** but **raises K$_m$ (Figure 5.16)**. In the presence of inhibitor, high concentrations of substrate are needed to approach that V$_{max}$.

The example of competitive inhibition

- **Methotrexate: Methotrexate**, drug used to treat cancer is a potent competitive inhibitor of the enzyme dihydrofolate reductase. Dihydrofolate reductase plays a role in biosynthesis of purines and pyrimidines. Methotrexate is a structural analog of dihydrofolate (substrate of dihydrofolate reductase).

- **Sulfonamide**, antibiotic is an analog of P-aminobenzoic acid (PABA) **(Figure 5.17)** and inhibits **dihydropteroate synthetase** enzyme required for the synthesis of **folic acid** in microorganisms. Since folic acid is involved in the biosynthesis of purines and thymine, sulfonamides inhibit growth of the pathogenic organisms. The drug is nontoxic to human, because human beings cannot synthesize folic acid. **Sulfonamide is** used to treat pneumonia, urinary tract infections, and shigellosis.

- **Physostigmine:** It inhibits **acetylcholine esterase** and use to treat glaucoma and myasthenia gravis.

- **Isoniazid [Isonicotinic acid Hydrazide (INH)]:** It is an antituberculous drug, an analog of nicotinamide **(Figure 5.18)**. Biosynthesis of NAD requires incorporation of nicotinamide moiety. Isoniazid an analog of nicotinamide interferes with the biosynthesis of NAD and restricts the growth of the organisms that cause human tuberculosis.

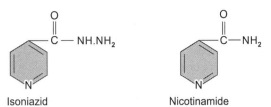

Figure 5.18: Structure of isoniazid and nicotinamide.

- **Dicumarol (Bishydroxy coumarin):** It is an anticoagulant drug that inhibits the formation of **prothrombin** in the liver. Dicumarol is an analog of vitamin K, which inhibit the enzyme **epoxide reductase** involved in liver **vitamin-K cycle *(see Figure 9.34).*** Dicumarol is used in the treatment of **thrombosis**, or **intravascular clotting**. This was the first drug to be used clinically to prolong the clotting time of blood by inhibiting the vitamin K activity.

- Drugs such an **ibuprofen** (anti-inflammatory drug), **statin** (cholesterol lowing drug) are competitive inhibitors of enzymes that involved in the inflammatory response and cholesterol synthesis respectively.

- Some competitive inhibitor which is not a drug is— **Malonate** inhibits an enzyme succinate dehydrogenase. Malonate compete with the substrate **succinate**.

> **The Medical Therapy for Methanol Poisoning based on Competitive Inhibition**
>
> The therapy for **methanol poisoning** is slow intravenous infusion of **ethanol** at a rate that maintains a controlled concentration in the bloodstream for several hours. This slows the formation of **formaldehyde**, lessening the danger while the kidneys filter out the methanol to be excreted harmlessly in the urine.
>
> The liver enzyme **alcohol dehydrogenase** converts methanol to formaldehyde, which is toxic to tissue. Ethanol competes effectively with methanol as an alternative substrate for alcohol dehydrogenase. The effect of ethanol is like that of a competitive inhibitor, with characteristic that ethanol is also a substrate for alcohol dehydrogenase and its concentration will decrease over time as the enzyme converts it to acetaldehyde.

Noncompetitive Inhibitors

Two types of noncompetitive inhibition are:

1. Reversible noncompetitive inhibition
2. Irreversible noncompetitive inhibition

Most of the noncompetitive inhibitions are irreversible, only few are reversible.

In noncompetitive inhibition, the inhibitor and substrate can bind simultaneously to an enzyme at sight distinct from the substrate-binding site and bear no structural resemblance to the substrate **(Figure 5.19)**. A noncompetitive inhibitor can bind **free enzyme** or the **enzyme substrate complex**.

In noncompetitive inhibition even after binding of inhibitor to enzyme, substrate can still bind to the EI complex. Formation of both EI and EIS complexes is

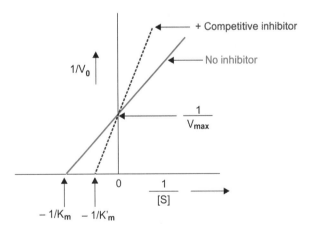

Figure 5.16: A double-reciprocal plot of enzyme kinetics in presence and absence of competitive inhibitor, V$_{max}$ is unaltered whereas K$_m$ is increased.

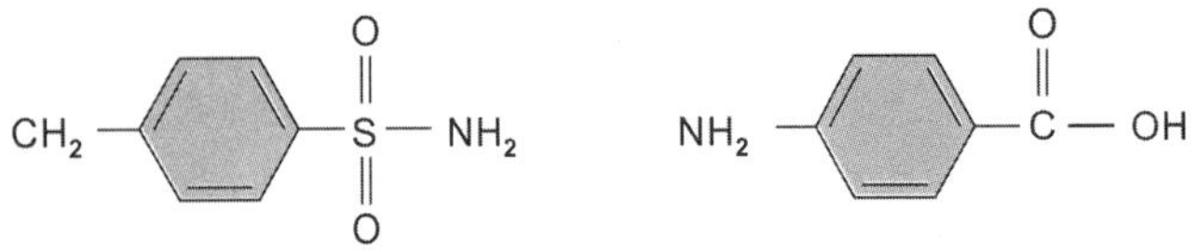

Figure 5.17: Structure of sulfonamide and para-aminobenzoic acid.

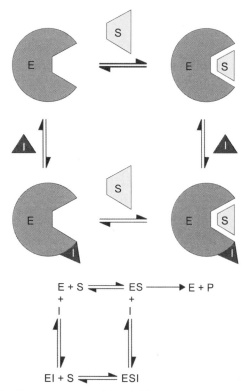

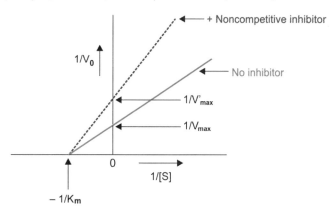

Figure 5.19: A noncompetitive inhibitor does not prevent the substrate from binding.

(E: Enzyme; S: Substrate; I: Noncompetitive inhibitor; P: Product)

Figure 5.20: A double-reciprocal plot of enzyme kinetics in presence and absence of noncompetitive inhibitor; K_m is unaltered by noncompetitive inhibitor, Whereas V_{max} is decreased.

therefore possible. E and EI possess identical affinity for the substrate. Noncompetitive inhibitor does not affect binding of the substrate to enzyme and thus the value of **K_m is unchanged** However, EIS complex does not continue to form product and the value of **V_{max} is decreased** **(Figure 5.20)**.

The example of noncompetitive inhibition

- **Doxycycline**, an antibiotic, functions at low concentrations as a noncompetitive inhibitor of a proteolytic enzyme, **collagenase**. It is used to treat periodontal disease.
- Most of the irreversible noncompetitive inhibitors are mostly poisonous agents **(Table 5.8)**. Almost all

TABLE 5.8: Irreversible noncompetitive inhibitors.	
Noncompetitive inhibitors	**Target enzymes**
Arsenite	Alpha ketoglutarate dehydrogenase
British anti-Lewisite	SH group of several enzymes
Cyanide	Cytochrome c oxidase
Fluoride	Enolase
Fluoroacetate	Aconitase
Iodoacetate	Glyceraldehyde-4-phosphate dehydrogenase
Diisopropyl fluorophosphate	Serine proteases

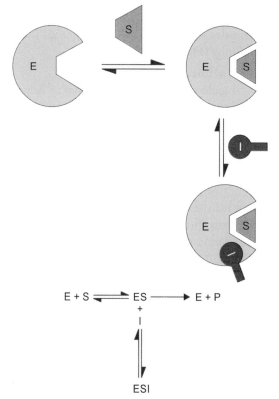

Figure 5.21: Uncompetitive inhibitor binds only to the enzyme-substrate complex.

(E: Enzyme; S: Substrate; I: Uncompetitive inhibitor; P: Product)

inhibitors of electron transport chain are examples of irreversible noncompetitive inhibition.

Uncompetitive Inhibitor

Uncompetitive inhibitor can bind only to the **enzyme-substrate (ES)** complex. The uncompetitive inhibitor's binding site is created only on interaction of the enzyme and substrate **(Figure 5.21)**. This enzyme-substrate-inhibitor complex, ESI does not continue to form any product and some unproductive ESI complex is formed.

The inhibitor causes a **decrease in V_{max}** because a fraction of the enzyme-substrate complex diverted by the inhibitor to the **inactive ESI complex**. Binding of the inhibitor and an increase in stability of the ESI complex may also affect the **dissociation of substrate**, causing

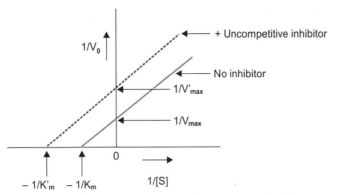

Figure 5.22: Effect of uncompetitive inhibitor on the double-reciprocal plot; it shows parallel lines with decrease in both V_{max} and K_m.

an apparent decrease in K_m, i.e., an apparent increase in substrate affinity **(Figure 5.22)**.

The example of uncompetitive inhibition:
- The herbicide **glyphosate**, also known as **Roundup**, is an uncompetitive inhibitor of an enzyme in the biosynthetic pathway for aromatic amino acids in bacteria but is fairly nontoxic in animals because they lack the enzyme.
- **Lithium compounds**, (lithium salts), used for the treatment of major **depressive disorder** inhibits the enzyme **inositol monophosphatase** by uncompetitive mechanism. Inositol monophosphatase is involved in degradation of inositol monophosphate to inositol. Lithium exerts its therapeutic action by interfering with phosphatidylinositol metabolism in brain.
- **Placental alkaline phosphatase** by **phenylalanine** is an example of uncompetitive inhibitions.

Suicide Inhibitor or Mechanism-based Inactivation

Suicide inhibitors or mechanism-based inhibitors are **irreversible inhibitors**, bind to the **active site of enzyme**. The inhibitor (which is initially unreactive) binds to the enzyme as a substrate and initially carries out the first few normal catalytic activities of the enzyme reaction. The

mechanism of catalysis then generates a chemically reactive intermediate that inactivates the enzyme through covalent modification.

Thus the enzyme participates in its own irreversible inhibition strongly. These are called mechanism-based inhibitors because they utilize the normal enzyme reaction mechanism to inactivate the enzyme. These inhibitors have potential as drugs for example **(Table 5.9)**.
- Penicillin
- Aspirin
- Disulfiram (antabuse)
- N,N-Dimethylpropargylamine
- (–) Deprenyl
- Clavulanic acid

Penicillin: Penicillin irreversibly inactivates an essential bacterial enzyme **glycopeptidyl transpeptidase** involved in the formation of bacterial cell wall. This in turn, blocks synthesis of the bacterial cell wall, and most bacteria die as the fragile inner membrane bursts under osmotic pressure.

Why often overuse of β-lactam antibiotics (e.g., penicillin and its derivatives) by human, the bacteria become resistant to the antibiotic

Penicillin, the first antibiotic was discovered in 1928 by Alexander Fleming. Penicillin consists of a thiazolidine ring fused to a β-lactam ring. A β-lactam ring is very labile. Penicillin interferes with the synthesis of peptidoglycan, the major component of the rigid cell wall that protects bacteria from osmotic lysis. Peptidoglycan consists of polysaccharide and peptides that are cross linked by transpeptidase. Penicillin binds to the active site of transpeptidase through β-lactam ring. The covalent complex between penicillin and the enzyme irreversibly inactivates the enzyme.

Use of penicillin and its derivatives by human has led to the evolution of strains of pathogenic bacteria that start producing β-lactamases enzymes that cleave β-lactam ring of antibiotics, making antibiotic inactive and thus by the often overuse of β-lactam antibiotics by human the bacteria become resistant to the antibiotic.

Drugs	Types of inhibition	Target enzymes	Therapeutic uses
Mevinolin and Lovastatin	Competitive	HMG-CoA reductase (3-hydroxy-3-methylglutaryl-CoA reductase)	Hypercholesterolemia
Allopurinol	Competitive	Xanthine oxidase	Gout
Methotrexate	Competitive	Dihydrofolate reductase	Cancer
Captopril and Enalapril	Competitive	Angiotensin-converting enzyme (ACE)	High blood pressure
5-fluorouracil	Suicide	Thymidylate synthase	Cancer
Aspirin	Suicide	Cyclo-oxygenase	Anti-inflammatory
Penicillin	Suicide	Bacterial transpeptidase	Antibacterial
N,N-Dimethylpropargylamine	Suicide	Monoamine oxidase	Antidepressant, Parkinson's disease
(-) Deprenyl	Suicide	Monoamine oxidase	Antidepressant, Parkinson's disease

TABLE 5.9: Commonly used drugs that are enzyme inhibitors.

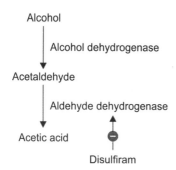

Alcohol

↓ Alcohol dehydrogenase

Acetaldehyde

↓ Aldehyde dehydrogenase

Acetic acid ⊖

Disulfiram

Figure 5.23: Action of disulfiram.

Aspirin: Aspirin inactivates an enzyme **cyclooxygenase** which catalyses the first reaction in the biosynthesis of prostaglandins from arachidonic acid. Aspirin is used as an anti-inflammatory, antipyretic and analgesic drug. Aspirin is also used prophylactically to inhibit platelet aggregation and coronary thrombosis.

Disulfiram: Disulfiram is a drug used in the treatment of alcoholism. It inhibits irreversibly **aldehyde dehydrogenase** enzyme resulting in accumulation of acetaldehyde in the body **(Figure 5.23)**. Accumulation of acetaldehyde in the tissue leads to alcohol avoidance.

Disulfiram is used to treat chronic alcoholism. It causes unpleasant effects when even small amounts of alcohol are consumed. These effects include **flushing of the face, headache, nausea, vomiting, chest pain, weakness, blurred vision, mental confusion, sweating, choking, breathing difficulty, and anxiety**.

N,N-Dimethylpropargylamine: An inhibitor of the enzyme **monoamine oxidase (MAO)** an enzyme deaminates neurotransmitters such as **dopamine** and **serotonin** and lowers their levels in the brain. Parkinson's disease is associated with low levels of dopamine and depression is associated with low levels of serotonin.

Monoamine oxidase requires a cofactor FAD. FAD of monoamine oxidase oxidizes the N, N-Dimethylpropargylamine which in turn inactivates the enzyme by binding covalently to N-5 of the flavin prosthetic group of FAD.

(–)Deprenyl: Deprenyl, a drug is used to treat **Parkinson's** disease and **depression**. It is a **suicide inhibitor** of monoamine oxidase.

Clavulanic acid: Clavulanic acid is a suicide inhibitor of β-lactamases. β-lactamase is an enzyme of pathogenic bacteria that cleave lactam ring in β-lactam antibiotics (e.g., penicillin), making inactive and resistant to the antibiotic.

Chemical Warfare between Humans and Bacteria

The cycle of chemical battle between humans and bacteria continues nonstop due to the evolution of strains of pathogenic bacteria. Human medicine responded with the clavulanic acid, a suicide inhibitor, which inactivates the β-lactamases (that cleave β-lactam ring of antibiotics, making antibiotic inactive).

Contd...

TABLE 5.10: Enzyme inhibitors as poisons.

Poisons	Enzyme inhibited	Impairment in pathway
Arsenate Fluoride	Glyceraldehyde-3-phosphate dehydrogenase Enolase	Inhibition of glycolysis
Cyanide	Cytochrome oxidase	Inhibition of ETC
Electron transport inhibitors Rotenone Antimycin Amobarbital Piericidin A	Inhibit transfer of reducing equivalents in ETC	Inhibition of ETC
Malonate	Succinate dehydrogenase	Inhibition of TCA cycle
Diisopropyl fluorophosphate (nerve gas)	Acetylcholinesterase	Impair nerve conduction
Melathione (organophosphorus insecticide)	Acetylcholinesterase	Impair nerve conduction

Contd...

Amoxicillin and clavulanic acid are combined with the trade name **Augmentin**. Strains of disease-causing bacteria that are resistant to both amoxicillin and clavulanic acids have been discovered. Mutations in β-lactamase within these strains make it unreactive to clavulanic acid.

Enzyme Inhibitors as Metabolic Poisons

Many **poisons** work by **inhibiting** the action of **enzymes** involved in **metabolic processes**, which hampers the metabolic pathways. Enzyme poisons are basically enzyme inhibitors. This inhibition can be reversible or irreversible. Most of the poisons, however act irreversibly. Some common examples of enzyme poisons are given in **Table 5.10**.

ISOENZYME: DEFINITION, EXAMPLES AND DIAGNOSTIC IMPORTANCE

Definition

Isoenzymes or isozymes are multiple forms (isomers) of the same enzyme, but catalyze the same reaction. The different isoenzymes catalyze the same chemical reaction but **differ in their primary structure and kinetic properties**. They are encoded by different genes located at different loci. Not all enzymes have isoenzymes. In fact, only those enzymes, which are **polymeric**, demonstrate isoenzyme.

Characteristics of Isoenzyme

Isoenzymes show different chemical and physical properties such as:

- Electrophoretic mobility.
- Kinetic properties
- Amino acid sequence
- Amino acid composition.

STRIKE A NOTE

Isoenzymes:
- ❖ They are encoded by different genes located at different loci
- ❖ Catalyse the same chemical reaction
- ❖ Same EC number
- ❖ Differ in structure
- ❖ Differ in electrophoretic mobility
- ❖ Differ in tissue location
- ❖ Differ in k_m value

Examples of Isoenzyme and Diagnostic Importance

Isoenzymes of lactate dehydrogenase (LDH) and creatine kinase (CK) (formerly called creatine phosphokinase, CPK) are discussed here. Some more examples of enzymes having isoenzyme forms are **acid phosphatase**, **alkaline phosphatase; amylase, hexokinase**, etc., are given in **Table 5.11**. The appearance of some isoenzymes in blood is a sign of tissue damage, useful for clinical diagnosis.

Lactate Dehydrogenase

Lactate dehydrogenase (LDH) is a **tetrameric** enzyme that catalyzes the oxidation of L-lactate to pyruvate.

- LDH has five isoenzymes: **LDH$_1$, LDH$_2$, LDH$_3$, LDH$_4$, and LDH$_5$.**
- LDH is made up of two types of polypeptide **M (*muscle*)** type and **H (*heart*)** type. Since LDH is a tetramer, five combinations are possible with varying ratios of two kinds of polypeptides **(Table 5.12)**.
- Five isoenzymes of LDH can be detected by electrophoresis as they have different electrophoretic mobility. **LDH$_1$** is the **fastest moving** fraction toward the anode and **LDH$_5$** is the **slowest moving** isoenzyme of LDH **(Figure 5.24)**.
- LDH isoenzyme content varies by tissue. Tissue-specific expression for the H and M genes determines the relative proportion of each subunit in different tissues. LDH$_1$ (H$_4$) predominates in cells of cardiac muscle and

TABLE 5.11: Examples of isoenzymes.

Enzymes	Isoenzyme forms
Lactate dehydrogenase (LDH)	LDH$_1$, LDH$_2$, LDH$_3$, LDH$_4$, LDH$_5$
Creatine kinase (CK)	CK$_1$, CK$_2$, CK$_3$
Acid phosphatase	Prostate, erythrocytes, platelets, liver, spleen, kidney and bone marrow
Alkaline phosphatase	Bone, liver, placenta, intestine and kidney
Amylase	Salivary and pancreatic
Hexokinase	Liver (glucokinase) and muscle

TABLE 5.12: Type, composition, location and diagnostic importance of lactate dehydrogenase (LDH).

Type	Composition	Location	Diagnostic importance (cause of elevated level)
LDH$_1$	HHHH	Heart, RBC	Myocardial infarction
LDH$_2$	HHHM	Heart, RBC	Kidney diseases, megaloblastic anemia
LDH$_3$	HHMM	Brain, kidneys	Leukemia, malignancy
LDH$_4$	HMMM	Lung, spleen	Pulmonary infarction
LDH$_5$	MMMM	Liver, muscle	Liver diseases, muscle damage/diseases

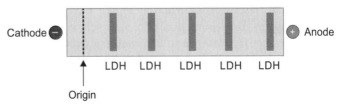

Figure 5.24: Electrophoretic separation of LDH isoenzyme.

erythrocytes, whereas LDH$_5$ (M$_4$) is most abundant form in the liver and skeletal muscle **(Table 5.12)**.

Normal Levels of LDH

Values for LDH activity in serum vary considerably, depending on the type of method used.
- The normal serum value is **100–200 U/L.**
- LDH level is 100 times more inside the RBC than in plasma and therefore hemolysis will give false result.

Diagnostic Importance of LDH

The LDH isoenzyme analysis may be useful in the following clinical situations **(Table 5.12)**:
- Significant elevation of LDH$_1$ and LDH$_2$ (LDH$_1$ > LDH$_2$) occurs within **24–48 hours** after **myocardial infarction** (MI). Normally LDH$_2$ is present in higher concentration than LDH$_1$. But this pattern is reversed in MI and called **flipped pattern** of LDH.
- **Megaloblastic anemia**, resulting from the deficiency of **folate** or **vitamin B$_{12}$**, cause the erythrocyte precursor cell to break down in the bone marrow resulting in the release of large quantities of LDH$_1$ and LDH$_2$ isoenzyme.
- Moderately increased LDH$_5$ activity is found in **muscular dystrophy**.
- Elevations of serum LDH$_5$ activity are found in **liver disease** especially in cases of toxic hepatitis with jaundice.
- Predominant elevation of LDH$_2$ and LDH$_3$ occur in **leukemia**. LDH$_3$ is the main isoenzyme elevated due to **malignancy** of many tissues.
- Especially high values of total LDH are associated with **Hodgkin's** disease and **abdominal** and **lung cancers**. The serum LDH level has been shown to correlate with

tumor mass in solid tumors and provides a prognostic indicator for disease progression.

Creatine Kinase

Creatin kinase (CK) catalyzes the reversible phosphorylation of creatine to creatine phosphate by ATP. Physiologically when muscle contracts, ATP are consumed to form ADP, and CK catalyzes the rephosphorylation of ADP to form ATP, using creatine phosphate as the phosphate donor.

- CK activity is greatest in striated muscle, brain, and heart tissue. **The liver and erythrocytes are essentially devoid of CK activity.** Other tissues, such as the kidneys and the diaphragm, contain significantly less activity.
- Creatine kinase isoenzymes are dimer that are made up of two types of polypeptide chains, which may be either **M (muscle)** type or **B (brain)** type, generating three isoenzymes **(Table 5.13)**:
  - **CK_1 (BB)** (present in brain)
  - **CK_2 (MB)** (present in cardiac tissue)
  - **CK_3 (MM)** (present in skeletal muscle and cardiac muscles).
- **Cardiac tissue** is the only tissue which has the **mixed MB (CK_2)** isoenzyme. Detection of **CK_2 (MB)** in serum is strongly suggestive of **myocardial damage**.

Normal Levels of CK

Normal serum value for total CK is:
- 15–100 U/L for males
- 10–80 U/L for females.

Diagnostic Importance of Creatine Kinase

Creatine kinase activity is elevated in many diseases, including those involving skeletal muscle, heart, central nervous system, and thyroid.

- CK-1 levels in CSF increase in neonates particularly in brain damaged or very low birth weight newborn and after certain types of neurological injury, e.g., **head injury**
- Increased level of **CK_2** in blood is characteristic of **damage of heart** tissue from myocardial infarction. In addition, serum CK_2 often is detected in those individuals with head injuries and in cases of

subarachnoid hemorrhage. **This appearance of CK_2 suggests myocardial damage after the cerebral accident.**

- Elevated levels of **CK_3** in serum occur in all types of **dystrophies** and **myopathies**.
- Serum CK activity shows an inverse relationship with thyroid activity. Hypothyroidism shows an elevation of CK activity. The major isoenzyme present is CK_3. In hyperthyroidism the serum CK activity tends to be at the low end of the normal values.

ALLOENZYMES

- Alloenzymes (or also called allozymes) are **variant forms** of an enzyme (due to mutation) which differs structurally but not functionally from other allozymes. They catalyse the same type of reaction.
- These are coded by **different alleles** (mutated forms of same gene) at the same locus
- These are opposed to **isozymes**, which are coded by **different genes located at different loci**
- For example, over 300 allelic variants of **glucose-6-phosphate dehydrogenase (G6PD)** have been identified; all of them are produced by the same locus.
- Though variant forms of alloenzyme are present, only one form will be present in one individual. However all the different forms will be seen in total population.
- WHO classifies these G6PD genetic variants into five classes according to the level of enzyme activity in the red cells.
  1. Class I includes severely deficient variants
  2. Class II variants have less than 10% of enzyme activity
  3. Class III variants have 10–60% enzyme activity
  4. Class IV variants have normal enzyme activity
  5. Class V the enzyme activity is increased

DIAGNOSTICALLY IMPORTANT SERUM ENZYMES

Enzymes are known as marker of **cellular damage** and **pathological conditions**. Their measurement in plasma is used in the investigation of diseases of **liver, cardiac**, and **skeletal muscle**, the **biliary tract**, and the **pancreas**. The enzymes that are found in plasma can be categorized into two major groups:
1. The plasma-specific enzyme
2. The plasma-nonspecific enzyme.

Plasma-specific Enzymes

The plasma-specific enzymes are those enzymes that have a definite and specific function in plasma. Plasma is their normal site of action, and they are present in higher concentration in plasma than in most tissues, e.g.,
- The enzymes involved in blood coagulation
- Lipoprotein lipase.

TABLE 5.13: Type, composition, location and diagnostic importance of creatine kinase (CK) isoenzymes.

Type	Composition	Location	Diagnostic importance (cause of elevated level)
CK_1	BB	Brain prostate, gland GI tract, lung, bladder, uterus	Neurological injury, tumor marker
CK_2	BM	Heart	Myocardial infarction
CK_3	MM	Skeletal muscle	Muscular dystrophies and myopathies

TABLE 5.14: Enzymes of diagnostic importance.		
Enzymes	**Locations**	**Clinical applications**
Acid phosphatase	Prostate, erythrocyte	Prostatic cancer
Alanine aminotransferase	Liver, skeletal muscle, heart	Hepatic parenchymal disease
Aldolase	Skeletal muscle, heart	Muscle diseases
Alkaline phosphatase	Liver, bone, kidney, intestinal mucosa, placenta	Bone disease, hepatobiliary disease
Amylase	Salivary glands, pancreas	Pancreatic diseases, peptic ulcer
Aspartate transaminase	Liver, skeletal muscle, heart, kidney, erythrocytes	Myocardial infarction, hepatic parenchymal disease, muscle disease, anemia
Cholinesterase	Liver	Organophosphorus insecticide poisoning, hepatic parenchymal diseases
Creatine kinase	Skeletal muscle, brain, heart, smooth muscle	Myocardial infarction, muscle diseases
γ-glutamyl transferase	Liver, kidney	Hepatobiliary disease, alcoholism
Lactate dehydrogenase	Heart, liver, skeletal muscle, erythrocytes, platelets, lymph nodes	Myocardial infarction, hemolysis, hepatic parenchymal diseases
5'-nucleotidase	Hepatobiliary tract	Hepatobiliary disease
Prostate specific antigen	Prostate	Prostate cancer
Trypsin	Pancreas	Pancreatic disease, cystic fibrosis

These enzymes are synthesized in liver and are constantly liberated into plasma. These enzymes are clinically of interest when their concentration decreases in plasma.

Plasma-nonspecific Enzymes

Plasma-nonspecific enzymes are those enzymes with no known function in plasma. The concentration of these enzymes in tissue is very high than in the plasma.

Pathological damage to a tissue increases permeability of the cell membrane and allows cytoplasmic enzymes to leak into the blood. A severe attack causing cell necrosis also disrupts the mitochondrial membrane, and both cytoplasmic and mitochondrial enzymes are detected in blood.

Not all intracellular enzymes are equally valuable as indicators of cellular damage. The main enzymes of established clinical value, together with their tissues of origin and clinical significances are listed in **Table 5.14**.

Classification of Diagnostically Important Enzymes

Diagnostically important enzymes can be categorized as follow:
1. Liver, cardiac and skeletal enzymes
2. Biliary tract enzymes
3. Digestive enzymes of pancreatic origin
4. Other enzymes of clinical utility and tumor marker enzymes.

Liver, Cardiac, and Skeletal Enzymes

Enzymes in this category include the:
- Aminotransferases or transaminases
- Alkaline phosphatase
- Creatine kinase
- Lactate dehydrogenase.

Aminotransferases or Transaminases

The aminotransferases are a group of enzymes that catalyze the interconversion of amino acids to keto acids by transfer of amino groups. The examples of aminotransferases of clinical interest are:
- Aspartate aminotransferase, also known as aspartate transaminase, (AST). It was known formerly as serum glutamate oxaloacetate transaminase (SGOT)
- Alanine aminotransferase, also known as alanine transaminase, (ALT). It was known formerly as serum glutamate pyruvate transaminase (SGPT)

Normal value of AST and ALT:
- The plasma AST normal value for adults is **10–30 U/L**
- The plasma ALT normal value for adults is **10–40 U/L**. Values for men slightly higher than those in women.

Clinical significance:
- **AST** is present in high concentrations in cells of **cardiac, liver, skeletal muscle** and **kidney**. Damage of any of these tissues may increase plasma AST.
- **ALT** is present in high concentration in **liver** and to a lesser extent in skeletal muscle kidney and heart.
- Both plasma AST and ALT levels are elevated in liver disease
- **Although serum levels of both AST and ALT become elevated in liver diseases, ALT is the more liver-specific enzyme.** Plasma ALT elevations are rarely observed in conditions other than liver disease. Moreover, elevations of ALT activity persist longer than do those of AST activity.

- **Increased AST level** occurs after **myocardial infarction** as heart muscles contain relatively high concentration of AST.
  - The plasma AST level starts increasing **after 6–8 hours** after the onset of chest pain with **peak values 18–24 hours** proportional to the extent of cardiac damage and the values fall to normal level by the fourth or fifth day, provided no new infarct has occurred.
  - **ALT levels** are within normal limits or only marginally increased in cases of uncomplicated myocardial infarction because the concentration of ALT in heart muscle is only a fraction of that of AST activity.
- AST (occasionally ALT) activity levels are increased (up 8 times normal) in progressive **muscular dystrophy** and **dermatomyositis**. They are usually normal in other types of muscle disease.
- Slight or moderate elevations of both AST and ALT activities have been observed after intake of alcohol and after administration of various drugs such as opiates, salicylates, or ampicillin.

Alkaline Phosphatase (ALP)

The ALPs are a group of enzymes that hydrolyzes organic phosphates at alkaline pH. They are present in most tissues but are in particularly high concentration in intestinal epithelial cell, kidney tubules, bone (osteoblast), liver, and placenta.

In adults plasma, ALP is derived mainly from bone and liver in approximately equal proportions. **Increased osteoblastic activity** increases the level of plasma ALP which may be physiological.

Normal value of ALP:
- Normal serum value for adults is 40–125 IU/L
- During pregnancy, the plasma total ALP level rises due to contribution of the placental isoenzymes.
- In children, the total activity is about 2.5 times more than the normal upper limit, because of the increased osteoblastic activity.

Clinical significance: Plasma ALP measurements are of particular interest in the investigation of **hepatobiliary disease**, and **bone disease** associated with increased osteoblastic activity.

Hepatobiliary disease:
- In extrahepatic obstruction (by stone or cancer of the head of the pancreas), the elevation of ALP is more significant than in intrahepatic obstruction, and usually return to normal on surgical removal of the obstruction
- Infectious hepatitis that affect liver parenchymal cells show normal plasma ALP level.

Bone diseases:
- Among bone diseases the highest levels (10–25 times the normal upper limit) of plasma ALP are seen with **Paget's disease**, a disease that disrupts the replacement of old bone tissue with new bone tissue. Plasma ALP

levels are elevated as a result of the action of the osteoblastic cells as they try to rebuild bone that is being resorbed by the uncontrolled activity of osteoclasts.
- Very high levels of plasma ALP occur in **bone cancer**
- Moderate rises are observed in **osteomalacia** and **rickets**
- Transient elevations may be found during healing of bone fractures.

STRIKE A NOTE

- ❖ *Regan isoenzyme* (named after the patient in whom it was detected) may occasionally be identified in plasma in patients with carcinoma of lung, liver and intestine.
- ❖ *Nago isoenzyme:* Variant of ALP of germ cell origin. Certain tumors also have produced ALPs called Nago isoenzyme that appear to be modified forms of nonplacental isoenzyme.
- ❖ *Kasahara isoenzyme:* Variant of ALP of fetal intestinal origin, seen in malignancy.

Creatine Kinase

Refer isoenzyme

Lactate Dehydrogenase

Refer isoenzyme

Biliary Tract Enzymes

Enzymes in this category include:
1. 5'-nucleotidase
2. γ-glutamyl transferase (GGT)

5'-Nucleotidase (Nucleotide Phosphatase, NTP)

NTP is distributed widely throughout the tissues and is localized in the cytoplasmic membrane of the cells in which it occurs. 5'-nucleotidase is a phosphatase that acts only on nucleoside 5'-phosphate such as AMP, releasing inorganic phosphates and adenosine.

Normal value:
- Normal serum NTP level is 2–17 U/L.
- Lower values have been reported in children.

Clinical significance:
- Increase in serum NTP (than ALP and GGT) occur in cholestasis (condition where bile cannot flow from the liver to the duodenum) due to mechanical blockage in the duct system that can occur from a gallstone or malignancy.
- Thus both NTP and ALP behave similarly in cases of hepatobiliary disease. But any significant rise in NTP is virtually specific for hepatobiliary disease because an increase in NTP activity is minimal in skeletal disease.

γ-Glutamyl Transferase

γ-Glutamyl transferase (GGT) is an enzyme found in many organs throughout the body, with the highest concentrations found in the liver. GGT catalyzes the transfer of the γ-glutamyl group from peptides to some acceptor. GGT is located in the cell membrane and may transport amino acids and peptides into the cell across the cell membrane in the form of γ-glutamyl peptides. GGT also involved in the synthesis of glutathione.

Normal serum value:
- For male 2–30 U/L
- For female 1–25 U/L.

Clinical significance:
- GGT is usually the first liver enzyme to rise in the blood by tumors or stones. This makes it the most sensitive liver enzyme test for detecting bile duct problems.
- However, the GGT test is not very specific and is not useful in differentiating between various causes of liver damage because it can be elevated with many types of liver diseases, such as liver cancer and viral hepatitis, as well as other nonhepatic conditions, such as acute coronary syndrome. For this reason, the GGT test is not recommended for routine use.
- GGT is often elevated in those who use alcohol or other liver-toxic substances to excess.
- The GGT test may be used in assessing someone for acute or chronic alcohol abuse.

Digestive Enzyme of Pancreatic Origin

The digestive enzymes such as, α-**amylase**, **lipase**, and **trypsin** secreted by pancreas are investigated for the diagnosis of pancreatic disease.

α-amylase (Calcium Metalloenzyme)

α-amylase, an enzyme that catalyzes the hydrolysis of α-1,4-glycosidic linkages in polysaccharides. The α-1,6 linkages at the branch points are not affected by the enzymes.
- α-amylase is the only enzyme normally found in urine because the enzyme is small enough to pass through the glomeruli and the kidneys.
- The greatest concentration is present in pancreas (**P-type**) synthesized by the acinar cells and then secreted into the intestinal tract via pancreatic duct system.
- The salivary glands also secrete α-amylase (**S-type**), which hydrolyzes starch in the mouth and esophagus.
- α-amylase activity also is found in semen, testes, ovaries, fallopian tubes, striated muscle, lungs, adipose tissue, colostrum, tears, and milk.

Normal serum value:
50–120 U/L.

Clinical significance:
- Assays of amylase activity in serum and urine are used primarily in the diagnosis of diseases of the **pancreas** and the investigation of **pancreatic function**.
- In cases of acute pancreatitis, a transient rise in serum amylase occurs.
- Ascitic and pleural fluids may contain amylase as a result of the presence of a tumor or pancreatitis.

- An increase in serum amylase may occur in some tumors of the lung.
- Hyperamylasemia occurs with salivary gland lesions caused by infection (mumps).

Lipase

Lipases enzymes hydrolyze triacylglycerol to β-monoglyceride and fatty acids. For catalytic activity of lipase, **bile salts** and cofactor called **colipase** are required. Most lipase found in serum is produced in the pancreas. Serum normal lipase value is 0.2–1.0 U/L.

Clinical significance:
- Lipase measurements on serum, plasma, ascitic and pleural fluid are used to investigate pancreatic disorders and pancreatitis.
- Acute pancreatitis may produce ascitic fluid, pleural fluid or both. These fluids may contain lipase activity.
- Obstruction of the pancreatic duct by a calculus or carcinoma of the pancreas may cause an increase in serum lipase activity.

Trypsin

Trypsin hydrolyzes the peptide bonds formed by the carboxyl groups of **lysine** or **arginine** with other amino acids. Natural trypsin inhibitors (α_1-antitrypsin) are present in pancreatic juice, serum, and urine. These inhibitors protect plasma and other proteins against hydrolysis by trypsin and other proteases. The absence of α_1-antitrypsin is associated with **emphysema** in early life.

Clinical significance:
- Determination of serum trypsin may be used to screen for **cystic fibrosis** during the first 6 weeks of life. Blockage of pancreatic ductules by sticky mucous secretion causes high serum trypsin concentrations. After about 6 weeks serum concentrations may fall as pancreatic insufficiency develops.
- Determination of trypsin in gastrointestinal secretions is used to evaluate pancreatic function and diagnose chronic pancreatitis and fibrocystic disease.

Other Enzymes of Clinical Utility and Tumor Marker Enzymes

It includes:
1. Acid phosphatase
2. Prostate-specific antigen
3. Tumor marker enzymes.

Acid Phosphatase

Acid phosphatase (ACP) hydrolyzes phosphoric acid ester at pH 5–6. It is found in different forms in the cells of the prostate, spleen, liver, erythrocytes, platelets, and bone. However, the ACP of greatest clinical importance is the one derived from the prostate.

STRIKE A NOTE

❖ Pancreatic isoenzyme (P-type) is not glycosylated, while salivary (S-type) may be glycosylated or deglycosylated.

❖ The ACPs particularly prostatic enzyme is unstable at room temperature above 37°C and at pH above 7.0 and more than 50% of the ACP activity may be lost in 1 hour at room temperature. Therefore, it should be transported to the lab rapidly.

❖ As ACP is present in very high concentration in semen, its measurement has become important in investigations of rape and similar offenses.

Normal values: Reference value for serum prostatic ACP is **0–0.6 U/L.**

Clinical significance:

● Prostatic acid phosphatase (PAP), also prostatic specific acid phosphatase (PSAP), is an **enzyme produced by the prostate**. It may be found in increased amounts in men who have prostate cancer or other diseases. The highest levels of acid phosphatase are found in metastasized prostate cancer.

● Although ACP once widely used to detect or monitor carcinoma of the prostate, determination of ACP level in serum now is used rarely for this purpose. It has been replaced by measurement of **prostate-specific antigen (PSA)**, a protein derived from prostate.

● Slight or moderate elevation in ACP level occurs in Paget's disease and bone cancer.

● Higher serum ACP level occurs in growing children, compared with adults due to increased osteoclastic activities in growing children.

● This enzyme is a useful marker of bone disorder.

Collection of sample for measurement of ACP

❖ Serum should be separated immediately from erythrocytes and stabilized by the addition of disodium citrate monohydrate at a level of 10 mg/mL of serum or 50 μL of acetic acid (5mol/L) per milliliter of serum is added to lower the pH to 5.4, at which the enzyme is stable.

❖ Under these conditions, activity is maintained at room temperature for several hours and for up to a week if the serum is refrigerated.

❖ Lipemic sera should not be used due to interference of turbidity with measurement.

Prostate-specific Antigen (Semenogelase)

Prostate specific antigen (PSA) is a **glycoprotein**, with mild **protease** activity. It is produced exclusively by normal, benign, hyperplastic and cancerous prostate glands but not by other tissues and involved in the liquification of the seminal coagulum formed after ejaculation. In the seminal fluid, PSA cleaves a seminal vesicle-specific protein into several low molecular weight proteins.

Clinical application:

● PSA is a tumor marker for prostate cancer. It is used to detect stage and monitor treatment of prostate cancer.

TABLE 5.15: Enzymes as tumor markers.

Enzymes	Types of cancer
Aldolase	Liver
Alkaline phosphatase	Bone, liver, leukemia, sarcoma
Placental alkaline phosphatase	Ovarian, lung, gastrointestinal, Hodgkin's disease
Amylase	Pancreatic
Creatine kinase	Prostate, lung, breast, colon, ovarian
γ-glutamyl transferase (GGT)	Liver
Lactate dehydrogenase (LDH)	Liver, lymphomas, leukemia
5'-nucleotidase	Liver
Prostate-specific antigen	Prostate
Prostatic acid phosphatase	Prostate

PSA is a better predictor than prostatic acid phosphatase (PAP) for the diagnosis of prostate cancer.

● In normal men only minute amounts of PSA circulate in the serum. Elevated blood levels of PSA occur in prostate cancer.

Normal values:

● Older men would have higher serum PSA levels than younger men.

● A serum PSA value of 3.5 μg/L might appear as normal on a lab test.

Enzymes as Tumor Marker

Enzymes were used historically as tumor markers before the discovery of oncofetal antigens and the advent of monoclonal antibodies. The abnormalities of enzymes as markers for cancer are either the expression of the fetal from of the enzyme (isoenzyme) or the ectopic production of enzymes.

Enzymes are present in much higher concentrations inside cells and are released into the systemic circulation as the result of tumor necrosis or a change in the membrane permeability of the cancer cells. By the time enzymes are released into the systemic circulation, the metastasis of tumors may have occurred. Most enzymes are not unique for a specific organ; therefore enzymes are most suitable as nonspecific tumor markers. Elevated enzyme levels may signal the presence of malignancy. **Table 5.15** summarizes various enzymes, their associated types of cancer.

▌SERUM ENZYME ASSAYS (PROFILE): MYOCARDIAL INFARCTION, LIVER DISEASES, AND PANCREATITIS

Enzyme Assays in Myocardial Infarction/Cardiac Markers

After myocardial infarction, a number of intracellular **enzymes** and **proteins** are released from the damaged cells. They have diagnostic importance and are called **cardiac markers**. Cardiac markers are useful in the detection of acute myocardial infarction (AMI) or minor myocardial injury.

- The cardiac markers of major diagnostic interest include enzymes such as:
  - Creatine kinase (CK)
  - Lactate dehydrogenase (LD)
  - Serum aspartate aminotransferase (AST) also called serum glutamate transaminase (SGOT).
- Nonenzyme proteins such as:
  - Myoglobin (Mb)
  - Cardiac troponin T and I (cTnT and cTnI).

In **Table 5.16** various cardiac markers with time course after onset of acute myocardial infarction is listed.

Plasma creatine kinase, (possibly with CK-MB isoenzyme) measurements are requested most often, less often, total LDH or LDH_1 (heart specific) may be requested, particularly if more than 36 hours have passed since the episode of chest pain. Clinical evidence has been shown that cardiac specific troponin, either cTnT or cTnI can be replaced CK-2 as the test of choice to rule in or rule out AMI.

- CK is the first enzyme to appear in serum in higher concentration after myocardial infarction and is probably the first to return to normal levels if there is no further coronary damage. The CK-MB isoenzyme starts to increase within 4 hours after an acute myocardial infarction (AMI) and reaches a maximum within 24 hours **(Figure 5.25)** CK-MB is a more sensitive and specific test for AMI than total CK.
- The serum activity of AST begins to rise about 6–12 hours after myocardial infarction and usually reaches its maximum value in about 24–48 hours. It usually returns to normal 4–6 days after the infarct.
- For patients having an AMI, serum total LDH values become elevated at 12–18 hours after onset of symptoms, peak at 48–72 hours and returns to normal after 6–10 days. The LDH_1 (heart specific) increase over LDH_2 in serum after AMI (the so called flipped pattern, in which the LDH_1/LDH_2 ratio becomes greater than 1). The use of LDH and LDH isoenzymes for detection of AMI is declining rapidly. Cardiac-specific

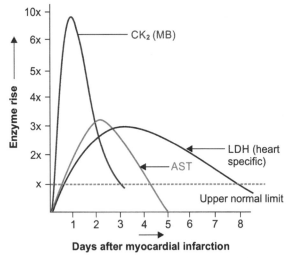

Figure 5.25: Typical rise in serum enzyme activities following a myocardial infarction.

troponin forms are currently the most sensitive and specific cardiac markers of AMI available.

- Serum concentrations of myoglobin rise above the normal values as early as 1 hour after the occurrence of an AMI with peak activity in the range of 4–12 hours. Myoglobin is cleared rapidly and thus has no clinical significance after 12 hours. The measurement of serum myoglobin has not been used extensively in clinical laboratories for the routine analysis of AMI because it is nonspecific, since it is raised following any form of muscle damage which may lead to the misdiagnosis of AMI.
- The initial rise in cardiac troponins (cTnI and cTnT) after myocardial infarction occurs at about the same time as CK and CK–MB, but this rise continues for longer than for most of the enzyme. The long time interval of cardiac troponin increase means it can replace the LDH isoenzyme assay in the detection of late presenting AMI individuals.

Enzyme Profile in Liver Diseases

- **Enzymes in hepatocyte damage:**
  - Aspartate aminotransferase (AST)
  - Alanine aminotransferase (ALT)

  AST and ALT are sensitive indicators of liver cell injury. Although serum levels of both AST and ALT become elevated in liver diseases, ALT is the more liver-specific enzyme.
- **Enzymes in cholestasis:**
  - Alkaline phosphatase (ALP)
  - 5'-nucleotidase
  - γ-glutamyl transferase (GGT)

Enzyme Profile in Pancreatitis

- **Amylase:** Serum amylase is not specific for pancreatic disease as its level is increased in parotitis (inflammation

TABLE 5.16: Enzymes in diagnosis of myocardial infarction and time course of plasma enzyme activity changes after myocardial infarction.

Markers	Abnormal activity detectable (hours)	Time for maximum rise (hours)	Time for return to normal (days)
CK-2 (MB)	3–10	10–24	2–3
AST/SGOT	6–12	24–48	4–6
LDH (heart specific)	8–16	48–72	7–12
Myoglobin (Mb)	1–3	6–9	1
Troponin I (cTnI)	3–8	24–48	3–5
Troponin T (cTnT)	3–8	72–100	5–10

(CK: Creatine kinase; LDH: Lactate dehydrogenase; SGOT: Serum glutamate transaminase; AST: Aspartate transaminase; cTnI: Cardiac specific troponin I; cTnT: Cardiac specific troponin T)

of a parotid gland, especially mumps) also. Apart from serum amylase level, urine amylase can also be estimated.

- **Lipase:** A serum lipase level measurement can be helpful in differentiating a pancreatic or nonpancreatic cause for hyperamylasemia.

STRIKE A NOTE

- ❖ **Enzyme profile for myocardial infarction:**
  - ➤ Creatine kinase (CKMB)
  - ➤ Aspartate transaminase (AST)
  - ➤ *Lactate dehydrogenase (LDH):* Not used now a days.
- ❖ **Enzyme profile for liver diseases:** Enzymes in hepatocyte damage:
  - ➤ Aspartate aminotransferase (AST)
  - ➤ Alanine aminotransferase (ALT)
- ❖ **Enzymes in cholestasis:**
  - ➤ Alkaline phosphatase (ALP)
  - ➤ 5'–nucleotidase
  - ➤ γ- glutamyl transferase (GGT)
- ❖ **Enzyme profile for pancreatitis:**
  - ➤ Serum amylase
  - ➤ Urine amylase
  - ➤ Lipase

Diagnostic use of Enzymes in Other Body Fluids

- ❖ *Lactate dehydrogenase in CSF, pleural fluid, ascitic fluid:* Suggestive of malignant tumor but not confirmatory
- ❖ *Adenosine deaminase in pleural fluid:* Suggestive of tuberculous pleural effusion
- ❖ *Amylase in urine:* Suggestive of pancreatitis

USE OF ENZYMES IN LABORATORY INVESTIGATIONS (ENZYME-BASED ASSAYS)

Enzymes can be used as **laboratory** *reagents* and *labels.*

- **Enzymes as laboratory reagent:** In addition to measurement of serum enzyme activity for the diagnosis and management of disease, enzymes are widely used in the clinical laboratory as reagents for the estimation of serum constituents. Some examples are given in **Table 5.17**.
- **Enzymes as labels:** Many enzymes have been used as the label in various immunoassays (enzyme-linked immunosorbent assay, ELISA) for determining the serum concentration of drugs, hormones or other compounds of interest. Commonly used enzymes are:
  - Glucose-6-phosphate dehydrogenase
  - Alkaline phosphatase
  - β-galactosidase
  - Peroxidase.

THERAPEUTIC USE OF ENZYMES

Some enzymes are used in the treatment of some diseases of human being. For example **(Table 5.18):**

TABLE 5.17: List of enzymes used in the clinical laboratory as reagents for investigations.

Enzymes as reagents	Investigations
Alcohol dehydrogenase	Ethanol
Lactate dehydrogenase	Lactate
Glucose oxidase and peroxidase	Glucose
Hexokinase and glucose-6-phosphate dehydrogenase	Creatine kinase
Uricase	Uric acid
Urease	Urea
Cholesterol oxidase and peroxidase	Cholesterol
Lipase, glycerol kinase, glycerol phosphate dehydrogenase	Triacylglycerol

TABLE 5.18: Some important therapeutic enzymes.

Enzymes	Uses
Asparaginase	Leukemia
Chymotrypsin	Inflammation and edema
Collagenase	Skin ulcers
Fibrinolysin	Blood clot
Glutaminase	Leukemia
Hyaluronidase	Heart attack
Lysozyme	Antibiotic
Rhodanase	Cyanide poisoning
Ribonuclease	Antiviral
β-lactamase	Penicillin allergy
Streptokinase	Blood clots
Trypsin	To dissolve the blood clot
Uricase	Gout
Urokinase	Blood clots

- **Asparaginase** is used in the treatment of some type of leukemia. Asparaginase hydrolyzes asparagine to aspartic acid. Asparagine is necessary for the formation of leukemic white cell.
- **Chymotrypsin:** Used in ophthalmology for dissolving ligaments of the lens during the extraction of cataract and to make inflammation and edema subside.
- **Collagenase:** Used for debridement (cleaning of wound by removing dead tissue) of dermal ulcers and severe burns.
- **Fibrinolysin:** It is used in the venous thrombosis, pulmonary and arterial embolism (blood clot carried by pulmonary artery).
- **Glutaminase:** It is used in the treatment of some type of leukemia.
- **Hyaluronidase:** It is used to promote the rapid absorption of drugs injected subcutaneously. It acts by depolymerizing hyaluronic acid (mucopolysaccharide) and increasing tissue permeability. It is used in the treatment of traumatic or postoperative edema.

- **β-lactamase:** It is used for penicillin allergy
- **Lysozyme** (an antibiotic) found in human tears and egg white, is used in the infection of eye. It has antibacterial action; it acts on cellulose of bacteria.
- **Penicillinase** (bacterial enzyme) is used for the treatment of persons who are allergic to penicillin, penicillinase destroys penicillin.
- **Rhodanese:** It is used for cyanide poisoning
- **Ribonuclease:** It is used as an antiviral.

- **Streptokinase:** Streptokinase and urokinase are used in myocardial infarction to dissolve blood clot or purulent material. It causes fibrinolysis.
- **Trypsin:** It is a proteolytic enzyme and is used to clean the wounds by dissolving purulent (containing pus) material and in the treatment of acute thrombophlebitis (a blood clot and inflammation in vein) to dissolve the blood clot.
- **Uricase:** It is used to treat gout.

ASSESSMENT QUESTIONS

▌STRUCTURED LONG ESSAY QUESTIONS (SLEQs)

1. Describe enzyme inhibitors under following headings:
   i. Types
   ii. Mechanism with diagram
   iii. Examples
2. Describe enzyme under following headings:
   i. Definition
   ii. IUBMB classification with suitable examples
   iii. Factors affecting enzyme activity
3. Describe clinical enzymology under following headings:
   i. Diagnostic importance of enzymes
   ii. Enzymes as therapeutic agents
   iii. Enzymes used in diagnostic assay
4. Describe isoenzymes under following headings:
   i. Definition
   ii. Examples
   iii. Diagnostic importance
5. Describe enzyme regulation under following headings:
   i. Short-term regulation
   ii. Long-term regulation

▌SHORT ESSAY QUESTIONS (SEQs)

1. Define enzyme and write IUBMB classification with suitable examples.
2. Write different models for mechanism of enzyme action.
3. Write various factors affecting enzyme kinetics
4. Define allosteric enzyme? Write mechanism of allosteric enzyme.
5. Write different classes of enzyme inhibition and give their effect on the kinetic parameter.
6. What is Lineweaver-Burk plot? Give its significance.
7. What are enzyme poisons? Enumerate poisons with the enzyme inhibited.
8. Write enzymes markers in diagnosis of myocardial infarction.
9. Write enzyme profile for liver diseases.
10. Define coenzyme. Write different types of coenzymes of vitamins with type of reaction they catalyze.
11. Define cofactor. Name enzymes requiring cofactor.

▌SHORT ANSWER QUESTIONS (SAQs)

1. What is optimum pH of an enzyme and its importance?
2. Give four examples of competitive inhibitors of enzymes and its importance.
3. Define isoenzymes with their diagnostic importance.
4. What is zymogen? Give examples of zymogen.
5. Name coenzymes of vitamin B complex with their corresponding vitamins.
6. Effect of competitive inhibitor on the kinetic parameter.
7. What is feedback of allosteric inhibition? Give one example.
8. What is regulation of enzymes by induction and repression?
9. List four examples of regulation of enzymes by covalent modification.
10. Write any four therapeutic uses of enzymes.
11. What is the analytical use of enzymes as reagents with examples?
12. Name any four enzymes requiring metal elements as a cofactor.
13. Write name of enzymes markers in diagnosis of liver disease.
14. What is suicide inhibition? Give an example.
15. What is ribozyme? Give an example.

▌MULTIPLE CHOICE QUESTIONS (MCQs)

1. **Enzymes, which are produced in inactive form in the living cells, are called:**
   a. Papain   b. Lysozymes
   c. Apoenzymes   d. Proenzymes

2. **The Michaelis constant (K_m) is:**
   a. Not changed by the presence of competitive inhibitor
   b. Equal to $1/2 \, V_{max}$
   c. The substrate concentration at $1/2 \, V_{max}$
   d. Changed by the presence of noncompetitive inhibitor

3. **Which of the following nonproteins can act as an enzyme?**
   a. DNA
   b. Ribozyme
   c. Phospholipid
   d. Glycolipid

4. The substrate concentration at which an enzyme exhibits half the maximum velocity is known as:
   a. V_{max}
   b. [S]
   c. K_m
   d. Keq

5. All of the following serum enzymes are elevated in myocardial infarction, *except*:
   a. Alkaline phosphatase
   b. Lactate dehydrogenase
   c. Aspartate transaminase
   d. Creatine kinase

6. Alcohol dehydrogenase comes under which class of enzyme?
   a. Oxidoreductase
   b. Dehydrogenase
   c. Hydrolase
   d. Oxidase

7. Enzyme activity in biological systems may be affected by the following:
   a. Negative modifiers
   b. Change in pH
   c. Change in temperature
   d. All of the above

8. Isoenzymes can be characterized as:
   a. Nonprotein part of enzyme
   b. Enzymes with same quaternary structure
   c. Called alloenzyme
   d. Multiple forms of given enzyme that catalyze same type of reactions

9. Transaminase enzymes belong to the class:
   a. Hydrolases
   b. Transferases
   c. Oxidoreductases
   d. Isomerases

10. Liver diagnostic enzyme is:
    a. Creatine kinase
    b. Acid phosphatase
    c. Alanine transaminase
    d. Amylase

11. Which of the following enzyme levels increases in obstructive jaundice?
    a. Lipase
    b. Amylase
    c. Acid phosphatase
    d. Alkaline phosphatase

12. The digestive enzymes belong to:
    a. Isomerases
    b. Transferases
    c. Hydrolases
    d. Ligases

13. The enzyme useful in the treatment of leukemia is:
    a. α-chymotrypsin
    b. Hyaluronidase
    c. Asparaginase
    d. Streptokinase

14. Earliest marker of myocardial infarction is:
    a. CK-1
    b. CK-2
    c. CK-3
    d. AST

15. Fischer's 'lock and key' model of the enzyme action implies that:
    a. The active site is complementary in shape to that of substance only after interaction.
    b. The active site is complementary in shape to that of substrate
    c. Substrates change conformation prior to active site interaction
    d. The active site is flexible and adjusts to substrate

16. In reversible noncompetitive enzyme inhibition:
    a. Inhibitor bears structural resemblance to substrate
    b. K_m is unaltered
    c. K_m is increased
    d. K_m is decreased

17. In competitive enzyme inhibition:
    a. K_m is decreased
    b. K_m is increased
    c. V_{max} is increased
    d. V_{max} is decreased

18. Coenzymes are:
    a. Heat stable, dialyzable, nonprotein organic molecules
    b. Soluble, colloidal, protein molecules
    c. Structural analog of enzymes
    d. Different forms of enzymes

19. An example of hydrogen transferring coenzyme is:
    a. CoA
    b. NAD^+
    c. Biotin
    d. TPP

20. The isoenzymes of LDH:
    a. Have similar electrophoretic mobility
    b. Differ in catalytic activity
    c. Exist in 5 forms depending on M and H monomer contents
    d. Occur as monomers

21. Translocase as per IUBMB system is classified as:
    a. EC-1
    b. EC-3
    c. EC-6
    d. EC-7

22. Enzymes involved in transport of molecules across the cell membrane belong to the class:
    a. Hydrolases
    b. Transferases
    c. Oxidoreductases
    d. Translocases

23. The type of enzyme inhibition (in which succinate dehydrogenase reaction is inhibited by malonate) is an example of:
    a. Competitive
    b. Uncompetitive
    c. Noncompetitive
    d. Allosteric

24. Nonfunctional enzymes are all, *except*:
    a. Alkaline phosphatase
    b. Acid phosphatase
    c. Lipoprotein lipase
    d. Gamma glutamyl transpeptidase

25. The predominant isozyme of LDH in cardiac muscle is:
    a. LDH-5
    b. LDH-2
    c. LDH-3
    d. LDH-1

26. In which of the following conditions the level of creatinine kinase-1 increases?
    a. Myocardial ischemia
    b. Brain ischemia
    c. Kidney damage
    d. Electrical cardioversion

27. In early stages of myocardial ischemia the most sensitive indicator is the measurement of the activity of:
    a. CPK   b. SGPT
    c. SGOT   d. LDH

28. Serum acid phosphatase level increases in:
    a. Metastatic carcinoma of prostate
    b. Myocardial infarction
    c. Wilson's disease
    d. Liver diseases

29. Serum alkaline phosphatase level increases in:
    a. Hypothyroidism
    b. Carcinoma of prostate
    c. Hyperparathyroidism
    d. Myocardial ischemia

30. Serum lipase level increases in:
    a. Liver disease
    b. Gaucher's disease
    c. Acute pancreatitis
    d. Diabetes mellitus

31. The isoenzymes LDH_5 is elevated in:
    a. Myocardial infarction
    b. Peptic ulcer
    c. Liver disease
    d. Infectious diseases

32. On the third day of onset of acute myocardial infarction the enzyme elevated is:
    a. Serum AST   b. Serum CK
    c. Serum LDH   d. Serum ALT

33. LDH_1 and LDH_2 are elevated in:
    a. Myocardial infarction   b. Liver disease
    c. Kidney disease   d. Brain disease

34. In acute pancreatitis, the enzyme raised in first five days is:
    a. Serum amylase
    b. Serum lactic dehydrogenase
    c. Urinary lipase
    d. Urinary amylase

35. An example of functional plasma enzyme is:
    a. Lipoprotein lipase
    b. Amylase
    c. Aminotransferase
    d. Lactate dehydrogenase

36. A nonfunctional plasma enzyme is:
    a. Pseudocholinesterase
    b. Lipoprotein lipase
    c. Proenzyme of blood coagulation
    d. Lipase

37. Zymogen is a:
    a. Vitamin   b. Enzyme precursor
    c. Modulator   d. Hormone

38. Enzyme inhibition caused by a substance resembling substrate molecule is:
    a. Competitive inhibition
    b. Noncompetitive inhibition
    c. Feedback inhibition
    d. Allosteric inhibition

39. Feedback inhibition of enzyme is influenced by:
    a. Enzyme
    b. External factors
    c. End product
    d. Substrate

40. If the amount of substrate is not limiting, the velocity of reaction is directly proportional to:
    a. pH
    b. Temperature
    c. Concentration of enzymes
    d. Concentration of products

41. Which one of the following statements concerning allosteric enzymes is correct?
    a. Allosteric effectors bind allosteric enzymes at their active sites
    b. Allosteric enzymes obey the Michaelis Menten behavior
    c. Allosteric control is irreversible
    d. Allosteric control with negative feedback is found in many metabolic pathways

42. Which of the following statement is not true about zymogen?
    a. Zymogen is inactive precursors of enzyme
    b. Zymogens are activated by cleavage of specific peptide bonds
    c. Pepsinogen is activated in stomach
    d. Pepsinogen is synthesized in pancreas

43. An example of enzyme as reagents in the clinical laboratory is:
    a. Glucose oxidase
    b. Urease
    c. Cholesterol oxidase
    d. All of the above

44. Elevation of serum amylase and lipase is commonly seen in:
    a. Acute pancreatitis
    b. Liver cirrhosis
    c. Bone disease
    d. Gallbladder disease

45. Enzymes belong to which group of biomolecules:
    a. Carbohydrates   b. Proteins
    c. Lipids   d. Phospholipids

46. The enzymes with different structures but the same catalytic function are called:
    a. Allosteric enzymes   b. Proenzymes
    c. Zymogens   d. Isoenzymes

47. The model that explains that the active site is flexible and shapes of the active site can be modify by the binding of the substrate is called, *except*:
    a. Induced fit model
    b. Hand-in-glove model
    c. Koshland model
    d. Lock and key model

48. The inhibitor that binds reversibly to active site of the enzyme is known as:
    a. Allosteric inhibitor
    b. Competitive inhibitor
    c. Noncompetitive inhibitor
    d. Suicide inhibitor

49. The site of the enzyme molecule into which the substrate binds is:
    a. Allosteric site
    b. Regulatory site
    c. Active site
    d. None of the above

50. Enzymes used as the treatment of some diseases of human being, *except*:
    a. Asparginase
    b. Penicillinase
    c. Alcohol dehydrogenase
    d. Hyaluronidase

51. Chymotrypsinogen is a:
    a. Zymogen
    b. Alloenzyme
    c. Coenzyme
    d. None of the above

52. Suicidal enzyme is:
    a. Lipoxygenase
    b. Cyclooxygenase
    c. Thromboxane synthase
    d. 5'-nucleotidase

53. Peroxidase enzyme is used in estimating:
    a. Hemoglobin   b. Ammonia
    c. Creatinine   d. Glucose

54. All of the following enzyme are involved in oxidation-reduction, *except*:
    a. Dehydrogenases   b. Hydrolases
    c. Oxygenases   d. Peroxidases

55. Enzyme which cleave C-C bond:
    a. Lyase   b. Oxidoreductase
    c. Ligase   d. Isomerase

56. Which of the following drug acts as competitive inhibitor?
    a. Statin   b. Allopurinol
    c. Lovastatin   d. All of the above

57. In which type of inhibition, both V_{max} and K_m are decreased?
    a. Competitive   b. Noncompetitive
    c. Both   d. None of the above

58. In which type of inhibition, inhibitor only binds to the ES complex?
    a. Competitive   b. Noncompetitive
    c. Uncompetitive   d. All of the above

59. Methotrexate is the drug for which disease?
    a. Cancer   b. Gout
    c. Hypertension   d. Renal failure

60. Which of the following is a lyase?
    a. Aldolase B
    b. Acetyl-CoA synthetase
    c. Fatty Acyl-CoA dehydrogenase
    d. Acetyl-CoA carboxylase

61. All are true about oxygenases, *except*:
    a. Can incorporate 2 atoms of O, in a substance
    b. Can incorporate 1 atom of O, in a substance
    c. Important in hydroxylation of steroids
    d. Catalyze carboxylation of drugs

62. Coenzyme in decarboxylation reaction:
    a. Niacin   b. Biotin
    c. Pyridoxine   d. Riboflavin

63. In noncompetitive antagonism which of the following is correct?
    a. V_{max} decreases
    b. K_m decreases
    c. No change in V_{max}
    d. Both K_m and V_{max} increases

64. The type of enzyme inhibition in which succinate dehydrogenase reaction is inhibited by malonate is an example of:
    a. Noncompetitive
    b. Uncompetitive
    c. Competitive
    d. Allosteric

65. Features of competitive inhibition is/are:
    a. V_{max} increases   b. K_m increases
    c. V_{max} decreases   d. K_m decreases
    e. V_{max} constant

66. Noncompetitive reversible inhibitors:
    a. Raise K   b. Lower K
    c. Lower V_{max} d. Raise both V and K_m
    e. Do not affect either V or K

67. True about competitive antagonism:
    a. V_{max} increased
    b. Substrate analog
    c. Reversible
    d. K_m increased
    e. V_{max} decreased

68. K_m changes and V remains the same. What is the type of enzyme inhibition?
    a. Competitive inhibition
    b. Noncompetitive inhibition
    c. Uncompetitive inhibition
    d. Suicide inhibition

69. Allosteric regulation true is:
    a. Binds to site other than active site
    b. Regulated by acting on catalytic site
    c. Follow Michaelis Menten kinetics
    d. Substrate and modifier are structural analogs

70. All of the covalent modification regulate enzyme kinetics, *except*:
    a. Phosphorylation
    b. Acetylation
    c. ADP ribosylation
    d. Glycosylation

71. The following affect enzyme activity, *except*:
    a. Methylation
    b. Acetylation
    c. Induction
    d. Phosphorylation

72. Biomarker of alcoholic hepatitis:
    a. ALP   b. AST
    c. LDH   d. GGT
73. What happens to LDH 1 and 2 ratio in MI?
    a. LDH1 > LDH2
    b. LDH2 > LDH1
    c. LDH1 = LDH2
    d. Remains the same
74. True about isoenzymes is:
    a. Catalyse the same reaction
    b. Same quaternary structure
    c. Same distribution in different organs
    d. Same enzyme classification with same number and name
75. Not raised in liver disorder is/are:
    a. Lipase   b. Urease
    c. ALP   d. AST

ANSWERS FOR MCQs

1. d	2. c	3. b	4. c	5. a
6. a	7. d	8. d	9. b	10. c
11. d	12. c	13. c	14. b	15. b
16. b	17. b	18. a	19. b	20. c
21. a	22. d	23. a	24. c	25. b
26. b	27. a	28. a	29. c	30. c
31. c	32. c	33. a	34. a	35. a
36. d	37. b	38. a	39. c	40. c
41. d	42. d	43. d	44. a	45. b
46. d	47. d	48. b	49. c	50. c
51. a	52. b	53. d	54. b	55. a
56. d	57. d	58. c	59. a	60. a
61. d	62. c	63. a	64. c	
65. b and e		66. c	67. b,c,d	68. a
69. a	70. d	71. c.	72. d	73. a.
74. a	75. a and b			

6 CHAPTER

Chemistry of Nucleic Acids

Competency	Learning Objectives
BI 7.1: Describe the structure and functions of DNA and RNA and outline the cell cycle.	1. Describe structure and functions of nucleotides. 2. Describe the biologically important free nucleotides and their importance. 3. Describe the major types of synthetic analogs of nucleotides (antimetabolites) and their clinical significance. 4. Describe structure and functions of DNA. 5. Describe DNA organization in the cell. 6. Describe structure and functions of RNA.

■ OVERVIEW

Nucleic acids are macromolecules present in all living cells in combination with proteins to form **nucleoproteins**. The protein is usually basic in nature, e.g., protamines and histones containing high concentration of basic amino acids. Nucleic acids have a variety of roles in organisms. Genetic information is encoded in a nucleic acid molecule. The cell interprets this information as sequences of amino acids in protein and peptide molecules.

Nucleic acids are polymers of a specific sequence of subunits or monomers called **nucleotides,** they are therefore called **polynucleotides**. The nucleic acids are of two main categories **deoxyribonucleic acid** or **DNA and ribonucleic acid** or **RNA**.

DNA is present in nuclei and small amounts are also present in **mitochondria**, whereas 90% of the RNA is present in cell **cytoplasm** and 10% in the **nucleolus**. This chapter provides the chemical nature and function of the nucleotides and nucleic acids.

■ STRUCTURE AND FUNCTIONS OF NUCLEOTIDES

Nucleotides are the building block of **nucleic acid**. Nucleotides have three characteristic components:
1. Nitrogen containing base
2. Pentose sugar
3. One or more phosphates.

The molecule without phosphate group is called **nucleoside**. The nitrogenous bases of nucleic acids are derivatives of two parent compounds, **purine** and **pyrimidine**.

Purine Bases

Two principal purine bases found in DNAs, as well as RNAs are **(Figure 6.1)**:
1. Adenine (A)
2. Guanine (G)

Pyrimidine Bases

The major pyrimidine bases are **(Figure 6.2)**:
1. Cytosine (C)
2. Uracil (U)
3. Thymine (T)

Cytosine and **uracil** are found in **RNAs** and **cytosine** and **thymine** in **DNAs**. Both DNA and RNA contain the pyrimidine cytosine but they differ in their second pyrimidine base. DNA contains thymine whereas RNA contains uracil.

Sugar Present in RNA and DNA

Nucleic acids have two kinds of **pentoses** both types of pentoses are in their β-**isomeric** form **(Figure 6.3)**.
1. Deoxyribonucleotides of DNA contain β-2′-**deoxy-D-ribose**
2. Ribonucleotides of RNA contain β-**D-ribose**.

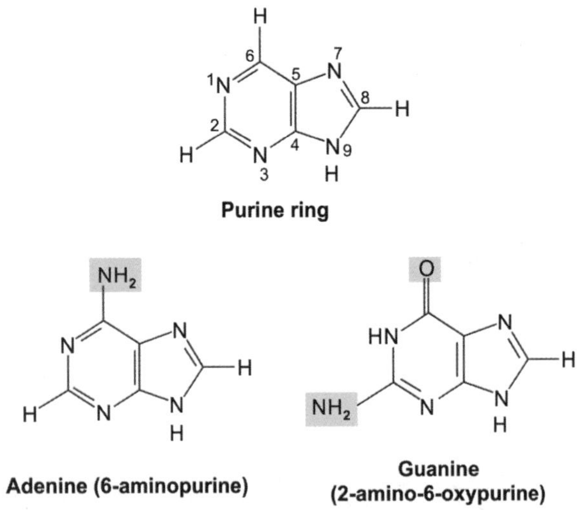

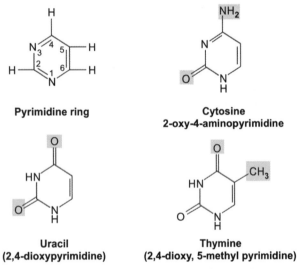

Figure 6.1: Structure of purine ring and purine bases.

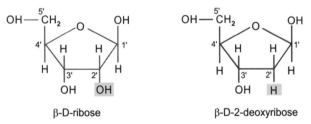

Figure 6.2: Structure of pyrimidine ring and pyrimidine bases.

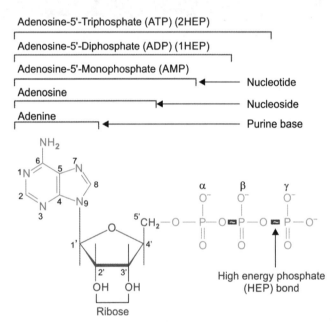

Figure 6.3: Structure of sugars present in nucleic acid.

The atoms of the nitrogenous base (purines and pyrimidines) in nucleotides are given **cardinal numbers**, whereas the carbon atoms of the **sugars** are given **primed numbers** as shown in **Figure 6.4** to distinguish sugar from those of the nitrogenous base.

The nitrogenous base of nucleotide is linked covalently to pentose sugar by β **N-glycosidic bond**. This linkage joins **N-9** of the purine base or **N-1** of the pyrimidine base with **1′-carbon** of the pentose sugar **(Figure 6.4)**. The β N-glycosidic bond is formed by removal of a molecule of

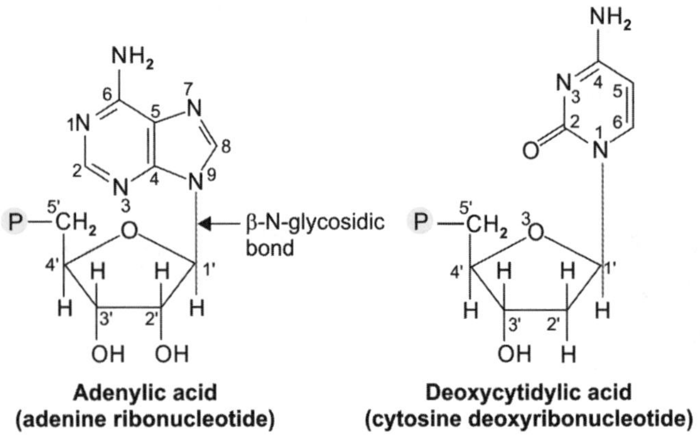

Figure 6.4: Structures of nucleotide.

Figure 6.5: Structure of ATP and its components.

water (a hydroxyl group from the pentose and hydrogen from the base).

Attachment of Phosphate to Pentose Sugar

The phosphate group is esterified to **5′-carbon** of pentose sugar **(Figure 6.4)**. Cells also contain nucleotides with phosphate groups in position other than on the 5′-carbon.

● Other variations are adenosine 3′,5′-cyclic monophosphate (cAMP) and guanosine 3′,5′-cyclic monophosphate (cGMP) which are considered later in this chapter.

● If an additional phosphate group is attached to the preexisting phosphate of mononucleotide, a dinucleotide (e.g., ADP) or trinucleotide (e.g., ATP) results **(Figure 6.5)**.

Different major bases with their corresponding nucleoside and nucleotide is summarized in **Table 6.1**. Nucleoside and nucleotide are generic terms that include both ribo and deoxyribo forms.

TABLE 6.1: Different major bases with their corresponding nucleoside, nucleotide, and nucleic acids.

	Base	Nucleoside	Nucleotide	Nucleic acid
Purines	Adenine	Adenosine	Adenylate	RNA
		Deoxyadenosine	Deoxyadenylate	DNA
	Guanine	Guanosine	Guanylate	RNA
		Deoxyguanosine	Deoxyguanylate	DNA
Pyrimidines	Cytosine	Cytidine	Cytidylate	RNA
		Deoxycytidine	Deoxycytidylate	DNA
	Thymine	Thymidine or deoxythymidine	Thymidylate or deoxythymidylate	DNA
	Uracil	Uridine	Uridylate	RNA

Importance of Nucleotides

Nucleotides are activated precursors of DNA and RNA. In addition to their roles as the subunit of nucleic acids, nucleotides have a variety of other functions in every cell as:

- **High energy carriers**, e.g., *ATP, GTP, CTP, and UTP*:
  - **Component of enzyme cofactors**, e.g., adenine nucleotides are components of three major coenzymes **NAD⁺**, and **FAD⁺**. **NAD⁺** and **FAD** functions in oxidation reduction reactions.
  - **Metabolic regulators** and **chemical messengers**, e.g., **cAMP** and **cGMP**.
  - **Activation of metabolic intermediates**, e.g., UDP-glucose and CDP-diacylglycerol are precursors for glycogen and phosphoglyceride synthesis.

Minor Purine and Pyrimidine Bases

In addition to the major bases present in DNAs and RNAs of both prokaryotes and eukaryotes, both DNA and RNA also contain considerably smaller quantities of additional purine and pyrimidine bases called *minor* or *unusual* or *rare* or **modified** *bases* (**Figure 6.6**). These bases are functionally important and therefore not of minor physiologic importance. Unusual or altered bases of DNA molecules often have roles in regulating and protecting the genetic information.

- In DNA the most common of these are methylated forms of the major bases, e.g.,
  - 5-Methylcytosine
  - 7-Methylguanine
  - Dimethyladenine, etc.

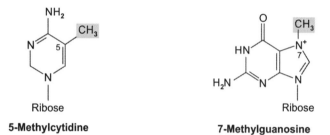
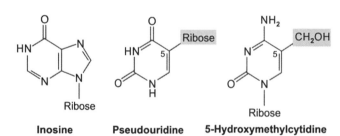

Figure 6.6: Unusual (minor) naturally occurring purine and pyrimidine bases.

- Some minor bases present in tRNAs are:
  - **Inosine** which contains the base **hypoxanthine**.
  - **Pseudouridine**, like uridine it contains uracil but is distinct in the point of attachment to the ribose. In uridine uracil is attached through N-1, the usual attachment point for pyrimidines, in pseudouridine it is through C-5.

Methylated derivatives of xanthine present in foods (**Figure 6.7**)
- ❖ Caffeine of coffee (Trimethyl xanthine)
- ❖ Theophylline of tea (Dimethyl xanthine)
- ❖ Theobromine of cocoa. (Dimethyl xanthine)

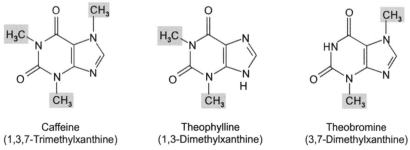

Figure 6.7: Plant bases present in foods.

■ BIOLOGICALLY IMPORTANT FREE NUCLEOTIDES

Besides being the structural components of nucleic acids, several free nucleotides such as **ATP, ADP, cAMP, SAM, PAPS, GTP, GDP, cGMP, UDP, CTP, CDP,** etc. participate in several biochemical and physiological functions. Free nucleotides involved in a various biochemical processes. Nucleotides involved in a various biochemical processes are discussed below.

Nucleotides of Adenine

- Adenosine triphosphate (ATP)
- Adenosine monophosphate (AMP)
- Cyclic adenosine monophosphate (cAMP)
- Phospho adenosine phospho sulphate (PAPS) and
- S-adenosyl methionine (SAM).
- Nicotinamide adenine dinucleotide (NAD$^+$) and flavin adenine dinucleotide (FAD$^+$).

Adenosine Triphosphate

Adenosine triphosphate (*see* **Figure 6.5**) serves as the main biological source of energy in the cell. ATP is required as a source of energy in several metabolic pathways, e.g., fatty acid synthesis, glycolysis, cholesterol synthesis, protein synthesis, gluconeogenesis, etc., and in physiologic functions such as muscle contraction, nerve impulse transmission, etc.

Adenosine Monophosphate

Adenosine monophosphate (*see* **Figure 6.5**) is the component of many coenzymes such as NAD$^+$, NADP$^+$, FAD, coenzyme A, etc. These coenzymes are essential for the metabolism of carbohydrate, lipid, and protein.

Cyclic Adenosine 3′, 5′-Monophosphate

Cyclic adenosine monophosphate (**Figure 6.8**) is formed from ATP by the action of **adenylate cyclase**.

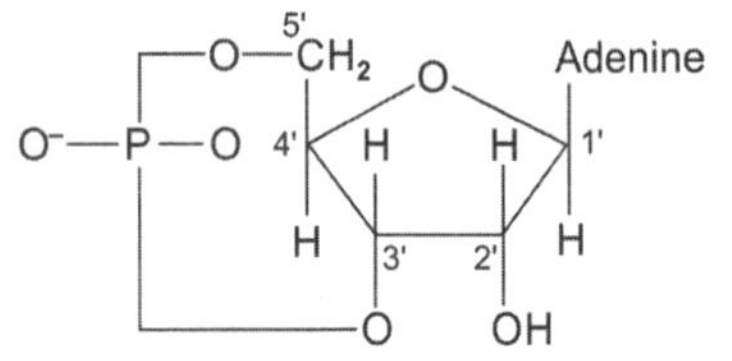

Adenosine 3′,5′-cyclic monophosphate (cyclic AMP; cAMP)

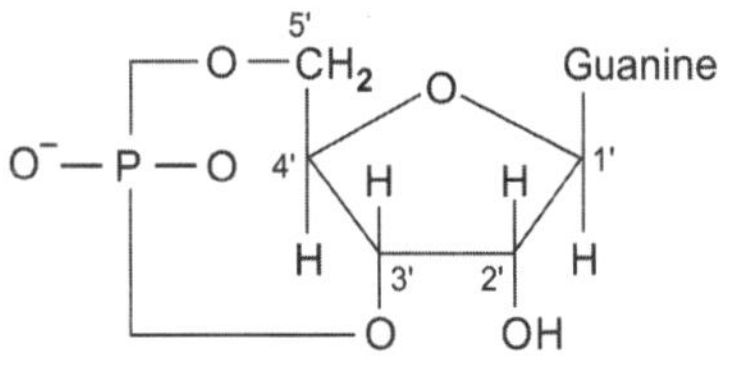

Guanosine 3′,5′-cyclic monophosphate (cyclic GMP; cGMP)

Figure 6.8: Structure of regulatory nucleotides.

TABLE 6.2: Hormones using c-AMP as a second messenger.

- Calcitonin
- Chorionic gonadotropin
- Corticotropin
- Epinephrine
- Follicle stimulating hormone
- Glucagon
- Luteinizing hormone
- Melanocyte stimulating hormone
- Norepinephrine
- Parathyroid hormone
- Thyroid stimulating hormone
- Vasopressin

- cAMP acts as a second messenger for many hormones, e.g., **epinephrine**, **glucagon** (Table 6.2).
- cAMP affects a wide range of cellular processes by acting as a **second messenger**. For example:
  - It enhances the degradation of storage fuels like fat and glycogen by stimulating lipolysis, glycogenolysis.
  - It inhibits the aggregation of blood platelets.
  - cAMP increases the secretion of acid by the gastric mucosa.

Phospho Adenosine Phospho Sulphate (PAPS, "Active Sulfate")

- Phosphoadenosine phosphosulfate is a derivative of adenosine monophosphate that is phosphorylated at the 3′ position and has a sulfate group attached to the 5′ phosphate.
- It is the most common coenzyme in sulfotransferase reactions.
- PAPS, is **a sulfate donor in the synthesis of sulfur-containing mucopolysaccharides as well as in the detoxification of sterols, steroids, and other compounds**.

S-adenosyl Methionine

- SAM is an intermediate product formed in the metabolic pathway of **methionine**.
- It is **made from ATP and methionine by methionine adenosyltransferase**.
- SAM is used in many biological reactions and serves as a regulator of a variety of processes.
- It is a commonly used **methyl donor** in numerous biologically important methylation reactions, including DNA methylation, RNA methylation, and protein methylation.

It is commonly used commercially to treat depression. SAM increases turnover of serotonin and may increase levels of dopamine and norepinephrine.

Nicotinamide Adenine Dinucleotide and Flavin Adenine Dinucleotide

Adenine nucleotides are components of two major coenzymes **NAD$^+$**, and **FAD$^+$**. **NAD$^+$** and **FAD** functions in oxidation reduction reactions.

Nucleotides of Guanine

- Guanosine diphosphate (GDP)
- Guanosine triphosphate (GTP) and
- Cyclic guanosine monophosphate (cGMP)

Guanosine Diphosphate and Guanosine Triphosphate

- These guanosine nucleotides participate in the conversion of **succinyl-CoA** to **succinate**, a reaction which is coupled to the **substrate level phosphorylation** of GDP to GTP in **citric acid cycle**.
- GTP is required for activation of adenylate cyclase by some hormones. GTP serves as an energy source for **protein synthesis**.

Cyclic Guanosine 3′, 5′-Monophosphate

Cyclic guanosine monophosphate P **(Figure 6.8)** is formed from GTP by **guanylyl cyclase**.

- cGMP is an intracellular signal or **second messenger** that can act antagonistically to cAMP.
- cGMP is involved in relaxation of smooth muscle and vasodilation.

Nucleotides of Uracil

- Uridine diphosphate sugar derivatives like; **UDP-glucose** and **UDP-galactose** act as sugar donors for **biosynthesis of glycogen** and for synthesis of **lactose** and **cerebrosides**.
- UDP-sugar derivatives participate in sugar epimerization such as the interconversion of glucose-1-phosphate and galactose-1-phosphate.
- UDP-sugars like UDP-galactose, UDP-glucuronate UDP-N-acetylgalactosamine, etc., act as sugar donors for biosynthesis of the glycoproteins and proteoglycans.
- UDP-glucuronate act as a glucuronyl donor for **detoxification processes** of bilirubin or drugs such as aspirin and for biosynthesis of **mucopolysaccharides** such as heparin, hyaluronic acid, etc.

Nucleotides of Cytosine

Cytidine Triphosphate (CTP) and **Cytidine Diphosphate (CDP)** are required for the biosynthesis of some **phospholipids**. CDP-choline is involved in the synthesis of sphingomyelin.

STRIKE A NOTE

- ❖ The Viagra increases cGMP concentration by inhibiting its catabolic enzyme phosphodiesterase and prolong the responses of cGMP which causes relaxation of the smooth muscle in the corpus cavernosum.
- ❖ Sildenafil citrate (Viagra) selectively inhibits phosphodiesterase type-V, which acts on cGMP.

SYNTHETIC ANALOGS OF NUCLEOTIDES OR ANTIMETABOLITES

Chemically synthesized analogues of purines and pyrimidines, their nucleosides and their nucleotides have therapeutic applications in medicine. An analogue is prepared either by altering the heterocyclic ring of a base (purine or pyrimidine) or sugar moiety. These are used **chemotherapeutically** (treatment of disease by the use of chemical substances) to control **cancer** or **infections**.

Action of Synthetic Analogs on Cancer Cells

Since a characteristic of cancerous tissue is its **uncontrolled cell division**, an increased synthesis of DNA and RNA is involved. Inhibition of the elevated synthesis of nucleic acids helps to restrict the growth of cancerous tissue. In nucleic acids normal bases are substituted by their analogues. Substitution of a base analogue will result in altered base pairings and structural changes that affect **DNA replication** and **transcription of genes**. Unfortunately, these drugs often also suppress normal cell division and therefore can be toxic.

Analogues of purines and pyrimidines used in the treatment of infections or in cancer chemotherapy are:

- **5-fluoro** or **5-iodo derivatives of uracil** or deoxyuridine which serves as thymine or thymidine analogues respectively.
- **6-mercaptopurine** and **6-thioguanine** are structural analogues of inosine and guanine respectively.
- Analogues such as **5** or **6-azauridine**, **5-** or **6-azacytidine** and **8-azaguanine** in which a nitrogen atom replaces carbon atoms of the heterocyclic ring.
- The nucleoside **cytarabine (arabinosylcytosine; ara-c)** in which arabinose replaces ribose is used in the chemotherapy of cancer and viral infections.
- The purine analogue **4-hydroxypyra zolopyrimidine (allopurinol)** used in treatment of hyperuricemia and gout.
- **Azidothymidine (AZT)** is a structural analogue of thymidine used in the treatment of acquired immunodeficiency syndrome (AIDS), a disease caused by the human immunodeficiency virus (HIV). AZT terminates DNA synthesis catalyzed by the reverse transcriptase of retroviruses.
- **Azathioprine**, which is catabolized to 6-mercaptopurine is an immunosuppressive agent that is used during organ transplantation to suppress events involved in immunologic rejection.
- **5-iododeoxyuridine**, a nucleoside analogue has antiviral activity and is used in the treatment of herpetic keratitis, an infection of the cornea by herpes virus. The structure of some drugs (analogues) commercially used in chemotherapy are shown in **Figure 6.9**.

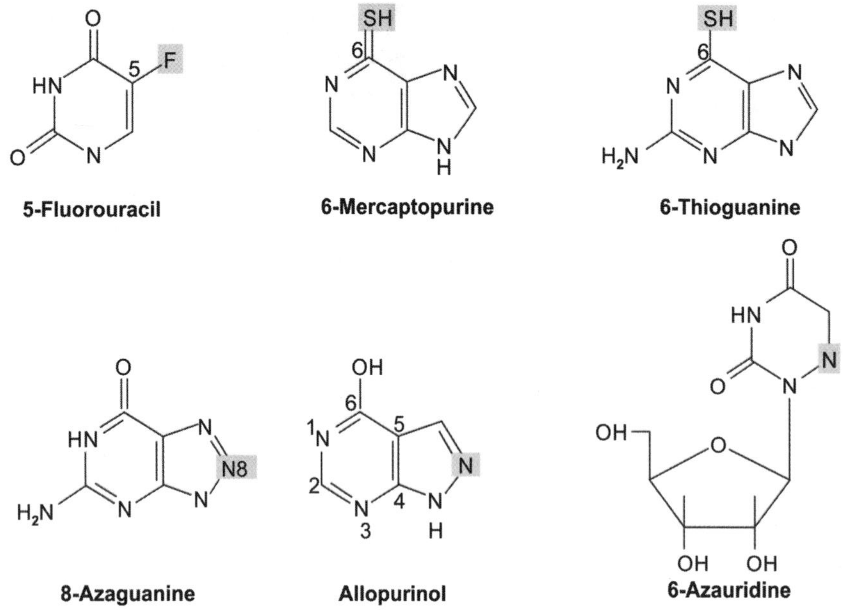

Figure 6.9: Selected commercially used purine and pyrimidine analogs.

DNA STRUCTURE AND FUNCTION

- Most of the DNA of **eukaryotes** is found in the **nucleus**, where DNA is folded and tightly packed with histones and nonhistone proteins to form **chromosomes**.
- DNA is present also in **mitochondria** (less than 0.1% of the total DNA) and in **chloroplast** of plants. Many viruses also contain DNA as their genetic material.
- Mitochondrial DNA (mtDNA) is very small molecule compared with the nuclear chromosomes. Human **mitochondrial DNA contains circular DNA** and **is not associated with histones**.
- Mitochondrial DNA also codes for, 13-proteins (These include part of the respiratory enzyme complex of the inner mitochondrial membrane), 2-rRNAs and, 22-tRNAs.

The structure of DNA is described in terms of **primary** and **secondary** levels.

Primary Structure of DNA

Deoxyribonucleic acid (DNA) is a polymer of repeating subunits called **deoxyribonucleotides**. In the polymer, nucleotides are joined to one another by **3′,5′-phosphodiester bonds** in which the 5′-phosphate group of one nucleotide unit is joined to the 3′-hydroxyl group of the next nucleotides **(Figure 6.10)**. The primary structure of a nucleic acid refers to the sequence of its nucleotide residues. Each deoxyribonucleotide subunit is composed of three components:

1. **Five carbon, pentose sugar:** Deoxyribose sugar
2. **Nitrogenous base:**
   - **Purines:** Adenine (A) and Guanine (G)
   - **Pyrimidines:** Thymine (T), Cytosine (C)

Each nitrogenous base is covalently linked to one molecule of deoxyribose sugar. In a deoxyribonucleotide, the C-1 carbon atom of deoxyribose is bonded to N-1 of pyrimidine or N-9 of purine **(see Figure 6.4)** by N-glycosidic linkage.

3. **The phosphate group (PO$_4$)**
   - Phosphate gives DNA the property of an acid at physiological pH, hence the name "nucleic acid". The phosphate groups are completely ionized and **negatively charged at pH 7**, and the negative charges are generally neutralized by ionic interactions with positive charges on proteins.
   - The hydroxyl group on the 3′ carbon of the deoxyribose sugar of one nucleotide forms an ester bond with the phosphate on 5′ carbon of the deoxyribose sugar of another nucleotide. This covalent bond is called **3′, 5′-phosphodiester** bond.

The backbone of DNA consists of many deoxyribonucleotides linked covalently by **3′,5′-phosphodiester bonds (Figure 6.10)**. The sequence of bases along a polynucleotide chain is not restricted in any way; the precise sequence of bases carries the genetic information.

The resulting long, unbranched DNA chain has polarity. One end of the chain has a **5′-phosphate group** and the other a **3′-hydroxy group** that is not linked to another nucleotide **(Figure 6.10)**. The symbol 5′ refers to the carbon in the sugar to which a phosphate (PO$_4$) group is attached. The symbol 3′ refers to the carbon in the sugar ring to which a hydroxyl (OH) group is attached. By convention, a DNA or RNA sequence is written from 5′ end of the chain to the 3′ end in the direction (5′→ 3′ direction).

Secondary Structure of DNA

In DNA, secondary structure relates to the helix formed by the interaction of two DNA strands.

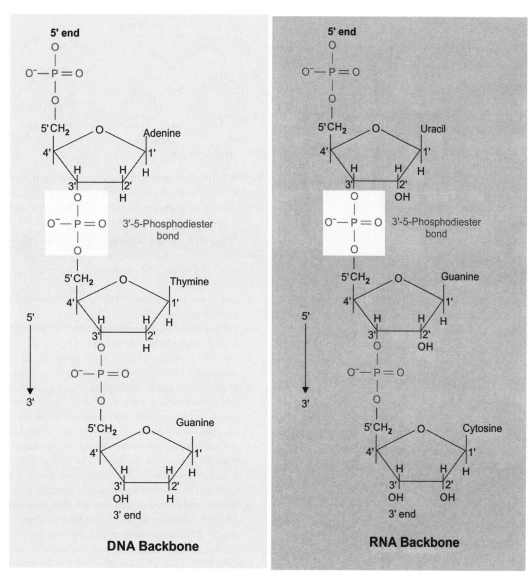

Figure 6.10: Phosphodiester linkages in the covalent backbone of DNA and RNA.

- It consists of two helical DNA chains wound around the same axis to form a **right handed double helix**. The chains are paired in an antiparallel manner, that is, the 5'- end of one strand is paired with the 3'- end of the other strand.

- The **hydrophilic deoxyribose** and **phosphate** groups of backbone of each chain are on the outside of the double helix, whereas the **hydrophobic purine** and **pyrimidine** bases of both strands are stacked inside the double helix **(Figure 6.11)**.

- The overall structure resembles a **twisted ladder**. The spatial relationship between the two strands in the helix creates a major (wide) groove and a minor (narrow) groove **(Figure 6.12)**. These grooves provide access for the binding of regulatory proteins along the DNA chain.

Certain anticancer drugs, such as dactinomycin (actinomycin D), exert their cytotoxic effect by interacting in to the narrow groove of the DNA double helix, thus interfering with DNA and RNA synthesis.

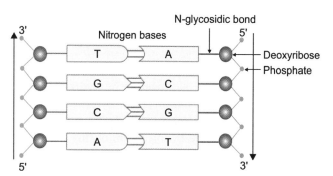

Figure 6.11: Backbones of DNA. Hydrophilic deoxyribose and phosphate groups are on the outside whereas the hydrophobic purine and pyrimidine bases of both strands are stacked inside.

- The bases of one strand of DNA are paired with bases of the second strand so that **A (Adenine)** is always paired with T **(Thymine)** and **G (Guanine)** is always paired with C **(Cytosine)**. Therefore, one polynucleotide chain of the DNA double helix is always the complement of the other.

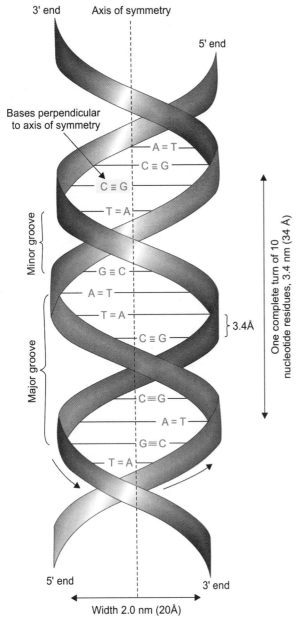

Figure 6.12: The double-helical structure of DNA.

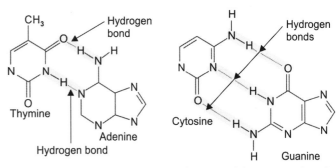

Figure 6.13: Base pairing between adenine and thymine involves the formation of two hydrogen bonds and base pairing between cytosine and guanine involves the formation of three hydrogen bonds.

Specificity of the Pairing of Bases and Chargaff's Rule

Erwin Chargaff and his colleagues in the late 1940s led to the following conclusions.

❖ The base composition of DNA generally varies from one species to another.

❖ DNA specimens isolated from different tissues of the same species have the same base composition.

❖ The base composition of DNA in a given species does not change with an organism's age, nutritional state or changing environment.

❖ In all cellular DNAs, regardless of the species, the number of adenosine residues is equal to the number of thymidine residues (A = T) and the number of guanosine residues is equal the number of cytidine residues (G = C). From these relationships it follows that the sum of the purine residues equals the sum of the pyrimidine residues; that is, A + G = T + C. The ratio of purine to pyrimidine bases in the DNA is always one, i.e. A + G/T + C = 1. These quantitative relationships is called Chargaff's rules.

❖ Watson and Crick deduced that adenine must pair with thymine and guanine with cytosine, because of stearic and hydrogen bonding factors adenine cannot pair with cytosine and guanine cannot pair with thymine. Thus, one member of a base pair in a DNA must always be a purine and the other a pyrimidine. This base pairing restriction explains that in a double stranded DNA molecule, the content of A equals that of T and the content of G equals that of C.

- The base pairs are held together by **hydrogen bonds**. Adenine is always paired with thymine in DNA by formation of **two hydrogen bonds**; guanine is always paired with cytosine by formation of **three hydrogen bonds (Figure 6.13)**. This is the reason why separation of DNA strands is more difficult having higher ratio of G ≡ C to A = T base pairs.
- The **hydrogen bonds**, plus **base stacking interactions** (the hydrophobic interaction between the stacked bases) stabilize the structure of the double helix.
- The specific base pairing in DNA leads to the **Chargaff rule**: i.e. in any sample of DNA the amount of adenine equals the amount of thymine; the amount of guanine equals to amount of cytosine, and the total amounts of purines equals the total amount of pyrimidines.

Functions of DNA

- DNA is the **store of genetic information**.
- The information is stored among 46 (23 pairs) chromosomes. These chromosomes are made up of thousands of shorter segments of DNA, called **genes**.
- Each gene stores directions for the synthesis of all protein molecules of the cell. Proteins act as enzymes, structural support, hormones, and other functional molecules.

▌ DNA ORGANIZATION

The DNA in a single human cell, if stretched to its full length, is 1.74 meters. To get DNA into a nucleus of the cells, it must have a very compact form. The structural flexibility of DNA allows it to form more compacted structures than simple linear B-form structure.

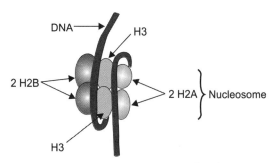

Figure 6.14: Diagrammatic representation of nucleosome in which DNA is wrapped around histone octamer consisting of two each of histones H2A, H2B, H3, and H4.

- Eukaryotic DNA is organized into **chromatin**, a compact form of DNA. In chromatin DNA is tightly bound to a group of small basic proteins called **histone**.
- Chromatin is made up of repeating units, each containing 200 BP of DNA and **histone octamer** containing two copies each of four histone proteins H2A, H2B, H3, and H4.
- Histones are positively charged **proteins** (because histone is rich in arginine or lysine) that strongly adhere to negatively-charged DNA and form complexes called **nucleosomes (Figure 6.14)**. Each nucleosome is composed of DNA wound around eight **histone proteins**. Around histone octamer a segment of the DNA double helix is wound nearly twice.
- The repeating units of the histone Octamer and the associated DNA are known as **nucleosomes**.
- In addition to the net shortening of a DNA strand produced by winding of it around the histones, additional shortening packaging of eukaryotic DNA is brought about by an orderly helical arrangement of **six nucleosomes** per turn called **solenoid (Figure 6.15)**.
- The solenoids are further folded into supercoiled loops which are attached to the nuclear lamina to form chromosomes.
- The packing of DNA in a chromosome represents a 10,000 fold shortening of its length from primary B-form DNA.
- The number of chromosomes varies from organism to organism; a human has 46 chromosomes or 23 pairs of chromosomes.
- When a eukaryotic cell is not actively dividing, its nucleus is occupied by chromatin **(Figure 6.16)**
- During cell division, chromatin organizes itself into chromosomes (a complex of proteins and DNA molecules that is visible during cell division) **(Figure 6.16)**.

Different Structural forms (Polymorphism) of DNA

- ❖ DNA is a very flexible molecule and has the ability to exist in various forms based on the environmental conditions, a feature known as **structural polymorphism**. The three different types of structural conformations of DNA are:

Contd...

Contd...

- ➢ A-DNA
- ➢ B-DNA
- ➢ Z-DNA
- ❖ Among these three types, the most abundant type of DNA is **B-DNA**, commonly known as **Watson-Crick Model** of DNA double helix.
- ❖ A and B forms of DNA are the right handed forms whereas Z-DNA is the left handed form.
- ❖ When hydrated the DNA generally adopts B-form. The A-form is found under dehydrating conditions.
- ❖ The formation of Z-DNA occurs with the methylation of deoxycytosine residues.
- ❖ Important structural features of A-DNA, B-DNA, and Z-DNA are given in **Table 6.3**.

Genetical Types of DNA

- ❖ In human genetics, there are four genetically types of DNA. These are the
  1. Autosomal
  2. Mitochondrial
  3. X chromosome
  4. Y chromosome
- ❖ **The autosomal DNA** makes up the 22 out of the 23 chromosome pairs in a human. The autosomes are the genetic material that humans inherit from their parents, who inherit theirs from their parents, and so on. Each autosome goes through a genetic process that randomly pairs up the autosomes from each parent, called "recombination," after which the newly paired autosomes are passed down to the children. This is why children tend to look like their parents, or even their great-grandparents, because the autosomes are imprinted with all the genetic blueprints from each of the preceding generations. The autosomal DNA is very important in finding out a person's ancestry and parentage, especially for people who question who their parents are.
- ❖ **Mitochondrial DNA** is another type that is contained inside the mitochondria. Unlike autosomes that pass down genes from both parents, the mitochondria follow a maternal line, although a mother also passes down her mitochondrial DNA to her sons. This makes mitochondrial testing less accurate if a person wants to trace her family tree, although it may be more effective to use a maternity test to determine a person's biological mother.
- ❖ **X and Y chromosomal DNA:** Of all the 23 chromosome pairs that make up a human being, only **one pair** is allocated to determine the sex of the child. This particular pair is called the **allosomal pair**, which contains the **X and Y chromosome DNA**. Females generally have **two X chromosomes**, while males have one each of the **X and Y chromosomes**. During fertilization, the mother passes down one of her X chromosomes to her offspring, regardless of its sex. The father's sperm, on the other hand, donates his X chromosome to make another female offspring, while passing down his Y chromosome to a male offspring.

■ RNA STRUCTURE AND FUNCTION

RNA is similar to DNA. The successive nucleotides of both DNA and RNA are covalently linked through **phosphate**

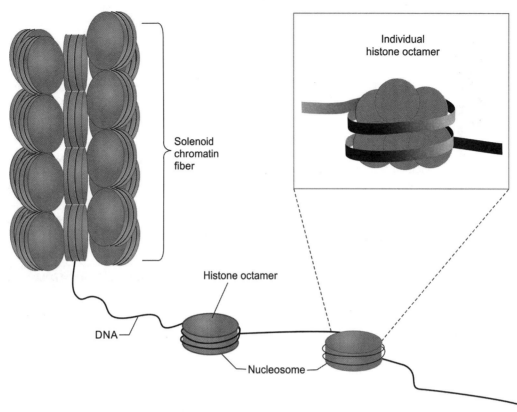

Figure 6.15: DNA wrapped around clusters of histone proteins to form nucleosomes, which are coiled to form solenoids, the basis of the chromatin fiber that makes up chromosomes.

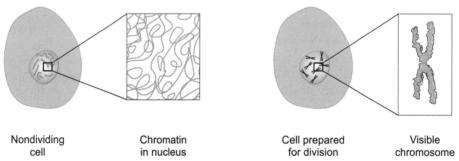

Figure 6.16: Chromatin in nondividing cell and chromosome in cell prepared for division.

TABLE 6.3: Comparison of the structural features of A-DNA, B-DNA, and Z-DNA.

Structural features	A-DNA	B-DNA	Z-DNA
Helix turn	Right hand	Right hand	Left hand
Helical diameter	26 Å	20 Å	18 Å
Height of helical turn (helical pitch)	28.6 Å	34 Å	44Å
Number of base pairs per helical turn	11.6	10	12
Distance between each base pair (helical rise/base pair)	2.9 Å	3.4 Å	7.4 Å
Tilt of the base pairs relative to the helical axis	20°	6°	7°
Major grove	Narrow and deep	Wide and deep	Flat major groves
Minor grove	Wide and shallow	Narrow and deep	Narrow and deep

group, in which the **5′-phosphate group** of one nucleotide unit is joined to the **3′-hydroxyl group** of the next nucleotides creating a **3′-5′ phosphodiester linkage (Figure 6.10)**. The four major bases in RNA are: **purine bases** are Adenine (A) and Guanine (G) and **pyrimidine bases** are Cytosine (C), and Uracil (U).

Although RNA shares many features with DNA, RNA possesses several different features. These are:

- In RNA, the sugar is **ribose** rather than **2′-deoxyribose** of DNA
- It does not possess **thymine** except in the rare case. Instead of thymine, RNA contains **uracil**.
- In RNA **adenine** pairs with **uracil** rather than thymine.
- Unlike DNA, RNA is a single stranded and does not exhibit the equivalence of adenine with uracil and cytosine with guanine.
- RNA molecules do contain regions of double helical structure that are produced by the formation of hairpin loops. RNA is capable of folding back on itself like a hairpin and thus acquiring double stranded characteristics.

Types of RNA

Cell contains three major types of RNA:
1. Messenger RNA (mRNA)
2. Transfer RNA (tRNA)
3. Ribosomal RNA (rRNA).

All of these are involved in some aspects in the process of protein biosynthesis. Each differs from the others by size and function.

Messenger RNA

Structure of mRNA

The mRNA comprises only about 5 to 10% of total cellular RNA. mRNA is synthesized in the nucleus as **heterogeneous RNA (hnRNA)**, which are processed into functional mRNA. The mRNA carries the genetic information in the form of **codons**. Codons are a group of three adjacent nucleotides that code for the amino acids of protein.

In eukaryotes mRNAs have some unique characteristics, e.g:
- The 5′ end of mRNA is **capped** by a **7-methyl-guanosine triphosphate**. The cap is involved in the recognition of mRNA in protein biosynthesis and it helps to stabilize the mRNA by preventing attack of 5′-exonucleases.
- **A poly (A) tail** is attached to the other 3′-end of mRNA. This tail consists of series of **adenylate residues**, 20 to 250 nucleotides in length joined by 3′ to 5′ phospho-diester bonds **(Figure 6.17)**. The function of poly A tail is not fully understood, but it seems that it helps to stabilize mRNA by preventing the attack of 3′-exonuclease.

Function of mRNA

The mRNAs serve as **template** for protein biosynthesis and transfer genetic information from DNA to protein synthesizing machinery.

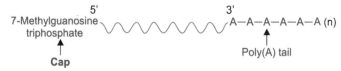

Figure 6.17: Schematic structure of mRNA.

If the mRNA codes for only one peptide, the mRNA is **monocistronic**. If it codes for two or more different polypeptides, the mRNA is **polycistronic**. In eukaryotes most mRNA are monocistronic but in prokaryotes it is polycistronic.

Transfer RNA

Structure of tRNA

The structure of tRNA appears like a **clover leaf**. tRNA molecules vary in length from 74 to 95 nucleotides. There are at least **20 different tRNA** molecules one for each of the amino acids that is used in the synthesis of proteins. Many amino acids have more than one tRNA.

All tRNAs contain four main **arms**. The arms have base paired stems and unpaired **loops** as shown in **Figures 6.18**. The four arms of tRNA are:
1. The acceptor arm
2. The D arm
3. The anticodon arm
4. The TΨ C arm.
    - The **acceptor arm** consists of a base paired stem that terminates in the sequence CCA (5′→ 3′) at the 3′ end, is the attachment site for the amino acid that is carried by the tRNA.
    - The **D arm** is named for the presence of the base dihydrouridine (D).
    - **The anticodon arm** contains the anticodon that base pairs with the codon on mRNA. Anticodon has nucleotide sequence complementary to the codon of mRNA and is responsible for the specificity of the tRNA.
    - The TΨC arm contains both ribothymidine (T) and pseudouridine (ψ psi). The extra arm also known

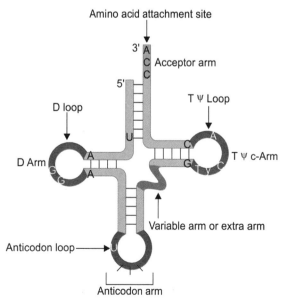

Figure 6.18: The clover leaf structure of transfer RNA. Bases that commonly occur in a particular position are indicated by letters. Base pairing in stem regions is indicated by lines between strands.

as variable arm because it varies in size, is found between the anticodon and TψC arms.

The secondary structure of tRNA molecules is maintained by the base pairing in these arms or stem regions. The acceptor arms have 7-bp (base pairing). TψC and anticodon arms have 5-bp and D arm has 3 or 4-bp.

Function of tRNA

tRNA carries amino acids in an activated form to the ribosome for the biosynthesis of protein.

Unusual Nucleotides
In eukaryotic cells, 10 to 20% of the nucleotides of tRNA may be modified and known as unusual nucleotides (**Figure 6.19**), e.g: ❖ **Dihydrouridine (D)**, in which one of the double bonds of the base is reduced   ❖ **Ribothymidine (T)** in which methyl group is added to uracil to form thymine   ❖ **Pseudouridine** (ψ psi), in which uracil is attached to ribose by a carbon-carbon bond rather than a nitrogen bond.

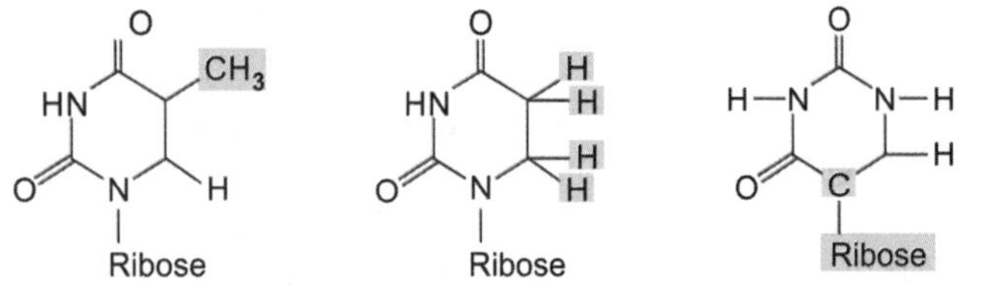

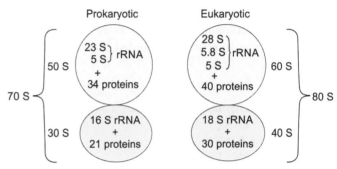

Ribothymidine (T)   **Dihydrouridine (D)**   **Pseudouridine (ψ)**

Figure 6.19: Three unusual (modified) nucleosides present in tRNA.

Figure 6.20: The components of prokaryotic and eukaryotic ribosomal subunits.

Ribosomal RNA

The RNA of the ribosomes is called the rRNA. Ribosomes are minute particles consisting of RNA and proteins that function to synthesize proteins from the mRNA template. Ribosomes can be found floating within the **cytoplasm** or attached to the **endoplasmic reticulum**.

- The ribosome is a spheroidal particle and is composed of a **large** and a **small** subunit.
- Ribosomes from prokaryotic and eukaryotic cells are characterized by having sedimentation coefficients of **70S** and **80S**, respectively.
- The 70S ribosome yields 50S and 30S, whereas 80S ribosome yields 60S and 40S subunits.
- Each subunit is composed of one or more strand of rRNA and numerous protein molecules.
- Prokaryotic ribosomes contain **three RNA** molecules, **16S rRNA** in the small subunit, and **23S** and **5S** in the large subunit.
- In the eukaryotes there are **four rRNAs, 18S** in the small subunit, and **28S, 5.8S,** and **5S** in the large subunits **(Figure 6.20)**.

- ❖ A sedimentation coefficient is a measure of rate of sedimentation of a macromolecule in a high speed centrifuge (ultracentrifuge).
- ❖ It is expressed in **Svedberg unit (S)**.
- ❖ Sedimentation rate depends on **shape** as well as **mass**. And isn't directly proportional to molecular weight.
- ❖ Sedimentation coefficient is not additive because sedimentation rate depends on shape as well as mass. And isn't directly proportional to molecular weight.
- ❖ A long organelle sediments slower, than a round globe shaped one, even if they have the same mass.

Functions of rRNA

- Ribosomes are the workplaces of protein biosynthesis, the process of translating mRNA into protein. Ribosomal RNA necessary to **maintain ribosomal structure**.
- Ribosomal RNAs also provide some of the **catalytic activities** and function as an enzyme a *ribozyme.*
- The RNA components of ribosomes have **peptidyl transferase** activity that is responsible for formation of peptide bonds during protein biosynthesis in an elongation process.
- Small nuclear RNA with proteins catalyzes **splicing of exons** (coding region).

Other Nuclear and Cytoplasmic RNAs

Besides mRNA, tRNA and rRNA eukaryotes have some other RNAs. These are:
- Heterogeneous RNAs (hnRNAs)
- Small cytoplasmic RNAs (scRNAs)
- Small nuclear RNAs (snRNAs)
- Micro RNA (miRNA)
- Small interfering RNA (siRNA)

Various RNAs and their functions are given in **Table 6.4**.

Heterogeneous RNAs (hnRNAs)

The nucleus contains a special type of RNA that **turns over very rapidly during protein synthesis** called **heterogeneous nuclear RNA (hnRNA)**, which consists of a mixture of very long RNA molecules. The hnRNAs are much longer than mRNA. The hnRNAs are precursors of mRNA, i.e., mRNAs are formed from longer hnRNAs. They are subsequently modified by attachment of a long poly-A tail at 3′ end and mehtylguanosine cap at the 5′ end.

TABLE 6.4: Different types of cellular RNAs and their functions.

Types of RNA	Functions
mRNA (messenger RNA)	Carriers the genetic information from DNA to the cytosol, where it is used as the template for proteins synthesis
tRNA (transfer RNA)	Serves as an "adaptor" molecule that carries its specific amino acid to the site of protein synthesis
rRNA (ribosomal RNA)	In association with protein serve as the sites for protein synthesis. Provide catalytic activities (peptidyl transferase activity)
hnRNA (heterogeneous nuclear RNA)	Serves as precursor for mRNA
sc-RNA (small cytoplasmic RNA)	Involved in recognition of signal sequence in protein synthesis on membrane bound ribosomes
snRNA (small nuclear RNA)	Aid excising introns and splicing exons
miRNA (Micro RNA)	Play a key role in gene expression to control diverse biological processes such as cellular growth, differentiation, development, and apoptosis
siRNA (small interfering RNA)	It interferes with the expression of specific genes by degrading mRNA after transcription, preventing translation

Small Cytoplasmic RNAs (scRNA)

The scRNA is of 294 nucleotides, present in cytoplasm and is associated with **signal recognition protein**. The scRNA is involved in recognition of signal sequence in protein synthesis on membrane bound ribosomes.

Small Nuclear RNAs (snRNA)

The nucleus contains many types of small RNA molecules with less than 300 nucleotides, referred to as snRNAs (small nuclear RNAs).

- These RNA molecules are associated with specific proteins to form complex termed **snRNPs** (small nuclear ribonucleoproteins particles). Some of them are designated **U1, U2, U4, U5,** and **U6,** etc. snRNAs are involved in the process of removal of introns and splicing of successive exons of mRNA precursor.
- Intron is noncoding sequences that interrupt the coding portions of a gene (exons). After transcription, they are removed to prepare mRNA for translation.

MicroRNA (miRNA)

- MicroRNAs (miRNAs) are **a class of noncoding RNAs which are 19–25 nucleotides in size**.
- **They play important roles in** post-transcriptional regulation of gene expression.
- miRNAs have a key role in gene expression to control diverse biological processes such as **cellular growth**, **differentiation**, **development**, and **apoptosis**.
- MicroRNAs are regulators of gene expression that are involved in **carcinogenesis**, **metastasis**, and **invasion**.
- Thus, miRNAs are likely to be useful as diagnostic and prognostic biomarkers and for cancer therapy.
- MicroRNAs are informative biomarkers for early cancer detection and treatment decisions.

Small Interfering RNA (siRNA)

- **Small interfering RNA**, sometimes known as **short interfering RNA** or **silencing RNA**, is a class of double-stranded RNA molecules, 20–25 nucleotides in length.
- It interferes with the expression of specific genes by degrading mRNA after transcription, preventing translation.
- Artificially synthesized 19–23 nucleotide long double-stranded siRNA molecules are routinely used in molecular biology to "silence" or turn off the production of specific genes that cause disease or that contribute to disease.

ASSESSMENT QUESTIONS

▌SHORT ESSAY QUESTIONS (SEQs)

1. What is synthetic analogue of nucleotide? Give its clinical application with examples.
2. Give structure and function of DNA.
3. Give types, structure, and functions of RNA.
4. Give different types and functions of biologically important nucleotides of adenine.
5. How DNA is organized?

▌SHORT ANSWER QUESTIONS (SAQs)

1. Write importance of cyclic AMP.
2. What is nucleotide? Name biologically important free nucleotides.
3. Draw and label the structure of tRNA. Write functions of tRNA.
4. Which are the unusual naturally occurring purine and pyrimidine bases?

5. Name the bases found in nucleic acids and their nucleotides.
6. Name four hormones using cAMP as a second messenger.
7. What is miRNA? Give its importance in medicine
8. Which are unusual nucleotides of tRNA?
9. DNA is negatively charged at physiological pH. Justify.
10. Which are the genetical types of DNA?

■ MULTIPLE CHOICE QUESTIONS (MCQs)

1. **Triple bonds are found between which base pairs:**
   a. A-T
   b. C-G
   c. A-G
   d. C-T

2. **Chargaff rule state that:**
   a. A + G = T + C
   b. A/T = G/C
   c. A = U = T = G = C
   d. A + T = G + C

3. **Thymine is present in which of the following:**
   a. Ribosomal RNA
   b. Messenger RNA
   c. Transfer RNA
   d. None of the above

4. **Unusual nucleotide pseudouridylic acid is present in:**
   a. mRNA
   b. tRNA
   c. rRNA
   d. hnRNA

5. **A nucleoside can be composed of, *except*:**
   a. Purine base
   b. Pentose sugar
   c. Phosphate group
   d. Pyrimidine base

6. **Nucleotides perform all of the following functions, *except*:**
   a. Structural units of DNA and RNA
   b. Catalytic in nature
   c. Regulators of metabolic reactions
   d. Components of certain coenzymes

7. **Which of the following is not a feature of Watson-Crick Model of DNA?**
   a. Helical
   b. Two strands are held by hydrogen bond
   c. A + T = C + G
   d. Two strands are right handed

8. **The number of hydrogen bonds between guanosine and cytosine in DNA are:**
   a. One
   b. Two
   c. Three
   d. Four

9. **DNA is present in:**
   a. Only nucleus
   b. Only mitochondria
   c. Both nucleus and mitochondria
   d. Cytoplasm

10. **RNA is present in:**
    a. Nucleus
    b. Only cytoplasm
    c. Mitochondria
    d. Cytoplasm and nucleolus

11. **In a double stranded molecule of DNA the ratio of purines to pyrimidines is:**
    a. 1:1
    b. 1:2
    c. 2:1
    d. Variable

12. **In DNA base adenine is always paired with:**
    a. Guanine
    b. Cytosine
    c. Uracil
    d. Thymine

13. **Which of the following is a correct description of the chemistry of DNA and RNA?**
    a. Uracil is a purine base that occurs in RNA but not in DNA
    b. Cytosine is a pyrimidine base that occurs in both RNA and DNA
    c. Ribose is a pentose sugar that occurs in DNA and RNA
    d. Thymine is a pyrimidine base that occurs in RNA but not in DNA.

14. **Which of the following does not involved in the formation of DNA?**
    a. Deoxyribose
    b. Pyrimidine
    c. Phosphate
    d. Uracil

15. **Which of the following nitrogenous bases is found in DNA but is not found in RNA?**
    a. Adenine
    b. Thymine
    c. Cytosine
    d. Uracil

16. **In nucleic acids, the purine nitrogenous bases are:**
    a. Guanine and thymine
    b. Cytosine and guanine
    c. Thymine and cytosine
    d. Adenine and guanine

17. **Which element occurs in nucleic acids?**
    a. Calcium
    b. Phosphorus
    c. Manganese
    d. Sulphur

18. **The groups of molecules called nucleotides contain:**
    a. Phosphate groups
    b. Pyrimidine and purine
    c. Pentose sugar
    d. All of the above

19. **Nucleotides have a nitrogenous base attached to a sugar at the:**
    a. 1' carbon of sugar
    b. 2' carbon of sugar
    c. 3' carbon of sugar
    d. 5' carbon of sugar

20. **The two strands of a DNA double helix are held together by:**
    a. Ionic bonds
    b. Hydrogen bonds
    c. Nonpolar covalent bonds
    d. Polar covalent bonds

21. **At the physiological pH the DNA molecules are:**
    a. Positively charged
    b. Negatively charged
    c. Neutral
    d. Amphipathic

22. **True about mitochondrial DNA:**
    a. Maternal inheritance
    b. Not highly conserved and has high mutation rate
    c. Mitochondrial diseases is associated mostly with mutation and some have deletion
    d. All of the above

23. **True about mitochondrial DNA, *except*:**
    a. UGA codes for tryptophan
    b. Codes for 13 protein
    c. Paternal inheritance
    d. Circular double stranded DNA
    e. Mitochondrial disease occur due to point mutation and large-scale rearrangements

24. **True about histone protein:**
    a. Ribonucleoprotein
    b. Present inside the nucleus
    c. Acidic
    d. Glycoprotein

25. Components of chromosome are:
    a. DNA
    b. tRNA
    c. mRNA
    d. rRNA
    e. Histones

26. The protein rich in basic amino acids, which function in the packaging of DNA in chromosomes, is:
    a. Histone
    b. Collagen
    c. Hyaluronic acid binding protein
    d. Fibrinogen

27. Nucleosome consists of:
    a. Histone
    b. DNA
    c. RNA
    d. DNA and RNA both
    e. Carbohydrate

28. True about nucleosome:
    a. Use only one type of histone protein
    b. Each complex is separated from each other by non-histone proteins
    c. Regular repeating structure of DNA and histone proteins
    d. None of the above

29. Which one of the following nucleotide base is not present in codons?
    a. Adenine
    b. Guanine
    c. Thymine
    d. Cytosine

30. Nucleoside is made up of:
    a. Pyrimidine
    b. Histone
    c. Sugar
    d. Purine
    e. Phosphate

31. A synthetic nucleotide analogue, 4-hydroxypyrazolopyrimidine is used in the treatment of:
    a. Acute nephritis
    b. Gout
    c. Cystic fibrosis of lung
    d. Multiple myeloma

32. A synthetic nucleotide analogue, used in the chemotherapy of cancer and viral infections is:
    a. Arabinosyl-cytosine
    b. 4-Hydroxypyrazolopyrimidine
    c. 6-Mercaptopurine
    d. 6-Thioguanine

33. ATP is a:
    a. Nucleoside
    b. Nucleotide
    c. Vitamin
    d. Nucleic acid

34. Which of the following free nucleotide act as a second messenger?
    a. AMP
    b. cAMP
    c. ADP
    d. ATP

35. Which of the following free nucleotide involved in relaxation of smooth muscle?
    a. AMP
    b. cAMP
    c. cGMP
    d. GMP

36. Which of the following free nucleotide involved in detoxification?
    a. ADP
    b. UDP
    c. GDP
    d. CDP

37. Pyrimidine is a part of:
    a. Adenosine
    b. Cytidine
    c. Uridine
    d. Cysteine
    e. Guanosine

38. Apart from occurring in nucleic acid, pyrimidines are also found in:
    a. Theophylline
    b. Theobromine
    c. Flavin mononucleotide
    d. Thiamin

39. Which of the following is not a nitrogenous base?
    a. Adenine
    b. Guanosine
    c. Cytosine
    d. Thymine

40. A nucleic acid was analyzed and found to contain 32% adenine, 18% guanine, 17% cytosine and 33% thymine. The nucleic acid must be:
    a. Single-stranded RNA
    b. Single-stranded DNA
    c. Double-stranded RNA
    d. Double-stranded DNA

41. Choose the true statement about mitochondrial DNA:
    a. Few mutation compared to nuclear DNA
    b. It has 3 x 10" base pairs
    c. It receives 23 chromosomes from each parent
    d. It codes for less than 20% of the proteins involved in respiratory chain

42. All are true about mitochondrial DNA, *except*:
    a. Contains 37 gene
    b. Transmit from mother to offsprings
    c. Transmit in classical Mendelian fashion
    d. Cause Leber hereditary optic neuropathy

43. Mitochondrial DNA is:
    a. Closed circular
    b. Nicked circular
    c. Linear
    d. Open circular

ANSWERS FOR MCQs

1. b	2. a	3. c	4. b	5. c
6. b	7. c	8. c	9. c	10. d
11. a	12. d	13. b	14. d	15. b
16. d	17. b	18. d	19. a	20. b
21. b	22. d	23. c	24. b	
25. a and e		26. a	27. a and b	
28. c	29. c	30. a,c, and d		31. b
32. a	33. b	34. b	35. c	36. b
37. b and c		38. d	39. b	40. d
41. d	42. c	43. a		

Chemistry of Hemoglobin and Hemoglobinopathies

Competency	Learning Objectives
BI 6.11: Describe the functions of heme in the body and describe the processes involved in its metabolism and describe porphyrin metabolism. **BI 6.12:** Describe the major types of hemoglobin and its derivatives found in the body and their physiological/pathological relevance.	1. Describe structure and functions of hemoglobin. 2. Describe the binding sites for oxygen, hydrogen (H⁺) and carbon dioxide (CO_2) with hemoglobin. 3. Describe cooperative oxygen binding of hemoglobin. 4. Describe effect of 2,3-bisphosphoglycerate on binding of oxygen to hemoglobin. 5. Describe the types of normal human hemoglobin. 6. Describe derivatives of hemoglobin. 7. Describe and discuss hemoglobinopathies.

■ OVERVIEW

Hemoglobin is conjugated proteins, with a prosthetic group heme. Hemoglobin found in red blood cell, carries oxygen from lungs to the tissues and carries carbon dioxide from tissues to the lungs. The red color of blood is due to the hemoglobin content of the erythrocytes.

■ STRUCTURE AND FUNCTIONS OF HEMOGLOBIN

Hemoglobin is a globular, oligomeric protein made up of **heme** and **globin**.

Heme

The heme is iron-containing compound belonging to the class of compounds **porphyrin**. Porphyrin is composed of four pyrrole rings which are linked by methane (=CH) bridge to form tetrapyrrole ring (porphyrin). Four methyl, two vinyl and two propionate side chain groups are attached to the porphyrin ring called **protoporphyrin IX** (derivative of porphyrin). This substituent can be arranged in 15 different ways. But only one of this isomer called **protoporphyrin IX** is biologically active.

The iron (Fe^{2+}) is held in the center of the protoporphyrin molecule by coordination bonds with the four nitrogen of

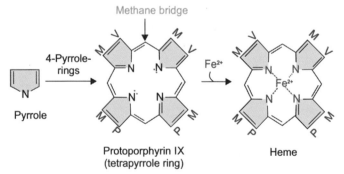

Figure 7.1: Structure of heme. Side chains of the pyrrole rings are designated.
(M: methyl, V: Vinyl, P: propionic acid)

the protoporphyrin ring **(Figure 7.1)**. The iron atom has six coordination bonds.

- Four bonds are formed between the iron and nitrogen atoms of the porphyrin ring system
- Fifth bond is formed between nitrogen atoms of histidine residue of the globin polypeptide chain, known as **proximal histidine (F-8) (eighth residue of F helix)**.
- Sixth bond is formed with oxygen.

The oxygenated form of hemoglobin is stabilized by the **hydrogen bond** between oxygen and side chain of another histidine residue of the chain, known as **distal histidine (F-7) (seventh residue of F helix) (Figure 7.2)**. The distal

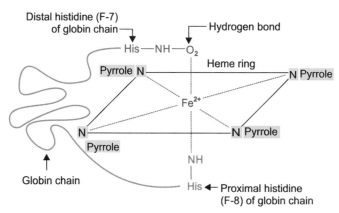

Figure 7.2: Coordination bonds of iron.

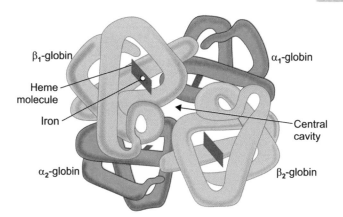

Figure 7.3: Quaternary structure of hemoglobin.

histidine is not directly involved with the heme group but helps to stabilize the binding of oxygen to the heme molecule. The proximal (F-8) and distal (F-7) histidine residues lie on opposite sides of the heme ring.

Globin

Globin belongs to the class of protein called **globulins**. Globin molecule contains four polypeptide chains, **two alpha (α)** chains (141 amino acid residues each) and **two beta (β)** or **two gamma (γ)** or **two delta (δ)** or **two epsilon (ϵ)** as per the type of hemoglobin (refer normal hemoglobin). The β, γ, δ and ϵ chains have 146 amino acid residues each.

With each polypeptide chain one molecule of heme is attached. A hemoglobin molecule therefore has four heme molecules. Four globin polypeptide chains with four heme molecules are held together in a definite arrangement or conformation to constitute a characteristic quaternary structure of hemoglobin (**Figure 7.3**), which is stabilized by:

- Hydrogen bonds
- Salt bridges
- Van der Waals forces

There is a central open channel or cavity in hemoglobin molecule.

Importance of Globin

The globin chains of hemoglobin form a protective hydrophobic pocket for binding of heme (**Figure 7.4**) that protects the reduced form of iron (Fe^{2+}) of heme from oxidizing to the ferric (Fe^{3+}) form, from the aqueous environment and permits reversible binding of oxygen with Fe^{2+} ion of heme. Exposure of heme iron to water result in oxidation of Fe^{2+} to Fe^{3+} form and loss of oxygen binding capacity.

Functions of Hemoglobin

- Transport of O_2 from lungs to tissues
- Transport of CO_2 and H^+ from tissues to lungs and kidney
- Acts as an intracellular buffer and is thus involved in acid-base balance

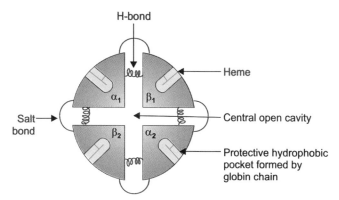

Figure 7.4: Schematic representation of quaternary structure of hemoglobin.

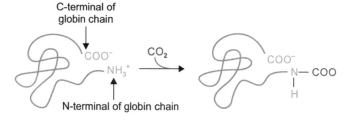

Figure 7.5: Binding site for carbon dioxide with globin chain of Hb.

BINDING SITES FOR OXYGEN, HYDROGEN (H$^+$) AND CARBON DIOXIDE (CO$_2$) WITH HEMOGLOBIN

- Oxygen is bound to the ferrous (Fe^{2+}) atoms of the heme (**Figure 7.2**) to form oxyhemoglobin.
- Hydrogen is bound to R-groups (side chain) of histidine residues in α- and β-chains
- Carbon dioxide is bound by the α-amino group of N-terminal end of each of the polypeptide chains of hemoglobin to form carbaminohemoglobin (**Figure 7.5**).

COOPERATIVE OXYGEN BINDING OF HEMOGLOBIN

The binding of the first oxygen to heme of the hemoglobin enhances the binding of oxygen to the remaining heme of the same molecule of hemoglobin. Oxygenation of hemoglobin is

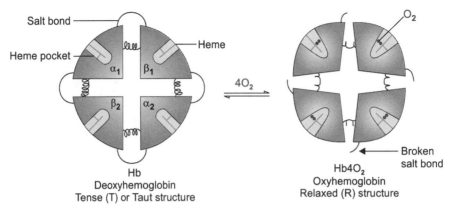

Figure 7.6: Schematic representation of changes during oxygenation of deoxyhemoglobin.

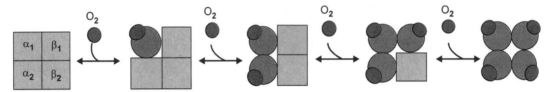

Figure 7.7: Cooperative binding of O_2 to hemoglobin: The binding of molecular oxygen to α-subunit of Hb changes the conformation of that particular subunit. This transition affects the affinity of the other subunit for oxygen.

accompanied by conformational changes in the tertiary and quaternary structure of hemoglobin **(Figure 7.6)**.

- A molecule of O_2 bound first by the α-chain whose heme pockets are more readily accessible than those of the β-chains as heme pockets of the β-**chains are blocked by valine residue**.
- Binding of oxygen is accompanied by the rupture of salt bonds of all four subunits and **protons** are generated.
- These changes alter hemoglobin's secondary, tertiary and quaternary structures and widening of heme pockets of the remaining subunits occurs and facilitates the binding of O_2 to these subunits

Thus as O_2 binds to some site of hemoglobin, the binding of more O_2 to hemoglobin becomes easier. In other words, we can say O_2 binds **cooperatively to hemoglobin (Figure 7.7)**.

- The cooperative binding of O_2 by hemoglobin enhances oxygen transport.
- The shape of O_2 binding curve of hemoglobin is **sigmoidal (S-shaped) (Figure 7.8)** because oxygen binding is cooperative. This shape indicates that the affinity of hemoglobin for binding the first molecule of oxygen is relatively very low, but subsequent oxygen molecules are bound with a very much higher affinity (almost 500-fold) accounting for the **steeply rising portion of the S-shaped curve (Figure 7.8)**.
- Because of cooperativity between O_2 binding sites, hemoglobin delivers more O_2 to tissues than would a noncooperative protein myoglobin **(see Figure 7.7)**. The cooperative binding of oxygen by hemoglobin enables it to deliver **1.7 times** more as much oxygen as it would if the binding sites were independent.

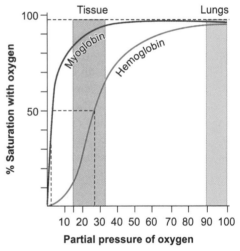

Figure 7.8: Oxygen binding curves for hemoglobin and myoglobin (the curve for hemoglobin is sigmoidal while that myoglobin is hyperbolic).

EFFECT OF 2,3-BISPHOSPHOGLYCERATE ON BINDING OF OXYGEN TO HEMOGLOBIN

2,3-bisphosphoglycerate (2,3-BPG) is formed as an intermediate in RBC by glycolysis **(see Figure 10.8)**. 2,3-BPG regulates the binding of O_2 to hemoglobin. The BPG significantly reduces the affinity of hemoglobin for oxygen. This reduced affinity allows hemoglobin to release oxygen efficiently at the partial pressure found in tissues.

- One molecule of 2,3-BPG binds in a pocket formed by **β-globin chains** in the central cavity of deoxygenated hemoglobin. This pocket contains several positively charged amino acid that form ionic bonds with the

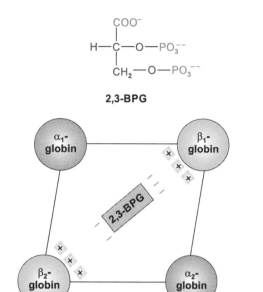

Figures 7.9: Structure of 2,3-BPG, and schematic representation of binding of 2,3-BPG to the hemoglobin.

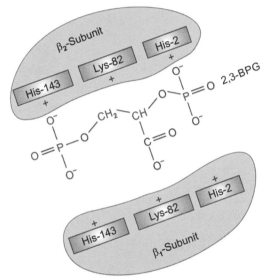

Figure 7.10: Binding of 2,3-BPG to β-globin chains of deoxyhemoglobin through ionic bonds with His-143, Lys-82 and His-2.

negatively charged phosphate groups of 2,3-BPG, cross linking β-chains **(Figure 7.9)**.

- In HbA the binding site is made up of **six positively** charged side chains of amino acid of β-globin chains. There 2,3-BPG interacts with **three positively** charged groups of His-143, His-2 and lys-82 on each β-chain **(Figure 7.10)**.
- Without 2,3-BPG, hemoglobin would be an extremely inefficient oxygen transporter, releasing only 8% of its oxygen in the tissue and the oxygen saturation curve of hemoglobin would approach that of myoglobin.

Clinical Importance of 2,3-BPG

The concentration of BPG in RBC can change by as much as **15–25%**. The number of 2,3-BPG molecules in each red blood is approximately **equal to the number of hemoglobin** molecules (about 2.2 mM).

- Its erythrocyte concentration is responsive to various physiological and pathological conditions.
- When there is a chronic tissue deprivation of oxygen, the level of 2,3-BPG increases, such compensatory increase occurs in:
  - Individuals who live at high altitudes
  - Patients with chronic obstructive pulmonary disease (COPD) like emphysema
  - Anemia
  - Cardiac failure.
- Elevated BPG levels lower the oxygen affinity of hemoglobin, permits greater unloading of oxygen in the capillaries of the hypoxic tissues.

STRIKE A NOTE

- ❖ 2,3-BPG plays an important role in blood that has been stored for transfusion. The concentration of 2,3-BPG in the stored red blood cells can fall from 2.2 mM to one-tenth of this concentration within a few days, resulting in a decreased ability of transfused blood to deliver O_2 to tissues.
- ❖ The problem cannot be solved by incorporating 2,3-BPG into the medium because this polar molecule cannot be transferred across the cell membrane.
- ❖ The decrease can be prevented by storing blood in the presence of inosine (hypoxanthine-ribose) that is converted to BPG by RBC. Inosine can enter RBC, where its ribose moiety is released from purine base and ribose can then be phosphorylated and enter the hexose monophosphate pathway and eventually being converted to 2,3-BPG via glycolysis.

▮ TYPES OF NORMAL HUMAN HEMOGLOBIN

Several different forms of hemoglobin can be found in adult humans and during human development, each containing four polypeptide subunits, made up of various combinations of six different polypeptide chains. They are designated:

1. Alpha (α)
2. Beta (β)
3. Gamma (γ)
4. Delta (δ)
5. Epsilon (ε)
6. Zeta (ζ)

Most forms of hemoglobin contain two α-chains plus two other chains usually β, γ, δ and ε **(Table 7.1)**.

Human Fetal Hemoglobin

Human fetal hemoglobin (HbF) is the major hemoglobin found in a fetus and a newborn:

- The first hemoglobin formed during embryogenesis is a tetramer of **two zeta** and **two epsilon** subunits ($\zeta_2\varepsilon_2$)
- Through the first 6 months of development the zeta subunits are replaced by alpha subunits and the epsilon subunits are replaced by the gamma subunits forming

TABLE 7.1: Normal type of Hb.

Type	Hemoglobin	Structure	Comment
Adult hemoglobin	HbA	$\alpha_2\beta_2$	Comprises 98% of adult Hb
	HbA2	$\alpha_2\delta_2$	Comprises 2% of adult Hb (Elevated in β-thalassemia)
Fetal hemoglobin	HbF	$\alpha_2\gamma_2$	Normal Hb in fetus (Increased in β-thalassemia)
Embryonic hemoglobin	HbE Portland	$\zeta_2\gamma_2$	Present at low levels during embryonic and fetal life
	HbE Gower I	$\zeta_2\epsilon_2$	Present only during embryonic life, and is the primary embryonic hemoglobin
	HbE Gower II	$\alpha_2\epsilon_2$	Present at low levels during embryonic and fetal life

HbF ($\alpha_2\gamma_2$). This type of hemoglobin is having a greater affinity for oxygen than adult hemoglobin. Therefore, the growing fetus is able to take its mother's oxygen from her bloodstream.

- Through later embryonic development and after birth, the gamma (γ) subunits are replaced by beta (β) chains and become $\alpha_2\beta_2$ (HbA1).

Adult Hemoglobin

After birth, the gamma (γ) subunits are replaced by beta (β) chains and become $\alpha_2\beta_2$ (HbA1). Hemoglobin F remains in the child's blood until it is around six months old and then almost all of it is replaced with adult hemoglobin. The two types of adult hemoglobin are:

1. **Hemoglobin A1 (HbA1, $\alpha_2\beta_2$):** It consists of **two alpha** and **two beta** chains and designated as $\alpha_2\beta_2$. Approximately 98% of the total hemoglobin of a normal adult is this type.
2. **Minor component of normal adult Hemoglobin A2 (HbA2, $\alpha_2\delta_2$):** It consists of **two alpha** and **two delta** chains and is designated as ($\alpha_2\delta_2$). It is present usually to the extent of 2.5% of the total.

Why HbF has High Affinity for O_2 than HbA1?

- ❖ **HbF** of fetal red blood cells has a higher oxygen affinity than that of maternal HbA1 of red blood cells because fetal hemoglobin does not bind 2,3-BPG as maternal hemoglobin does. 2,3-bisphosphoglycerate regulates the binding and release of oxygen from hemoglobin.
- ❖ Fetal hemoglobin tetramers include two α-chains and two γ-chains. In the γ-chain one of the basic amino acid **His-143** of the β-chain (of the BPG binding site) has been replaced by **neutral serine amino acid** and reduces the affinity of fetal Hb for 2,3-BPG, thereby increasing the oxygen binding affinity of fetal Hb relative to that of maternal (adult) hemoglobin **(Figure 7.11)**.
- ❖ This difference in oxygen affinity of hemoglobin allows oxygen to be effectively transferred from maternal to fetal red blood cells. This is one of the physiological adaptations in order to attract oxygen from maternal blood (at the lower PO_2 of the placenta) and deliver it to the fetus.

■ TYPES OF DERIVATIVES OF HEMOGLOBIN

Hemoglobin readily combines with any gas or other substances to form some products which are called the

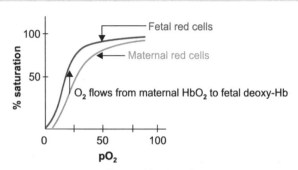

Figure 7.11: Oxygen affinity of fetal and maternal red blood cell.

derivatives of hemoglobin. These can be grouped into—**normal derivatives** and **abnormal derivatives**.

- **Normal hemoglobin derivatives**
  - Oxyhemoglobin
  - Reduced hemoglobin
  - Carbaminohemoglobin or carbhemoglobin
  - Glycated hemoglobin (HbA1c)
- **Abnormal hemoglobin derivatives**
  - Methemoglobin
  - Sulfhemoglobin
  - Carboxyhemoglobin
- The derivatives of hemoglobin give **characteristic absorption bands** in the solar spectrum by which they may be identified.
- Abnormal hemoglobin derivatives are compounds of clinical importance.
- Measurement of these abnormal hemoglobin derivatives can be helpful in the diagnosing and monitoring exposure to the toxic compounds.
- Abnormal hemoglobin derivatives reduce the oxygen carrying capacity of the blood.

Normal Hemoglobin Derivatives

The normal hemoglobin derivatives are:

- Oxyhemoglobin
- Reduced hemoglobin
- Carbaminohemoglobin or carbhemoglobin.

Oxyhemoglobin and Reduced Hemoglobin

- Oxyhemoglobin is a derivative of hemoglobin with **oxygen**.
- Oxygen is bound to the ferrous (Fe^{2+}) atoms of the heme to form **oxyhemoglobin**. Oxyhemoglobin is an unstable compound

- Oxygen can be released from this compound. When oxygen is released from oxyhemoglobin, it is called **reduced hemoglobin**.
- The iron remains in ferrous (Fe^{2+}) state in this compound

$$Hb + 4O_2 \rightleftharpoons Hb + 4O_2$$
$$\text{Reduced Hb} \qquad \text{Oxy-Hb}$$

Carbaminohemoglobin or Carbhemoglobin

It is a derivative of hemoglobin with carbon dioxide.

- Carbon dioxide is bound by the α-amino group of N-terminal end of each of the polypeptide chains of hemoglobin **(Figure 7.5)**.
- Carbon dioxide can be released easily from carbhemoglobin.
- The affinity of hemoglobin with CO_2 is 20 times more than for oxygen.

Glycated Hemoglobin (HbA1C)

- Blood glucose that enters the erythrocytes can react nonenzymatically with amino groups of N-terminal residue (valine) of β-chains of hemoglobin, a process referred to as glycation. The derivative formed is known as glycated hemoglobin (HbA1c) **(Figure 7.12)**.
- Unlike glycosylation, (a post-translational modification) glycation is not enzyme catalyzed.
- Normally the concentration of HbA1C in blood is very low, to the extent of about 5% of the total hemoglobin. Formation of HbA1C is proportional to blood glucose concentration.

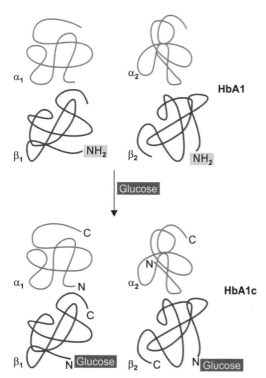

Figure 7.12: Nonenzymatic formation of glycated hemoglobin (HbA1c).

- Increased amounts of HbA1C are found in patients with diabetes mellitus, where the blood sugar level is high. The concentration of HbA1C may reach 12% or more, of the total hemoglobin.
- Measurement of HbA1C provides information useful for the management of diabetes mellitus, since RBCs have a life span of about 120 days, the content of HbA1C is an indicator of how effectively blood glucose levels have been regulated over the previous 2–3 months.

STRIKE A NOTE

- ❖ **Glycosylation** is a post-translational modification mediated by enzymes, in which a defined carbohydrate molecule is added to a predetermined region of the protein. Protein glycosylation is a controlled mechanism that confers defined properties to living cells.
- ❖ On the other hand **glycation** (sometimes incorrectly mentioned as glycosylation) is a random nonenzymatic mechanism that occurs in the bloodstream. The reducing ends of free glucose covalently attach to proteins, creating glycated products. Glycated proteins have reduced functionality.
- ❖ Old textbooks and articles use the glycosylated hemoglobin to describe glycated hemoglobin (HbA1C).

Abnormal Hemoglobin Derivatives

Acquired hemoglobinopathies are due to variations of the hemoglobin molecule by toxins. Hemoglobin readily combines with any toxic gas or other substances to form some products which are called the **abnormal hemoglobin derivatives, for example**:

- Methemoglobin
- Sulfhemoglobin
- Carboxyhemoglobin

Methemoglobin

Methemoglobin is **oxidized hemoglobin**. The iron normally present in heme in ferrous (Fe^{2+}) state is replaced by **ferric (Fe^{3+}) state** in methemoglobin which cannot transport oxygen. The ferrous of hemoglobin is oxidized to ferric state by:

- Superoxide
- Certain drugs
- Oxidizing agents

Amount of methemoglobin present in normal blood is less than 1% of the total hemoglobin. Erythrocyte has two mechanisms for detoxification of methemoglobin.

1. The first mechanism is by reducing oxidant compounds such as hydrogen peroxide or superoxide before they react with hemoglobin to form methemoglobin by enzyme **(Figure 7.13A)**.
    - Catalase
    - Glutathione peroxidase
    - Reduced glutathione
    - NADPH

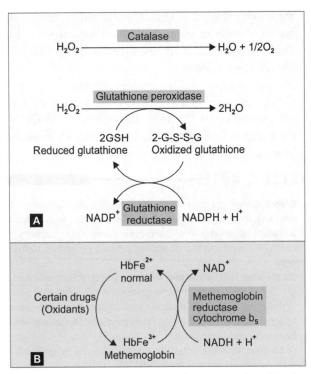

Figures 7.13A and B: Erythrocyte mechanisms for detoxification of methemoglobin.

2. Second mechanism of erythrocyte is the **NADH-cytochrome b$_5$ methemoglobin reductase system**, for reducing heme ferric (Fe^{3+}) back to the ferrous (Fe^{2+}) state. This system consists of:
   - NADH
   - Flavoprotein named cytochrome b$_5$ reductase (known as methemoglobin reductase)
   - Cytochrome b$_5$ **(Figure 7.13B)**.

Methemoglobinemia

Excess methemoglobin may be present in blood because of increased production or diminished ability to convert it back to hemoglobin and cause **methemoglobinemia**. This results in a decreased availability of oxygen to the tissues.

- Methemoglobinemia usually arises following the ingestion of large amounts of drugs, e.g., **phenacetin**, **sulfonamides** or chemicals like **aniline**, **excess of nitrites** or certain **oxidizing agents** present in the diet.
- Methemoglobinemia can be **inherited**. Inherited methemoglobinemia is usually due to:
  - Deficient activity of **methemoglobin reductase**, transmitted in an autosomal recessive manner
  - Due to mutation of amino acid residue **histidine** to which heme is attached is replaced by **tyrosine** residue, which stabilizes iron in oxidized ferric form and thus affecting its affinity for O$_2$ **(Figure 7.14)**.

Symptoms of Methemoglobinemia

Cyanosis (bluish discoloration of the skin and mucous membrane) is the sign in both types.

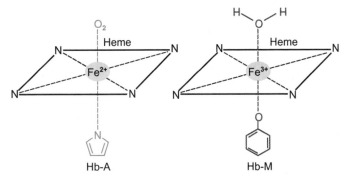

Figure 7.14: Proximal histidine is substituted by tyrosine, results in the formation of HbM. Water rather than O$_2$ is bound at the sixth coordination position in HbM.

Diagnostic Tests

Diagnosis is made by spectroscopic analysis of blood, which gives characteristic absorption spectrum of methemoglobin at **630 nm**.

Treatment

- Ingestion of reducing agents like **methylene blue** or **ascorbic acid** is used to treat mild methemoglobinemia due to enzyme deficiency
- Acute severe methemoglobinemia due to ingestion of chemicals should be treated by intravenous injection of methylene blue.

Sulfhemoglobin

- Many drugs that cause methemoglobinemia also stimulate production of **sulfhemoglobin**, a greenish derivative.
- Sulfhemoglobin is formed by **irreversible oxidation of hemoglobin** by drugs (such as sulfanilamides, phenacetin, nitrites, and phenylhydrazine) or exposure to sulfur-containing compounds either occupationally or from air pollution.
- Sulfhemoglobin is formed by the addition of a **sulfur atom** to the **pyrrole ring** of **heme**.
- Sulfhemoglobin cannot act as oxygen carrier and leads to **cyanosis**.
- Sulfhemoglobin cannot be converted to normal HbA; it persists for the life of the cell.
- **Treatment** is to wait until the affected red blood cells are destroyed as part of their normal life cycle and avoidance of the offending agent.
- Sulfhemoglobin has a similar peak to methemoglobin on a spectral absorption instrument.
- The sulfhemoglobin spectral curve, however, does not shift when cyanide is added, a feature that distinguishes it from methemoglobin.

Carboxyhemoglobin (COHb)

- **Carbon monoxide** combines with the heme moiety in hemoglobin. It combines at the same position in the hemoglobin molecule as oxygen but with an affinity about 210 times greater than oxygen.

- As a result, even small quantities of CO in the inspired air cause the formation of relatively large amounts of carboxyhemoglobin (COHb), with a corresponding reduction in the O_2 carrying capacity of the blood. Even as little as 1% CO in inspired air can be fatal in minutes.
- Some carboxyhemoglobin is produced endogenously, but it normally comprises less than 2% of total hemoglobin.
- Exogenous carbon monoxide is derived from the exhaust of automobiles, tobacco smoke and from industrial pollutants, such as coal, gas and charcoal burning.
- In smokers, COHb levels may be as high as 15%. As a result, smokers may have a higher hematocrit and polycythemia (increased concentration of hemoglobin) to compensate for the hypoxia.
- Carbon monoxide has been termed the *silent killer* because it is an odorless and colorless gas, and victims may quickly become hypoxic.

Symptoms of Carbon Monoxide Toxicity

Toxic effects, such as headache, dizziness, and disorientation, begin to appear at blood levels of 20–30% COHb. Levels of more than 40% of total hemoglobin may cause coma, seizure, hypotension, cardiac arrhythmias, pulmonary edema, and death.

Diagnostic Tests

Carboxyhemoglobin may be detected by spectral absorption instruments at 540 nm.

Treatment

One treatment for carbon monoxide poisoning is administration of 100% oxygen, often at pressures greater than atmospheric pressure; this treatment referred to as **hyperbaric oxygen therapy**. With this therapy, the partial pressure of oxygen in the blood becomes sufficiently high to increase substantially the rate of carbon monoxide displacement from hemoglobin.

■ HEMOGLOBINOPATHIES

Hemoglobinopathies are a group of disorders due to alterations in hemoglobin structure or impaired synthesis of polypeptide chains. Hemoglobinopathies can be categorized into two major groups **(Table 7.2)**.

1. **Structural hemoglobinopathies** (hemoglobins with altered amino acid sequences)
   - It occurs when amino acid sequence of a globin chain is altered due to mutations. Change in the amino acid sequence of a globin chain, alters the physiologic properties of the variant hemoglobin and results in deranged function, e.g., **(Table 7.3)**

TABLE 7.2: Classification of hemoglobinopathies.

Type	Cause	Example
Structural hemoglobinopathies	Altered amino acid sequence of a globin chain due to mutation	HbS, HbC, HbM
Quantitative hemoglobinopathies	Defective biosynthesis of globin chain due to mutation	α-thalassemia β-thalassemia

TABLE 7.3: Abnormal type of Hb.

Type of hemoglobinopathy	Abnormal hemoglobin	Structure	Comment
Structural (due to abnormal chain structure)	HbS	$\alpha_2\beta^S_2$	Substitution of valine for glutamic acid in position 6 of β-chain
	HbC	$\alpha_2\beta^C_2$	Substitution of lysine for glutamic acid in position 6 of β-chain
	HbM	$\alpha_2\beta_2$	Substitution of tyrosine for histidine either of α or β-chains, which bound with iron in the heme molecule
Quantitative (due to abnormal chain production)	HbH	β_4	Found in α-thalassemia biologically useless
	Hb Barts	γ_4	Comprises 100% of Hb in homozygous α-thalassemia

   i. Sickle cell disease (HbS)
   ii. Hemoglobin C (HbC)
   iii. Hemoglobin M (HbM).
   - There are large varieties of hemoglobin variants, not all of which are harmful.
2. **Quantitative hemoglobinopathies**
   - Quantitative hemoglobinopathies lead to reduced amounts of one type of globin chain due to mutations, affecting the rate of synthesis normal hemoglobin, e.g., thalassemias.
   - Thalassemias are a group of disorders that result from a reduced rate of synthesis of one or more globin chains and consequently a reduced rate of synthesis of the hemoglobin.
     - α-**Thalassemia** indicates a reduced rate of synthesis of α globin chain; similarly
     - β-**Thalassemia** indicates a reduced rate of synthesis of the β-globin chain respectively.

Structural Hemoglobinopathies

Since α, β, γ and δ chains of the globin of hemoglobin are synthesized from amino acids under genetic control, mutations in the genes that code for globin chains can affect their formation and biological function of hemoglobin. Such hemoglobin is called **abnormal hemoglobin** or **variant hemoglobin (Table 7.3)**. Some of the clinically significant abnormal forms of hemoglobin are: **HbS, HbC, HbM**.

Sickle Hemoglobin (Hemoglobin S)

Hemoglobin S is the predominant hemoglobin in people with **sickle cell disease**. Production of HbS is due to **mutation in the β-globin gene** which codes for β-globin chain. The mutant β-globin chain of HbS has an altered amino acid sequence. **Glutamic acid** residue normally present in the **sixth position of β-chain** of **HbA** is replaced by a **valine** residue as a result of mutation in the β-globin chain occur. The alpha chain of HbS is normal.

```
 1    2    3    4    5    6    7    8
Val—His—leu—Thr—Pro—Glu—Glu—Lys—(β-chain of HbA)
Val—His—leu—Thr—Pro—Val—Glu—Lys—(β-chain of HbS)
```

Sickle hemoglobin deforms the red blood cells which look like the **blade of a sickle (Figure 7.15)**. Hence, the cell is called sickle cell.

Cause of Distortion of Erythrocyte to Sickle Shaped

- When HbS deoxygenated, it becomes **insoluble** and forms polymers of **deoxy-HbS**. Normal hemoglobin (HbA) remains soluble on deoxygenation.
- Polymerization of deoxy-HbS forms insoluble long tubular fiber. The insoluble fibers of deoxygenated

HbS extended across the red blood cells and deform the red blood cells, which look like the **blade of a sickle**.

- The altered properties of HbS (insolubility) result from a single amino acid substitution, a **nonpolar, hydrophobic, Valine (Val) instead** of a **polar, hydrophilic Glutamic acid (Glu)** residue at position 6 in the two β-chains.
- In HbS, replacement of the hydrophilic glutamic acid at position 6 in the β-globin chains by the hydrophobic valine residue makes hydrophobic area (patch) at position 6 of the β-chain on the outer surface of the molecule.
- This hydrophobic patch interacts with other hydrophobic patch formed by **Phe 85** and **Leu 88** on the β-globin chain of another deoxy-HbS molecule **(Figure 7.16)** forming the long, fibrous aggregates which distort the shape of RBC to sickle shaped.
- A single hemoglobin S fiber is formed from **14 chains** of multiple interlinked hemoglobin molecules. Sickle-shaped hemoglobin clog small capillaries and impair blood flow
- Stiffening and fragility of sickle cell RBC explain vaso-occlusion and hemolytic anemia, respectively.

Why Aggregates are not form when Hemoglobin S is Oxygenated?
In oxyhemoglobin-S, the residues Phe 85 and Leu 88 of the β-chain are largely buried inside the hemoglobin. Without a complementary hydrophobic patch with which to interact, the surface Val residue in position 6 is benign.

Classification of Sickle Cell Disease

Sickle cell disease may be **(Table 7.4)**.
1. **Homozygous** called **sickle cell anemia or**
2. **Heterozygous** called **sickle cell trait**

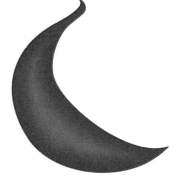

Figure 7.15: Sickle red blood cells.

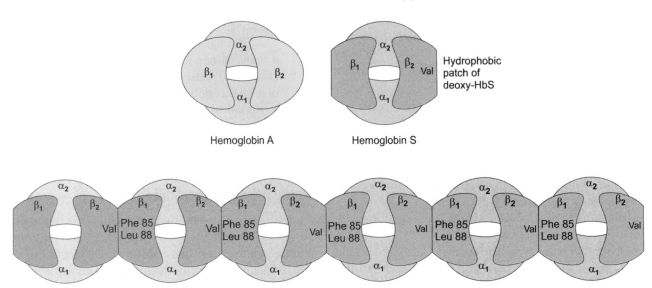

Fiber formation

Figure 7.16: Schematic representation of polymerization of deoxyhemoglobin-S molecules and formation of tubular fibrous structure.

TABLE 7.4: Classification of sickle cell disease.

Class	Type	State	Structure
Sickle cell anemia	Homozygous	Both genes are abnormal/ defective	Hb SS
Sickle cell trait	Heterozygous	One gene is abnormal One gene is normal	HbAS

- **Sickle cell anemia** is a **homozygous** disorder in which the individual has **inherited two mutant globin genes (HbSS)** one from each parent. It is characterized by chronic hemolytic anemia, tissue damage and pain and increased susceptibility to infections. Such patients usually die in their adult age.
- **Sickle cell trait** is a **heterozygous** state, in which individuals have received the abnormal mutated β-globin gene from only one parent and have one normal gene (HbAS). They do not show any clinical symptoms and have normal lifespan.

STRIKE A NOTE

- ❖ Subjects who inherit one normal and one abnormal gene are heterozygotes. The heterozygous state is usually referred to as the trait, e.g., sickle cell trait/HbS trait/ HbAS.
- ❖ Subjects who inherit two identical abnormal genes are homozygotes. The homozygous state is usually referred to as the disease, e.g., sickle cell disease/HbS disease/ HbSS.
- ❖ Subjects who inherit two different genes are double heterozygotes, e. g. HbSC; HbS-β-thalassemia, etc.
- ❖ Person with sickle cell trait is resistant to malaria caused by *Plasmodium falciparum*. This parasite spends an essential part of its life cycle in the red blood cell. Since the sickle red blood cells have a shorter lifespan than normal red blood cell, the parasite cannot complete its life cycle.

Clinical Manifestations

- **Hemolytic anemia:** Hemolysis occurs because the spleen destroys the abnormal red blood cells. Red blood cells in sickle cell anemia have a much shorter lifespan than normal cells (20 days compared with 120 days, one sixth of normal). The sickled red blood cells lose water (due to potassium leakage and calcium influx) become fragile leading to lysis of the red blood cells and results in **hemolytic anemia.**
- **Vaso-occlusion crises:** The more serious consequence is that, small blood capillaries in different organs become blocked by the long abnormally shaped red cell. This interrupts the supply of oxygen and leads to **anoxia** (oxygen deprivation) which causes ischemic (deficiency of blood supply) infarcts of various organs and pain crises.
- Sickle cell trait does not show any clinical symptoms and have normal lifespan.

Factors Affecting Severity of Sickling

The extent of sickling and severity of disease are increased by any variable that increases the proportion of deoxy-HbS such as:

- Decrease oxygen tension caused by high altitude
- Increase CO_2 concentration
- Decrease pH
- Increase concentration of 2,3-BPG in erythrocytes.

Diagnosis

Sickle cell disease is suspected on the basis of:

- Hemolytic anemia, RBC morphology (the elongated and crescent-shaped red blood cells seen on smear)
- Intermittent episodes of ischemic pain
- Diagnosis is confirmed by:
  1. **Hemoglobin electrophoresis:** Demonstrate two bands of HbS and HbA. HbS can be separated and identified from HbA by electrophoresis. During electrophoresis at alkaline pH, HbS migrate more slowly toward the anode (+ve electrode) than does HbA. This altered mobility of HbS is due to the absence of two negatively charged glutamate residues **(Figure 7.17)**.
  2. **Sickling test:** Sickling is induced by adding reducing agent like 2% **sodium metabisulphite** or **sodium dithionate** to blood. (HbS in a reducing solution gives a turbid appearance because of precipitation of HbS, whereas normal Hb gives a clear solution).
- Family study to differentiate whether patient is homozygous or heterozygous.
- Genetic counseling. Genotyping of family members and potential parental partners.

Management

- Folic acid treatment
- Rest, analgesics and hydration
- Blood transfusion
- Bone marrow transplantation.

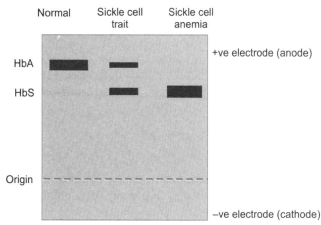

Figure 7.17: Electrophoresis pattern of normal, sickle cell trait and sickle cell anemia person.

HbC Disease or Cooley's Hemoglobin

- In HbC, the **glutamic acid** at position 6 in the β-chain is mutated.
- In HbC, the **glutamic acid** at position 6 in the β-**chain** is replaced by **a lysine** residue.
- The red blood cells of people with HbC do not sickle; however, crystals of HbC may form within the cell.
- Both **homozygous** and **heterozygous** individuals of the disease are known.
- This disease is characterized by a **mild hemolytic anemia**.
- Clinically, heterozygous individuals are asymptomatic.

HbM Diseases

- The letter **'M'** of HbM signifies that the affected chains are in the **methemoglobin** (ferric hemoglobin) form.
- HbM disease is due to mutation in **histidine** residue of either α- or β-chains, which bound with the iron in the heme molecule.
- In HbM **histidine** is replaced by **tyrosine**.
- The side chain of tyrosine is ionized and iron is stabilized in the ferric (Fe^{3+}) form instead of ferrous (Fe^{2+}) form (**Figure 7.14**) which cannot bind oxygen and leads to **cyanosis**.
- Only patients who are heterozygous for these mutations have been found affected by HbM diseases. Presumably homozygosity is lethal.

Thalassemia

Thalassemia is a group of genetically transmitted disorder of hemoglobin synthesis, due to **lack or decreased synthesis of α or β globin** chains. Because the synthesis of one globin chain is reduced, there is a relative excess synthesis of the other globin chains. These globin chains may precipitate in the cell causing hemolysis, resulting in a **hypochromic anemia**.

The name of this group of diseases comes from the Greek word **'thalasa'**, meaning **'sea'**, because this disorder occurs more commonly among people living near the Mediterranean Sea.

Types of Thalassemia

Depending upon whether the genetic defect lies in synthesis of α- or β-**globin** chains, thalassemias are classified into:
- α-**thalassemia**
- β-**thalassemia**

α-thalassemia

In this condition, synthesis of α-globin chain is defective. α-globin chains are coded by **four copies of α-globin gene**. The α-thalassemia results from genetic defect in one or more copies of α-globin genes (located on chromosome 16) and is characterized by either decreased or total absence of

TABLE 7.5: Types of α-thalassemia.

Type	Genetic defect	Level of HbA1%	HbH (β4)%
Silent α-thalassemia	1 α gene loci deleted	98–100	0
Thalassemia trait	2 α gene loci deleted	85–95	Rare blood cell inclusion
HbH disease	3 α gene loci deleted	70–95	5–30
Hydrops fetalis	All the four loci deleted	0	5–10 (90–95 % is Hb Barts, γ4)

synthesis of α-globin chains. The α-thalassemia is of four types (**Table 7.5**). These are:

1. **Silent carrier type of α-thalassemia:** In this type of α-thalassemia, only one of the four copies of α-globin gene is mutated. Since the patients of this disorder can synthesize sufficient α-globin chains, they do not show any clinical symptoms of thalassemia. They are only carriers of α-thalassemia.

2. **α-thalassemia trait:** In this type of α-thalassemia, two of the four copies of α-globin genes are mutated. They usually have only mild anemia and is not fatal.

3. **Hemoglobin H disease:**
   - In this type of α-thalassemia three of the four copies of α-globin genes are mutated. With only one normal α-globin gene, the synthesis of α-chain is markedly reduced, and **tetramers of β-globin**, called **HbH**, form.
   - HbH has an extremely high affinity for oxygen and therefore is not useful for oxygen delivery, leading to **tissue hypoxia**.
   - Additionally, HbH is prone to oxidation, which causes it to precipitate and causes moderately severe anemia

4. **Hydrops fetalis:**
   - This is a fatal condition. In hydrops fetalis, all four copies of α-globin genes are mutated and unable to produce any α-globin chains leading to failure of synthesis of HbA, HbF, or HbA2.
   - In the fetus, an excess number of γ-globin chains join together to form unstable **tetramer γ 4** known as **Hb Barts**.
   - It is moderately insoluble, and therefore accumulates in the red blood cells.
   - Hb Barts has an extremely high affinity for oxygen, so it cannot release oxygen to the tissue and a fetus will develop **hydrops fetalis** and normally die before or shortly after birth.

β-thalassemia

In β-thalassemia, synthesis of β-**globin chain** is impaired due to genetic defect in β-globin genes. In β-thalassemia, codon 17 of the β-chain is changed from UGG (tryptophan) to UGA (stop codon).

β-globin chains are coded by **two copies of β-globin genes** and are characterized by decreased or total absence of synthesis of β-globin chains. The β-thalassemia is of two types. These are:

1. **β-thalassemia minor (also known as β-thalassemia trait):** In this condition, one of the two copies of β-globin genes is mutated. It is a **heterozygous** state. The presence of one normal gene in the heterozygous allows enough normal globin chain synthesis, so that affected individuals are usually asymptomatic. The individual may be completely normal or has a mild anemia

2. **β-thalassemia major:** β-thalassemia major is **homozygous state**, carrying two mutated β-globin genes. Thalassemia major leads to **severe anemia**. They regularly need blood transfusion. Bone marrow transplant has been introduced as a remedy.

ASSESSMENT QUESTIONS

▮ STRUCTURED LONG ANSWER QUESTION (SLAQ)

1. Describe hemoglobinopathies under the following headings:
   i. Major types and their subtypes
   ii. Causes
   iii. Manifestations

▮ SHORT ESSAY QUESTIONS (SEQs)

1. What is thalassemia? Write its causes, types and clinical manifestations.
2. What is sickle cell anemia? Write its causes, types and clinical manifestations.
3. Write normal and abnormal derivatives of hemoglobin.
4. What is cooperative oxygen binding of hemoglobin? Give its significance.
5. Give structure of hemoglobin with its functions.
6. Give types of normal hemoglobin.

▮ SHORT ANSWER QUESTIONS (SAQs)

1. Write normal forms of hemoglobin with their constituent polypeptide chains.
2. What is the role of 2,3-BPG in transport of oxygen by hemoglobin?
3. Write binding sites for oxygen, hydrogen (H^+) and carbon dioxide (CO_2) with hemoglobin.
4. What is cooperative oxygen binding of hemoglobin?
5. Why HbF has high affinity for O_2 than HbA?
6. What is glycated hemoglobin (HbA1C)? Give its clinical significance.
7. Why does a person with sickle cell trait show an increased resistance to malaria?
8. Give factors affecting severity of sickling.
9. Write diagnostic tests for sickle cell disease.
10. What is methemoglobin? Write mechanism involved in detoxification of methemoglobin.

▮ CASE VIGNETTE-BASED QUESTIONS (CVBQs)

Case Study

1. **A 20-year-old male complaining of severe back pain was hospitalized and sickle cell anemia was diagnosed.**

   Questions
   a. What is sickle cell anemia?
   b. Give its biochemical cause.
   c. Give cause for the sickling of RBC.
   d. Why does a person with sickle cell trait show an increased resistance to malaria?

2. **A 6-month-old infant was admitted to hospital for episodes of breathing difficulty and vomiting. The infant's skin and mucous membrane were bluish, indicating cyanosis. Analysis of arterial blood revealed a chocolate brown color, a normal pO_2, an O_2 saturation of 60% and a methemoglobin level of 40%. The tentative cause of acute toxic methemoglobinemia was found to be well water contaminated by a nitrate/nitrite.**

   Questions
   a. What is methemoglobin?
   b. How will you treat the acquired methemoglobinemia of the infant?
   c. What is the cause of genetic form of methemoglobinemia?
   d. What is the diagnostic test for methemoglobin?
   e. How methemoglobin is get detoxified in the body?

▮ MULTIPLE CHOICE QUESTIONS (MCQs)

1. **2,3-BPG binds Hb by salt bonds by cross linking:**
   a. β_1, β_2
   b. α_1, α_2
   c. β_1, α_1
   d. β_2, α_2

2. **HbF has high affinity for O_2 than HbA due to presence of:**
   a. β-chain
   b. γ-chain
   c. δ-chain
   d. ε-chain

3. The following are the normal forms of hemoglobin, *except*:
   a. HbA2
   b. HbF
   c. HbA1
   d. HbS

4. Which of the following is not true for hydrops fetalis?
   a. It is a β-thalassemia
   b. It is an α-thalassemia
   c. Neither HbF nor HbA can be synthesized
   d. Death occurs before birth

5. Persons with sickle cell trait show an increased resistance to:
   a. Typhoid
   b. Cancer
   c. Malaria
   d. Diabetes

6. Hb Bart consists of:
   a. α_4
   b. β_4
   c. γ_4
   d. δ_4

7. Iron in heme is linked to globin through:
   a. Histidine
   b. Arginine
   c. Glycine
   d. Cysteine

8. Which of the following has a protective effect against malaria?
   a. HbF
   b. HbM
   c. HbS
   d. Hb Bart

9. Porphyrin is formed by joining pyrrol rings by:
   a. Methene bridge
   b. Hydrogen bond
   c. Phosphate bond
   d. Glycosidic bond

10. Normal adult hemoglobin (HA$_1$) has the following chains:
    a. $\alpha_2\beta_2$
    b. $\alpha_2\delta_2$
    c. $\alpha_2\gamma_2$
    d. $\alpha_2\varepsilon_2$

11. Hemoglobin is a:
    a. Monomeric protein
    b. Trimeric protein
    c. Tetrameric protein
    d. Dimeric protein

12. Which type of α-thalassemia results from mutation of three genes and produces a moderate hemolytic anemia?
    a. Silent carrier type α-thalassemia
    b. Hemoglobin H disease
    c. α-thalassemia trait
    d. Hydrops fetalis

13. In silent carrier type α-thalassemia how many α-genes are mutated?
    a. 1
    b. 2
    c. 3
    d. 4

14. Which hemoglobin contains two alpha and two gamma chains and has high affinity for oxygen:
    a. HbF
    b. HbA2
    c. HbA1C
    d. Hb Bart's

15. HbA1c is:
    a. Glucose to C terminal β-globin
    b. Glucose to N terminal valine residue of β-globin
    c. Glucose to glutamine residue of β-globin
    d. Glucose to N terminal valine residue of α-globin

16. Porphyrin ring in hemoglobin molecules have in center an atom of
    a. Magnesium
    b. Iron
    c. Zinc
    d. Cobalt

17. If iron in hemoglobin is oxidized to Fe^{3+}, what disease may occur?
    a. Sickle cell anemia
    b. Methemoglobinemia
    c. Carbon monoxide poisoning
    d. Cystic fibrosis

18. A point mutation in the beta-globin gene changing the codon from glutamate to valine will likely cause what disease?
    a. Sickle cell anemia
    b. Methemoglobinemia
    c. Thalassemia
    d. Cooley Hb

19. In the binding of oxygen to myoglobin, can best be described graphically as:
    a. Hyperbolic
    b. Linear
    c. Sigmoidal
    d. None of the above

20. Each hemoglobin molecule has how many heme group(s) and globin molecule(s).
    a. 1, 2
    b. 1, 4
    c. 4, 4
    d. 4, 2

21. In carboxyhemoglobin carbon monoxide is attached to:
    a. Porphyrin ring
    b. Iron atom of heme at the same position as oxygen
    c. N-terminal of globin chain
    d. C-terminal of globin chain

22. In carboxyhemoglobin carbon dioxide is attached to:
    a. Porphyrin ring
    b. Iron atom of heme at the same position as oxygen
    c. N-terminal end of each of the polypeptide chains of hemoglobin
    d. C-terminal end of each of the polypeptide chains of hemoglobin

23. 2,3-BPG binds to site in Hb and cause in oxygen affinity:
    a. Four, increases
    b. Two, increases
    c. Four, decreases
    d. One, increase

ANSWERS FOR MCQs

1. a	2. b	3. d	4. a	5. c
6. c	7. a	8. c	9. a	10. a
11. c	12. b	13. a	14. a	15. b
16. b	17. b	18. a	19. a.	20. c
21. b	22. c	23. b		

8 CHAPTER

Biological Oxidation

Competency	Learning Objectives
BI 6.6: Describe the biochemical processes involved in generation of energy in cells.	1. Describe free energy and redox potential. 2. Describe the biochemical processes involved in generation of ATP in cells. 3. Describe the enzymes, coenzymes and electron carriers involved in biological oxidation. 4. Describe the mitochondrial electron transport chain. 5. Describe oxidative phosphorylation and its mechanism. 6. Describe inhibitors of electron transport chain and oxidative phosphorylation. 7. Describe brown adipose tissue metabolism. 8. Explain shuttle systems for oxidation of extra-mitochondrial NADH. 9. Describe disorders of mitochondrial electron transport and oxidative phosphorylation.

OVERVIEW

Chemically, **oxidation** is defined as the removal of electrons and **reduction** as the gain of electrons. Thus, oxidation is always accompanied by reduction of an electron acceptor. This principal of oxidation-reduction applies to biochemical systems.

The energy requirements of aerobic cells are met by the energy released in the oxidation of carbohydrates, fatty acids, and amino acids by molecular oxygen. In these oxidative processes, the reducing equivalents [electrons, hydrogen atom ($H^+ + e^-$) or a hydride ion ($:H^-$), i.e., $2H^+ + 2e^-$] from substrates are transferred to NAD^+, flavin mononucleotide (FMN) or flavin adenine dinucleotide (FAD).

The reducing equivalents are removed catalytically from NADH and reduced flavin nucleotides, ($FADH_2$) and transferred through a series of coupled reduction-oxidation (redox) reactions to oxygen. The reduced oxygen is then converted to water. Oxygen serves as the ultimate electron acceptor. The entire process is known as **cell respiration** and the reaction sequence which takes place in the inner mitochondrial membrane is called **electron transport respiratory chain**.

During this electron flow a portion of the free energy liberated is conserved in the form of ATP. Since the energy is conserved in the phosphate bond of ATP through phosphorylation of ADP to ATP, the overall coupled process is known as **oxidative phosphorylation**.

FREE ENERGY AND REDOX POTENTIAL

Free energy (ΔG) is that portion of total energy change in a system that is available for executing a task, i.e., it is the actual useful amount of energy, also known as the **chemical potential**. In oxidation and reduction reactions, the **free energy change** is proportionate to the tendency of reactants to donate or accept electrons.

- If ΔG is negative in sign, it means that the products contain less free energy than the reactants and reaction proceeds spontaneously with loss of free energy and reaction is called **exergonic** reactions.
- If ΔG is positive in sign, it means that the products of the reaction contain more free energy than the reactants and reaction proceeds only if free energy can be gained and this is known as **endergonic reactions**.

TABLE 8.1: The redox potential (E°) of redox couples of components of electron transport chain.

Redox couple components of electron transport chain	Redox potential (E°) in volt
$2H^+/H_2$	– 0.414
NAD/NADH	– 0.32
FMN/FMNH$_2$	– 0.30
Ubiquinone (ox)/Ubiquinone (red)	+ 0.045
Cytochrome b (ox)/Cytochrome b (red)	+ 0.077
Cytochrome c$_1$ (ox)/Cytochrome c$_1$ (red)	+ 0.22
Cytochrome c (ox)/Cytochrome c (red)	+ 0.254
Cytochrome a (ox)/Cytochrome a (red)	+ 0.29
Cytochrome a$_3$ (ox)/Cytochrome a$_3$ (red)	+ 0.35
$1/2O_2 + 2H^+/H_2O$	+ 0.8166

- If ΔG is zero, it means that the system is at equilibrium and no net change takes place.

  This free energy changes are expressed as **Redox potential (E'°)**. The redox potentials of some redox systems of electron transport chain are shown in **Table 8.1**.

- Increasing negative values of a system have an increasing tendency to lose electrons and increasingly positive values of a system have an increasing tendency to accept electrons.
- Thus, electrons tend to flow from redox couple to another redox couple in the direction of the more positive system.
- The E'° values of various redox couples allow us to predict the direction of flow of electrons from one redox couple to another.

BIOCHEMICAL PROCESSES INVOLVED IN GENERATION OF ATP IN CELLS

ATP acts as the energy source of the cell. ATP is the primary **high energy phosphate compound (~p)** produced by catabolism, in the process of:

1. Oxidative phosphorylation
2. Substrate level phosphorylation:
   - Glycolysis
   - Citric acid cycle.
3. Hydrolysis of phosphagens (phosphocreatine)

- **Oxidative phosphorylation:** It is the greatest quantitative source of ATP in aerobic cells. ATP is generated in the mitochondrial matrix as O_2 is reduced to H_2O by electron passing down the respiratory chain.
- **Substrate level phosphorylation:** When formation of ATP directly coupled with individual steps of certain metabolic reaction without involvement of electron transport chain and molecular O_2, is called the **production of ATP at the substrate level**. Examples of substrate level phosphorylation **(Figure 8.1)**:
   1. 1,3-bisphosphoglycerate to 3-phosphoglycerate
   2. Phosphoenolpyruvate to pyruvate
   3. Succinyl-CoA to succinate
- **Hydrolysis of phosphagens:** Phosphagens are energy storing compounds that are chiefly found in **muscle** and **nervous tissue**. A common phosphagen used by humans is **phosphocreatine** or **creatine phosphate**. Phosphagens supply immediate but limited energy.
   - At rest, ATP is hydrolyzed to ADP and the phosphate is transferred to creatine to make **phosphocreatine** by the enzyme creatine kinase. This occurs in **mitochondria**, where ATP levels are high.
   - During exercise, phosphocreatine is hydrolyzed and the phosphate is released to make ATP from ADP. This occurs in muscles, where ADP levels will be high **(Figure 8.2)**.

ENZYMES, COENZYMES AND ELECTRON CARRIERS INVOLVED IN BIOLOGICAL OXIDATION

Biological oxidation is brought about with different enzymes, coenzymes and electron carriers.

Enzymes and Coenzymes

The enzymes involved in oxidation and reduction reactions are called **oxidoreductase** and are classified into four groups as follows.

1. **Oxidases:** They catalyze the removal of hydrogen from a substrate in the form of H_2O or H_2O_2 (hydrogen peroxide), using oxygen as a hydrogen acceptor, e.g., cytochrome oxidase (cytochrome aa$_3$), L-amino acid oxidase, xanthine oxidase, etc.

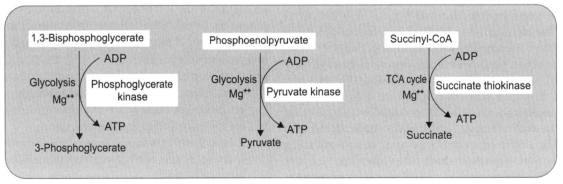

Figure 8.1: Substrate level phosphorylation.

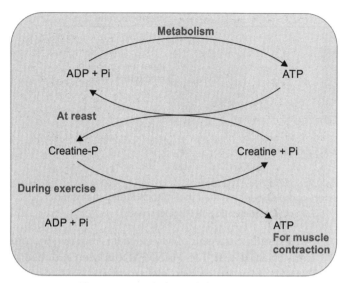

Figure 8.2: Hydrolysis of phosphagens.

2. **Dehydrogenases:** They catalyze the removal of hydrogen from a substrate but are not able to use oxygen as a hydrogen acceptor. These enzymes, therefore, require specific **coenzymes** as acceptor of hydrogen atoms. The coenzymes of dehydrogenases may be either nicotinamide coenzymes (NAD^+ or $NADP^+$) or flavin coenzymes (FMN or FAD).

3. **Hydroperoxidases:** They use hydrogen peroxide or organic peroxide as substrate. There are two types of hydroperoxidases, **peroxidases** and **catalases**.

> Hydroperoxidases protect the body against harmful peroxides. Accumulation of peroxides can lead to generation of free radicals, which in turn disrupt membranes and cause diseases like cancer and atherosclerosis.

4. **Oxygenases:** They catalyze the direct transfer and incorporation of oxygen into a substrate molecule. The two types of oxygenases are **dioxygenases** which catalyze the incorporation of both atoms of molecular oxygen into substrate and **mono-oxygenases**, this enzyme incorporate only one atom of molecular oxygen into the substrate in the form of hydroxyl group, while the other oxygen atom of O_2 is reduced to H_2O_2 by reducing equivalents donated by coenzymes.

> **Cytochrome P450** is mono-oxygenases (mixed function oxidase) important for the detoxification of many drugs and for the hydroxylation of steroids.

Electron Carriers

The cytochromes are **iron-containing** electron transferring **hemoproteins** in which the iron atom oscillates between Fe^{3+} and Fe^{2+} during oxidation and reduction reactions. There are three classes of cytochromes **a**, **b** and **c** having differences in their light absorption spectra.

- Several cytochromes occur in the respiratory chain are **cytochrome b, cytochrome c_1, cytochrome c** and **cytochrome aa_3.**
- In the respiratory chain, they are involved as carriers of electrons from flavoprotein to cytochrome oxidase.
- Cytochrome aa_3 are also called **cytochrome oxidases;** and are **copper-containing heme proteins**.
- The cytochromes in the respiratory chain are arranged in the sequence $b \rightarrow c_1 \rightarrow c \rightarrow aa_3$.
- Of these, only **cytochrome c** is **water soluble** and easily diffusible, whereas cytochromes b, c_1, and aa_3 are lipid soluble and therefore, are fixed components of the membrane.

■ MITOCHONDRIAL ELECTRON TRANSPORT CHAIN

The **electron transport chain** or **respiratory chain** is the final common pathway in aerobic cells by which electrons (reducing equivalents) derived from various substrates are transferred to oxygen.

- Electron transport chain is a series of highly organized oxidation reduction **enzymes**, **coenzymes** and **electron carrier cytochromes**.
- The electron transport chain is present in the **inner mitochondrial membrane**
- The enzymes of the electron transport chain are embedded in the inner membrane in association with the enzymes of oxidative phosphorylation, **F_0F_1 ATPase**.

The energy liberated during oxidation of carbohydrates, fatty acids and amino acids is made available within the mitochondria as **reducing equivalents (H^+ or e^-)**. The mitochondria which contain respiratory chain transport these reducing equivalents and hands them over to their final acceptor, **oxygen** to form **water**. Liberated free energy is trapped as high energy phosphate **ATP** in the mitochondria by **oxidative phosphorylation**.

Components and Structural Organization of the Respiratory Chain

Components of the Respiratory Chain

The major components of the respiratory chain include:

- Nicotinamide adenine dinucleotide (NAD^+) of various dehydrogenases.
- Flavin mononucleotide (FMN)
- Flavin adenine dinucleotide (FAD).
- Ubiquinone or coenzyme Q (CoQ) or simply Q.
- Two different types of **iron-sulfur proteins**.
  1. **Iron-sulfur (Fe-S) protein** in which iron is present in association with inorganic sulfur atoms or with the sulfur atoms of cysteine residues of the protein or both.

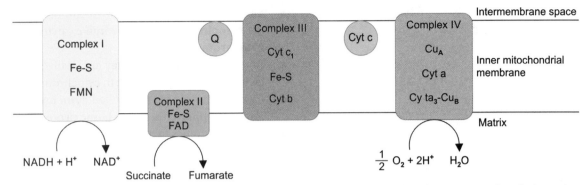

Figure 8.3: Organization of the components of the electron transport complexes within the inner mitochondrial membrane.
(Fe-s: Iron-sulfur center; Q: Coenzyme Q (ubiquinone) b, c_1, c, a, a_3: Cytochromes; Cu_A, Cu_B: Copper centers)

2. **Rieske iron-sulfur proteins** (named after their discoverer, John S. Rieske) in Rieske iron-sulfur proteins one Fe atom is coordinated to two histidine residue rather than two cysteine residues.

- Cytochromes (heme proteins), **b, c, c_1** and **aa_3**.

> ❖ Except coenzyme Q, all members of this chain are proteins. Coenzyme Q is a fat-soluble quinone and is a constituent of mitochondrial lipids.
> ❖ All iron-sulfur proteins transfers one electron, in which one iron atom of the iron-sulfur cluster is oxidized or reduced.
> ❖ Cytochrome c is the only water-soluble cytochrome and easily diffusible, also play a role in programmed cell death (apoptosis)

Structural Organization of Components of Respiratory Chain

Components of the respiratory chain are arranged in order of increasing redox potential **(Table 8.1)**.

- The reducing equivalents flow through the chain from the components of **more negative redox potential to the components of more positive redox potential.**
- The electron carriers of the respiratory chain are organized into **four enzyme complexes**, each capable of catalyzing transfer of electron **(Figure 8.3)**.
  1. **Complex I:** NADH-Q oxidoreductase (transfers electrons from NADH to Q).
  2. **Complex II:** Succinate-Q reductase (transfers electrons from $FADH_2$ to Q).
  3. **Complex III:** Q-Cytochrome c oxidoreductase (transfers electrons from Q to cytochrome **c**).
  4. **Complex IV:** Cytochrome c oxidase-O_2 (transfers electrons from cytochrome c to oxygen and get reduced to H_2O).

Reactions of Electron Transport (Respiratory) Chain

Complex I: NADH-Q Oxidoreductase

NADH-Q oxidoreductase complex also called **NADH dehydrogenate complex**, is a large enzyme consisting of **FMN** and at least **six iron-sulfur (Fe-S) centers (proteins)**. Complex-I catalyzes two simultaneous and obligatory coupled processes **(Figure 8.4)**:

1. The exergonic transfer of two electrons and two protons from **(NADH + H⁺)** to FMN. FMN is then reduced to $FMNH_2$ from which two electrons are pass through Fe-S proteins and finally to coenzyme Q to form QH_2.
2. The second process is the endergonic **transfer of four protons (4H⁺) from the matrix to the intermembrane space**. The flow of two electrons form NADH to coenzyme Q through NADH-Q oxidoreductase leads to the **pumping of four hydrogen ions** out of the matrix of the mitochondrion.

Complex II: Succinate-Q Reductase

- Complex II contains **succinate dehydrogenase** and its **iron-sulfur** proteins
- In complex-II, $FADH_2$ is formed during the conversion of **succinate** to **fumarate** in the citric acid cycle and electrons are then passed via several Fe-S centers to coenzyme Q to form QH_2 **(Figure 8.5)**.

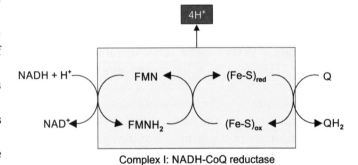

Complex I: NADH-CoQ reductase

Figure 8.4: Transfer of electrons through complex I: NADH-CoQ reductase.

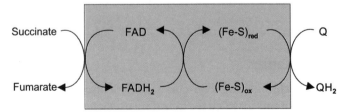

Complex II: Succinate-CoQ reductase

Figure 8.5: Transfer of electrons through complex II: Succinate-CoQ oxidoreductase.

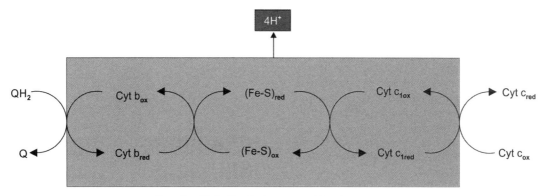

Complex III: CoQ-cytochrome c oxidoreductase

Figure 8.6: Transfer of electrons through complex III: CoQ-cytochrome c reductase.

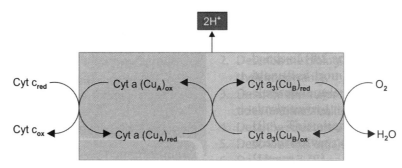

Complex IV: Cytochrome c oxidase-O_2

Figure 8.7: Transfer of electrons through complex IV: Cytochrome c oxidase-O_2.

- **Glycerol-3-phosphate** (breakdown product of triacylglycerol and glycolysis) and **acyl-CoA** also pass electrons to Q via $FADH_2$.
- Complex II in contrast with complex I **does not pump protons** from one side of the membrane to the other. Consequently, less ATP is formed from the oxidation of $FADH_2$ than from NADH.

Complex III: Q-Cytochrome c Oxidoreductase

- Complex III also called **cytochrome bc_1 complex**. It contains **cytochrome b, cytochrome c_1** and **Rieske iron-sulfur protein**.
- Rieske protein is unusual in that one of the irons is linked to two **histidine** residues rather than two **cysteine** residues and stabilizes the protein so that it can readily accept electrons from QH_2.
- The function of Q-cytochrome c oxidoreductase is to catalyze the transfer of electrons from QH_2 to cytochrome c, with **transfer of four protons ($4H^+$) from the matrix to the intermembrane space (Figure 8.6)**.

Complex IV: Cytochrome c Oxidase-O_2

- Complex IV also called **cytochrome c oxidase** is the terminal component of the respiratory chain. In the final step of the respiratory chain, complex IV carries electrons from cytochrome c to the molecular oxygen, reducing it to H_2O.

- Complex IV is a large enzyme of inner mitochondrial membrane. It consists of four redox centers: **Cytochrome a, cytochrome a_3, Cu_A center** (contain two Cu ions linked to protein) and **Cu_B center** which is linked to heme a_3.
- Cu centers resemble the Fe-S center and like iron atoms, the copper ions functions as **one electron carrier**.
- Cytochrome c oxidase catalyzes the transfer of electrons from reduced form of cytochrome c to molecular oxygen, with the concomitant reduction of O_2 to two molecules of H_2O **(Figure 8.7)**.
- Electron transfer through complex IV is from cytochrome c to Cu_A center, to cytochrome a, to cytochrome a_3-Cu_B center and finally to O_2.
- For every pair of electrons passing down the chain from NADH or $FADH_2$, **$2H^+$ are pumped across the membrane by complex IV (Figure 8.7)**.

> The O_2 remains tightly bound to complex IV until it is fully reduced to water, and this minimizes the release of incompletely reduced potentially damaging intermediates such as hydrogen peroxide, or hydroxyl free radicals (which are formed when O_2 accepts one or two electrons respectively) would damage cellular components.

STRIKE A NOTE

- ❖ Complex II: Succinate-Q reductase in contrast with the other complexes does not pump protons.

Contd...

Contd...

- ❖ Complexes I, II and III are termed **respirasome** (super molecular complex); facilitate the rapid transfer of substrate and prevent the release of reaction intermediates.
- ❖ Cardiolipin, the lipid that is especially abundant in the inner mitochondrial membrane, may be critical to the integrity of respirasome. Absence of cardiolipin results in defective mitochondrial electron transport.
- ❖ Complex II has also been reported to contain a specific cytochrome; cytochrome b558 is not in the direct path of electron transfer. It provides binding site for coenzyme Q.
- ❖ Human with point mutations in complex II subunits near cytochrome b558 coenzyme Q binding site suffer from hereditary **paraganglioma**. This hereditary condition is characterized by benign tumors of the head, and neck. These mutations result due to excess production of ROS during succinate oxidation.

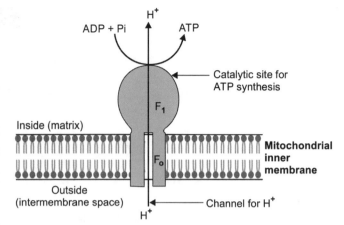

Figure 8.8: F_0F_1 ATPase (ATP synthase) showing catalytic site for ATP synthesis and H^+ channel.

Oxidative Phosphorylation

During the transport of electrons through respiratory chain a portion of free energy liberated is conserved by an energy transducing system by which electrical energy is change to chemical energy. Since the energy is conserved in the form of ATP through phosphorylation of ADP to ATP by an enzyme F_0F_1 **ATPase**, the overall coupled process is known as **oxidative phosphorylation**.

Energy Conserving or Coupling Sites

There are **three energy conserving** or coupling sites of the electron transport chain these are **complex I**, **complex III** and **complex IV** that provides the energy required to make ATP from ADP and inorganic phosphate by an enzyme F_0F_1 **ATPase** in the process of oxidative phosphorylation.

Electrons that enter the chain through NADH pass through all three energy conserving or coupling sites and thus yield **2.5 ATPs**. However, electrons that enter the chain through $FADH_2$ pass through only two energy conserving sites, as they bypass site-I, they yield **1.5 ATPs (Figure 8.3)**.

F_0F_1 ATPase

- The enzyme complex F_0F_1ATPase that synthesizes ATP is also called **ATP synthase**.
- 'F' is for protein factor. F_0F_1 ATPase is composed of two protein subunits, F_0 and F_1. F_0 and F_1 are embedded in the inner membrane and extend across it **(Figure 8.8)**.
- F_0 **complex** is hydrophobic in nature and forms channel or path through which hydrogen ions pass across the membrane. **Oligomycin** is an inhibitor of this enzyme and thus **oxidative phosphorylation**. The subscript 'O' is not zero, but the letter 'O' to denote that it is the portion of ATP synthase that binds the toxic antibiotic Oligomycin.
- F_1-**complex** is subscript 1 indicating this was the first of several factors isolated form mitochondria. It is hydrophilic in nature and tightly bound to F_0 subunits.

It projects into the mitochondrial matrix from inner mitochondrial membrane. It contains catalytic site for ATP synthesis (phosphorylation mechanism). ADP and Pi are taken up sequentially to from ATP.

Mechanism of Oxidative Phosphorylation

Chemiosmotic Theory

The **chemiosmotic coupling hypothesis** is the most accepted theory. The chemiosmotic theory which was proposed by the **British biochemist Peter Mitchell** explains the mechanism of oxidative phosphorylation.

- The theory states that the energy released from oxidation generates the **electrochemical potential** by the pumping of protons across the inner mitochondrial membrane and the energy of electrochemical potential can be converted into ATP.
- There are three basic principles of the theory **(Figure 8.9)**.
  1. When electrons are passed from one carrier to another allows proton to be pumped across the inner mitochondrial membrane from the matrix to the intermembrane space,.
  2. The inner mitochondrial membrane is impermeable to protons, so that their pumping results in the generation of the **electrochemical potential**.
     - ◆ Protons once pumped to the cytosolic side of the membrane, cannot diffuse back through the membrane into the matrix.
     - ◆ Thus, pumping of protons creates a much higher concentration of protons outside of the mitochondrion than inside, resulting in the generation of **electrochemical potential gradient (proton motive force)** across the inner mitochondrial membrane.
  3. Due to this electrochemical potential or proton motive force, the H^+ ions ejected out by electron transport, flow back into the mitochondrial matrix down its electrochemical gradient through a specific **H^+ channels or pore (F_0)** of the F_0F_1**ATPase** molecule

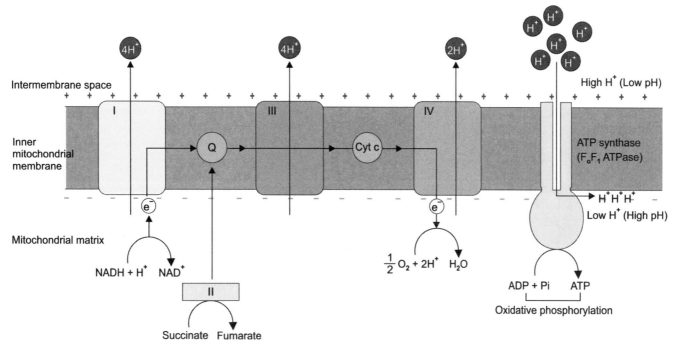

Figure 8.9: The chemiosmotic mechanism of oxidative phosphorylation. Complexes I, III and IV acts as proton pumps generating electrochemical gradient. The proton motive force generated drives the synthesis of ATP by flowing protons back into the matrix through ATP synthase (F_0F_1 ATPase) enzyme.

(Figure 8.9). The free energy is released as H^+ ions flow back through the F_0F_1ATPase into the zone of lower H^+ concentration. The free energy released is coupled with the **phosphorylation of ADP** to ATP. The F_1 of F_0F_1ATPase catalyzes the addition of inorganic phosphate to ADP to form ATP.

P:O Ratios for Mitochondrial Electron Transport and Oxidative Phosphorylation

The P:O ratio (ratio of phosphate incorporated into ATP to atoms of O_2 utilized) is a number of inorganic phosphates utilized for ATP production for every atom of oxygen consumed.

- The transfer of two electrons from NADH to O_2 results in the translocation of 10 protons across the membrane, **four** each from complexes I and III and **two** from

complex IV. **The number of protons required to make the synthesis of an ATP molecule is 4.**

- If 10 protons are pumped out per NADH and 4 must flow in to produce one ATP, the **P:O ratio** is:
  - 2.5 (10/4) for NADH as the electron donor
  - 1.5 (6/4) for $FADH_2$ as the electron donor.

INHIBITORS OF ELECTRON TRANSPORT CHAIN AND OXIDATIVE PHOSPHORYLATION

Many poisons inhibit the electron transport (respiratory) chain. They may be classified into four groups **(Table 8.2)**:
1. Inhibitors of the respiratory chain **(Figure 8.10 and Table 8.2)**
2. Inhibitors of (F_0F_1 ATPase) oxidative phosphorylation
3. Uncouplers of oxidative phosphorylation
4. Ionophores

TABLE 8.2: Inhibitors of electron transport chain and oxidative phosphorylation.

Type of inhibitors	Site of action	Inhibitors	Site or mode of action
Inhibitors of electron transport chain	Complex-I	• Amobarbital • Piericidin A • Rotenone • Myxathiazole	Block transfer of electrons from Fe-S of FMN to ubiquinone
	Complex-II	• Malonate • TTFA • Carboxin	Inhibit succinate dehydrogenase. Prevent transfer of electrons from $FADH_2$ to CoQ
	Complex-III	• Dimercaprol • Antimycin A • British Anti-Lewisite	Prevent transfer of electrons from cyt b to cyt c_1

Contd...

Contd...

Type of inhibitors	Site of action	Inhibitors	Site or mode of action
	Complex-IV	• Cyanide • Carbon monoxide • H_2S • Sodium azide	Prevent transfer of electrons from cyt aa_3 to molecular oxygen by inhibiting cytochrome oxidase
Inhibitors of oxidative phosphorylation (F_0F_1 ATPase)	F_0-complex	• Oligomycin • DCCD (Dicyclo hexyl carbo di imide) • Venturicidin	Inhibit activity of an enzyme $F_0 F_1$ ATPase by blocking proton flow through F_0 channel
	F_1-complex	Aurovertin	Inhibits F_1
	ATP-ADP transporter	Atractyloside	Inhibition of ATP export. ATP-ADP translocase enzyme is inhibited
Uncouplers of oxidative phosphorylation		• Dinitrophenol (DNP) • Chlorocarbonyl cyanide (CCCP) • Salicylate	Prevent the formation of proton gradient across inner mitochondrial membrane by transporting protons across the membrane
	Physiological uncouplers	• Thermogenin • Thyroxine • Long chain fatty acids • Unconjugated bilirubin	Form proton conducting pores in inner mitochondrial membrane and prevent the formation of proton gradient
Ionophores		• Valinomycin • Gramicidin	Carry cations other than H^+ through the mitochondrial membrane and discharge the membrane potential

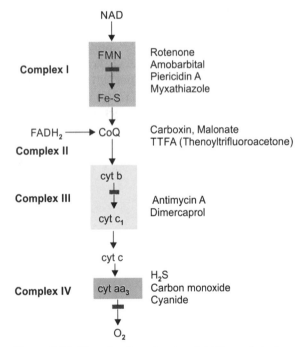

Figure 8.10: Sites of action of various inhibitors of electron transport chain.

Inhibitors of the Respiratory Chain

Many poisons inhibit the electron transport (respiratory) chain. Some of these are **(Figure 8.10)**.

Barbiturates such as amobarbital, an antibiotic piericidin-A, the insecticide rotenone and myxathiazole inhibit electron transport via **Complex I** by blocking the transfer from **Fe-S** to **Q**.

- **Complex II** is inhibited by malonate, carboxin fungicide, **TTFA (Thenoyltrifluoroacetone)**.

- Malonate is a competitive inhibitor of **succinate dehydrogenase**
- Thenoyltrifluoroacetone is a chemical compound used pharmacologically as a chelating agent. It is an inhibitor of cellular respiration by blocking the respiratory chain at complex II.

- Dimercaprol and Antimycin A, British Anti-Lewisite inhibit respiratory chain at **Complex III** by blocking the transfer from **cytochrome b** to **cytochrome c₁**.
- **Cyanide**, **Carbon monoxide** and **H_2S** inhibit **Complex IV** by inhibiting cytochrome oxidase which block the transfer from cyt aa_3 to molecular oxygen and therefore totally arrest respiration.

Inhibitors of Oxidative Phosphorylation

Another set of inhibitors do not inhibit special complexes. Instead, these, compounds block phosphorylation directly by inhibiting **$F_0 F_1$ ATPase** enzyme. For example:

- Antibiotic **oligomycin, dicyclohexylcarbodiimide (DCCD)**, **Venturicidin** and **Aurovertin** completely block oxidation and phosphorylation blocking the flow of protons through an enzyme F_0F_1 ATPase.
- **Atractyloside** inhibits oxidative phosphorylation by inhibiting the transfer of ADP into the mitochondria and of ATP out of the mitochondrion by inhibiting ATP-ADP translocase enzyme.

Uncouplers of Oxidative Phosphorylation

- Uncouplers dissociate oxidation from phosphorylation.
- These compounds are toxic, and lipophilic (lipid soluble), which readily diffuses through the mitochondrial membrane.

- Thus, these compounds make the inner mitochondrial membrane abnormally permeable to protons.
- Uncouplers allow transport of H^+ ion across the membrane toward the side with the lower H^+ ion concentration, thus, preventing the formation of **proton gradient** which is required for the formation of ATP.
- The energy produced by the transport of electrons is released as heat rather than being used for synthesis of ATP. Examples of uncouplers include:
  - **2,4-Dinitrophenol (DNP)** which was once used as a weight loss drug, but was banned by the Food and Drug Administration in the USA because of its toxicity.
  - **Dicumarol** (an anticoagulant)
  - **Carbonyl cyanide chlorophenylhydrazone** (CCCP, is a protonophore which is a widely used uncoupler of mitochondrial oxidative phosphorylation. CCCP disrupts ATP synthesis by transporting protons across the mitochondrial inner membrane, interfering with the proton gradient).
  - **Salicylate**, a metabolite of aspirin
  - **Physiological uncouplers**, thermogenin, thyroxine, bilirubin, and free fatty acids. However, these compounds normally are not present in concentrations high enough to act as uncouplers.

Ionophores: Inhibitors of Oxidative Phosphorylation

- Ionophore means **ion carrier molecules**. Oxidative phosphorylation can be prevented by certain ionophores.
- They are lipid-soluble substances, capable of binding and carrying specific cations (other than H^+) through the mitochondrial membrane.
- They differ from uncoupling agents in that they promote the transport of cations other than H^+ through the membrane and **abolish the membrane potential** and/or **pH gradient** across the membrane and phosphorylation is therefore completely inhibited. For example:
  - The toxic antibiotic **valinomycin** which allows penetration of K^+ through the mitochondrial membrane, discharging the membrane potential across inner membrane.
  - **Gramicidin** also acts as an ionophore for K^+ and Na^+ and several other monovalent cations through the inner mitochondrial membrane, and abolishes the membrane potential and/or pH gradient across the membrane and phosphorylation is therefore completely inhibited.

BROWN ADIPOSE TISSUE METABOLISM

Most newborn mammals, including humans have a type of adipose tissue called **brown adipose tissue (BAT)**. In which fuel oxidation serves not only to produce ATP but also to generate heat to keep them newborn warm. This specialized adipose tissue is brown because of the presence of large numbers of mitochondria and thus high concentrations of cytochromes, with heme groups that are strong absorbers of visible light.

- The mitochondria of brown fat have a unique protein in their inner membrane: **thermogenin** also called the **uncoupling protein 1 (UCP 1)**. This protein transports protons back into the matrix, without passing through the F_0F_1 ATPase complex.
- As a result, the energy of oxidation is not conserved by ATP formation, but is dissipated as heat, which is used to maintain the body temperature.
- Until recently, adult humans were believed to lack brown fat tissue. However, new studies have established that adults, women especially, have brown adipose tissue in the neck and upper chest regions that is activated by cold.
- Obesity leads to a decrease in brown adipose tissue.

SHUTTLE SYSTEMS FOR OXIDATION OF EXTRAMITOCHONDRIAL NADH

Most of the NADH and $FADH_2$ entering the mitochondrial electron transport chain arises from **Krebs cycle** and **β-oxidation** of fatty acids, located in the mitochondria itself. Since the inner mitochondrial membrane is not permeable to cytoplasmic NADH, how can the NADH generated by glycolysis, which take place outside of the mitochondria, be oxidized to NAD by respiratory chain located in mitochondria. Special shuttle systems carry **reducing equivalents** from **cytosolic NADH** into the mitochondria by an indirect route. This transport of reducing equivalents as NADH regardless of sources by enzymatic processes called **shuttle mechanisms**. Two such mechanisms that can lead to the transport of reducing equivalent from the cytoplasm into mitochondria are:

1. Malate shuttle system
2. Glycerophosphate shuttle

Malate Shuttle System

Malate-aspartate shuttle is the most active **NADH shuttle** which functions in liver, kidney and heart mitochondria, which is mediated by **two membrane carriers** and **four enzymes (Figure 8.11)**.

- The reducing equivalents of cytosolic NADH are first transferred to cytosolic oxaloacetate to yield malate by **cytosolic malate dehydrogenase**.
- Malate, which carries the reducing equivalents, is transported across the inner membrane by **malate-α-ketoglutarate transport** system.
- The reducing equivalents carried by malate are then transferred to mitochondrial NAD^+ by **mitochondrial malate dehydrogenase** and malate itself gets reoxidized

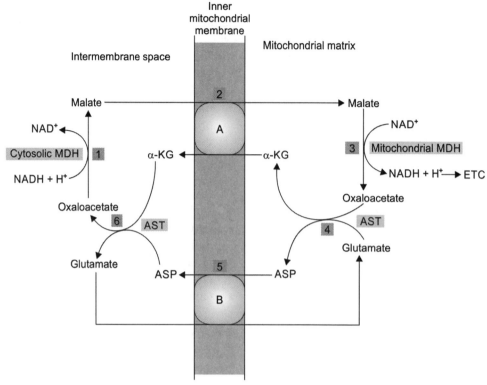

Figure 8.11: Malate shuttle.

(A: malate/α-KG transporter; B: aspartate/glutamate transporter; α-KG: α-ketoglutarate; ASP: aspartate; MDH: malate dehydrogenase; ETC: electron transport chain; AST: aspartate aminotransferase)

to oxaloacetate. The resulting mitochondrial NADH is oxidized by the mitochondrial electron transport chain, leading to formation of 2.5 molecules of ATP per electron pair.

- The oxaloacetate so formed cannot pass through the membrane from the mitochondrion back into cytosol, so it is converted to **aspartate**. Oxaloacetate in mitochondria undergoes transamination reaction, with glutamate, catalyzed by aspartate aminotransferase to yield α-ketoglutarate and amino acid aspartate.
- Aspartate is transported to the cytosolic side via amino acid transport system.
- In the cytosol, a reversal of the aspartate aminotransferase reaction gives rise to oxaloacetate and glutamate, thereby completing the "shuttle like" process.

Glycerophosphate Shuttle

Skeletal muscle and brain use a different NADH shuttle, the **glycerol-3-phosphate shuttle (Figure 8.12)**. It differs from the malate-aspartate shuttle in that it delivers the reducing equivalents form NADH to coenzyme Q and thus into complex III, not complex I synthesizing **1.5 ATP** molecules per pair of electrons.

- The first step in this shuttle is the transfer of a pair of electrons from cytosolic NADH to dihydroxyacetone phosphate to from glycerol-3-phospate catalyzed by cytosolic glycerol-3-phosphate dehydrogenase enzyme.

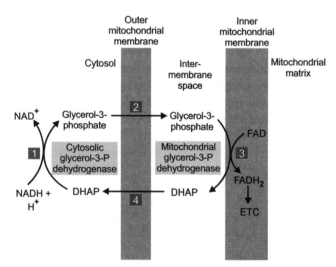

Figure 8.12: Glycerophosphate shuttle.

(DHAP: dihydroxyacetone phosphate)

- Glycerol-3-phosphate in turn diffuses through the outer mitochondrial membrane into the intermembrane space of the mitochondria.
- Here glycerol-3-phosphate is reoxidized to dihydroxyacetone phosphate on the outer surface of the inner mitochondrial membrane by a membrane bound FAD containing isoenzyme of glycerol-3-phosphate dehydrogenase. An electron pair from glycerol-3-phosphate is transferred to an FAD of the enzyme to from $FADH_2$. $FADH_2$ then transfers its electrons to the respiratory

chain through CoQH$_2$. Since the mitochondrial enzyme is linked to the respiratory chain via FAD rather than NAD, only **1.5** molecules rather than **2.5** molecules of ATP are formed per atom of oxygen consumed.

- The dihydroxyacetone phosphate returns to the cytosol and can be reused for reduction of glycerol-3-phosphate.

DISORDERS OF MITOCHONDRIAL ELECTRON TRANSPORT AND OXIDATIVE PHOSPHORYLATION

Disorders involving components of oxidative phosphorylation referred to as **OXPHOS diseases**. OXPHOS diseases are caused due to mutation in **mitochondrial DNA (mtDNA)**. Mitochondrial DNA has a high rate of mutation than nuclear DNA may be due to inadequate repair mechanisms. The mtDNA encodes 13 proteins required for oxidative phosphorylation. These are:

- Seven proteins of ETC complex I (NADH-dehydrogenase complex).
- One protein of complex III (cytochrome b, c$_1$ complex).
- Three proteins of complex IV (cytochrome oxidase).
- Two subunits of the ATP synthase complex.
- In addition mtDNA encodes the necessary components of its translation, e.g., large and small r-RNA gene and 22 t-RNAs.
- **Mutations in mtDNA are maternally inherited** because almost all of the mitochondrial genes in the zygote are contributed by the ovum.
- Mitochondria from the sperm cell do not enter the zygote. No affected male transmit the disease.
- Organs that are highly dependent on oxidative phosphorylation, such as, CNS and heart muscle are most affected by mutations in mtDNA.

TABLE 8.3: Inherited defects of oxidative phosphorylation (OXPHOS).

Disease	Causes	Clinical features
LHON (Leber's hereditary optic neuropathy)	mtDNA mutations to the NADH-CoQ oxidoreductase of component-I of ETC	Blindness, tremor, ataxia
MELAS (Mitochondrial encephalopathy, lactic acidosis and stroke)	A neuromuscular disease due to mutation of mtDNA gene that encodes for the tRNA for amino acid leucine	Deafness, diabetes mellitus, stroke like episodes, lactic acidosis, dementia
MERRF (Myoclonic epilepsy and ragged red fiber) disease, so called because, of the unusual form of the fiber seen in muscle biopsy	Defect in mtDNA	Abnormal eye movement, deafness, lactic acidosis ragged red muscle fibers in muscle and progressive dementia

- Most mitochondrial mutations result in, accumulation of **lactic acid**, a product of anaerobic metabolism of glucose and impaired ATP production, which may result in cell death, especially in skeletal muscle (myopathies), cardiac muscles (cardiomyopathies) and nerve tissues (encephalopathies), which are dependent on oxidative phosphorylation.
- Decreased production of ATP also increases the production of reactive oxygen species (ROS), which may lead to cancer.

Some of the mitochondrial myopathies that result from mutation in mtDNA are listed in **Table 8.3**. Diagnosis of these diseases involves muscle biopsy and isolation of mitochondria for morphological, biochemical and genetic analysis.

ASSESSMENT QUESTIONS

STRUCTURED LONG ESSAY QUESTIONS (SLEQs)

1. Describe the electron transport chain under the following headings:
   i. Structural organization of components of complexes with diagram
   ii. Reactions of each complex with diagrams
   iii. Inhibitors of each complex
2. Describe oxidative phosphorylation under the following headings:
   i. Mechanism (Chemiosmotic theory) with diagram
   ii. P:O ratio
   iii. Inhibitors and uncouplers
3. Describe shuttle pathways for transport of NADH across mitochondrial membranes under following headings:
   i. Malate-aspartate shuttle
   ii. Glycerol phosphate shuttle

SHORT ESSAY QUESTIONS (SEQs)

1. Define biological oxidative phosphorylation. Write its mechanism.
2. Define biological oxidation and mechanism of ATP synthesis.
3. Mechanism of synthesis of ATP in ETC.
4. Write enzymes, coenzymes and electron carriers of biological oxidation.
5. Give inhibitors of ETC with their site of action.
6. Give inhibitors and uncouplers of oxidative phosphorylation.
7. Write brown adipose tissue metabolism.
8. Write malate-aspartate shuttle.
9. Write glycerol phosphate shuttle.

SHORT ANSWER QUESTIONS (SAQs)

1. What are ionophores? Give two examples.
2. Diagrammatic representation of mitochondrial ETC and location of ATP formation sites.
3. Name components of the respiratory chain in order.
4. What is the difference between uncoupling agent and Ionophores?
5. What is substrate level phosphorylation? Give two examples.
6. What is P:O ratio?
7. Name the poisons of respiratory chain. Write mechanism of cyanide poisoning.
8. Mention inhibitors of ETC with their site of action.
9. What are cytochromes? Enumerate cytochromes in ETC.
10. What are OXPHOS (Oxidative phosphorylation) diseases? Give any two examples.

MULTIPLE CHOICE QUESTIONS (MCQs)

1. **All of the following are true regarding mitochondrial cytochromes, *except*:**
   a. They all contain heme groups
   b. All are bound to protein components
   c. Iron must remain in the ferrous state to function in electron transport
   d. They accept or donate one electron at a time

2. **Which one of the following respiratory chain components reacts directly with molecular oxygen?**
   a. Coenzyme Q
   b. Cytochrome b
   c. Cytochrome aa$_3$
   d. Cytochrome c

3. **In oxidative phosphorylation, the oxidation of one molecule of FADH$_2$ produces:**
   a. 3 ATP molecules
   b. 1.5 ATP molecules
   c. 1 ATP molecule
   d. No ATP at all

4. **All of the following statements are true regarding ETC, *except*:**
   a. Located in inner mitochondrial membrane
   b. Components are organized in decreasing order of redox potential
   c. Involved with ATP synthesis
   d. Cyanide inhibits electron flow

5. **The oxidation and phosphorylation of intact mitochondria is blocked by:**
   a. Puromycin
   b. Oligomycin
   c. Streptomycin
   d. Erythromycin

6. **Respiratory chain is found in:**
   a. Mitochondria
   b. Cytoplasm
   c. Nucleus
   d. Endoplasmic reticulum

7. **In oxidative phosphorylation, the oxidation of one molecule of NADH produces:**
   a. 2 ATP molecules
   b. 2.5 ATP molecules
   c. 4 ATP molecules
   d. 1 ATP molecule

8. **Which of the following vitamin is involved in ETC?**
   a. Thiamine
   b. Folic acid
   c. Riboflavin
   d. Cobalamin

9. **Which of the following trace elements has role in ETC?**
   a. Iron and copper
   b. Iodine
   c. Iron
   d. Fluoride

10. **An uncoupler of oxidative phosphorylation:**
    a. Inhibits electron transport and ATP synthesis
    b. Allows electron transport to occur without ATP formation
    c. Inhibits electron transport without impairment of ATP synthesis
    d. Inhibits transfer of electrons from cytochrome aa$_3$ to molecular oxygen

11. **Energy currency of the cell is:**
    a. High energy phosphate (~P)
    b. S-adenosyl methionine (SAM)
    c. Creatine phosphate
    d. Glucose-6-phosphate

12. **The enzyme that synthesizes ATP in oxidative phosphorylation is:**
    a. Hexokinase
    b. NADH dehydrogenase
    c. Cytochrome oxidase
    d. F$_0$F$_1$ ATPase

13. **A naturally occurring uncoupler is:**
    a. Dicumarol
    b. 2,4-DNP
    c. Thermogenin
    d. Salicylate

14. **A biochemical substance that can act as an uncoupler is:**
    a. Bilirubin
    b. Free fatty acid
    c. Thyroxine
    d. All of the above

15. **Which of the following is an ionophore?**
    a. 2,4-dinitrophenol
    b. Valinomycin
    c. Thermogenin
    d. Oligomycin

16. **Which of the following is not an ATP synthesizing site in respiratory chain?**
    a. Complex I
    b. Complex II
    c. Complex III
    d. Complex IV

17. **Which of the following is true during the transfer of electrons to O$_2$ via the electron transport chain?**
    a. The energy is used directly in the addition of Pi to ADP to form ATP
    b. The energy released is used to translocate protons across the inner membrane
    c. A proton gradient is generated with the matrix now being more positive than the intermembrane space
    d. Pumping of protons across the membrane occurs each time electrons are removed

18. **All of the following statements are correct for ATP synthase which consists of two domains F$_1$ and F$_0$, *except*:**
    a. F$_1$ and F$_0$ are both associated with the outer mitochondrial membrane
    b. F$_0$ unit forms a channel through which [H$^+$] pass across the membrane
    c. F$_1$ contains the catalytic site for ATP synthesis
    d. Oligomycin inhibits this enzyme

19. Which of the following statement is true for complex I?
    a. It is one of the ATP synthesizing sites of respiratory chain
    b. Transfers electrons directly from NADH to ubiquinone
    c. Does not contain Fe-S center
    d. Can transfer electrons from $FADH_2$ of succinate dehydrogenase as well as from NADH

20. Cyanide inhibits the electron transport chain by preventing transfer of electrons from:
    a. Cyt aa_3 to molecular O_2
    b. Cyt b to $Cytc_1$
    c. From $FMNH_2$ to ubiquinone
    d. From $FADH_2$ to ubiquinone

21. In Rieske iron-sulfur center of ETC is linked to:
    a. Histidine   b. Cysteine
    c. Methionine   d. Glycine

22. Following passes electrons to coenzyme Q via $FADH_2$, *except*:
    a. α-ketoglutarate   b. Succinate
    c. Glycerol-3-phosphate d. Acyl-CoA

23. Which of the following is a physiological uncoupler?
    a. Thyroxine   b. Glucagon
    c. Epinephrine   d. Insulin

24. Mechanism of cyanide poisoning:
    a. Inhibition of cytochrome oxidase
    b. Inhibition of carbonic anhydrase
    c. Inhibition of cytochrome c
    d. Inhibition of ATP synthase

25. Transport of ADP in and ATP out of mitochondria is inhibited by:
    a. Atractyloside   b. Oligomycin
    c. Rotenone   d. Cyanide

26. The electron flow in cytochrome c oxidase can be blocked by:
    a. Rotenone   b. Antimycin-A
    c. Cyanide   d. Actinomycin

27. Cytosolic cytochrome c mediates:
    a. Apoptosis   b. Electron transport
    c. Krebs cycle   d. Glycolysis

28. Which component transfers four protons?
    a. NADH-Q oxidoreductase
    b. Cytochrome-c oxidase
    c. Cytochrome c -Q oxidoreductase
    d. Succinate Q reductase

29. The specialized mammalian tissue/organ in which fuel oxidation serves not a produce ATP but to generate heat is:
    a. Adrenal gland   b. Skeletal muscle
    c. Brown adipose tissue d. Heart

30. Electron transport chain involves all, *except*:
    a. NADP   b. NAD
    c. Coenzyme Q   d. FAD

31. F_0-F_1 complex, ATP synthase inhibitor is:
    a. Atractyloside   b. Oligomycin
    c. Antimycin   d. Rotenone

32. Phenobarbital inhibits which complex of ETC:
    a. Complex I   b. Complex II
    c. Complex III   d. Complex IV

33. Final acceptor of electrons in ETC is:
    a. Cyt c   b. Oxygen
    c. $FADH_2$ d. CoQ

ANSWERS FOR MCQs

1. c	2. c	3. b	4. b	5. b
6. a	7. b	8. c	9. a	10. b
11. a	12. d	13. c	14. d	15. b
16. b	17. b	18. a	19. a	20. a
21. a	22. a	23. a	24. a	25. a
26. c	27. a	28. a,c	29. c	30. a
31. b	32. a	33. b		

9 CHAPTER

Vitamins

Competency	Learning Objectives
BI 6.5: Describe the biochemical role of vitamins in the body and explain the manifestations of their deficiency.	1. Define, classify vitamins and enumerate the difference between fat soluble and water soluble vitamins. 2. Describe water soluble vitamins: Structure, metabolism, active/coenzyme form, sources, biochemical functions, nutritional requirement and deficiency manifestations and toxicity of excessive intakes. 3. Describe fat soluble vitamins: Structure, metabolism, active/coenzyme form, sources, biochemical functions, nutritional requirement and deficiency manifestations and toxicity of excessive intakes.

■ OVERVIEW

The name **'Vitamine'** was proposed in 1911 by Polish chemist Casimir Funk for the nutrient compound required to prevent the nutritional deficiency disease **beriberi**, because of its vital (vita = life) need and because chemically it was found to be an **amine**. Later, after a number of other essential organic nutrients were discovered, the **"e"** was dropped, when it was found that not all of them are amines. The term **'Vitamin'** has now been adopted universally and applied to a group of biologically essential compounds that includes 14 compounds, which cannot be synthesized by human beings. They must, therefore, be supplied through food.

Since their chemical nature was unknown letter designations were applied for their nomenclature, e.g., vitamins A, B, and C. Later, vitamin B was shown to consist of several substances and subscripts were added, i.e., vitamin B_1, B_2, B_6, etc., and collectively called **vitamin B-complex**.

■ DEFINITION AND CLASSIFICATION OF VITAMINS

Definition

A vitamin is defined as an organic compound that is required in the diet in small quantities (in micrograms to milligram quantities per day) for the maintenance of normal metabolic integrity. They may be water or fat soluble.

Vitamins generally cannot be synthesized by the body and must, therefore, be supplied by the diet. Deficiency causes a specific disease, which is cured or prevented only by restoring the vitamins to the diet.

However, vitamin D which is formed in the skin from 7-dehydrocholesterol on exposure to sunlight, and niacin which can be formed from the essential amino acid tryptophan; do not strictly fulfil with this definition.

Classification

The vitamins are grouped into two categories based on their solubility:
● Water soluble vitamins.
● Fat soluble vitamins

Water soluble vitamins which include:
● Vitamin B complex, e.g.,
  ■ Thiamine (vitamin B_1)
  ■ Riboflavin (vitamin B_2)
  ■ Niacin (vitamin B_3)
  ■ Pantothenic acid (vitamin B_5)
  ■ Pyridoxine (vitamin B_6)
  ■ Biotin
  ■ Folic acid
  ■ Cobalamin (vitamin B_{12})
● Vitamin C or ascorbic acid.

Fat soluble vitamins, which include:

- Vitamin A or retinol
- Vitamin D or cholecalciferol
- Vitamin E or tocopherol
- Vitamin K.

Table 9.1 summarizes the best food sources, dietary allowances, the active coenzyme forms, the principal metabolic functions and the major clinical manifestations of deficiencies of the water soluble and fat soluble vitamins.

Difference between Fat Soluble and Water Soluble Vitamins

- Water soluble vitamins function as precursor for coenzymes and antioxidants while fat soluble vitamins function as coenzymes, hormones, and antioxidants.
- Water soluble vitamins are usually **nontoxic** (except B_3, B_6, B_{12}) since excess amounts of these vitamins are excreted in the urine, while fat soluble vitamins are **toxic** (vitamin E is east toxic in fat soluble vitamins) and even lethal when taken in excessive quantities.
- Water soluble vitamins are not stored extensively **except vitamin B_{12}**, and so their intake has to be more frequent than that of other fat soluble vitamins which are stored.

We shall first examine nature and functions of the water soluble vitamins that include vitamin B-complex and vitamin C (ascorbic acid).

WATER SOLUBLE VITAMINS: STRUCTURE, METABOLISM, ACTIVE/COENZYME FORM, SOURCES, BIOCHEMICAL FUNCTIONS, NUTRITIONAL REQUIREMENT AND DEFICIENCY MANIFESTATIONS AND TOXICITY OF EXCESSIVE INTAKES

Thiamine (Vitamin B_1)

Structure

Thiamine consists of a pyrimidine ring attached to a thiazole ring **(Figure 9.1)** by methylene bridge.

Absorption, Transport, and Metabolism

- Thiamine is absorbed readily in the small intestine by a carrier mediated active transport process as long as intake is less than 5 mg/day. At higher intake levels passive diffusion contributes to absorption.
- **Phosphorylation** takes place in the jejunal mucosa to yield **thiamine pyrophosphate (TPP)**.
- Thiamine is carried by the portal blood to the liver. The free vitamin occurs in the blood but the coenzyme form, TPP predominates in the cellular components. About half the body's stores is found in skeletal muscles, the remainder in the heart, liver, kidneys, and nervous tissue.

TABLE 9.1: Summary of the best food sources, dietary allowances, the active coenzyme forms, the principal metabolic functions and the major clinical manifestations of deficiencies of the water soluble and fat soluble vitamins.

Name	Active form	Sources	Daily requirements	Function	Deficiency manifestations
Water soluble vitamins					
Thiamine (vitamin B_1)	TPP	Cereals, meat, nuts green vegetables, eggs	1.0–1.5 mg	Coenzyme for oxidative decarboxylation and transketolase reactions	Beriberi, Wernicke-Korsakoff syndrome
Riboflavin (vitamin B_2)	FMN, FAD	Yeast, germinating seeds, green leafy vegetables, milk, eggs, liver, meat	1.3–1.7 mg	Coenzyme for oxidation reduction reactions	Cheilosis, glossitis, dermatitis vascularization of cornea
Niacin (vitamin B_3)	NAD^+ and $NADP^+$	Yeast, legumes, liver, meat	15–20 mg	Coenzyme for oxidation reduction reactions	Pellagra
Pantothenic acid (vitamin B_5)	Coenzyme A (CoA SH)	Wheat germs, cereals, yeast, liver, eggs	5–10 mg	Acyl carrier	Burning feet syndrome
Pyridoxine (vitamin B_6)	PLP	Yeast, unrefined cereals, pulses, vegetables, meat, fish, egg yolk	1.6–2 mg	Coenzyme for transamination, decarboxylation, nonoxidative deamination, trans-sulfuration reactions	Epileptic convulsions, dermatitis, hypochromic microcytic anemia
Biotin (vitamin B_7)	Biocytin (enzyme-bound biotin)	Liver, kidney, egg yolk, vegetables	150–300 μg	Coenzyme for carboxylation reactions	Rare dermatitis
Folic acid (vitamin B_9)	Tetrahydrofolic acid (THF)	Green leafy vegetables, liver, yeast	200 μg	• Carrier of one carbon unit • Synthesis of methionine, purines and pyrimidines	Megaloblastic anemia, Neural tube defects
Cynocobalamin (vitamin B_{12})	Methylcobalamin, deoxyadenosylcobalamin	Only animal origin, meat, egg, liver, fish	3 μg	*Coenzyme for reactions:* • Homocysteine to Methionine • Methylmalonyl-CoA to Succinyl-CoA	Pernicious anemia Megaloblastic anemia Neuropathy (dementia) Methylmalonic aciduria

Contd...

Contd...

Name	Active form	Sources	Daily requirements	Function	Deficiency manifestations
Ascorbic acid (vitamin C)	Ascorbic acid	Citrus fruits, Amla, leafy vegetables, tomatoes	60–70 mg	Antioxidant, involved in hydroxylation reactions in the synthesis collagen, steroid hormones, adrenaline, etc., facilitates absorption of iron from intestine	Scurvy
Fat soluble vitamins					
Vitamins A (retinol)	Retinol-Retinal, Retinoic acid	Fish liver oils, milk, milk products, green leafy vegetables, carrots, yellow and red fruits	800–1000 retinol equivalents	Retinal and retinol are involved in vision. Retinoic acid regulates the expression of gene during growth and development. Antioxidant	Night blindness xerophthalmia formation of Bitot's spots, dry, rough and scaly skin. Retardation of growth in children
Vitamins D (cholecalciferol)	1,25 Dihydroxy cholecalciferol	Cool liver oil, sunlight induced synthesis of vitamin D$_3$ in skin, egg yolk	200–400 IU	Regulations of the plasma level of calcium and phosphorus, calcification of bone	• Rickets (in children) • Osteomalacia (in adults)
Vitamin E (α-tocopherol)	α-Tocopherol	Soya and corn oils, germ oil, fish oil, eggs, alfalfa	8–10 mg	Natural antioxidant and acts as a scavenger of free radicals. Protects the RBCs from hemolysis Prevents peroxidation of PUFA in cell membrane	Hemolytic anemia. Retrolental fibroplasia (RLF) in premature infants
Vitamin K	Phylloquinone (Vitamin K$_1$) Menaquinone (Vitamin K$_2$)	Green leafy vegetables, tomatoes, cheese, meat, egg yolk	70–140 µg	Required for activation of blood clotting factors. Required for γ carboxylation of glutamic and residue in clotting and osteocalcin proteins	Hemorrhagic disorder, increased clotting time

- Thiamine and several of its catabolites are excreted into the urine.

Active/Coenzyme Form of Thiamine

Thiamine pyrophosphate is an active coenzyme form of vitamin thiamine **(Figure 9.2)**. Dietary thiamine is readily absorbed and phosphorylated to its active form TPP in the jejunal mucosa.

Sources

- It is present in all natural foods but particularly good dietary sources are unrefined cereals, meat, nuts, green vegetables, eggs, etc.
- White bread and polished rice are very poor sources of the vitamins.

Functions

Thiamine is required mainly for **carbohydrate metabolism**. Thiamine pyrophosphate is a coenzyme involved in several enzymatic reactions mainly for **oxidative decarboxylation** and **transketolase** reactions as follows:

- TPP is a coenzyme for **pyruvate dehydrogenase complex**, which catalyzes the conversion of pyruvate into acetyl-CoA by oxidative decarboxylation (*see* **Figure 10.12**). Acetyl-CoA is a substrate for tricarboxylic acid cycle, precursor for the synthesis of the **neurotransmitter, acetylcholine** and also for the

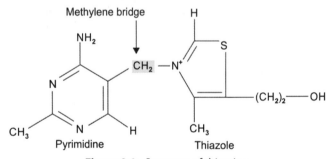

Figure 9.1: Structure of thiamine.

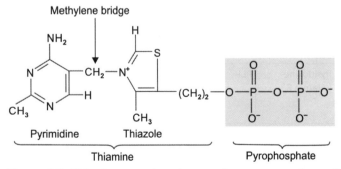

Figure 9.2: Thiamine pyrophosphate, active coenzyme form of thiamine.

(OH-group of thiazole is replaced by pyrophosphate)

synthesis of lipid including **myelin**. Thus, thiamine is required for the **normal functioning of the nervous system**.

- TPP is a coenzyme for α-**ketoglutarate dehydrogenase**, which catalyzes the conversion of α-ketoglutarate to succinyl-CoA by oxidative decarboxylation in TCA cycle (*see* **Figure 10.15**). Malfunctioning of TCA in absence of thiamine results in **defective energy metabolism**.
- It is also involved in **decarboxylation** reactions in the metabolism of **branched chain amino acids** (*see* **Figure 10.15**).
- TPP is a coenzyme for the enzyme **transketolase** in the pentose phosphate pathway of glucose oxidation (*see* **Figure 10.34**) which produces **ribose sugars** and supplies **NADPH** which is necessary for a wide variety of biosynthetic reactions and detoxification reactions.

Nutritional Requirements

- Nutritional research council recommends daily intake of **1.0 to 1.5 mg** of thiamine for adults.
- Thiamine requirement is increased with increased muscular activity, dietary carbohydrates and in pregnancy and lactation.

Deficiency Manifestations

- Most dietary deficiency of thiamine worldwide is the result of poor dietary intake. Thiamine deficiency occurs primarily in people whose caloric or carbohydrate intake is disproportionately high compared to their thiamine intake. Such an imbalance occurs in:
  - Populations that depend on a diet consisting of mainly of polished rice, which lacks the hulls in which most of the thiamine of rice found. The processing of rice removes the thiamine.
  - People who habitually consume large amount of alcohol can also develop thiamine deficiency, because much of their dietary intake consists of the vitamin free "empty calories". As well as alcohol interferes directly with the absorption of thiamine and with the synthesis of thiamine pyrophosphate.
- Thiamine deficiency leads to failure of carbohydrate metabolism, resulting in decreased production of ATP and thus impaired cellular functions of brain and heart. Brain and heart usually obtains all its energy from the aerobic oxidation of glucose in a pathway that necessarily includes oxidation of pyruvate. Thiamine deficiency affects the nervous system and the heart.
- In the absence of thiamine, pyruvate is converted to lactate, and results in increased plasma concentration of **lactate** which may cause life threatening **lactic acidosis**.
- Thiamine deficiency in its early stage induces anorexia and nonspecific symptoms, e.g., irritability, decrease in short-term memory.
- Prolonged thiamine deficiency causes **beriberi**.

Beriberi

Beriberi is characteristically categorized as **dry beriberi** and **wet beriberi**.

Dry Beriberi

- **Dry beriberi** develops when the diet chronically contains slightly less than the thiamine requirement. Dry beriberi primarily affects the **nervous system**, leading to the degeneration of the nerves. Patients with dry beriberi present with:
  - Peripheral neuropathy
  - Tingling or loss of sensation
  - Numbness in hands and feet.
- The neuropathy affects the legs most markedly, and patients have difficulty rising from a squatting (bending) position.

Wet Beriberi

- **Wet beriberi** develops when the deficiency is more severe. This mainly affects the **cardiovascular system**, causing poor circulation and fluid accumulation in the tissues. The cardiovascular symptoms are due to **impaired myocardial energy metabolism**. Patients present with:
  - Enlarged heart
  - Tachycardia
  - High-output heart failure
  - Peripheral edema, and
  - Peripheral neuritis.

Both forms of beriberi may overlap to a varying degree and patients of beriberi may die due to heart failure, if not treated.

Wernicke-Korsakoff Syndrome (Cerebral Beriberi)

The syndrome is more common among people with **alcoholism** than in general population.

- Heavy alcohol consumption interferes with the intestinal **absorption of thiamine** and with the synthesis of **thiamine pyrophosphate**. The syndrome can be worse by a **mutation of the gene** for **transketolase** that results in reduced affinity of transketolase for TPP.
- **Alcoholic patients** with chronic thiamine deficiency may also have central nervous system (CNS) manifestations known as **Wernicke's encephalopathy** characterized by:
  - Anorexia
  - Cerebellar ataxia
  - Depression
  - Loss of memory
  - Mental confusion
  - Peripheral paralysis
  - Muscular weakness
  - Horizontal nystagmus
  - Double vision
  - Ophthalmoplegia (weakness of one or more extraocular muscles), cerebellar ataxia, and mental impairment.
- When there is an additional loss of memory and a confabulatory psychosis (memory error, production

of fabricated, distorted, or misinterpreted memories about oneself or the world), the syndrome is known as **Wernicke-Korsakoff syndrome**.

> Wernicke is a region of the brain that contains motor neurons involved in the comprehension of speech. This area was first described in 1874 by German neurologist Carl Wernicke.

Infantile Beriberi

Maternal thiamine deficiency can lead to **infantile beriberi** in breast-fed children. It is characterized by cardiac dilation (enlargement of heart), tachycardia, convulsions, edema, and GI disturbances such as vomiting, abdominal colic, etc. In acute condition, the infant may die due to cardiac failure.

STRIKE A NOTE

- ❖ Thiamine can be destroyed if the diet contains **thiaminase**.
- ❖ Thiaminase is present in raw fish and seafood.
- ❖ **Whole blood** or **erythrocyte transketolase** activity is used as a measure of thiamine deficiency.
- ❖ The reference interval for transketolase activity is:
  - ➤ Whole blood = 9–12 µmol/hour/mL (150–200 U/L)
  - ➤ Erythrocyte = 0.75–1.30 U/g of hemoglobin.

Toxicity

No adverse effects have been recorded from either food or supplements at high doses.

Riboflavin (Vitamin B$_2$)

Structure

Riboflavin is a yellow compound (Flavus = **yellow** in Latin) consisting of an **isoalloxazine ring** with a **ribitol** (sugar alcohol) side chain **(Figure 9.3)**. Riboflavin is relatively **heat stable** but decomposes in the presence of visible light (photosensitive).

Absorption, Transport, and Metabolism

- Riboflavin is ingested in the form of **flavoprotein**. During digestion the flavin adenine dinucleotide (FAD) and flavin mononucleotide (FMN) components are released from the protein complex in the stomach and free riboflavin is released in the intestine from which it is absorbed by an active transport process.
- After transport through blood in protein-bound complexes, conversion of riboflavin to coenzymes occurs within the cellular cytoplasm of most tissue, but particularly in the small intestine, liver, heart, and kidney.
- The main storage form of the vitamin, found mainly in the liver, is fad, where it forms complexes mainly with numerous flavoprotein dehydrogenases and oxidases. Because only small amounts of riboflavin are stored in this manner, the urinary excretion reflects dietary intake.

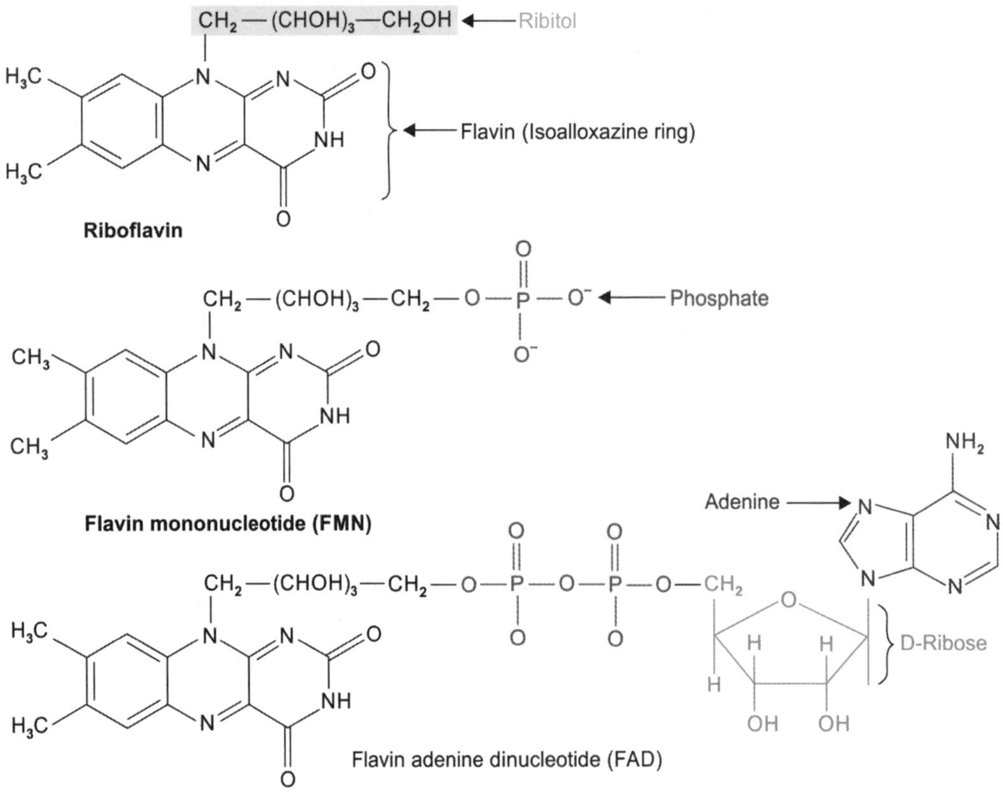

Figure 9.3: Structure of riboflavin and its active coenzyme forms FMN and FAD.

Active/Coenzyme Form of Riboflavin

The active or coenzyme forms of the riboflavin are:
- Flavin mononucleotide
- Flavin adenine dinucleotide
  Riboflavin is converted to FMN in the intestinal mucosal cells, then to FAD in the liver.

Sources

- The main dietary sources of riboflavin are yeast, germinating seeds, green leafy vegetables milk and milk products, eggs, liver, meat etc.
- Cereals are a poor source.

Functions

- Riboflavin is a precursor of coenzymes **FMN** and **FAD**, which are required by several **oxidation-reduction** reactions in metabolism.
- FMN and FAD serve as coenzymes for oxidoreductase enzymes involved in carbohydrate, protein, lipid, nucleic acid metabolism, and electron transport chain. Some examples are given in **Table 9.2**.

TABLE 9.2: Examples of enzymes requiring FMN or FAD as a coenzyme (flavoprotein enzymes) and reaction where they are involved.

Flavoprotein enzyme	Pathway/reaction
Amino acid oxidase	Deamination of amino acids
Xanthine oxidase	Purine degradation
Mitochondrial glycerol-3-phosphate dehydrogenase	Transfer of reducing equivalents from cytosol into mitochondria
Succinate dehydrogenase	Citric acid cycle
Acyl-CoA dehydrogenase	Fatty acid oxidation
NADH dehydrogenase	Respiratory chain into mitochondria
Pyruvate dehydrogenase and α-ketoglutarate dehydrogenase	Oxidative decarboxylation of pyruvate and α-ketoglutarate

- The vitamin also plays a role in drug and steroid metabolism, including detoxification reactions.
- It is needed for maintenance of mucosal epithelial and the ocular tissues.

Nutritional Requirements

- The RDA for vitamin B_2 is **1.3 to 1.7** mg for adults.
- The requirement of riboflavin does not appear to be related to caloric requirement or to muscle activity, but it is related to protein use and increases during growth, pregnancy, lactation, and wound healing.

Deficiency Manifestations

- Riboflavin deficiency is quite rare as it has a wide distribution in food stuffs. Manifestations of riboflavin deficiency are nonspecific and are usually seen along with deficiencies of other vitamins of B-complex group, and condition is called **ariboflavinosis** or **avitaminosis**.
- Riboflavin deficiency most commonly seen in:
  - Chronic alcoholics.
  - Drugs such as **barbiturates** by inducing microsomal oxidation of vitamin.
  - **Newborn infants** with **hyperbilirubinemia**, who are treated by phototherapy, because of its light sensitivity
- Riboflavin deficiency symptoms are relatively mild and not life threatening. Riboflavin deficiency is manifested by lesions of mucocutaneous surfaces of mouth and skin
  - *Cheilosis:* Fissures at the angles of the mouth **(Figure 9.4)**
  - *Glossitis:* Inflammation of tongue that becomes swollen and magenta colored
  - *Dermatitis*: Rough and scaly skin
  - Corneal vascularization **(Figure 9.4)**
- In addition to the mucocutaneous lesions **anemia** also occur with riboflavin deficiency.

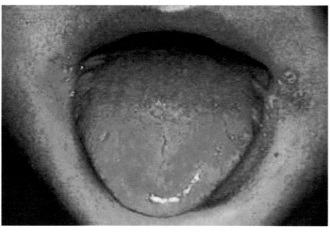
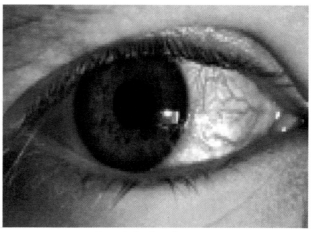

Glossitis and chelosis

Vascularization of cornea

Figure 9.4: Clinical manifestation of deficiency of riboflavin.

- Severe riboflavin deficiency affect:
  - Conversion of vitamin B$_6$ to its coenzyme and
  - Inhibit conversion of tryptophan to niacin.

Toxicity

Because the capacity of the gastrointestinal tract to absorb riboflavin is limited (approximately 20 mg if given in one oral dose), riboflavin toxicity has not been described.

Riboflavin Assay

Laboratory diagnosis of riboflavin deficiency can be made by measurement of red blood cell or urinary riboflavin concentrations or by measurement of erythrocyte glutathione reductase activity.

The reference interval for:

- Erythrocyte riboflavin by use of flurometric method is 10 to 15 µg/dL (266–1330 nmol/L)
- Serum or plasma levels of riboflavin is 4 to 24 µg/dL (106–638 nmol/L)

Niacin (Vitamin B$_3$)

Structure

The term *niacin* refers to nicotinic acid and nicotinamide and their biologically active derivatives.

Niacin is a general name for the **nicotinic acid** and **nicotinamide (Figure 9.5)** either of which may act as a source of the vitamin in the diet. Niacin is a simple derivative of **pyridine**. Niacin is related chemically to nicotine but has very different physiological properties.

Absorption, Transport, and Metabolism

- The coenzymes of niacin are hydrolyzed in the intestinal tract, and both the acid and amide forms of the vitamin are absorbed readily.
- Both compounds are converted to the coenzyme forms in the blood cells, kidney, brain, and liver and present as nicotinamide in NAD and NADP.
- Humans excrete through urine, 2-pyridone and 2-methyl nicotinamide as the primary metabolites of niacin, measurements of which are used in diagnosis of niacin deficiency.

Active/Coenzyme Form

Active forms of niacin are:

- Nicotinamide adenine dinucleotide (NAD$^+$)
- Nicotinamide adenine dinucleotide phosphate (NADP$^+$) **(Figure 9.5)**.

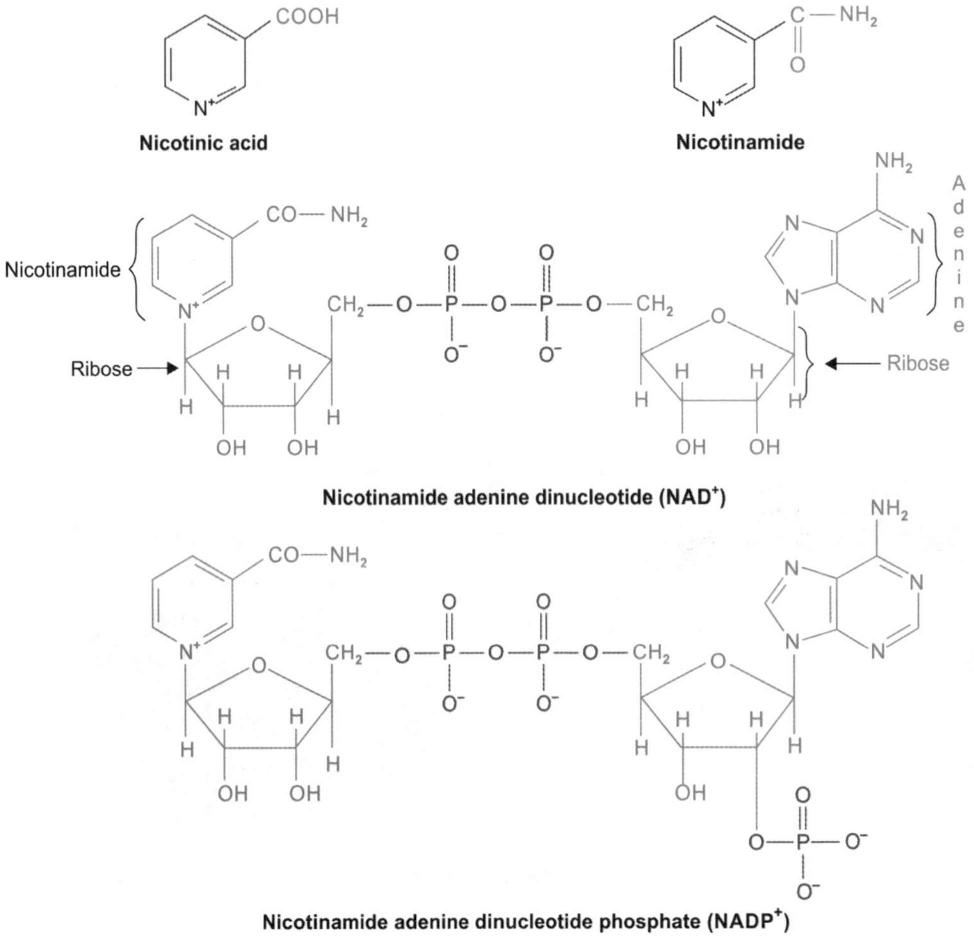

Figure 9.5: Structure and active coenzyme forms of niacin.

TABLE 9.3: Examples of enzymes requiring NAD⁺ or NADP⁺ or NADPH and reaction where they are involved.

Enzyme	Pathway/reaction
NAD dependent	
Glyceraldehyde-3-phosphate dehydrogenase	Glycolysis: Glyceraldehyde-3 phosphate to 1,3-bisphosphoglycerate
Pyruvate dehydrogenase	Oxidative decarboxylation of pyruvate to acetyl-CoA
α-ketoglutarate dehydrogenase	TCA cycle: α-ketoglutarate to succinyl-CoA
β-hydroxy acyl-CoA dehydrogenase	β-oxidation of fatty acid: β-hydroxy acyl-CoA to β-keto acyl-CoA
NADP dependent	
Glucose-6-phosphate dehydrogenase gluconolactone	Pentose phosphate pathway: Glucose 6-phosphate to 6-phospho gluconolactone
Malic enzyme	Transfer of acetyl-CoA from mitochondria to cytosol
NADPH dependent	
3-ketoacyl reductase	Fatty acid synthesis: 3-ketoacyl enzyme to 3-hydroxyacyl enzyme
HMG CoA reductase	Cholesterol synthesis: HMG-CoA to mevalonate

Sources

- Yeast, liver, legumes, and meats are major sources of niacin.
- Limited quantities of niacin can also be obtained from the metabolism of tryptophan.
- **For every 60 mg of tryptophan, 1 mg equivalent of niacin can be generated**.

Functions

- Niacin is a precursor of coenzymes, **NAD⁺** and **NADP⁺**.
- NAD⁺ and NADP⁺ are involved in various **oxidation** and **reduction reactions** catalyzed by dehydrogenases in metabolism **(Table 9.3)**.
- They are, therefore involved in many metabolic pathways of carbohydrate, lipid, and protein. Generally, **NAD⁺** linked dehydrogenases catalyze **oxidation-reduction** reactions in oxidative pathways, e.g., citric acid cycle and glycolysis.
- Whereas **NADP⁺** linked dehydrogenases or reductases are often found in pathways concerned with **reductive synthesis**, e.g., synthesis of cholesterol, fatty acid and pentose phosphate pathways. Selected examples of enzymes and the reactions they catalyze are given in **Table 9.3**.
- In addition to its coenzyme role, NAD also seems to play a role in **DNA repair**.
- NAD is a source of ADP-ribose for the **ADP-ribosylation** of proteins and poly ADP-ribosylation of nucleoproteins involved in a DNA repair, cell proliferation and differentiation and calcium mobilization.

Nutritional Requirement

- The RDA for niacin is **15 to 20 mg**
- **Tryptophan** can only provide about **10%** of the total **niacin** requirement
- Lowered conversion of tryptophan to niacin occurs in vitamin B₆ deficiency, or in the presence of isoniazid.

Deficiency Manifestation

Niacin deficiency causes **pellagra**:

- When diet is poor in both available **niacin** and **tryptophan** leads to deficiency of niacin.
- Niacin deficiency mostly found in:
  - Populations dependent on maize (corn) or sorghum (jawar) as the staple food. In maize, niacin is present, but it is a bound unavailable form that is **niacytin**. Sorghum is also pellagragenic due to high content of **leucine**. Excess of leucine can bring about niacin deficiency by inhibiting, quinolinate phosphoribosyl transferase key enzyme in the conversion of tryptophan to niacin **(Figure 9.6)**.
  - Deficiency of riboflavin or vitamin B₆, which are required for synthesis of nicotinamide from tryptophan **(Figure 9.6)**.
  - In patients with congenital defects of intestinal and kidney absorption of tryptophan **(Hartnup disease)**
  - In patients with **carcinoid syndrome**, where there is increased conversion of tryptophan to serotonin.

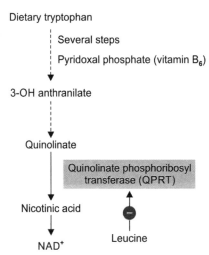

Figure 9.6: The conversion of tryptophan into nicotinic acid.

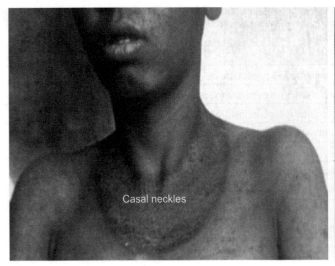
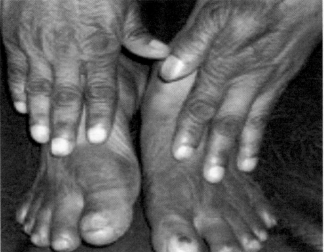

Scaly pigmented skin rash

Figure 9.7: Clinical manifestation of deficiency of niacin.

Pellagra

- Niacin deficiency causes pellagra, a disease involving the:
  - Skin
  - Gastrointestinal tract
  - Central nervous system.
- Pellagra is characterized by:
  - Dermatitis (Photosensitive, resembles sunburn)
  - Diarrhea
  - Depression and dementia
  - Untreated pellagra is fatal leading to death.
- The four *D*s: *D*ermatitis, *d*iarrhea, and *d*ementia leading to death

Symptoms of Pellagra

- The early symptoms of pellagra include loss of appetite, generalized weakness and irritability, abdominal pain, and vomiting.
- Bright red glossitis then followed by a characteristic skin rash that is pigmented and scaling, particularly in skin areas exposed to sunlight **(Figure 9.7)**.
- This rash is known as **Casal's necklace** because it forms a ring around the neck; it is seen in advanced cases **(Figure 9.7)**
- Vaginitis and esophagitis may also occur.

Pellagra can occur Despite an Adequate intake of Tryptophan and Niacin

A number of genetic diseases that result in defects of tryptophan metabolism are associated with the development of pellagra, despite an adequate intake of both tryptophan and niacin. For example:
- ❖ **Hartnup disease** is a rare genetic condition in which there is defect of the membrane transport mechanism for tryptophan, resulting in intestinal malabsorption and failure of renal reabsorption of tryptophan.

Contd...

Contd...

- ❖ **Carcinoid syndrome**, (liver cancer of enterochromaffin cells, which synthesize 5-hydroxytryptamine, serotonin) in which about 60% of the body's tryptophan metabolism is diverted to formation of serotonin causing pellagra because of the diversion away from NAD synthesis.

Therapeutic Uses of Niacin

High doses of nicotinic acid (2 g/d) are used for the treatment of elevated cholesterol, LDL cholesterol and VLDL triglyceride in patients with **hyperlipoproteinemias** which inhibits adipose tissue lipolysis, thus reducing the free fatty acid flux to the liver.

Toxicity

- Niacin when taken as a supplement or as therapy for dyslipidemia has undesirable side effects, mainly **vasodilation**, **flushing**, **nausea**, **vomiting**, and **abdominal pain**, and **liver damage**.
- Hepatic toxicity is the most serious toxic reaction due to niacin and may present as jaundice with elevated **aspartate aminotransferase (AST)** and **alanine aminotransferase (ALT)** levels.

Pantothenic Acid (Vitamin B₅)

The name pantothenic acid is derived from the Greek word **'pantothene,'** meaning from **"everywhere"** and gives an indication of the wide distribution of the vitamin in foods.

Structure

Pantothenic acid is formed by a combination of **pantoic acid** and β-**alanine (Figure 9.8)**.

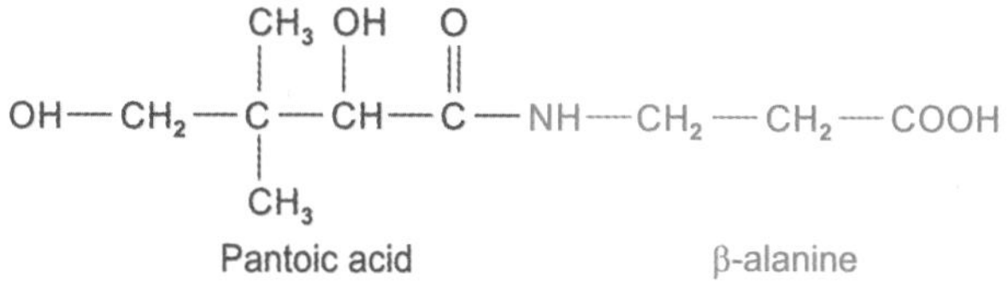

$$OH-CH_2-\underset{\underset{CH_3}{|}}{\overset{\overset{CH_3}{|}}{C}}-\underset{\overset{|}{OH}}{CH}-\underset{\overset{||}{O}}{C}-NH-CH_2-CH_2-COOH$$

Pantoic acid   β-alanine

Figure 9.8: Structure of pantothenic acid.

Active/Coenzyme Form

Active forms of pantothenic acid are:
- Coenzyme-A (CoA-SH)
- Acyl carrier protein (ACP).

Source

Eggs, liver, yeast, wheat germs, cereals, etc., are important sources of pantothenic acid, although the vitamin is widely distributed.

Absorption, Transport, and Metabolism

- CoA, the form in which pantothenic acid is ingested, is hydrolyzed by intestinal enzymes to pantetheine, and is absorbed into portal circulation.
- About 80% of the vitamin in tissues is in CoA form, with the rest existing mainly as phosphopantetheine and phosphopantethenate.
- Enzymes hydrolyze the phosphate moieties from pantothenate releasing β-mercaptoethylamine, which is excreted in urine. Only a small fraction of pantothenate is secreted into milk and even less into colostrum.

Functions

Pantothenic acid is a component of **coenzyme-A (CoA-SH)** and **phosphopantetheine** of acyl carrier protein (ACP). The thiol (-SH) groups of CoA-SH and ACP act as a carrier of **acyl groups**.
- Coenzyme-A involved in reactions concerned with:
  - Citric acid cycle
  - Fatty acid synthesis and oxidation
  - Acetylation reactions of drugs
  - Synthesis of cholesterol
  - Synthesis of steroid hormones
  - Utilization of ketone bodies.
- ACP participates in reactions concerned with fatty acid synthesis.

Nutritional Requirement

The RDA of pantothenic acid is not well established. A daily intake of about **5 to 10 mg** is advised for adults.

Deficiency Manifestations

The vitamin is abundant in the food supply. No clear cut case of pantothenic acid deficiency has been reported. Human pantothenic acid deficiency has been established in experimental feeding of diets low in pantothenic acid.

- The symptoms of pantothenic acid deficiency are nonspecific and include:
  - Gastrointestinal disturbance
  - Depression
  - Muscle cramps
  - Paresthesia
  - Ataxia and
  - Hypoglycemia
- Pantothenic acid deficiency is believed to have caused the **burning feet syndrome** seen in prisoners of war during World War II.

Toxicity

No toxicity of this vitamin has been reported.

Pyridoxine (Vitamin B$_6$)

Structure

Vitamin B$_6$ consists of a mixture of three different closely related pyridine derivatives **(Figure 9.9)** namely:
- Pyridoxine
- Pyridoxal
- Pyridoxamine.

All the three have equal vitamin activity, as they can be interconverted in the body.

Active/Coenzyme Form of Vitamin B$_6$

Pyridoxal phosphate (PLP) is the active form of vitamin B$_6$ **(Figure 9.10)**. PLP is formed from phosphorylation of all three forms of vitamin B$_6$.

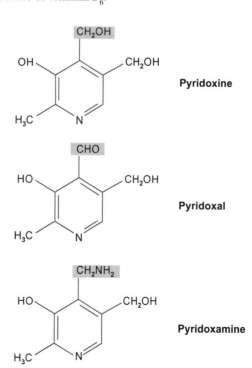

Figure 9.9: Structure of three different forms of vitamin B$_6$.

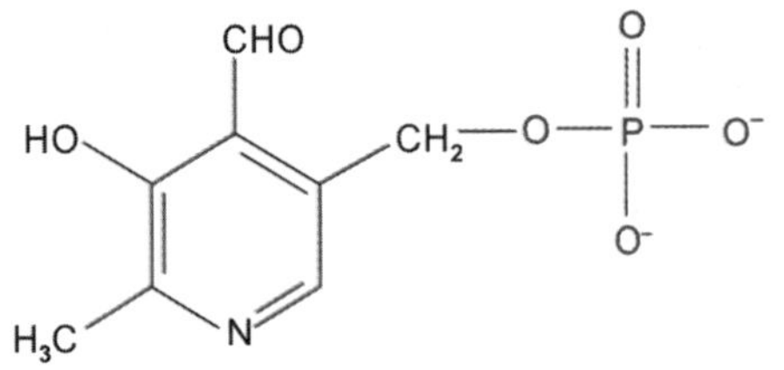

Figure 9.10: Structure of pyridoxal phosphate an active form of vitamin B$_6$.

Sources

- Pyridoxine occurs mainly in plants, whereas pyridoxal and pyridoxamine are present mainly in animal products.
- Major dietary sources of vitamin B$_6$ are meat, poultry fish, potatoes, and vegetables.
- Dairy products and grains contribute lesser amounts.
  The predominant food form is PLP which is readily lost in food processing.

Absorption, Transport, and Metabolism

- The three B$_6$ vitamins are released by dephosphorylation from their phosphate esters by intestinal alkaline phosphatase.
- These vitamins are absorbed readily by the mucosal cells, which contain cytoplasmic pyridoxal kinase responsible for catalyzing the rephosphorylation of all three vitamin forms.
- Most cells contain a cytosolic FMN-dependent oxidase enzyme responsible for catalyzing the conversion of PLP and pyridoxamine phosphate to PLP.
- PLP is transported in the blood bound to albumin.
- Most of the body stores of pyridoxine are associated with the enzyme **glycogen phosphorylase** in the skeletal muscle for which it is a coenzyme.

Functions

- Active form of vitamin B$_6$, PLP acts as coenzyme in large number of reactions of amino acid metabolism. For example:
  - Transamination
  - Decarboxylation
  - Nonoxidative deamination
  - Trans-sulfuration
  - Condensation reactions of amino acids
  - Other PLP-dependent reactions
- **Transamination reactions:** Transamination reactions are catalyzed by transaminases and PLP acts as coenzyme converting amino acid to keto acid, e.g., aspartate transaminase (AST) and alanine transaminase (ALT) (*see* **Figure 12.7**).
- **Decarboxylation reaction:** PLP acts as coenzyme in decarboxylation of some amino acids. The amino acids are decarboxylated to corresponding amines.

The important biogenic amines synthesized by PLP decarboxylation are given here (*see* **Figure 12.56**).

- ■ **γ-Amino butyric acid (GABA):** It is an inhibitory neurotransmitter derived from glutamate on decarboxylation hence in vitamin B$_6$ deficiency underproduction of GABA leads to convulsions (epileptic seizures) in infants and children.
- ■ **Serotonin and melatonin:** These are produced from tryptophan. Serotonin is a neurotransmitter and stimulates the cerebral activity. Melatonin is a sleep inducing substance and is involved in regulation of **circadian rhythm** of body.
- ■ **Histamine:** Histamine produced by decarboxylation of histidine. It is a vasodilator and lowers blood pressure. It is involved in allergic reactions.
- ■ **Catecholamines** (dopamine, norepinephrine and epinephrine) Synthesis of catecholamines from tyrosine requires PLP-dependent DOPA decarboxylase. Catecholamines are neurotransmitters and involved in metabolic and nervous regulation.
- **Nonoxidative deamination:** Hydroxyl group containing amino acids (serine, threonine) are nonoxidatively deaminated to α-keto acids and ammonia, which requires PLP (*see* **Figure 12.11**).
- **Trans-sulfuration reaction:** PLP is a coenzyme for **cystathionine synthase** involved in synthesis of cysteine from methionine (*see* **Figure 12.37**). In these reactions transfer of sulfur from methionine to serine occurs to produce cysteine.
- **Condensation reactions:** Pyridoxal phosphate is required for the condensation reaction of L-glycine and succinyl CoA to form δ-aminolevulinic acid, a precursor of heme (*see* **Figure 14.2**)
- Other PLP-dependent reactions are:
  - ■ Synthesis of niacin coenzyme (NAD$^+$/NADP$^+$) from tryptophan (*see* **Figure 12.34**).
  - ■ Synthesis of glycine from serine (*see* **Figure 12.20**).
  - ■ Synthesis of glycogen. PLP is the cofactor of glycogen phosphorylase.
  - ■ Synthesis of sphingosine, a component of sphingomyelin.
  - ■ PLP is necessary for the conversion of homocysteine to cystathionine.

Nutritional Requirement

The RDA for vitamin B$_6$ is **1.6** to **2.0** mg. Requirements increase during pregnancy and lactation.

Deficiency Manifestations

- As pyridoxine occurs in most foods, the dietary deficiency of vitamin B$_6$ is rare. The most common cause of pyridoxine deficiency is:
  - ■ **Drug antagonism (interference with the action of PLP), e.g., isoniazid (INH),** used in the treatment of

tuberculosis and **penicillamine** used in the treatment of Wilson's disease and rheumatoid arthritis can combine with PLP forming an inactive derivative with PLP.

- **Alcoholism:** Alcoholics may be deficient due to metabolism of ethanol to acetaldehyde, which stimulates hydrolysis of the phosphate of the PLP.
- The main clinical symptoms of deficiency are:
  - Vitamin B_6 deficiency causes neurological disorders such as **depression, nervousness**, and **irritability**. These symptoms are due to decreased production of neurotransmitters, catecholamines, GABA, and serotonin.
  - Severe deficiency of pyridoxine causes **epileptic seizures (convulsions)** in infants due to reduced production of GABA.
  - **Demyelination of nerves** causes peripheral **neuropathy**. Since vitamin B_6 is required for synthesis of sphingolipids needed for myelin formation.
  - Vitamin B_6 deficiency causes **hypochromic microcytic anemia** due to decreased heme synthesis. Since PLP is required for the synthesis of heme.
  - Since vitamin B_6 is necessary for the conversion of homocysteine to cystathionine, it is possible that chronic lowgrade vitamin B_6 deficiency may result in **hyperhomocysteinemia** and increased risk **of cardiovascular disease**.

STRIKE A NOTE

- ❖ Activities of blood **transaminases** have been used frequently as indirect measurements of vitamin B_6 status.
- ❖ Erythrocyte levels of aspartate and alanine aminotransferase provide better information of vitamin B_6 status.

Therapeutic Uses

Pyridoxine is used for the treatment of:
- Schizophrenia
- **Down's syndrome**, a state of mental subnormality (incomplete development of mind) due to chromosome defect.
- **Autism**, psychiatric disorder of childhood.
- **Premenstrual tension syndrome** (PMS).

Toxicity

The safe upper limit for vitamin B_6 has been set at 100 mg/day, although no adverse effects have been associated with high intakes of vitamin B_6 from food sources only. When toxicity occurs, it causes a severe sensory neuropathy, leaving patients unable to walk. Some cases of photosensitivity and dermatitis have also been reported.

> Vitamin B_6 supplements should not be taken by Parkinson's disease patients being treated with L-dopa as vitamin B_6 can diminish the effects of dopa in the brain.

Biotin

Biotin, also called vitamin B_7.

Structure

Biotin is an imidazole derivative **(Figure 9.11)**. It consists of a **tetrahydrothiophene** ring bound to an imidazole ring and a **valeric acid** side chain.

Sources

- It is widely distributed in foods.
- Liver, kidneys, vegetables, soy protein, beans, yeast, and egg yolk are the important sources of biotin.
- Biotin is also synthesized by intestinal bacteria.

Absorption, Transport, and Metabolism

- Biotin is widely distributed in many foods as biocytin (ε-amino-biotinyl lysine), which is released on proteolysis which is absorbed readily.
- Biotin is cleared from the circulating blood and taken up by liver and muscle.
- Because it is synthesized by intestinal flora in excess of requirements, urinary excretion of biotin often exceeds dietary intake with fecal excretion as much as three to six times greater than dietary intake.

Active/Coenzyme Form of Biotin

Enzyme-bound biotin, **biocytin** is an active form of biotin. Biotin is covalently bound to ε-amino group of lysine of an enzyme to form **biocytin**.

Functions

- Biotin is a coenzyme of carboxylase reactions, where it is a carrier of CO_2. The carboxylation reactions requiring biotin are given here.
  - Conversion of acetyl-CoA into malonyl-CoA catalyzed by **acetyl-CoA carboxylase** in fatty acid synthesis (*see* **Figure 11.32**).
  - Conversion of pyruvate into oxaloacetate, catalyzed by **pyruvate carboxylase** in gluconeogenesis (*see* **Figure 10.24**).

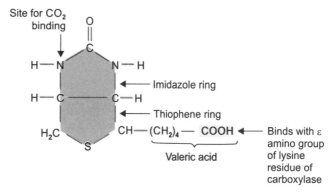

Figure 9.11: Structure of biotin.

- Conversion of propionyl-CoA to D-methyl malonyl-CoA catalyzed by propionyl-CoA carboxylase in the pathway of conversion of propionate to succinate (**see Figure 11.22**).
- It is also involved in the catabolism of branched chain amino acid catalyzed by β-**methyl-crotonyl-CoA carboxylase** (*see* Figure 12.24).

- Biotin also has a role in regulation of the **cell cycle**, acting to **biotinylate** key nuclear proteins.

Biotin Independent Carboxylation Reaction

There are few carboxylation reactions which do not require biotin. For example:

❖ Formation of carbamoyl phosphate by **carbamoyl phosphate synthetase** in urea cycle.

❖ Addition of CO_2 to form C_6 in purine ring.

❖ Conversion of pyruvate to malate by malic enzyme.

Nutritional Requirements

A daily intake of about **150 to 300 µg** is recommended for adults. Biotin is synthesized by intestinal microorganisms in such a large quantity that a dietary source is probably not necessary.

Deficiency Manifestation

- Since biotin is widely distributed in plant and animal foods and intestinal bacterial flora supply adequate amounts of biotin. Biotin deficiency due to low dietary intake is rare. Deficiency of biotin occurs in:
  - The people with the unusual dietary habit of consuming large amounts of uncooked eggs. Egg white contains the **glycoprotein avidin**, which binds the imidazole group of biotin and prevents biotin absorption.
  - Use of antibiotics, that inhibit the growth of intestinal bacteria, eliminates this source of biotin and leads to deficiency of biotin.
- The experimentally induced symptoms of biotin deficiency are:
  - In the adult, biotin deficiency results in mental changes (depression, hallucinations), paresthesia, anorexia, and nausea.

- A scaling, seborrheic, and erythematous rash may occur around the eyes, nose, and mouth as well as on the extremities.
- In infants, biotin deficiency presents as hypotonia, lethargy, and apathy.
- In addition, the infant may develop alopecia and a characteristic rash that includes the ears.

Antimetabolites

Egg white contains the protein **avidin**, which strongly binds the vitamin and reduces its bioavailability.

Folic Acid (Vitamin B$_9$)

The word folate is related to folium which means leaf in Latin. The term "folate" includes all naturally occurring as well as synthetic compounds of folic acid

Structure

Folic acid consists of three components, **pteridine ring**, **p-amino benzoic acid (PABA)**, and **L-glutamic acid (Figure 9.12)**. In a folic acid molecule, the number of glutamic acid residues varies from one to seven. Folic acid usually has one glutamic acid residue.

Source

- Folates occur in most foods; high amounts are present in liver, kidney, green leafy vegetables like spinach and cabbage, yeast, nuts and fruits.
- Milk and eggs are poor in folate.
- It is easily destroyed by cooking, particularly if large volumes of water and high temperature are used.
- Vitamin C protects it from oxidative destruction.
- Although some folate is synthesized by bacteria in the large intestine, it is not available to the body.

Absorption, Transport, and Metabolism

- Folate is found mainly in green vegetables, liver and whole grains. Ninety percent of food folates are polyglutamates and 10% are monoglutamates. Polyglutamate forms of folate present in food are first converted to monoglutamates by glutamyl hydrolase in the intestinal mucosa.

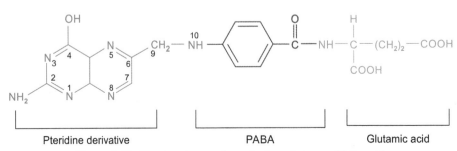

Figure 9.12: The structure and numbering of atoms of folic acid.

- During absorption, monoglutamates are converted to methyl tetrahydrofolate and enters the circulation as N5-methyl-tetrahydrofolate (N5-THF).
- In blood, folate is transported as methyl tetrahydrofolate bound to protein.
- Serum folate binding capacity increases in individuals with leukemia, acute hepatitis, cirrhosis and uremia and in pregnant women.

Active/Coenzyme form of Folic Acid

Tetrahydrofolate (THF) is the active form of folic acid. Folate is enzymatically reduced in a two stage process in tissues to yield the dihydro and then tetrahydrofolate, which requires vitamin C **(Figure 9.13)**.

Functions

- THF acts as a carrier of **one carbon units** (*see* **Figure 12.44**). The one carbon units are:
  - Methyl CH_3
  - Methylene CH_2

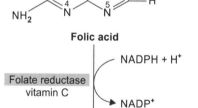

Folic acid

Folate reductase
vitamin C

Dihydrofolate (DHF)

Folate reductase
vitamin C

Tetrahydrofolate (THF)

Figure 9.13: Formation of tetrahydrofolate from folic acid.

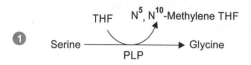

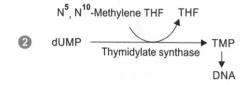

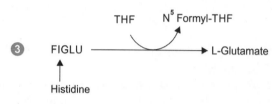

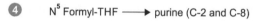

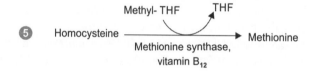

Figure 9.14: Role of vitamin folic acid as THF in one carbon metabolism.

(dUMP: deoxyuridine monophosphate; FIGLU: formimino glutamate; PLP: pyridoxal phosphate; THF: tetrahydrofolate; TMP: thymidine monophosphate)

- Methenyl   CH
- Formyl   CHO
- Formimino   CH = NH
- The THF coenzymes serve as acceptors or donors of one carbon units in a variety of reactions involved in amino acid and nucleic acid metabolism. One carbon unit binds to THF through N5 or N10 or both N5, N10 position. Five of the major reactions in which THF is involved are given here **(Figure 9.14)**.

1. **Conversion of serine to glycine:** The conversion of serine to glycine is accompanied by the formation of N5, N10-methylene THF.

2. **Synthesis of thymidylate (pyrimidine nucleotide):** The enzyme **thymidylate synthase** that converts deoxyuridylate (dUMP) into thymidylate (TMP) uses N5, N10-methylene THF as the methyl donor for this reaction. Thus, folate coenzyme plays a central role in the biosynthesis of **nucleic acids**.

3. **Catabolism of histidine:** Histidine in the course of its catabolism is converted into **formiminoglutamate (FIGLU)**. This molecule can donate the formimino group to THF to produce N5-formimino THF. In case of folic acid deficiency, FIGLU accumulates and is excreted in urine.

4. **Synthesis of purine:** N5-Formyl THF intermediate formed in histidine catabolism is used in the biosyn-

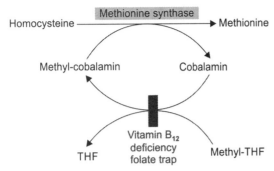

Figure 9.15: Combined role of vitamin B_{12} and folic acid and folate trap.

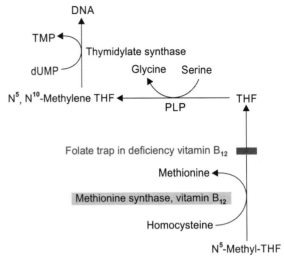

Figure 9.16: Role of folic acid and vitamin B_{12} in the synthesis of DNA.

thesis of purine and therefore in the formation of both DNA and RNA.

5. **Synthesis of methionine from homocysteine:** Homocysteine is converted to methionine in presence of N^5-methyl THF, and vitamin B_{12}. In this reaction the methyl group bound to cobalamin (Vitamin B_{12}) is transferred to homocysteine to form methionine and the cobalamin then removes the methyl group from N^5-methyl THF to form THF **(Figure 9.15)**. This step is essential for the liberation of free THF and for its repeated use in one carbon metabolism.

In B_{12} deficiency, conversion of N^5-methyl THF to free THF is blocked. Thus, most of THF of the body is irreversibly "trapped" as its methyl derivative (N^5-methyl THF), which leads to the deficiency of free THF although the tissue folate levels are adequate or high.

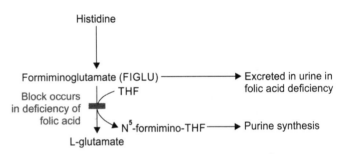

Figure 9.17: Excretion of **FIGLU** in folic acid deficiency.

Vitamin B_{12} Deficiency causes Functional Folate Deficiency: The Folate Trap

❖ Methylation of homocysteine to methionine depends on vitamin B_{12} and N^5-methyl THF. When vitamin B_{12} is deficient N^5-methyl THF cannot be converted to free THF. Thus, most of THF of the body is irreversibly "trapped" as its methyl derivative (N^5-methyl THF), which leads to the deficiency of free THF **(Figure 9.15)**.

❖ Folate trap creates folate deficiency and an adequate supply of free THF is not available for the synthesis of purine and pyrimidine bases. Thus, a B_{12} deficiency can lead to a folate deficiency. Although the tissue folate levels are adequate or high, there is a functional folate deficiency due to the lack of THF.

Nutritional Requirements

The minimum daily requirement is 100 to 200 µg for adults, but may be increased several-fold during periods of increased metabolic demands such as pregnancy.

Deficiency Manifestations

Folate deficiency frequently occurs particularly in pregnant women and in alcoholics. Clinical symptoms of folic acid deficiency include:

- **Megaloblastic or macrocytic anemia:** The deficiency of folic acid leads to impairment of synthesis of DNA **(Figure 9.16)**. Impaired DNA synthesis impairs the

maturation of erythrocytes. Consequently, megaloblasts are formed instead of normoblast. These megaloblasts are accumulated in the bone marrow which is destroyed by spleen resulting in anemia.

- **Accumulation and excretion of FIGLU in the urine:** Folate deficiency blocks the last step of histidine catabolism, due to lack of THF. This results in accumulation of FIGLU in body, which leads to increased excretion of FIGLU in urine **(Figure 9.17)**.

- **Hyperhomocysteinemia:** Due to folic acid deficiency the methylation of homocysteine to methionine is impaired which leads to accumulation of homocysteine (hyperhomocysteinemia). Increased level of homocysteine is a risk factor for cardiovascular disease.

- **Neural tube defect in fetus:** Since, folate is required for the formation of **neural tube** in early stage of gestation; the folate deficiency during early stage of pregnancy increases the risk of neural tube defect. Folic acid deficiency promotes birth defects such as spina bifida (improper closure of the neural tube). Spina bifida is characterized by the incomplete or incorrect formation of the neural tube early in development (3 to 4 weeks after conception).

- When folic acid deficiency is severe, it leads to **heart disease**, **cancer**, and some types of **brain dysfunction**.

Folic acid deficiency leads to reduction of thymidylate synthesis (*see* **Figure 9.16**). Reduction of thymidylate synthesis causes abnormal incorporation of uracil into DNA. Uracil is recognized by DNA repair pathways and is cleaved from the DNA. The presence of high levels of uracil in DNA leads to strand breaks that can greatly affect the function and regulation of nuclear DNA; ultimately causing impaired function of the heart and brain, as well as increased mutagenesis that leads to cancer.

Therapeutic Uses

Folic acid supplements reduce the risk of **neural tube defects** and **hyperhomocysteinemia**, and may reduce the incidence of **cardiovascular disease** and some **cancers**.

Cobalamin (Vitamin B₁₂)

The term "vitamin B_{12}" is used as generic descriptor for the **cobalamins**; cobalt containing compounds.

Structure

Vitamin B_{12} bears a complex **corrin ring** (containing pyrrole similar to porphyrin), linked to a **cobalt atom** held in the center of the corrin ring, by four coordination bonds with the nitrogen of the pyrrole groups. The remaining coordination bonds of the cobalt are linked with the nitrogen of **dimethylbenzimidazole nucleotide** and sixth bond is linked to either **methyl** or **5′-deoxyadenosyl** or **hydroxy** group to form **methylcobalamin**, **adenosylcobalamin** or **hydroxycobalamin** respectively (**Figure 9.18**). Thus, cobalamin exists in three forms that differ in the nature of the chemical group attached to cobalt. **Cynocobalamin is the commercial available form of vitamin B_{12}**.

Active/Coenzyme Form of Vitamin B₁₂

- The two active forms of vitamin B_{12} coenzymes are:
  - **5-deoxyadenosylcobalamin** (the major intracellular form) and
  - **Methylcobalamin** (the predominant form in plasma, the transport form), occur in normal human tissues. Both are unstable in light.
- The commercially available stable forms of vitamin B_{12} are **cyanocobalamin** and **hydroxycobalamin**. The latter binds more tightly to plasma proteins and is retained in the body about three times better; hence it is used therapeutically.

Sources

- Vitamin B_{12} is exclusively present in foods of animal origin.
- Meat, liver, eggs, dairy products, and yeast contain adequate amounts of the vitamin.
- Vegetable sources do not contain vitamin B_{12}; therefore, vegans (persons who do not take any form of animal foods or dairy products) suffer from B_{12} deficiency.

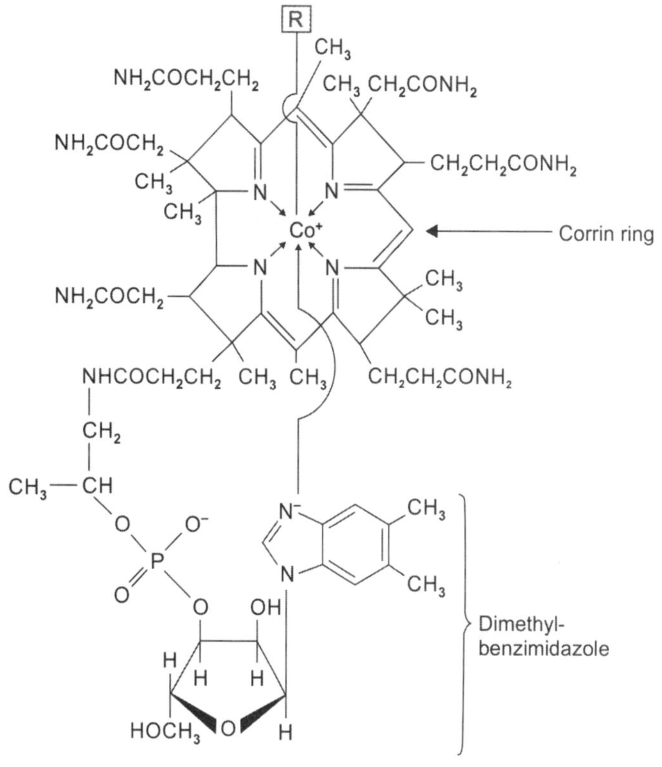

Figure 9.18: Structure of cobalamin (vitamin B_{12}).
(R: either methyl or deoxyadenosyl or hydroxy group)

- Vitamin B_{12} is synthesized in human colon by normal bacterial flora but it is not absorbed. Therefore, man is dependent on dietary sources for vitamin B_{12}.

Absorption, Transport, and Storage

- The intestinal absorption of vitamin B_{12} requires an **intrinsic factor (IF)**, a glycoprotein secreted by parietal cells of the stomach. In stomach IF binds the dietary vitamin B_{12} to form **vitamin B_{12}-IF complex**. This complex binds to specific receptors on the surface of the mucosal cells of the ileum. After binding to the receptor, the bound vitamin B_{12} is released from the complex and enters the illeal mucosal cells through a Ca^{2+} dependent process.
- The vitamin in mucosal cell is converted into its main plasma transport form to **methylcobalamin**. It is then transported by a vitamin B_{12} binding protein known as **transcobalamin** (TC-I and TC-II). Methylcobalamin which is in excess is taken up by the liver, **stored in deoxyadenosyl B_{12}** form. Vitamin B_{12} is the only water soluble vitamin that is stored in significant amounts in the liver.

Functions

- Vitamin B_{12} plays a vital role in the **synthesis of DNA** in every biological cell. It is particularly necessary for normal **haemopoiesis** and for the maintenance of **integrity of the nervous system**.

- Further, it helps in preventing (folate trap) deficiency of functional folate and helps in adequate supply of free THF for synthesis of purine and pyrimidine bases.
- In human, the enzyme systems that are known, to require vitamin B_{12} coenzyme are:
  - *Isomerization of methylmalonyl CoA to succinyl CoA:* Propionyl CoA is produced as catabolic end product of some aliphatic amino acids and in β-oxidation of odd chain fatty acids. The propionyl CoA is then converted to succinyl CoA. During conversion of propionyl-CoA to succinyl-CoA vitamin B_{12} coenzyme, deoxyadenosyl cobalamin is required for the isomerization of L-methylmalonyl CoA to succinyl CoA. In vitamin B_{12} deficiency methylmalonyl CoA accumulates and is excreted in urine as methylmalonic acid **(Figure 9.19)**.
  - *Conversion of homocysteine to methionine:* Methylcobalamin is a coenzyme in the conversion of homocysteine to methionine, which joins the metabolic roles of vitamin B_{12} and those of folic acid (*see* **Figure 9.15**). This is the only mammalian reaction known to require both vitamins.

Nutritional Requirements

The daily requirement of vitamin B_{12} is 2–3 µg for an adult with higher allowances for pregnancy and lactating women.

Deficiency Manifestations

Deficiency of vitamin B_{12} is seen in:
- Inadequate intake of cobalamin and folate in the diet.
- Impaired absorption of the vitamin by the small intestines (malabsorption).
- Increased demands as in pregnant women, women who are breastfeeding.
- Strict vegetarians, since the vitamin found only in foods of animal origin or in microorganisms.

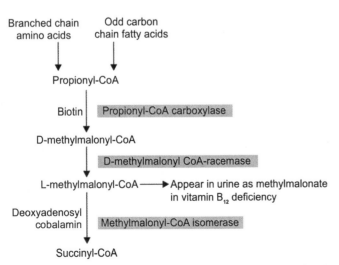

Figure 9.19: Role of vitamin B_{12} in isomerization of methylmalonyl CoA to succinyl CoA.

- Pernicious anemia due to lack of intrinsic factor, a protein that binds with cobalamin and aids in its absorption by the small intestines. Without enough intrinsic factor, the body cannot absorb enough cobalamin.

Deficiency of vitamin B_{12} leads to:
- Megaloblastic anemia
- Methylmalonic aciduria
- Subacute combined degeneration (SCD)

Megaloblastic Anemia

- Megaloblastic anemia is a condition in which the bone marrow produces unusually large, structurally abnormal, immature nucleated red blood cells (megaloblasts).
- Megaloblastic anemia has several different causes. Deficiencies of either cobalamin (vitamin B_{12}) or folate (vitamin B_9) are the two most common causes. These vitamins play an essential role in the production of red blood cells. This condition is due to impaired DNA synthesis, which inhibits nuclear division.
- In most cases, megaloblastic anemia develops slowly and affected individuals may remain asymptomatic for many years. Symptoms common to anemia usually develop at some point and may include fatigue, paleness of the skin, shortness of breath, dizziness, muscle weakness and a fast or irregular heartbeat.
- Megaloblastic anemia resulting from cobalamin deficiency may also be associated with **neurological symptoms**. The initial neurological symptom may be **tingling or numbness** in the hands or feet. In vitamin B_{12} deficiency neurological symptoms are due to degeneration of **myelinated nerves**.
- Additional symptoms develop over time including balance problems, vision loss due to degeneration (atrophy) of the nerve that transmits impulses from the retina to the brain (optic nerve), and mental confusion or memory loss.
- A variety of psychiatric abnormalities has also been reported in individuals with cobalamin deficiency including depression, insomnia, lethargy, and panic attacks.

Methylmalonic Aciduria

- Methylmalonic acidemia is a disorder of amino acid metabolism, involving a defect in the conversion of **methylmalonyl-CoA to succinyl-CoA.**
- Because vitamin B_{12} is necessary for the conversion of methylmalonic acid to succinic acid, individuals deficient in vitamin B_{12} excrete excess amounts of methylmalonic acid in the urine **(Figure 9.19)**.
- Symptoms include vomiting, dehydration, tachypnea (abnormally rapid breathing), lethargy, failure to thrive, developmental delay, hypotonia (abnormally low level of muscle tone) and encephalopathy (impaired brain function).

Subacute Combined Degeneration (SCD)

- Subacute combined degeneration is a degenerative disease of the **central** and **peripheral nervous system** that is caused by vitamin B$_{12}$ deficiency. SCD predominantly involves the spinal cord and peripheral nerves.
- In vitamin B$_{12}$ deficiency neurological symptoms are due to degeneration of **myelinated nerves**.
- Degeneration of myelinated nerves is due to accumulation of L-methylmalonyl-CoA, which impairs the myelin sheath formation.
- The neurological symptoms include numbness and tingling of fingers and toes, mental confusion, poor muscular coordination and dementia and spasticity, and paralysis.

Vitamin C (Ascorbic Acid)

Vitamin C is also called ascorbic acid.

Structure

Ascorbic acid (vitamin C) **(Figure 9.20)** is one of the essential substances, which cannot be synthesized in the body and must be supplied by the diet. It cannot be stored well within the body. It is water-soluble, rapidly destroyed by exposure to air, heat, and processing.

Active Form of Ascorbic Acid

Both ascorbic acid and dehydroascorbic acid have vitamin activity.

Sources

- The main dietary sources of vitamin C are green leafy vegetables and fruits, especially citrus fruits, strawberries, tomatoes, spinach, and potatoes.
- Cereals contain no vitamin C.
- Animal tissues and dairy products are very poor sources.

Absorption, Transport, and Metabolism

- Absorption of vitamin C occurs readily from the stomach, where some of the ascorbic acid is converted to the dehydro form.

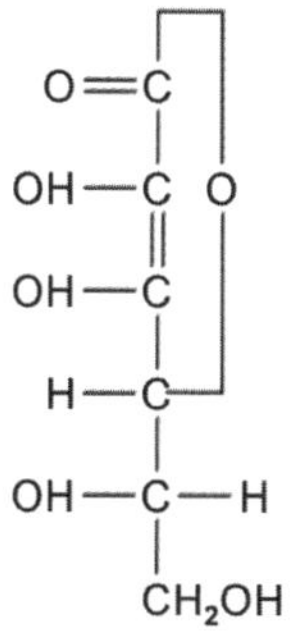

L-ascorbic acid

Figure 9.20: Structure of ascorbic acid.

- Vitamin C is found in highest concentrations in the adrenals, the pituitary, and the retina than in plasma.
- The half-life for vitamin C in the human is approximately 16 days. In addition to the presence of ascorbate and dehydroascorbic acid, lesser amounts of a number of catabolites also are excreted in urine.

Functions

- Ascorbic acid is essential for the normal health of **connective tissues**. Vitamin C is involved in **collagen biosynthesis**. Ascorbic acid is necessary for the **hydroxylation of proline** (by proline hydroxylase) and **lysine** (by lysine hydroxylase) of collagen. Hydroxyproline and hydroxylysine are essential for the collagen cross-linking and collagen strength and stability.
- Since vitamin C is required for collagen formation, vitamin C is also involved in **bone** and **dentin formation** as well as **wound healing process**. The deficient formation of collagen results in delayed wound healing and changes in the growth of bones in infants and children.
- The error in formation of collagen makes the small blood vessels more susceptible to even minor trauma and probably is the cause of bleeding.
- Proline hydroxylases is also required in the formation of **osteocalcin** and the **C1q** a complement protein of the innate immune system. C1q is rich in hydroxyproline.
- **Dopamine β-hydroxylase** is a **copper containing** enzyme involved in the synthesis of the **catecholamines (norepinephrine and epinephrine)** from tyrosine in the adrenal medulla and central nervous system. During hydroxylation ascorbate is required for the reduction of Cu^{2+} to Cu$^+$. In its absence, the metabolism of tyrosine is disturbed and the metabolites appear in the urine.
- Ascorbic acid helps in the transformation of **folic acid** to its active form **tetrahydrofolate**. Its deficiency may contribute to **macrocytic anemia**.
- Ascorbic acid stimulates iron absorption by keeping iron in reduced state, more soluble ferrous form.
- **Ascorbic acid is a water soluble antioxidant**
  - It reduces oxidized vitamin E (tocopherol) to regenerate functional vitamin E.
  - Vitamin C, thought to be involved in the prevention of atherosclerosis and coronary heart disease by preventing oxidation of LDL.
  - Antioxidant property of vitamin C is also associated with prevention of cancer by inhibiting nitrosamine formation from naturally occurring nitrates during digestion.

Nutritional Requirements

- The recommended daily allowance is about **60 to 70 mg.**

- Additional intakes are recommended for women during pregnancy and lactation.
- Cigarette smoking can increase ascorbic acid turn over due to free radical scavenging by the vitamin C.

Deficiency Manifestation

- Deficiency has been observed in infants receiving unsupplemented cow's milk and in infants receiving breast milk from deficient mother.
- Deficiency occurs most commonly in the elderly, especially those who do not eat fresh fruits and vegetables and who tend to cook in frying pans, the combination of heat and large area of food in contact with air irreversibly oxidizes the vitamin and loses its biological activity.
- Deficiency also can occur in iron overload.
- Deficiency of ascorbic acid causes **scurvy**.

Scurvy

- Vitamin C is required for formation of collagen, where it is needed for the hydroxylation of **proline** and **lysine** residues of collagen. Hydroxyproline and hydroxylysine are essential for the collagen cross-linking and collagen strength and stability. Since vitamin C is required for normal collagen formation, vitamin C is also involved in bone and dentin formation as well as wound healing process.
- Symptoms of scurvy are related to **deficient collagen formation**. These include:
  - Fragility of vascular walls causing bleeding tendency, muscle weakness, soft spongy, swollen bleeding gums, loosening of teeth **(Figure 9.21)**.
  - Abnormal bone development and osteoporosis. In children bone formation is impaired.
  - Poor wound healing.
  - Anemia due to impaired erythropoiesis.
  - Milder forms of vitamin C deficiency are more common and manifestations of such include **easy bruising (contusion) (Figure 9.21)** and **formation of**

petechiae (small hemorrhages under the skin), both due to **increased capillary fragility**.

- Laboratory diagnosis of vitamin C deficiency is made on the basis of low plasma or leukocyte levels.

Therapeutic Uses

Use of vitamin C in preventing cold and cancers has not been scientifically supported. Although the incidence of common cold is not reduced by vitamin C, the duration of cold episodes and severity of symptoms can be decreased. Vitamin C may act by reacting with free radicals.

Toxicity

- Taking more than 2 g of vitamin C in a single dose cannot be absorbed from the intestine and can cause in abdominal pain, diarrhea, and nausea and deposition of oxalate stones in kidneys (as vitamin C may be metabolized to oxalate).
- High doses of vitamin C can induce hemolysis in patients with glucose-6-phosphate dehydrogenase deficiency, and doses more than 1 g/day can cause interfere with tests for urinary glucose.
- High doses may interfere with certain drugs.

FAT SOLUBLE VITAMINS: STRUCTURE, METABOLISM, ACTIVE/COENZYME FORM, SOURCES, BIOCHEMICAL FUNCTIONS, NUTRITIONAL REQUIREMENT AND DEFICIENCY MANIFESTATIONS AND TOXICITY OF EXCESSIVE INTAKES

Vitamin A

Structure

Vitamin A contains a single 6-membered ring to which is attached an 11-carbon side chain **(Figure 9.22)**. Vitamin A is an **alcohol (retinol)**, but can be converted into an **aldehyde (retinal)**, or an **acid (retinoic acid)**.

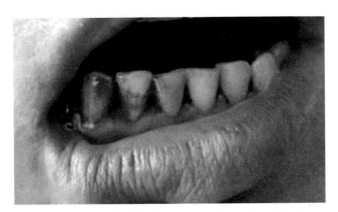

Soft spongy, swollen bleeding gums, and loosening of teeth

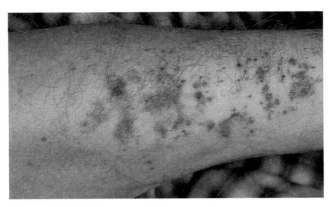

Skin bruising and formation of petechiae

Figure 9.21: Clinical manifestations of vitamin C deficiency, scurvy.

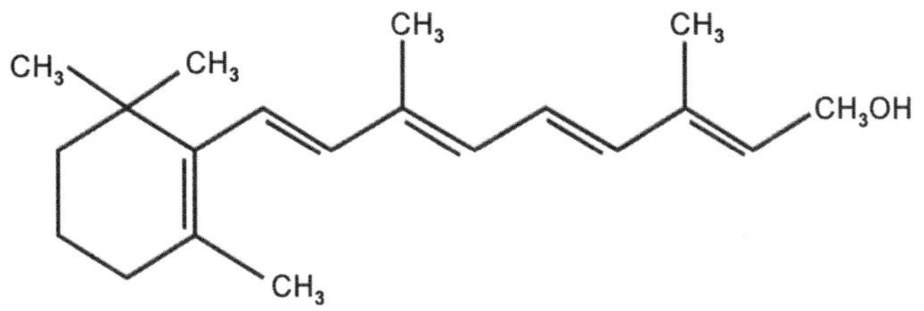

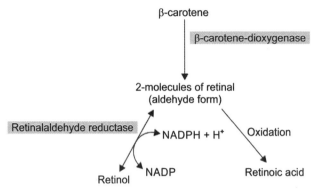

Figure 9.22: Structure of vitamin A, retinol.

β-carotene

β-carotene-dioxygenase

2-molecules of retinal
(aldehyde form)

Retinalaldehyde reductase

NADPH + H⁺   Oxidation

Retinol   NADP   Retinoic acid

Figure 9.23: Conversion of β-carotene (provitamin) to biologically active forms of vitamin A.

Active Form

Vitamin A consists of three biologically active molecules which are collectively known as **retinoids**.

1. **Retinol:** Primary alcohol (CH_2OH) containing form
2. **Retinal:** Aldehyde (CHO) containing form
3. **Retinoic acid:** Carboxyl (COOH) containing form

Each of these compounds is derived from the plant precursor molecule, β-**carotene** (a member of a family of molecules known as carotenoids). β-carotene which consists of two molecules of retinal linked at their aldehyde ends is also referred to as the **provitamin** form of vitamin A. The retinol and retinal are interconverted by enzyme **retinal aldehyde reductase**. The retinoic acid is formed by oxidation of retinal. The retinoic acid cannot be reduced to either retinol or retinal **(Figure 9.23)**.

Absorption, Transport, and Storage

Ingested β-carotene is cleaved in the intestine by β-**carotene dioxygenase** to yield retinal. Retinal is reduced to retinol by **retinaldehyde reductase**, an NADPH requiring enzyme within the intestine **(Figure 9.23)**.

- Retinol is esterified with palmitic acid incorporated into chylomicrons together with dietary lipid and delivered to the liver for storage.
- Transport of retinol from the liver to extrahepatic tissues, occurs by binding of retinol to retinol binding protein (RBP).
- Transport of retinoic acid is accomplished by binding to albumin.

Dietary Sources

- Vitamin A is widely distributed in animal foods, as preformed vitamin A (retinol) and in plant foods as provitamin, carotenes. Moderate cooking of vegetables enhances carotenoid release for uptake in the gut.
- Liver, fish, and eggs are excellent food sources for preformed vitamin A.
- Vegetable sources of provitamin A carotenoids include dark green and yellow and red fruits (melon, papaya, apricot, and mango) and vegetables, such as carrots, tomatoes, and peaches.

Functions of Vitamin A

- Vitamin A is required for a variety of functions such as, for normal vision, **cell differentiation** and **growth**, **mucus secretion**, and **maintenance of epithelial cells**. Vitamin A also plays a role to enhance immune functions and to protect against infections and probably some cancers
- Different forms of the vitamin have different functions.
  - Retinal and retinol are involved in vision.
  - Retinoic acid is involved in normal morphogenesis, growth, and cell differentiation and metabolic processes. Retinoic acid does not function in vision
  - β-carotene is involved in antioxidant function.

Role of Vitamin A in Vision

The role of vitamin A in vision has been known through the studies of **G Wald**, who received the Nobel Prize in 1943 for this work. The cyclic events occur in the process of vision, known as **rhodopsin cycle** or **Wald's visual cycle** **(Figure 9.24)**. Both rod and cone cells of retina contain photochemicals; **Rhodopsin** or **visual purple** in their membrane. **Rhodopsin** or **visual purple**, of rod cells in the retina consists of **11-cis-retinal** bound to protein **opsin**.

- When rhodopsin absorbs light, the 11-cis-retinal is converted to all-transretinal.
- The isomerization is associated with a conformational change in the protein opsin.

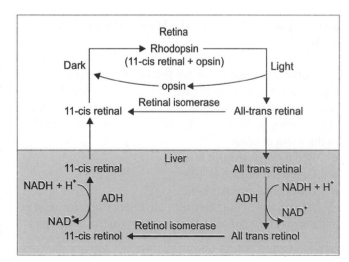

Figure 9.24: Wald's visual cycle in rod cells of retina, involving the pigment rhodopsin (visual purple). Similar cycle is found in cone cells of retina, utilizing color sensitive pigments porphyropsin (red), iodopsin (green) and cyanopsin (blue) and resulting in color vision.

- Conformational changes in opsin generate a nerve impulse that is transmitted by the optic nerve to the brain.
- This is followed by dissociation of the all-transretinal from opsin.
- The all-transretinal is immediately isomerized by retinal isomerase to 11-cis-retinal.
- This combines with opsin to regenerate rhodopsin and complete the visual cycle.

The conversion of all-trans retinal to 11-cis-retinal is incomplete and therefore remaining all-trans retinal which is not converted to 11-cis-retinal is converted to all-trans retinol by **alcohol dehydrogenase** and is stored in the liver. When needed, retinol re-enters the circulation and is taken up by the retina, where it is converted back to 11-cis-retinal which combines with opsin again to form rhodopsin **(Figure 9.24)**.

Dark adaptation time: In ocular physiology, **adaptation** is the ability of the eye to adjust to various levels of light. When a person enters from bright light to dark there is difficulty in seeing due to depletion of rhodopsin, but after few minutes the vision improves. During these few minutes, rhodopsin is resynthesized, and vision is improved.

The time taken for regeneration of rhodopsin is known as **dark adaptation time**. This adaptation period depends on the regeneration of photopigments to restore retinal sensitivity. Dark adaptation time is increased in vitamin A deficient individuals.

Color Vision

While vision in dim light is mediated by rhodopsin of the rod cells, color vision is mediated by three different retinal containing pigments in the cone cells, the three pigments are called **porphyropsin**, **iodopsin**, and **cyanopsin**. Porphyropsin, iodopsin and cyanopsin are sensitive to the three essential colors: **red**, **green**, and **blue** respectively. All these pigments consist of **11-cis-retinal** bound to protein **opsin**.

Thus, when light strikes the retina, it bleaches one or more of these pigments, depending on the color quality of the light. The pigments are converted to all-transretinal, and the protein moiety opsin is released as in the case of rhodopsin. This reaction gives rise to the nerve impulse that is read out in the brain as color:

- Red if porphyropsin is split
- Green if iodopsin is split
- Blue if cyanopsin is split.

If mixtures of the three are converted, the color read out in the brain depends on the proportions of the three split.

Cellular Differentiation and Metabolic Effect

Retinoic acid is an important regulator of **gene expression** especially during growth and development. Retinoic acid is essential for normal gene expression during embryonic development such as cell differentiation in spermatogenesis and in the differentiation of epithelial cells. Retinoic acids exert a number of metabolic effects on tissues. These include:

- Control of biosynthesis of membrane **glycoproteins** and **glycosaminoglycans** (mucopolysaccharide) necessary for mucus secretion. The normal mucus secretion maintains the epithelial surface moist and prevents keratinization of epithelial cell.
- Control of biosynthesis of **cholesterol**.

Antioxidant Function

β-carotene (provitamin A) is an antioxidant and may play a role in trapping peroxy free radicals in tissues. The antioxidant property of lipid soluble vitamin A may account for its possible anticancer activity. High levels of dietary carotenoids have been associated with a decreased risk of cardiovascular disease.

Nutritional Requirements

The retinol activity equivalent (RAE) is used to express the vitamin A value of food. 1 retinol activity equivalent = 1 mg retinol = 12 mg β-carotene. The recommended daily intake of retinol equivalent (RAE) is:

- 800–1000 µg for adults,
- 1200 µg for pregnant and lactating women, and
- 300 to 600 µg for children.

Deficiency Manifestation

Vitamin A is stored in the liver and deficiency of the vitamin occurs only after prolonged lack of dietary intake. Clinically, degenerative changes in **eyes** and **skin** are observed commonly in individuals with vitamin A deficiency. Vitamin deficiency may be **primary** (dietary insufficiency) or **secondary**. Vitamin A deficiency can be prevented by adequate intake of animal fats and dark-green leafy vegetables. The causes of secondary deficiency may include:

- Impaired absorption of lipids, as in celiac disease, tropical sprue, gastrectomy or obstructive jaundice.
- Failure to synthesize apo B-48 and therefore inability to form chylomicrons into which vitamin A is normally incorporated after absorption.
- Lack of lipase, as in pancreatitis.
- Failure in converting β-carotene to retinol; because of an enzyme defect.
- Impaired storage in hepatic cell in liver disease.
- Failure to synthesize retinol binding proteins, thus affecting transport to target tissues.

Effect on Vision

The earliest symptoms of vitamin A deficiency is:

- Impaired dark adaptation or night blindness (nyctalopia)

- Poor vision in dim light
- Xerophthalmia.

Night Blindness (Nyctalopia)

- Night blindness is one of the earliest symptoms of vitamin A deficiency. This is characterized by loss of vision in night (in dim or poor light) since **dark adaptation time** is increased. Prolonged deficiency of vitamin A leads to an irreversible loss of visual cells. Severe vitamin A deficiency causes dryness of cornea and conjunctiva, a clinical condition termed as **xerophthalmia** (dry eyes).
- If this situation prolongs, **keratinization** and **ulceration** of cornea takes place. This result in destruction of cornea, in which the cornea becomes soft and milky (opaque) in appearance due to ulceration and necrosis of the cornea finally resulting in permanent loss of vision (blindness), a clinical condition termed as **keratomalacia (Figure 9.25)**. Xerophthalmia and keratomalacia are commonly observed in children.
- Later white opaque spots (plaques) developed due to xerophthalmia on either side of cornea are known as **Bitot's spot (Figure 9.25)**. Bitot's spot are consisting of layers of keratinized epithelial cells resulting from deficiency of mucous secretion due to vitamin A deficiency.

> Rods are **responsible for vision at low light levels**. They do not mediate color vision. Cones are active at higher light levels are capable of color vision.

Effect on Skin and Epithelial Cells

Vitamin A deficiency causes keratinization of epithelial cells of skin which leads to **keratosis** of hair follicles, and dry, rough and scaly skin. **Keratinization of epithelial cells** of respiratory, urinary tract makes them susceptible to infections.

Other Symptoms of Vitamin A Deficiency

- Failure of growth in children.
- Faulty bone modeling producing thick cancellous (spongy) bones instead of thinner and more compact ones.
- Abnormalities of reproduction, including degeneration of the testes, abortion or the production of malformed offspring.
- Increased pressure of cerebrospinal fluid, independent or associated with deformity in skull bones.
- Abnormalities of reproduction, including degeneration of the testes, abortion or the production of malformed offspring.
- Certain forms of skin disease.

> Because maternal hepatic accumulation of vitamin A in fetus occurs during the last trimester of pregnancy, preterm infants are relatively deficient in vitamin A at birth. Therefore provision of a daily oral intake of vitamin A that meets the RDA of 375 retinol equivalent (RE) is important. Infants with birth weights of less than 1500 g (those less than 30 weeks gestation) have virtually no hepatic vitamin A stores and are at risk for vitamin A deficiency.

Therapeutic Use of Vitamin A

The use of **retinoic acid** preparations, in the treatment of **psoriasis**, **acne** and several other **skin diseases**, is related to its involvement with epithelial cell differentiation and integrity. Some precancerous lesions seem to respond to treatment with carotenoids.

Hypervitaminosis A (Toxicity of Excessive Intake of the Vitamin A)

There is only limited capacity to metabolize vitamin A, and excessive intakes lead to accumulation beyond the capacity of intracellular binding proteins. Unbound vitamin A causes membrane lysis and tissue damage. Symptoms of toxicity affect:

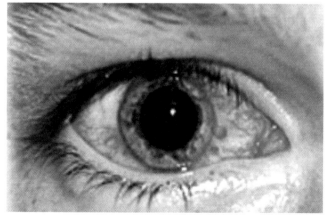

Xerophthalmia and keratinization

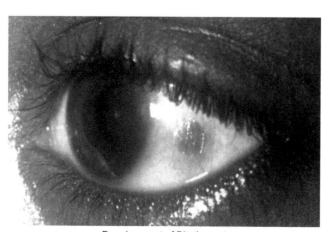

Development of Bitot's spot

Figure 9.25: Clinical manifestations of vitamin A deficiency.

- The central nervous system and leads to headache, nausea, ataxia, and anorexia. These all associated with increased cerebrospinal fluid pressure.
- **The liver:** Hepatomegaly with histological changes and hyperlipidemia
- **Calcium homeostasis:** Thickening of the long bones, hypercalcemia, and calcification of soft tissues, bone, and joint pain
- **The skin:** Loss of hair (alopecia), scaly and rough skin.
- In pregnant women, the hypervitaminosis A may cause congenital malformation in growing fetus (teratogenic effect).
- The excess intake of carotenoids is not toxic like vitamin A.

Why Vitamin A is Considered as a Hormone?
Within cells both retinol and retinoic acid function by binding to specific receptor proteins present in the nucleus of target tissues like other endocrine hormones. Following binding, the **receptor-vitamin complex** interacts with several genes involved in growth and differentiation and affects expression of these genes. In this capacity, retinol and retinoic acid are considered as hormones.

Vitamin D (Cholecalciferol)

Vitamin D is also known as **calciferol** because of its role in calcium metabolism and **antirachitic factor** because it prevents rickets.

Why Vitamin D is Considered as a Hormone?
Vitamin D could be thought of as a hormone rather than a vitamin because:
❖ As it can be synthesized in the body
❖ It is released in the circulation
❖ Has distinct target organs
❖ Action of vitamin D is similar to steroid hormones. It binds to a receptor in the cytosol. Following binding, the **receptor-vitamin complex** interacts with DNA to stimulate the synthesis of calcium binding protein.

Structure

Vitamin D is a steroid compound. There are two forms of vitamin D. These two forms are differing slightly in the structure of their side chains.

1. The naturally produced **vitamin D₃ or cholecalciferol (Figure 9.26)** is the form obtained from animal sources in the diet, or made in the skin by the action of ultraviolet light from sunlight on **7-dehydrocholesterol (Figure 9.27)**
2. Artificially produced form **vitamin D₂ or ergocalciferol**, is the form made in the laboratory by irradiating the plant sterol, **ergosterol (Figure 9.27)** and it is the form most readily available for pharmaceutical use.

   Both **cholecalciferol** and **ergocalciferol** are converted about equally in humans to hormonally active dihydroxy forms.

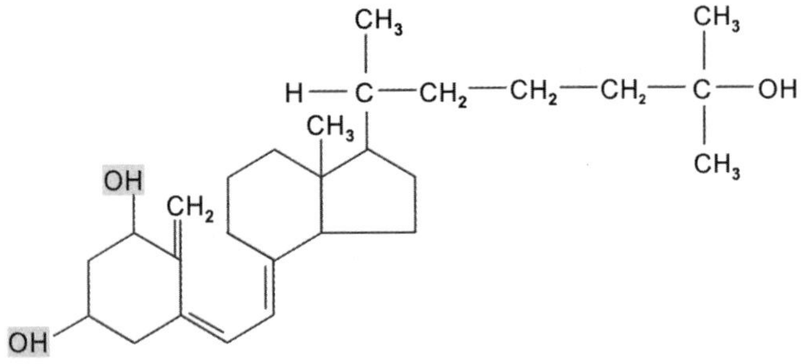

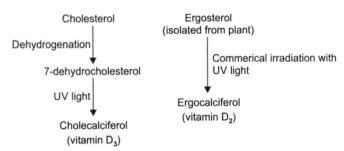

Figure 9.26: Structure of 1,25 dihydroxycholecalciferol an active form of vitamin D₃.

Figure 9.27: The formation of vitamin D₃ in the body and vitamin D₂ commercially.

Absorption, Transport, and Activation

Exogenous or dietary vitamin D is absorbed in the duodenum along with lipids. It is transported to the liver in chylomicron remnants. **Cholecalciferol is a prohormone**, as it needs further metabolism to produce the active form of the hormone. It is not clear how cholecalciferol is transported from the skin to the liver. Its circulating form is bound to **"vitamin D-binding protein,"** a α-globulin produced in the liver.

Active Form of Vitamin

- Cholecalciferol is an **inactive** form of vitamin D. It needs further metabolism to produce the active form of the vitamin.
- **1, 25 dihydroxycholecalciferol** also known as **calcitriol** is an active form of vitamin D.

Formation of Active Vitamin D

- The naturally produced **vitamin D₃** or **cholecalciferol** is the form obtained from animal sources in the diet, or made in the skin by the action of ultraviolet light from sunlight on **7-dehydrocholesterol** is an inactive form of vitamin D. The steps involved in activation are given in **Figure 9.28**.
1. The first step is the conversion of cholecalciferol to 25-hydroxycholecalciferol. The **25-hydroxylation occurs in liver** and is catalyzed by **cytochrome P₄₅₀ dependent hydroxylase**, which requires oxygen and NADPH.
2. The 25-hydroxycholecalciferol formed transported in the plasma, bound to a specific α-globulin to

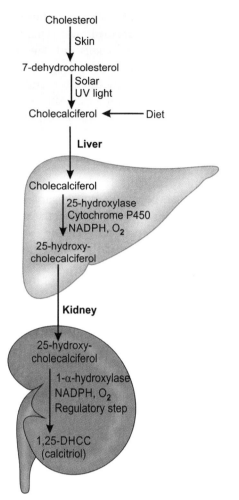

Figure 9.28: Sites of formation of vitamin D₃ to its metabolically active form 1,25 dihydroxycholecalciferol.

(1,25 DHCC: 1,25 dihydroxycholecalciferol)

the kidney, where it is further hydroxylated by **1, α-hydroxylase** to 1:25 dihydroxycholecalciferol (**Figure 9.28**). This hydroxylation reaction is also dependent on NADPH, O_2, and cytochrome P_{450}. It is an important site of regulation of activation of vitamin D.

- The activity of **1-α-hydroxylase** in the kidney is strictly controlled. 25-hydroxycholecalciferol entering the kidney is normally metabolized to 24, 25 dihydroxycholecalciferol unless the **1-α-hydroxylase** is active.
- The activity of the 1-α-hydroxylase depends on:
  - **Parathyroid hormone:** A low level of plasma calcium stimulates 1, α-hydroxylase through the secretion of parathyroid hormone.
  - **Plasma calcium:** High concentration of calcium in plasma **inhibits** the activity of 1, α-hydroxylase.
  - **Plasma phosphate:** Reduced plasma phosphate concentration also activates the 1, α-hydroxylase but independent of parathyroid hormone. High concentration of plasma phosphate inhibits the activity of 1, α-hydroxylase.

- **Insulin**, **growth hormone**, **prolactin** and **estrogen** are also known to affect (increase) the production of active form of vitamin D.
- The most potent **inhibitor** of the **1, α-hydroxylation** is the product of the reaction; **1:25 dihydroxycholecalciferol**. As the concentration of 1:25 dihydroxycholecalciferol increases, its production is halted allowing more of the inactive form hormone 24:25 dihydroxycholecalciferol to be produced. This allows accurate control to be exerted over plasma calcium concentration.

Sources

- Fatty fish and their liver oils contain large amounts of vitamin D.
- Sunlight-induced synthesis of vitamin D in skin is the best source.
- Butter and eggs contain much smaller quantities.
- Milk has a very small content of 0.125 µg or 5 IU/100 mL.
- Human milk has been shown to contain considerable amounts of water-soluble vitamin D sulphate.
- Cereals, vegetables and fruits do not contain any, while meat contains only negligible amount.

Functions

Vitamin D itself is metabolically inactive, and it exerts its effects through **1:25 dihydroxycholecalciferol** called **Calcitriol**. The main function of vitamin D (1:25 dihydroxycholecalciferol/Calcitriol) is to **regulate calcium homeostasis**. It maintains the normal plasma level of calcium and phosphorus by acting on **intestine**, **kidneys** and **bones** (**Figure 9.29**).

- **Action of calcitriol on intestine:** It increases the plasma calcium and phosphorus concentration by stimulating the absorption of calcium and phosphorus from the

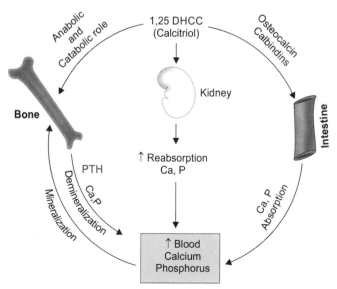

Figure 9.29: Role of vitamin D in homeostasis of calcium and phosphorus.

intestine by enhancing the synthesis of calcium binding proteins **calbindins** and **osteocalcin**. These proteins increase the calcium uptake by the intestine.

- **Action of calcitriol on kidney:** It stimulates the reabsorption of calcium and phosphorus through renal tubules and decreases their excretion.
- **Action of calcitriol on bone:** It is believed that calcitriol has both anabolic and catabolic role on bone.
  - Calcitriol promotes the mineralization of bones by deposition of calcium and phosphorus.
  - Calcitriol along with PTH enhances bone resorption (mobilization of calcium and phosphorus from bone).

Vitamin D increases serum calcium and phosphate through all these actions.

Nutritional Requirement

- The daily requirement of vitamin D is **200 to 400 IU**.
- During growth, pregnancy, and lactation, 400 IU daily is the minimum requirement.
- With adequate exposure to sunlight, no dietary supplements are needed.
- When the entire body is exposed to sufficient sunlight to cause mild erythema, the increase in the blood vitamin D is equivalent to consuming an oral dose of 10,000 IU (1 IU = 0.025 µg) of vitamin D_3.
- There is a need for dietary supplementation only when skin irradiation is insufficient to produce the required quantities of vitamin D_3 is

Higher intakes of Vitamin D may be Beneficial
There is growing evidence that intake of higher levels than reference range of vitamin D is protective against various cancers, including prostate and colorectal cancer and also against prediabetes and the metabolic syndrome.

Deficiency Manifestation

Deficiency of vitamin D may occur due to the following reasons:

- The natural diet contains small amount of vitamin D, and inadequate exposure to ultraviolet light is the critical factor in the causation of rickets and osteomalacia.
- Repeated pregnancies and lactation impose a considerable drain on the bone mineral reserves and vitamin D stores of the mother, causing osteomalacia.
- Age-related impaired intestinal absorption of calcium and deficient synthesis and supply of vitamin D precipitate osteomalacia in elderly women.
- Congenital (neonatal) rickets may occur in babies born to osteomalacic mothers who had completely exhausted their bone mineral and vitamin D reserves.

Vitamin D deficiency produces defective mineralization of bone, leading to **rickets** in children and **osteomalacia** in adults. Both rickets and osteomalacia have the same cause. In rickets and osteomalacia there is impaired mineralization of bone of newly formed organic matrix of the skeleton due to deficiency of vitamin D.

Vitamin D-deficiency rickets and osteomalacia can be prevented by:

- Adequate dietary intake of vitamin D and calcium
- Exposure to sunlight (2 to 4 hours per day)
- Appropriate supplementations of calcium and vitamin D to growing children and pregnant and lactating mothers.

Rickets

- In rickets, the **growing skeleton** is involved and defective mineralization occurs not only in bone but also in the cartilaginous matrix of the growth plate.
- It is characterized by formation of soft and flexible bones due to poor mineralization and calcium deficiency. The humerus, radius and ulna are bent and deformed due to softness. The deformity is more apparent on the weight bearing bones the femur, tibia, and fibula especially when the child begins to stand, resulting in the characteristic bowing of legs **(Figure 9.30)**.
- The main features of the rickets are, a large head with protruding forehead, pigeon chest, bow legs, (curved legs), knock knees and abnormal curvature of the spine (kyphosis) **(Figure 9.30)**.

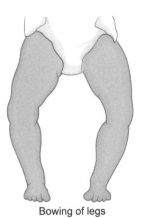
Bowing of legs

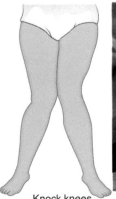
Knock knees

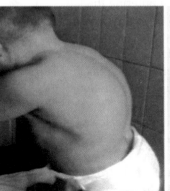
Kyphosis

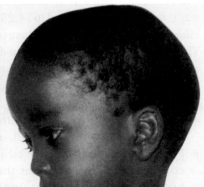
Large head with protruding forehead

Figure 9.30: Clinical manifestations of vitamin D deficiency.

- Affected (rachitic) children are usually anemic or prone to infections. They have low plasma levels of calcium and phosphorus and high alkaline phosphatase activity.
- Rickets can be fatal when severe.

Osteomalacia (Adult Rickets)

- Osteomalacia characterized by **demineralization of previously formed bones**. Demineralization of bones makes them soft and susceptible to fractures.
- Muscular weakness, bone pains and tenderness, backache, difficulty in walking or climbing, and deformities of the spine and pelvis are the most common features of osteomalacia.
- Inability to stand unaided or the tendency to prop on self while rising up from the floor is an important clue to the diagnosis of osteomalacia.
- Severe and long-standing cases may develop ankylosis (abnormal stiffening and immobility of a joint due to fusion of the bones).

Renal Rickets (Renal Osteodystrophy)

In chronic renal failure synthesis of calcitriol in kidney is impaired. As a result, the deficiency of calcitriol occurs which leads to hypocalcemia and hyperphosphatemia. It can be treated by oral or intravenous administration of calcitriol (active form of vitamin D).

Vitamin D Resistant Rickets

As the name implies, this is a disease which does not respond to treatment with vitamin D. There are various possible causes of this condition and all involve a defect in the metabolism or mechanism of action of 1,25 dihydroxycholecalciferol. The causes are as follows:

- Due to **defective vitamin D receptor**
- Due to a **defective 1, α-hydroxylase activity in kidney**
- Due to liver disease and kidney failure as the production of 25-hydroxycholecalciferol and 1,25 dihydroxycholecalciferol respectively will be inefficient in the damaged tissue.

> Vitamin D and calcium deficiencies have been shown to be associated with an increased incidence of colon and breast cancers. Studies on breast cells *in vitro* have shown that vitamin D analogs inhibit the proliferation of these cells.

Vitamin D Intoxication

High doses of vitamin D over a long period are toxic. Hypervitaminosis D can occur because of excessive consumption of vitamin D, abnormal conversion of vitamin D to its biologically active metabolites, or when the sensitivity of the target to vitamin D alters.

- The early symptoms of hypervitaminosis D include nausea, vomiting, anorexia, diarrhea, drowsiness, muscular weakness, headache, profuse sweating, polyuria, increased thirst, loss of weight, and vertigo occur in mild cases because of associated hypercalcemia and hypercalciuria. Hypercalcemia is seen due to increased bone resorption and intestinal absorption of calcium.
- The prolonged hypercalcemia causes calcification of soft tissues and organs such as kidney and may lead to formation of stones in the kidneys.

Therapeutic Use

Vitamin D analogs have been used in the treatment of psoriasis, a disease of abnormal epidermal growth and differentiation.

Vitamin E (Tocopherol)

Vitamin E is a collective name for four tocopherols (alpha, beta, gamma, and delta) and four tocotrienols (alpha, beta, gamma, and delta) which differ in the number and position of the methyl groups on the ring.

- The **α-tocopherol** is the most active form **(Figure 9.31)**.
- Tocotrienols have unsaturated isoprenoid side chain with **three carbon-carbon double bonds** while tocopherols have saturated side chain.

Sources

- The tocopherols are fat-soluble and are distributed primarily in plants and to a lesser degree in animal tissues, so that the major portion of human dietary intake of vitamin E is derived from vegetable oils, such as soyabean, corn, sunflower oil, safflower oil, and wheat germ oil.
- Vitamin E is also found in meats, nuts, and cereal grains, and small amounts are present in fruits and vegetables.
- Coconut and olive oils are relatively low in vitamin E content (1–10 mg/100 g).

Absorption, Transport, and Storage

Vitamin E is absorbed from intestine together with dietary lipid. It is incorporated in chylomicrons. It is delivered to the liver via chylomicron. The liver can export vitamin E into very low density lipoprotein (VLDL) to target cells. In cells, tocopherols are distributed where antioxidant activity

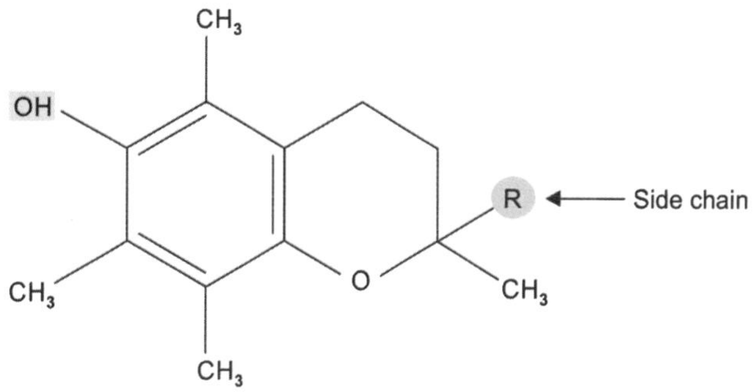

Figure 9.31: Structure of α-tocopherol.

is required. **The major site of vitamin E storage is in the adipose tissue.**

Nutritional Requirements

- The RDA for vitamin E is 10–15 mg/day (or 15–22.5 IU) for all adults.
- Diets high in polyunsaturated fatty acids may require a slightly higher intake of vitamin E.
- One mg of α-tocopherol is equal to 1.5 IU.

Functions

- Vitamin E acts as an antioxidant that prevents oxidation of LDL cholesterol, polyunsaturated fatty acids in cell membranes and protects from coronary artery disease.
- Vitamin E terminates free radical lipid peroxidation by donating single electron to form the stable fully oxidized tocopheryl quinine **(Figure 9.32)**
- Vitamin E acts collectively along with other natural antioxidants such as vitamin C, glutathione and beta-carotene. Other antioxidants, e.g., vitamin C, glutathione, and enzymes maintains vitamin E in a reduced state **(Figure 9.32)**
- Protection of erythrocyte membrane from oxidant is the major role of vitamin E in humans. It protects the RBCs from hemolysis
- Vitamin E also inhibits prostaglandin synthesis and the activities of protein kinase C and phospholipase A_2.
- Vitamin E supplements seem to have beneficial effects in chronic diseases like diabetes mellitus, coronary artery disease, hypertension, chronic interstitial mastitis.
- In food it prevents rancidity of fats.

Deficiency Manifestation

Vitamin E deficiency in humans is rare. Since vitamin E is absorbed from the intestine in chylomicrons, any fat malabsorption disease like **abetalipoproteinemia** can lead to **vitamin E deficiency**.

- The major symptom of vitamin E deficiency in human is **hemolytic anemia** due to increased red blood cell fragility

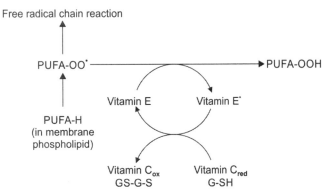

Figure 9.32: Role of vitamin E as an antioxidant.

- Another symptom of vitamin E deficiency is **retrolental fibroplasia (RLF)** observed in some premature infants of low birth weight.
- Children with this defect show **neuropathy**.

Premature and low birth weight infants are particularly susceptible to development of vitamin E deficiency, because placental transfer is poor and these infants have limited adipose tissue, where much of the vitamin normally is stored.

Toxicity/Hypervitaminosis E

Unlike other fat soluble vitamins such as A and D, vitamin E does not seem to have toxic effects from administration of large doses of vitamin E.

Vitamin K

Vitamin K is called an **anti-hemorrhagic factor** as its deficiency produced uncontrolled hemorrhages. Vitamin K consists of a number of related compounds known as quinones. There are two naturally occurring forms of vitamin K have same general activity **(Figure 9.33)**.

- **Vitamin K_1** also known as **phylloquinone** derived from vegetable and animal.
- **Vitamin K_2** or **menaquinones**, produced by intestinal bacteria and found in hepatic tissue
- **Vitamin K_3** or menadione is a synthetic product, which is an alkylated form of vitamin K_2.

Dietary Sources

- Vitamin K is present in green leafy vegetables such as spinach, cabbage, and cauliflower.
- Vitamin K is present in vegetable oils; olive, and soybean oils are particularly rich sources.
- The vitamin is also synthesized by microorganisms in the intestinal tract. Approximately 50% of the daily requirement is derived from plant sources and the rest from bacterial synthesis.

Absorption, Transport, and Storage

- The naturally occurring vitamin K derivatives are absorbed only in the **presence of bile salts**, like other lipids. It is transported to the liver in the form of chylomicrons, where it is stored.
- Menadione (synthetic vitamin K), being water soluble, is absorbed even in the absence of bile salt, passing directly into the hepatic portal vein. Stores of vitamin K in the body are very small

Nutritional Requirements

- Since the efficiency of absorption of vitamin K varies from 10 to 70%, a total requirement for vitamin K, from both dietary and intestinal bacterial synthesis, has been estimated from these data to be about 1 mg/kg body weight.
- The suggested intake for adults is **50 to 100 µg/day**.

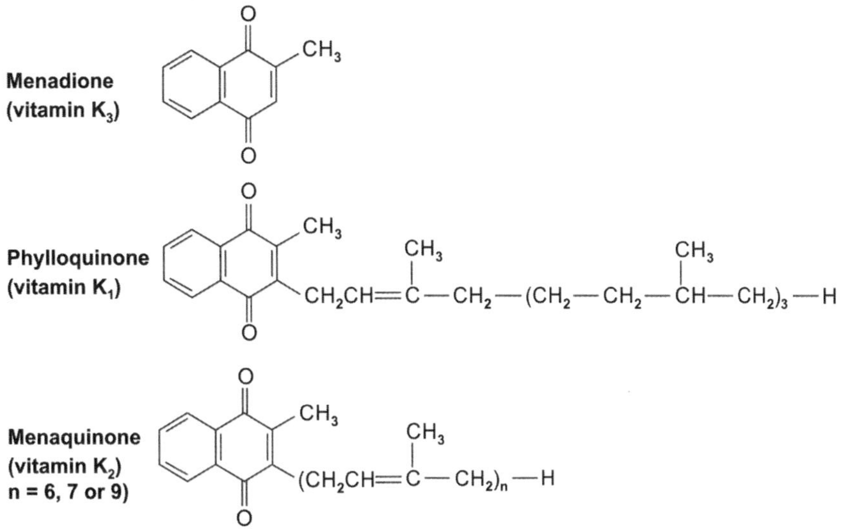

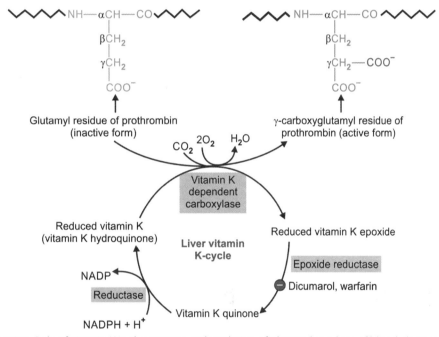

Figure 9.33: Structure of vitamin K.

Figure 9.34: Role of vitamin K in the gamma-carboxylation of glutamyl residues of blood-clotting factors.

Functions of Vitamin K

- Vitamin K plays an important role in **blood coagulation**. Vitamin K is required for the activation of blood clotting factors, prothrombin (II), factor VII, IX, and X. These blood clotting proteins are synthesized in liver in inactive form, and are converted to active form by **vitamin K dependent carboxylation** reaction.
- In this, vitamin K dependent carboxylase enzyme adds the extra carboxy group at γ-carbon of glutamic acid residues of inactive blood clotting factors **(Figure 9.34)**. In this reaction vitamin K as a coenzyme regenerated by epoxide reductase. This post-translational carboxylation of glutamic acid is necessary for calcium binding to γ-carboxylated proteins such as prothrombin (factor II); factors VII, IX, and X.
- Vitamin K is also required for the carboxylation of glutamic acid residues of osteocalcin, a Ca^{2+} binding protein present in bone.

> Anticoagulants, **dicumarol** and **warfarin** are structurally similar to vitamin K and inhibit γ-carboxylation by preventing the conversion of vitamin K to its active hydroquinone form.

Deficiency Manifestation

- Vitamin K deficiency is associated with **hemorrhagic disease**. In vitamin K deficiency, clotting time of blood is increased. Uncontrolled hemorrhages occur on minor injuries as a result of reduction in prothrombin and other clotting factors.

- Vitamin K is widely distributed in nature and its production by the intestinal microflora ensures that dietary deficiency does not occur. Vitamin K deficiency, however, is found in:
    - **Patients with liver disease** and **biliary obstruction**. Biliary obstruction inhibits the entry of bile salts to the intestine.
    - **In newborn infants**, because the placenta does not pass the vitamin to the fetus efficiently, and the gut is sterile immediately after birth.
    - Broad-spectrum antibiotic treatment; by reducing gut bacteria which synthesize menaquinones.
    - In patients with warfarin therapy, the antiobesity drug; due to vitamin K malabsorption.
    - **In fat malabsorption**, that impairs absorption of vitamin K.
- The diagnosis of vitamin K deficiency usually is made on the basis of an elevated prothrombin time or reduced clotting factors.
- If an elevated prothrombin time does not improve on vitamin K therapy, it can be assumed that it is not the result of vitamin K deficiency.
- Patients with liver disease may have an elevated pro-thrombin time because of liver cell destruction as well as vitamin K deficiency.

Toxicity/Hypervitaminosis K

Excessive doses of menadione and its derivatives produce a hemolytic anemia and kernicterus in infants with low birth weights. This toxic effect appears to result from an increased break down of erythrocytes and undeveloped capacity for its conjugation. Vitamin K_1 seems to be free from these side effects.

Therapeutic Use

An important therapeutic use of vitamin K is an antidote (drug that counteracts the effects of a poison) to poisoning by dicumarol type drugs.

STRIKE A NOTE

- ❖ In most outbreaks of pellagra, twice as many women as men are affected, probably the result of inhibition of tryptophan metabolism by estrogen metabolites.
- ❖ In vitamin B_6 deficiency, there is increased sensitivity to the actions of low concentrations of estrogens, androgens, cortisol, and vitamin D. Increased sensitivity to steroid hormone action may be important in the development of **hormone-dependent cancer** of the breast, uterus, and prostate, and vitamin B_6 status may affect the prognosis.
- ❖ Biotin also has a role in regulation of the cell cycle, acting to biotinylate key nuclear proteins.
- ❖ Higher intakes of vitamin D may be beneficial. Higher vitamin D status is protective against various cancers, prediabetes and the metabolic syndrome.
- ❖ Although excess dietary vitamin D is toxic, excessive exposure to sunlight does not lead to vitamin D poisoning, because there is a limited capacity to form the precursor, 7-dehydrocholesterol, and prolonged exposure of provitamin D to sunlight leads to formation of inactive compounds.

ASSESSMENT QUESTIONS

▌STRUCTURED LONG ESSAY QUESTIONS (SLEQs)

1. Describe vitamin A under the following headings:
    i. Active form
    ii. Sources and nutritional requirements
    iii. Biochemical functions
    iv. Deficiency manifestations
    v. Toxicity of excess intake
2. Describe vitamin D under the following headings:
    i. Active form
    ii. Sources and nutritional requirements
    iii. Biochemical functions
    iv. Deficiency manifestations
    v. Toxicity of excess intake
3. Describe vitamin C under the following headings:
    i. Sources and nutritional requirements
    ii. Biochemical functions
    iii. Deficiency manifestations

4. Describe vitamin thiamine under the following headings:
    i. Active form
    ii. Sources and nutritional requirements
    iii. Biochemical functions
    iv. Deficiency manifestations
5. Describe vitamin riboflavin under the following headings:
    i. Active form
    ii. Sources and nutritional requirements
    iii. Biochemical functions
    iv. Deficiency manifestations
6. Describe vitamin niacin under the following headings:
    i. Active form
    ii. Sources and nutritional requirements
    iii. Biochemical functions
    iv. Deficiency manifestations
7. Describe vitamin pyridoxine under the following headings:
    i. Active form
    ii. Sources and nutritional requirements

iii. Biochemical functions
iv. Deficiency manifestations

8. Describe vitamin folic acid under the following headings:
   i. Active form
   ii. Sources and nutritional requirements
   iii. Biochemical functions
   iv. Deficiency manifestations

9. Describe vitamin cyanocobalamin under the following headings:
   i. Active form
   ii. Sources and nutritional requirements
   iii. Biochemical functions
   iv. Deficiency manifestations

SHORT ESSAY QUESTIONS (SEQs)

1. Write the functions and deficiency manifestations of vitamin A.
2. Role of vitamin A in vision.
3. Write active form of vitamin D and its biochemical role.
4. Write deficiency manifestations of thiamine.
5. Write active form and functions with examples of riboflavin
6. Write active form and functions with examples of niacin
7. Write deficiency manifestations of Niacin
8. Write coenzyme form of pyridoxine and reactions where it functions.
9. Write reactions where biotin acts as a coenzyme.
10. Write functions of Folic acid.
11. Write active coenzyme form of vitamin B_{12} and reactions where it functions.
12. Write the deficiency manifestations of vitamin B_{12}
13. Write the deficiency manifestations of vitamin C.

SHORT ANSWER QUESTIONS (SAQs)

1. What is pernicious anemia and name the vitamin involved?
2. Name any four B-complex vitamins and their active forms.
3. Give biochemical reactions involving cobalamin as coenzyme.
4. Write coenzyme form of pyridoxine and one reaction in which it functions.
5. Write coenzyme form of thiamin and one reaction in which it functions.
6. Write coenzyme form of riboflavin and one reaction in which it functions.
7. Write coenzyme form of niacin and one reaction in which it functions.
8. Write coenzyme form of Pantothenic acid and one reaction in which it functions.
9. Write coenzyme form of biotin and one reaction in which it functions.
10. Write coenzyme form of folic acid and one reaction in which it functions.
11. Write coenzyme form of vitamin B_{12} and one reaction in which it functions.
12. Outline the role of vitamin A in the visual process.
13. Vitamin D and vitamin A can be classified as a hormone. Justify.

14. Why folate and B_{12} deficiency leads to megaloblastic anemia.
15. Name water and fat soluble vitamins with an antioxidant function.
16. Why vitamin K is called antihemorrhagic factor?
17. Why vitamin D is called antirachitic factor?
18. List the vitamins that are required for the functioning of the citric acid cycle.

CASE VIGNETTE-BASED QUESTIONS (CVBQs)

Case Study

1. **A 15-year-old male has polished rice as a major component of his diet. He is hospitalized with symptoms of poor appetite, peripheral neuropathy, and muscular weakness.**
   Questions
   a. Name the probable disorder and its different types.
   b. Which factor is deficient in the diet?
   c. Give the active form of the deficient factor.
   d. Give any reaction where this factor is required.

2. **A male infant, 6 months of age, was admitted to the hospital in a coma. Blood investigation indicated that the child was anemic and that his vitamin B_{12} level was very low. A urine sample contained increased amount of methylmalonate and homocysteine.**
   Questions
   a. Why was the infant anemic?
   b. What are the sources of vitamin B_{12} in the diet?
   c. Explain the high level of methylmalonate and homocysteine in the infant's urine.
   d. Give active form of vitamin B_{12}.

3. **A 42-year-old woman with a chronic inflammatory bowel disease was on intravenous feeding containing fat free and carbohydrate rich diet. After 3 months, she began to complain of being unable to see appropriately in dim light.**
   Questions
   a. Name the probable disorder.
   b. Which factor is deficient in the diet?
   c. What is the daily requirement of this factor?
   d. Name the rich sources of this factor.

4. **A 6-year-old girl is hospitalized with symptoms of digestive disorders, dermatitis, depression, and dementia.**
   Questions
   a. Name the disorder.
   b. Disorder is due to deficiency of which biomolecule?
   c. Give active form of this biomolecule.
   d. Give any reaction requiring the active form of this biomolecule.

5. **A 10-year-old boy presented with spongy bleeding gums with loose teeth.**
   Questions
   a. What is the disease he is suffering from?
   b. What is the cause?
   c. What is the biochemical basis of the disease?
   d. Give RDA for the concerned biomolecule.

6. A small 3-year-old child was brought with bow legs, protruding forehead, pigeon chest, depressed ribs, and kyphosis.

   Questions
   a. Name the disease.
   b. Which biomolecule is deficient?
   c. What are the functions of the concerned biomolecule?
   d. RDA of the concerned biomolecule.

7. A 65-year-old woman was admitted to the hospital with complaints of numbness, tingling in the calves and feet, and weight loss. The physical examination revealed a slightly confused, depressed, pale woman. Her laboratory results showed decreased level of serum vitamin B_{12}.

   Questions
   a. What is the biologically active form of vitamin B_{12} in plasma?
   b. Which factor is required for the absorption vitamin B_{12} from intestine?
   c. What is the binding protein for vitamin B_{12}?
   d. List food substances that contain vitamin B_{12}.

8. A 56-year-old male belonging to poor socioeconomic strata presents with the history of forgetfulness, muscle weakness, poor appetite and tremors in hand and nystagmus (involuntary eye movements). He is a known alcoholic for past 20 years. On examination, he was found to have unsteady gait and fine tremors. He was found to have mental confusion too.

   Questions
   a. What is the probable diagnosis?
   b. What is the cause of your diagnosis?
   c. What is the effect of alcohol on your diagnosis?
   d. What investigation is done to confirm the diagnosis and what are the reference intervals for the investigated biomolecules?

9. A 35-year-old female came with history of increased pigmentation around the neck, bright reddish patches on the feet, ankles, and face which increased on exposure to sunlight. She complained of recurrent diarrhea. On examination, she was disoriented. Her staple diet was jowar and maize for several years.

   Questions
   a. What is the probable diagnosis?
   b. What is the cause of the above diagnosed case?
   c. Name the active forms and dietary sources of deficient biomolecule?
   d. What is the nutritional treatment?

10. A 14-month-old baby was brought to the hospital with history of bleeding in response to minor trauma. There was history of mucosal and subcutaneous bleeding, such as epistaxis (bleeding from the nose), hematuria, gum bleeding, and oozing from vaccination site. On investigation prothrombin time was prolonged.

    Questions
    a. What is the probable diagnosis?
    b. What is the cause of the above diagnosed case?

c. Name the dietary sources of deficient biomolecule?
d. What is the standard treatment?

11. A 42-year-old female presented with a sensation of cold, numbness, in the tips of the toes, fingertips, occasionally with lancinating pain. She also complained of constriction in the abdomen and chest, limb weakness, and ataxia. The symptoms were aggravating since past one year. She gave a history of frequent episodes of diarrhea and weight loss. She was a strict vegetarian and did not consume even milk and milk products. On examination she was anemic; tongue was beefy red, fissured and neurological examination revealed numbness in all extremities with decreased vibration senses. A peripheral blood smear showed megaloblasts.

    Questions
    a. What is the probable diagnosis?
    b. What is the cause of the above diagnosed case?
    c. Name the dietary sources of deficient biomolecule?
    d. Name the active forms of deficient biomolecule.

12. A 5-year-old child was brought to OPD with complaints of slow growth, pain in bones and history of late walking at 2 years of age. On examination the child was found malnourished and had frontal bossing, bowing of legs and knocked knees during walking.

    Questions
    a. What is your probable diagnosis?
    b. Which biomolecule is deficient? Write its active form?
    c. Write biochemical basis of the disease.
    d. Which biochemical investigations are needed to be carried out?

13. A 4-year-old child presents with history of decreased vision after sunset. Mother gives the history of repeated upper respiratory infection in the child. On examination, he was found to have follicular hyperkeratosis on the back of the arm. Eye examination revealed dry eye (xerophthalmia) and white patches on sclera.

    Questions
    a. Which biomolecule is deficient?
    b. What is the name given to the eye manifestation?
    c. What are the active form/forms of deficient molecule?
    d. Why this biomolecule is considered as a hormone?

14. A 42-year-old woman with a chronic inflammatory bowel disease was on intravenous feeding containing fat free and carbohydrate rich diet. After 3 months she began to complain of being unable to see appropriately in dim light.

    Questions
    a. Name the probable disorder.
    b. Which biomolecule is deficient in the diet?
    c. What is the cause of poor vision in dim light?
    d. What is the daily requirement of this biomolecule?
    e. Name the rich sources of this biomolecule.

MULTIPLE CHOICE QUESTIONS (MCQs)

1. Which of the following coenzymes is not derived from vitamins?
   a. CoASH
   b. TPP
   c. Pyridoxal phosphate (PLP)
   d. Coenzyme Q

2. A deficiency of vitamin B_{12} causes:
   a. Scurvy
   b. Rickets
   c. Pernicious anemia
   d. Beriberi

3. Rickets is due to deficiency of:
   a. Vitamin D
   b. Vitamin A
   c. Vitamin C
   d. Vitamin B_1

4. Which of the following vitamins would most likely become deficient in a person who developed a completely vegetarian lifestyle?
   a. Vitamin C
   b. Niacin
   c. Cobalamin
   d. Vitamin E

5. Pyridoxal phosphate is a coenzyme for the reactions, *except*:
   a. Transamination
   b. Deamination
   c. Decarboxylation
   d. Oxidation-reduction

6. Both folic acid and methylcobalamin are required in:
   a. Phosphorylation
   b. Deamination
   c. Methylation of homocysteine to methionine
   d. Conversion of pyruvate to acetyl-CoA

7. Beriberi is caused by a deficiency of:
   a. Thiamine
   b. Thymine
   c. Threonine
   d. Tyrosine

8. Precursor of CoA is:
   a. Folic acid
   b. Thiamine
   c. Riboflavin
   d. Pantothenic acid

9. Biotin is involved in:
   a. Oxidation-reduction
   b. Carboxylation
   c. Decarboxylation
   d. Dehydration

10. Antihemorrhagic vitamin is:
    a. Vitamin A
    b. Vitamin E
    c. Vitamin K
    d. Vitamin D

11. Both Wernicke's disease and beriberi can be treated by administering vitamin:
    a. Thiamine
    b. Niacin
    c. Riboflavin
    d. Ascorbic acid

12. Pellagra occurs due to deficiency of:
    a. Biotin
    b. Niacin
    c. Pantothenic acid
    d. Folic acid

13. All of the following vitamins have antioxidant property, *except*:
    a. β-carotene
    b. Ascorbic acid
    c. Tocopherol
    d. Cholecalciferol

14. Increased prothrombin time is observed in the deficiency of:
    a. Vitamin K
    b. Vitamin B
    c. Vitamin A
    d. Vitamin B_{12}

15. Thiamine pyrophosphate is required for the following enzymatic activity:
    a. Hexokinase
    b. Transketolase
    c. Transaldolase
    d. Glucose-6-phosphatase

16. Excretion of FIGLU in urine occurs in deficiency of:
    a. Thiamine
    b. Folic acid
    c. Ascorbic acid
    d. Nicotinic acid

17. Which of the following vitamin is required for collagen synthesis?
    a. Ascorbic acid
    b. Nicotinic acid
    c. Pantothenic acid
    d. Folic acid

18. Functionally active form of vitamin D is:
    a. 1,25-dihydroxycholecalciferol
    b. 24,25-dihydroxycholecalciferol
    c. 25-hydroxycholecalciferol
    d. 1,24-dihydroxycholecalciferol

19. Which of the following enzyme is used as a measure of thiamine deficiency?
    a. Pyruvate dehydrogenase
    b. Erythrocyte transketolase
    c. α-ketoglutarate dehydrogenase
    d. Decarboxylase

20. Which of the following is used as an assay of riboflavin status?
    a. Transketolase
    b. Glutathione reductase
    c. FIGLU
    d. Pyruvate dehydrogenase

21. Which of the following trace elements is an integral part of the vitamin B_{12} molecule?
    a. Zinc
    b. Iron
    c. Copper
    d. Cobalt

22. Deficiency of pyridoxine in the diet will impair the catalytic activity of:
    a. Glutamate dehydrogenase
    b. Glutamine synthetase
    c. Alanine amino transferase
    d. Glutaminase

23. Identify the correct statement about the vitamin whose deficiency results in the disorder, pernicious anemia:
    a. It is absorbed in the gut as a combination with folic acid
    b. Is the only water soluble vitamin can be stored in liver
    c. Found in large amounts in the diets of vegans
    d. It is synthesized in the parotid glands

24. Which of the following vitamins can be synthesized in the liver by a pathway that involves pyridoxal phosphate and an aromatic amino acid:
    a. Vitamin D
    b. Thiamine
    c. Folic acid
    d. Niacin

25. Protein in raw egg white avidin prevents the absorption of which of the following vitamins:
    a. Pantothenic acid
    b. Biotin
    c. Niacin
    d. Riboflavin

26. Deficiency of which one of these vitamins is a major cause of blindness worldwide:
    a. Vitamin A
    b. Vitamin C
    c. Vitamin D
    d. Vitamin K

27. Deficiency of which one of these vitamins may lead to hemolytic anemia:
    a. Vitamin B_4
    b. Vitamin E
    c. Vitamin K
    d. Vitamin D

28. Which of the following vitamins provides the cofactor for reduction reactions in fatty acid synthesis?
    a. Vitamin B_6
    b. Thiamin
    c. Niacin
    d. Riboflavin

29. Which one of these vitamins may mask the anemia due to vitamin B_{12} deficiency?
    a. Folic acid
    b. Riboflavin
    c. Biotin
    d. Pyridoxin

30. Which of the following vitamins provides the coenzyme for transamination of amino acids?
    a. Thiamine
    b. Vitamin B_6
    c. Niacin
    d. Folic acid

31. Deficiency of which of these vitamins lead to megaloblastic anemia:
    a. Vitamin D
    b. Vitamin B_6
    c. Vitamin B_{12}
    d. Vitamin E

32. Which of the following vitamins acts as a coenzyme for transfer of one carbon units?
    a. Niacin
    b. Thiamin
    c. Vitamin B_6
    d. Folic acid

33. For fatty acid synthesis which of the following vitamins as a coenzyme required:
    a. Biotin
    b. Riboflavin
    c. Folic acid
    d. Thiamin

34. For calcium homeostasis which of the following vitamins is involved:
    a. Vitamin C
    b. Vitamin A
    c. Vitamin D
    d. Vitamin E

35. Vitamin involved in blood clotting is:
    a. Vitamin K
    b. Vitamin E
    c. Vitamin C
    d. Vitamin D

36. Ascorbic acid is required for synthesis of:
    a. Phenylserine
    b. Homoserine
    c. Hydroxylysine
    d. Selenocysteine

37. Which vitamin is required for hydroxylation of proline?
    a. A
    b. B
    c. C
    d. D

38. Coenzyme form of pyridoxine is:
    a. ADP
    b. NAD
    c. PLP
    d. FAD

39. Methylmalonyl aciduria is seen in deficiency of:
    a. Vitamin B_{12}
    b. Vitamin B_6
    c. Vitamin C
    d. Folic acid

40. Which vitamin deficiency causes glossitis and cheilosis?
    a. Thiamine
    b. Riboflavin
    c. Folic acid
    d. Vitamin E

41. Only vitamin that help in carbon fixation:
    a. Folic acid
    b. Pantothenic acid
    c. Niacin
    d. Thiamine

42. Vitamin B_6 deficiency cause increased excretion of:
    a. Methylmalonyl CoA
    b. Xanthurenic acid
    c. Branched chain keto acids
    d. Ketone bodies

43. Vitamin deficiency associated with increased xanthurenic acid excretion in urine?
    a. Niacin
    b. Ascorbic
    c. Thiamine
    d. Pyridoxine

44. Riboflavin deficiency is characterized by:
    a. Cheilosis, desquamation
    b. Beriberi
    c. Pellagra
    d. Dementia

45. Transfer of one carbon units requires:
    a. Retinol
    b. Folic acid
    c. Niacin
    d. Riboflavin

46. Beta carotene is a provitamin of:
    a. Niacin
    b. Ascorbic
    c. Retinoid
    d. Pyridoxine

47. Which of the following statements is false about ascorbic acid?
    a. It shows antioxidant activity
    b. It is a strong reducing agent
    c. It can be synthesized in the body
    d. Involved in the hydroxylation of prolyl- and lysyl-residues of collagen

48. Which of the following vitamin functions as both, hormone and visual pigment?
    a. Thiamine
    b. Retinal
    c. Riboflavin
    d. Folic acid

49. Which of the following is the source of beta carotene?
    a. Liver
    b. Fish
    c. Eggs
    d. Yellow and red fruits

50. Which of the following is not the form of vitamin A?
    a. Retinol
    b. Retinal
    c. Riboflavin
    d. Retinoic acid

51. All are true about vitamin D, except:
    a. 1-alpha hydroxylation occur in kidney
    b. 25-alpha hydroxylation occur in liver
    c. 1-alpha hydroxylation occur in liver
    d. Synthesized from 7-dehydrocholesterol

52. All of the following have antioxidant action, except:
    a. Retinol
    b. Cholecalciferol
    c. Ascorbate
    d. Tocopherol

53. Vitamin K as coenzyme form is regenerated by:
    a. Pyruvate carboxylase
    b. Glutamate reductase
    c. Dihydrofolate reductase
    d. Epoxide reductase

54. Vitamin K is required for:
    a. Hydroxylation
    b. Chelation
    c. Transamination
    d. Carboxylation

55. Vitamin K is involved in the post-translational modification of:
    a. Glutamate
    b. Aspartate
    c. Lysine
    d. Proline

56. Tocopherol radical is converted to tocopherol by which vitamin?
    a. Vitamin D
    b. Vitamin B_3
    c. Vitamin E
    d. Vitamin C

57. Which coenzyme acts as reducing agent in anabolic reactions.
    a. $FADH_2$
    b. $FMNH_2$
    c. NADPH
    d. NADH

58. A middle aged woman with fissures in tongue angular stomatitis, tingling and numbness in hands. Investigation showed reduced glutathione reductase activity in RBC. Which vitamin deficiency causes this?
    a. Vitamin B_1
    b. Vitamin B_2
    c. Vitamin B_6
    d. Vitamin B_{12}

59. An alcoholic malnourished patient present to hospital with respiratory distress. His pulse rate is high, pedal edema, hypertension and systolic murmur along with bilateral crepitation. A diagnosis of congestive high output cardiac failure is made. Which vitamin deficiency can cause this?

a. Vitamin B_1
b. Vitamin C
c. Vitamin B_2
d. Vitamin B_6

60. A 50-year-male with symptoms of fatigue and he has swelling of feet and loss of sensations in legs and anemia. He also has dilatation of ventricle and high cardiac output state. What is the vitamin deficiency associated with this presentation?
    a. Vitamin B_1
    b. Vitamin B_2
    c. Vitamin B_{12}
    d. Vitamin B_3

■ ANSWERS FOR MCQs

1. d	2. c	3. a	4. c	5. d
6. c	7. a	8. d	9. b	10. c
11. a	12. b	13. d	14. a	15. b
16. b	17. a	18. a	19. b	20. b
21. d	22. c	23. b	24. d	25. b
26. a	27. b	28. c	29. a	30. b
31. c	32. d	33. a	34. c	35. a
36. c	37. c	38. c	39. a	40. b
41. a	42. b	43. d	44. a	45. b
46. c	47. c	48. b	49. d	50. c
51. c	52. b	53. d	54. d	55. a
56. d	57. c	58. b	59. a	60. a

Carbohydrate Metabolism

Competency	Learning Objectives
BI 3.2: Describe the processes involved in digestion and assimilation of carbohydrates and storage. **BI 3.3:** Describe and discuss the digestion and assimilation of carbohydrates from food. **BI 3.4:** Define and differentiate the pathways of carbohydrate metabolism, (glycolysis, gluconeogenesis, glycogen metabolism, HMP shunt). **BI 3.5:** Describe and discuss the regulation, functions and integration of carbohydrate along with associated diseases/disorders. **BI 3.6:** Describe and discuss the concept of TCA cycle as a amphibolic pathway and its regulation. **BI 3.7:** Describe the common poisons that inhibit crucial enzymes of carbohydrate metabolism (e.g., fluoride, arsenate). **BI 3.8:** Discuss and interpret laboratory results of analytes associated with metabolism of carbohydrates. **BI 3.9:** Discuss the mechanism and significance of blood glucose regulation in health and disease. **BI 3.10:** Interpret the results of blood glucose levels and other laboratory investigations related to disorders of carbohydrate metabolism.	1. Describe digestion, absorption, transport of carbohydrates and associated disorders. 2. Describe glycolysis: Pathway, energetics, significance, regulation and associated disorders. 3. Describe metabolic fates of pyruvate and associated disorders. 4. Describe TCA cycle: Pathway, energetics, regulation, and significance. 5. Describe gluconeogenesis: Pathway, regulation and significance. 6. Describe glycogen metabolism: Pathway, significance, regulation and associated disorders. 7. Describe hexose monophosphate pathway (HMP): Regulation, significance and associated disorders. 8. Describe uronic acid pathway and its significance. 9. Describe galactose metabolism: Pathway, significance and associated disorders. 10. Describe fructose metabolism: Pathway, significance and associated disorders. 11. Describe regulation of blood glucose level in fed and fasting state. 12. Describe diabetes mellitus: Types, symptoms, clinical features, and metabolic changes occur in diabetes mellitus. 13. Describe laboratory investigations for diagnosis of diabetes mellitus.

OVERVIEW

The major source of carbohydrates is found in plants. Glucose is the universal fuel for human cells. The glucose concentrations in the body are maintained within limits by various metabolic processes.

Carbohydrates are not essential to the diet because through gluconeogenesis the body can synthesize necessary carbohydrates from other metabolites. This chapter focuses on the chemical reactions involved in the:

- Digestion of dietary carbohydrate
- The storage of temporary excess of carbohydrate as glycogen
- Conversion of glucose to other molecules and control of these metabolic pathways
- Disorders related to glucose metabolism and laboratory investigation related to disorder.

DIGESTION, ABSORPTION, TRANSPORT OF CARBOHYDRATES AND ASSOCIATED DISORDERS

Digestion of Carbohydrates

The principal sites of carbohydrate digestion are the **mouth** and **small intestine**. The dietary carbohydrate consists of:

- **Polysaccharides:** Starch, glycogen and cellulose
- **Disaccharides:** Sucrose and lactose
- **Monosaccharides:** Mainly glucose and fructose

Monosaccharides need no digestion prior to absorption, whereas disaccharides and polysaccharides must be hydrolyzed to simple sugars before their absorption **(Figure 10.1)**.

Digestion in Mouth

Digestion of carbohydrates begins in the mouth. Salivary gland secretes α-**amylase (ptyalin)**, which initiates the hydrolysis of a **starch** and **glycogen**. This enzyme is endoglycosidase that hydrolyzes random internal α-(1 → 4) glycosidic bonds. It cannot catalyze the hydrolysis of α-(1 → 6) glycosidic bonds, found at the branch point of glycogen and starch.

During mastication salivary α-amylase acts briefly on dietary starch and glycogen in random manner breaking some α–(1 → 4) bonds. α-amylase hydrolyzes starch into **(Figure 10.2)**:

- Disaccharides, maltose
- Trisaccharides, maltotriose (trimer of glucose linked by α-(1 → 4) glycosidic bond)

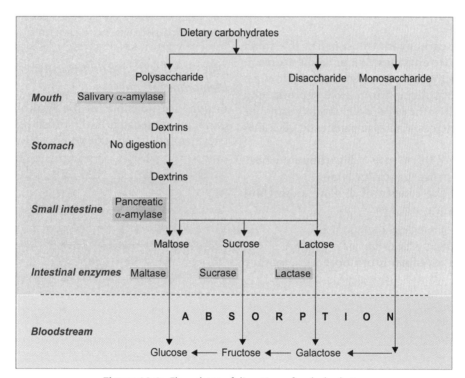

Figure 10.1: Flow sheet of digestion of carbohydrates.

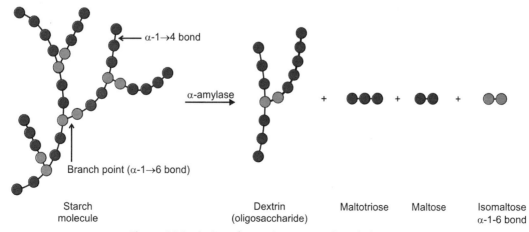

Figure 10.2: Action of α-amylase on starch and glycogen.

- Oligosaccharides (with one or more α-(1 → 6) glycosidic bonds of about 8 glucose residues in length called dextrins).

> Humans are unable to digest **cellulose** a polysaccharide of plant origin containing β-(1, 4) glycosidic bonds between glucose residues, due to absence of β-(1, 4) glucosidase enzyme in digestive juice. Undigested cellulose called roughage or fiber.
> ❖ Fiber aids intestinal motility and acts as a stool softer and prevents constipation.
> ❖ Dietary fibers are fermented in the large intestine by bacteria to form butyrate and other short chain fatty acids.
> ❖ There is some evidence that butyrate has anti-proliferative activity and prevents against colorectal cancer.

Digestion in Stomach

Carbohydrate digestion halts temporarily in the stomach because the high acidity inactivates the salivary α-amylase.

Digestion in Intestine

Further digestion of carbohydrates occurs in the small intestine by **pancreatic enzymes**. When acidic stomach contents (chyme) reach the small intestine, they stimulate mucosal cells of the duodenum to release **secretin** and **cholecystokinin (CCK)**, the two local peptide hormones that stimulate the pancreas to release pancreatic juice into the intestinal lumen.

- **Secretin** stimulates the release of **bicarbonate** whose function is to neutralize the acidic chyme
- **CCK** stimulates the release of digestive enzymes including pancreatic α-**amylase**.

There are two phases of intestinal digestion:
1. Digestion due to pancreatic α-amylase
2. Digestion due to intestinal brush border membrane enzymes.

> Salivary α-amylase and pancreatic α-amylase are isoenzyme forms. The pancreatic isoenzyme is not **glycosylated**, but the salivary isoenzyme may exist in both glycosylated and deglycosylated forms.

Digestion due to Pancreatic α-amylase

The function of pancreatic α-amylase is to degrade dextrins further. This degradation results in a mixture of **maltose**, **isomaltose** and α-**limit dextrin**. The α-limit dextrins are smaller oligosaccharides containing 3–5 glucose units.

What is Resistant Starch (RS)?

❖ All starches are composed of two types of polysaccharides: **amylose** and **amylopectin**. Most starches are broken down by **amylase** enzyme in small intestine into glucose, which is then absorbed into the blood. Resistant starch is a type of starch that is not fully broken down and absorbed in the small intestine. Instead, RS makes its way to the large intestine (colon), where intestinal bacteria ferment it. When RS is fermented in the large intestine, **short-chain fatty acids (SCFA)** such as **acetate**, **butyrate**, and **propionate**, along with gases are produced. Thus, resistant starch (RS) is so named because it resists digestion.

Contd...

> ➤ **Amylopectin** of starch is highly branched, leaving more surface area available for digestion. It is broken down quickly, and produces a larger rise in blood glucose and subsequently, a rise in insulin.
> ➤ **Amylose** is a straight chain, which limits the amount of surface area exposed for digestion. This predominates in resistant starch. Foods high in amylose are digested more slowly. They are less likely to raise blood glucose or insulin.
> ❖ The extent to which starch in foods is hydrolyzed by α-amylase is determined by its structure. The amount of amylose and amylopectin basically determines the digestibility of starch and thus glycemic index. The proportion of amylose and amylopectin can vary from one variety of starch to the other.
> ❖ Starches with lower amylose contain will have higher glycemic index; inversely starches with a higher amylose content will have low glycemic indexes.
> ❖ Foods that have a low glycemic index are considered to be more beneficial since they cause less fluctuation in insulin secretion.

Digestion due to Intestinal Brush Border Membrane Enzymes

Enzymes responsible for the final phase of carbohydrate digestion are located in the brush border membrane. The enzymes and the reactions they catalyze are as follows:

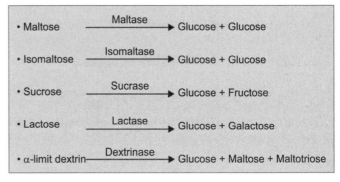

- All the above enzymes in the brush border membrane are disaccharidases except **dextrinase** which hydrolyzes α-(1 → 6) bonds at the branch points of the limit dextrins.
- The end products of carbohydrate digestion are **glucose**, **fructose** and **galactose** which are readily absorbed through the intestinal mucosal cells into the blood stream.

Dietary Fiber

❖ Dietary fiber is a type of carbohydrate that cannot be digested by our bodies' enzymes.
❖ It is found in edible plant foods such as cereals, fruits, vegetables, dried peas, nuts, lentils and grains.
❖ Fiber is grouped by its physical properties and is called **soluble**, **insoluble** or **resistant starch**.
❖ Most sources of dietary fiber tend to have a combination of both soluble and insoluble fiber in varying proportions.

Contd...

Contd...

Contd...

- ❖ All types of fibers have important roles to play.
  - ➤ Dietary fiber helps keep the gut healthy and is important in helping to reduce the risk of diseases such as diabetes, coronary heart disease and bowel cancer.
  - ➤ Fiber reaches the large bowel undigested where it is fermented by bacteria. The by-products of this fermentation are carbon dioxide, methane, hydrogen and short-chain fatty acids (SCFAs). The SCFAs are used by the body.
- ❖ Soluble fiber helps to:
  - ➤ Support the growth of probiotic bacteria needed to help maintain a healthy gut.
  - ➤ Reduce cholesterol absorption by binding to it in the gut.
  - ➤ Slow down the time it takes for food to pass through the stomach into the small intestine This helps slow down the absorption of glucose into the bloodstream and has the benefits of feeling fuller for longer, helping to control blood sugar levels, which are important for the management of diabetes.
- ❖ Insoluble fiber does not dissolve in water and is found in foods like whole meal bread, wheat bran, vegetables and nuts.
  - ➤ Insoluble fiber adds bulk to stools by absorbing water, and helps to prevent constipation.
  - ➤ It increases fluid intake as increase in fiber. Without fluid, the fiber stays hard, making it difficult to pass and causing constipation.

Absorption of Carbohydrates

Carbohydrates are absorbed as monosaccharides from the intestinal lumen through the mucosal epithelial cells into the blood stream of the portal venous system. Two mechanisms are responsible for the absorption of monosaccharides:

- **Active transport** against a concentration gradient (uphill process, i.e., from a low glucose concentration outside the cell to a higher concentration within the cell).
- **Facilitative transport**, with concentration gradient (downhill process, i.e., from a higher concentration to a lower one).

Active Transport Against Concentration Gradient

The transport of glucose and galactose across the brush border membrane of mucosal cells occurs by an active transport, energy requiring process that requires a specific transport protein and the presence of sodium ions **(Figure 10.3)**.

A sodium-dependent glucose transporter **(SGLT-1)** binds both glucose and Na^+ at separate sites and transports them both through the plasma membrane of the intestinal cell. The Na^+ is transported down its concentration gradient (higher concentration to lower concentration) and at the same time glucose is transported against its concentration gradient. The free energy required for this active transport is obtained from the hydrolysis of ATP linked to a **sodium pump** that expels Na^+ from the cell in exchange of K^+ **(Figure 10.3)**.

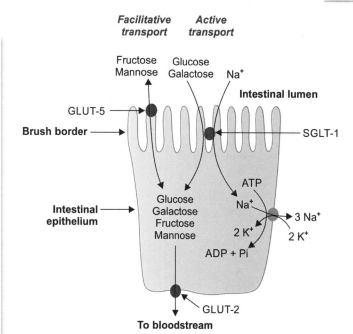

Figure 10.3: Transport of glucose, fructose, galactose and mannose. (SGLT: Sodium-dependent glucose transporter)

STRIKE A NOTE

- ❖ Cardiac glycoside **ouabain**; inhibits of Na pump.
- ❖ **Phlorizin** (glycoside) inhibits sodium-dependent glucose transporter by competing with D glucose binding sites of the carrier.
- ❖ Phloretin (Aglycan of Phlorizin) inhibits facilitated diffusion by inhibiting GLUT-1 or GLUT-4.

Facilitative Transport (with the Concentration Gradient)

Fructose and **mannose** are transported across the brush border by a Na^+ **independent facilitative diffusion** process, involving another specific glucose transporter, **GLUT-5**. Movement of sugar in facilitative diffusion is strictly downhill, going from a higher concentration to a lower one until it reaches equilibrium. The same transport can also be used by glucose and galactose if the concentration gradient is favorable.

Transport of Carbohydrate

The sodium-independent transporter, **GLUT-2** facilitates transport of sugars out of the mucosal cells and transported to the liver through portal circulation. Several glucose transporter proteins have been described in various tissues. The role of these glucose transporter proteins is shown in **Table 10.1**.

Disorders of Digestion and Absorption of Carbohydrate

Any condition that results in impaired ability to digest and absorb carbohydrate may result in bacterial fermentation in the large intestine with the production of H_2 and CO_2 **gases** and low molecular weight acids like **acetic acid**, **propionic acid** and **butyric acid** which are **osmotically active**.

TABLE 10.1: Glucose transporter.

Transporters	Occurrence	Function
Facilitative bidirectional transporters		
GLUT-1	Brain, kidney, colon, placenta and erythrocyte	Uptake of glucose
GLUT-2	Liver, pancreatic β-cell, small intestine, kidney	Rapid uptake and release of glucose
GLUT-3	Brain, kidney, placenta	Uptake of glucose
GLUT-4	Heart and skeletal muscle, adipose tissue	Insulin stimulated uptake of glucose
GLUT-5	Small intestine	Absorption of glucose
Sodium-dependent unidirectional transporter		
SGLT-1	Small intestine and kidney	Active uptake of glucose from lumen of intestine and reabsorption of glucose in proximal tubule of kidney against concentration gradient

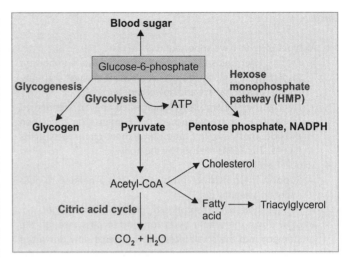

Figure 10.4: Metabolic pathways for glucose-6-phosphate in the liver.

Abdominal cramps and flatulence results from the accumulation of gases and the osmotically active products draw water from the intestinal cells into the lumen resulting in **diarrhea** and **dehydration**. Genetic deficiencies in most of the disaccharidases result in the symptoms described above.

Lactose Intolerance (Hypolactasia)

Many adults are unable to metabolize the milk sugar lactose and experience gastrointestinal disturbances if they drink milk. **Lactose intolerance** is the intolerance to lactose not to milk. **Lactose intolerance** or **hypolactasia** is the most common disorder due to deficiency of enzyme **lactase** which cleaves lactose into glucose and galactose.

- **Lactose intolerance**, common among adults of most human populations, is due to the disappearance after childhood of most or all of the **lactase** activity of the intestinal epithelial cells.
- Without intestinal lactase, lactose cannot be completely digested and absorbed in the small intestine, and it passes into the large intestine.
- The lactose is a good energy source for microorganisms in the colon and ferment it to lactic acid and toxic products such as methane CH_4 and hydrogen gas H_2 that cause abdominal cramps and diarrhea. The problem is further complicated because undigested lactose and its metabolites such as low molecular weight acids like **acetic acid**, **propionic acid** and **butyric acid** which are **osmotically active** increase the osmolarity of the intestinal contents, and draws water into the intestine resulting in diarrhea.
- The simplest treatment is to avoid the consumption of products containing much lactose. Alternatively, the enzyme lactase can be ingested with milk products.

Sucrase Deficiency Disorder

There is an inherited deficiency of the disaccharidases **sucrase** and **isomaltase**. These two deficiencies coexist, because sucrase and isomaltase occur together as a complex enzyme. Symptoms occur in early childhood and as the same as those described above.

Metabolic Fate of Carbohydrates

After being absorbed from the intestinal tract the monosaccharides are carried by the portal circulation directly to the liver. In the liver most of the entering free D-glucose is phosphorylated to **glucose-6-phosphate** and sugar is trapped within the cell and it cannot diffuse back out of the cell because its plasma membrane is impermeable to the glucose-6-phosphate. The rest of the glucose passes into the systemic blood supply.

Other dietary monosaccharides **D-fructose** and **D-galactose** are phosphorylated and may be converted into glucose in the liver. Glucose-6-phosphate is an intermediate in several metabolic pathways that uses glucose in the liver **(Figure 10.4)** depending upon the supply and demand includes:

- Glycolysis
- Hexose monophosphate pathway (HMP)
- Glycogenesis
- Glycogenolysis.

GLYCOLYSIS: PATHWAY, ENERGETICS, SIGNIFICANCE, REGULATION AND ASSOCIATED DISORDERS

Glycolysis (from the Greek **glykys**, "sweet or sugar", and lysis "splitting"), is the sequence of reactions that metabolizes one molecule of **glucose** to two molecules of **pyruvate** in the presence of **oxygen**. During the sequential reactions of glycolysis, some of the free energy released from glucose is

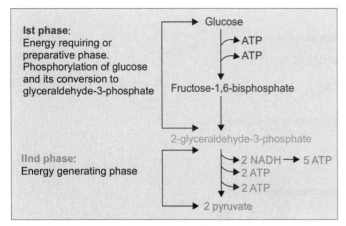

Figure 10.5: Phases of the glycolytic pathway.

conserved in the form of ATP and NADH. Pyruvate can be further processed **anaerobically** to **lactate**. Under aerobic conditions, pyruvate can be completely oxidized to CO_2, generating much more ATP.

The complete glycolytic pathway was elucidated by 1940. This pathway is also called **Embden-Meyerhof pathway**, after two pioneers of research on glycolysis.

It is a unique pathway since it can utilize oxygen if available, or it can function in the total absence of oxygen. Glycolysis is the major pathway for the utilization of glucose to virtually all cells, both prokaryotic and eukaryotic. In eukaryotic cells, glycolysis takes place in the **cytoplasm**.

Reactions of Glycolysis

The breakdown of six carbon glucose into two molecules of three carbon pyruvate occurs in 10 **steps** which can be divided into two phases **(Figure 10.5)**.

1. **Ist phase**, first 5 steps constitute the preparative phase (energy requiring phase). No ATP is generated in this phase.
2. **IInd phase**, energy generating phase.

Ist Phase, Energy Requiring Phase or Preparative Phase

First five reactions of glycolysis correspond to this phase where phosphorylated form of glucose and fructose are synthesized at the expense of **two moles of ATP** per glucose molecule. The hexose glucose is cleaved into two triose phosphates.

Reactions of Ist Phase

1. **Phosphorylation of glucose to glucose-6-phosphate (Figure 10.6):** Glucose enters cells through specific transport proteins. In the first step of glycolysis, glucose is activated for subsequent reactions by its phosphorylation at C-6 to yield **glucose-6-phosphate** with ATP by the enzyme **hexokinase**. ATP is required as a phosphate donor.

The strategy of this initial step in glycolysis is to trap the glucose in the cell. Hexokinase requires **Mg^{2+}** for its activity. The reaction is accompanied by a considerable loss of free energy as heat and therefore under physiologic conditions is regarded as **irreversible**.

Isoenzyme forms of Hexokinase

The human genome encodes four different hexokinases, I to IV all of which catalyze the same reaction. They differ with respect to their kinetic properties.

❖ Brain and kidney have chiefly the type I isoenzyme
❖ Skeletal muscle has type II
❖ Adipose tissue has both I and II
❖ Liver possesses all four isoenzyme of hexokinase. In liver, the principal form of hexokinase is type IV, commonly known as **glucokinase**.

The difference between muscle hexokinase and liver hexokinase, i.e., glucokinase is given in **Table 10.2**.

---

2. **Conversion of glucose-6-phosphate to fructose-6-phosphate:** The enzyme **phosphohexose isomerase** catalyzes the reversible of isomerization of glucose-6-phosphate an aldose, to **fructose-6-phosphate** a ketose.

3. **Phosphorylation of fructose-6-phosphate to fructose 1,6-bisphosphate:** Fructose-6-phosphate to fructose 1,6-bisphosphate is a second phosphorylation reaction of glycolysis. Phosphofructokinase-1 (PFK-1) catalyzes the transfer of a phosphoryl group from ATP to fructose-6-phosphate to yield **fructose 1,6-bisphosphate**. This step is **irreversible committed step** under physiological conditions.

- **Phosphofructokinase-1** is both **allosteric** and an **inducible** enzyme which is the **rate limiting, regulatory enzyme of glycolysis**.
- Its activity is increased whenever the cell's ATP supply is depleted or when the ATP breakdown products, ADP and AMP accumulate.
- The enzyme is inhibited whenever the cell has ample ATP. **Fructose 2,6-bisphosphate** is potent allosteric activator of PFK-1.

Fructose is more rapidly glycolyzed by the liver than glucose, because it bypasses the step in glucose metabolism catalyzed by phosphofructokinase, at which point metabolic control is exerted on the rate of catabolism of glucose.

4. **Cleavage of fructose-1,6-bisphosphate: Fructose-1,6-bisphosphate** is cleaved by **aldolase** to two triose phosphates, glyceraldehyde-3-phosphate an aldose, and dihydroxyacetone phosphate (DHAP), a ketose. Several tissue-specific isoenzymes of aldolase exist. Aldolase-A occurs in most tissues and aldolase-B occurs in liver and kidney.

5. **Interconversion of triose phosphate:** Dihydroxyacetone phosphate (DHAP) is isomerized to glyceraldehyde-3-phosphate by the enzyme **phosphotriose isomerase**,

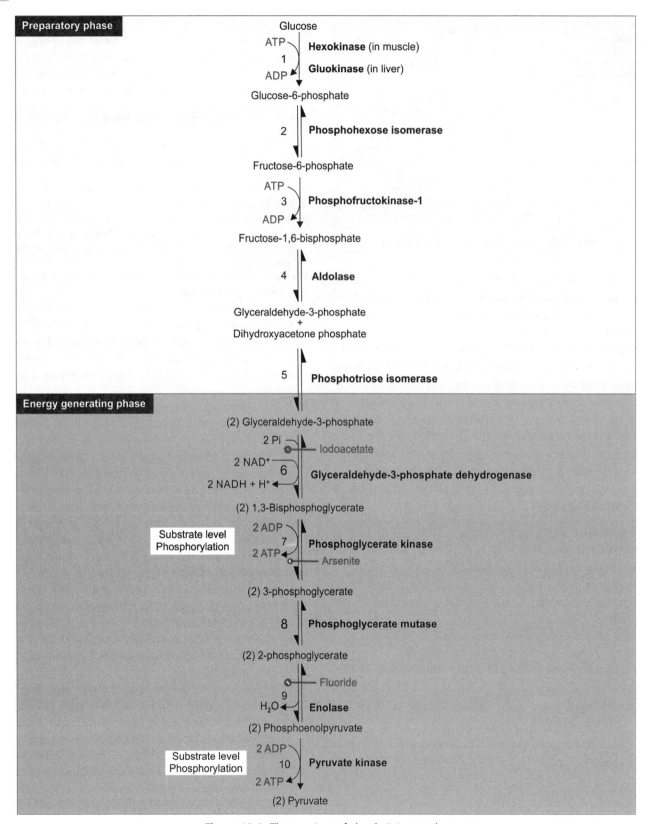

Figure 10.6: The reactions of glycolysis in muscle.

so that for every molecule of glucose entering glycolysis, 2 moles of glyceraldehyde-3-phosphate are formed. This reaction completes the preparative phase of glycolysis.

Phosphotriose isomerase enzyme deficiency, a rare condition, is the only glycolytic enzymopathy that is lethal. This deficiency is characterized by severe hemolytic anemia and neurodegeneration.

TABLE 10.2: Differences between muscle hexokinase and glucokinase (liver hexokinase).

Muscle hexokinase	Glucokinase (liver hexokinase)
Distributed in extrahepatic tissue	Present in liver and β-cells of pancreas
High affinity for its substrate glucose (low K_m)	Low affinity for its substrate glucose (high K_m)
Inhibited by its product glucose-6-phosphate, in an allosteric manner	No inhibition by its product glucose-6-phosphate
Its function is to ensure supply of glucose for the tissues irrespective of blood glucose concentration	Its function is to remove glucose from the blood, when the blood glucose level increases (following meal)
Catalyze the phosphorylation of other hexoses like fructose, galactose also	Specific for glucose
Its activity is not affected by insulin	It is an inducible enzyme that increases its synthesis in response to insulin

IInd Phase, Energy Generating Phase

In IInd phase of glycolysis, the chemical energy of glucose molecule is conserved in the form of ATP and NADH (**Figure 10.6**).

6. **Oxidation of glyceraldehyde-3-phosphate to 1,3-bisphosphoglycerate:** The first step in the energy generating phase is the oxidation of glyceraldehyde-3-phosphate to **1,3-bisphosphoglycerate**, catalyzed by **glyceraldehyde-3-phosphate dehydrogenase**. It is a reversible reaction. The reducing equivalents NADH + H+ formed are reoxidized by electron transport chain, to generate **2.5 ATP** molecules per NADH + H+.

7. **Phosphoryl transfer from 1,3-bisphosphoglycerate to ADP:** The **phosphoglycerate kinase** transfers the high energy phosphoryl group from 1,3-bisphosphoglycerate to ADP forming **ATP** and **3-phosphoglycerate**. This is the first step in glycolysis that generates **ATP**, an example of **substrate level phosphorylation**. Since two molecules of triose phosphate are formed per molecule of glucose undergoing glycolysis two molecules of ATP are generated at this stage per molecule of glucose.

> Arsenate is toxic to phosphoglycerate kinase reaction. Arsenate competes with inorganic phosphate (Pi) forming **1-arseno-3-phosphoglycerate**, which undergoes spontaneous hydrolysis to 1-phosphoglycerate without forming ATP.

8. **Conversion of 3-phosphoglycerate to 2-phosphoglycerate:** 3-phosphoglycerate to 2-phosphoglycerate is a reversible reaction catalyzed by **phosphoglycerate mutase**. It catalyzes reversible shift of the phosphoryl group between C-2 and C-3 of glycerate; Mg+ is essential for this reaction.

9. **Dehydration of 2-phosphoglycerate to phosphoenolpyruvate:** 2-phosphoglycerate to phosphoenolpyruvate (PEP) is catalyzed by **enolase**. Enolase promotes reversible removal of a molecule of water from 2-phosphoglycerate, raising the phosphate on position 2 to high energy state, thus forming phosphoenolpyruvate.

> Enolase is inhibited by fluoride, a property that can be made use in the estimation of glucose. When blood samples are taken for measurement of glucose, glycolysis in blood is inhibited by taking sample into the tubes-containing fluoride.

10. **Transfer of phosphoryl group from phosphoenolpyruvate to ADP:** The last step in glycolysis is the transfer of the phosphoryl group from phosphoenolpyruvate to ADP, catalyzed by **pyruvate kinase** which requires K+ and either Mg^{2+} or Mn^{2+}. This is an **irreversible** reaction. The high energy phosphate of phosphoenolpyruvate is transferred to ADP by the enzyme **pyruvate kinase** to generate ATP, **another example of substrate level phosphorylation**. **Pyruvate kinase** is an allosteric enzyme. Enol pyruvate formed in this reaction is converted spontaneously to the keto form of **pyruvate**.

Under aerobic conditions, pyruvate is transported into mitochondria and undergoes oxidative decarboxylation to acetyl-CoA then oxidation to CO_2 in the citric acid cycle.

> **Poisons that Inhibit Enzymes of Glycolysis**
>
> ❖ **Iodoacetate:** Inhibit glyceraldehyde-3-phosphate dehydrogenase.
> ❖ **Fluoride:** Inhibit enolase, a property that can be made use in the estimation of glucose. Glycolysis is inhibited by taking a sample into test tubes containing fluoride.
> ❖ **Arsenite:** Arsenate is toxic to phosphoglycerate kinase reaction. Arsenate competes with inorganic phosphate (Pi) forming 1-arseno-3-phosphoglycerate, which undergoes spontaneous hydrolysis to 3-phosphoglycerate without forming ATP.
> ❖ **Arsenite and mercuric ions** react with the –SH groups of lipoic acid (one component of pyruvate dehydrogenase) and inhibit pyruvate dehydrogenase and develops lactic acidosis.

Anaerobic Glycolysis

The availability of oxygen now determines which of the two pathways is followed.

● If anaerobic conditions prevail, the reoxidation of NADH to NAD+ by transfer of reducing equivalents through the respiratory chain to oxygen is prevented. Under these conditions **pyruvate** is reduced to **lactate**, by **lactate dehydrogenase** accepting electrons from NADH and thereby regenerating the NAD+ necessary for glycolysis to continue (**Figure 10.7**).

● Tissues that function under low oxygen conditions (hypoxia) produce lactate, e.g., vigorously contracting

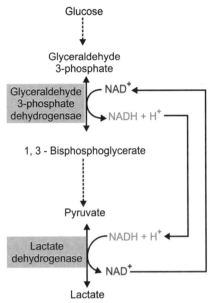

Figure 10.7: Anaerobic glycolysis. Conversion of pyruvate to lactate.

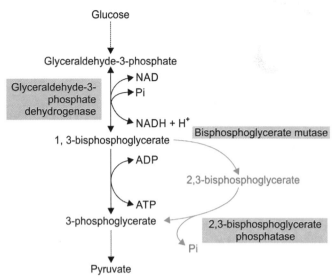

Figure 10.8: Rapoport-Luebering cycle of erythrocytes.

skeletal muscle. Certain tissues and cell types (retina and erythrocytes) coverts glucose to lactate even under aerobic conditions because of absence of mitochondria.

- Lactate production is increased in septic shock (a condition in which the body cannot supply enough blood to its tissues and organs, caused by damage to an organ by infection) and many cancers.

Clinical Significance of Blood Lactate
❖ Measurement of blood lactate is useful to assess the presence and severity of **septic shock** and to monitor the **patient's recovery**. ❖ In many disorders, levels of blood lactate provide rapid and early detection of **oxygen debt** in patients. ❖ Oxygen debt is the excess amount of oxygen required to recover from the anoxic episodes.

Additional Pathway of Glycolysis

Rapoport-luebering cycle: 2,3-Bisphosphoglycerate pathway in erythrocytes:

- In erythrocytes, the reaction of glycolysis catalyzed by **Phosphoglycerate kinase** may be bypassed to some extent and 1,3-bisphosphoglycerate is converted to **2,3-bisphosphoglycerate** by an enzyme **bisphosphoglycerate mutase**.
- Then 2,3-bisphosphoglycerate converted to 3-phosphoglycerate and inorganic phosphate (P_i) by 2,3-bisphosphoglycerate phosphatase **(Figure 10.8)**.
- This pathway is also called **Rapoport-Luebering cycle** or **bisphosphoglycerate shunt**.
- This alternative pathway involves **no net yield of ATP** from glycolysis as due to lack of mitochondria in erythrocytes glycolysis occur anaerobically to lactate.
- It supplies 2,3-bisphosphoglycerate for the **hemoglobin function** in oxygen transport. 2,3-bisphosphoglycerate

regulates the binding and release of oxygen from hemoglobin.

- 2,3-bisphosphoglycerate present in erythrocytes acts as a **buffer**. Organic phosphate (about 4.5 mmol/L) in the form of **2,3-bisphosphoglycerate** accounts for about 16% of the **noncarbonate buffer** value of erythrocyte fluid.

STRIKE A NOTE

- ❖ 2,3-BPG plays an important role in blood that has been stored for transfusion. The concentration of 2,3-BPG in the stored red blood cells can fall from 2.2 mM to one-tenth of this concentration within a few days, resulting in a decreased ability of transfused blood to deliver O_2 to tissues.
- ❖ The problem cannot be solved by incorporating 2,3-BPG into the medium because this polar molecule cannot be transferred across the cell membrane.
- ❖ The decrease can be prevented by storing blood in the presence of inosine (hypoxanthine-ribose) that is converted to BPG by RBC. Inosine can enter RBC, where its ribose moiety is released from purine base and ribose can then be phosphorylated and enter the hexose monophosphate pathway and eventually being converted to 2,3-BPG via glycolysis.

Significance of Glycolysis

- Glycolysis is the principal route for glucose metabolism for the production of ATP molecules.
- It also provide pathway for the metabolism of fructose and galactose derived from diet.
- Glycolysis has the ability to provide ATP in the absence of oxygen and allows tissues to survive anoxic episodes.
- It generates precursors for biosynthetic pathway, e.g.,
  - Pyruvate may be transaminated to amino acid **alanine**.
  - In the liver, pyruvate provides substrate, acetyl-CoA for **fatty acid** and **cholesterol** biosynthesis.

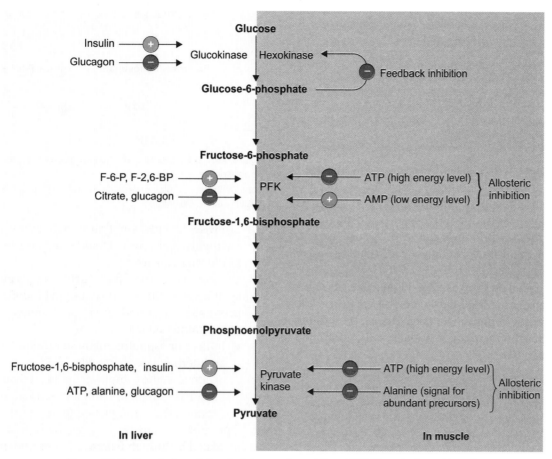

Figure 10.9: Regulation of glycolysis in muscle and liver. (PFK: Phosphofructokinase)

- Glycerol-3-phosphate derived from glycolytic pathway forms the backbone of **triacylglycerol** and **phospholipids**.
- In erythrocytes glycolysis supplies 2,3-BPG which is required for the hemoglobin function in the transport of oxygen.
- The reoxidation of NADH via lactate formation (anaerobic glycolysis) allows glycolysis to proceed in the absence of oxygen by regenerating sufficient NAD⁺ necessary for glycolysis to continue.
- Anaerobic glycolysis is an emergency source of ATP.
- In mammals, glucose is the only fuel that the brain uses under nonstarvation conditions and the only fuel that red blood cells can use at all.

Regulation of Glycolysis

- The glycolytic pathway has dual role. It degrades glucose to:
  - Generate ATP
  - Provide precursors for synthesis of fatty acids, cholesterol, triglyceride **(Figure 10.4)** and alanine.
- The rate of conversion of glucose into pyruvate is regulated to meet these two major cellular needs.
- Glycolysis is regulated at **3 irreversible** steps. These reactions are catalyzed by:

1. Hexokinase
2. Phosphofructokinase-1
3. Pyruvate kinase

- We will consider the control of glycolysis in two tissues: **muscle** and **liver**.

Regulation of Glycolysis in Muscle

Glycolysis in muscle is regulated to meet the **need of ATP**. Control of glycolysis in muscle depends on the ratio of **ATP** to **AMP (Figure 10.9)**.

1. **Phosphofructokinase-1 (PFK-1)** is the most important primary regulatory enzyme in glycolysis.
   - High levels of ATP allosterically inhibit the enzyme by lowering the **phosphofructokinase-1** enzyme's affinity for its substrate, fructose 6-phosphate.
   - AMP reverses the inhibitory action of ATP and so the activity of the enzyme increases when the ATP/AMP ratio is lowered.
   - A **decrease in pH** also **inhibits phosphofructokinase-1** activity. The pH might fall when muscles functioning anaerobically, producing excessive quantities of **lactic acid**. The inhibitory effect protects the muscle from damage that would result from the accumulation of too much of lactic acid.

Why is AMP and not ADP the Positive Regulator of Phosphofructokinase?

❖ When ATP is being utilized rapidly to ADP, the enzyme adenylate kinase can form ATP from ADP by the following reaction.

$$ADP + ADP \rightleftharpoons ATP + AMP$$

❖ Thus, some ATP is salvaged from ADP, and AMP becomes the signal for the low energy state.

---

2. **Hexokinase** is an allosteric enzyme catalyzing the first step of glycolysis in muscle is inhibited by its product **glucose-6-phosphate** in extrahepatic tissue.
   ▪ High concentration of glucose-6-phosphate signal that the cell no longer requires glucose for energy or for the synthesis of glycogen, a storage form of glucose.
   ▪ When phosphofructokinase-1 is inactive, the concentration of fructose-6-phosphate rises. In turn, the level of glucose-6-phosphate rises. Hence, the inhibition of phosphofructokinase-1 leads to the inhibition of hexokinase.

Phosphofructokinase rather than hexokinase is the most important primary regulatory enzyme of glycolysis, because, glucose-6-phosphate is not only a glycolytic intermediate. In muscle, glucose-6-phosphate can also be a precursor for the synthesis of glycogen.

---

3. **Pyruvate kinase** is the enzyme catalyzing the third irreversible step in glycolysis. This final step yields ATP and pyruvate that can be oxidized further or used as a precursor for synthetic reactions.
   ▪ **ATP allosterically inhibits pyruvate kinase** to slow glycolysis when energy level is high.
   ▪ **Alanine** synthesized from pyruvate in muscle also **allosterically inhibits pyruvate kinase** but in this case, it signals that precursors are abundant.

Regulation of Glycolysis in Liver

- The liver has more diverse biochemical functions than dose muscle:
   ▪ The liver maintains blood glucose levels:
      ♦ It stores glucose as glycogen when glucose is plentiful, and it releases glucose when it is low.
      ♦ It provides biosynthetic precursors
      ♦ It also uses glucose to generate NADPH.
- Although the liver has many of the regulatory features of muscle glycolysis, the regulation of glycolysis in the liver is more complex.

Liver Phosphofructokinase-1

- Liver phosphofructokinase-1 can be regulated by ATP as in muscle, but such regulation is not as important since the liver does not experience the sudden ATP needs that a contracting muscle does.

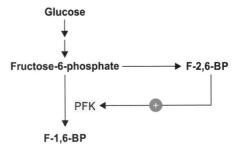

Figure 10.10: Regulation of phosphofructokinase by fructose-2,6-bisphosphate.
(F-1,6-BP: fructose-1,6-bisphosphate; F-2,6-BP: fructose-2,6-bisphosphate; PFK: Phosphofructokinase)

- Likewise, low pH is not an important metabolic signal for the liver enzyme, because lactate is not normally produced in the liver.
- Glycolysis in the liver furnishes **precursors** for synthetic reactions and so a signal indicating whether precursors are abundant or scarce should also regulate phosphofructokinase.
   ▪ In liver phosphofructokinase is inhibited by **citrate**, an intermediate in the citric acid cycle. A high level of citrate in the cytoplasm indicates that biosynthetic precursors are abundant, and so there is no need to degrade additional glucose for this purpose.
- One more means by which glycolysis in the liver is regulated is through **fructose 2,6-bisphosphate** (F-2,6-BP) a potent activator of **phosphofructokinase-1** (**Figure 10.10**). In the liver, the concentration of fructose-6-phosphate rises when blood glucose concentration is high, and the abundance of fructose-6-phosphate accelerates the synthesis of F-2, 6-BP. The binding of F-2, 6-BP increases the affinity of phosphofructokinase-1 for fructose-6-phosphate.
- Glycolysis is thus accelerated when glucose is abundant (**feed-forward stimulation**).

Regulation of Glucokinase (Liver Hexokinase)

- Glucokinase reaction is the same in the liver as in muscle. However, the liver is involved in regulation of blood glucose levels, possesses another specialized isoenzyme of hexokinase, called **glucokinase**, which is not inhibited by **glucose-6-phosphate**.
- Glucokinase phosphorylates glucose only when glucose is abundant because the affinity of glucokinase for glucose is about 50-fold lower than that of hexokinase. The role of glucokinase is to provide glucose-6-phosphate for the synthesis of **glycogen** and for the formation of **fatty acids**.
- The activity of glucokinase is thus **influenced by carbohydrate intake**:
   ▪ The activity increases with carbohydrate intake.
   ▪ Decreases during **starvation** and **diabetes mellitus**.
- Liver glucokinase is an **inducible enzyme** that increases its synthesis in response to **insulin** and decreases

in response to **glucagon**. Insulin signals the need to remove glucose from the blood for storage as glycogen or conversion into fat.

Pyruvate Kinase

- Fructose 1,6-bisphosphate allosterically stimulates the enzyme, while **ATP** and **alanine** are allosteric inhibitors.
- Liver **pyruvate kinase** is an **inducible enzyme** that increases its synthesis in response to **insulin** and decreases in response to **glucagon**. Glucagon, secreted in response to low blood glucose and insulin secreted when blood glucose levels are adequate.

Energetics of Glycolysis

- The net reaction of aerobic glycolysis of glucose into two molecules pyruvate generates:
  - Two molecules of NADH
  - Four molecules of ATP at substrate level phosphorylation.
  - Two molecules of ATP per mole of glucose are consumed for reactions of **hexokinase** and **phosphofructokinase**.
- The net gain is **2 moles of ATP** and **2 moles of NADH**.
- The NADH produced transported into the mitochondria, where these undergo oxidative phosphorylation with the release of **5 moles of ATP** (2.5 moles of ATP per mole of NADH).
- The total net ATP gain in aerobic glycolysis is **7 moles** of ATP per mole of glucose oxidized to pyruvate (**Table 10.3**).
- In anaerobic glycolysis, on the other hand, **only 2 moles of ATP** are produced per mole of glucose and no NADH is formed.

> Anaerobic tissues metabolize glucose much more rapidly than aerobic tissues do to compensate for this meager (scanty) energy gain.

- When the anaerobic glycolysis occur using glycogen as a starting compound, the net production of ATP is increased from 2 to 3 by glycolytic pathway. This is due to bypass of hexokinase reaction (1 ATP consuming reaction), because glycogen through glycogenolysis provides glucose-6-phosphate directly to glycolysis (*see* **Figure 10.26**). Thus, in muscles anaerobic glycolysis from **glycogen generates 3 ATPs** but not two.
- In aerobic conditions, pyruvate is converted to **acetyl-CoA** which enters the TCA cycle for complete oxidation to CO_2 and H_2O. Complete oxidation of glucose through **glycolysis plus citric acid cycle** will yield net 32 moles of ATP.

Disorders of Glycolysis

Pyruvate Kinase Deficiency

- Pyruvate kinase is a key enzyme in glycolysis, catalyzes the final step with formation of ATP. Genetic deficiency of pyruvate kinase in the erythrocyte leads to **hemolytic anemia** due to excessive erythrocyte destruction.
- The normal mature erythrocyte lacks mitochondria and is completely dependent on glycolysis for its energy in the form ATP. In erythrocytes deficiency of **pyruvate kinase** leads to reduced rate of glycolysis and the rate of ATP being inadequate to meet the energy needs of the cells and maintain the structural integrity of the erythrocyte membrane.
- Decreased ATP production affects the **cation pump** in the cell membrane. Ca^{2+} enters cells, while K^+ and H_2O leave the cell and cells become dehydrated and phagocytosed by cells in the spleen. The premature death and lysis of the red blood cells result in hemolytic anemia.

Hexokinase Deficiency

- Genetic defect in the **hexokinase** of erythrocyte reduces the amount of oxygen that is available for the tissues.
- Because hexokinase is the first enzyme in glycolysis, the red blood cells of these patients contain low concentration of **2,3-BPG** (glycolytic intermediate in erythrocytes) which normally allows hemoglobin to release oxygen in tissue.
- Consequently, due to low level of 2,3-BPG less oxygen is available for the tissue. This defect will result in anemia.

TABLE 10.3: Production of ATP in glycolysis.

Reaction	Reaction catalyzed by	Mechanism of ATP production	No. of ATP formed
Glyceraldehyde-3-phosphate to 1,3-bisphosphoglycerate	Glyceraldehyde-3-phosphate dehydrogenase	Respiratory chain oxidation of 2 NADH	+5*
1,3-bisphosphoglycerate to 3-phosphoglycerate	Phosphoglycerate kinase	Substrate level phosphorylation	+2
Phosphoenolpyruvate to pyruvate	Pyruvate kinase	Substrate level phosphorylation	+ 2
Consumption of ATP for reactions of hexokinase and phosphofructokinase			−2
			Net 7

*This assumes the NADH formed by glycolysis is transported into mitochondria by the **malate shuttle**.

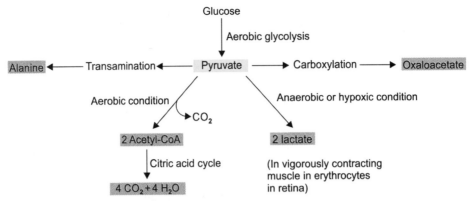

Figure 10.11: Catabolic fates of pyruvate.

Lactic Acidosis

- Lactic acidosis is the accumulation of lactic acid in the blood to levels that significantly affect the blood pH. The high concentration of lactate results in lowered blood pH (7.2).
- Under normal conditions, lactate is metabolized in the liver and the blood lactate level is in between 1 and 2 mM. With lactic acidosis, the blood lactate level may be **5 mM or more**.
- Lactate accumulation in the body fluids can be due to **increased formation** or **decreased utilization**.
    - A common cause of lactic acidosis is tissue **hypoxia** caused by **shock**, **cardiopulmonary arrest**, and **hypoperfusion**.
    - Inadequate blood flow leads to deprivation of oxygen. Oxygen deprivation leads to decreased ATP production and accumulation of NADH, which promotes conversion of pyruvate to **lactate**. In order to survive, the cells use anaerobic glycolysis for generating ATP with increased formation of lactic acid.
- Laboratory assessment includes measurements of **blood lactate**, **pyruvate**, **beta-hydroxybutyrate** and **acetoacetate**.
- Blood **lactate to pyruvate** ratio below 25 suggests defects in a **gluconeogenic enzyme** or **pyruvate dehydrogenase**.
- The primary treatment of lactic acidosis involves correcting the basic cause such as reversal of circulatory failure.

Glycolysis in Cancer Cell

In fast growing cancer cells, glycolysis proceeds at a high rate. Cancer cells stimulate glucose uptake and glycolysis. As cancer cells grow more rapidly, blood vessels cannot supply oxygen efficiently to fulfill the required demand of oxygen by rapidly grown tumor cells. For the survival of tumor cells, some metabolic adaptations occur.

- They begin to grow in hypoxic (absence of oxygen) condition.

- Under these conditions glucose is oxidized anaerobically to **lactic acid** and this pathway becomes primary source of ATP for tumor cells.
- Thus fast growing cancer cells, leads to **lactic acidosis**.

METABOLIC FATES OF PYRUVATE AND ASSOCIATED DISORDERS

During aerobic glycolysis glucose is converted to pyruvate. Pyruvate is also formed in degradation of amino acids and has several fates depending on the tissue and its metabolic state. It can be converted to **acetyl-CoA**, **lactate**, **alanine**, or **oxaloacetate** depending on the needs of the cell. The fates of pyruvate and types of reactions in which it participates are given in **Figure 10.11**.

1. **Conversion into acetyl-CoA:** Pyruvate is oxidized, with loss of its carboxyl group as CO_2 to yield **acetyl-CoA**.
2. **Conversion into lactate in muscle and RBC (Anaerobic glycolysis (Figure 10.7):** Pyruvate is reduced to **lactate**. Certain tissues and cell types (retina and erythrocytes for example) convert glucose to lactate even under aerobic conditions.
3. **Conversion into alanine, or oxaloacetate:** The oxidation of pyruvate is an important catabolic process, but pyruvate has anabolic fates as well. It can provide the carbon skeleton for the synthesis of the amino acid **alanine** or **oxaloacetate**.

Conversion of Pyruvate into Acetyl-CoA

Pyruvate formed in **cytosol** by glycolysis, is transported into the **mitochondrion** by a specific carrier protein present in the mitochondrial membrane. Inside the mitochondria, it is **oxidatively decarboxylated** to **acetyl-CoA** by a multienzyme complex, **pyruvate dehydrogenase**. Pyruvate dehydrogenase is a large complex of **three distinct enzymes** and **five coenzymes (Table 10.4)**.

- In this reaction, the **carboxyl group** is removed from pyruvate as a molecule of CO_2 and the two remaining carbons become the acetyl group of **acetyl-CoA** with the generation of a molecule of **NADH (Figure 10.12)**.

TABLE 10.4: Enzymes, coenzymes and vitamins required for pyruvate dehydrogenase complex.

Enzymes	• Pyruvate dehydrogenase • Dihydrolipoyl transacetylase • Dihydrolipoyl dehydrogenase
Coenzymes	• Thiamine pyrophosphate (TPP) • Flavin adenine dinucleotide (FAD) • Coenzyme A (Co-A or denoted as CoA-SH) • Nicotinamide adenine dinucleotide (NAD⁺) • Lipoamide (Lipoic acid)
Vitamins	• Thiamine (in TPP) • Riboflavin (in FAD) • Niacin (in NAD⁺) • Pantothenic acid (in CoA)

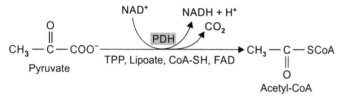

Figure 10.12: Oxidative decarboxylation of pyruvate by the pyruvate dehydrogenase complex.

- The transfer of electrons from NADH to oxygen ultimately generates **2.5 molecules of ATP** per molecule of pyruvate.
- Pyruvate dehydrogenase is regulated by **feedback inhibition**. Pyruvate dehydrogenase is inhibited by its product **acetyl-CoA** and **NADH**.
- It is also regulated by **phosphorylation** and **dephosphorylation** (covalent modification) of pyruvate dehydrogenase multienzyme complex. By phosphorylation active pyruvate dehydrogenase enzyme is converted to its inactive form.

❖ Lipoic acid is an organosulfur compound synthesized by humans and plants in mitochondria from octanoic acid and cysteine and is essential for aerobic metabolism.
❖ α- Lipoic acid is found in small amounts in spinach, broccoli, peas, and potatoes.
❖ It acts as a cofactor for **pyruvate dehydrogenase** and **α-ketoglutarate dehydrogenase** activity.

Significance of Pyruvate to Acetyl-CoA Pathway

- The conversion of pyruvate to acetyl-CoA is a central step, linking the glycolytic pathway with citric acid cycle **(Figure 10.13)** hence called **link reaction**.
- Acetyl-CoA is also an important intermediate in lipid metabolism, cholesterol biosynthesis and acetylation reactions.
- Different metabolic sources and fates of acetyl-CoA are shown in **Figure 10.14**.
- Fates of acetyl-CoA generated in the mitochondrial matrix include:
  1. Complete oxidation of the acetyl group in the TCA cycle for energy generation.

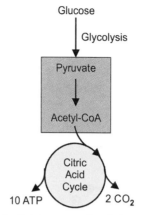

Figure 10.13: The link between glycolysis and final common pathway citric acid.

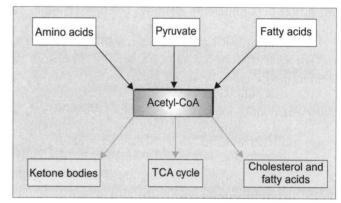

Figure 10.14: Metabolic fates of acetyl-CoA.

2. In liver, conversion of excess acetyl-CoA into the ketone bodies, acetoacetate, and β-hydroxybutyrate.
3. Transfer of acetyl units as citrate to the cytosol for the synthesis of long chain fatty acids and cholesterol.

Abnormalities of Pyruvate Dehydrogenase Activity

- **Thiamine deficiency** causes decreased pyruvate oxidation leading to accumulation of pyruvate and lactates in blood and brain and is accompanied by impairment of cardiovascular, nervous and gastrointestinal systems. Thiamine in the form of **thiamine pyrophosphate (TPP)** acts as a coenzyme of **PDH** as well as for **transketolase** activity in **pentose phosphate pathway**. Deficiency of TPP inhibits PDH enzyme as a result pyruvate is unable to oxidize normally to acetyl-CoA and pyruvate is converted to lactate, leading to **lactic acidosis** and **neurological disorders**.
- Many alcoholics are thiamine deficient because alcohol inhibits the transport of thiamine through the intestinal mucosal cells as well as much of their dietary intake consists of vitamin free "empty calories" of alcohol.
- **Inherited deficiency of PDH** is accompanied by **lactic acidemia** and **abnormalities of nervous system**, e.g., ataxia and psychomotor retardation. Nervous system

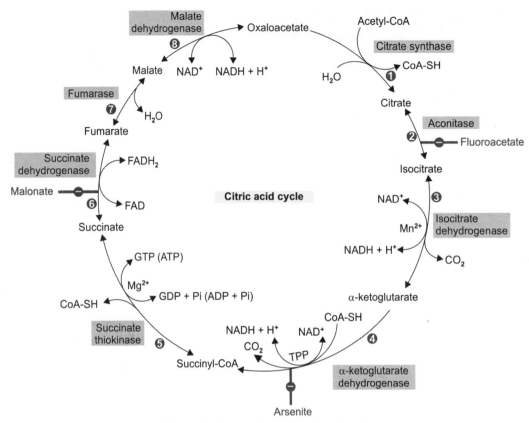

Figure 10.15: Reactions of citric acid cycle.

abnormalities may be due to diminished synthesis of neurotransmitters rather than to inadequate synthesis of ATP. In pyruvate dehydrogenase complex deficiency, diminished levels of acetyl-CoA cause decreased production of **acetylcholine.** Ketogenic diets have been beneficial in pyruvate dehydrogenase complex deficiency, since they provide the product of the deficient reaction, i.e., acetyl-CoA. Administration of large doses of thiamine may be of benefit because mutations of pyruvate dehydrogenase complex may give rise to decreased affinity for thiamin pyrophosphate (TPP).

- **The toxicity of arsenate and mercuric ions** is due to their ability to bind functional –SH groups of pyruvate dehydrogenase complex and may develop lactic acidosis. In earlier times arsenicals were used in the treatment of syphilis, however due to their toxicity it has been replaced with better drugs such as penicillin.

CITRIC ACID CYCLE: PATHWAY, ENERGETICS, REGULATION AND SIGNIFICANCE

The citric acid cycle is the final common pathway for the oxidation of fuel molecules; **carbohydrates, fatty acids,** and **amino acids.** Most fuel molecules enter the cycle as **acetyl coenzyme A.** In eukaryotes, the reactions of citric acid cycle take place in the matrix of the mitochondria in contrast with those of glycolysis, which take place in cytoplasm.

- The citric acid cycle is a series of reactions in mitochondria that bring about the catabolism of **acetyl-CoA** to CO_2 and H_2O, liberating reducing equivalents, which, upon oxidation through respiratory chain of mitochondria, generate **ATP.**
- Citric acid cycle is also called **Krebs cycle** or **Tricarboxylic Acid Cycle (TCA):**
  - It is called **citric acid cycle** because citrate was one of the first compounds known to participate.
  - It is called **Krebs cycle,** because its reaction was formulated into a cycle by **Sir Hans Krebs.**
  - The most common name for this pathway is the **Tricarboxylic acid cycle** or **TCA cycle,** due to involvement of the tricarboxylate **citrate** and **isocitrate.**

Location of Citric Acid Cycle

The enzymes of citric acid cycle are located in the **mitochondrial matrix,** which facilitates the transfer of reducing equivalents to the respiratory chain, situated in the inner mitochondrial membrane.

Reactions of Citric Acid Cycle

The citric acid cycle has **eigh**t steps **(Figure 10.15).**

1. **Formation of citrate:** The first reaction of cycle is the condensation of acetyl-CoA with oxaloacetate to yield citrate, catalyzed by **citrate synthase.**

2. **Formation of isocitrate via cis-aconitate:** Citrate is converted to isocitrate through the intermediary formation of the tricarboxylic acid **cis-aconitate** by an enzyme **aconitase** (aconitate hydratase), which contains iron in the Fe^{2+} state. This conversion takes place in two steps, dehydration to cis-aconitate, and rehydration to isocitrate. The reaction is inhibited by **fluoroacetate**.

3. **Oxidation of isocitrate to α-ketoglutarate and CO_2:** Isocitrate undergoes oxidative decarboxylation catalyzed by **isocitrate dehydrogenase** to form α-ketoglutarate. The formation of **NADH** and liberation of CO_2 occurs at this stage.

4. **Oxidation of α-ketoglutarate to succinyl-CoA and CO_2:** The next step is another oxidative decarboxylation in which α-ketoglutarate is converted to succinyl-CoA and CO_2 catalyzed by a multienzyme system, **α-ketoglutarate dehydrogenase**, similar to that described for the conversion of pyruvate to acetyl-CoA.
   - α-ketoglutarate dehydrogenase complex also requires identical cofactors to that of pyruvate dehydrogenase complex, e.g., thiamine pyrophosphate (TPP), lipoate, NAD, FAD and coenzyme A. The energy of oxidation of α-ketoglutarate is conserved in the formation of thioester (a high energy bond of succinyl-CoA.
   - This reaction is physiologically **irreversible**.
   - At this stage **second NADH is produced** along with **liberation of second CO_2 molecule**.

5. **Conversion of succinyl-CoA to succinate:** Succinyl-CoA is converted to succinate by the enzyme **succinate thiokinase** (succinyl-CoA synthetase). The energy conserved from the previous step in the succinyl-CoA as the thioester bond is now liberated in the form of **GTP** or **ATP**. The GTP can donate its terminal phosphoryl group to ADP to form ATP. This is the only example in citric acid cycle of generation of ATP at the **substrate level**.

Isoenzymes of Succinate Thiokinase: One Specific for ADP and the other for GDP

- Tissues in which gluconeogenesis occurs (the liver and the kidney) contains two isoenzymes of succinate thiokinase; one specific for ADP and the other for GDP.
- The GTP formed is used for the decarboxylation of oxaloacetate to phosphoenolpyruvate in gluconeogenesis, and provides a regulatory link between citric acid cycle activity and the withdrawal of oxaloacetate for gluconeogenesis.
- Nongluconeogenic tissues have only the isoenzyme that uses ADP.
- ATP and GTP are energetically equivalent.

---

6. **Oxidation of succinate to fumarate:** Succinate formed from succinyl-CoA is metabolized further by flavoprotein enzyme, **succinate dehydrogenase**, catalyzes a reversible dehydrogenation of succinate to fumarate.
   - This enzyme contains three different iron-sulfur clusters and one molecule of FAD.
   - The reaction results in the production of $FADH_2$.

7. **Hydration of fumarate to malate:** Next **fumarase** catalyzes the addition of water to fumarate to give L-malate. Malate is freely permeable to the mitochondrial membrane.

8. **Oxidation of malate to oxaloacetate:** Malate is converted to oxaloacetate by **malate dehydrogenase**, and requires NAD^+.
   - **The third synthesis of NADH occurs at this stage**.
   - The oxaloacetate is regenerated which can combine with another molecule of acetyl-CoA and continue the cycle.

Genetic defect in the fumarase gene lead to tumors of smooth muscle (leiomyoma) and kidney. Mutations in succinate dehydrogenase lead to tumors of the adrenal gland (pheochromocytomas).

Poisons that Inhibit Enzymes of TCA Cycle

- ❖ **Arsenite and mercuric ions** inhibit pyruvate dehydrogenase enzyme by reacting with the functional –SH groups of the enzyme and may develop lactic acidosis.
- ❖ *Fluoroacetate:* Inhibit aconitase
- ❖ *Arsenite:* Inhibit α-ketoglutarate dehydrogenase system
- ❖ *Malonate:* Inhibit succinate dehydrogenase

Generation of ATP in Citric Acid Cycle per Turn

- As a result of oxidation of acetyl-CoA to H_2O and CO_2 by citric acid cycle **three molecules of NADH** and **one $FADH_2$** are produced for each molecule of acetyl-CoA catabolized in one turn of the cycle. These reducing equivalents are transferred to respiratory chain in the inner mitochondrial membrane:
  - During passage along the chain three molecules of NADH generate **3×2.5 ATP = 7.5 ATP**.
  - However $FADH_2$ generate **1.5 ATP** molecules.
- One molecule of ATP is generated at **substrate level** during the conversion of succinyl-CoA to succinate.
- Thus, **10 ATP** molecules are generated for each turn of the cycle **(Table 10.5)**.

Significance of Citric Acid Cycle

- The primary function of the citric acid cycle is to provide energy in the form of **ATP**.
- Citric acid cycle provides substrate for the respiratory chain. During the course of oxidation of acetyl-CoA in the cycle, reducing equivalents are formed; these then enter the respiratory chain where ATPs are generated in the process of oxidative phosphorylation.
- Citric acid cycle is the final common pathway for the oxidation of **carbohydrate**, **lipids**, and **protein** as glucose, fatty acids and many amino acids are all metabolized to acetyl-CoA or intermediates of the cycle.

TABLE 10.5: Production of ATP in TCA cycle per turn.

Reaction	Reaction catalyzed by	Mechanism of ATP production	No. of ATP formed
Isocitrate to α-ketoglutarate	Isocitrate dehydrogenase	NADH: Respiratory chain oxidation of	+2.5
α-ketoglutarate to succinyl-CoA	α-ketoglutarate dehydrogenase	NADH: Respiratory chain oxidation of	+2.5
Succinyl-CoA to succinate	Succinyl thiokinase	Substrate level phosphorylation	+1
Succinate to fumarate	Succinate dehydrogenase	FADH$_2$: Respiratory chain oxidation of	+1.5
Malate to oxaloacetate	Malate dehydrogenase	NADH: Respiratory chain oxidation of	+2.5
			Net 10

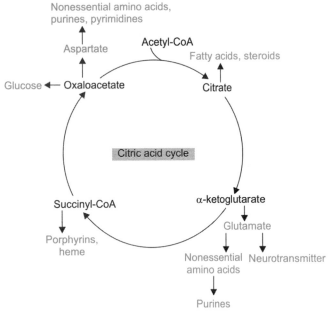

Figure 10.16: Anabolic role of the citric acid cycle.

- Citric acid cycle is an **amphibolic pathway**, i.e., it plays roles in both oxidative (catabolic) and synthetic (anabolic) processes **(Figure 10.16)**. Some metabolic pathways end in the constituent of the citric acid cycle while other pathways originate from the cycle, e.g.,
  - Gluconeogenesis
  - Transamination
  - Fatty acid synthesis
  - Porphyrin synthesis.
- All major members of the citric acid cycle from citrate to oxaloacetate are glucogenic. They can give rise to glucose in the liver or kidney, the organs that contain a set of enzymes necessary for gluconeogenesis.
- Aminotransferase (transaminase) reactions produce:
  - Pyruvate from alanine
  - Oxaloacetate from aspartate
  - α-ketoglutarate from glutamate.
  As these reactions are reversible the intermediates of the cycle also serves as a source of carbon skeleton for the synthesis of nonessential amino acid.
- Acetyl-CoA is the precursor for the synthesis of **long-chain fatty acids**. Since formation of acetyl-CoA in the mitochondria and the enzymes responsible for fatty

acid synthesis are extramitochondrial, the cell needs to transport acetyl-CoA through the mitochondrial membrane which is impermeable to acetyl-CoA. This is accomplished by allowing acetyl-CoA to form citrate in citric acid cycle; transporting citrate out of the mitochondria and making acetyl-CoA available in the cytosol by cleaving citrate into acetyl-CoA and oxaloacetate (*see* **Figure 11.31**).

- **Succinyl-CoA** together with **glycine** is a substrate for the biosynthesis of porphyrins and therefore essential in the production of **hemoglobin**, **cytochromes** and other **heme proteins**.

Regulation of Citric Acid Cycle

- The rate of citric acid cycle is specifically regulated to meet cell's needs for ATP. The cycle is regulated primarily by the concentration of **ATP** and **NADH**.
  - High ratios of ATP/ADP, acetyl-CoA/CoA and NADH/NAD⁺ will serve as signals to inhibit the cycle.
  - An excess of ATP, NADH and acetyl-CoA occurs when energy supply is sufficient for the cell.
  - As energy is used, the ratio of ATP/ADP declines and the inhibition of the cycle is relieved.
- The primary control points are the allosteric enzymes **isocitrate dehydrogenase** and α-**ketoglutarate dehydrogenase (Figure 10.17)**.
  - The enzyme isocitrate dehydrogenase, the first control site is allosterically stimulated by **ADP**, which enhances the enzyme's affinity for substrate. In contrast, **ATP** and **NADH** inhibit the enzyme.
  - A second control site is α-**ketoglutarate dehydrogenase** which is inhibited by **ATP**, **succinyl-CoA** and **NADH**, the product of the reaction that it catalyzes. Thus, the rate of the cycle is reduced when the cell has a high level of ATP.
- In a tissue such as **brain**, which is largely dependent on carbohydrate to supply acetyl-CoA, control of the citric acid cycle may occur at **pyruvate dehydrogenase** which is inhibited by **ATP**, **acetyl-CoA** and **NADH** and stimulated by **ADP** and **pyruvate**.
- All these dehydrogenases are activated by Ca²⁺ which increases in concentration during contraction of muscles and secretion by other tissues, when there is increased energy demand.

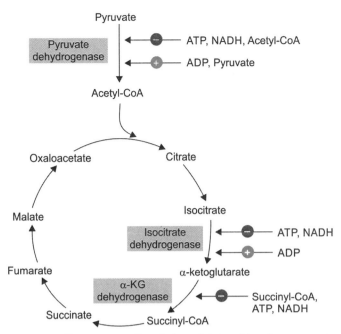

Figure 10.17: Regulation of citric acid cycle.

> **Isocitrate dehydrogenase** and **α-ketoglutarate dehydrogenase** integrates the citric acid cycle with other pathways. For example:
> ❖ The inhibition of **isocitrate dehydrogenase** leads to an accumulation of citrate. Citrate can be transported to the cytoplasm, where it signals **phosphofructokinase** to stop glycolysis and where citrate can serve as a source of acetyl-CoA for fatty acid synthesis.
> ❖ The **α-ketoglutarate** that accumulates when **α-ketoglutarate dehydrogenase** is inhibited can be used as a precursor for the synthesis of several amino acids and the purine bases.

Role of Vitamins in Citric Acid Cycle

Four water-soluble vitamins of B-complex have a specific role in the functioning of the citric acid cycle **(Table 10.6)**.

Amphibolic Nature of Citric Acid Cycle

Citric acid cycle has a dual function; it functions in both catabolism (of carbohydrates, fatty acids and amino acids) and anabolism **(Figure 10.16)**. It provides intermediates

TABLE 10.6: Vitamin B-complex involved in citric acid cycle.		
Vitamin	**Coenzyme form**	**Coenzyme for**
Riboflavin	FAD	α-ketoglutarate dehydrogenase and succinate dehydrogenase
Niacin	NAD⁺	Isocitrate dehydrogenase, α-ketoglutarate dehydrogenase, and malate dehydrogenase
Thiamine	TPP	α-ketoglutarate dehydrogenase (for decarboxylation)
Pantothenic acid	Coenzyme-A	A cofactor attached to active carboxylic acid residues such as acetyl-CoA and succinyl-CoA

for the biosynthesis of many compound required for the body, for example, most of the carbon atoms in porphyrins come from succinyl-CoA. Many of amino acids are derived from α-**ketoglutarate** and **oxaloacetate** and hence the cycle is said to be an amphibolic (Greek amphi, "both").

Anaplerotic Reactions

Certain intermediates of the citric acid cycle (particularly α-ketoglutarate, succinate and oxaloacetate) can be removed from the cycle to serve as precursors of many compounds needed by the body, e.g.,

- Succinate is removed for heme or porphyrin synthesis.
- In nervous tissue α-ketoglutarate is removed for the formation of glutamate and then to γ-aminobutyric acid (GABA), a neurotransmitter.
- Many of the amino acids are derived from α-ketoglutarate and oxaloacetate.

When this happens, the rate of citric acid cycle would be expected to decline because the drain of its intermediates would result in lowering their concentration in the cell. However, the intermediates of the citric acid cycle can be replenished again by the action of another enzymatic reaction. The special enzymatic reactions by which the pool of citric acid cycle intermediate can be replenished are called **anaplerotic** (of Greek origin, meaning to fill up) **reactions**. When the citric acid cycle is deficient in oxaloacetate or any other intermediates, following anaplerotic reactions occurs **(Figure 10.18)**.

1. One of the major anaplerotic reactions is the conversion of **pyruvate** and **CO₂** to **oxaloacetate** by **pyruvate carboxylase**, which requires biotin, ATP and Mg²⁺.

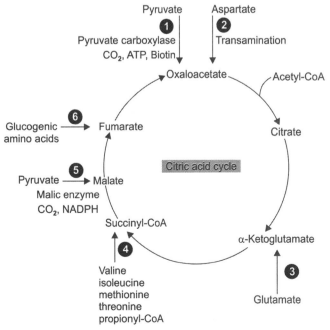

Figure 10.18: Major anaplerotic pathways of citric acid cycle.

2. **Transamination of aspartate** and **glutamate** to produce oxaloacetate and α-ketoglutarate respectively.
3. **Deamination of glutamate** by **glutamate dehydrogenase** in which glutamate is reversibly converted to α-ketoglutarate.
4. Formation of succinyl-CoA from carbon skeletons of amino acids valine, isoleucine, methionine and threonine and odd chain fatty acid propionyl-CoA.
5. A cytoplasmic enzyme, **malic enzyme**, also converts pyruvate to malate, which can then enter the mitochondria as a substrate for the citric acid cycle.
6. Other glucogenic amino acids are also degraded to fumarate and oxaloacetate

Significance of Anaplerotic Reactions

Under normal circumstances the reactions by which the cycle intermediates are drained away and those by which they are replenished are in dynamic balance, so that the concentrations of the citric acid cycle intermediates in mitochondria usually remain relatively constant.

GLUCONEOGENESIS: PATHWAY, REGULATION AND SIGNIFICANCE

The formation of glucose or glycogen from noncarbohydrate precursors is called **gluconeogenesis** (i.e., synthesis of new glucose). The major noncarbohydrate substrates for gluconeogenesis are **(Figure 10.19)**:

- Lactate
- Glycerol
- Glucogenic amino acids
- Propionate
- Intermediates of the citric acid cycle

- **Lactate** produced by anaerobic glycolysis after vigorous exercise in skeletal muscle and oxidation of glucose by erythrocytes is transported to the liver where it is converted to glucose and moves back to muscle via circulation for oxidation in the tissue. This cycling of lactate between muscle and liver is known as the **Cori cycle** or **lactic acid cycle (Figure 10.20)**.

> In vigorously contracting skeletal muscle, the rate of glycolysis far exceeds that of citric acid cycle, and much of the pyruvate formed is reduced to lactate which flows to the liver where it is converted into glucose by Cori cycle. Cori cycle shifts part of the metabolic burden of muscle to the liver.

- **Glycerol** is released during hydrolysis of triacylglycerol in adipose tissue, which cannot be utilized by adipose tissue due to poor content of enzyme **glycerol kinase**. Therefore, it diffuses out into the blood and is delivered to the liver and kidney, where it is used solely as a substrate for gluconeogenesis **(Figure 10.21)**.
- **Amino acids** are derived from proteins in the diet and during starvation from the breakdown of proteins in

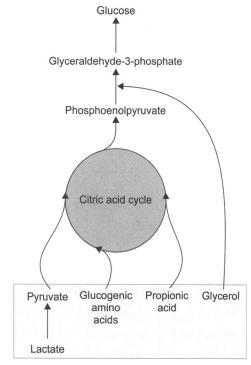

Figure 10.19: Major noncarbohydrate substrates and their entry points into gluconeogenesis.

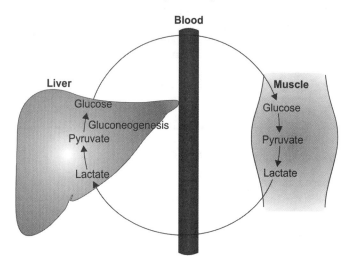

Figure 10.20: Pathway of Cori cycle or Lactic acid cycle.

skeletal muscle. Alanine is the predominant amino acid released from muscle to liver during fasting by **glucose-alanine cycle (Figure 10.22)**. As muscle is incapable of synthesizing urea, most of the ammonia formed by protein catabolism is transferred to pyruvate to form **alanine** by transamination reaction.

- Alanine enters the blood and is taken up by the liver. In the liver, the amino group of alanine is removed by transamination and the resulting pyruvate is converted to glucose by gluconeogenesis which is then transported to the muscle, where it is oxidized to pyruvate. The pyruvate acts again as the acceptor for another amino group. These reactions transport amino groups from muscle to the liver in the form

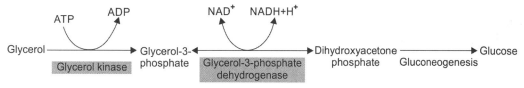

Figures 10.21: Conversion of glycerol to dihydroxyacetone phosphate.

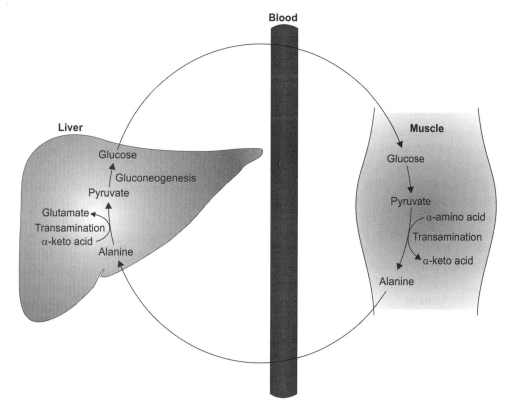

Figure 10.22: Glucose alanine cycle or Cahill cycle.

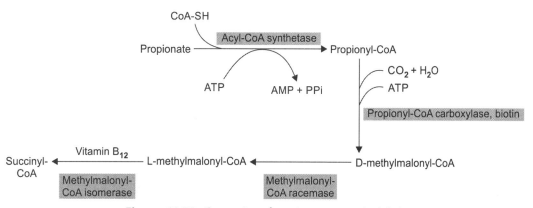

Figures 10.23: Conversion of propionate to succinyl-CoA.

of **alanine**. This cycle is called the **glucose-alanine cycle** or **Cahill cycle (Figure 10.22)**.

- In addition to alanine, **glutamine** is another important amino acid released from muscle to the blood and taken up by the kidneys and the intestine. In this case ammonium ions are coupled with **glutamate** to yield **glutamine**.
- In addition to alanine, many other amino acids are converted to **pyruvate or citric acid cycle intermediates**, which are metabolized to oxaloacetate, an intermediate of gluconeogenesis.

- **Fatty acids** with an odd number of carbons and carbon skeleton of some amino acids produce **propionyl-CoA**. These are minor precursors of gluconeogenesis in humans. Propionate enters the main gluconeogenic pathway via citric acid cycle after conversion of succinyl-CoA **(Figure 10.23)**.

Why Conversion of Acetyl-CoA to Glucose is not Possible in Human Being?

❖ The pyruvate dehydrogenase reaction is essentially nonreversible which prevents the direct conversion of acetyl-CoA to pyruvate.

❖ Secondly, there cannot be a net conversion of acetyl-CoA to oxaloacetate via citric acid cycle, since one molecule of oxaloacetate is consumed to condense with acetyl-CoA and only one molecule of oxaloacetate is regenerated (*see* **Figure 10.15**), which is not formed denova (new) when acetyl-CoA is oxidized by citric acid cycle.

Site of Gluconeogenesis

Gluconeogenesis takes place mainly in the **liver** and to a lesser extent in **kidney (renal cortex)** and in the epithelial cells that line the inside of the **small intestine**. Enzymes catalyzing the reactions of gluconeogenesis are distributed between the **mitochondria** and the **cytoplasm**.

The kidney contributes up to 40% of total glucose synthesis in fasting state and more in starvation. The key gluconeogenic enzymes are expressed in the small intestine, but it is unclear whether or not there is significant glucose production by the intestine in the fasting state.

Characteristics of Gluconeogenesis

- Gluconeogenesis involves **glycolysis**, the **citric acid cycle** plus some **special reactions**.
- **Glycolysis** and **gluconeogenesis** share the same pathway but are not identical pathways, running in opposite directions.
- Seven of the ten reactions of gluconeogenesis are reverse of glycolytic reactions. However, three reactions of glycolysis are essentially irreversible and cannot be used in gluconeogenesis. These are:
  - Conversion of phosphoenolpyruvate to pyruvate by **pyruvate kinase**
  - Phosphorylation of fructose 6-phosphate to fructose 1,6-bisphosphate by **phosphofructokinase-1.**
  - Conversion of glucose to glucose-6-phosphate by **hexokinase.**
- In gluconeogenesis, the irreversible steps are bypassed by a separate set of enzymes which are:
  - Pyruvate carboxylase and phosphoenolpyruvate carboxykinase
  - Fructose-1,6-bisphosphatase
  - Glucose-6-phosphatase.

Reactions of Gluconeogenesis

We begin by considering the three bypass reactions of gluconeogenesis (irreversible bypass glycolytic reactions) **(Figure 10.24)**.

1. **Conversion of pyruvate to p hosphoenolpyruvate:** The first of the bypass reactions in gluconeogenesis is the conversion of **pyruvate** to **phosphoenolpyruvate**. This reaction cannot occur by simple reversal of the pyruvate kinase reaction of glycolysis which is irreversible under physiological conditions. Conversion of pyruvate to phosphoenolpyruvate requires two special reactions:

   - **Carboxylation of pyruvate to oxaloacetate:** Pyruvate is first transported from the cytosol into mitochondria. Then **pyruvate carboxylase**, a mitochondrial enzyme in presence of ATP, coenzyme **biotin** and CO_2 converts pyruvate to **oxaloacetate** in mitochondria. **Pyruvate carboxylase** is the first regulatory enzyme in gluconeogenic pathway requiring acetyl-CoA as a positive effector. Oxaloacetate, formed in mitochondria, must enter the cytosol, where the other enzymes of gluconeogenesis are located. However, as oxaloacetate is unable to cross the inner mitochondrial membrane directly, it must be reduced to malate by mitochondrial **malate dehydrogenase**, at the expense of **NADH**, which can be transported from the mitochondria to the cytosol. In the cytosol, malate is reoxidized to oxaloacetate with the production of cytosolic NADH.

   - **Decarboxylation of cytosolic oxaloacetate to phosphoenol pyruvate (PEP):** Oxaloacetate is then decarboxylated to phosphoenolpyruvate (PEP) in the cytosol by **phosphoenolpyruvate carboxykinase**. High energy phosphate in the form of **GTP** is required in this reaction. PEP then enters the reversed reaction of glycolysis until it reaches fructose-1,6-bisphosphate.

2. **Conversion of fructose-1,6-bisphosphate to fructose-6-phosphate:** The second glycolytic reaction that cannot participate in gluconeogenesis is the phosphorylation of fructose-6-phosphate by phosphofructokinase-1, because this reaction is irreversible. The formation of fructose-6-phosphate from fructose-1,6-bisphosphate is catalyzed by fructose-1,6-bisphosphatase (FBPase). **Fructose-1,6-bisphosphatase is an allosteric enzyme which is the major regulatory enzyme in gluconeogenesis**.

3. **Conversion of glucose-6-phosphate to glucose:** Hydrolysis of glucose-6-phosphate to glucose by **glucose-6-phosphatase** is the third and final bypass reaction of **gluconeogenesis**. It bypasses the irreversible hexokinase reaction of glycolysis. Glucose-6-phosphatase is found in liver and kidney but not in other tissues. Thus, glucose produced by gluconeogenesis in liver and kidney is provided to other tissues. Muscle cannot provide blood glucose by gluconeogenesis due to lack of enzyme **glucose-6-phosphatase**.

Energetics of Gluconeogenesis

- Gluconeogenesis is energetically expensive process. For each molecule of glucose formed from pyruvate, **six high energy phosphate** groups are required.

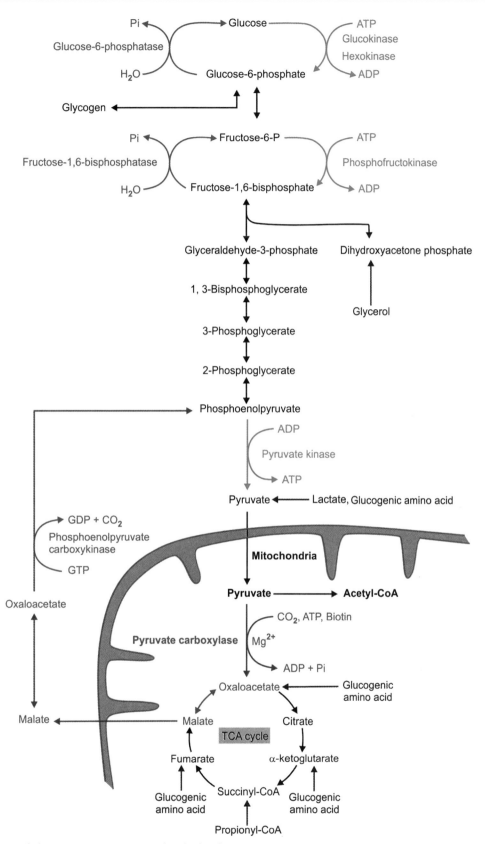

Figure 10.24: Pathway of gluconeogenesis compared with glycolysis:

- Special reactions and enzymes of gluconeogenic pathway are shown in red.
- Irreversible reactions of glycolysis are shown in green.
- Remaining reactions which are common to glycolysis and gluconeogenesis are shown in black.
- The entry points of substrate are shown in blue.

- ■ Four from ATP
- ■ Two from GTP
- ■ In addition two molecules of NADH are required for the reduction of two molecules of 1,3-bisphospho-glycerate.
- ● Conversion glucose to pyruvate by glycolysis would require only two molecules of ATP.

Regulation of Gluconeogenesis

As glycolysis and gluconeogenesis share the same pathway but in opposite direction, they are regulated reciprocally. Glycolysis and gluconeogenesis are coordinated so that, within a cell, one pathway is relatively inactive while the other is highly active **(Figure 10.25)**. The basic principle of reciprocal regulation is that:

1. When energy is needed glycolysis will predominate.
2. When there is a surplus of precursors, gluconeogenesis will take place.
3. Glucose precursors will be surplus in presence of **glucagon** and **epinephrine**

- ● Gluconeogenesis is regulated by four key enzymes. The four key enzymes are:
  1. Pyruvate carboxylase
  2. Phosphoenolpyruvate carboxykinase
  3. Fructose-1,6-bisphosphatase
  4. Glucose-6-phosphatase.
- ● The first important regulation site is the interconversion of fructose-1,6-bisphosphate to fructose-6-phosphate:
  - ■ High levels of ATP and citrate indicates that the energy is high. ATP and citrate inhibit phospho-fructokinase, whereas citrate activates fructose-1,6-

bisphosphatase. Under these conditions, glycolysis is nearly inhibited and gluconeogenesis is promoted.
  - ■ AMP stimulates phosphofructokinase of glycolysis but inhibits fructose-1,6-bisphosphatase of gluconeogenesis. Thus, when glycolysis is turned on gluconeogenesis is inhibited.
  - ■ Fructose-2,6-bisphosphate strongly stimulates phosphofructokinase and inhibits fructose-1,6-bisphosphatase
- ● The second regulation site is the interconversion of pyruvate to phosphoenolpyruvate:
  - ■ Pyruvate carboxylase, which catalyzes the first step in gluconeogenesis from pyruvate, is inhibited by ADP. Likewise ADP inhibits phosphoenolpyruvate carboxykinase.
  - ■ Pyruvate carboxylase is activated by acetyl-CoA, which like citrate, indicates that the citric acid cycle is producing energy.
- ● The hormones **glucagon** and **insulin** have long-term effects on hepatic glycolysis and gluconeogenesis by **induction** and **repression** of key enzymes of both pathways.
  - ■ Glucagon stimulates gluconeogenesis by inducing the synthesis of the key enzymes, **phosphoenolpyruvate carboxykinase**, **fructose-1,6-bisphosphatase**, and **glucose-6-phosphatase**.
  - ■ **Insulin** inhibits the gluconeogenesis by repressing the synthesis of the key enzymes.
- ● During starvation and in diabetes mellitus, a high level of glucagon stimulates gluconeogenesis. However, in well-fed state, insulin suppresses the gluconeogenesis.

Significance of Gluconeogenesis

- ● Gluconeogenesis occurs primarily in the liver, where its role is to provide glucose to other tissues when glycogen stores are exhausted and when no dietary glucose is available. Liver glycogen stores can meet these needs for only **8–12 hours** in the absence of dietary intake of carbohydrate. As the glycogen store starts depleting, gluconeogenesis takes place, which ensure a continuous supply of glucose to the brain and other tissues.
- ● Gluconeogenesis provides glucose to some tissues such as the brain, erythrocytes, lens, and cornea of the eye and kidney medulla which require a continuous supply of glucose as a source of energy.
- ● Gluconeogenic mechanisms are used to clear the products of the metabolism of other tissues from the blood, e.g.,
  - ■ Lactate, produced by muscle and erythrocytes
  - ■ Glycerol produced by adipose tissue
  - ■ Propionyl-CoA produced by oxidation of odd carbon number fatty acids and carbon skeleton of some amino acids.

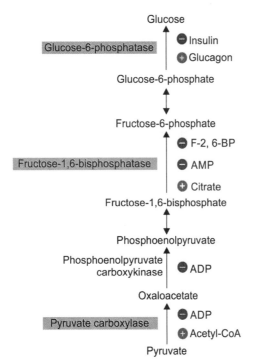

Figure 10.25: Regulation of gluconeogenesis.

GLYCOGEN METABOLISM: PATHWAY, SIGNIFICANCE, REGULATION AND ASSOCIATED DISORDERS

Glycogen is the major readily mobilized storage form of **glucose** mainly in the **liver** and **skeletal muscle**, although most of the cells may store minute amounts. Glycogen is a very large, branched polymer of glucose residues that can be broken down to yield glucose molecules when energy is needed. A glycogen molecule contains approximately **55000 glucose** residues. Most of the glucose residues in glycogen are linked by α-**1,4 glycosidic bonds**. Branches at about every 12 residues are created by α-**1,6 glycosidic bonds**.

- The concentration of liver glycogen is greater than in muscle (10% versus 2% by weight). However, because muscle tissue comprises a large mass, its total capacity to storage is four to five times that of the liver.
- Liver glycogen serves as a reservoir of glucose for other tissues when dietary glucose is not available (between meals or during fast); this is especially important for the brain, which cannot use fatty acids as fuel, except during prolonged starvation. Liver glycogen can be depleted in 8–12 hours.
- In contrast in muscle, glycogen provides a quick source of energy for either aerobic or anaerobic metabolism to meet the needs of the muscle itself. Muscle glycogen can be exhausted in less than an hour during vigorous activity.
- The synthesis, **glycogenesis** and degradation, **glycogenolysis** occurs by different pathways **(Figure 10.26)** thereby allowing each pathway to operate independently of the other.
- Glycogenesis and glycogenolysis are both **cytosolic** processes.

Why Store Glucose as Glycogen?

Glucose cannot be stored because high concentrations of glucose disrupt the osmotic balance of the cell, which would cause cell damage or death. Glucose is stored in its polymeric form, the **glycogen** which is not osmotically active.

Why not Store our Excess Glucose Calories Entirely as Fat Instead of Glycogen?

❖ Fat cannot be mobilized as rapid as glycogen
❖ Fat cannot be used as a source of energy in the absence of oxygen. As it cannot be catabolized anaerobically.
❖ Fat cannot be converted to glucose to maintain blood glucose levels required by the brain.

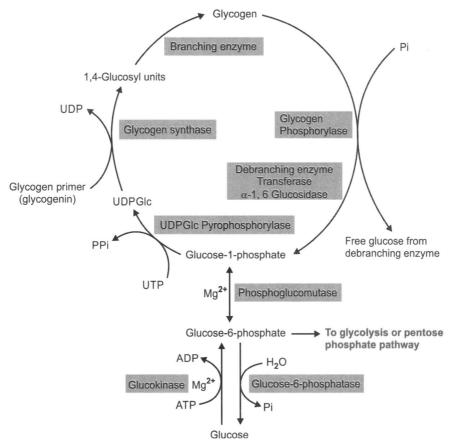

Figure 10.26: Pathway of glycogenesis and glycogenolysis in liver.
(UTP: Uridine triphosphate; UDP: Uridine diphosphate; UDPGlc: Uridine diphosphate glucose)

Glycogenesis

Glycogenesis is the pathway for the formation of **glycogen** from glucose. Glycogenesis is a **cytosolic** process occurs in muscle and in liver when glucose is abundant. With modest amount it occurs in **brain** also.

Glycogen is synthesized by a pathway that utilizes **uridine diphosphate glucose (UDP-glucose)** as the activated glucose donor.

Reactions of Glycogenesis

1. Glucose is phosphorylated to glucose-6-phosphate catalyzed by **hexokinase** in muscle and **glucokinase** in liver.
2. Glucose-6-phosphate is converted to glucose-1-phosphate by the enzyme **phosphoglucomutase**.
3. Glucose-1-phosphate reacts with uridine triphosphate (UTP) to form **uridine diphosphate glucose (UDP-Glu)**. The reaction is catalyzed by the enzyme **UDP-glucose pyrophosphorylase**. Pyrophosphate (PPi), the second product of the reaction, is hydrolyzed to two inorganic phosphates (Pi) by pyrophosphatase.
4. By the action of the enzyme **glycogen synthase** the C_1 of the activated glucose of UDP-Glu forms a glycosidic bond with C_4 of a terminal glucose residue of **pre-existing glycogen molecule (glycogen primer, called glycogenin)**, liberating uridine diphosphate (UDP). Thus, pre-existing glycogen molecule must be present to initiate this reaction.
5. In the above reaction, a new α-1,4 linkage is established between carbon atom one of incoming glucose and carbon 4 of the terminal glucose of a glycogen primer **(Figure 10.27)**.
6. Glycogen synthase catalyzes only the synthesis of α-1,4 linkages. It cannot form α-1,6 linkages, a branching point of glycogen. Glycogen synthase can produce only a straight chain polymer of glucose. Another enzyme, **glycogen branching enzyme** is required to form the α-1,6 linkages. The **glycogen branching enzyme**, is also called **amylo-1,4 to 1,6-trans-glycosylase or (4,6) transferase**.

7. Once a straight chain polymer of glucose of at least 11 residues has been formed, a branching enzyme removes a part of about 6 or 7 glucosyl residues from a growing chain and transfers it to another chain to form **α-1,6-linkage**, thus establishing a branching point in the molecule **(Figure 10.27)**. The branches grow by further additions of 1,4-glycosyl units and further branching. The new branch point must be at least 4 residues away from a pre-existing one.

Glycogenolysis

Glycogenolysis is the degradation of glycogen to **glucose-6-phosphate** in muscle and **glucose** in liver. Glycogenolysis is not the reverse of the glycogenesis but is a separate pathway **(Figure 10.26)**. Glycogenolysis is **cytosolic** processes occurs in muscle and in liver.

Reactions of Glycogenolysis

1. **Glycogen phosphorylase** catalyzes cleavage of glycogen by the addition of inorganic phosphate (Pi) to release **glucose-1-phosphate**. The cleavage of a bond by the addition of phosphate is referred to as **phosphorolysis**.

> This reaction is different from that of hydrolysis of glycosidic bonds by α-amylase during intestinal degradation of glycogen and starch, in which α-amylase uses water rather than inorganic phosphate (P_i) to cleave α-1,4-glycosidic bonds of glycogen and starch.

2. **Glycogen phosphorylase** is the **key enzyme** in glycogenolysis. It catalyzes the sequential removal of glucosyl residues from the nonreducing ends of the glycogen molecule until approximately four glucose residues remain on either side of a branch point.
3. Glycogen phosphorylase is specific for α-1,4-glycosidic linkages. The enzyme can break α-1,4-glycosidic bonds but the α-1,6-glycosidic bonds at the branch points of glycogen are not cleaved by phosphorylase.
4. **Pyridoxal phosphate** is an essential cofactor in the glycogen phosphorylase reaction. This is an unusual

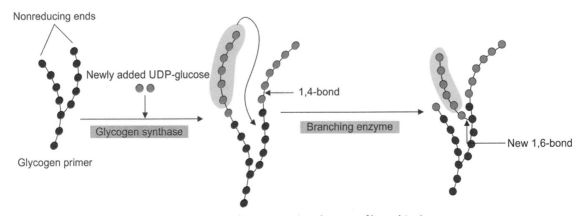

Figure 10.27: Glycogenesis (mechanism of branching).

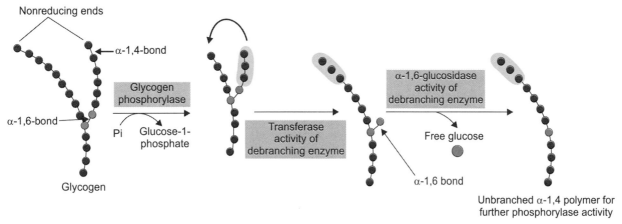

Figure 10.28: Glycogenolysis (mechanism of debranching).

role for pyridoxal phosphate. It's more typical role is as a cofactor in amino acid metabolism

5. Glycogen phosphorylase degrades glycogen to a limited extent because of the α-1,6-glycosidic bonds at the branches. Phosphorylase stops cleaving α-1,4-glycosidic bonds when it reaches a residue which is four residue away from a branch point **(Figure 10.28)**.

6. Further degradation by glycogen phosphorylase can occur only after the action of **debranching enzyme**, which catalyzes two successive reactions by **transferase** and α-**1, 6-glucosidase**.

   ▪ First, debranching enzyme acts as **transferase** and transfers block of three glucosyl residues from one branch to the other. This exposes the α-1,6 branch point **(Figure 10.28)**.

   ▪ In the second step, the hydrolytic splitting of the α-1, 6 linkages occurs by the action of α-**1,6-glucosidase**. This step releases **free glucose**. Thus, transferase and α-1,6-glucosidase convert the branched structure into a linear one, which further cleaved by the action of phosphorylase.

   The combined action of **phosphorylase**, and **debranching enzyme (transferase and α-1,6-glucosidase)** leads to the complete breakdown of glycogen with the formation of **glucose-1-phosphate** and **free glucose** (from hydrolytic cleavage of the 1,6-glycosidic bond).

7. Next, glucose-1-phosphate is converted to glucose-6-phosphate by **phosphoglucomutase**. The glucose-6-phosphate derived from the breakdown of glycogen has three possible fates **(Figure 10.29)**

   ▪ The glucose-6-phosphate formed from glycogen in liver, can be converted into **free glucose** by an enzyme **glucose-6-phosphatase**. It releases **glucose** into the blood when the blood glucose level drops (between meals and during muscle activity). The enzyme **glucose-6-phosphatase**, present in liver and kidney but not in muscles.

   ▪ The glucose-6-phosphate formed from glycogen in **skeletal muscle** can enter glycolysis and serve as an energy source in muscle itself. Because muscle

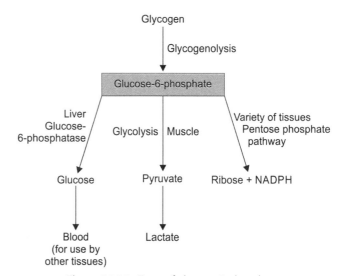

Figure 10.29: Fates of glucose-6-phosphate.

and adipose tissue lack **glucose-6-phosphatase**, they cannot convert glucose-6-phosphate formed by glycogen breakdown to glucose, and these tissues therefore do not contribute glucose to the blood. The glucose-6-phosphate is not transported out of cell.

   ▪ It can be processed by the pentose phosphate pathway to yield **NADPH** and **ribose** in a variety of tissues.

Lysosomal Degradation of Glycogen

● A small amount of glycogen is continuously degraded by the **lysosomal enzyme**, α-**1,4-glucosidase (acid maltase)** to glucose.

● The significance of this pathway is that this is important in glucose homeostasis in neonates.

● However, a deficiency or genetic lack of acid maltase causes accumulation of glycogen in the cytosol resulting in **glycogen storage diseases type II Pompe's disease**.

Regulation of Glycogenolysis and Glycogenesis

Glycogen breakdown and glycogen synthesis are regulated **reciprocally**. It means that when the control mechanism

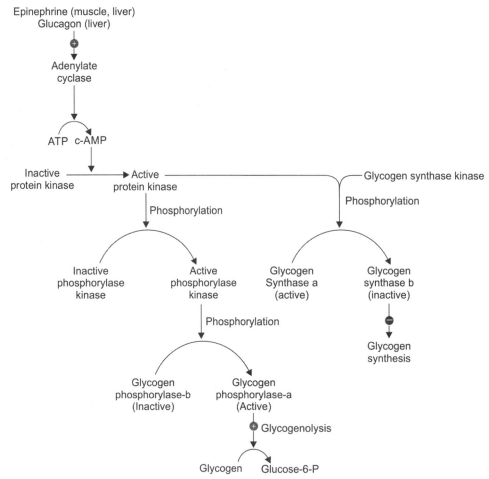

Figure 10.30: Hormone triggered coordinated regulation of glycogen metabolism.

inhibits glycogen synthesis at the same time it stimulates glycogen breakdown. The key enzymes controlling glycogen metabolism are **glycogen phosphorylase** (for breakdown of glycogen) and **glycogen synthase** (for synthesis of glycogen). These enzymes are regulated by **reversible phosphorylation** and **dephosphorylation.**

Note that phosphorylation has opposite effects on the enzymatic activities of glycogen synthase and glycogen phosphorylase. **Phosphorylated** form of glycogen synthase is **inactive**, whereas **phosphorylated** form of **glycogen phosphorylase** is **active**. Phosphorylation and dephosphorylation of enzymes depends on the **hormones** such as **epinephrine** and **glucagon**. The **glucagon** (in liver) and **Epinephrine** (in liver and muscle) stimulate glycogen breakdown and simultaneously inhibits glycogen synthesis **(Figure 10.30).**

The control of glycogen phosphorylase differs between **liver** and **muscle**. These differences are due to the fact that in muscle the role of glycogen is to provide **glucose 6-phosphate** for **glycolysis** in response to the need for ATP for **muscle contraction;** however in liver the role of glycogen is to provide free **glucose** to **maintain blood glucose homeostasis**.

● Low blood levels of glucose lead to the secretion of the hormone **glucagon**. Fear or the excitement or exercise will increase the levels of the hormone **epinephrine (adrenaline).**

● The rise in glucagon and epinephrine levels results in **phosphorylation** of the enzymes **glycogen phosphorylase** to its active form **(glycogen phosphorylase-a)** and **glycogen synthase** to its inactive form **(glycogen synthase-b)** in liver and muscle.

● **Glucagon** and **Epinephrine** control both glycogen breakdown and glycogen synthesis through **protein kinase A** as follows **(Figure 10.30).**

■ **Epinephrine** and **glucagon** activate **adenylate cyclase**. This enzyme catalyzes the formation of the second messenger **cyclic AMP (cAMP)** from ATP.

■ The elevated level of cAMP activates **protein kinase A**. Active protein kinase A phosphorylates **phosphorylase kinase**. Active phosphorylase kinase eventually phosphorylates **glycogen phosphorylase b** to its active form **glycogen phosphorylase a**. Active form of **glycogen phosphorylase a** stimulate breakdown of glycogen to **glucose-6-phosphate** in muscle.

■ At the same time **protein kinase-A** and **glycogen synthase kinase**, (which is under the control of **insulin**) phosphorylates **glycogen synthase**, but phosphorylation of glycogen synthase leads to inhibition of enzymatic activity. Inactive form of **glycogen synthase** inhibits the synthesis of glycogen.

The cAMP cascade **(Figure 10.30)** highly amplifies the effects of hormones. The binding of a small number of hormone molecules to cell surface receptors leads to the release of a very large number of glucose from stored glycogen within seconds. In this way glycogen breakdown and synthesis are reciprocally regulated. Now we will see how the enzymatic activity is reversed so that glycogen breakdown halts and **glycogen synthesis** begins.

● When glucose needs have been satisfied, secretion of epinephrine and glucagon ceases. When secretion of the hormones **epinephrine** and **glucagon** ceases, the activation of **glycogen phosphorylase** is shut down automatically. **Phosphodiesterase** which is always present in the cell converts cAMP into AMP (inactive form). Simultaneously, glycogen synthesis is activated as follows **(Figure 10.30)**:

■ **Protein phosphatase-1** reverses the regulatory effect of kinases on glycogen metabolism. **Protein phosphatase-1 (PP-1)** plays key role in regulating glycogen metabolism. **Protein phosphatase-1** catalyzes the **dephosphorylation. Phosphorylase kinase** and **glycogen phosphorylase** are inactivated by dephosphorylation by **protein phosphatase-1 (PP-1)**. PP-1 decreases the rate of glycogen breakdown and reverses the effects of the phosphorylation cascade.

■ Moreover PP-1 also dephosphorylates **glycogen synthase** to convert it into the active **glycogen synthase** form and accelerate glycogen synthesis **(Figure 10.31)**.

● When blood glucose levels are high, **insulin** stimulates the synthesis of glycogen by **inactivating glycogen**

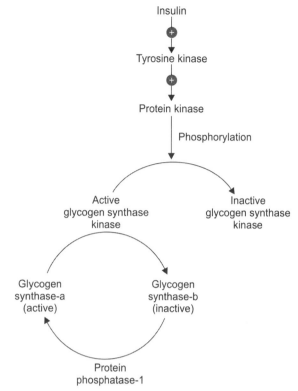

Figure 10.32: Inactivation of glycogen synthase kinase by insulin.

synthase kinase, the enzyme that maintains glycogen synthase in its phosphorylated, inactive form **(Figure 10.32)**.

■ The insulin activates **protein kinase** through **tyrosine kinase**. Protein kinase then phosphorylates and inactivates **glycogen synthase kinase**.

■ The **inactive glycogen synthase kinase** no longer maintains glycogen synthase in its phosphorylated, inactive form, and the **protein phosphatase-1** dephosphorylates glycogen synthase, thereby activating the enzyme and allowing glycogen synthesis.

Significance of Glycogenolysis and Glycogenesis

Glycogen is the major readily mobilized storage form of **glucose**. Glucose cannot be stored because high concentrations of glucose disrupt the osmotic balance of the cell, which would cause cell damage or death. Glucose is stored in its polymeric form, the **glycogen** which is not osmotically active. The functional role of glycogen differs considerably from tissue to tissue, for example:

In Liver

Following a meal, excess glucose is removed from the portal circulation and stored as glycogen by glycogenesis. Conversely, between meals, blood glucose levels are maintained within the normal range by release of glucose from liver glycogen by glycogenolysis. Liver glycogen serves as a reservoir of glucose for other tissues when dietary

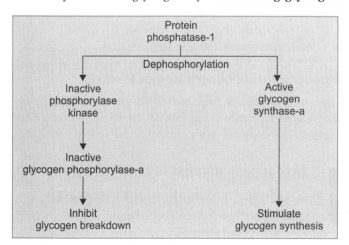

Figure 10.31: Regulation of glycogen synthesis by protein phosphatase-1 (PP1).

glucose is not available (between meals or during fast); this is especially important for the brain, which cannot use fatty acids as fuel, except during prolonged starvation. Liver glycogen can be depleted in 8–12 hours.

In Muscle

The function of muscle glycogen is to act as a readily available source of glucose for glycolysis within the muscle itself. Moreover the readily mobilized glucose from glycogen is a good source of energy for sudden, strenuous activity. Unlike fatty acids, the released glucose can be metabolized in the absence of oxygen and can thus supply energy for anaerobic activity.

The muscle cannot release glucose into the blood, because of the absence of **glucose-6-phsophatase** that hydrolyses glucose 6-phosphate to glucose, therefore muscle do not contribute glucose to the blood. However, muscle glycogen stores are used exclusively by muscle. Muscle glycogen can be exhausted in less than an hour during vigorous activity.

Glycogen Storage Disease

This is a group of genetic diseases that result from a defect in an enzyme required for either glycogen synthesis or degradation and characterized by deposition of either normal or abnormal glycogen in the specific tissues. There are at least 13 types of glycogen storage disease here we will discuss some of the more common forms of these diseases and their characteristics. All glycogen storage diseases (GSDs) are autosomal recessive. The most common types are type I, II, III, IV, V, VI and VII. These seven types are also known by other names. The more common forms of these diseases and their defective enzymes are given in **Table 10.7**.

Symptoms of GSD

Children with glycogen storage disease cannot effectively catabolize glycogen. Glycogen is thus stored in huge quantities in the liver. GSD mostly affects the **liver** and the **muscles**. Symptoms vary based on the type of GSD.

TABLE 10.7: Types of glycogen storage diseases and affected enzymes.

Types	Names	Affected enzymes
Type I	Von Gierke's disease	Glucose-6-phosphatase
Type II	Pompe's disease	Acid maltase
Type III	Cori's or Forbes disease	Debranching enzyme
Type IV	Anderson's disease	Branching enzyme
Type V	McArdle's disease	Muscle glycogen phosphorylase
Type VI	Her's disease	Hepatic glycogen phosphorylase
Type VII	Tauri's disease	Phosphofructokinase

Mnemonic for the order of the disease: Very poor carbohydrate affects muscle and hepatic tissue

- Type I, III, IV and VI **(Hepatic forms)** may cause:
  - Storage of glycogen in liver (hepatomegaly)
  - Reduction of glucose in blood (hypoglycemia)
- Type V and VII **(Myopathic forms)** may cause:
  - Glycogen deposition in muscle
  - Muscle weakness, pain and cramp after exercise
  - Exercise induced lactic acidosis due to block in glycolysis.
  - There may be myoglobinemia
- **Type II (Pompe's disease):** Generalized form may cause
  - Accumulation of glycogen in lysosome. Infantile form is very severe and the infant dies with few months due to cardiac failure.

Metabolic Features

- Glucose-6-phosphate cannot be converted to glucose which leads to severe hypoglycemia with accumulation of glucose-6-phosphate. There is metabolic block in formation of free glucose from liver glycogen due to deficiency of glucose-6-phosphatase enzyme.
- Accumulated glucose-6-phosphate undergoes glycolysis and generates pyruvate and then lactate. Lactate cannot be recycled to gluconeogenesis in liver which causes **lactic acidosis**.
- Lactic acidosis inhibits urinary excretion of uric acid and leads to **hyperuricemia**.
- Glucose-6-phosphate undergoes HMP shunt and generates excessive ribose-5-phosphate which generates purine nucleotides and degraded into uric acid and causes **hyperuricemia**.
- Increased glycolysis and decreased gluconeogenesis leads to increased NADH, NADPH, glycerol and acetyl-CoA causes **hypertriglyceridemia**.
- Malonyl-CoA derived from acetyl-CoA inhibits carnitine acyltransferase which inhibit beta-oxidation of fatty acid.

Investigations for Glycogen Storage Diseases

- Enzyme activity in blood leukocytes (all except type I GSD) and liver (type I GSD) and/or
- Molecular analysis of appropriate gene.

Management of Glycogen Storage Diseases

Ingestion of regular high carbohydrate meals during the day and continuous feeds during the night (or uncooked cornstarch, a slow release form of glucose, every 4–6 hours).

HEXOSE MONOPHOSPHATE PATHWAY (HMP): REGULATION, SIGNIFICANCE AND ASSOCIATED DISORDERS

The **pentose phosphate pathway** is an alternative route for the oxidation of glucose. The major catabolic fate of glucose-

TABLE 10.8: Tissues most enriched in pentose phosphate pathway enzymes and their functions.

Tissues	Functions
Adrenal gland	Steroid synthesis
Testes	Steroid hormone synthesis
Ovaries	Steroid hormone synthesis
Liver	Fatty acid, cholesterol and bile acid synthesis
	P450-dependent detoxification reactions
Adipose tissue	Fatty acid synthesis
Mammary gland	Fatty acid synthesis
Red blood cell	Maintenance of reduced glutathione
Neutrophils	Generation of superoxide

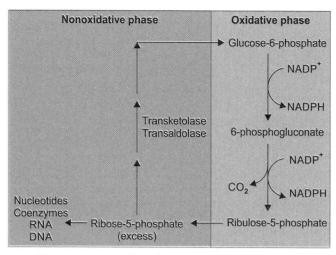

Figure 10.33: Outline of pentose phosphate pathway.

6-phosphate is glycolytic breakdown to pyruvate. The pentose phosphate pathway is the other catabolic pathway for glucose-6-phosphate. Major purpose of this pathway is generation of **NADPH** for use in reductive biosynthesis and **pentose phosphates** for nucleotide synthesis. **It does not generate ATP**. The pentose phosphate pathway is also called the **phosphogluconate pathway** or the **hexose monophosphate pathway**.

The pentose phosphate pathway occurs in **cytoplasm**. The pathway is found in all cells. Tissues most enriched in enzymes of the pentose phosphate pathway are those that have the greater demand for NADPH **(Table 10.8)**.

Reactions of the Pentose Phosphate Pathway

The reactions of the pathway are divided into two phases: **(Figure 10.33)**:
1. **Phase I:** Oxidative, generates pentose phosphates and NADPH
2. **Phase II:** Nonoxidative recycles excess pentose phosphates to glucose-6-phosphate.

Oxidative Phase

- The first reaction of the pentose phosphate pathway is the dehydrogenation of glucose-6-phosphate to 6-phosphoglucono-δ-lactone, with generation of **NADPH** catalyzed by **glucose-6-phosphate dehydrogenase**. This enzyme is highly specific for NADP **(Figure 10.34)**.
- The next step is the hydrolysis of 6-phosphoglucono-δ-lactone by specific **lactonase** to give 6-phosphogluconate.
- The subsequent oxidative decarboxylation of 6-phosphogluconate is catalyzed by **6-phosphogluconate dehydrogenase**, to produce **ribulose-5-phosphate, CO_2** and second molecule, of **NADPH**.

Nonoxidative Phase

The above reactions yield two molecules of NADPH and one molecule of ribulose-5-phosphate for each molecule of glucose-6-phosphate oxidized. Ribulose-5-phosphate formed in the phase I now serves as substrate for two different enzymes; **phosphopentose isomerase** and **phosphopentose epimerase (Figure 10.34)**:
- Ribulose-5-phosphate is subsequently isomerized to **ribose-5-phosphate** by **phosphopentose isomerase**.
  - Ribose-5-phosphate and its derivatives are component of RNA, DNA, as well as ATP, NAD, FAD, and coenzyme A. In some tissues, pentose phosphate pathway ends at this point.
  - Many cells require mainly NADPH for reductive biosynthesis **(Table 10.7)** much more than they need ribose-5-phosphate for the formation of nucleotides. In these cases, ribulose-5-phosphate produced in the Ist oxidative phase of the pathway recycled into glucose-6-phosphate.
- First ribulose-5-phosphate is epimerized to **xylulose-5-phosphate** by **phosphopentose epimerase**. Then, in a series of rearrangements of the carbon skeletons of five carbon sugar phosphates are converted into the glycolytic intermediates to fructose-6-phosphate and glyceraldehyde-3-phosphate by **transketolase** and **transaldolase**. The pentose phosphate pathway and glycolysis are linked by **transketolase** and **transaldolase** enzymes. They create a reversible link between the pentose phosphate pathway and glycolysis by catalyzing three successive reactions.
1. **Transketolase** catalyzes the transfer of two carbon units from xylulose-5-phosphate to ribose-5-phosphate, producing a 7-carbon, sedoheptulose-7-phosphate and glyceraldehyde-3-phosphate. The reaction requires coenzyme **thiamine pyrophosphate (TPP)** and Mg^{2+} ions.

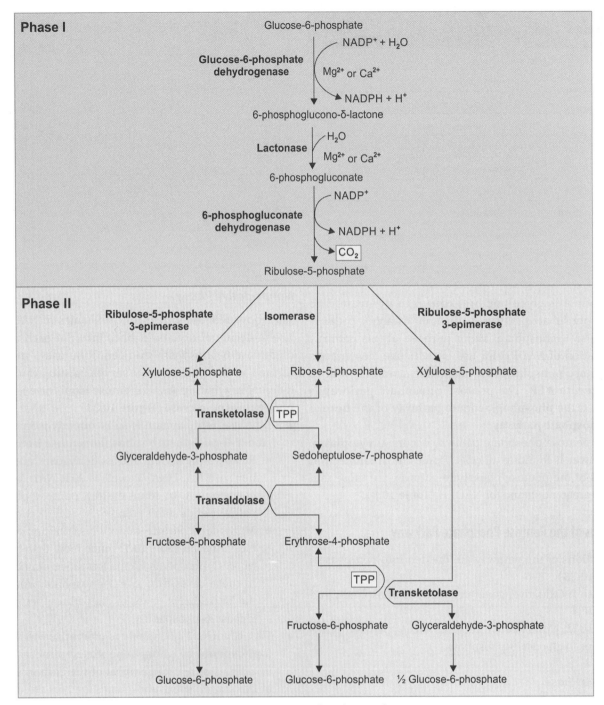

Figure 10.34: Pentose phosphate pathway.
(TPP: Thiamine pyrophosphate)

2. **Transaldolase** catalyzes the transfer of a three carbon dihydroxyacetone group from sedoheptulose-7-phosphate to glyceraldehyde-3-phosphate to form fructose-6-phosphate and the 4-carbon, erythrose-4-phosphate.

3. Further reaction again involves **transketolase**, which catalyzes the transfer of the two carbon units from xylulose-5-phosphate to erythrose-4-phosphate producing fructose-6-phosphate and glyceraldehyde-3-phosphate.

STRIKE A NOTE

❖ The pentose phosphate pathway and glycolysis are linked by **transketolase** and **transaldolase** enzymes.

❖ The transketolase activity of red blood cells is used to measure nutritional status of thiamine and to diagnose the presence of thiamine deficiency.

❖ Excess ribose-5-phosphate formed by the pentose phosphate pathway can be completely converted into glycolytic intermediates.

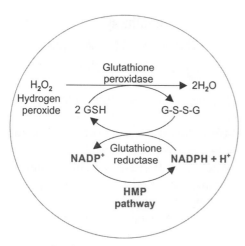

Figure 10.35: Role of NADPH and glutathione in protecting cells against free radicals when exposed to oxidants.

Significance of Pentose Phosphate Pathway

Pentose phosphate pathway is a source of **Ribose-5-phosphate** and **NADPH**. Moreover, any ribose ingested in the diet can be processed into glycolytic intermediates by this pathway.

- Rapidly dividing cells, such as those of bone marrow, skin, and intestinal mucosa, and those of tumors, use **ribose-5-phosphate** for synthesis of RNA, DNA and coenzymes as ATP, NAD, FAD and coenzyme A.
- **NADPH** needed for reductive biosynthesis as well as for protection against oxidative stress, to counter the damaging effects of oxygen radicals.
  - Tissues that carry out extensive fatty acid synthesis (liver, adipose tissue, lactating mammary gland) or very active biosynthesis of cholesterol and steroid hormones (like liver, adrenal glands, gonads) require large amount of NADPH which are provided by pentose phosphate pathway.
  - Erythrocytes and the cells of the cornea and lens are directly exposed to oxygen which generates the damaging free radicals. In such cells by maintaining a reducing atmosphere (high ratio of **NADPH** to **NADP⁺** and high ratio of **reduced** to **oxidized glutathione**) can prevent oxidative damage to proteins, lipids and DNA.
  - The reduced glutathione (GSH) protects the RBC membrane from toxic effect of H_2O_2 by reducing H_2O_2 to H_2O. Regeneration of GSH from its oxidized form (G-S-S-G) requires the NADPH provided by pentose phosphate pathway **(Figure 10.35)**.

Regulation of Pentose Phosphate Pathway

1. In the **oxidative phase** of pentose phosphate pathway the first step, catalyzed by **glucose-6-phosphate dehydrogenase (G-6-PD)** is the **rate limiting** step under physiological conditions and serves as the control site for the oxidative phase of pentose phosphate pathway. The activity of this enzyme is regulated by cellular concentration of NADPH.

- An increased concentration of NADPH decreases the activity of G-6-PD, for example:
  - Under well fed condition the ratio of NADPH/NADP⁺ decreases and pentose phosphate pathway is stimulated.
  - In starvation and diabetes, the ratio NADPH/NADP⁺ is high and inhibits the pathway.
- Insulin is also involved in the regulation of pentose phosphate pathway. It enhances the pathway by inducing the enzyme G-6-PD and 6-phosphogluconate dehydrogenase.
2. The nonoxidative phase of pentose phosphate pathway is controlled mainly by the availability of substrate.

Disorder of Pentose Phosphate Pathway

Glucose-6-Phosphate Dehydrogenase Deficiency

Glucose-6-phosphate dehydrogenase deficiency causes a **drug-induced hemolytic anemia**. The gene is on the **X-chromosome**, so it is mainly males who are affected but most are **asymptomatic**.

Only when people deficient in G-6-PD are exposed to **oxidative stress**, due to drugs such as **antimalarial primaquine**, **sulfa drugs**, certain **herbicides** or when they have eaten **fava beans (Favism)** produces the clinical manifestations. The defect is manifested as **hemolytic anemia**.

G-6-PD catalyzes the first step in **pentose phosphate pathway** which produces **NADPH**. NADPH protects cells from oxidative damage by H_2O_2 and reactive oxygen species (free radicals) which are generated as metabolic byproducts and through the action of drugs such as primaquine and natural products such as **divicine** (the toxic ingredients of fava beans). In G-6-PD deficient individuals, the **NADPH production is diminished** and detoxification of H_2O_2 is inhibited. Cellular damage results due to **lipid peroxidation** and **oxidation** of **proteins** and **DNA**.

The rate of occurrence for G-6-PD deficiency is high among Americans of African heritage. The geographic distribution of this deficiency is similar to that of **sickle cell trait** and is also associated to the resistance against the *Plasmodium falciparum* **malarial parasite**. This suggests that deficiency of G-6-PD may be advantageous under certain environmental conditions.

The malarial parasite infects the red blood cell, where it depends on the reduced glutathione and products of the pentose phosphate pathway for its optimum growth. Therefore, person with G-6-PD deficiency cannot support growth of this parasite and thus are less susceptible to malaria than the normal population.

Wernicke-Korsakoff Syndrome

Wernicke-Korsakoff syndrome is a disorder caused by a severe deficiency of thiamine, a component of **thiamine** pyrophosphate **(TPP)**. The syndrome is more common among people with alcoholism than in general population, because chronic heavy alcohol consumption interferes with the intestinal absorption of thiamine. The syndrome can be worse by a **mutation** in the gene for **transketolase** that results in an enzyme with much **reduced affinity for TPP**.

The result is a slowing down of the whole pentose phosphate pathway. In people with Wernicke-Korsakoff syndrome this results in a deteriorating of symptoms, such as memory loss, mental confusion and partial paralysis.

URONIC ACID PATHWAY AND ITS SIGNIFICANCE

A pathway in liver for the conversion of glucose to glucuronic acid, ascorbic acid (except in humans and other primates as well as in guinea pigs) and pentoses is referred to as the uronic acid pathway. It is also an alternative oxidative pathway for glucose but does not generate ATP.

Reactions of Uronic Acid Pathway

- Glucose-6-phosphate is converted to glucose-1-phosphate catalyzed by **phosphoglucomutase (Figure 10.36)**.

- Glucose-1-phosphate then reacts with uridine triphosphate (UTP) to form uridine diphosphate glucose (UDP-Glc). This reaction is catalyzed by the enzyme **UDP-glucose pyrophosphorylase**.

- UDP-glucose is oxidized to glucuronate via UDP-glucuronate, catalyzed by an NAD-dependent **UDP-glucose dehydrogenase**.

- Glucuronate is reduced to L-gulonate by the NADPH-dependent enzyme **gulonate dehydrogenase**.

- L-gulonate is the precursor of ascorbate (vitamin C) in those animals capable of synthesizing this vitamin. In humans and other primates, as well as in guinea pigs, ascorbic acid cannot be synthesized because of the **absence of the enzyme L-gulonolactone oxidase**.

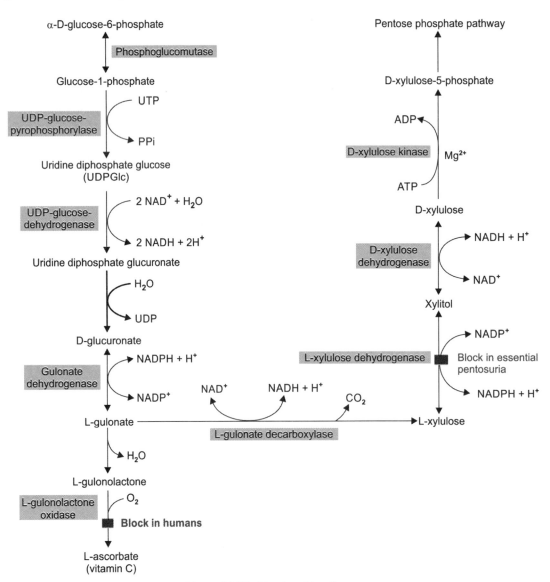

Figure 10.36: Uronic acid pathway.

- L-gulonate is oxidized and decarboxylated to the pentose L-xylulose by the enzyme **L-gulonate decarboxylase**.
- L-xylulose is reduced to xylitol catalyzed by NADPH-dependent **L-xylulose dehydrogenase**.
- Xylitol is oxidized to D-xylulose (isomer of L-xylulose) by an NAD-dependent **D-xylulose dehydrogenase** enzyme.
- D-xylulose, in turn, is phosphorylated by ATP in the presence of **xylulose kinase** to yield xylulose-5-phosphate, which is further metabolized in pentose phosphate pathway and leads to formation of glucose.

Significance of Uronic Acid Pathway

The uronic acid pathway is a source of **UDP-glucuronate**.
- UDP-glucuronate is a precursor in biosynthesis of **proteoglycans** (glycosaminoglycans) and **glycoproteins**.
- UDP-glucuronate is involved in **detoxification** reactions that occur in liver. Many naturally occurring waste substances (like bilirubin and steroid hormones) as well as many drugs (like morphine, methanol, salicylic acid, etc.) are eliminated from the body by conjugating with UDP-glucuronate **(Figure 10.37)**.
- The uronic acid pathway is a source of **UDP-glucose**, which is used for **glycogen** formation.
- The uronic acid pathway provides a mechanism by which dietary D-xylulose can enter the central metabolic pathway.

Disorder of Glucuronic Acid Pathway

Essential Pentosuria

It is a benign (harmless) inborn error of metabolism in which the sugar L-xylulose is excreted in the urine in excess due to defect in NADP+ linked **L-xylulose dehydrogenase**, one of the enzymes in the **uronic acid** pathway **(Figure 10.36)**. L-xylulose dehydrogenase is necessary to accomplish reduction of L-xylulose to xylitol.

GALACTOSE METABOLISM: PATHWAY, SIGNIFICANCE AND ASSOCIATED DISORDERS

Galactose is derived from disaccharide, lactose (the milk sugar) of the diet. It is important for the formation of:
- Glycolipids
- Glycoproteins
- Proteoglycans
- Lactose during lactation.

Galactose is readily converted in the liver to glucose **(Figure 10.38)**. **The ability of the liver to convert galactose to glucose is used as a liver function test (galactose tolerance test)**.

Reactions of the Pathway

- The first reaction in galactose metabolism in the liver is phosphorylation of galactose to galactose-1-phosphate, by the enzyme **galactokinase**, using ATP as phosphate donor.
- Galactose-1-phosphate reacts with UDP-glucose to form UDP-galactose and glucose-1-phosphate, catalyzed by **galactose-1-phosphate uridyl transferase**. In this reaction, galactose displaces glucose of UDP-glucose.
- The conversion of UDP-galactose to UDP-glucose is catalyzed by an **UDP-galactose-4-epimerase**.
- Finally, glucose is liberated from UDP-glucose via formation of glycogen by glycogenesis followed by glycogenolysis **(Figure 10.38)**.

Disorder of Galactose Metabolism

Galactosemia

It is an inborn error of galactose metabolism, caused by deficiency of enzyme **galactose-1-phosphate uridyl transferase (Figure 10.38)**. The inherited deficiencies of

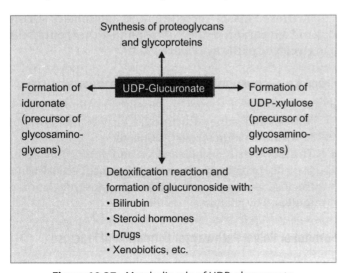

Figure 10.37: Metabolic role of UDP-glucuronate.

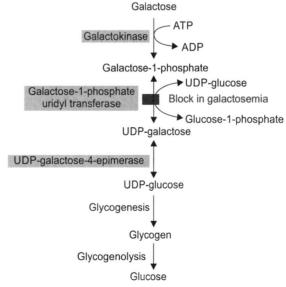

Figure 10.38: Pathway for conversion of galactose to glucose in the liver.

galactokinase and **UDP-galactose-4-epimerase** also lead to minor types of galactosemia. They all interfere with the normal metabolism of galactose, causing a rise in blood and urine galactose.

The most common and most severe enzymatic defect is due to **galactose-1-phosphate uridyl transferase** deficiency which prevents conversion of galactose to glucose and leads to accumulation of galactose and galactose-1-phosphate in blood, liver, brain, kidney and eye lenses. In these organs, the galactose is reduced to galactitol (dulcitol) by the enzyme **aldose reductase**.

Clinical Findings

- Infants suffering from galactosemia fail to thrive. They show following clinical features:
  - Vomiting or have diarrhea after consuming milk
  - Enlargement of the liver
  - Jaundice is common, sometimes progressing to cirrhosis.
- The accumulation of galactitol and galactose-1-phosphate in:
  - Liver causes liver failure (hepatomegaly followed by cirrhosis)
  - Brain it causes mental retardation
  - Eye lenses, it leads to cataract formation. Galactitol is a osmotically active substance due to which water will diffuse from the lens to maintain osmotic balance, causing the development of cataract.
- The blood galactose level is markedly elevated, and galactose is found in the urine.

Treatment

The most common treatment is to remove galactose (lactose) from the diet. Sufficient galactose required for body can be synthesized endogenously as UDP-galactose.

FRUCTOSE METABOLISM: PATHWAY, SIGNIFICANCE AND ASSOCIATED DISORDERS

D-fructose, present in free form in many fruits and formed by hydrolysis of sucrose in the small intestine. There is no catabolic pathway for metabolizing fructose, so it is converted into a metabolite of glucose. **Figure 10.39**, shows how fructose is channeled into the glycolytic pathway.

Reactions of Fructose Metabolism

Liver is the main site of fructose metabolism.

Fructose-1-phosphate Pathway in the Liver

- Fructose is phosphorylated to fructose-1-phosphate by **fructokinase** in the liver. This enzyme will not phosphorylate glucose and unlike glucokinase, its activity is not affected by fasting or by insulin and that is why fructose disappears from the blood of diabetic patients at a normal rate.

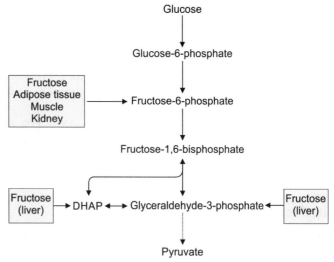

Figure 10.39: Entry points of fructose in glycolysis.

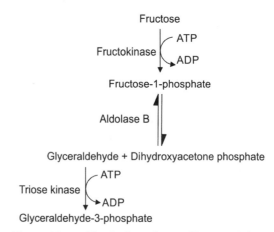

Figure 10.40: Metabolic pathway of fructose in liver.

- Fructose-1-phosphate is split into **glyceraldehyde** and **dihydroxyacetone phosphate (DHAP)** an intermediate in glycolysis by a specific **fructose-1-phosphate aldolase (Aldolase B)**.
- Glyceraldehyde is then phosphorylated to **glyceraldehyde-3-phosphate** a glycolytic intermediate by **triose kinase**. These two triose phosphates (DHAP and glyceraldehyde-3-phosphate) then enter the **glycolytic pathway (Figure 10.40)**.

Fructose-6-phosphate Pathway in Extrahepatic Tissues

- In extrahepatic tissues, especially the adipose tissues, muscles and kidney, fructose can be phosphorylated by hexokinase to fructose-6-phosphate.
- This however is a slow reaction and occurs only in the presence of high concentration of fructose because when fructose is present with glucose, its phosphorylation is inhibited by glucose.

Sorbitol or Polyol Pathway for Formation of Fructose

The sorbitol (polyol) pathway is for the formation of fructose from glucose **(Figure 10.41)**.

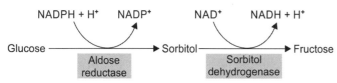

Figure 10.41: Sorbitol or polyol pathway.

- **Aldose reductase** reduces glucose to sorbitol (glucitol). It is found in many tissues such as lens, retina, peripheral nerve cells, kidney, placenta, red blood cells, ovaries and seminal vesicles. But it is not present in liver.
- In liver, ovaries and sperm cells, there is a second enzyme, **sorbitol dehydrogenase** that oxidizes the sorbitol to fructose.
- The pathway from sorbitol to fructose in the liver provides a mechanism by which dietary sorbitol is converted into fructose which can enter glycolysis.

Effect of Hyperglycemia on Sorbitol Metabolism

- ❖ Because insulin is not required for entry of glucose into the cells (such as lens, retina and nerve) large amounts of glucose may enter these cells during hyperglycemia, e.g., in uncontrolled diabetes.
- ❖ Elevated intracellular glucose concentrations cause increase in the amount of sorbitol, which, unlike glucose, cannot diffuse efficiently through cell membrane and therefore accumulates inside the cell.
- ❖ This is exaggerated when sorbitol dehydrogenase is low or absent, e.g., in retina, lens, kidney, and nerve cells causing osmotic damage, leading to cataract formation, peripheral neuropathy, retinopathy and nephropathy.
- ❖ Drugs inhibiting aldose reductase improve the peripheral nerve function in diabetes.

STRIKE A NOTE

- ❖ Fructokinase in the liver will not phosphorylate glucose and unlike glucokinase its activity is not affected by fasting or by insulin and that is why fructose disappears from the blood of diabetic patients at a normal rate.
- ❖ In extrahepatic tissues, especially the adipose tissues, muscles and kidney, fructose can be phosphorylated by hexokinase to fructose-6-phosphate.
- ❖ Fructose is more rapidly glycolyzed by the liver than glucose. Because fructose bypasses the most important regulatory step in glycolysis catalyzed by phosphofructokinase.
- ❖ Because insulin is not required for entry of glucose into the cells (such as lens, retina and nerve) large amounts of glucose may enter these cells during hyperglycemia, e.g., in uncontrolled diabetes.
- ❖ Elevated intracellular glucose concentrations cause increase in the amount of sorbitol, which, unlike glucose, cannot diffuse efficiently through cell membrane and therefore accumulates inside the cell.
- ❖ This is overloaded when sorbitol dehydrogenase is low or absent which causes osmotic damage, leading to cataract formation, peripheral neuropathy, retinopathy and nephropathy.
- ❖ Drugs inhibiting aldose reductase improve the peripheral nerve function in diabetes.

Disorders of Fructose Metabolism

Essential Fructosuria

Essential fructosuria is a rare and benign genetic disorder caused by a deficiency of the enzyme **fructokinase**. In this disorder fructose cannot be converted to **fructose-1-phosphate**. This is benign because no toxic metabolites of fructose accumulate in the liver and the patient remains nearly asymptomatic with excretion of fructose in urine.

There is no renal threshold for fructose, so that the appearance of fructose in urine (fructosuria) does not require a high fructose concentration in the blood.

Hereditary Fructose Intolerance

It is due to deficiency of the enzyme *aldolase-B.* Fructose-1-phosphate cannot be converted to **dihydroxyacetone phosphate** and glyceraldehyde and therefore **fructose-1-phosphate** accumulates. This results in the inhibition of *fructokinase* and an impaired clearance of fructose from the blood. Hereditary fructose intolerance is characterized by intense **hypoglycemia** due to inhibition of glycogenolysis and gluconeogenesis and vomiting after consumption of fructose (or sucrose which yield fructose after digestion).

Clinical Findings

Accumulation of fructose-1-phosphate leads to liver and kidney damage. Hypoglycemia occurs due to inhibition of glycogenolysis (because fructose-1-phosphate allosterically inhibits liver glycogen phosphorylase) and gluconeogenesis.

Treatment

Elimination of foods containing fructose from the diet.

REGULATION OF BLOOD GLUCOSE LEVEL IN FED AND FASTING STATE

The **liver** is the organ primarily responsible for controlling the concentration of glucose in the blood. It can rapidly **take up** and **release** glucose in response to the **concentration of blood glucose**. The uptake and release of glucose by liver is regulated by **hormones**.

- The blood glucose level must be maintained within the narrow limits of **70–100 mg/dL**.
- After the ingestion of a carbohydrate meal, it may rise to **120–140 mg/dL**.
  - A level above the normal range is termed **hyperglycemia**
  - A level below the normal range is called **hypoglycemia**.
- Factors involved in the **homeostasis** of blood glucose are:
  - *Hormones:* The two major hormones controlling blood glucose levels are; **insulin (hypoglycemic**

hormone) and **glucagon (hyperglycemic hormone)** **(Figure 10.42)**
- Metabolic processes
- Renal mechanism

Maintenance of Glucose in Fed State (Hyperglycemic Condition)

Normally, there is an **increased blood glucose** level shortly after each meal, a **postprandial hyperglycemia**. Increased level of circulating glucose releases **insulin** by β-cells of the islets of the Langerhans. This hormone reduces the blood glucose level in a number of ways as follows **(Figure 10.43)**:
- By stimulating the **active transport** of glucose across cell membranes of muscle and adipose tissue by stimulating **GLUT-4 transporter** but not the liver. **Glucose is rapidly taken up into liver as it is freely permeable to glucose via GLUT-2 transporter** (*see* Table 10.1)
- In the liver insulin increases the use of glucose by **glycolysis** by inducing the synthesis of key glycolytic enzymes:
  - Glucokinase
  - Phosphofructokinase
  - Pyruvate kinase
- **Glucokinase is important in regulating blood glucose after meal**. Like hexokinase (of extrahepatic tissue) glucokinase of the liver is not inhibited by glucose-6-phosphate. Glucokinase increases in activity whenever

blood glucose concentration is higher than normal levels and seems to be specifically concerned with glucose uptake into the liver after a carbohydrate meal.
- In the muscle and the liver insulin stimulates **glycogenesis** by stimulating **glycogen synthase** (by reducing elevated cAMP levels) and thereby leading to suppression of **glycogenolysis**.
- Insulin inhibits **gluconeogenesis** by suppressing the action of key enzymes of gluconeogenesis, e.g.,
  - Pyruvate carboxylase
  - Phosphoenolpyruvate carboxykinase
  - Fructose 1,6-bisphosphatase
  - Glucose-6-phosphatase
- In adipose tissue, glucose is converted to the glycerol-3-phosphate, required for the formation of triacylglycerol (lipogenesis) and inhibits the lipolysis by inhibiting **hormone sensitive lipase**.
- Insulin increases **protein synthesis** and decreases protein catabolism, thereby decreases release of amino acids required for gluconeogenesis.

All these mechanisms are responsible for a drop in glucose level (hypoglycemia).

Maintenance of Blood Glucose in Fasting State (Hypoglycemic Condition)

After meal blood glucose level rises to maximum (120–140 mg %) at half to 1 hour. One hour after a meal, blood glucose levels begin to fall and by 2 hours the level returns to the fasting range (70–100 mg/dL) and leads to hypoglycemia. For the brain, the erythrocytes, the bone marrow, the renal medulla and peripheral nerves glucose is the major fuel and which has to be supplied for their energy needs. Therefore, it is essential to maintain the blood glucose level within normal range. The blood glucose level is maintained within normal range by the following ways.

The decrease in blood glucose causes:
- Decrease in **insulin** secretion
- Stimulate secretion of **glucagon** and other hyperglycemic hormones like **epinephrine**, **glucocorticoids**, **anterior pituitary hormones**, **growth hormone**, **adrenocorticotropic hormone (ACTH)**, and **thyroxin**.

Glucagon

Just as **insulin** signals the **hyperglycemic state**, **glucagon** signals **hypoglycemia state**. Glucagon opposes the actions of insulin. Glucagon is secreted by α-cells of the pancreas in response to low blood sugar level in the fasting state. The main target organ of glucagon is the liver. Glucagon causes an increase in blood glucose concentration in several ways **(Figure 10.44)**.
- In the liver, it stimulates **glycogen breakdown** and inhibits glycogen synthesis by triggering c-AMP **(Figure 10.30)**. The glucose formed by breakdown of glycogen

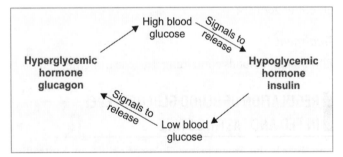

Figure 10.42: Reciprocal control of insulin and glucagon on the homeostasis.

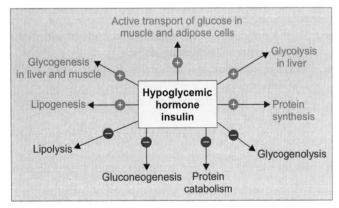

Figure 10.43: Various metabolic systems affected by insulin.

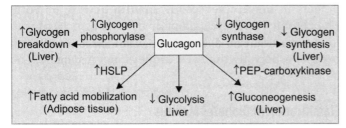

Figure 10.44: Various metabolic systems affected by glucagon. (HSLP: Hormone sensitive lipoprotein lipase; PEP: Phosphoenol pyruvate)

is then released from the liver into the blood. The liver glycogen is capable of maintaining the blood glucose concentration at normal values for **8–12 hours**.

- Glucagon does not have an effect on muscle phosphorylase due to lack of receptors require for glucagon.
- Glucagon enhances **gluconeogenesis** from **amino acids** and **lactate** by inducing the action of key enzymes of gluconeogenesis.
    - **Alanine** is the predominant amino acid released from muscle to liver by glucose alanine cycle (*see* **Figure 10.22**).
    - **Lactate** formed by oxidation of glucose in skeletal muscle is transported to the liver by **lactic acid (Cori) cycle** (*see* **Figure 10.20**).

Epinephrine or Adrenaline

- Epinephrine is secreted by adrenal medulla. It stimulates **glycogenolysis** in the liver and the muscle by stimulating phosphorylase activity via **cAMP (Figure 10.30)**.
- In **muscle** as a result of the **absence of glucose-6-phosphatase**, glycogenolysis results with the formation of **lactate**, whereas in the **liver** glucose is the main product, leading to **increase in blood glucose**.

Glucocorticoids

- These hormones are secreted by adrenal cortex, which causes increased:
    - Gluconeogenesis
    - Protein catabolism to provide glucogenic amino acid for gluconeogenesis
    - Activity of aminotransferase
    - Hepatic uptake of amino acids for gluconeogenesis
    - Activity of enzymes of gluconeogenesis.
- In addition, glucocorticoids inhibit the utilization of glucose in extrahepatic tissues. Thus, all the actions of glucocorticoids are antagonistic to insulin.

Anterior Pituitary Hormones

- Growth hormone and ACTH antagonize the action of insulin by elevating the blood glucose level.
- Growth hormone decreases glucose uptake in the muscle and ACTH decreases glucose utilization by the tissue.

Thyroxine

- It is secreted by thyroid gland. Thyroxine accelerates hepatic glycogenolysis with consequent rise in blood glucose.
- It may also increase the rate of absorption of hexoses from the intestine.

Renal Control Mechanism

When blood glucose rises to relatively high levels, the kidney also exerts a regulatory effect. Glucose is continuously filtered by the glomeruli but is normally reabsorbed completely in renal tubules. The capacity of the tubular system to reabsorb glucose is limited to a rate of about **350 mg/min** which is known as tubular maximum for glucose **(TmG)**.

- If the blood glucose level is raised above **180 mg/100 mL**, complete tubular reabsorption of glucose does not occur and the extra amount appears in the urine causing **glycosuria**.
- The 180 mg/100 mL is the limiting level of glucose in the blood, above which tubular reabsorption does not occur which is known as **renal threshold value for glucose**.
- Thus, by excreting extra amount of sugar in the urine during hyperglycemic state and reabsorbing sugar during the hypoglycemic state, the kidney helps in regulating the level of glucose in blood.

Glycosuria

Normally the urine contains about 0.05 gm% of sugar. Such a small quantity cannot be detected by Benedict's test, but under certain circumstances a considerable amount of glucose or other sugar may be excreted in the urine.

Excretion of detectable amount of sugar in urine is known as **glycosuria**. Glycosuria is a general term used for *"sugar in the urine"*.

- The term **glucosuria, fructosuria, galactosuria, lactosuria** and **pentosuria** *are* applied specifically to the urinary excretion of **glucose, fructose, galactose, lactose** and **pentose** respectively.
- In normal individuals, glucose is the only sugar present in the blood and thus glucosuria being the most important type of glycosuria. Glucosuria results from the rise of blood glucose above its renal threshold level (180 mg%).
- Glucosuria may be due to various reasons on the basis of which it is classified into the following groups:
    - Alimentary (lag storage) glucosuria.
    - Renal glucosuria.
    - Diabetic glucosuria.

Alimentary (Lag Storage) Glucosuria

- Alimentary glycosuria is a temporary condition, when a high amount of carbohydrate is taken; it is rapidly absorbed above the normal renal threshold (180 mg/dL) in some individuals after meal and results in glucosuria.

- This is due to an increased rate of absorption of glucose from the intestine. This is called alimentary glucosuria since alimentary canal (GI-tract) is involved.
- Characteristic feature of this glucosuria is that usually high blood glucose level returns to normal at 2 hours after a meal. This type of glucosuria is benign (harmless).

Renal Glucosuria

Normally, the body excretes glucose in the urine only when glucose levels in the blood are very high, such as in uncontrolled diabetes mellitus. In normal people, glucose that is filtered from the blood by the kidneys is completely reabsorbed back into the blood.

- In renal glucosuria, glucose is excreted in the urine in spite of normal levels of glucose in the blood. This happens because of a **defect in the tubular cells of the kidneys** that decreases the reabsorption of glucose.
- Renal glucosuria may be hereditary or it may be acquired.
- Hereditary renal glucosuria is due to defects in the kidney such as in **Fanconi syndrome**. Fanconi syndrome is a rare disorder of **kidney tubule function** that results in excess amounts of glucose, bicarbonate, phosphates, uric acid, potassium, and certain amino acids being excreted in the urine.
- The acquired form can be caused by certain drugs or diseases that damage the kidney tubules. It may occur temporarily in pregnancy without symptoms of diabetes.
- Renal glucosuria has no symptoms. It is a benign condition, unrelated to diabetes.
- It is diagnosed when a routine urine test detects glucose in the urine even though glucose levels in the blood are normal.
- No treatment is needed.

Diabetic Glucosuria

- Diabetic glucosuria is a pathological condition and is due to deficiency or lack of insulin which causes diabetes mellitus.
- Although, the renal threshold is normal, as blood glucose level exceeds the renal threshold, the excess glucose passes into the urine to produce glucosuria.

▌DIABETES MELLITUS: TYPES, SYMPTOMS, CLINICAL FEATURES AND METABOLIC CHANGES OCCUR IN DIABETES MELLITUS

Definition

Diabetes mellitus is a metabolic disease characterized by **hyperglycemia**, caused by inherited and/or acquired defects in **insulin secretion**, **insulin action**, or **both**. The chronic hyperglycemia of diabetes is associated with long-term damage, dysfunction, and failure of different organs, especially the eyes, kidneys, nerves, heart, and blood vessels.

Classification of Diabetes Mellitus

Diabetes mellitus is broadly divided into two groups namely **(Figure 10.45)**:

1. Type 1 diabetes mellitus or insulin-dependent diabetes mellitus (IDDM).
2. Type 2 diabetes mellitus or noninsulin-dependent diabetes mellitus (NIDDM).

The comparison between two types of diabetes mellitus is given in **Table 10.9**.

Type 1 Diabetes Mellitus

Type 1 diabetes also called insulin-dependent diabetes mellitus (IDDM) or juvenile onset diabetes.

Cause

- It is caused by lack of insulin secretion due to destruction of pancreatic beta cells. The cause of β-cell destructions may be due to:
- Viral infection

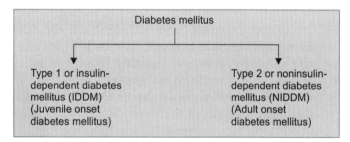

Figure 10.45: Classification of diabetes mellitus.

TABLE 10.9: Comparison of two types of diabetes mellitus.		
Features	**Type 1 insulin dependent diabetes mellitus**	**Type 2 noninsulin-dependent diabetes mellitus**
Frequency	5–10%	90–95%
Age of onset	Early during childhood or puberty usually <20 years	Later after age of 40 years
Onset of symptoms	Abrupt and severe	Gradual, insidious
Plasma insulin	Low or absent	Normal to high
Body weight	Low to normal	Obese
Blood glucose	Increased	Increased
Insulin sensitivity	Normal	Reduced
Ketosis	Common	Rare
Acute complications	Ketoacidosis	Hyperosmolar coma
Treatment with insulin	Necessary	Usually not required

- Autoimmune disorder
- There may be hereditary tendency for β-cell degeneration.

Onset

The usual onset of type-1 diabetes occurs at about 14 years of age and for this reason it is called juvenile diabetes mellitus.

Symptoms

Symptoms are developed very abruptly.
- Hyperglycemia with glycosuria
- Polyuria (osmotic diuresis, loss of water and electrolytes and frequent urination)
- Polydipsia, dehydration and thirst
- Polyphagia (excessive hunger due to negative energy balance)
- Ketoacidosis
- Loss of body weight, weakness, and tiredness

Treatment

Since patients of IDDM (type-1) fail to secrete insulin, administration of exogenous insulin is required.

Type 2 Diabetes Mellitus

Type 2 diabetes mellitus is also called, noninsulin dependent diabetes mellitus (NIDDM) or adult onset diabetes mellitus.

Cause

It is caused by decreased sensitivity (decreased response to insulin) of target tissues to insulin. This reduced sensitivity of insulin is often referred to as **insulin resistance**. This is perhaps due to **inadequate insulin receptors** on the cell surfaces of the target tissues.

Onset

Onset of the type 2 diabetes occurs after age 40 and the disorder develops gradually. Therefore, this syndrome is referred to as adult onset diabetes.

Symptoms

This syndrome is often found in **obese person**. The symptoms are developed gradually similar to that of type 1 as follows:
- Hyperglycemia with glycosuria
- Polyuria (osmotic diuresis, loss of water and electrolytes and frequent urination)
- Polydipsia, dehydration and thirst
- Polyphagia (excessive hunger due to negative energy balance)
- Loss of body weight, weakness, and tiredness.
- Ketoacidosis (less common in type 2 diabetics compared to type 1 diabetics because these patients are insulin resistant rather than insulin lacking.

Treatment

- It can be treated in early stages by **diet control**, **exercise** and **weight reduction** and no exogenous insulin administration is required. Regular exercise, including walking, can help people with type 2 diabetes lower their blood glucose levels. Physical activity also reduces body fat, lowers blood pressure, and helps prevent cardiovascular disease. It is recommended that people with type 2 diabetes get 30 minutes of moderate exercise on most days.
- Oral medication is recommended for people with type 2 diabetes who cannot adequately control their blood sugar with diet and exercise. Drugs that **increase insulin sensitivity** or drugs that cause **additional release of insulin** by the pancreas may be used.
  - **Thiazolidinedione** and **metformin** increase insulin sensitivity.
  - **Sulfonylureas** cause additional release of insulin by the pancreas.
- In the later stages insulin administration is required. If insulin is not produced in "beta-cell failure," in response to elevated blood glucose insulin treatment is necessary.
- There are other noninsulin drugs given in injection form that are used to treat type 2 diabetes. Examples are pramlintide (Symlin), exenatide (Byetta), and liraglutide (Victoza). These drugs stimulate the release of insulin.

Metabolic Changes and Clinical Features of Diabetes Mellitus

In diabetes mellitus, the metabolic changes occur due to a **deficiency of insulin** and relative **excess of glucagon**. These changes in hormonal levels most profoundly affect metabolism in three tissues; **liver**, **muscle** and **adipose tissue**.

Since insulin is a major **anabolic hormone** in the body, deficiency of insulin results in a **catabolic state** that affects not only glucose metabolism but also fat and protein metabolism. The major metabolic changes occur in diabetes mellitus **(Figure 10.46)** are:

1. Inability to utilize glucose and overproduction of glucose (hyperglycemia)
2. Increased protein catabolism and diminished protein synthesis
3. Increased lipolysis resulting in hyperlipidemia hence there is rapid muscle wasting and weight loss

- Due to lack of insulin activity in diabetes mellitus, transfer of glucose from the blood into muscle and adipose tissue is diminished or abolished and leads to **hyperglycemia**. The body responds as it were in the fasting state with stimulation of catabolic processes:
  - Glycogenolysis, storage of glycogen in liver and muscle is depleted by glycogenolysis

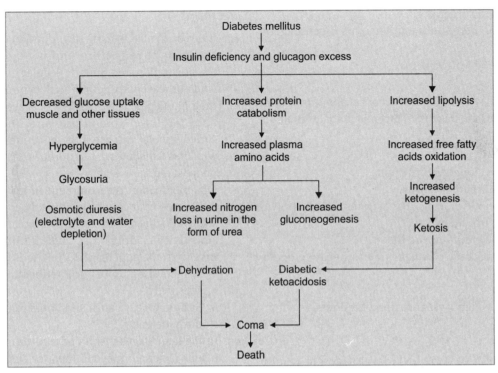

Figure 10.46: Metabolic changes occur in diabetes mellitus.

- Lipolysis, hyperlipidemia
- Proteolysis
- Gluconeogenesis, synthesis of glucose from amino acids.
- The resultant hyperglycemia exceeds the glucose renal threshold for reabsorption, and **glycosuria** results.
- The glycosuria induces an **osmotic diuresis** which leads to profound loss of water and electrolytes; consequently resulting in, **polyuria**, **dehydration** and **thirst (polydipsia)**.
- An **increase in glucagon** favors **lipolysis** in adipose tissue. Increased lipolysis leads to increased mobilization of fatty acids from adipose tissue to liver, where they are converted to **ketone bodies;** β-hydroxybutyrate, acetoacetate and acetone.
- Increased utilization of fats for energy causes metabolic acidosis, due to release of keto acids into the plasma more rapidly than can be taken up and oxidized by the tissue cells. As a result, these moderately strong acids are buffered when present in blood or other tissues and that leads to loss of buffer cation (HCO_3^-) that progressively depletes the alkali reserve, causing ketoacidosis. This may be fatal in uncontrolled diabetes mellitus (*see* **Figure 10.46**).
- Due to lack of insulin, the synthesis of the enzyme **lipoprotein lipase**, required for the degradation of VLDL is decreased. Decreased synthesis of lipoprotein lipase leads to elevated levels of plasma VLDL, resulting in **hypertriglyceridemia**.
- Deficiency of insulin in diabetes mellitus stimulates **catabolism of protein**. Increased rate of proteolysis

stimulates mobilization of **glucogenic amino acids** from muscles. The amino acids released from muscle are converted to glucose by **gluconeogenesis**.
- Stimulation of protein breakdown to provide amino acids for gluconeogenesis results in the muscle wasting and weight loss.
- The combined result of severe **ketoacidosis**, **hyperglycemia** and **hyperosmolarity** and **electrolytes disturbance** impairs **cerebral function**, producing **diabetic ketoacidotic coma**. This is quite distinct than the hypoglycemic coma, that may also be found in diabetic patients; this is due to insulin over dosage, and has entirely different clinical features.
- The catabolism of proteins and fats tends to induce a negative energy balance which in turn leads to **increasing appetite (polyphagia)**. Despite the increased appetite, catabolic effects result in **weight loss** and **muscle weakness**.
- **Secondary effects:** Chronic high glucose concentration causes tissue injury, when blood glucose is poorly controlled over long periods in diabetes mellitus, e.g., the functions of blood vessels in multiple tissues is impaired that result in inadequate blood supply to the tissues. This in turn leads to increased risk for:
  - Heart attack
  - Stroke (cerebral arterial occlusion)
  - Nephropathy
  - Retinopathy and blindness
  - Peripheral neuropathy
  - Cataract
  - Hypertension secondary to renal injury

■ Atherosclerosis secondary to abnormal lipid metabolism.

Gestational Diabetes Mellitus

Hyperglycemia first detected at any time during pregnancy should be classified as either:

- Diabetes mellitus in pregnancy
- Gestational diabetes mellitus (GDM)

Worldwide, one in 10 pregnancies is associated with diabetes, 90% of which are GDM. Gestational diabetes mellitus is a condition in which a woman without diabetes develops high blood sugar levels during pregnancy. Diabetes mellitus in pregnancy differs from GDM in that the hyperglycemia is more severe and does not resolve after pregnancy as it does with GDM. Gestational diabetes mellitus has occurred as a global public health problem.

- Gestational diabetes mellitus is defined as impaired glucose tolerance (IGT) with onset or first recognition during pregnancy. Gestational diabetes is associated with intermediate hyperglycemia, impaired glucose tolerance and impaired fasting glycemia (IFG).
- Undiagnosed or inadequately treated GDM can lead to significant maternal and fetal complications. Moreover, women with GDM and their offsprings are at increased risk of developing type 2, diabetes later in life.
- Maternal risks of GDM include polyhydramnios (excess of amniotic fluid), pre-eclampsia (disorder of pregnancy characterized by the onset of high blood pressure and often a significant amount of protein in the urine), prolonged labor, obstructed labor, infection and progression of retinopathy which are the leading global causes of maternal mortality.
- Fetal risks include spontaneous abortion, intrauterine death, stillbirth, congenital malformation, birth injuries, neonatal hypoglycemia and infant respiratory distress syndrome.
- Gestational diabetes mellitus should be diagnosed at any time in pregnancy if one or more of the following criteria are met:
  - Fasting plasma glucose 92–125 mg/dL (5.1–6.9 mmol/L)
  - 2-hour plasma glucose 153–199 mg/dL (8.5–11.0 mmol/L) following a 75 g oral glucose load.

LABORATORY INVESTIGATION FOR THE DIAGNOSIS OF DIABETES

The following investigations are helpful in diagnosis of diabetes mellitus:

- Urine testing
- Blood glucose estimation
- Glucose tolerance test
- Glycated hemoglobin estimation.

Urine Testing

Urine tests can be used for diagnosing and monitoring diabetes. Urine testing is less accurate than blood testing but is useful as a screening test for people who already know they have diabetes. In diabetes urine is tested for the presence of three parameters: **glucose**, **ketones**, and **protein** (microalbumin).

Glucose Test

Glucose is not normally found in urine, but it can pass from the kidneys into the urine in people who have diabetes. **Urine glucose** measurements are less reliable than blood glucose measurements and are not used to diagnose diabetes or evaluate treatment for diabetes. They may be used for screening purposes. Urine glucose can also be analyzed in the people who are undiagnosed. Urine is tested for the presence of glucose by **Benedict's qualitative** test or **dipstick test**.

Ketone Test

This test detects the presence of ketones in urine. Ketones are formed from fat when there is insufficient insulin to allow glucose to be used for fuel. At high levels of ketones, ketoacidosis may occur.

Ketones can be detected by **Rothera's qualitative test (nitroprusside reaction)**, or by **dipstick test**, by dipping a test strip into a sample of urine. A color change on the test strip signals the presence of ketones in the urine.

Ketones occur most commonly in people with type 1 diabetes but uncommonly, people with type 2 diabetes may test positive for ketones. The presence of ketones in a person with diabetes may indicate a high blood glucose level.

Microalbumin Test

A urine microalbumin test is a test to detect very small levels of a blood protein (albumin) in urine. A microalbumin test is used to detect early signs of kidney damage in people who are at risk of developing kidney disease. Protein is present in the urine when there is damage to the kidneys. The level of microalbumin can be detected by **special albumin-specific urine dipsticks**.

> The urine test used may be referred to as the **"dipstick test"** as it involves dipping a strip into the urine and reading the results using a color chart. A strip will be dipped into the urine sample during the test. The different blocks of color change indicate levels of glucose, ketones, and protein in the urine.

Blood Glucose Estimation

In symptomatic cases, the diagnosis can be confirmed by finding **glucosuria** and a **blood glucose** concentration. Fasting blood glucose is directly proportional to the severity of diabetes mellitus.

- An enzymatic method, using the highly specific enzyme **glucose oxidase**, is used for the routine determination of blood glucose level. Blood sugar level estimated at:
    - Any time of the day without any prior preparations is known as **random blood sugar (RBS)**.
    - In the morning after an overnight fast of 8–12 hours is called **fasting blood sugar (FBS)**.
    - At two hours after a meal is called post lunch or **postprandial blood sugar** (PLBS or PPBS). Prandial in Latin means after food.
- Random blood sugar level of 200 mg/dL higher suggests diabetes.
- Fasting blood sugar level less than 100 mg/dL is normal.
- A fasting blood sugar level from 100 to 125 mg/dL is considered prediabetes. If it's 126 mg/dL or higher is considered diabetes.

Glucose Tolerance Test

In symptomatic cases, the diagnosis of diabetes can be confirmed by finding **glucosuria** and a **blood glucose** concentration. But the problem arises in asymptomatic cases, which have normal fasting blood glucose level but are suspected to have diabetes on other grounds. Such individuals are diagnosed by glucose tolerance test (GTT). Glucose tolerance test (GTT) is performed in asymptomatic cases.

The glucose tolerance is the ability of the body to utilize glucose. It is indicated by the nature of **blood glucose curve** following the administration of glucose. GTT can be performed by two ways:
1. Oral GTT
2. Intravenous GTT.

Oral Glucose Tolerance Test

- The patient who is scheduled for oral GTT is instructed to eat a high carbohydrate diet for at least 3 days prior to the test, and come after an overnight fast on the day of the test.
- A fasting blood glucose sample is first drawn.

- Then 75 g of glucose (or 1.75 g per kg body weight) dissolved in 300 mL of water is ingested.
- Blood and urine specimens are collected at half hourly intervals for at least 2 hours.
- Blood glucose content is measured and urine is tested for glucosuria.
- A curve is plotted for time against blood glucose concentration and is called glucose tolerance curve.

Intravenous Glucose Tolerance Test

- The intravenous glucose tolerance test is often used for persons with malabsorptive disorders or previous gastric or intestinal surgery.
- Glucose is administered intravenously over 30 minutes using 20% solution. A glucose load of 0.5 g/kg of body weight is used.

Types of Glucose Tolerance Curve

- Normal glucose tolerance curve **(Figure 10.47)**
- Abnormal glucose tolerance curve may be due to:
    - Diminished glucose tolerance or
    - Increased glucose tolerance
- Lag type glucose tolerance curve

Normal Glucose Tolerance Curve

Normal response to glucose load is as follows:
- Initial fasting glucose is within the normal fasting limits (70–100 mg %).
- Blood glucose level rises to a peak (120–140 mg %) at half to 1 hour.
- The blood glucose level then returns rapidly to the fasting normal limits in about 2 hours.
- Glucose should not be present in any of the urine specimens collected for 2 hours.

Diminished Glucose Tolerance

Diminished glucose tolerance means decreased ability of the body to utilize glucose. In diminished glucose tolerance:
- Fasting glucose is higher than normal limits.

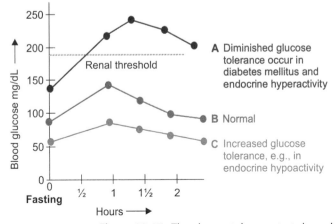

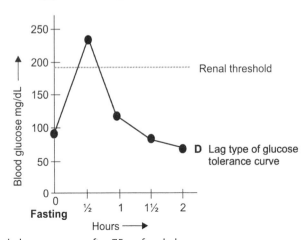

Figure 10.47: The glucose tolerance test shows blood glucose curves after 75 g of oral glucose.

- The blood glucose level rises above 180 mg/100 mL (renal threshold) after ingestion of glucose.
- The blood glucose remains high for a longer time and may not return to fasting level even after 3 hours.
- The urine samples corresponding to blood glucose level over 180 mg/100 mL may show urine Benedict's test positive (glucosuria).
- Diminished glucose tolerance occurs in diabetes mellitus and certain endocrine disorders like:
  - Hyperthyroidism
  - Hyperpituitarism
  - Hyperadrenalism (Cushing's syndrome).

Increased Glucose Tolerance

Increased glucose tolerance means increased ability of the body to utilize glucose. In increased glucose tolerance:

- Fasting blood glucose is lower than normal.
- Only small rise in blood glucose level may be observed (not more than 100 mg%) even after glucose administration.
- A flatter type of curve is obtained.
- No appearance of glucose in urine.
- This type of curve is obtained in endocrine hypoactivity like:
  - Hypothyroidism (myxoedema, cretinism)
  - Hypoadrenalism (Addison's disease)
  - Hypopituitarism.

Lag Type of Glucose Tolerance Curve (Figure 10.47)

In lag type of glucose tolerance curve:

- Fasting blood glucose is within the normal limits.
- The temporary rise in blood glucose level, after the ingestion of glucose is due to a delay in insulin mechanism coming into action.
- Blood glucose level returns to normal limits in the usual time.
- As peak of the curve is above the normal renal threshold, a transient glucosuria may result.

Significance of GTT

Glucose tolerance test (GTT) is not necessary in symptomatic or in known cases of hyperglycemic patients. In such cases determination of fasting or postprandial glucose is usually sufficient for the diagnosis.

- GTT is most important in the investigation of asymptomatic hyperglycemia or glucosuria such as renal glucosuria and alimentary glucosuria.
- This test may contribute useful information in some cases of endocrine dysfunctions.
- It is also helpful in recognizing milder cases of diabetes.

Glycated Hemoglobin (HbA1c) Estimation

All above tests provide information about the patient's glucose concentration only at that time and may be unrepresentative of overall control. Glycated hemoglobin is better than fasting glucose for determining long-term glycemic control and is a reliable biomarker for the diagnosis and prognosis of diabetes.

- HbA1c test tells about average level of blood sugar over the past 2–3 months.
- Estimation of HbA1c levels in blood is used as a guide to the degree of control over a long period.
- The red blood cells of all people contain a small proportion of HbA1c (3–5% of the total hemoglobin) (*see* **Chapter 7**).
- The rate of its formation is proportional to the glucose levels and so persons with diabetes have a higher proportion of HbA1c than do normal individuals (6–15% compared with 3–5%).
- Once formed, glycated Hb stays within the red cell for its lifetime, 120 days.
- An elevated HbA1c which indicates poor control of blood glucose level in the previous 2–3 months, and can guide the physician in selection of appropriate treatment.
- Diagnostic criteria for diabetes as per WHO is given in **Table 10.10**.

TABLE 10.10: WHO diabetes diagnostic criteria.			
Conditions	**2-hour glucose**	**Fasting glucose**	**HbA1c**
Normal	<140 mg/dL (<7.8 mmol/L)	<110 mg/dL (<6.1 mmol/L)	<6.0 %
Impaired fasting glycemia	<140 mg/dL (<7.8 mmol/L)	≥110 mg/dL and <126 mg/dL (≥6.1 mmol/L) and (<7.0 mmol/L)	6.0–6.4%
Impaired glucose tolerance	≥140 mg/dL (≥7.8 mmol/L)	<126 mg/dL (<7.0 mmol/L)	6.0–6.4%
Diabetes mellitus	≥200 mg/dL (≥11.1 mmol/L)	≥126 mg/dL (≥7.0 mmol/L)	≥6.5

ASSESSMENT QUESTIONS

◼ STRUCTURED LONG ESSAY QUESTIONS (SLEQs)

1. Describe pathway of glycolysis under the following headings:
   i. Definition
   ii. Pathway with diagram
   iii. Energetics
   iv. Regulation
   v. Significance
2. Describe pathway of citric acid cycle under the following headings:
   i. Pathway with diagram
   ii. Energetics
   iii. Regulation
   iv. Amphibolic role
   v. Significance
3. Describe pathway of gluconeogenesis under the following headings:
   i. Definition
   ii. Sources
   iii. Pathway with diagram
   iv. Regulation
   v. Significance
4. Describe pathway of HMP pathway under the following headings:
   i. Reactions with diagram
   ii. Regulation
   iii. Significance
   iv. Disorders associated with the pathway
5. Describe pathway of glycogenesis under the following headings:
   i. Definition
   ii. Reactions with diagram
   iii. Regulation
   iv. Significance
   v. Name the glycogen storage diseases
6. Describe pathway of glycogenolysis under the following headings:
   i. Definition
   ii. Reactions with diagram
   iii. Regulation
   iv. Significance
   v. Name the glycogen storage diseases
7. Describe diabetes mellitus under the following headings:
   i. Types
   ii. Cause
   iii. Clinical features
   iv. Metabolic changes
   v. Laboratory investigations for the diagnosis
8. Describe the homeostasis of blood glucose level under the following headings:
   i. Normal blood glucose level
   ii. Definition of hyperglycemia and hypoglycemia
   iii. Maintenance of glucose in fed state
   iv. Maintenance of glucose in fasting state

◼ SHORT ESSAY QUESTIONS (SEQs)

1. Write different types of glycogen storage diseases with their defective enzyme and clinical manifestations.
2. What is glycosuria? Give different types and causes.
3. What is galactosemia? Write its causes, and clinical manifestations.
4. How carbohydrates are digested and absorbed in the body?
5. What is glucose tolerance test? Write different types of glucose tolerance curve with its clinical importance.
6. What is Rapoport-Luebering cycle? Give its significance.
7. What is Cori cycle? Write its pathway and significance.
8. What is lactose intolerance? Write its cause and clinical manifestations.
9. Write formation of 2,3 BPG and its role.
10. Give the energetics of complete oxidation of 1 mole of glucose to CO_2 and H_2O under aerobic and anaerobic conditions.
11. Write gluconeogenesis, with reference to definition, substrates, sites and importance in the body.
12. What is the importance of the pentose phosphate pathway in the body?
13. What is glycated hemoglobin? Give its reference value in blood and its clinical importance.

◼ SHORT ANSWER QUESTIONS (SAQs)

1. Compare and contrast starch and glycogen.
2. Mention any four glycogen storage diseases with their deficient enzymes.
3. What is the role of liver in regulation of blood sugar?
4. Why TCA cycle is an amphibolic pathway, justify?
5. What is Cori cycle? Draw Cori cycle.
6. What is the importance of uronic acid pathway in the body?
7. Give significance of sorbitol or polyol pathway.
8. Write significance of glycolysis.
9. Name key enzymes of glycolysis and gluconeogenesis.
10. What is the fate of pyruvate and its significance?
11. What is the role of TCA in transamination reactions?
12. Why does fructose disappear from the blood of a diabetic patient at a normal rate?
13. What is the cause of lactic acidosis in cancer?
14. List the laboratory investigations for diagnosis of diabetes mellitus?
15. What is resistant starch? Give its clinical importance.
16. Give coenzymes and vitamins involved in pyruvate dehydrogenase reaction.
17. What is the cause and clinical manifestation of fructose intolerance
18. What is the cause and clinical manifestation of lactose intolerance
19. Name the insulin-dependent glucose transporters and their tissue distribution.

20. List 4 differences between hexokinase and glucokinase.
21. Write significance of Rapoport-Luebering cycle.
22. Give reaction where substrate level phosphorylation occurs in glycolysis and TCA cycle.
23. Write various fate of glucose-6-phosphate.
24. Write inhibitors/poisons of glycolysis with their inhibiting enzyme.
25. Write inhibitors/poisons of citric acid cycle with their inhibiting enzyme.
26. Give significance of HMP shunt.
27. What is the clinical manifestation of deficiency of glucose-6-phosphate dehydrogenase?
28. Write enzyme defect and commonest clinical feature in Von Gierke's disease?
29. Enumerate hyperglycemic hormones.
30. What are the actions of insulin in maintenance of blood glucose?
31. What is glycated hemoglobin? Write its clinical importance.
32. What are the causes for abnormal GTT curves?
33. WHO criteria for diagnosis of diabetes mellitus.
34. What is the biochemical basis of development of cataract in diabetes mellitus?
35. What are the consequences of diabetic ketosis?
36. Enumerate the vitamin B-complex involved in citric acid cycle.
37. Write anaplerotic pathways of citric acid cycle.
38. Write entry points gluconeogenic substrates.
39. Why conversion of acetyl-CoA to glucose is not possible?
40. Compare between type 1 and type 2 diabetes mellitus

CASE VIGNETTE-BASED QUESTIONS (CVBQs)

Case Study

1. **A 12-year-male had complained of abdominal discomfort, a feeling of being bloated, increased passage of urine and development of diarrhea after taking milk.**

   Questions
   a. Name the probable disorder.
   b. Cause of disorder.
   c. What will you suggest the patient to relieve the symptoms?

2. **The following are the findings in a patient brought to the hospital in a coma state.**

Findings	Patient	Normal
Blood sugar (Fasting)	270 mg%	70–100 mg%
Urine Benedict's test	Positive	Negative
Urine Rothera's test	Positive	Negative
Plasma pH	7.20	7.35–7.45

   Questions
   a. Name of the disorder.
   b. Why is patient's plasma pH lower than normal?
   c. What does positive Rothera's test indicate?
   d. What is the renal threshold value for glucose?

3. **A 20-year-old male suffering from malaria was treated with chloroquine and manifested as hemolytic anemia. Provisional diagnosis of glucose-6-phosphate dehydrogenase (G-6-PD) deficiency was made.**

   Questions
   a. Which reaction is catalyzed by the enzyme G-6-PD?
   b. How does deficiency of G-6-PD produce hemolytic anemia?
   c. Name the pathway in which this reaction occurs.

4. **A chronically cranky, irritable and lethargic baby girl has an extended abdomen, resulting from an enlarged liver and was diagnosed of having Von Gierke's disease.**

   Questions
   a. Which enzyme is deficient in Von Gierke's disease?
   b. Name the pathways where the enzyme is required.
   c. Give manifestations of the disorder.

5. **A 6-month-old infant was presented with elevated blood and urine galactose.**

   Questions
   a. Name the disease.
   b. Give the biochemical steps related to the disease and point out the metabolic defect.
   c. What is the clinical manifestation of the disease?

6. **An obese person came to the hospital with complaints of polyuria, thirst, weakness and increased appetite. On investigations, he was diagnosed having diabetes mellitus.**

   Questions
   a. What is the cause of diabetes mellitus?
   b. Give names of different types of diabetes mellitus.
   c. What is glucosuria? Name different types of glucosuria.
   d. What is the normal blood sugar level?

7. **A 28-year-old man has complained of chronic leg muscle pains and cramps during exercise. This patient suffers from McArdle syndrome.**

   Questions
   a. What is McArdle syndrome? To metabolism of which biomolecule is it related?
   b. What is the cause of this syndrome?
   c. Name different types of disorders related to the concerned biomolecule.

8. **A 13-year-old diabetic boy visits a diabetic clinic for a check-up. He tells the doctor that he complies with all the dietary advice and never misses insulin. His random blood glucose level is within normal limit but his HbA1c concentration is 10% (normal 4–6%). He has no glucosuria or ketone bodies in his urine.**

   Questions
   a. What does normal blood glucose and urine glucose indicate?
   b. What does elevated level of HbA1c suggest?
   c. Name the type of diabetes the boy is suffering.
   d. What is HbA1c?

9. A 3-year-old patient with mild mental retardation was found to have cataract. Biochemical investigations show high blood concentrations of a sugar alcohol and galactose.

   Questions
   a. Name the probable disease.
   b. Name enzyme most likely to be defective.
   c. What is the cause of development of cataracts?
   d. What is the treatment?

10. A fasting glucose and glycosylated hemoglobin were performed for three consecutive quarters on a patient. The results are as follows:

Quarter	Plasma glucose fasting mg/dL	Glycosylated hemoglobin %
1	280	7.8
2	85	15.3
3	91	8.5

    Questions
    a. In which quarter was the patient's glucose best controlled?
    b. What is the normal fasting blood glucose?
    c. What is the normal level of glycosylated Hb?
    d. What is glycosylated hemoglobin?

11. A 13-year-old girl was admitted to hospital. Her mother mentioned that her daughter had been losing weight and had polyuria. Doctor noticed a fruity breath. On admission following biochemical parameters of urine and blood were obtained.
    – Urine pH 5.5
    – Urine glucose 4+
    – Urine ketones moderate
    – Blood glucose 480 mg/dL
    – Blood ketones positive.

    Questions
    a. Identity this patient's type of diabetes.
    b. What is the cause of fruity breath?
    c. What is the cause of weight loss?
    d. Name ketone bodies.

12. A diabetic 22-year old patient comes to the emergency department. She gives a 3 days history of vomiting and abdominal pain. She is drowsy and her breathing is deep and rapid. There is fruity smell from her breath.

    Questions
    a. What is the most likely diagnosis?
    b. Which bedside tests could you do to confirm this diagnosis?
    c. Which laboratory tests would you request?

13. A 23-year-old African boy was brought with history of fever and chills and rigors for which he was given antimalarial drug Primaquine. Fever subsided but the patient was fatigued with breathlessness. Presently, he is presenting with mild yellow discoloration of conjunctiva.

On examination, skin and mucous membrane were pale. Following are the investigations done:
– Hb   7 g%
– Total bilirubin   4 mg/dL
– Direct bilirubin   1 mg/dL
– Indirect bilirubin   3 mg/dL
– Fouchet's test   Negative
Liver enzymes are normal.

Questions
a. What is the probable diagnosis?
b. Name the pathway concerned with your diagnosis.
c. What is the importance of the pathway?
d. What is the cause of your diagnosis? Justify.

14. A 40-year-old woman, weighing about 80 kg, came to the OPD of a hospital, complaining of weakness and lethargy for the last 2–3 months. She also noticed that she felt very thirsty. In the night she gets up 4–5 times for urination. When asked about the family history for such symptoms, she said that her mother had such symptoms for which she had been started with some treatment. On physical examination, she appeared dehydrated with dryness of tongue, and had mild rise of BP (146/96 mm Hg). There was no other finding.
The following were the results of investigations done.
– Blood sugar (fasting)   152 mg/dL
– Blood sugar (postprandial)   246 mg/dL
– HbA1c   14%
– Cholesterol   270 mg/dL
– Urea   36 mg/dL
– X-ray chest and ECG were normal.

Questions
a. What is your diagnosis?
b. Why is the patient lethargic?
c. What is the cause of frequent urination?
d. What is the significance of the HbA1c?

■ MULTIPLE CHOICE QUESTIONS (MCQs)

1. Which of the following enzymes produce a product used for synthesis of ATP by substrate level?
   a. Phosphofructokinase
   b. Aldolase
   c. 1,3-bisphosphate mutase
   d. Enloase

2. 2,3-bisphosphoglycerate is:
   a. A high energy substrate
   b. Involved in substrate level phosphorylation
   c. An intermediate in pentose phosphate pathway
   d. An allosteric effector that decreases the O_2 affinity of Hb

3. Muscle glycogen is not available for maintenance of blood glucose concentration because:
   a. Muscle lacks glucose-6-phosphatase activity
   b. There is insufficient glycogen in muscle
   c. Muscle lacks glucose transporter GLUT-4
   d. Muscle lacks glucagon receptors

4. The primary metabolic fate of lactate released from muscle during intense exercise is:
   a. Excretion of lactate in urine
   b. Transported to liver for replenishment of blood glucose by gluconeogenesis
   c. Conversion to pyruvate
   d. Gradual reuptake in muscle during the recovery phase following exercise

5. Which of the following statement is true of TCA cycle?
   a. It requires coenzyme biotin, FAD, NAD and coenzyme A
   b. Two NADH are produced per turn
   c. It participates in the synthesis of glucose from pyruvic acid
   d. Enzymes are located in cytosol

6. Which of the following vitamins does not participate in the oxidative decarboxylation of pyruvate to acetyl-CoA?
   a. Thiamine   b. Biotin
   c. Niacin   d. Riboflavin

7. The following enzymes catalyze a decarboxylation reaction, *except*:
   a. α-ketoglutarate dehydrogenase
   b. Pyruvate dehydrogenase
   c. Pyruvate carboxylase
   d. Isocitrate dehydrogenase

8. The principal source of glucose after an overnight fast is:
   a. Gluconeogenesis
   b. Glycolysis
   c. Glycogenolysis
   d. HMP pathway

9. Which of the following cannot take place in the human body?
   a. Transformation of lactate into glucose
   b. Transformation of glycerol into glucose
   c. Transformation of propionyl-CoA into glucose
   d. Transformation of acetate into glucose

10. In a patient with galactosemia who is on a galactose free diet, the D-galactose that is required for cell membrane and other biopolymers is formed by:
    a. Isomerization of glucose-1-phosphate
    b. Epimerization of UDP-glucose
    c. Epimerization of D-fructose
    d. Epimerization of glucose-6-phosphate

11. Gluconeogenesis, must bypass irreversible reactions of glycolysis, *except*:
    a. Hexokinase
    b. Phosphohexose isomerase
    c. Pyruvate kinase
    d. Phosphofructokinase

12. In skeletal muscle, glycogen synthesis occurs during:
    a. Contraction
    b. Relaxation
    c. Well-fed state
    d. Increased level of insulin

13. The following hormones have hyperglycemic effect, *except*:
    a. Glucagon   b. Thyroid
    c. Epinephrine   d. Insulin

14. Rate controlling steps in the citric acid cycle include all of the following, *except*:
    a. Isocitrate dehydrogenase
    b. Citrate synthase
    c. Fumarase
    d. α-ketoglutarate dehydrogenase

15. Gluconeogenesis can proceed from all of the following, *except*:
    a. Pyruvate   b. Palmitic acid
    c. Propionyl-CoA   d. Oxaloacetate

16. The following are the functions of pentose phosphate pathway, *except*:
    a. Interconverts hexoses and pentoses
    b. Produces NADPH
    c. Supplies ribose-5-phosphate
    d. Converts glucose to galactose

17. People with diabetes mellitus are prone to develop cataracts because their elevated blood glucose concentration:
    a. Inhibit gluconeogenesis
    b. Increase glycosylate hemoglobin
    c. Increase glycogen synthesis within the lens
    d. Allow aldose reductase to reduce glucose to sorbitol

18. Both glycolysis and gluconeogenesis involve which of the following enzymes:
    a. Pyruvate carboxylase
    b. Hexokinase
    c. Aldolase
    d. Phosphofructokinase

19. Glucose-6-phosphate is involved in which of the following pathways:
    a. Glycolysis
    b. Gluconeogenesis
    c. Pentose phosphate pathway
    d. All of the above

20. Gluconeogenesis occurs in which of the following:
    a. Heart   b. Erythrocytes
    c. Liver   d. Lungs

21. Von Gierke's disease is characterized by deficiency of the enzyme:
    a. Glucokinase
    b. Glucose-6-phosphatase
    c. Phosphoglucomutase
    d. Glycogen synthase

22. McArdle syndrome involves a deficiency of which of the following enzymes:
    a. Hepatic phosphorylase
    b. Muscle phosphorylase
    c. Debranching enzyme
    d. Hepatic glycogen synthase

23. Deficiency of glucose-6-phosphate dehydrogenase causes:
    a. Cataract   b. Hypoglycemia
    c. Hemolytic anemia   d. Galactosemia

24. Essential pentosuria is due to metabolic defect in:
    a. Glycolysis   b. HMP-shunt
    c. Uronic acid pathway d. Glycogenolysis

25. Rapoport Luebering cycle in RBC produces:
    a. ATP
    b. NADPH
    c. 2,3-bisphosphoglycerate
    d. 1,3-bisphosphoglycerate

26. The first loss of carbon in the metabolism of glucose takes place as CO_2 in the formation of:
    a. Acetyl-CoA   b. Pyruvate
    c. 2,3 BPG   d. Fructose 1,6-bisphosphate

27. Anaerobic glycolysis from glycogen generates:
    a. 3 moles of ATP   b. 2 moles of ATP
    c. 8 moles of ATP   d. 6 moles of ATP

28. The net production of ATP when glycolysis occurs via Rapoport-Luebering route:
    a. Two   b. Six
    c. Eight   d. Zero

29. In erythrocytes, the end product of glycolysis is:
    a. Pyruvate   b. Acetyl-CoA
    c. Lactate   d. 2,3-bisphosphoglycerate

30. Which of the following step is not involved in substrate level phosphorylation?
    a. Dihydroxyacetone phosphate to glyceraldehyde-3-phosphate
    b. 1,3-diphosphoglycerate to 3-phosphoglycerate
    c. Succinyl-CoA to succinate
    d. Phosphoenol pyruvate to pyruvate

31. How many ATP molecules are produced in the citric acid cycle itself?
    a. One   b. Two
    c. Ten   d. Fifteen

32. CO_2 is not produced in the reaction catalyzed by the enzyme.
    a. Pyruvate dehydrogenase
    b. Succinate dehydrogenase
    c. Isocitrate dehydrogenase
    d. α-ketoglutarate dehydrogenase

33. Which of the following statements is not true of HMP shunt pathway?
    a. CO_2 is not produced in it
    b. NADPH is produced
    c. Pentoses are produced
    d. Does not produce ATP

34. They utilize fructose but not glucose.
    a. Ovum   b. Spermatozoa
    c. Adipose tissue   d. Mammary gland

35. The uronic acid pathway is unique as it provides to man.
    a. Ascorbic acid   b. Xylulose
    c. Glucuronic acid   d. All of these.

36. The hormone does not stimulate hepatic glycogenolysis:
    a. Thyroxine   b. Adrenaline
    c. Glucagon   d. Cortisol

37. Suggest a test to distinguish a case of renal glucosuria from diabetic glucosuria:
    a. Benedict's test   b. Blood sugar
    c. Urine sugar   d. GTT

38. NADPH serves to regenerate in red cells to prevent their lysis:
    a. Cholesterol
    b. Glutathione
    c. NADP
    d. Cysteine

39. The G-6-PD deficiency causes hemolytic anemia due to lack of:
    a. NADPH   b. NADP
    c. Pentoses   d. Cholesterol

40. How many ATP molecules are produced on complete oxidation of acetyl-CoA in the citric acid cycle?
    a. Six   b. Nine
    c. Ten   d. Fifteen

41. Which of the following enzyme is not involved in gluco-neogenesis?
    a. Pyruvate carboxylase
    b. Phosphoenolpyruvate carboxykinase
    c. Glucose 6-phosphatase
    d. Hexokinas

42. The most important initial source of blood glucose during fasting is:
    a. Muscle glycogen
    b. Muscle protein
    c. Liver triglyceride
    d. Liver glycogen

43. The major fate of glucose-6-phosphate in tissues in a well-fed state is:
    a. Hydrolysis of glucose
    b. Conversion to glycogen
    c. Isomerization to fructose-6-phosphate
    d. Conversion to ribulose-5-phosphate

44. The major fuel for the brain after prolonged starvation is:
    a. Glucose   b. Fatty acids
    c. Ketone bodies   d. Glycerol

45. The monosaccharide most rapidly absorbed from the intestine is:
    a. Glucose   b. Fructose
    c. Mannose   d. Galactose

46. Lactose intolerance is due to:
    a. ADH deficiency
    b. Deficiency of bile
    c. Lactase deficiency
    d. Malabsorption syndrome

47. In contrast to liver, muscle glycogen does not contribute directly to blood glucose level because:
    a. Muscles lack glucose-6-phosphatase
    b. Muscles contain no glucokinase
    c. Muscles lack glycogen
    d. Muscles contain no glycogen phosphorylase

48. Which of the following statement is true regarding the α-amylase?
    a. Breaks glucose from one end of the carbohydrate
    b. Cleaves only α-1,4 linkages
    c. Cleaves only α-1,6 linkages
    d. All of the above

49. When blood glucagon rises, which of the following hepatic enzyme activities fall?
    a. Protein kinase
    b. Glycogen synthase
    c. Glycogen phosphorylase
    d. Adenylyl cyclase

50. Glucose 6-phosphatse is necessary for the production of blood glucose from:
    a. Lactose
    b. Amino acids
    c. Liver glycogen
    d. All of the above

51. Insulin promotes hypoglycemia by a mechanism including all of the following, *except*:
    a. Repressing the synthesis of key gluconeogenic enzymes.
    b. Decreasing levels of C-AMP
    c. Stimulating glycogen phosphorylase enzyme
    d. Inducing the synthesis of key glycolytic enzymes.

52. The most severe form of galactosemia is due to:
    a. A genetic deficiency of a galactose-phosphate uridyl transferase
    b. Deficiency of epimerase
    c. Defect in galactokinase
    d. None of the above

53. UDP glucuronate is required for:
    a. Synthesis of proteoglycans and glycoproteins
    b. Formation of iduronate
    c. Detoxification of bilirubin
    d. All of the above

54. Which of the following hormones promotes glycolysis?
    a. Growth hormone
    b. Glucagon
    c. Insulin
    d. ACTH

55. Hyperglycemic hormone secreted by pancreas:
    a. Insulin   b. Glucagon
    c. Epinephrine   d. Growth hormone

56. Cori's cycle involves the conversion of:
    a. Liver glucose to lactate
    b. Pyruvate to lactate in muscle
    c. Muscle lactate to glucose in the liver
    d. Pyruvate to glucose in the liver

57. Identity the amino acid that is the major contributor of hepatic gluconeogenesis:
    a. Alanine   b. Glutamine
    c. Leucine   d. Lysine

58. What is the preferred specimen for glucose analysis?
    a. EDTA plasma
    b. Serum
    c. Fluoride oxalate plasma
    d. Heparinized plasma

59. Glucose-6-phosphatase catalyzes the formation of:
    a. Glucose-6-phosphate
    b. Glucose + Pi
    c. Glucose-1-phosphate
    d. Fructose-6-phosphate

60. Enzyme hexokinase catalyzes the formation of:
    a. Glucose-6-phosphate
    b. Glucose-1-phosphate
    c. Acetyl-CoA
    d. None of the above

61. Irreversible steps of glycolysis are catalyzed by:
    a. Hexokinase, phosphofructokinase, pyruvate kinase
    b. Glucokinase, pyruvate kinase, glyceraldehyde 3 phosphate dehydrogenase
    c. Hexokinase, phosphoglycerate kinase, pyruvate kinase
    d. Pyruvate kinase, fructose-1,6-bisphosphatase, Phosphofructokinase

62. Which enzyme is active when insulin: glucagon ratio is low?
    a. Glucokinase
    b. Hexokinase
    c. Glucose-6-phosphatase
    d. Phosphofructokinase

63. The reason for ketosis in von Gierke's disease are all *except*:
    a. Hypoglycemia
    b. Oxaloacetate is necessary for gluconeogenesis
    c. Low blood glucose less than 40 mg%
    d. Fatty acid mobilization is low

64. A child with low blood glucose is unable to do glycogenolysis or gluconeogenesis. Which of the following enzyme is missing in the child?
    a. Fructokinase
    b. Glucokinase
    c. Glucose-6-phosphatase
    d. Transketolase

65. Enzyme responsible for complete oxidations of glucose to CO_2 and water is present in:
    a. Cytosol
    b. Mitochondria
    c. Lysosomes
    d. Endoplasmic reticulum

66. Glycolysis occurs in:
    a. Cytosol
    b. Mitochondria
    c. Nucleus
    d. Lysosome

67. Irreversible step(s) in glycolysis is/are, *except*:
    a. Hexokinase
    b. Phosphofructokinase
    c. Pyruvate kinase
    d. Glyceraldehyde-3-phosphate dehydrogenase

68. Which of the following metabolic pathway does not generate ATP?
    a. Glycolysis
    b. TCA cycle
    c. Fatty acid oxidation
    d. HMP pathway

69. In which of the following tissue, is glycogen incapable of contributing directly to blood glucose?
    a. Liver   b. Muscle
    c. Both   d. None

70. Common enzyme for gluconeogenesis and glycolysis is:
    a. Glyceraldehyde-3-phosphate dehydrogenase
    b. Hexokinase
    c. Pyruvate kinase
    d. Pyruvate carboxylase

71. The enzyme which released free glucose in glycogenolysis:
    a. Glucan Transferase
    b. α-1,6-glucosidase
    c. Glycogen phosphorylase
    d. α-1,4-glucosidase

72. Reduced NADPH produced from which pathway?
    a. Krebs cycle
    b. Anaerobic glycolysis
    c. Uronic acid pathway
    d. Hexose monophosphate pathway

73. Not a substrate for gluconeogenesis
    a. Acetyl-CoA   b. Lactate
    c. Glycerol   d. Propionyl-CoA

74. Which of the following reaction takes place in two cellular compartments?
    a. Gluconeogenesis
    b. Glycolysis
    c. Glycogenesis
    d. Glycogenolysis

75. Substrate level phosphorylation is by
    a. Pyruvate kinase
    b. Phosphofructokinase
    c. Hexokinase
    d. ATP synthase

76. An example of anaplerotic reaction of TCA cycle is:
    a. Pyruvate to oxaloacetate
    b. Pyruvate to lactate
    c. Pyruvate to acetyl-CoA
    d. Pyruvate to acetaldehyde

77. In which step of TCA cycle ATP is generated?
    a. Succinate dehydrogenase
    b. Fumarase
    c. Succinate thiokinase
    d. Malate dehydrogenase

78. Which of the following is not an intermediate of TCA CYCLE?
    a. Acetyl-CoA   b. Citrate
    c. Succinyl-CoA   d. Alpha ketoglutarate

79. First substrate of Krebs cycle
    a. Oxaloacetate   b. Pyruvate
    c. Malate   d. Lipoprotein

80. Which of the following is not correct for hemoglobin A1c?
    a. Less than 6% of HbA1c is normal
    b. More than 6.5% of HbA1c occurs in diabetes mellitus
    c. Not present in normal person
    d. Value depends on the level of blood glucose

81. Which of the following are tests for the diagnosis for diabetes?
    a. Urine testing
    b. Glucose tolerance test
    c. Glycated hemoglobin estimation
    d. All of the above

82. In diminished glucose tolerance all of the following is true, *except*:
    a. Fasting glucose is higher than normal limits
    b. Blood glucose level returns to fasting normal limits in about 2 hours
    c. Blood glucose level rises above 180 mg/100 mL after ingestion of glucose
    d. Blood glucose remains high and may not return to fasting level even after 3 hours

83. Diminished glucose tolerance occurs in:
    a. Hyperpituitarism   b. Hypopituitarism
    c. Hypoadrenalism   d. Hypothyroidism

84. Patient with Type I Diabetes mellitus, with complains of polyuria. Which of the following will occur normally in his body?
    a. Glycogenesis in muscle
    b. Increased protein synthesis
    c. Increased conversion of fatty acid to Acetyl-CoA
    d. Decreased in Cholesterol synthesis

85. A baby is hypotonic and shows increased ratio of Pyruvate to Acetyl CoA. Pyruvate cannot form Acetyl CoA in fibroblast. He also shows features of lactic acidosis. Which of the following can revert the situation?
    a. Biotin   b. Pyridoxine
    c. Free fatty acid   d. Thiamin

86. A child with low blood glucose is unable to do glycogen-olysis or gluconeogenesis. Which of the following enzyme is missing in the child?
    a. Fructokinase
    b. Glucokinase
    c. Glucose 6 Phosphatase
    d. Transketolase

87. A genetic disorder renders fructose 1,6-bisphosphatase in liver less sensitive to regulation by fructose 2,6-biphosphate. All of the following metabolic changes are observed in this disorder, *except*:
    a. Level of fructose 1,6-biphosphate is higher than normal
    b. Level of fructose 1,6-biphosphate is lower than normal
    c. Less pyruvate is formed
    d. Less ATP is generated

88. A male patient came with pain in calf muscles in exercise. On biopsy glycogen was present in the muscle. What is the enzyme eficiency?
    a. Branching enzyme
    b. Phosphofructokinase I
    c. Debranching enzyme
    d. Glucose 6 phosphatase

89. A four-year-old child presented with exercise intolerance. On investigation blood pH 7.3, FBS 60 mg%, hypertri-glyceridemia, ketosis and lactic acidosis occur. The child had hepatomegaly and renomegaly. Biopsy of liver and kidney showed increased glycogen content. What is the diagnosis?
    a. Mc Ardle's disease
    b. Cori's disease
    c. Von Gierke's disease
    d. Pompe's disease

90. A female infant appeared normal at birth but developed signs of liver disease one month of age and muscle weakness at 3 months and severe hypoglycemia on early morning awakening. Examination revealed hepatomegaly; laboratory analysis showed ketoacidosis, pH 7.2, increased AST and ALT over 1000 IU. Intravenous administration glucagon followed by meals normalized blood levels, but glucose levels did not rise when glucagon was administered overnight fast. Liver biopsy was done and glycogen constituted (8%) of wet weight. With the above clinical picture which of the following enzyme is deficient?
    a. Debranching enzyme
    b. Glucose 6 phosphatase
    c. Muscle phosphorylase
    d. Branching enzyme

91. A child with low blood glucose is unable to do glycogenolysis or gluconeogenesis. Which of the following enzyme is missing in the child?
    a. Fructokinase
    b. Glucokinase
    c. Glucose 6 Phosphatase
    d. Transketolase

92. A 5 years old boy presents with hepatomegaly, hypoglycemia, ketosis. The diagnosis is:
    a. Mucopolysaccharidoses
    b. Glycogen storage disorder
    c. Lipopolysaccharidosis
    d. Diabetes mellitus

93. An infant has hepatosplenomegaly, hypoglycemia, hyperlipidemia, acidosis and normal structured glycogen deposition in liver. What is the diagnosis:
    a. Her's disease   b. Von Gierke's disease
    c. Cori's disease   e. Pompe's disease
    d. Anderson's disease

94. A baby boy 10-month old comes with vomiting severe jaundice, hepatomegaly and features of irritability on starting weaning with fruit juice. Which of the following enzymes is defective?
    a. Aldolase B
    b. Fructokinase
    c. Glucose 6 phosphatase
    d. Galactose 1 Phosphate Uridyl transferase

95. A newborn baby refuses breast milk since the second day of birth, vomits on force-feeding but accepts glucose-water, develops diarrhea on third day, by fifth day she is jaundiced with liver enlargement and eyes show cataract. Urinary reducing sugar was positive but blood glucose estimated by glucose oxidation method was found low. The most likely cause is deficiency of:

a. Galactose 1-phosphate uridyl transferase
b. Beta galactosidase
c. Glucose 6-phosphate
d. Galactokinase

96. A child presents with hepatomegaly and bilateral lenticular opacities. Deficiency of which of the following enzymes will not cause such features?
    a. Galactose-1-phosphate uridyl transferase
    b. UDP galactose 4-epimerase
    c. Galactokinase
    d. Lactase

97. A chronic alcoholic have low energy production because of thiamine deficiency as it is:
    a. Acting as a cofactor for alpha ketoglutarate dehydrogenase and pyruvate dehydrogenase
    b. Acting as cofactor for transketolase in pentose phosphate pathway
    c. Interferes with energy production from amino acids
    d. Act as cofactor for oxidation reduction

98. A child ingested cyanide and rushed to the emergency room. Which of the following of citric acid cycle is inhibited at the earliest?
    a. Citrate synthase
    b. Aconitase
    c. Acetyl CoA production
    d. NAD+ donor

ANSWERS FOR MCQs

1. d	2. d	3. a	4. b	5. c
6. b	7. c	8. a	9. d	10. b
11. b	12. b	13. d	14. c	15. b
16. d	17. d	18. c	19. d	20. c
21. b	22. b	23. c	24. c	25. c
26. a	27. a	28. d	29. c	30. a
31. c	32. b	33. a	34. b	35. c
36. b	37. d	38. b	39. a	40. c
41. d	42. d	43. b	44. c	45. d
46. c	47. a	48. b	49. b	50. d
51. c	52. a	53. d	54. c	55. b
56. c	57. a	58. c	59. b	60. a
61. a	62. c	63. c	64. c	65. b
66. a	67. d	68. d	69. b	70. a
71. b	72. d	73. a	74. a	75. a
76. a	77. c	78. a	79. a	80. c
81. d	82. b	83. a	84. c	85. d
86. c	87. a	88. b	89. c	90. a
91. c	92. b	93. b	94. a	95. a
96. d	97. a	98. d		

Lipid Metabolism

Competency	Learning Objectives
BI 4.2: Describe the processes involved in digestion and absorption of dietary lipids and also the key features of their metabolism. **BI 4.3:** Explain the regulation of lipoprotein metabolism and associated disorders. **BI 4.4:** Describe the structure and functions of lipoproteins, their functions, interrelations and relations with atherosclerosis. **BI 4.5:** Interpret laboratory results of analytes associated with metabolism of lipids. **BI 4.6:** Describe the therapeutic uses of prostaglandins and inhibitors of eicosanoid synthesis. **BI 4.7:** Interpret laboratory results of analytes associated with metabolism of lipids.	1. Describe digestion, absorption, and transport of dietary lipids with associated abnormalities. 2. Describe lipoprotein metabolism and associated disorders. 3. Describe triacylglycerol metabolism: Synthesis, breakdown, regulation and associated disorder. 4. Describe fatty acid metabolism: β-oxidation, energetics, regulation and associated disorders. 5. Describe ketone bodies metabolism: Synthesis, breakdown, regulation, significance and associated disorders. 6. Describe biosynthesis of fatty acids. 7. Describe cholesterol metabolism: Synthesis, regulation, metabolic fates, excretion and associated disorders. 8. Describe eicosanoids: Types, functions, synthesis, inhibitors of synthesis and therapeutic uses of prostaglandins. 9. Describe lipid profile tests and interpretations with various disorders.

OVERVIEW

The lipids, present in the various cells of the human body, constantly undergo changes. They are continually being oxidized for energy, converted to other essential tissue constituents or stored as reserve fat in adipose tissue. Lipids include a wide variety of chemical substances such as:

- Neutral fat (triacylglycerol or triglycerides)
- Fatty acids and their derivatives
- Phospholipids
- Glycolipids
- Sterols
- Fat soluble vitamins (A, D, E, and K).

An adult ingests about 60 to 150 g of lipids per day, of which more than 90% fat intake in the diet is as **triacylglycerols**, with the remainder consisting of **cholesterol**, **cholesterol ester**, **phospholipid** and **free fatty acid**.

We begin this chapter with a brief discussion on digestion, absorption and transport of lipids. We then focus on metabolism of the major classes of lipids, fatty acids, triacylglycerols, phospholipids, lipoproteins, and cholesterol. In addition ketone body metabolism is reviewed. Several metabolic control mechanisms are also discussed throughout the chapter.

DIGESTION, ABSORPTION, AND TRANSPORT OF DIETARY LIPIDS WITH ASSOCIATED ABNORMALITIES

Digestion of Lipids

The digestion of lipid presents a problem not raised by other constituents of the diet, since lipid molecules are completely immiscible with water and enzymes are soluble in aqueous medium. **Enzymes cannot act on water insoluble substance**. This problem is solved by the

emulsification of lipids by **bile salts**. Before fat digestion can occur, it must be dispersed in fine droplets as an **emulsion**, which facilitates the digestion of lipids. Little or no digestion occurs in the mouth or stomach since:

- No significant amount of lipase is present in the secretion of mouth or stomach
- No mechanism for emulsification of lipid exists
- The acid pH of gastric secretion is not helpful to lipid digestion.

The major site of lipid digestion is the small intestine, where dietary lipid undergoes its major digestive processes using enzymes secreted by pancreas.

Digestion in Mouth

A lingual lipase is secreted by the dorsal surface of the tongue, but this enzyme is not of such significance in humans as it is in the rat and the mouse.

Digestion in Stomach

The stomach secretes a **gastric lipase**, lingual lipase and gastric lipase, which are active only at neutral pH; preferentially hydrolyze short and medium chain fatty acids (containing 12 or fewer carbon atoms) from dietary triacylglycerols. Therefore, they are most active in infants and young children, whose stomach pH is nearer to neutrality and diets often contain milk lipids (cow's milk) which contains triacylglycerols with a high percentage of short and medium chain fatty acids. *Overall, in adults, where the stomach pH is acidic, dietary lipids are not digested to any extent in the stomach or in the mouth.*

The released hydrophilic short and medium chain fatty acids are absorbed via the stomach wall and enter the portal vein, whereas longer chain fatty acids dissolve in the fat droplets and pass on into the duodenum.

Digestion in Small Intestine

The acidic stomach contents called **chyme**; containing dietary fat leaves the stomach and enters the small intestine, in the duodenum. Entrance of the acidic chyme from the stomach into the duodenum stimulates the secretion of enteric hormones called **secretin** and **cholecystokinin (pancreozymin)** by duodenal mucosa.

- **Cholecystokinin** acts on the gallbladder, causing it to contract and release bile into the small intestine. Cholecystokinin also acts on the exocrine cells of the pancreas, causing them to release digestive enzymes containing lipase. Cholecystokinin also decreases gastric motility, resulting in a slower release of the gastric contents into the small intestine.
- **Secretin** causes the pancreas to release a solution enriched in bicarbonate that helps neutralize the pH of the acidic chyme and changes the pH to the alkaline side, which is necessary for the activity of pancreatic

and intestinal enzymes. Pancreatic juice and bile enter the upper small intestine, the duodenum, by way of the pancreatic and bile ducts respectively. The major function of bile is to provide the emulsifying agents, the bile salts and phosphatidylcholine. Both these are powerful emulsifying agents. They emulsify the triacylglycerols into small droplets of 200 to 5000 nm in diameter.

Action of Pancreatic Enzymes on Dietary Lipids in the Small Intestine

Three lipid digestive enzymes secreted by pancreas are:
- Pancreatic lipase
- Cholesterol esterase and
- Phospholipase-A_2.

Hydrolysis of Dietary Triacylglycerols

Emulsified triacylglycerols are readily attacked by **pancreatic lipase**.

Lipase hydrolyses fatty acid in the 1 and 3 positions of the triacylglycerol, producing 2-monoacylglycerols and two molecules of fatty acids. Subsequent slow isomerization of the 2-monoacylglycerol to 1 or 3 monoacylglycerols occurs and these are then hydrolyzed to **glycerol** and a third molecule of **fatty acid (Figure 11.1)**.

However, under most conditions in the digestive tract, minimal formation of glycerol occurs, most of the hydrolyzed triacylglycerol forms monoacylglycerols.

Hydrolysis of Dietary Phospholipids

Dietary glycerophospholipids are digested by pancreatic **phospholipase-A_2**. This enzyme catalyzes the hydrolysis of fatty acid residues at the 2-position of the glycerophospholipids, leaving lysophospholipids **(Figure 11.2)** which being **detergents**, **aid emulsification**, and **digestion of lipids**.

The lysophospholipids either enter the mucosal cells or are degraded further by lysophospholipase enzyme secreted by intestinal cells, which catalyzes the removal of the remaining fatty acid residue.

Hydrolysis of Cholesterol Ester

Cholesterol esters are hydrolyzed by pancreatic **cholesterol ester hydrolase (cholesterol esterase)**, which produces cholesterol plus free fatty acid.

Products of Lipid Digestion (Micelle Formation)

The primary products of dietary lipid digestion are:
- Free fatty acids
- Free cholesterol
- 2-monoacylglycerol
- Small amount of 1-monoacylglycerol and
- Lysophospholipid.

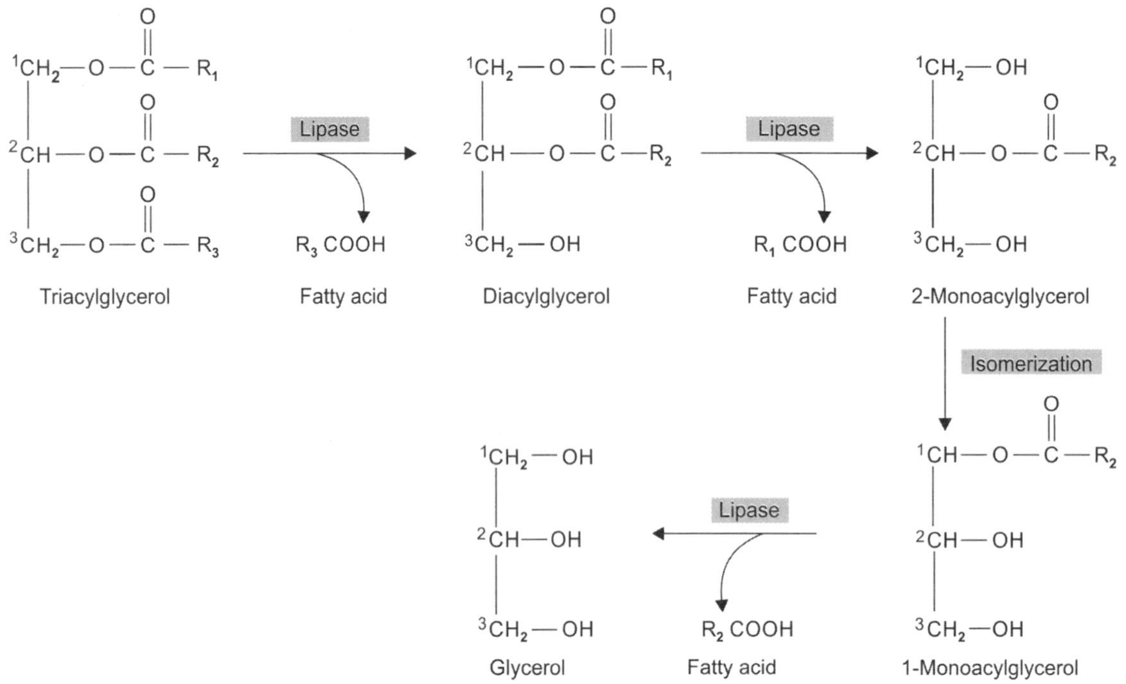

Figure 11.1: Hydrolysis of triacylglycerol by lipase in intestine.

These, together with bile salts, form **mixed micelles**. Micelles are of very much smaller dimensions than emulsion globules. Fat soluble vitamins A, D, E, and K are also packaged in these micelles and are absorbed from the micelles along with the primary products of dietary lipid digestion.

Absorption of Lipids by Intestinal Mucosal Cells

The mixed micelles approach the brush border membrane of the intestinal mucosal cells. There the lipid components from mixed micelles pass through and are absorbed into the mucosal cells of the jejunum and ileum by diffusion. The net result is the transfer of monoacylglycerols, fatty acids, cholesterol, and lysophospholipid molecules into the cell. After absorption within the intestinal wall, the following events occur:

- 1-monoacylglycerols are further hydrolyzed to produce free glycerol and fatty acids by an **intestinal lipase (glycerol ester hydrolase)**.
- 2-monoacylglycerols are reconverted to triacyl-glycerols. The fatty acids are required for this synthesis. The utilization of fatty acids for resynthesis of, triacylglycerols first requires their conversion to active form acyl-CoA by the action of **acyl-CoA synthetase** (thiokinase) **(Figure 11.3)**.
- The absorbed lysophospholipids and cholesterol are also reacylated with acyl-CoA to regenerate phospholipids and cholesterol esters.
- The free glycerol released in the intestinal lumen is not reutilized but passes directly to the portal vein, however, the glycerol-3-phosphate, formed within the intestinal cells by the glucose, can be reutilized for triacylglycerol synthesis.

Bile salts of the micelles are not absorbed at this point. They are reabsorbed in the lower part of the small intestine and return to the liver by the portal vein for resecretion into the bile. This is known as enterohepatic circulation of bile salts.

Short and medium chain triacylglycerols can be absorbed as such and are then hydrolyzed by an **intestinal lipase**, also known as **glycerol ester hydrolase**, which is distinct from pancreatic lipase. This enzyme has importance in patients, who are suffering from pancreatic lipase deficiency and who are fed on medium chain triacylglycerols.

Short and medium chain fatty acids (C_4 to C_{12}) do not require bile salts for their absorption. They are absorbed directly into intestinal epithelial cells. Because they do not need to be packaged into chylomicrons, they enter the portal blood rather than lymph and are transported to the liver bound to serum albumin.

Transport of Dietary Lipids

Triacylglycerol, phospholipid, cholesterol esters synthesized in the intestinal mucosa and absorbed fat soluble vitamins are transported from the mucosal cells into the **lymph** in the form of lipoprotein globule known as **chylomicrons (Figure 11.3)**. Chylomicrons are composed of:

- Triacylglycerols (85 to 90%)
- Cholesterol and cholesterol ester (5%)
- Phospholipids (7%)
- Protein (apolipoprotein B-48, 1–2%).

After a meal there is a transient elevation of blood lipids called **alimentary hyperlipemia**. The peak level of lipid in blood plasma usually occurs after 1/2 to 3 hours and returns to normal in 5 to 6 hours. The **chylomicrons** are responsible

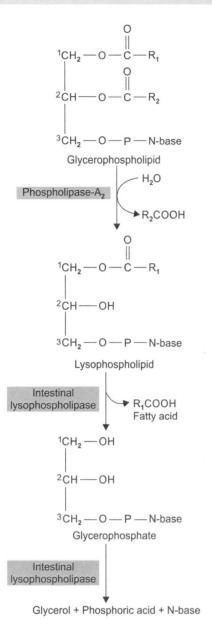

Figure 11.2: Hydrolysis of glycerophospholipid by phospholipase A_2 in intestine.

for the turbid or milky appearance of the plasma after a meal rich in fat.

Fat absorbed from the diet and fat synthesized by the liver and adipose tissue must be transported between the various tissues and organs for utilization and storage. Since lipids are insoluble in water, the problem arises of how to transport them in an aqueous environment of the blood plasma. Lipids are nonpolar and insoluble in water. To facilitate their transport, they are carried in the blood as **lipoproteins**.

Abnormalities in Lipid Digestion and Absorption

Lipid Malabsorption

Lipid malabsorption results in a loss of lipid as much as 30 g/day including the fat soluble vitamins and essential

fatty acids in the feces. Conditions in which the feces contain large amounts of fat and fatty acids, commonly **stearic acid** therefore called **steatorrhea**, (Greek, steato = fat). **Steatorrhea** caused by a number of conditions. The most common causes are:
- Bile salt deficiency occurs in liver disease or due to obstruction in the bile duct.
- Pancreatic enzyme deficiency occurs in pancreatitis or cystic fibrosis.
- Defective chylomicron synthesis occurs in congenital **abetalipoproteinemia**.

LIPOPROTEIN METABOLISM AND ASSOCIATED DISORDERS

- Lipoproteins are water miscible complexes of proteins and lipids which have a hydrophobic, nonpolar **core of triacylglycerol** and **cholesterol ester**, wrapped in a hydrophilic coating containing amphipathic, polar lipids such as the **phospholipid** and **free cholesterol** and specially synthesized proteins called **apoprotein** or **apolipoprotein** (*see* **Figure 3.17; Chemistry of Lipids**). The phospholipid, free cholesterol and apolipoprotein solubilize the particle in an aqueous plasma medium. No free fatty acid is found in any of the lipoproteins. Fatty acids are transported mainly in association with plasma albumin.
- Four major groups of lipoproteins are (**Table 11.1**).
  1. **Chylomicron:** Formed from intestinal absorption of dietary lipid (exogenous lipid). It transports dietary lipids from intestine to peripheral tissues.
  2. **Very low density lipoproteins (VLDL, pre-beta lipoprotein):** Formed in liver for the transport of endogenous triacylglycerol from liver to peripheral tissues.
  3. **Low density lipoprotein (LDL, beta lipoprotein):** Formed from VLDL. It transports cholesterol from liver to peripheral tissues.
  4. **High density lipoprotein (HDL, alpha lipoprotein):** Formed in liver and intestine. It transports free cholesterol from peripheral tissues to the liver where it can be catabolized (reverse cholesterol transport)
- **Triacylglycerol** is the predominant lipid in **chylomicron** and **VLDL**, whereas **cholesterol** is the predominant lipids in **LDL** and **phospholipid** is the predominant lipids in **HDL**.
- Each class of lipoproteins has a specific function, determined by its point of synthesis, lipid composition, and apolipoprotein content.
- **Apolipoprotein** is protein component of the lipoproteins. There are four major classes of apolipoproteins designated by letters A, B, C, and E, with subgroups given in roman numerals I, II, III, etc. At least 10 distinct

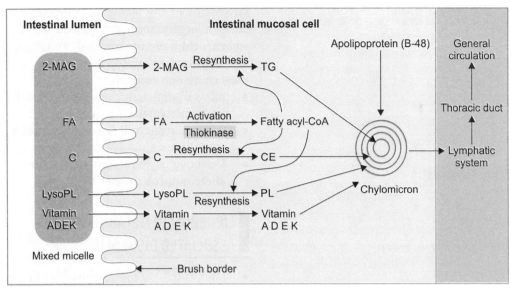

Figure 11.3: Absorption and transport of lipid from intestinal lumen.
(2-MAG: 2-monoacylglycerol; FA: fatty acid; C: cholesterol; LysoPL: lysophospholipid; TG: triacylglycerol; CE: cholesterol ester)

Lipoprotein	Main apolipoprotein	Major lipid content	Site of synthesis	Function
Chylomicrons	B-48, A, C, E	Dietary triacylglycerol	Intestine	Transport of dietary lipids from intestine to peripheral tissues
Very low density lipoprotein (VLDL)	B-100, C, E	Endogenous triacylglycerol	Liver	Transport endogenous triacylglycerol from liver to peripheral tissues
Low density lipoprotein (LDL)	B-100	Endogenous cholesterol esters	Plasma VLDL	Transport cholesterol from liver to peripheral tissues
High density lipoprotein (HDL)	A, C, and E	Phospholiplids	Liver and intestine	• Transport free cholesterol from peripheral tissues to the liver where it can be catabolized (reverse cholesterol transport) • Reservoir of apoC-II and apoE required for the metabolism of chylomicrons and VLDL

TABLE 11.1: Plasma lipoproteins and their properties and mode of catabolism.

apolipoproteins found in lipoproteins of human plasma. The characteristics and main known functions of the major apolipoproteins are summarized in *see* **Table 3.5**.

- These protein components act as signals, targeting lipoproteins to specific tissues or activating enzymes that act on the lipoproteins.

The pathways of lipoprotein metabolism are complex and include ten steps.

Metabolism of Chylomicrons

1. Chylomicrons are synthesized from dietary fats in the small intestine. Then these together with apoA, apoB-48 (unique to chylomicrons), move through the lymphatic system and enter the bloodstream as **nascent chylomicron (Figure 11.4)**.
2. Shortly after entering the circulation they acquire apoC-II and apoE from circulating HDL. ApoC-II activates **lipoprotein lipase** in the capillaries of adipose, heart, skeletal muscle, and lactating mammary tissues. Lipoprotein lipase hydrolyzes triacylglycerol to free fatty acids (FFA) and glycerol. The free fatty acids are taken up by these tissues, thus chylomicrons carry dietary fatty acids to tissues where they will be consumed or stored as fuel. The glycerol component enters the hepatic glycolytic pathway. Simultaneously, some of the **phospholipids** and **apoA**, **apoC-II** are transferred from the chylomicron onto HDL.
3. As the chylomicrons loses triacylglycerol (approximately 90% of the triacylglycerol of chylomicrons), the resulting chylomicron becomes smaller but still containing cholesterol, apoE, and apoB-48, called **chylomicron remnants**. These remnants are taken up by the liver. Receptors in the liver bind to the apoE in the chylomicron remnants and mediate uptake of these remnants by endocytosis.
4. In the liver, the remnants release their cholesterol and may be utilized to form cell membrane components or bile salts or may be excreted in the bile. Thus, the liver helps in dispersing dietary cholesterol.

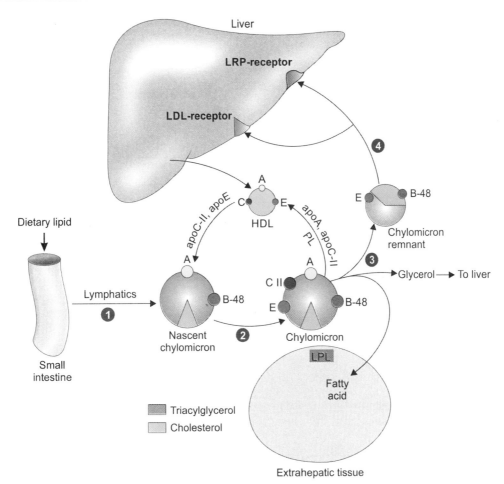

Figure 11.4: Metabolism of chylomicron.

(LPL: lipoprotein lipase; PL: phospholipid)

Chylomicron remnant receptors, called, **LDL receptor-related protein (LRP)** and the **LDL (apoB-100/E) receptor**; it is so designated because it is specific for apoB-100 but not B48.

Metabolism of VLDL and LDL the Endogenous Pathway

5. When the diet contains more fatty acids and cholesterol than are needed immediately as fuel or precursors to other molecules, they are converted to triacylglycerols or cholesterol esters in the liver and packaged with specific apolipoproteins into very **low density lipoprotein (VLDL)**. Excess carbohydrate in the diet can also be converted to triacylglycerols in the liver and exported as VLDL. Hepatic cholesterol can either be derived from chylomicron remnants via the exogenous pathway or by de novo synthesis of cholesterol by hepatocytes.

The endogenously made triacylglycerol and cholesterol are packaged and transported in the form of **nascent VLDL (Figure 11.5)**. In addition to triacylglycerols and cholesteryl esters, VLDL contains **apoB-100, apoE** and small amount of **apoC-II**. Additional apoC-II and apoE

are transferred after secretion from HDL within the circulation to convert nascent VLDL to VLDL.

6. VLDL is transported in the blood from the liver to muscle and adipose tissue. In the capillaries of these tissues, apoC-II activates **lipoprotein lipase**. Like chylomicrons VLDL-triacylglycerol is hydrolyzed by lipoprotein lipase in the peripheral tissues with the release of **free fatty acids**. Adipocytes take up these fatty acids, reconvert them to triacylglycerols, and stored them in adipose tissues instead to oxidize to supply energy.

■ During the hydrolysis of VLDL triacylglycerol, the apoC-II is transferred back to HDL. Finally, some triacylglycerol are transferred from VLDL to HDL in an exchange reaction that concomitantly transfers some cholesteryl ester from HDL to VLDL.

■ This exchange is catalyzed by **cholesterol ester transfer protein (Figure 11.6)**.

■ The loss of triacylglycerol converts some VLDL to **VLDL remnants**, also called **intermediate density lipoprotein IDL**.

■ IDL contains cholesterol and triacylglycerol as well as apoB-100 and apoE. Formation of IDLs is transient which are not normally present in plasma.

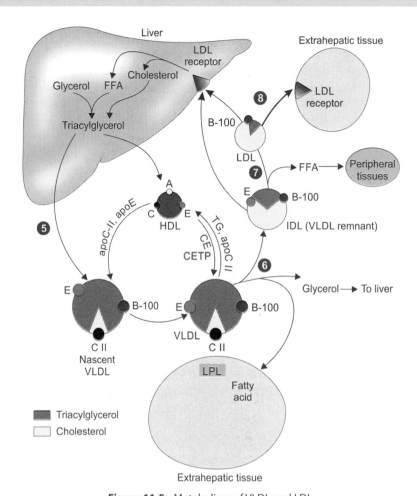

Figure 11.5: Metabolism of VLDL and LDL.

(TG: triacylglycerol; CE: cholesterol ester; FFA: free fatty acids; LP: lipoprotein lipase)

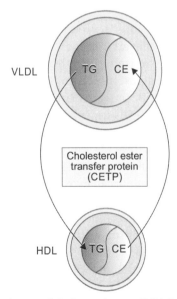

Figure 11.6: Exchange of cholesterol ester of HDL for triacylglycerols of VLDL.

(TG: triacylglycerol; CE: cholesterol ester)

7. IDL is either taken up by the liver directly via LDL receptor (in humans hepatocytes remove about 50% of the IDL) or it undergoes a further hydrolysis, in which most of the remaining triacylglycerol are removed and all apolipoproteins except B-100 are transferred to other lipoproteins. Further removal of triacylglycerol from IDL (remnants) produces **low density lipoprotein (LDL)**, rich in **cholesterol** and **cholesteryl esters**, and containing **apoB-100** as its major apolipoprotein.

8. LDL carries cholesterol to extrahepatic tissues such as muscle, adrenal glands, and adipose tissue. These tissues have plasma membrane LDL receptors that recognize apoB-100 and mediate uptake of cholesterol and cholesteryl esters.

- LDL not taken up by peripheral tissues and cells returns to the liver and is taken up via LDL receptors in the hepatocyte. Cholesterol that enters hepatocyte by this path may be incorporated into membranes, converted to bile acids, or re-esterified by **acyl-CoA-cholesterol acyltransferase** (ACAT) for storage within the cell. Approximately 30% of LDL is degraded in extra hepatic tissues and 70% in the liver.

- Accumulation of excess intracellular cholesterol is prevented by reducing the rate of cholesterol synthesis when sufficient cholesterol is available from LDL in the blood.

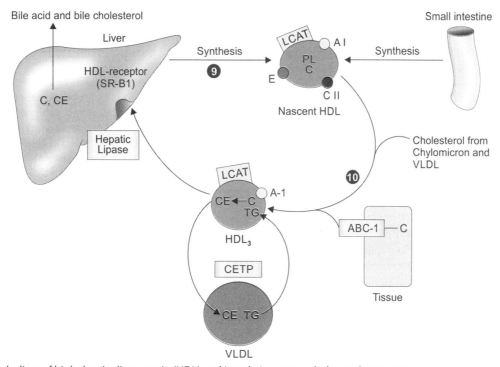

Figure 11.7: Metabolism of high density lipoprotein (HDL) and its role in reverse cholesterol transport.

(CE: cholesterol ester; C: cholesterol; TG: triacylglycerol; PL: phospholipid; LCAT: lecithin-cholesterol acyltransferase; SR-B1: scavenger receptor B1; ABC-1: ATP binding cassette transporter-1)

9. **High density lipoprotein (HDL)**, originates in the liver and small intestine as small protein-rich nascent particles that contain primarily **phospholipids** (largely phosphatidyl choline also known as lecithin), relatively little cholesterol and **apoA-1** as the main apolipoproteins together with **apoC-II** and **apoE (Figure 11.7)**. However, apoC-II and apoE are synthesized in the liver and transferred from liver HDL to intestinal HDL when later enters the plasma.

- These **nascent HDL** particles are nearly **devoid** of **cholesterol ester** and **triacylglycerol**.
- After secretion of nascent HDL into the plasma, the enzyme synthesized by liver, **lecithin-Cholesterol acyltransferase (LCAT**, pronounced **'el cat')** binds to the nascent HDL, which catalyzes transfer of an **acyl** group (fatty acid residue) from lecithin to cholesterol, forming a **cholesterol ester** in plasma and lecithin is converted to **lysolecithin (Figure 11.8)**.

Absence of LCAT leads to block in reverse cholesterol transport. HDL remains as nascent disks incapable of taking up and esterifying cholesterol.

10. Nascent HDL picks up cholesterol from other lipoproteins and from tissues. It accepts cholesterol from the tissue via the **ATP binding cassette protein-1 (ABC-1)**. ABC-1 is a transport protein that transports cholesterol across the membrane. This cholesterol is

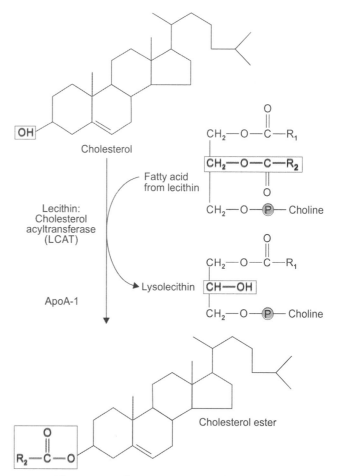

Figure 11.8: The reaction catalyzed by lecithin: Cholesterol acyltransferase.

converted to **cholesterol esters** by the action of **LCAT**. This hydrophobic, nonpolar cholesterol ester moves into the hydrophobic interior core of the HDL. As the nascent HDL fill with cholesterol ester the size of the nascent HDL increases and become spherical in shape. The HDL particle is now called **mature HDL** or **HDL$_3$**.

- HDL$_3$ enriched in cholesterol ester, transfers some of its cholesterol esters to lipoproteins like LDL and VLDL (apoB-100 containing lipoproteins) in exchange of triacylglycerol via **Cholesterol ester transfer proteins (CETP)** which is then taken up by the liver through specific LDL-receptors (*see* **Figure 11.7**)

- Mature HDL then returns to the liver where cholesterol esters are selectively taken up by **hepatic HDL receptors** known as the **scavenger receptor B-1 (SR-B-1)**. HDL binds to these receptors via apoA-I, and cholesterol ester is selectively delivered to the liver cells but apoA-I, is not taken up.

- Much of this cholesterol is excreted through the **bile** either as **cholesterol** or after conversion to **bile salts**. The bile salts are stored in the gallbladder and excreted into the intestine when a meal is ingested.

- The process of transport of cholesterol from tissues to the liver is known as **reverse cholesterol transport**. This aids the removal of excess unesterified cholesterol from **lipoproteins** and **tissues**.

Significance of Reverse Cholesterol Transport

- ❖ By reverse cholesterol transport cellular and lipoprotein cholesterol is delivered back to the liver. This is important because the steroid nucleus of cholesterol cannot be degraded; and the liver is the only organ that can clear the excess cholesterol of body by secreting it in the bile either as **cholesterol** or after conversion to **bile acids** for excretion in the feces.

- ❖ Reverse cholesterol transport prevents deposition of cholesterol in the tissues and is thought to be antiatherogenic and an elevated HDL cholesterol (good cholesterol) level has been shown to confer a decreased risk of coronary heart disease.

Metabolic Significance of LCAT

- ❖ The HDL takes up free cholesterol released from peripheral tissues. The cholesterol that is taken up is converted to cholesterol ester by LCAT. If the cholesterol is not esterified within the HDL particle, the free cholesterol can leave the particle by the same route that it entered.

- ❖ To trap the cholesterol within the HDL core, LCAT catalyzes the transfer of a fatty acid from the second carbon of lecithin (phosphatidylcholine) to the 3-hydroxyl group of cholesterol, forming a cholesterol ester (*see* **Figure 11.8**). The cholesterol ester migrates to the core of the HDL particle and is no longer free to return to the cell.

- ❖ As cholesterol in HDL becomes esterified by LCAT activity, it creates a concentration gradient and draws in free cholesterol from tissues and from other lipoproteins, and delivers it to the liver. Thus esterification by LCAT serves to trap cholesterol within the lipoprotein, preventing it from deposition in the tissues.

Mechanism for Removal of LDL from Blood

LDL is removed from the circulation by two processes, **one is regulated** and other is **unregulated**.

- ❖ **Regulated mechanism for removal of LDL from blood** involves the binding of LDL to specific **LDL receptor (B-100/E)** located in the cell membrane of hepatocytes and other peripheral tissue cells. The LDL receptor recognizes and binds **apoB-100 of LDL** and brings it into cell by the process of **endocytosis**. This receptor is defective in **familial hypercholesterolemia**. Inside the cell the particle fuses with lysosomes, apoB is then broken down and the cholesterol esters are hydrolyzed, thereby making unesterified cholesterol available to the cell.

  - ➤ The cells may use this cholesterol to maintain their **cell membranes**.

  - ➤ In specific tissue such as adrenal cortex, or gonads this cholesterol is utilized in **steroid hormone** synthesis.

  - ➤ Hepatocytes use this cholesterol for synthesis of **bile acids**.

- ❖ **The unregulated mechanism for removal of LDL from blood:** Some cells, particularly the **phagocytic macrophages**, have non-specific receptors known as **"scavenger" receptors**, which recognize LDL that has been chemically modified, such as **oxidized LDL**.

  - ➤ The scavenger receptors are unregulated it allows the cell to take up oxidatively modified LDL long after which results in elevated intracellular levels of LDL-cholesterol.

  - ➤ When the macrophages become engorged with cholesterol ester, they are called **foam cell (Figure 11.9)** and are considered the earliest components of the **atherosclerotic lesion**.

  - ➤ These mechanisms are active when plasma cholesterol concentration is increased as is the case with **familial hypercholesterolemia**. Two thirds of LDL normally is removed by LDL receptors and the remainder by the scavenger cell system.

Diagnostic Importance of Lipoproteins

The blood levels of certain lipoproteins have diagnostic importance. The **ratio of HDL cholesterol to that in the LDL cholesterol** can be used to evaluate susceptibility to the development of **heart disease**.

- ❖ For healthy person **LDL/HDL ratio is 3:5**.

- ❖ Raised plasma LDL-cholesterol concentration is associated with an increased risk of ischemic heart disease.

- ❖ Whereas raised plasma concentration of HDL cholesterol is associated with a decreased risk of ischemic heart disease and seems to have protective effect.

- ❖ LDL cholesterol is called bad cholesterol and HDL cholesterol is called **good cholesterol**.

Good and Bad Cholesterol

- ❖ **HDL cholesterol** is considered to be the **"good cholesterol,"** because it scavenges excess cholesterol from peripheral tissues and transport it to the liver where it is degraded or excreted in the bile. HDL thus tends to lower blood cholesterol level.

- ❖ On the other hand, **LDL cholesterol** is called **"bad cholesterol,"** because it transports cholesterol from liver to the peripheral tissue. A positive correlation exists between the incidence of coronary atherosclerosis and blood concentration of LDL cholesterol.

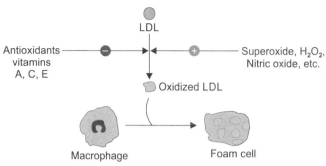

Figure 11.9: Formation of foam cells by macrophage by receptor independent mechanism of LDL uptake.

Disorders of Plasma Lipoproteins (Dyslipoproteinemias)

Lipoproteins are transport form of lipid. Lipoprotein disorders result from abnormal synthesis, processing, or catabolism of plasma lipoprotein. Inherited defects in lipoprotein metabolism lead to either:

- Familial hypercholesterolemia
- Hyperlipoproteinemia
- Hypolipoproteinemia.

Familial Hypercholesterolemia

- Hypercholesterolemia is **autosomal dominant** disorder caused by **mutation** of **LDL receptors gene. Homozygotes** have almost **no functional receptors** for LDL, whereas heterozygotes have about half the normal number.
- Due to mutation there may be **absence** or **deficiency** of **functional LDL receptors** and impairs the uptake of LDL into liver and other cells. Impaired uptake leads to elevated levels of LDL cholesterol in blood.
- Furthermore, less IDL enters liver cells because IDL entry, too, is mediated by the LDL receptor. Consequently IDL remains in the blood longer in hypercholesterolemia

and more of it is converted into LDL than in normal individual.

- Endogenous cholesterol synthesis continues because extracellular cholesterol cannot enter cells to regulate intracellular synthesis (feedback regulation).
- Because of high concentration of LDL cholesterol in blood, **cholesterol is deposited** in various tissues.
- Elevated LDL cholesterol levels lead to formation of **nodules of cholesterol** called **xanthomas** (yellow patches of cholesterol) around eyelids and within the tendons of the elbows, hands, knees, and feet **(Figure 11.10 xanthoma)**.
- Severely elevated LDL cholesterol levels also lead to **atherosclerotic plaque** deposition in the coronary arteries at an early age, leading to an increased risk for **cardiovascular disease** which may manifest as **angina** and **myocardial infarction**.

Hyperlipoproteinemia

In practice hyperlipoproteinemias are classified as follows:

- Primary hyperlipoproteinemia (genetic) when the disorder is not due to some other disorders or
- Secondary hyperlipoproteinemia when the disorder is manifested due to some other disease.

Primary Hyperlipoproteinemia

- Primary hyperlipoproteinemia is due to genetic defect in, lipoprotein formation, transport, or degradation. There are several types of hyperlipoproteinemia.
- The **WHO** or **Fredrickson classification** is the most widely accepted for primary hyperlipidemia. Latest Frederickson classification is based on concentrations of type of lipoproteins in plasma rather than genetics **(Table 11.2)**. The major advantage of this classification is that it is widely accepted and gives some guidance for treatment.

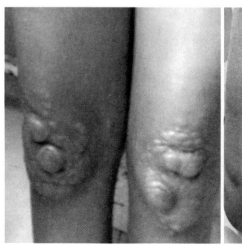
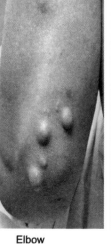
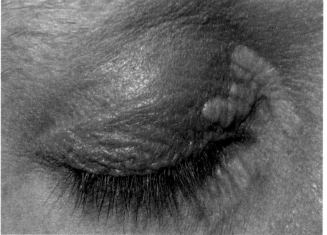

knees   Elbow   Eyelid

Figure 11.10: Formation of nodules of cholesterol (xanthomas) around eyelids and within the tendons of the elbows, and knees.

TABLE 11.2: Frederickson classification of hyperlipoproteinemia.

Name	Type	Defect	Lipoprotein increased	TGs	Cholesterol	Risk
Hyperchylomicronemia	I	Lipoprotein lipase deficiency or ApoC-II deficiency	Chylomicron ↑↑ VLDL ↑↑	↑↑	Normal	Pancreatitis
Familial hypercholesterolemia	IIa	LDL receptor or ApoB-100	LDL ↑↑	Normal	↑↑	CHD
Familial combined hyperlipoproteinemia	IIb	Unknown	VLDL ↑ LDL ↑	↑	↑	CHD
Dysbeta-lipoproteinemia or Broad beta disease	III	ApoE	Chylomicron remnant ↑↑ VLDL remnant ↑	↑↑	↑↑	CHD
Familial hypertriglyceridemia	IV	ApoA-V	VLDL ↑	↑	Normal or ↑	CHD
Familial hypertriglyceridemia	V	ApoA-V and GPIHB 1	Chylomicron ↑ VLDL ↑	↑↑	Normal or ↑	CHD

- The six types of hyperlipoproteinemia defined in Frederickson classification are not equally common.
- Types I and V are rare, while types IIa, IIb, and IV are common.
- Type III hyperlipoproteinemia, is also known as **familial dysbetalipoproteinemia is** intermediate in frequency.
- Nearly all of the primary conditions are due to defect at a stage in lipoprotein formation, transport, or degradation.
- Not all of the abnormalities are harmful. Some primary disorders of dyslipoproteinemias, their defects are given below:
  1. **Familial chylomicronemia (Type I hyperlipoproteinemia):** Hypertriacylglycerolemia due to deficiency of LPL, abnormal LPL, or apoC-II. Lipoprotein lipase (LPL) is required for hydrolysis of triglycerides (TGs) in chylomicrons and VLDL. ApoC-II is the cofactor for LPL.
  2. **Familial hypercholesterolemia (FH) (type IIa hyperlipoproteinemia):** Elevated LDL levels and hypercholesterolemia, resulting in atherosclerosis and coronary disease. LDL is not cleared from blood due to defective LDL receptors due to mutation.
  3. **Dysbeta-lipoproteinemia or Broad beta disease (Type III hyperlipoproteinemia):** Due to abnormality in apoE, impairs clearance of remnant by the liver. Increase in chylomicron and VLDL remnants causes hypercholesterolemia, xanthomas, and atherosclerosis.
  4. **Familial hypertriacylglycerolemia (type IV and V hyperlipoproteinemia):** Loss of function due to mutation of ApoA-V causes accumulation of chylomicrons and VLDL. ApoA-V facilitates association of VLDL and chylomicron with LPL. Mutation in GPIHBP-I (glycosylated phosphatidyl inositol HDL binding protein-I) causes defect in transport of LPL to vascular endothelium.

TABLE 11.3: Common clinical features of primary hyperlipoproteinemia and interpretation.

Clinical feature	Interpretation
Tendon xanthoma	Cholesterol increased
Eruptive xanthoma	TG increased
Palmer and tubero eruptive xanthoma	Chylomicron remnant VLDL remnant
Milky plasma	Chylomicron increased
Acute pain abdomen (acute pancreatitis)	TG increased

TABLE 11.4: Some common causes of secondary hyperlipoproteinemia.

Disease	Lipid abnormality
Nephrotic syndrome	Hypercholesterolemia
Hypothyroidism	Hypercholesterolemia
Chronic renal failure	Hypertriglyceridemia
Alcohol abuse (excess)	Hypertriglyceridemia
Diabetes mellitus	Hypertriglyceridemia
Use of contraceptive containing estrogen	Hypertriglyceridemia

This type of pattern is commonly associated with coronary heart disease, type 2 diabetes mellitus, obesity, alcoholism.

- Common clinical features of primary hyperlipoproteinemia are given in **Table 11.3**. The mechanism by which hypertriglyceridemia causes pancreatitis is not completely understood.

Secondary Hyperlipoproteinemia

- Secondary causes of hyperlipoproteinemia are common and include **(Table 11.4)**:
  - Renal failure
  - Nephrotic syndrome
  - Cirrhosis of the liver
  - Hypothyroidism
  - Alcohol abuse
  - Estrogen therapy

- Renal failure especially that associated with proteinuria is accompanied by abnormalities of lipoprotein transport. Impaired clearance of chylomicrons and VLDL has appeared as the dominant factor for the increased serum triglyceride and cholesterol concentration.
- Hypercholesterolemia in **hypothyroidism** is mainly due to reduction in **low-density lipoprotein (LDL) receptor** activity and reduced clearance of LDL.
- Estrogen treatment can aggravate hypertriglyceridemia by **increasing VLDL secretion** and **reducing hepatic lipase**.
- In diabetes mellitus increased insulin resistance causes reduced LPL activity which causes reduced clearance of chylomicron and VLDL. This results in hypertriglyceridemia.
- The most common effect of alcohol is to increase plasma triglyceride levels. Alcohol get metabolized into acetyl-CoA which is converted to fatty acids in the liver, fatty acids esterified to form triacylglycerols and secreted in to liver as VLDL.

Hypolipoproteinemia

Hypolipoproteinemia is also classified as:
- Primary hypolipoproteinemia is due to reduced synthesis of protein, e.g.
  - Abetalipoproteinemia
  - Tangier disease
  - Fish-eye disease
  - ApoA-I (LCAT activator) deficiency
- Secondary hypoliporoteinemia is due to reduced synthesis of protein which occurs in, e.g.
  - Kwashiorkor in children
  - Severe malabsorption
  - Some forms of chronic liver disease.

Abetalipoproteinemia

- Abetalipoproteinemia is an autosomal recessive defect due to mutation in the gene encoding microsomal **triglyceride transfer protein (MTP)**
- MTP transfers lipids to nascent chylomicrons in the intestine and VLDLs in the liver.
- Since microsomal triglyceride transfer protein is defective TG is not incorporated into VLDL and chylomicrons. As a result, chylomicrons, VLDL are not produced and LDL (beta lipoprotein) which is formed from VLDL also is not produced.
- Plasma levels of cholesterol and triglyceride are extremely low in this disorder

Clinical Features

- Fat malabsorption occurs in abetalipoproteinemia because chylomicrons cannot be formed by intestine.
- Due to malabsorption fat soluble vitamins are not absorbed, causing mental and physical retardation.

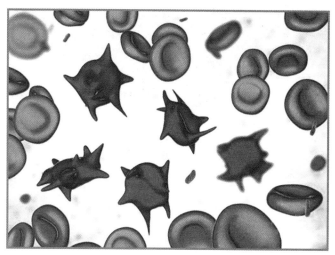

Figure 11.11: Acanthocytes: Formation of abnormal red blood cells with spikes on cell surface.

- Blindness may occur as a result of degenerative changes in retina.
- Acanthocytes (formation of abnormal red blood cells with spikes on cell surface) **(Figure 11.11)** may occur.

Tangier Disease

- It was first described in patients from Tangier Island in North West Africa. It is relatively benign autosomal dominant condition.
- The biochemical defect is the absence of ATP-Binding Cassette Transpoter-1 (ABC-1) due to mutation in the gene encoding ABC-1, a cellular transporter that facilitates efflux (flowing out) of unesterified cholesterol and phospholipids from cells to apoA-I.
- In the absence of ABCA1, formation of the nascent HDL hampered which leads to reduction of HDL (alpha lipoprotein) levels in the blood. So plasma HDL is low and alpha band is not seen in electrophoresis.
- Cholesterol is accumulated in the reticuloendothelial system.

Clinical Features

- Hepatosplenomegaly
- Enlarged, yellow or orange tonsils are seen due to deposition of cholesterol **(Figure 11.12)**.
- Atherosclerosis
- Intermittent peripheral neuropathies.

TRIACYLGLYCEROL METABOLISM: SYNTHESIS, BREAKDOWN, REGULATION AND ASSOCIATED DISORDER

Triacylglycerol is the body's major fuel storage reserve. Triacylglycerols are esters of glycerol and fatty acids. It contains a glycerol backbone to which 3-fatty acids are esterified **(Figure 11.13)**.

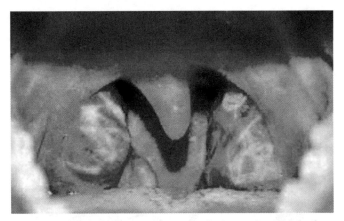

Figure 11.12: Yellow or orange tonsils due to deposition of cholesterol.

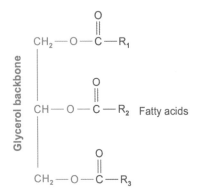

Figure 11.13: Structure of triacylglycerol.

- Human can store only few hundred grams of glycogen in liver and muscle, hardly enough to supply the body's energy needs for **12 hours**. In contrast, the total amount of stored triacylglycerol in 70 kg man is about 15 kg, enough to support basal energy needs for as long as **12 weeks**. Triacylglycerols have the highest energy content of all stored nutrients. Whenever carbohydrate ingested in excess of the body's capacity to store glycogen, the excess is converted to triacylglycerol and stored in adipose tissue.

- Most of the fatty acids synthesized or ingested have one of two fates.
  1. Incorporation into triacylglycerol or
  2. Incorporation into phospholipid components of membranes.

- These alternative fates depend on the body's current needs. During rapid growth synthesis of new membranes requires the production of membrane phospholipids, in contrast when the body has a plentiful food supply but is not actively growing then most of its fatty acids are stored in the **adipose tissue** in the form of **triacylglycerol**, called as **"neutral fat"**.

- Triacylglycerol stored in the **adipose tissue** serves as **"depot fat"** ready for mobilization when the body requires it for fuel. The triacylglycerol stored in adipose tissue are continually undergoing lipolysis (hydrolysis)

and re-esterification through **triacylglycerol cycle**, discussed later (*see* **Figure 11.16**).

> **Why Triacylglycerols are highly Concentrated energy Stores than Glycogen?**
>
> ❖ Triacylglycerols are highly concentrated energy stores because they are **reduced** and **anhydrous**. As fatty acids of triacylglycerol are more reduced (having more hydrogen atoms) it yield 9 kcal/g from its complete oxidation in contrast with about 4 kcal/g for carbohydrates and proteins.
>
> ❖ As triacylglycerols are **nonpolar** they are stored in nearly anhydrous form, whereas much polar proteins and carbohydrates are more highly hydrated. One gram of dry glycogen binds about 2 g of water. Consequently, a gram of nearly anhydrous fat stores more than six times as much energy as a gram of hydrated glycogen.

Biosynthesis of Triacylglycerols

The major sites of endogenous triglyceride synthesis are the **liver** and **adipose tissue**. The precursors for the synthesis of triacylglycerol are **fatty acid** and **glycerol-3-phosphate**.

1. First stage in the biosynthesis of triacylglycerol is activation of fatty acids to **acyl-CoA** by **acyl-CoA synthetase (Figure 11.14)**.
2. Then two molecules of acyl-CoA combine with glycerol-3-phosphate to form **1,2-diacylglycerol phosphate** more commonly called phosphatidic acid or phosphatidate **(Figure 11.15)**.
   - Mainly glycerol-3-phosphate is derived from the glycolytic intermediate **dihydroxyacetone phosphate (DHAP)** by the action of the cytosolic NAD-linked **glycerol-3-phosphate dehydrogenase** in liver and kidney. A small amount of glycerol-3-phosphate is also formed from the phosphorylation of glycerol by **glycerol kinase** in liver.
   - Adipose tissue lacks glycerol kinase and can produce glycerol-3-phosphate only from glucose via dihydroxy acetone phosphate (DHAP) by glycolysis. Thus adipose tissue can store fatty acids only when glycolysis is activated, i.e., in the fed state.
3. In the pathway phosphatidic acid is hydrolyzed by **phosphatidic acid phosphatase** (also called lipin) to form a **1,2-diacylglycerol**.
4. A further molecule of acyl-CoA is esterified with diacylglycerol to form **triacylglycerol**.

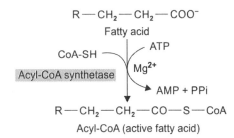

Figure 11.14: Activation of fatty acid to acyl-CoA.

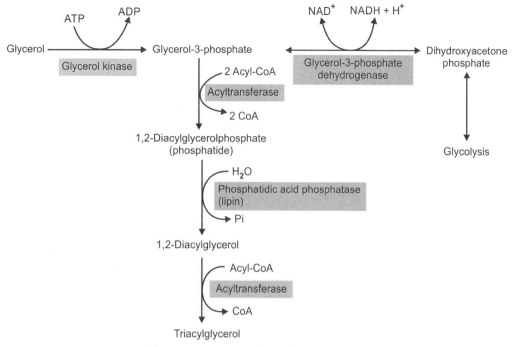

Figure 11.15: Biosynthesis of triacylglycerol.

Breakdown of Triacylglycerol

- The triacylglycerol stored in adipose tissue are continually undergoing lipolysis (hydrolysis) and re-esterification through **triacylglycerol cycle (Figure 11.16)**.
- The triacylglycerol stored in adipose tissue undergoes hydrolysis by a **hormone sensitive lipase** to form free **fatty acids** and **glycerol (Figure 11.17)**. Some of the fatty acids released from hydrolysis of triacylglycerol are transported in blood by binding with serum **albumin** and made available as:
  - A fuel for several tissues, including muscle, where it is oxidized to provide energy, and
  - Some are taken up by the liver and remainder are used for
  - Resynthesis of triacylglycerol in adipose tissues through **triacylglycerol cycle (Figure 11.16)**.

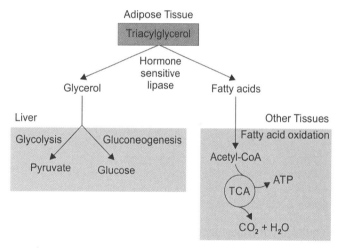

Figure 11.17: Mobilization of fatty acids from triglyceride.

- Much of the fatty acid taken up by liver is not oxidized but is recycled to **triacylglycerol** and exported again into the blood in the form of **VLDL** back to **adipose tissue**, where the fatty acids released from hydrolysis of TG of VLDL by the action of **lipoprotein lipase**, taken up by adipocytes, and reesterified into triacylglycerol **(Figure 11.16)**.
- The glycerol, released in adipose tissue, cannot be metabolized by adipocytes because they lack **glycerol kinase** enzyme. Glycerol formed by lipolysis is transported to the liver where it is phosphorylated, and oxidized to dihydroxyacetone phosphate and then isomerized to glyceraldehydes-3-phosphate. Glyceraldehy-3-phosphate can be converted to pyruvate by glycolysis or glucose by gluconeogenesis in the

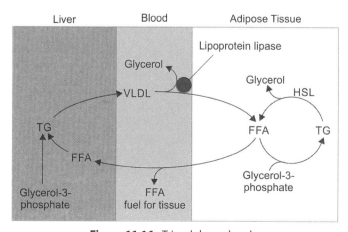

Figure 11.16: Triacylglycerol cycle.
(TG: triacylglycerol; FFA: free fatty acid; HSL: hormone-sensitive lipase)

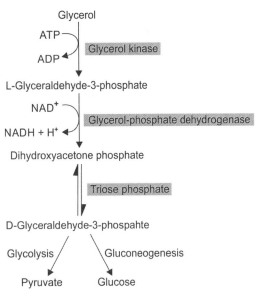

Figure 11.18: Metabolism of glycerol.

liver depending on the metabolic circumstances (**Figure 11.18**).

Difference between Lipoprotein Lipase and Hormone-sensitive Lipase
❖ The main difference between lipoprotein lipase and hormone-sensitive lipase is that the lipoprotein lipase (LPL) is attached to the surface of the endothelial cells in the capillaries (extracellular) of the tissue whereas the hormone-sensitive lipase (HSL) occurs inside the adipocyte (intracellular).
❖ Lipoprotein lipase and hormone-sensitive lipase are two types of lipases that mainly occur in the adipose tissue. They are water-soluble enzymes, which hydrolyze triglycerides. Furthermore, insulin activates lipoprotein lipase while insulin inhibits hormone-sensitive lipase.

Regulation of Triacylglycerol Metabolism

Carbohydrate, fat, or protein consumed in excess of energy needs is stored in the form of triacylglycerols that can be drawn upon for energy, enabling the body to withstand periods of fasting.

- The rate of biosynthesis and degradation of triacylglycerols depends on the **metabolic resources** and **requirements of the moment**. The rate of triacylglycerol biosynthesis is regulated by the action of hormones.
  - **Insulin** stimulates the conversion of dietary carbohydrates and proteins to triacylglycerol.
  - In the presence of insulin, **hormone-sensitive lipase** is dephosphorylated and becomes inactive and inhibits breakdown of triacylglycerol.
  - When the mobilization of fatty acids is required to meet energy needs, breakdown of triacylglycerol and thus release of fatty acids from adipose tissue is stimulated by the hormones **glucagon** and **epinephrine**.

- **Epinephrine**, and **glucagon**, stimulates **hormone-sensitive lipase** by increasing *cAMP* and **phosphorylation**.
- Simultaneously, these hormonal signals decrease the rate of glycolysis and increase the rate of gluconeogenesis in the liver.

People with severe diabetes mellitus, due to failure of insulin secretion or action, not only are unable to use glucose properly but also fail to synthesize fatty acids from carbohydrates or amino acids. If the diabetes is untreated, these individuals have increased rates of fat oxidation and ketone body formation and therefore lose weight.

Hormones Secreted by Adipose Tissue
❖ In addition to its central function as a fuel depot, adipose tissue plays an important role as an **endocrine organ**, producing and releasing hormones that signal the state of energy reserves and coordinate metabolism of fats and carbohydrates throughout the body.
❖ Adipose tissue secretes hormones such as **adiponectin**, which controls glucose and lipid metabolism and **leptin**, which regulate energy homeostasis.
❖ **Adiponectin** enhances insulin sensitivity and has **antiatherogenic** properties, reduces hepatic glucose production, and diminishes gluconeogenesis.
❖ Current evidence suggests that the main role of **leptin** in humans is to suppress appetite when food intake is sufficient. If it is lacking, food intake may be uncontrolled, causing obesity.
❖ Leptin thus helps to regulate energy balance by inhibiting hunger, which in turn diminishes fat storage in adipocytes.

Disorder of Triacylglycerol Metabolism

Fatty Liver

Fatty liver is the excessive accumulation of fat primarily **triacylglycerol** in the liver parenchymal cells, fat is mainly stored in **adipose tissue**. Liver is not a storage organ; it contains about 5% fat. In pathological conditions, this may go up to 25 to 30% and is known as **fatty liver** or **fatty infiltration** of liver.

When accumulation of lipid in the liver becomes chronic, inflammatory and fibrotic changes occur in cells which can progress to liver diseases including **cirrhosis**, **hepatocarcinoma**, and **liver failure**. Fatty liver occurs in conditions in which there is an imbalance between hepatic **triacylglycerol synthesis** and the **secretion of VLDL**. Fatty liver falls into two main categories:

1. The first type is associated with the increased levels of **plasma free fatty acids** resulting from mobilization of fat from adipose tissue or from the hydrolysis of lipoprotein triacylglycerol by lipoprotein lipase in extra hepatic tissues. The increasing amounts of free fatty acids are taken up by the liver and esterified to triacylglycerol, but the production of VLDL does not match with the increasing entry of free fatty acids,

allowing triacylglycerol to accumulate which in turn causes fatty liver. This occurs during **starvation** and **feeding high fat diet**.

2. The second type of fatty liver is due to impairment in the **biosynthesis** of **plasma lipoproteins**, which in turn impair the transport of triacylglycerol from liver, thus allowing triacylglycerol to accumulate in the liver. This defect may be due to:
   - A block in **apolipoprotein** synthesis
   - A block in the **synthesis of lipoprotein** from lipid and apolipoprotein
   - Defect in the synthesis of **phospholipids** that are found in lipoproteins
   - A failure in the **secretory mechanism** itself.

Factors that Cause Fatty Liver

- **High fat diet:** Due to increased supply of free fatty acids from the diet, capacity of liver for lipoprotein formation is outweighed.
- **Starvation or uncontrolled diabetes mellitus or insulin insufficiency:** Due to increased mobilization of free fatty acids from adipose tissue.
- **Alcoholism:** Due to increased hepatic triacylglycerol synthesis and decreased fatty acid oxidation.
- **Dietary deficiency of:**
  - **Lipotropic factors:** Deficiency of lipotropic factors like choline, betaine, methionine, and lecithin may cause fatty liver. Choline is required for the formation of phospholipid lecithin, which, in turn, is an essential component of lipoprotein. Betaine and methionine possessing labile methyl groups can be used to synthesize choline from ethanolamine
  - **Essential fatty acids:** Essential fatty acids are required for the formation of phospholipid. A deficiency of essential fatty acids leads to decreased formation of phospholipids
  - **Essential amino acids:** Essential amino acids are required for the formation of apolipoprotein and lipotropic factor choline
  - **Vitamin E and selenium:** Deficiency of vitamin E or selenium enhances the hepatic necrosis. They have protective effect against lipid peroxidation
  - **Protein deficiency:** For example, in **Kwashiorkor** deficiency of protein impairs formation of apolipoprotein
  - **Vitamin deficiency:** Deficiency of pyridoxine and pantothenic acid decrease the availability of ATP, needed for protein biosynthesis.
- **High cholesterol diet:** Excess amount of cholesterol in diet competes for essential fatty acids for esterification.
- **Use of certain chemicals:** For example, puromycin, chloroform, carbon tetrachloride, leads and arsenic inhibits protein biosynthesis and impairs formation of, apolipoprotein.

Lipotropic Factors

The substances that prevent the accumulation of fat in the liver are known as **lipotropic factors**. The phenomenon is said to be **lipotropism**. Dietary deficiency of these factors can result in fatty liver. The various lipotropic agents are **choline**, **methionine**, **betain**, etc.

- Choline is the principal lipotropic factor, and other lipotropic agents are involved in the formation of choline in the body, e.g., betain and methionine possessing labile methyl groups is donated to ethanolamine to form choline.
- Choline is required for the formation of **phospholipid**, **lecithin**, which, in turn, is an essential component of lipoprotein. And formation of lipoprotein is important in the disposal of triacylglycerol.
- Dietary deficiency of choline or precursors of choline, i.e., the **amino acids** such as **glycine**, **serine**, and **methionine** may cause fatty liver.
- **Vitamin B$_{12}$** and **folic acid** are also able to produce lipotropic effect, as these are involved in the formation of **methionine** from **homocysteine**.
- **Casein** and other proteins also possess lipotropic activity.

FATTY ACID OXIDATION: β-OXIDATION, ENERGETICS, REGULATION AND ASSOCIATED DISORDERS

Fatty acids are ***amphipathic*** compounds containing a long hydrocarbon chain and a terminal carboxylate group (R-COOH). For the utilization of fatty acids in the tissues these are first activated to **fatty acyl-CoA** and transported into **mitochondria** for degradation. Fatty acyl-CoA degraded by beta-oxidation into **acetyl-CoA**, which is then oxidized in the citric acid cycle.

Activation and Transport of Fatty Acids into Mitochondria

Fatty acid oxidation occurs in the mitochondrial matrix but in order to enter the mitochondria, the fatty acids are first activated through the formation of a thioester linkage between the fatty acid carboxyl group and the thiol (sulfydryl) group of coenzyme-A to yield a **fatty acyl-CoA**. This reaction is coupled with the cleavage of ATP to AMP and PPi (*see* **Figure 11.14**).

- The activation reaction takes place in the **outer mitochondrial membrane**, where it is catalyzed by **acyl-CoA synthetase** (also called **fatty acid thiokinase**).
- Fatty acids are activated on the outer mitochondrial membrane, whereas they are oxidized in the mitochondrial matrix.
- A special transport mechanism is needed to carry activated long chain fatty acids across the inner mitochondrial membrane. These fatty acids are carried across the inner mitochondrial membrane by **carnitine**.

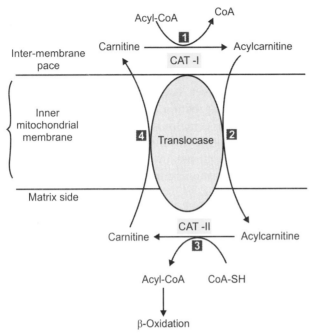

Figure 11.19: Activation and transport of fatty acids into mito-chondria by carnitine shuttle.

(CAT-I: carnitine acyltransferase-I; CAT-II: carnitine acyltransferase-II)

Carnitine (β-hydroxy γ-trimethyl ammonium butyrate) is an alcohol with both positive and negative charge (a zwitter ion) formed from lysine and methionine in liver and kidney.

Activation and transport of fatty acid occurs in four steps **(Figure 11.19)** as follows:

1. The acyl group of acyl-CoA is transferred from coenzyme-A to the hydroxyl group of carnitine to form **acyl carnitine**. This reaction is catalyzed by **carnitine acyltransferase-I (CAT-I)** also called carnitine palmitoyl transferase 1 **(CPT 1)**, which is bound to the outer mitochondrial membrane.

2. Acyl-carnitine is then shuttled across the inner mitochondrial membrane by an enzyme **translocase**.

3. The acyl group is transferred back to coenzyme A on the matrix side of the mitochondrial membrane by the enzyme **carnitine acyltransferase-II (CAT-II) also**

called carnitine palmitoyltransferase 2 **(CPT 2)**. This reaction is simply the reverse of the reaction that takes place in cytoplasm.

4. Finally, the **translocase returns** carnitine to the cytoplasmic side in exchange for an incoming acyl carnitine.

Carnitine mediated entry process is the rate limiting step for oxidation of fatty acids in mitochondria.

The fatty acids with chain lengths of 12 or fewer carbons enter mitochondria without the help of membrane transporters. Those with 14 or more carbons cannot pass directly through the mitochondrial membranes. They must first undergo the four enzymatic reactions of the **carnitine shuttle**.

Oxidation of Fatty Acyl-CoA

- Saturated fatty acids are oxidized by following pathways:
  - β-oxidation (principal pathway)
  - α-oxidation
  - ω-oxidation
  - Peroxisomal fatty acid oxidation
- Unsaturated fatty acids are oxidized by modified β-oxidation pathway.

β-Oxidation of Fatty Acids

Beta-oxidation of fatty acids occur in mitochondria. In β-oxidation two carbons are cleaved sequentially at a time from acyl-CoA molecules, starting from the carboxyl terminal end. The chain of acyl-CoA molecule is broken at β **carbon** (between α, C_2 and β, C_3, hence the name β-**oxidation**) by removing **successive** two-carbon units in the form of acetyl-CoA **(Figure 11.20)**.

Sequence of Reactions of β-oxidation

A saturated fatty acyl-CoA is degraded by a repeated sequence of four reactions **(Figure 11.21)**.

1. Oxidation by FAD
2. Hydration
3. Oxidation by NAD
4. Thiolysis (cleavage)

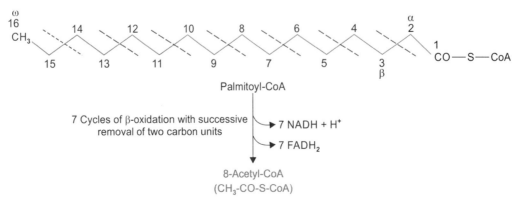

Figure 11.20: Overall process of β-oxidation.

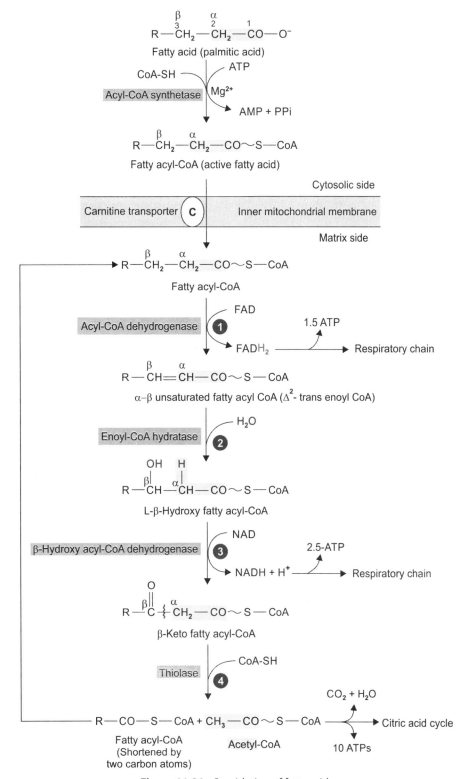

Figure 11.21: β-oxidation of fatty acids.

- **Oxidation by FAD:** The first reaction is the oxidation of fatty acyl-CoA by **acyl-CoA dehydrogenase** to give Δ²-transenoyl-CoA (*trans* double bond between C_2 and C_3) also called α-β-unsaturated fatty acyl-CoA. The coenzyme for the dehydrogenase is FAD which is converted to **FADH₂**.

- **Hydration:** The next step is the hydration (addition of water) of the double bond between C_2 and C_3 by Δ²-**enoyl-CoA hydratase** to form L (+) β-hydroxy acyl-CoA. Hydration of the enoyl-CoA is stereospecific. Only L-isomer of β-hydroxyl-CoA is formed when the Δ²-trans double bond is hydrated.

- ***Oxidation by NAD:*** The β-hydroxy derivative undergoes second oxidation reaction catalyzed by ***β-hydroxyacyl-CoA dehydrogenase*** to form corresponding **β-keto fatty acyl-CoA** compound and generates **NADH**.
- ***Thiolysis (cleavage):*** Finally 3-ketoacyl-CoA is split at the β-carbon (between α and β position) by *thiolase* involving another molecule of CoA-SH to yield acetyl-CoA and a fatty acyl-CoA which is shorter by two carbon atoms than the original fatty acyl-CoA that underwent oxidation.
  - The shortened fatty acyl-CoA (containing two carbons less than the original), formed in the cleavage reaction re-enters the oxidative pathway at reaction catalyzed by acyl-CoA dehydrogenase.
  - In this way, a long chain fatty acid may be degraded completely to acetyl-CoA.
  - In this way the **C-16 palmitic acid** would be converted to **eight acetyl-CoA** molecules after seven cycles of β-oxidation.
  - The overall result of β-oxidation of 16 carbons palmitic acid is shown in **Figure 11.20**.
  - Acetyl-CoA can be oxidized further to CO_2 and H_2O via citric acid cycle in mitochondria and thus oxidation of fatty acids is completed.

Oxidation of a Fatty Acid with an Odd Number of Carbon Atoms

- Fatty acids, having an odd number of carbon atoms, are oxidized by the pathway β-oxidation described above producing acetyl-CoA until a three-carbon, **propionyl-CoA** residue remains. Thus in the oxidation of odd carbon fatty acids, the **propionyl-CoA** and **acetyl-CoA**, rather than two molecules of acetyl-CoA are produced in the final round of degradation.
- Propionyl-CoA is converted to **succinyl-CoA** (**Figure 11.22**), a constituent of citric acid cycle.

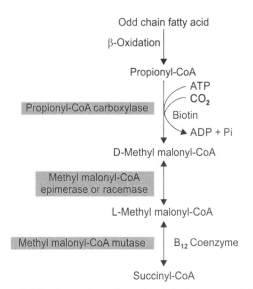

Figure 11.22: Conversion of propionyl-CoA to succinyl-CoA.

> Propionyl residue from an odd chain fatty acid which is the only part of fatty acid is glucogenic.

- Propionyl-CoA is first carboxylated at the expense of an ATP to yield the D-isomer of methylmalonyl-CoA; catalyzed by **propionyl-CoA carboxylase**, which requires the coenzyme **biotin** enzyme.
- The D-isomer of methylmalonyl-CoA is epimerized to its L-isomer by **methylmalonyl-CoA epimerase**.
- The L-methylmalonyl-CoA then undergoes an intramolecular rearrangement to form **succinyl-CoA** which can enter the citric acid cycle. This rearrangement is catalyzed by **methylmalonyl-CoA mutase**, which requires **vitamin B$_{12}$** as a coenzyme.

Energy Yield from the β-oxidation of Fatty Acids

Complete β-oxidation of palmitoyl CoA (16 carbon acid) occurs through 7 cycles of β-oxidation yielding finally **8 acetyl-CoA, 7 FADH$_2$, and 7 NADH** (*see* **Figure 11.20**).

- **2.5 ATP** molecules are generated when each of these **NADH** is oxidized by mitochondrial respiratory chain.
- **1.5 ATP** molecules are formed for each **FADH$_2$**.
- The oxidation of **acetyl-CoA** by the **citric acid cycle** yields **10 ATPs**. Therefore, the number of ATPs formed in the oxidation of palmitoyl-CoA is:
  - 10.5 ATPs from the 7 FADH$_2$
  - 17.5 ATPs from the 7 NADH
  - 80 ATPs from the oxidation of 8 molecules of acetyl-CoA in TCA cycle
  - **Total of 108 ATPs**.
- In the activation of fatty acid palmitate, the equivalents of two high energy phosphate bonds are consumed in which a molecule of ATP is split into **AMP and PPi**.
- Thus, the net yield from the complete oxidation of palmitate is 108 ATPs minus 2 ATPs = 106 ATPs **(Table 11.5)**.

Regulation of β-oxidation

- Rate limiting step in the β-oxidation pathway is the formation of **fatty acyl-carnitine** as catalyzed by **carnitine acyltransferase-I (CAT-I)**. Once fatty acyl-CoA has entered the mitochondria, it is committed to oxidation to yield acetyl-CoA.
- CAT-I is an **allosteric enzyme**. **Malonyl-CoA** is an **inhibitor** of CAT-I. Malonyl-CoA is the first intermediate in the biosynthesis of long-chain fatty acids from acetyl-CoA.
  - Malonyl-CoA increases in well fed state, which inhibits **CAT-I** and inhibits the oxidation of fatty acids.
  - In starvation, due to decrease in the [insulin]/[glucagon] ratio due to increase in glucagon, **acetyl-CoA carboxylase** is inhibited and concentration of malonyl-CoA decreases, releasing the inhibition of CAT-I and allowing more acyl-CoA to be oxidized **(Figure 11.23)**.

TABLE 11.5: Yield of ATP during β-oxidation of one molecule of palmitoyl CoA to CO_2 and H_2O.

Enzyme catalyzing oxidation step	Number of NADH and $FADH_2$ formed	Number of ATP formed
Acyl-CoA dehydrogenase	7 $FADH_2$	10.5
β-Hydroxyacyl-CoA dehydrogenase	7 NADH	17.5
Isocitrate dehydrogenase	8 NADH	20
α-Ketoglutarate dehydrogenase	8 NADH	20
Succinyl-CoA synthase (substrate level phosphorylation)		08
Succinate dehydrogenase	8 $FADH_2$	12
Malate dehydrogenase	8 NADH	20
Total (Two must be subtracted for the initial activation of the fatty acids)		108–2
Net gain		106

These calculations assume that mitochondrial oxidative phosphorylation produces 1.5 ATP per $FADH_2$ and 2.5 ATP per NADH oxidized.

Disorders Associated with β-Oxidation of Fatty Acid

Carnitine Transport System Disorders

- A number of diseases have been found due to deficiency of:
  - Carnitine
  - Carnitine acyltransferase or
  - Translocase
- **Carnitine deficiency** limits the transfer of longer chain fatty acids to the interiors of mitochondria, where in muscle; fatty acids provide a major source of energy. In general, functioning of the muscle, kidney, and heart is mainly impaired.
  - The symptom of carnitine deficiency is muscle cramps and even death.

- Inability to synthesize carnitine may be a causative factor to the development of autism in males.
- Muscle weakness during prolonged exercise is an important characteristic of a deficiency of **carnitine acyltransferase** because muscles depend on fatty acids as long-term source of energy. Medium chain (C_8 to C_{10}) fatty acids are oxidized normally in these patients because these fatty acids do not require carnitine to enter the mitochondria.

Genetic Defects in Fatty Acyl-CoA Dehydrogenases

- A mutation in the gene encoding the **medium chain acyl-CoA dehydrogenase (MCAD)** is unable to oxidize fatty acids of 6 to 12 carbons.
- The disease is characterized by fat accumulation in the liver, high blood levels of **octanoic acid**, **hypoglycemia**, **sleepiness**, **vomiting**, and **coma**.
- Urine commonly contains high levels of 6 to 10 carbons dicarboxylic acids produced by ω-oxidation and low levels of urinary ketone bodies.
- If the genetic defect is detected shortly after birth, the infant can be started on a low fat, high carbohydrate diet.

α-Oxidation

Although β-oxidation represents the major pathway for metabolism of fatty acids, two other pathways also exist. These are **α-oxidation** and **ω-oxidation** which **do not require CoA intermediates**.

Oxidation occurs at α-carbon of fatty acid in which one carbon is removed from the carboxyl end of the fatty acid chain and released as CO_2. The remaining carbons of the fatty acid can repeat the process. It does not require CoA

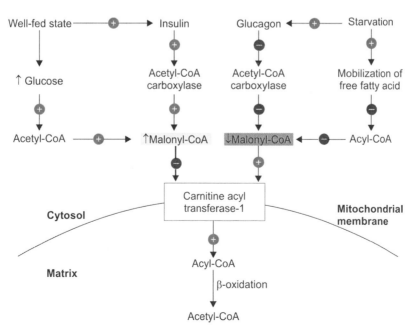

Figure 11.23: Regulation of long chain fatty acid oxidation in the liver.

intermediates and does not generate ATP. This process occurs in **brain** and **other nervous tissues**.

Significance of α-oxidation

In α-oxidation, oxidative decarboxylation eliminates one carbon and converts the even numbered fatty acid to odd carbon numbered, which are constituent of complex lipids of the brain. A fatty acid that can be metabolized by α-oxidation is phytanic acid, is a C_{20} fatty acid, a major component of chlorophyll and is present in almost all vegetables as well as ruminant's milk.

ω-Oxidation

Fatty acids may be, oxidized at the ω-carbon (ω-carbon is a carbon furthest from the carboxyl end) of the chain. The enzymes unique to ω-oxidation are located in the **endoplasmic reticulum**, of liver and kidney, and the preferred substrates are fatty acids of 10 or 12 carbon atoms.

In mammals ω-oxidation is normally a minor pathway for fatty acid degradation but when β-oxidation is defective (because of mutation or a carnitine deficiency) it becomes more important.

- The ω-methyl group is first oxidized to an alcohol (CH_2OH) by hydroxylase that uses **cytochrome P$_{450}$** molecular oxygen and NADPH in the endoplasmic reticulum.
- The alcoholic group is subsequently oxidized to –COOH by dehydrogenase producing a fatty acid with a carboxyl group at each end. At this point, either end can be attached to coenzyme-A, and the molecule can enter the mitochondria and undergo β-oxidation by the usual route releasing acetyl-CoA and dicarboxylic acids of 12, 10, 8, 6, and 4 carbons. The four carbon acid, **succinic acid**, can enter the citric acid cycle.
- Short chain dicarboxylic acid such as **pimelic acid**, a precursor of **biotin** is formed by ω-oxidation.

Peroxisomal Fatty Acid Oxidation

Peroxisomes are subcellular organelles found in all nucleated cells. They are principal sites of metabolism of H_2O_2 in the cell.

- Peroxisomal fatty acid oxidation is modified form of β-oxidation found in peroxisomes and leads to the breakdown of very long chain fatty acids containing 20 to 26 carbons with the formation of acetyl-CoA and H_2O_2. **Catalase** an enzyme present in peroxisomes converts H_2O_2 to water and molecular oxygen. There is no generation of ATP. The enzymes in peroxisomes do not attack shorter chain fatty acids.
- When very long chain fatty acids are reduced to octanoyl CoA, (8 carbons fatty acyl chain) it halts further oxidation. It serves to shorten very long chains to make them better substrates of β-oxidation

in mitochondria. They leave the peroxisomes and transported into mitochondria where they undergo β-oxidation to complete the oxidation.

- Another role of peroxisomal β-oxidation is to shorten the side chain of cholesterol in bile acid formation. Peroxisomes also take part in the synthesis of plasmalogens (ether lipids), cholesterol and dolichol (a long chain alcohol which takes part in glycoprotein synthesis).

> Clofibrate, a drug used to treat certain types of hyperlipoproteinemia, stimulates the proliferation of peroxisomes and causes induction of the peroxisomal fatty acid oxidation system.

Oxidation of Unsaturated Fatty Acids

Oxidation of unsaturated fatty acid occurs by modified β-oxidation pathway. The CoA esters of unsaturated fatty acids are degraded by the enzymes normally responsible for β-oxidation with two additional enzymes **isomerase** and **reductase** to move the double bonds of these fatty acids into proper positions, so that β-oxidation can occur.

Disorder of Fatty Acid Oxidation

Fatty acid oxidation disorders (FAODs) are inborn errors of metabolism resulting in failure of:
1. Carnitine transport defect
2. Alpha oxidation
3. Peroxisomal oxidation

Carnitine Transport Defect

- A number of diseases have been found due to deficiency of:
  - Carnitine
  - Carnitine acyltransferase (CPT-I and CPT-II)
  - Translocase
- Carnitine deficiency occurs particularly in newborn and in preterm infants due to inadequate biosynthesis or renal leakage.
- The symptoms of carnitine deficiency include lipid accumulation with **muscle cramps**. Carnitine deficiency limits the transfer of longer chain fatty acids to the interiors of mitochondria, where in muscle fatty acids are major source of energy. In general, functioning of the muscle, kidney, and heart are mainly impaired.
- Treatment is oral supplementation of carnitine.
- Inherited CPT-I and CPT-II deficiency affects liver and skeletal muscle resulting in reduced fatty acid oxidation and ketogenesis, with hypoglycemia.
- Muscle weakness during prolonged exercise is an important characteristic of a deficiency of **carnitine acyltransferase** because muscles depend on fatty acids as long-term source of energy. Medium chain (C_8 to C_{10}) fatty acids are oxidized normally in these patients

because these fatty acids do not require carnitine to enter the mitochondria.

- The sulfonylurea drugs (glyburide and tolbutamide), used in the treatment of type 2 diabetes mellitus, reduce fatty acid oxidation by inhibiting CPT-I.

Refsum's Disease (Phytanate Storage Disease)

- Refsum's disease is a rare inherited inborn disorder of fatty acid oxidation. It is characterized by accumulation of phytanic acid in the nerve tissue causing severe neurological defects, including blindness and deafness. It was first described by Sigvald Refsum in 1945.
- There is defective **alpha oxidation of phytanic acid**, a branched chain fatty acid present in a wide range of foodstuffs, including dairy food, meat, and fish.
- There is a genetic deficiency in **phytanoyl-CoA hydroxylase** required for the hydroxylation of phytanic acid. Phytanic acid contains a methyl group on C_3 that blocks β-oxidation. Therefore, it undergoes α-oxidation.
- Normally, an initial α-oxidation removes the methyl group but persons with Refsum's disease have an inherited defect in α-oxidation that leads to accumulation of phytanic acid
- Treatment involves elimination of dietary sources of phytol. Fish, beef, lamb, and dairy products should be avoided.

Zellweger Syndrome (Cerebrohepatorenal Syndrome)

A rare inborn error of peroxisomal fatty acid oxidation is due to inherited absence of **functional peroxisomes** in all tissues. As a result, the long chain fatty acids (C_{26} to C_{38} polyenoic acids) are not oxidized in peroxisomes and accumulate in tissues, particularly in brain, liver, kidney, and muscle. The disease causes severe neurologic symptoms and most patients die in the first year of life. It also exhibits a generalized loss of peroxisomal functions, e.g., impaired bile acid and ether lipid synthesis.

X-linked Adrenoleukodystrophy

In X-linked Adrenoleukodystrophy (XALD), peroxisomes fail to oxidize very long chain fatty acids, due to lack of a **functional transporter** for these fatty acids in the peroxisomal membrane. This leads to accumulation of very long chain fatty acids in blood. XALD affects young boys before the age of 10 years, causing loss of vision, behavioural disturbances and death within few years.

KETONE BODIES METABOLISM: SYNTHESIS, BREAKDOWN, REGULATION, SIGNIFICANCE AND ASSOCIATED DISORDERS

The acetyl-CoA formed in fatty acid oxidation enters the citric acid cycle only if fat and carbohydrate degradation

is appropriately balanced. However, if fat breakdown predominates, acetyl-CoA in the liver undergoes a different fate.

The reason is that the entry of acetyl-CoA into citric acid cycle depends on the availability of **oxaloacetate** for the formation of citrate. Oxaloacetate is normally formed from pyruvate, the product of glucose degradation in glycolysis, by pyruvate carboxylase. If carbohydrate is unavailable or improperly utilized the concentration of oxaloacetate is lowered and acetyl-CoA cannot enter the citric acid cycle. The dependency of fat for its metabolism on carbohydrate is the molecular basis of the proverb, ***"Fats Burn in the Flame of Carbohydrates".***

In fasting or in diabetes, oxaloacetate is used to form glucose by gluconeogenic pathway and hence is unavailable for the first step of the citric acid cycle (condensation of oxaloacetate with acetyl-CoA). Under these conditions, acetyl-CoA undergo to the formation of **acetoacetate** and **β-hydroxybutyrate**.

- **Acetoacetate**, **β-hydroxybutyrate**, and **acetone**, these three substances are collectively known as ketone bodies **(Figure 11.24)**. Acetoacetate and acetone are true ketones, while β-hydroxybutyrate does not possess a keto group. The term "bodies" is an historical tag.
- These are water soluble energy yielding substances. Acetone is, however, an exception, since it cannot be metabolized and is readily exhaled through lungs. Acetone is a waste product as it is volatile.
- Acetoacetate and β-hydroxybutyrate are interconverted by the mitochondrial enzyme β-**hydroxybutyrate dehydrogenase**.
- Acetoacetate continually undergoes spontaneous nonenzymatic decarboxylation to yield acetone **(Figure 11.25)**.
- The concentration of total ketone bodies in the blood of well-fed condition does not normally exceed **0.2 mmol/L**.

Synthesis of Ketone Bodies

Synthesis of ketone bodies occurs in the **liver** and transferred to other organs as fuel. Enzymes responsible for ketone body formation are associated mainly with the mitochondria. Acetoacetate, β-hydroxybutyrate, and

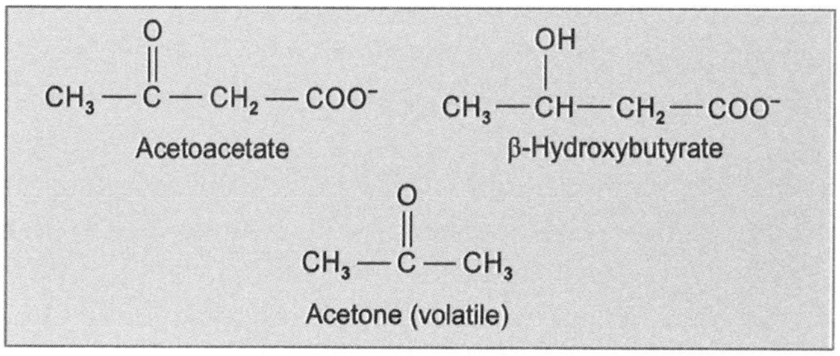

Figure 11.24: Ketone bodies.

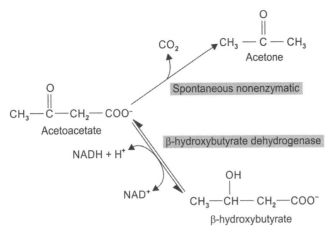

Figure 11.25: Interconversion of ketone bodies.

Acetone are formed from acetyl-CoA in following steps **(Figure 11.26)**:

- Two molecules of acetyl-CoA condense to form **acetoacetyl-CoA**. This reaction, catalyzed by **thiolase**, is a reversal of thiolysis step in the oxidation of fatty acids.
- Acetoacetyl-CoA then condenses with another molecule of acetyl-CoA to give β-**hydroxy-β-methylglutaryl-CoA (HMG-CoA)**, catalyzed by **HMG-CoA synthase**.
- β-HMG-CoA is then cleaved to acetyl-CoA and **acetoacetate** by the enzyme **HMG-CoA lyase**.
- β-hydroxybutyrate is formed by the reduction of acetoacetate in the mitochondrial matrix by the enzyme β-**hydroxybutyrate dehydrogenase**. The ratio of β-hydroxybutyrate to acetoacetate in blood varies between 1:1 to 10:1. This ratio depends on the mitochondrial NADH/NAD$^+$ ratio, i.e., the redox state.
- Acetoacetate also undergoes a slow, nonenzymatic spontaneous decarboxylation to acetone. Acetone is volatile and imparts a characteristic odour. The odour of acetone may be detected in the breath of a person who has a high level of acetoacetate in blood.

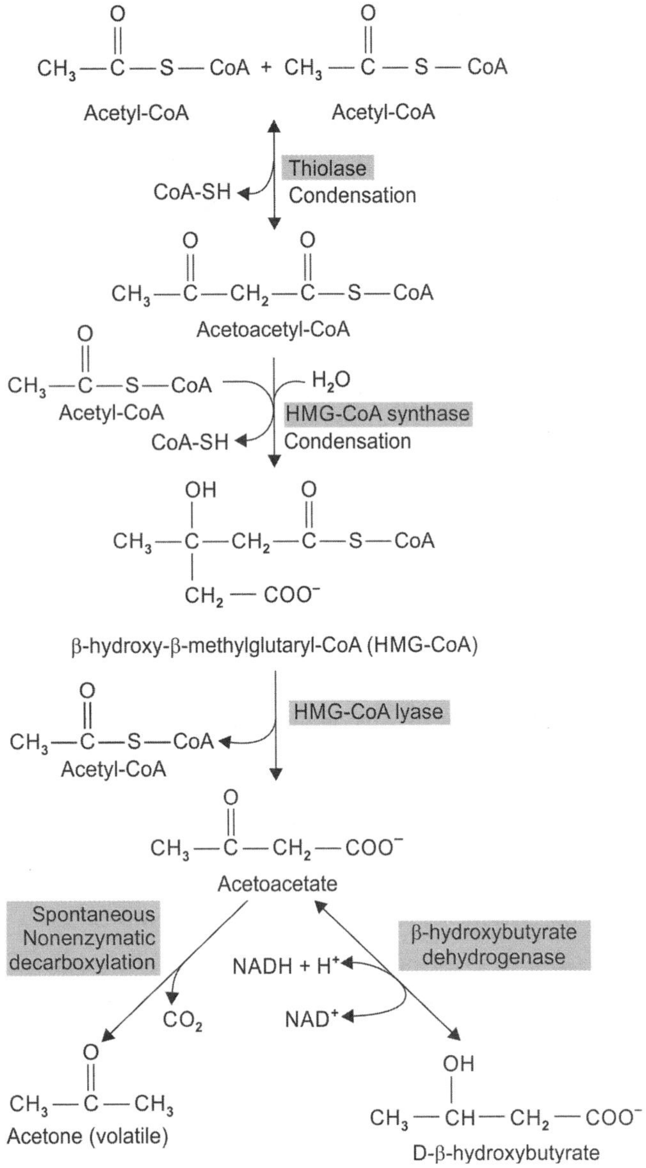

Breakdown of Ketone Bodies

The site of production of ketone bodies is exclusively the **liver**, as liver is equipped with an active enzymatic mechanism for production of acetoacetate from acetoacetyl-CoA. But the liver cannot utilize ketone bodies because it lacks the particular enzyme **CoA-transferase** which is required for the activation of ketone bodies.

Acetoacetate, β-hydroxybutyrate and acetone diffuse from the liver mitochondria into the blood and are transported to peripheral tissues. In these, the β-hydroxybutyrate is converted to acetoacetate and the acetoacetate is then activated to acetoacetyl-CoA as follows:

- In extra hepatic tissues the β-hydroxybutyrate is first converted to acetoacetate by β-**hydroxybutyrate dehydrogenase (Figure 11.27)**.

Figure 11.26: Pathway for formation of ketone bodies.

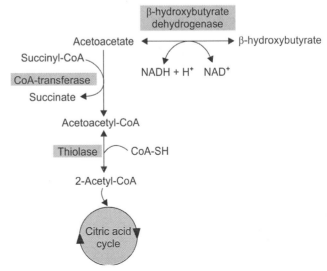

Figure 11.27: Activation and utilization of ketone bodies.

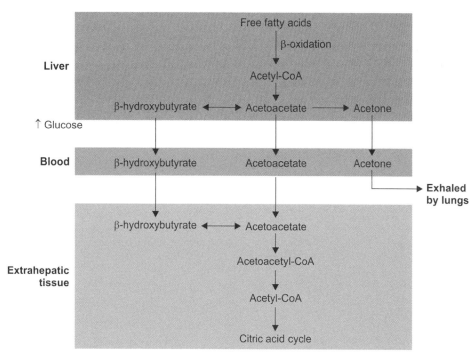

Figure 11.28: Schematic representation of metabolism (formation and fate) of ketone bodies.

- The acetoacetate is then activated to acetoacetyl-CoA by transfer of CoA from succinyl CoA, an intermediate of the citric acid cycle, in a reaction catalyzed by **β-ketoacyl-CoA transferase**.
- Acetoacetyl-CoA, formed by these reactions, is then cleaved by **thiolase** to yield two molecules of acetyl-CoA which can be oxidized in the citric acid cycle to H_2O and CO_2.
- Further metabolism of acetone does not readily occur. Because acetone is volatile, it is expired by the lungs. Schematic representation of overall metabolism (synthesis and breakdown) of ketone bodies is shown in **Figure 11.28**.

Significance of Ketogenesis

- The production and export of ketone bodies from the liver to extra hepatic tissues allows continued oxidation of increasing quantities of fatty acids in the liver when acetyl-CoA is not being oxidized in the citric acid cycle. During **starvation** intermediates of citric acid cycle are being drain off for glucose synthesis by gluconeogenesis slows oxidation of acetyl-CoA by citric acid cycle diverting them to ketone body formation.
- During deprivation of carbohydrate as in starvation and diabetes mellitus, acetoacetate and β-hydroxybutyrate serve as an alternative source of energy for extrahepatic tissues such as skeletal muscle, heart muscle, renal cortex, etc.
- In prolonged starvation 75% of the energy needs of the brain are supplied by ketone bodies reducing its need for glucose

- Moreover the liver contains only a limited amount of coenzyme-A, and when most of it is tied up in acetyl-CoA, β-oxidation slows for want of the free coenzyme-A. The formation and export of ketone bodies releases coenzyme-A, allowing continued fatty acid oxidation.
- Ketone bodies can be regarded as water soluble transportable form of derivatives of acetyl-CoA. Therefore, they do not need to be incorporated into lipoproteins or carried by albumins as do the other lipids.
- Acetoacetate also has a regulatory role in lipid metabolism. High levels of acetoacetate in the blood specify an abundance of acetyl units and lead to a decrease in the rate of lipolysis in adipose tissue.

Regulation of Ketogenesis

Ketogenesis is regulated at three important steps **(Figure 11.29)**:

1. Free fatty acids are the precursors of ketone bodies in the liver. Free fatty acids arise from lipolysis of triacylglycerols in adipose tissue. Therefore, the factors regulating mobilization of free fatty acids from adipose tissue are involved in controlling ketogenesis.
2. Upon uptake by the liver free fatty acids have two major pathways open to them after they are activated to acyl-CoA:
   - Oxidation in mitochondria to acetyl-CoA or to ketone bodies
   - Esterification to triacylglycerol.

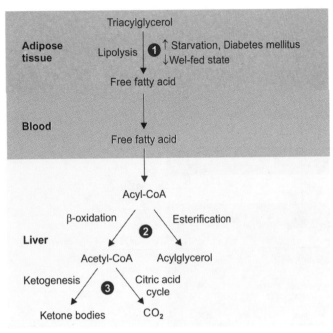

Figure 11.29: Steps of regulation of formation of ketone bodies

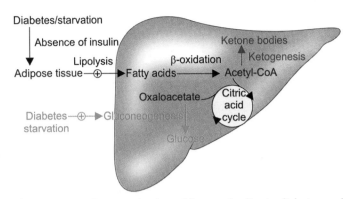

Figure 11.30: Over production of ketone bodies in diabetes and starvation. Drain off oxaloacetate for glucose synthesis, slows oxidation of acetyl-CoA by citric acid pathway, diverting acetyl-CoA to the formation of ketone bodies.

Which pathway is taken depends upon the entry of acyl-CoA (active fatty acid) into mitochondria via carnitine (*see* Figure 11.23).

- **Carnitine-acyl-transferase-l (CAT-I)** activity regulates the entry of long chain fatty acyl group into mitochondria prior to β-oxidation
- Its activity is low in **fed state**, leading to depression of fatty acid oxidation and stimulation of esterification of triacylglycerol. Its activity is high in **starvation** allowing fatty acid oxidation to increase with decrease in esterification of triacylglycerol.

3. The acetyl-CoA, formed in β-oxidation in liver mitochondria, has two possible fates;
   - It may be oxidized to CO_2 via the citric acid cycle
   - It enters the pathway of ketogenesis to form ketone bodies.

The entry of acetyl-CoA into citric acid cycle depends on the availability of **oxaloacetate** for the formation of citrate. When oxaloacetate concentration is very low, little acetyl-CoA enters the citric acid pathway, and ketone body formation is then favored. Concentration of oxaloacetate is lowered if carbohydrate is unavailable or improperly utilized, e.g., in fasting or in diabetes. Under these conditions, acetyl-CoA is diverted to the formation of acetoacetate.

Disorders of Ketone Body Metabolism

Ketosis and Ketoacidosis

Normally the concentration of ketone bodies in blood is very low **less than 0.2 mmol/L** but in fasting and in diabetes mellitus it may reach extremely high levels.

During starvation gluconeogenesis depletes citric acid cycle intermediates, diverting acetyl-CoA to ketone body production **(Figure 11.30)**.

- In untreated diabetes, when the insulin level is insufficient, extrahepatic tissues cannot take up glucose efficiently from the blood either for fuel or for conversion to triacylglycerol. Under these conditions, levels of malonyl-CoA (a precursor for fatty acid synthesis) fall.
- Decreased level of **malonyl-CoA** releases the inhibition of **carnitine acyltransferase-I** and fatty acids enter the mitochondria and degraded to acetyl-CoA; which cannot enter the citric acid cycle because, oxaloacetate, an intermediate of the cycle has been drawn off for synthesis of glucose by gluconeogenesis.
- The resulting accumulation of acetyl-CoA converted to **ketone bodies** beyond the capacity of extrahepatic tissues to oxidize them. The increased blood levels of acetoacetate and β-hydroxybutyrate **lower the blood pH**, the condition is called **ketoacidosis**. Extreme acidosis can lead to **coma** and **death**.
- Since acetoacetate and β-hydroxybutyrate are moderately strong acids, increased levels of these ketone bodies decrease the pH of the blood and cause **metabolic acidosis**. The acidosis caused by over production of ketone bodies is termed as **ketoacidosis**.
- Acetoacetate and β-hydroxybutyrate when present in high concentration in blood are buffered by HCO_3^- (alkali) fraction of bicarbonate buffer. The excessive use of HCO_3^- **depletes the alkali reserve** causing **ketoacidosis**. Ketoacidosis is seen in type I diabetes mellitus, whereas in type II diabetes ketoacidosis is relatively rare. Ketoacidosis is partly compensated by hyperventilation with reduction of pCO_2 and therefore reduction of H_2CO_3 concentration.
- An increased in concentration of ketone bodies in blood is called **ketonemia** and eventually leads to excretion of ketone bodies into the urine called **ketonuria**.

The overall condition (ketonemia and ketonuria) is called **ketosis**.

STRIKE A NOTE

❖ Ketone bodies in the blood and urine of patient with untreated diabetes can reach levels; in **blood 90 mg/100 mL** (normal is <3 mg/100 mL) and **urinary excretion of 5000 mg/24 hours** (normal rate of ≤25 mg/24 hour).

❖ Diets that promote ketone body formation, called **ketogenic diets** are frequently used as a therapeutic option for children with **drug resistant epilepsy**. Ketogenic diets are rich in fats and low in carbohydrates, with adequate amounts of protein. Basically, the body is forced into starvation mode, where fats and ketone bodies become the main fuel source. How such diets reduce the seizures suffered by the children is currently unknown.

■ BIOSYNTHESIS OF FATTY ACIDS

The majority of fatty acids required by the body are supplied by the diet. Fatty acids are synthesized whenever there is a caloric excess in the diet. Excess amounts of carbohydrate and protein obtained from the diet can be converted to fatty acids which are stored as **triacylglycerol**.

- In humans fatty acid synthesis occurs mainly in the **liver** and **lactating mammary glands** and, to a lesser extent, in **adipose tissue**, **kidney**, and **brain**.

- Fatty acids are both synthesized from **acetyl-CoA** and oxidized to acetyl-CoA. Although the starting material of one process is identical to the product of the other, fatty acid biosynthesis is not the simple reversal of fatty acid oxidation, but an entirely different process taking place in a separate compartment of the cell.

- Fatty acid oxidation takes place in **mitochondria**. In contrast fatty acid biosynthesis takes place in the *cytosol*. Some important features of the pathways for the biosynthesis and degradation of fatty acids are, listed in **Table 11.6**.

- **Acetyl-CoA** is the immediate substrate for fatty acid synthesis. The initial two carbons incorporated into fatty acids are donated by acetyl-CoA and are found at the ω-**end** of the fatty acid (carbon atoms 15 and 16 of palmitate). All other carbon atoms are donated by **malonyl-CoA** formed from acetyl-CoA. The synthesis of palmitate C-16 saturated fatty acid requires the input of **8 molecules of acetyl-CoA, 14 NADPH**, and **7 ATP**.

Phases of De Novo Fatty Acid Synthesis

Fatty acid synthesis occurs in three phases.

1. Transport of **acetyl-CoA** a substrate from mitochondria to cytosol
2. Carboxylation of acetyl-CoA to **malonyl-CoA**
3. Reactions of fatty **acid synthase complex**.

TABLE 11.6: Important features of the biosynthesis and degradation pathways of fatty acid.

Biosynthesis of fatty acids	Degradation of fatty acids
Occurs in cytosol	Occurs in mitochondrial matrix
Intermediates are covalently linked to the sulfhydryl group of an acyl carrier protein (ACP)	Intermediates are covalently linked to the sulfhydryl group of coenzyme-A (CoA-SH)
Enzymes are joined in a single polypeptide chain to form a multienzyme complex called fatty acid synthase	Enzymes do not seem to be associated
Reducing equivalent involved is NADPH	Reducing equivalents involved are NAD and FAD
Fatty acids are synthesized by an elongation process in which two carbon units (acetyl-CoA) are added in the form of malonyl-CoA sequentially to the carboxyl end of the growing fatty acid chain	Fatty acids are degraded by sequential removal of the two carbon units, acetyl-CoA
CO_2 participates in the formation of malonyl-CoA from acetyl-CoA	No participation of CO_2
Stereoisomeric form of hydroxyl acyl group is D (–)	Stereoisomeric form of hydroxyl acyl group is L (+)

Transport of Acetyl-CoA from Mitochondria to Cytosol

Fatty acids are synthesized in the **cytosol**, whereas acetyl-CoA is formed from pyruvate in mitochondria, hence, acetyl-CoA must be transferred from mitochondria to the cytosol. Mitochondria, however, are not readily permeable to acetyl-CoA. **The barrier to acetyl-CoA is bypassed by citrate, which carries acetyl-CoA across the inner mitochondrial membrane (Figure 11.31).**

- Citrate is formed in the mitochondrial matrix by the condensation of acetyl-CoA with oxaloacetate (first reaction in the citric acid cycle).

- Then citrate is transported to the cytosol by **translocase**, where it is cleaved by **citrate lyase** to oxaloacetate and acetyl-CoA.

- Oxaloacetate formed in this reaction must be returned to the mitochondria. The inner mitochondrial membrane is impermeable to oxaloacetate. Therefore, oxaloacetate is reduced to malate, catalyzed by cytosolic **malate dehydrogenase**. Then malate is oxidatively decarboxylated to pyruvate by **NADP-linked malic enzyme**. NADPH and CO_2 regenerated in this reaction.

- Both (NADPH and CO_2) of them are utilized for fatty acid synthesis.

- The pyruvate formed in this reaction readily diffuses into mitochondria, where it is carboxylated to oxaloacetate by **pyruvate carboxylase**.

Thus, one NADPH is generated for each acetyl-CoA that is transferred from mitochondria to the cytosol. Consequently, eight NADPHs are formed when eight molecules of acetyl-CoA are transferred to the cytosol for the synthesis of palmitate. The additional **six NADPH** required for synthesis of palmitate come from the **pentose phosphate pathway**.

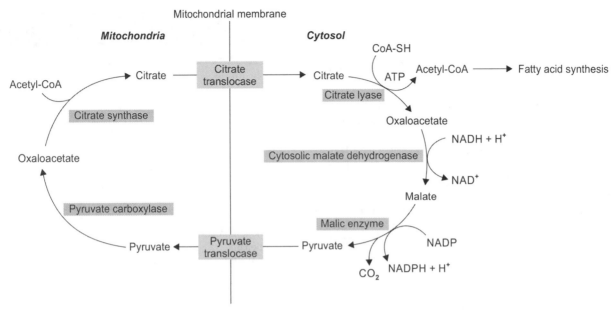

Figure 11.31: Transfer of acetyl-CoA from mitochondria to the cytosol with liberation of NADPH.

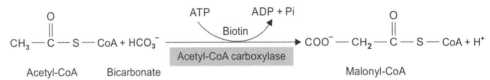

Figure 11.32: Biosynthesis of malonyl-CoA.

Carboxylation of Acetyl-CoA to Malonyl-CoA

- Carboxylation of acetyl-CoA to malonyl-CoA is catalyzed by an enzyme complex, **acetyl-CoA carboxylase** that contains biotin (prosthetic group) and utilizes **bicarbonate** (as a source of CO_2) in presence of ATP **(Figure 11.32)**.

- It is the **rate limiting reaction in fatty acid synthesis**. **Acetyl-CoA carboxylase** is an **allosteric enzyme** that is activated by **citrate** and inhibited by its end product **palmitoyl-CoA**. In addition to allosteric control, a high carbohydrate and low fat diet stimulates the synthesis of the enzyme.

Reactions of Fatty Acid Synthase Complex

Once malonyl-CoA is formed from acetyl-CoA, the de novo synthesis of palmitic acid is carried out in cytosol by **fatty acid synthase complex**. Malonyl-CoA is the substrate for **fatty acid synthase complex**. Fatty acid synthase sequentially adds two carbon units from malonyl-CoA to the growing fatty acyl chain to form palmitate. Fatty acid synthase complex is a multienzyme complex possessing 6 different enzymes and one **acyl carrier protein (ACP)** molecule **(Figure 11.33)**. The six enzymes are:

1. Malonyl/acetyl transacylase (MAT)
2. Ketoacyl synthase (KS)
3. Ketoacyl reductase (KR)
4. Dehydratase (DH)
5. Enoyl reductase (ER)
6. Thioesterase (TE)

- The fatty acid synthase (FAS) enzyme is a **dimmer** of identical subunits (homodimer). Each subunit contains all of the six enzymes, as well as an acyl carrier protein (ACP) linked to the complex in the sequence as shown in **Figure 11.33**. Even though each subunit possesses all enzymes required for fatty acid synthesis, the **monomers are not active**. A dimmer is required for the synthesis.

- The ACP segment contains the vitamin **pantothenic acid** in the form of **4'-phosphopantetheine**. 4'-phosphopantetheine provides the **sulfhydryl (–SH)** group to which the growing fatty acid chain is attached as it is synthesized.

- Fatty acid synthase has one more **sulfhydryl (–SH)** group which is furnished by a specific **cysteine residue** of **3-ketoacyl synthase** enzyme. Both –SH groups participate in fatty acid biosynthesis. One SH group is from cysteine residue of 3-ketoacyl synthase and another SH group is from 4'-phosphopantetheine of ACP of second monomer **(Figure 11.34)**. Both SH group never be from same monomer in an active enzyme.

Reactions de novo Fatty Acid Synthesis

1. Initially, a molecule of **acetyl-CoA** combines with a **cysteine–SH** group while **malonyl-CoA** combines with the adjacent **pantothein–SH** of **ACP** of the other

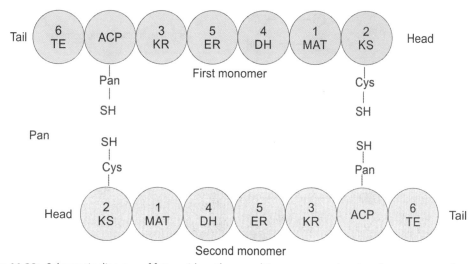

Figure 11.33: Schematic diagram of fatty acid synthase multienzyme complex showing sequence of enzymes.
(MAT: malonyl/acetyl transacylase; KS: ketoacyl synthase; KR: ketoacyl reductase; H: hydratase; ER: enoyl reductase; TE: thioesterase; ACP: acyl carrier protein)

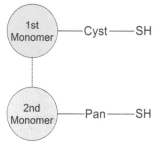

Figure 11.34: Diagrammatically representation of active dimer. (Cys-SH group from one monomer, while ACP-SH group from second monomer).

monomer **(Figure 11.35)**. These reactions are catalyzed by **malonyl-acetyl transacylase**, to form **acetyl-malonyl enzyme**.

2. The acetyl and malonyl groups, covalently bonded to –SH groups of the fatty acid synthase, undergo a condensation reaction, simultaneously a molecule of CO_2 set free, forming **3-ketoacyl enzyme (acetoacetyl enzyme)**. This reaction is catalyzed by **3-ketoacyl synthase**. Here acetyl group is transferred from the **cysteine –SH group** to the malonyl group which is on the –SH of pantetheine of ACP making **cysteine –SH group** free. The CO_2 formed in this reaction is the same CO_2 that was originally introduced into malonyl-CoA by the acetyl-CoA carboxylase reaction (*see* **Figure 11.32**). Thus, CO_2 is not permanently fixed in covalent linkage during fatty acid biosynthesis. The loss of CO_2 from the malonyl group momentarily makes the remaining two carbon portion reactive, enabling it to react readily with the acetyl group.

3. The 3-ketoacyl enzyme (acetoacetyl enzyme) undergoes reduction at the 3-keto group, at the expense of **NADPH** as electron donor to form **D (–) 3-Hydroxyacyl enzyme**, catalyzed by **3-ketoacyl reductase**. The D (–) 3-hydroxyacyl group is not the same stereoisomeric

form as the L (+) 3-hydroxyacyl intermediate in fatty acid oxidation. The main source of NADPH for fatty acid synthesis is the pentose phosphate pathway and from malic enzyme **(Figure 11.31)**.

4. D (–) 3-hydroxyacyl enzyme is dehydrated by **3-hydroxyacyl hydratase** to yield **unsaturated acyl (enoyl) enzyme**.

5. Unsaturated acyl (enoyl) enzyme is reduced or saturated to form corresponding **saturated acyl enzyme** containing 4-carbon, by the action of **enoyl reductase** and **NADPH** is the electron donor. This acyl group (4 carbons) is now transferred from Pan –SH group to the Cys –SH group. To lengthen the chain by another 2-carbon unit, the sequence of reactions is repeated, a new malonyl residue being incorporated during each sequence to Pan –SH group, until a saturated 16-carbon palmitic acid has been assembled.

6. Thus, after a total of **seven** such cycles, **palmitoyl enzyme** is formed, which is liberated from the enzyme complex by the activity of a sixth enzyme in the complex **thioesterase (deacylase) (Figure 11.35)**.

> The acetyl-CoA used as a primer, for a synthesis of long chain fatty acids having an even number of carbon atoms. Propionyl-CoA acts as a primer for a synthesis of long chain fatty acids having an odd number of carbon atoms.

Regulation of Fatty Acid Synthesis

When a cell has more than enough metabolic fuel to meet its energy needs, the excess is generally converted to **fatty acids** and stored as **triacylglycerols**. The reaction catalyzed by **acetyl-CoA carboxylase** is the **rate limiting step** in the biosynthesis of fatty acids and this enzyme is an important site of regulation. The acetyl-CoA carboxylase is regulated by following mechanisms **(Figure 11.36)**.

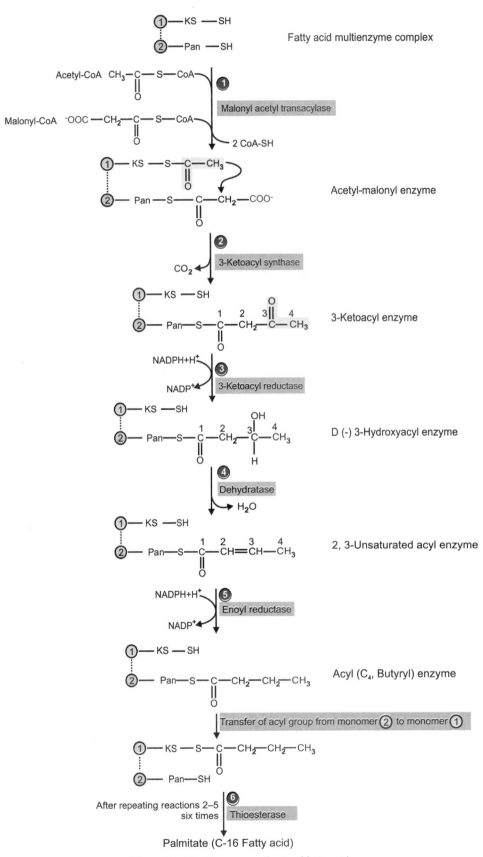

Figure 11.35: De nova synthesis of fatty acids.

(KS: ketoacyl synthase; ACP: acyl carrier protein)

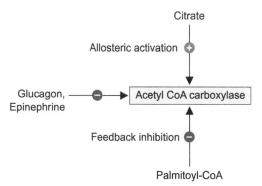

Figure 11.36: Regulation of fatty acid synthesis by allosteric mechanism and covalent modification.

- **Allosteric mechanism**
  - Acetyl-CoA carboxylase is an **allosteric enzyme**, **palmitoyl-coA**, the principle product of fatty acid synthesis, is a **feedback inhibitor** of the enzyme.
  - **Citrate** is an allosteric **activator** of **acetyl-CoA Carboxylase**. When the concentrations of mitochondrial acetyl-CoA and ATP increase, citrate is transported out of mitochondria. In cytosol citrate then becomes both the precursor of cytosolic acetyl-CoA and an allosteric activator of acetyl-CoA carboxylase.
- **Covalent modification of enzyme**
  - Acetyl-coA carboxylase is also regulated by **phosphorylation and dephosphorylation**. Acetyl-CoA carboxylase is **active** in **dephosphorylated** form and **inactive** in **phosphorylated** form.
  - **Glucagon** and **epinephrine** inactivate acetyl-CoA carboxylase by phosphorylating the enzyme and thereby reduces fatty acid synthesis.
  - Insulin activates acetyl-CoA carboxylase by dephosphorylating the enzyme.

Fates of acyl-CoA

- ❖ Esterification into triacylglycerol.
- ❖ Chain elongation to produce very long chain fatty acids.
- ❖ Desaturation to produce unsaturated fatty acids.
- ❖ Esterified with cholesterol to form cholesterol ester.

Chain Elongation and Unsaturation of Fatty Acids

Elongation and unsaturation of fatty acids occurs in the **endoplasmic reticulum (microsomal system)** and **mitochondria**. The major product of the fatty acid synthase is **palmitate**. Longer fatty acids are formed by elongation reactions catalyzed by microsomal **fatty acid elongase** enzyme.

- Palmitate is first activated, forming palmitoyl-CoA. The palmitoyl-CoA can be elongated by two carbons at a time by a series of reactions that occur in endoplasmic reticulum. **Malonyl-CoA** serves as the donor of the

two carbon units, and **NADPH** provides the reducing equivalents. The series of elongation reaction resembles those of fatty acid synthesis, except that the fatty acyl chain is attached to coenzyme-A, rather than to phosphopantetheine group of ACP.

- The major elongation reaction that occurs in the body involves the conversion of palmitoyl-CoA (C_{16}) to stearoyl-CoA (C_{18}).
- Very long chain fatty acids (C_{22} and C_{24}) are also produced, particularly in the brain. Elongation of stearoyl-CoA in brain increases rapidly during myelination in order to provide C_{22} and C_{24} fatty acids that are present in sphingolipids.
- Fatty acids can be elongated in mitochondria, but mitochondrial elongation of fatty acids is less active. In this case, the source of the two carbon units is acetyl-CoA and the substrates are usually fatty acids containing less than 16 carbons, mainly short and medium chain fatty acids.

Synthesis of Unsaturated Fatty Acids

- **Endoplasmic reticulum** systems also synthesize unsaturated fatty acids by introducing double bonds into long chain acyl-CoA by **acyl-CoA desaturase**, which requires **molecular oxygen**, **NADH cytochrome-b$_5$ reductase**, and **cytochrome-b$_5$**.
- Palmitic and stearic acids in turn serve as precursors of the two monounsaturated fatty acids, namely, palmitoleic (C_{16}) acid and oleic acid (C_{18}), each of which has a single cis double bond in the C_9 position.

- ❖ Humans lack the enzymes to introduce double bonds at carbon atoms beyond C_9 in the fatty acid chain. Therefore, humans cannot synthesize **linoleic acid**, ω-6 ($\Delta^{9,12}$) and **linolenic acid**, ω-3 ($\Delta^{9,12,15}$).
- ❖ Linoleic and linolenic are the two essential fatty acids. The term essential means that, they must be supplied in the diet because they are required and cannot be endogenously synthesized.
- ❖ Arachidonic acid is listed in other textbooks as an essential fatty acid. Although it is an ω-6 fatty acid, it is not essential in the diet, if linoleic acid is present because arachidonic acid can be synthesized from dietary linoleic acid.

CHOLESTEROL METABOLISM: SYNTHESIS, REGULATION, METABOLIC FATES, EXCRETION AND ASSOCIATED DISORDERS

Cholesterol is the major sterol in human and has a steroid (**cyclopentano-perhydro-phenanthrene** ring) nucleus as a parent structure (**Figure 11.37**). Cholesterol is the most **advertised**, **notorious lipid** because the strong correlation between **high levels of cholesterol** in blood and the incidence of human **cardiovascular diseases**.

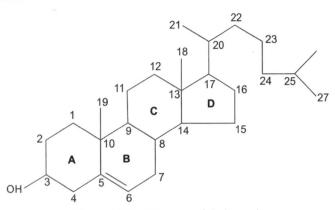

Figure 11.37: Structure of cholesterol.

- Cholesterol is an **amphipathic** lipid which can be synthesized by most cells of the body and it is obtained from the diet in foods of animal origin.
- **It is not synthesized in plants**.
- The major source of dietary cholesterol is egg yolk and meat, particularly liver.
- Unlike other biomolecules, cholesterol does not degrade to generate energy.
- An abnormality in either cholesterol metabolism or transport through the plasma appears to be related to the development of **atherosclerosis** that can lead to **myocardial infarction** or **stroke**.

Synthesis of Cholesterol

Cholesterol is synthesized by a pathway that occurs in most cells of the body. **Liver** and **intestine** are major sites of cholesterol synthesis.

- All 27 carbon atoms of cholesterol are derived from the acetyl-CoA.
- The enzyme system of cholesterol synthesis presents in **cytosolic** and **endoplasmic reticulum fractions**.
- The reactions of cholesterol biosynthesis occur into **five stages (Figure 11.38)**.
  1. Condensation of 3-molecules of acetyl-CoA to **mevalonate**
  2. Conversion of mevalonate to activated **isoprene units**
  3. Polymerization of six isoprene units to form **squalene**
  4. Cyclization of squalene to form parent steroid **nucleus lanosterol**
  5. Formation of **cholesterol** from lanosterol.

The first two stages take place in the **cytoplasm** and next three in the **endoplasmic reticulum**.

  1. **Synthesis of mevalonate from Acetyl-CoA:** The first stage in cholesterol biosynthesis leads to the formation of intermediate mevalonate.
     - First, two molecules of acetyl-CoA condense to form acetoacetyl-CoA, catalyzed by a cytosolic **thiolase** enzyme.

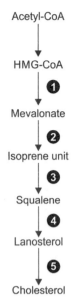

Figure 11.38: Five stages of cholesterol biosynthesis.

- Next, a third molecule of acetyl-CoA condenses with **acetoacetyl-CoA** to form β-hydroxy-β-methylglutaryl-CoA (HMG-CoA), catalyzed by **HMG-CoA synthase**. These sequences of reactions in the cholesterol synthesis are similar to those for the synthesis of ketone bodies (*see* **Figure 11.26**) except that ketone body synthesis occurs in mitochondria and cholesterol is in the cytoplasm.
- The cytosolic HMG-CoA synthase in this pathway is distinct from the mitochondrial isoenzyme that catalyzes HMG-CoA synthesis in ketone body formation.
- The third reaction is the **principle regulatory step** in the cholesterol synthesis, is catalyzed by **HMG-CoA reductase** enzyme. This enzyme reduces HMG-CoA to **mevalonate** by **NADPH** as the reducing agent and releases CoA-SH **(Figure 11.39)**. This is the **principle regulatory step** in the cholesterol synthesis and is the site of action of the cholesterol lowering drugs, the **statins**, which are HMG-CoA reductase inhibitors.

  2. **Conversion of mevalonate to activated isoprene units:** Mevalonate is phosphorylated by ATP and subsequently decarboxylated to form **activated isoprene units**.

Isoprene units are also the precursor to many other isoprenoid compounds, e.g., vitamin-A, vitamin-K, carotenoids, ubiquinone (a component of electron transport chain) or dolichol (a compound used to transfer branched oligosaccharides during glycoprotein synthesis).

  3. **Polymerization of six isoprene units to squalene:** Six isoprene molecules condense with loss of their pyrophosphate groups to yield the linear hydrocarbon **squalene** (30-carbon atoms compound) **(Figure 11.39)**.

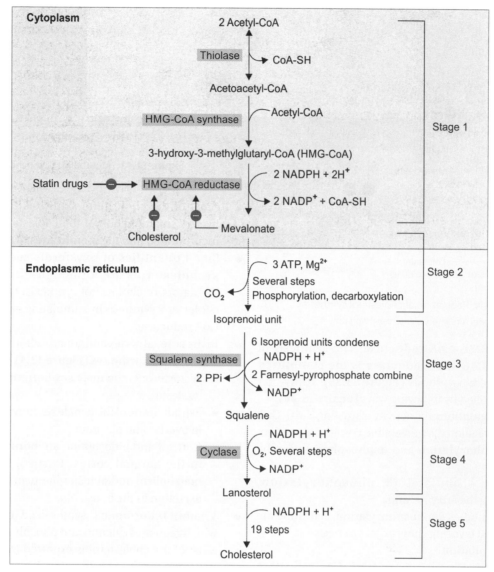

Figure 11.39: Biosynthesis of cholesterol, showing its 5 stages.

Squalene was first isolated from the liver of sharks of genus squalus.

4. **Cyclization of squalene to form parent steroid nucleus lanosterol:** Squalene undergoes a series of complex enzymatic reactions, in which its linear structure is folded and cyclized to form **lanosterol**, which has the four condensed rings that form the steroid nucleus of cholesterol.

5. **Formation of cholesterol from lanosterol:** Lanosterol is finally converted to cholesterol in a series of about 20 reactions that include the migration of methyl groups and the removal others. The conversion of lanosterol to cholesterol is a multistep process, resulting in the,

- Shortening of the carbon chain from 30 to 27
- Removal of the three methyl groups at C_4
- Migration of the double bond from C_8 to C_5
- Reduction of the one double bond between C_{24} and C_{25} by NADPH.

All these enzymes catalyzing this conversion are located in the endoplasmic reticulum.

Energy cost of Cholesterol Synthesis

Cholesterol biosynthesis is a complex and energy-expensive process. ATP is consumed only in the steps that convert **mevalonate** to the activated **isoprene units**. **Three ATP** molecules are used to create each of the six activated isoprenes required to construct squalene, for a total cost of **18 ATP** molecules.

Regulation of De Novo Synthesis of Cholesterol

In humans cholesterol production is regulated by:
- Hormonal regulation
- Feedback regulation

A major site of regulation of cholesterol biosynthesis is conversion of **HMG-CoA** to **mevalonate**. The reaction

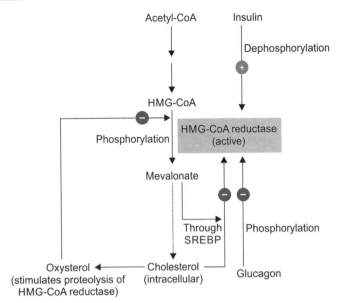

Figure 11.40: Regulation of cholesterol synthesis.
(SREBP: sterol regulatory element-binding protein)

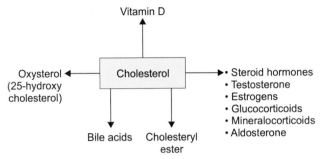

Figure 11.41: Metabolic fate of cholesterol.

is catalyzed by **HMG-CoA reductase**. The synthesis of mevalonate by **HMG-CoA reductase** is the **committed step** in cholesterol biosynthesis **(Figure 11.39)**. HMG-CoA reductase is controlled by following ways **(Figure 11.40)**:

- **Hormonal regulation:** The activity of existing **HMG-CoA reductase** is regulated by reversible covalent alteration, i.e., by **phosphorylation** and **dephosphorylation** by hormones:
  - **Glucagon** stimulates its **phosphorylation**, inactivating the enzyme, and
  - **Insulin** promotes **dephosphorylation**, activating the enzyme and favoring cholesterol synthesis.
- **Feedback regulation**
  - The number of molecules of **HMG-CoA reductase** is increased or decreased in response to cellular concentrations of cholesterol and mevalonate.
  - Regulation of synthesis of HMG CoA reductase by mevalonate and cholesterol is mediated by **transcriptional regulation** of the HMG-CoA gene.
  - Mevalonate and cholesterol **repress transcription** of the **HMG-CoA reductase** via activation of a transcription factor, **sterol regulatory element-binding protein (SREBP)** and thus decreases the cholesterol synthesis.
- Small quantities of **oxysterols** such as 25-hydroxycholesterol are formed in the liver and act as regulators of cholesterol synthesis. Oxysterols inhibits cholesterol synthesis by stimulating proteolysis of **HMG-CoA reductase**.

Metabolic Fates of Cholesterol

Cholesterol biosynthesis is a complex and energy-expensive process. Excess cholesterol cannot be catabolized for use as fuel and must be excreted. Cholesterol has several fates.

- Most of the cholesterol synthesis takes place in the liver. A small fraction of the cholesterol made there, is incorporated into the **membranes of the hepatocytes**.
- Small quantities of **oxysterols** such as, **25-hydroxycholesterols** are formed in the liver and act as regulators of cholesterol synthesis. Oxysterols inhibits cholesterol synthesis by stimulating proteolysis of HMG-CoA reductase.
- In the adrenal cortex and gonads, cholesterol is converted into **steroid hormones (Figure 11.41)** for example:
  - Testosterone, the male sex hormone, is produced in the testes.
  - Estradiol, one of the female sex hormones, is produced in ovaries and placenta.
  - Cortisol and aldosterone are hormones synthesized in the adrenal cortex. Cortisol regulate glucose metabolism and aldosterone regulate water and salt excretion in the body.
- **Vitamin D hormone** is synthesized in liver and kidney, which regulates calcium and phosphorus metabolism.
- Most of the cholesterol is exported from liver in one of the three forms, as **bile acids**, **biliary cholesterol**, or **cholesteryl ester**.
  - **Bile acids** one of the three forms of cholesterol exports from liver, are the principle components of **bile**, a fluid stored in the gallbladder and excreted into the small intestine to aid in the digestion of fat containing meals.
  - The 7α-hydroxylation of cholesterol is the first and principal regulatory step in the biosynthesis of bile acids and is catalyzed by cholesterol 7α-hydroxylase, a microsomal enzyme. It requires oxygen; NADPH and cytochrome P_{450} **(Figure 11.42)**.
  - The primary bile acids synthesized in the liver from cholesterol are **cholic acid** (found in largest amount) and **chenodeoxy cholic acid**. Before the bile acids leave the liver, they are conjugated to a molecule of either **glycine** or **taurine** to form bile salts: **Glycocholic** or **glycochenodeoxycholic acids** and **taurocholic** or **taurochenodeoxycholic** acids. In alkaline bile, the bile acids and their conjugates are assumed to be in a salt form, hence the term **'bile salts'**.

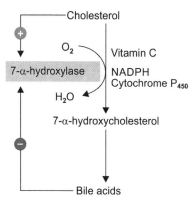

Figure 11.42: Synthesis of bile acid and its regulation.

- Primary bile acids are further metabolized in the intestine by the activity of the intestinal bacteria, producing secondary bile acids, **deoxycholic** acid and **lithocholic acid**.
  - **Biliary cholesterol:** Bile also contains much smaller amounts of cholesterol called biliary cholesterol.
- **Cholesteryl esters** are formed in the liver by the action of **acyl-CoA-cholesterol acyltransferase (ACAT)**. This enzyme catalyzes the transfer of a **fatty acid** from fatty acyl-CoA to the hydroxyl group of cholesterol, converting the cholesterol to a more hydrophobic form and preventing it from entering membranes. Cholesteryl esters are transported through lipoprotein particles to other tissues that use cholesterol, or they are stored in the liver in lipid droplets.

Importance of Bile Acids

- ❖ The bile acids aid in the emulsification of the ingested lipids and facilitate the enzymatic digestion and absorption of dietary lipids.
- ❖ Bile acid production is the most important catabolic pathway for cholesterol. Continuous conversion of cholesterol into bile acid in the liver prevents the body from becoming overloaded with cholesterol.
- ❖ As steroidal nucleus cannot be degraded in the body, the excretion of bile salts serves as a major route for removal of the steroid nucleus from the body.

Excretion of Cholesterol

Excess cholesterol cannot be catabolized for use as fuel and must be excreted. Cholesterol is excreted in feces. Unlike many other metabolites, cholesterol cannot be destroyed by oxidation to CO_2 and H_2O, because absence of enzymes capable of catabolizing the steroid nucleus. However, for excretion, cholesterol must enter the liver.

- It is excreted in the bile either as cholesterol or after conversion to bile acids.
- About 1 g of cholesterol is eliminated from the body per day. Roughly, half is excreted in the form of bile acids and half is in the form of intact sterol. Moreover, some dietary cholesterol is excreted in feces without being absorbed.
- Some of the cholesterol in the intestine is acted on by intestinal bacterial enzymes and converted to neutral sterols, coprostanol, and cholestanol and excreted through feces.

Disorder Associated with Cholesterol Metabolism

Atherosclerosis

Atherosclerosis (athero = fatty and **sclerosis = scaring or hardening)** is due to dysregulation of cholesterol metabolism. **Atherosclerosis** is the general term for **hardening of the arteries**, due formation of **plaque** initiated by an injury to endothelial cells of arteries which leads to narrowing of the lumen **(Figure 11.43)**.

- The injury to endothelial cells of arteries may be caused by:
  - Elevated plasma levels of LDL and modified LDL (oxidized LDL; LDL containing partially oxidized fatty acyl groups)
  - Oxidized LDL is **potentially harmful cholesterol** that is produced in the body when normal LDL cholesterol is damaged by chemical interactions with free radicals.
  - Free radicals (e.g., caused by cigarette smoking)
  - Diabetes mellitus
  - Hypertension
  - Elevated plasma homocysteine levels (that leads to desquamation of endothelial cells)
  - Genetic factors.
- Atherosclerotic lesions cause ischemia, which can result in infarction of the heart (myocardial infarction) or brain (stroke) due to thrombus formation.
- **Plaque** formation in blood vessels is initiated when oxidized LDL adheres to and accumulates in the epithelial cells lining arteries.

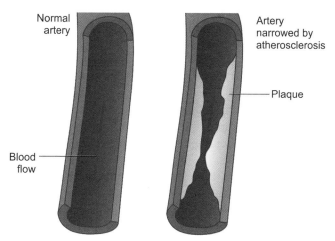

Figure 11.43: Narrowing of blood vessel due to formation of plaque.

- Accumulated oxidized LDL and cholesterol is taken up by **macrophages**. Macrophages cannot limit their uptake of cholesterols, and with the increasing accumulation of cholesteryl esters and free cholesterol the macrophages become **foam cells (*see* Figure 11.9)**.

- The foam cells form yellow patches on the arterial wall that are called **fatty streaks**. Over long periods of time, arteries become gradually occluded as plaques become larger that cause arterial narrowing.

- Occasionally, a plaque burst out from the site of its formation and is carried through the blood to a narrowed region of an artery in the brain or heart causing a stroke or heart attack.

- In familial hypercholesterolemia, blood levels of cholesterol are extremely high and severe atherosclerosis develops in childhood. These individuals have defective **LDL receptors** and lack receptor mediated uptake of LDL cholesterol. Consequently cholesterol is not cleared from the blood and accumulates in foam cells and leads to the formation of atherosclerotic plaques. Endogenous cholesterol synthesis continues despite the excessive cholesterol in the blood, because extracellular cholesterol cannot enter cells to regulate intracellular synthesis.

Factors Responsible for Development of Atherosclerosis

- **Age:** Aging brings about changes in the blood vessel wall due to decreased metabolism of cholesterol. As age advances, the elasticity of the vessel wall decreases and leads to a turbulent flow of blood and injury to endothelium of arteries.

- **Sex:** Males are affected more than females, female incidence increases after menopause. Sex incidence is equal after age 65 years, suggesting that male sex hormone might be atherogenic or conversely that female sex hormones might be protective.

- **Genetic factor:** Hereditary genetic derangement of lipoprotein metabolism leads to high blood lipid level and familial hypercholesterolemia.

- **Hyperlipidemia**: Hyperlipidemia is the major risk factor in patients under 45 years of age.

- **Lipoprotein (a) (LPa):** Some people have a special type of LDL called LP (a) containing an additional protein, **apoprotein-a**. Elevated LPa levels are associated with an increased risk of coronary heart disease. It interferes with activation of plasminogen to plasmin. Hence, fibrin clot is not lysed and susceptible to intravascular thrombosis.

- **Level of HDL:** Low level of HDL is associated with atherosclerosis.

- **Hypertension:** Hypertension is the major risk factor in patients over 45 years of age. It acts probably by mechanical injury of the arterial wall due to increased blood pressure.

- **Cigarette smoking:** Ten cigarettes per day increases the risk three-fold due to reduced level of HDL and accumulating carbon monoxide that may cause endothelial cell injury. Cessation of smoking decreases risk to normal after one year.

- **Diabetes mellitus:** The risk is due to the coexistence of other risk factors such as obesity, hypertension, and hyperlipidemia.

- Elevated plasma **homocysteine** levels, that leads to desquamation of endothelial cells.

- **Minor factors:** The risk is due to increased LDL and decreased HDL levels. These include lack of exercise, stress, obesity, high caloric intake, diet containing large quantities of saturated fats, use of oral, contraceptive, alcoholism, and hyperuricemia, etc.

Prevention of Atherosclerosis

- The most important preventive measure against the development of atherosclerosis is to eat a low fat diet that contains mainly unsaturated fat with low cholesterol content.

- Since oxidized LDL is an important and possibly an essential component in the pathogenesis of atherosclerosis, the inhibition of LDL oxidation by variety of antioxidants has been considered in treating coronary artery disease. Natural antioxidants such as vitamin E, C or β-carotene may decrease the risk of cardiovascular disease by protecting LDL against oxidation. The antioxidants also help to maintain normal endothelial function by preserving endothelial derived nitric oxide production.

- **Moderate alcohol consumption may** elevate of HDL concentration due to increased synthesis of **apoA-I** and changes in activity of **cholesterol ester transfer protein** (CETP).

- Regular exercise lowers plasma LDL but raises the level of HDL. HDL is associated with a protein that has **esterase activity** which degrades and destroys the oxidized LDL, accounting for HDLs ability to protect against heart attacks.

- HDL has protective effect against atherosclerosis. HDL participates in **reverse transport of cholesterol**, i.e., it transports cholesterol from cells to the liver for excretion in the bile. The higher the level of HDL, the lower is the risk of ischemic heart disease. Consequently, high ratio of HDL/LDL reduces the development of atherosclerosis. There is an inverse relationship between cardiovascular risks and HDL concentration.

Drug Therapy

- A class of drugs **statins**, (e.g., lovastatin, clofibrate, cholestyramine) is used to treat patients with familial hypercholesterolemia and other conditions involving elevated plasma cholesterol. Statin resemble mevalonate and are **competitive inhibitors** of **HMG CoA reductase** which inhibit cholesterol synthesis.

- Activation of **liver X receptor (LXR)** is another approach to control serum cholesterol level, which has an overall effect of decreasing cholesterol absorption in the small intestine and promoting its excretion. This is the mode of action of drug called **ezetimibe**. Ezetimibe is recommended as second line therapy for those intolerant of statins or unable to achieve target cholesterol levels on statins alone. Ezetimibe (brand name zetia) is an intestinal cholesterol absorption inhibitor.

- **Liver X receptor (LXR)** is a nuclear receptor, an important regulator of cholesterol homeostasis.

EICOSANOIDS: TYPES, FUNCTIONS, SYNTHESIS, INHIBITORS OF SYNTHESIS AND THERAPEUTIC USES OF PROSTAGLANDINS

The eicosanoids are a diverse group of hormone like molecules produced in most mammalian tissues. They include the **prostaglandins, thromboxane, leukotrienes**, and **lipoxins**. Together the eicosanoids mediate a wide variety of physiological functions.

Types of Eicosanoids

- Eicosanoids are usually designated by their abbreviations. The first two letters indicate the type of eicosanoids:
  - PG = Prostaglandins
  - TX = Thromboxane
  - LT = Leukotriene
  - LX = Lipoxins.

- Eicosanoids are derived from **arachidonic acid**, **(Figure 11.44)** a polyunsaturated fatty acid containing 20 carbon atoms from which they take their general name (Greek: eikosi means twenty).

- They are not synthesized in advance and stored, instead the precursor, arachidonic acids are stored in tissues. Arachidonic acid is stored in tissues attached to the C-2 of phospholipids. When needed, the phospholipids

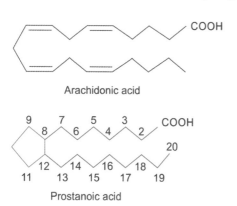

Figure 11.44: Structure of arachidonic acid and prostanoic acid.

hydrolyzed by phospholipase A_2 to release arachidonic acid.

- Eicosanoids are produced in small amounts and remain active for short periods (in seconds or minutes).

Prostaglandins (PG)

- By convention prostaglandins are abbreviated PG. Prostaglandins (PG) derive their name from the tissue in which they were first recognized (the prostate gland) but they are now known to be present in almost all tissues.

- All PGs are structurally related to **prostanoic acid**, **(Figure 11.44)** having:
  - Cyclopentane (5 carbon) ring and
  - Two aliphatic side chains, R_1 and R_2 attached to the cyclopentane ring (at C8 and C12 respectively) of the prostanoic acid.

- In addition to cyclopentane ring, each of the biological active prostaglandin has a hydroxyl group at carbon 15, a double bond between carbons 13 and 14 and various substituents on the ring.

Classification of PGs

- They are classified into nine major classes, designated as: PGA, PGB, PGC, PGD, PGE, PGF, PGG, PGH, and PGI depending on the substituents on the cyclopentane ring **(Figure 11.45)**.

- These are subclassified by a subscript number 1, 2 or 3 corresponding to the number of double bonds in the side chains, but not the cyclopentane ring. Prostaglandin of the:
  - Series 1: One double bond between carbons 13 and 13.
  - Series 2: Two double bond between 13 and 14 and between 5 and 6.
  - Series 3: Three double bond between 13 and 15, 15 and 16, 17 and 18.

- The Greek letter subscript "α" found in the **F-series**, indicates the configuration of a C-9 OH group. In the α-series the hydroxyl group at C-9 projects below the plane of the ring.

- Sixteen naturally occurring prostaglandins have been described but only seven are found commonly throughout the body. These are termed the **primary prostaglandins (Table 11.7)**.

Functions of Prostaglandins

Prostaglandins have hormone like actions. They exert very short lived effects and are catabolized rapidly. They alter the activities of the cells in which they are synthesized and adjoining cells **(Table 11.8)**. Prostaglandins in many tissues act by regulating the synthesis of the intracellular messenger molecule 3′, 5′ cyclic-AMP (cAMP). cAMP mediates the action of many hormones. Some of these are:

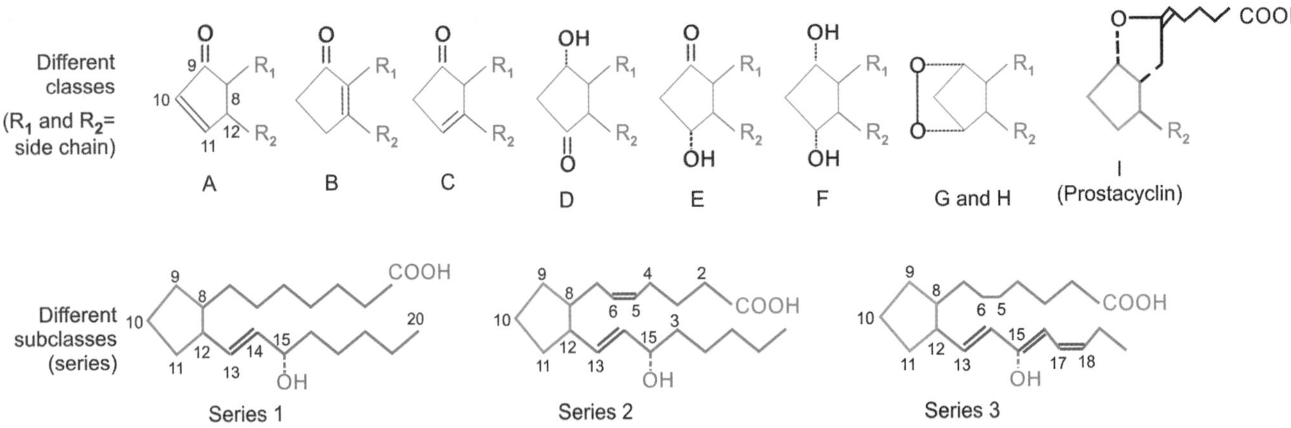

Figure 11.45: Different classes of classification of prostaglandins.

TABLE 11.7: Naturally occurring prostaglandins.

Primary PG	Other PG
PGE$_1$	PGA$_1$
PGF$_{1\alpha}$	PGA$_2$
PGE$_2$	19α—OH PGA$_1$
PGF$_{2\alpha}$	19α—OH PGA$_2$
PGG$_2$	PGB$_1$
PGH$_2$	PGB$_2$
PGI$_2$	19α—OH PGB$_2$
	PGE$_3$
	PGF$_{3\alpha}$

TABLE 11.8: Functions of some important prostaglandins, thromboxanes and leukotrienes.

Type	Site of formation	Function
PGE$_2$	Most tissues	Vasodilation
		• Smooth muscle relaxation • Labor inducer • Increase cAMP • Inflammatory response • Promote platelet aggregation • Suppress gastric acid secretion • Regulation of body temperature • Regulation of sodium excretion and GFR • Decrease blood pressure
PGF$_{2\alpha}$	Most tissues	• Vasoconstriction • Bronchoconstriction • Smooth muscle contraction • Stimulates uterine contraction
PGI$_2$	Endothelium of vessels	• Vasodilation • Inhibits platelet aggregation • Increase cAMP
TXA$_2$	Platelets	• Increase platelet aggregation • Vasoconstriction • Mobilizes intracellular calcium • Smooth muscle contraction • Bronchoconstriction
LT	Leukocytes platelets, Mast cells, Heart and lung vascular tissues	• Increase chemotaxis (movement of cell in response to stimuli) of polymorphonuclear leukocytes contraction of smooth muscle • Bronchoconstriction • Vasoconstriction • Increase vascular permeability • Release of lysosomal enzyme components of slow–reacting substance of anaphylaxis (SRS-A)
LX	Leukocytes	Anti-inflammatory agent

- **Smooth muscle contraction and relaxation:** Some PGs stimulate contraction of smooth muscle of the uterus during menstruation and labor. For example, in pregnancy PGF$_{2\alpha}$ are produced in response to oxytocin and act to promote uterine contraction. Because of this effect, they have been used to terminate unwanted pregnancies. PGE$_2$ are involved in relaxation of bronchial smooth muscle.
- **Platelet aggregation:** Prostaglandins have an effect on platelet aggregation. PGE$_2$ promote aggregation and are thus, involved in the blood clotting whereas PGI$_2$ inhibits platelet aggregation.
- **Blood pressure regulation:** PGE$_2$ decrease blood pressure through their vasodilator effect.
- **Regulation of gastric secretion:** PGE$_2$ suppress **gastric secretion**, increases **bicarbonate ion** and **mucus** secretion. It keeps balance between gastric acid secretion and HCO$_3$ and mucus secretion. By increasing HCO$_3$ and mucus secretion gastric acid secretion can be controlled. All these three processes controlled by PGE$_2$.
- **Inflammatory response:** During any inflammatory condition PGs are synthesized by COX-2 which is having pathological roles. These can produce pain, increase fever (hyperthermia) as well as they can induce inflammation. COX-1 play important role in physiological systems. They have some productive action in the body. COX-2 have pathological role.

Thromboxane

- Thromboxane (TX) is produced by platelets (also called thrombocytes) and act in the formation of blood clots and the reduction of blood flow to the site of clot. The term thromboxane refers to their thrombus forming action.

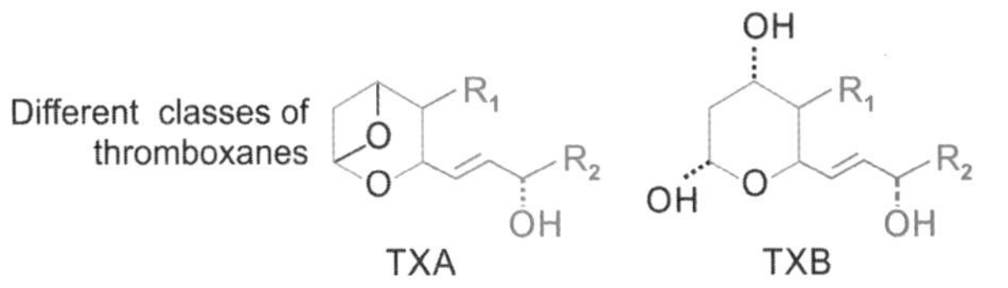

Different classes of thromboxanes

TXA   TXB

Figure 11.46: Different classes of classification of thromboxane.

- Thromboxanes are abbreviated as **TX**. In thromboxane the cyclopentane ring is replaced by a six membered oxygen containing (oxane) ring. Different capital letters are used to designate different substituents of the ring **(Figure 11.46)**. A subscript if present denotes the number of double bonds, e.g., the most common thromboxane TXA_2 having two double bonds.

Functions of Thromboxane

- TXA_2 promotes **platelet aggregation** and **vasoconstriction**. Platelet aggregation initiates thrombus formation at sites of vascular injury. Vasoconstriction of TXA_2, raises the blood pressure.
- Effects of TXA_2 are exactly opposite of those caused by prostacyclin (PGI_2). Prostacyclin inhibits platelet aggregation, relaxes the arterial wall and lowers the blood pressure.
- Thus, TXA_2 and PGI_2 are antagonistic in activity and regulate thrombi formation to sites of vascular injury. TXA_2 after its action is rapidly converted to its inactive metabolite TXB_2.

Leukotrienes (LT)

- Leukotrienes (LT) first found in **leukocytes**, contain **three conjugated double bonds (alternate double bond)**, hence the name.
- Leukotrienes are linear noncyclic molecules derived from arachidonic acid with the help of enzyme **lipooxygenase**.
- All leukotrienes are abbreviated as **LT**. These are grouped into **five classes (A to E)** based on the type of substituents attached to the parent compound.
- The leukotrienes found in humans have a subscript '4' to denote that they contain four double bonds **(Figure 11.47)**.

Functions of Leukotrienes

- The leukotrienes are powerful chemotactic agents, i.e., they attract immune system cells to damaged tissue.
- They also induce **vasoconstriction** and **bronchoconstriction**. Leukotriene D4 induces contraction of the smooth muscle lining the airways to the lung. Over production of leukotrienes causes asthmatic attacks.
- Leukotrienes **LTC_4, LTD_4, and LTE_4** have been identified as components of **slow reacting substances of**

anaphylaxis **(SRS-A)** which causes smooth muscle contraction.

> Like leukotrienes **lipoxins** are linear eicosanoids. Their distinguishing feature is the presence of several hydroxyl groups along the chain. These compounds are potent anti-inflammatory agents.
> Because their synthesis is stimulated by low dose (81 mg) of aspirin taken daily, this low dose is commonly prescribed for individuals with cardiovascular disease.

Biosynthesis of Prostaglandins, Thromboxane and Leukotrienes

In response to a hormonal or other stimulus a specific **phospholipase A_2** present in most types of cells attacks **membrane phospholipids** releasing **arachidonic acid**. Phospholipase A_2 is specific for the carbon-2 (sn-2) position of the phospholipids, to which arachidonic acid is attached. After arachidonic acid is released into the cytosol, it can follow one of the two pathways.

1. The **cyclooxygenase (COX) pathway**, which produces the prostaglandins and thromboxanes **(Figure 11.48)**.
2. The **lipooxygenase pathway**, which produces leukotrienes **(Figure 11.49)**.

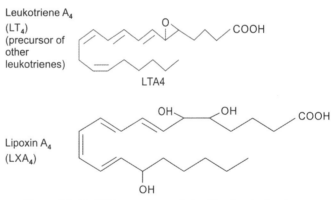

Leukotriene A_4 (LT_4) (precursor of other leukotrienes)

LTA4

Lipoxin A_4 (LXA_4)

Figure 11.47: Different classes of classification leukotrienes.

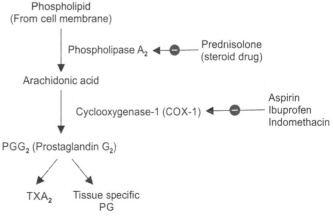

Phospholipid (From cell membrane)

Phospholipase A_2 ← Prednisolone (steroid drug)

Arachidonic acid

Cyclooxygenase-1 (COX-1) ← Aspirin Ibuprofen Indomethacin

PGG_2 (Prostaglandin G_2)

TXA_2 Tissue specific PG

Figure 11.48: Cyclooxygenase pathway for synthesis of prostaglandins and thromboxanes.

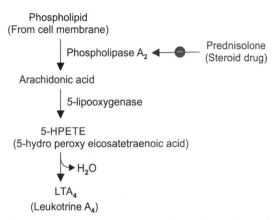

Figure 11.49: Lipooxygenase pathway for synthesis of leukotrienes.

Isoforms of Cyclooxygenase

- Two isoforms of cyclooxygenase (COX) are known as:
  - COX-1 and
  - COX-2.
- COX-1 is constitutively expressed and thus the level of it is rather constant in cells, whereas **COX-2** is an **inducible enzyme** synthesized in response to inflammation. COX-2 levels are usually low in healthy tissue but increased levels occur in inflamed tissue.
- COX-1 synthesizes PGs which have productive action. They are required for maintenance of healthy gastric tissue, renal homeostasis, and platelet aggregation.
- **COX-2** synthesizes PGs which are responsible for the **inflammatory response**, and can produce pain, heat, redness, swelling, and fever due to infections.

Inhibitors of Eicosanoid Synthesis

The synthesis of prostaglandins can be inhibited by a number of compounds.

- The **cyclooxygenase enzyme (both COX-1 and COX-2)** is inhibited by all **nonsteroidal anti-inflammatory drugs (NSAIDs)**, such as aspirin, naproxen, ibuprofen, indomethacin, etc. **(Figure 11.48)**.
- NSAIDs are used to reduce inflammation, fever, pain and blood clotting. At the same time NSAIDs inhibit the productive function and increase gastric acid secretion and leads to gastric ulcer.
- Regular use of **low dose of aspirin** can reduce the risk of heart attacks.
- At low dosage, it inhibits **platelet COX-1** preventing formation of **TXA2**, and **thrombus** formation and is effective in prevention of **acute myocardial infarction**.
- At higher doses, **aspirin** acts as an **anti-inflammatory** drug.
- Steroid drugs, such as **prednisolone**, have both **anti-pyretic** and **anti-inflammatory** action by inhibiting **phospholipase A$_2$**, the enzyme responsible for release of arachidonic acid from membrane phospholipid.

- **Lipooxygenases** are not affected by NSAID. It is inhibited by steroid drugs, such as **prednisolone**.
- **Inhibitors of lipooxygenase** are used in the treatment of **asthma**.

At sufficiently high dose NSAIDs inhibit activity of both isoforms COX-1 and COX-2 and have nephrotoxic and ulcerogenic side effects and impaired clotting of blood. The adverse effect of NSAIDs is due to inhibition of COX-1, which is required for maintenance of healthy gastric tissue, renal homeostasis, and platelet aggregation.

Therapeutic Uses of Prostaglandins

- Prostaglandins may be used therapeutically as follows:
  - PGF$_{2\alpha}$ is used in the induction of labor, in termination of pregnancy as they induce uterine smooth muscle contraction.
  - PGE$_2$ is used for prevention of conception.
  - PGE$_2$ (a bronchodilator) is used in the treatment of bronchial asthma and nasal congestion.
  - PGE, PGA and PGI$_2$ are vasodilators used to control inflammation and blood pressure.
  - PGE is used to prevent and treat peptic ulcers.
  - PGE$_1$ is used as ophthalmic solution in treatment of glaucoma. It reduces pressure inside the eye (intraocular pressure) by increasing the outflow of aqueous humor in the eye.
  - PGD$_2$ is a potent sleep-promoting substance.

LIPID PROFILE TESTS AND INTERPRETATIONS WITH VARIOUS DISORDERS

Lipid Profile Tests

Lipid profile tests are used to estimate increased risk of cardiovascular disease which includes measurement of:

- Total serum cholesterol
- Serum triglycerides
- HDL cholesterol
- LDL cholesterol.

Total Serum Cholesterol

Enzymatic Method for Estimation of Cholesterol

Commercially available cholesterol reagents commonly combine all enzymes and other required components into a single reagent. The reagent usually is mixed with 3 to 10 μL aliquot of serum or plasma, incubated under controlled conditions for color development and absorbance is measured at about 500 nm. The reagents typically use a bacterial **cholesterol ester hydrolase** to hydrolyze cholesterol esters to cholesterol and fatty acids **(Figure 11.50)**. The 3-OH group of cholesterol is then oxidized to a ketone derivative and H$_2$O$_2$ by cholesterol oxidase. H$_2$O$_2$, is then measured in a peroxidase catalyzed reaction that forms dye.

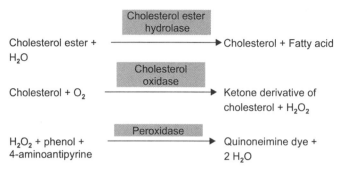

Figure 11.50: Reaction occurs in enzymatic method of total serum cholesterol estimation.

Normal Values and Interpretation of Cholesterol

- The normal range for healthy young adults is less than **200 mg/dL**
- It may be lower in children
- The concentration increases with age
- The concentration in the women is generally somewhat lower than in men up to the time of menopause but then increase and may exceed that in men of the same age.

Increased Concentration of Cholesterol

- The total concentration is increased in:
  - Hypothyroidism
  - Uncontrolled diabetes mellitus
  - Nephrotic syndrome
  - Extrahepatic obstruction of the bile ducts
  - Various hyperlipidemias.
- Long time elevated cholesterol concentration (more than 240 mg/dL) is a high-risk factor for the development of coronary artery disease.
- Lowering of plasma cholesterol concentration reduces the incidence of coronary heart diseases.
- National Cholesterol Education Program (NCEP) defined the levels of serum cholesterol believed to be desirable, tolerable or a high-risk factor for development of coronary artery disease. The report classifies total cholesterol concentration **(Table 11.9)** which is applicable to all individuals over 20 years of age and sex.

Decreased Concentration of Cholesterol

Hypocholesterolemia is usually present in:
- Hyperthyroidism
- Hepatocellular disease
- Certain genetic defects, e.g., abetalipoproteinemia.

Serum Triglycerides

Enzymatic Method for Estimation of Triglycerides (TG)

Single reagents that consist of all the required enzymes, cofactors and buffers generally are used. The first step is the hydrolysis of triglycerides to glycerol and fatty acid by lipase. Glycerol is then oxidized to dihydroxyacetone and H_2O_2 by

TABLE 11.9: Classification of serum cholesterol and serum triglycerides concentration according to the NCEP.

Category	Serum cholesterol mg/dL	Serum triglycerides mg/dL	Serum LDL-cholesterol mg/dL
Normal (desirable, safer side)	Below 200	Below 200	Below 130
Borderline high-risk	200–240	200–400	130–160
High-risk	Above 240	400–1000	Above 160

NCEP = National Cholesterol Education Program. All values are in mg/dL; to convert to mml/L, multiply by 0.259.

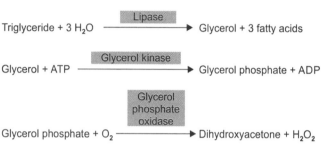

Figure 11.51: Reaction of enzymatic estimation of triglycerides.

TABLE 11.10: Ratio of total cholesterol: HDL cholesterol and LDL cholesterol: HDL cholesterol for the assessment of risk of coronary artery disease.

	Total cholesterol/HDL cholesterol		LDL cholesterol/HDL cholesterol	
Category	Men	Women	Men	Women
Safer side	3.40	3.25	1.00	1.45
Borderline high-risk	4.95	4.45	3.50	3.20
High-risk	9.50	7.00	6.25	5.00

glycerophosphate oxidase enzyme. The H_2O_2 formed in the reaction subsequently is measured as described in enzymatic method for total serum cholesterol **(Figure 11.51)**.

Normal Value and Clinical Interpretation

The normal range of serum triglycerides is **40 to 145 mg/dL**. Mean values rise slowly with age after the third decade.

Increased Concentration of Serum Triglycerides

- Elevated concentration is often found in disturbances of lipid metabolism and in atherosclerosis and coronary artery disease. The classification of triglyceride concentration according to the NCEP is listed in **Table 11.10**.
- The serum triglyceride concentration is greatly elevated in hyperlipoproteinemia type I and V and moderately increased in type II b and III.
- The cause of hyperlipoproteinemia is a genetic origin but hypertriglyceridemia occur commonly secondary to the following pathologic conditions:

- Hypothyroidism
- Nephrotic syndrome
- Alcoholism
- Obstructive liver diseases
- Acute pancreatitis
- Uncontrolled diabetes mellitus
- Glycogen storage disease (type I).

Decreased Concentration of Triglycerides (TG)

The plasma triglyceride concentration is low in the rare disease, **abetalipoproteinemia (absence of low density lipoproteins)**.

HDL Cholesterol

Method for HDL cholesterol Estimation

Commercial kits are available for the HDL cholesterol determination.
Principle: LDL, VLDL and chylomicrons are precipitated by polyanions in the presence of magnesium ions to leave HDL in solution. The cholesterol content of the supernatant fluid is then determined by an enzymatic method.

Normal Values and Clinical Significance of HDL Cholesterol

- Serum level of HDL cholesterol for:
  - Men is 30 to 60 mg/dL
  - For women 40 to 80 mg/dL which is 20 to 30% higher than men.
- Studies have indicated that when the HDL cholesterol value is lower than 45 mg/dL in men and lower than 55 mg/dL in women there is an increased risk for heart disease and the relative risk increases with lower HDL cholesterol concentrations.
- Higher HDL cholesterol concentrations may be associated with decreased risk of coronary disease. Thus, HDL cholesterol levels are inversely related to the risk of cardiovascular disease. HDL cholesterol level above 60 mg/dL indicates very low risk for coronary artery

disease (CAD). HDL below 35 mg/dL increases the risk of CAD.
- The ratio of total cholesterol to HDL cholesterol gives a more accurate and definite assessment of heart disease risk **(Table 11.10)**.
- Decreased levels are associated with stress, obesity, androgens, cigarette smoking and diseases like diabetes mellitus, augments the risk of coronary artery disease. HDL cholesterol is very low in genetic disorder, **Tangier disease**.

LDL Cholesterol

The value of LDL cholesterol may be calculated, if the concentrations of total and HDL cholesterol and triglycerides are measured. In practice, LDL can be measured indirectly by use of **Friedewald equation** assuming that total cholesterol is composed primarily.

Total cholesterol = Cholesterol in (VLDL + LDL + HDL).

LDL cholesterol = Total cholesterol – [HDL cholesterol + 1/5 × Triglyceride (TG)].

The concentrations of all constituents should be expressed in the same units mg/dL or mg/L. 1/2.22 × TG is used when LDL cholesterol is expressed in mmol/L. The factor 1/5 × TG is an estimate of the VLDL cholesterol concentration.

Normal Values and Clinical Interpretation

- The LDL cholesterol in women is somewhat lower than in men but increase after menopause
- Low levels of LDL cholesterol lower the risk
- Values above 160 mg/dL indicate high risk
- Values between 130 and 160 mg/dL are in borderline risk
- Values below 130 mg/dL are safer side **(Table 11.10)**.

Thus, the risk of cardiovascular disease is correlated directly with a high concentration of LDL cholesterol. The highest correlations have been obtained as a risk factor by the ratio of LDL cholesterol to HDL cholesterol **(Table 11.10)**.

ASSESSMENT QUESTIONS

■ STRUCTURED LONG ESSAY QUESTIONS (SLEQs)

1. Describe lipoprotein metabolism under the following headings:
   i. Types of lipoproteins
   ii. Metabolism of VLDL and LDL with diagram
   iii. Atherosclerosis
2. Describe lipoprotein metabolism under the following headings:
   i. Types of lipoproteins
   ii. Metabolism of chylomicrons with diagram
   iii. Familial hypercholesterolemia
3. Describe Lipoprotein metabolism under the following headings:
   i. Types of lipoproteins
   ii. Metabolism of HDL with diagram
   iii. Importance of reverse cholesterol transport
   iv. Metabolic significance of LCAT
4. Describe pathway of cholesterol metabolism under the following headings:
   i. Five stages of de novo synthesis
   ii. Regulation of synthesis with diagram
   iii. Metabolic fates
   iv. Good cholesterol and bad cholesterol

5. Describe β-oxidation of palmitic acid under the following headings:
   i. Pathway with diagram
   ii. Energetics
   iii. Regulation
   iv. Disorders
6. Describe the metabolism of ketone bodies under the following headings:
   i. Name ketone bodies
   ii. Synthesis (ketogenesis)
   iii. Utilization (ketolysis)
   iv. Significance
   v. Regulation
   vi. Related disorders
7. Describe de novo syntheses of fatty acids under the following headings:
   i. Fatty acid synthase multienzyme complex
   ii. Reactions with diagram
   iii. Regulation
8. Describe triacylglycerol metabolism under the following headings:
   i. Biosynthesis with diagram
   ii. Fate
   iii. Regulation
   iv. Disorder

SHORT ESSAY QUESTIONS (SEQs)

1. What is fatty liver? Write its biochemical basis, factors that cause fatty liver.
2. What is ketosis? Write its causes, biochemical basis and clinical manifestations.
3. What is atherosclerosis? Write its biochemical basis, factors that cause development of atherosclerosis.
4. Fredrickson's classification of hyperlipoproteinemias.
5. What is reverse cholesterol transport? Write its importance.
6. Write types and causes of hypolipoproteinemia.
7. Write biomedical importance of derivatives of cholesterol.
8. Write digestion and absorption of lipids.
9. What is carnitine? Write its role in fatty acid oxidation.
10. Write synthesis, regulation, and biological role bile acids.
11. What are prostaglandins? Give different types and functions.
12. Describe lipid profile tests and interprets laboratory results of analytes with various disorders.

SHORT ANSWER QUESTIONS (SAQs)

1. Define lipotropic factor. Write any four lipotropic factors.
2. Describe the metabolic fate of glycerol of triacylglycerol in adipose tissue.
3. Why does ketogenesis occur during fasting and starvation?
4. Justify "fats burn in the flame of carbohydrates".
5. Draw schematic diagram of fatty acid synthase multienzyme complex.
6. Write four differentiating features of β-oxidation and biosynthesis of fatty acids?
7. What is reverse cholesterol transport?

8. Write the causes of hypercholesterolemia.
9. Write types of lipases with their role.
10. What is the function of lipoprotein lipase?
11. What is steatorrhea? Write its cause.
12. Mention the types of fatty acid oxidation with their importance.
13. Write metabolism of propionyl-CoA.
14. What is Refsum's disease? Write its cause.
15. What is Zellweger's syndrome? Write its cause.
16. Key enzyme of cholesterol synthesis and its regulation.
17. Name the derivatives of cholesterol.
18. What is the mechanism of action of statins? What is the therapeutic use of this group of drugs?
19. Write significance of lecithin cholesterol acyltransferase (LCAT).
20. Write role of ApoC-II.
21. What is the biochemical basis of fatty liver?
22. What are the products of arachidonic acid?
23. Name essential fatty acids. Why arachidonic acid is not considered 'purely' an essential fatty acid?
24. Write inhibitors of prostaglandins with its importance

CASE VIGNETTE-BASED QUESTIONS (CVBQs)

Case Study

1. **Despite strict dietary control, a 55-year-old man had elevated serum cholesterol level. He started to take simvastatin and 3 months later his cholesterol was normal.**

   Questions
   a. Which enzyme of cholesterol biosynthesis is inhibited by simvastatin?
   b. What is the role of that enzyme in cholesterol biosynthesis?
   c. What is the normal serum cholesterol level?
   d. Name precursors of cholesterol synthesis.

2. **A 32-year-old heavy smoker developed a sudden crushing chest pain. He was admitted to the casualty department. Myocardial infarction was confirmed.**

   Questions
   a. Is there any relationship between smoking and myocardial infarction? If yes, what is it?
   b. What are the preventive measures against the development of heart disease?
   c. Name the lipoproteins that have protective effect against development of myocardial infarction.
   d. Name the enzymes likely to be elevated in myocardial infarction.

3. **A 50-year-old male, with history of chronic alcoholism, had fatty liver.**

   Questions
   a. What is fatty liver?
   b. What are the causes of fatty liver?
   c. What are lipotropic factors? Name any two.
   d. What is the nutritional therapy for fatty liver?

4. A 19-year-old girl was referred to a medical center because of poor exercise tolerance and muscle weakness. After biochemical investigations carnitine deficiency was confirmed.

   Questions
   a. What is carnitine?
   b. What is the role of carnitine?
   c. What is cause of muscle weakness?

5. A 60-year-old woman was referred to a hospital. She was noted to have hypertension. The plasma cholesterol level was 390 mg/dL. An angiogram of the right carotid artery demonstrated a narrowed lumen and the concentration of LDL was elevated.

   Questions
   a. What is your probable diagnosis?
   b. What is the normal plasma cholesterol level?
   c. By which enzyme is cholesterol biosynthesis regulated?
   d. Which lipoprotein has protective effect against the disorder?

6. A 35-year-old female was admitted to the hospital. Analysis of her plasma lipid levels revealed an elevated amount of cholesterol and almost no measurable cholesterol esters. No lecithin-cholesterol acyltransferase (LCAT) activity was detected in the patient's plasma.

   Questions
   a. Where does the LCAT reaction occur?
   b. What is the role of LCAT?
   c. What is the normal percentage of plasma cholesterol ester and free cholesterol?
   d. Name the other enzyme that esterifies cholesterol in tissues.

7. A 30-year-old woman was hospitalized, with an acute myocardial infarction. Her plasma cholesterol and LDL level were highly elevated. She was found to have familial hypercholesterolemia.

   Questions
   a. How are LDL formed?
   b. What apoprotein does LDL contain?
   c. What is the function of LDL?
   d. Why LDL is called bad cholesterol?

8. A male infant was admitted to the hospital. Examination revealed the presence of Gaucher's disease.

   Questions
   a. What is sphingolipidoses?
   b. What is the cause of Gaucher's disease?
   c. Name the defective enzyme.
   d. What are the clinical symptoms?

9. A 7-year-old boy was brought to the OPD with whitish and firm eruptions on his right elbow. They were identified as subcutaneous xanthomas. His mother said that his father had similar symptoms and had died at the age of 32 years of a heart attack. The mother was worried about her son and wanted to ensure that he does not develop heart disease.

The following were the results of investigations done:
– Fasting blood sugar   84 mg/dL
– Total cholesterol   486 mg/dL
– LDL cholesterol   318 mg/dL
– HDL cholesterol   25 mg/dL
– TG   118 mg/dL

Questions
a. What is the probable diagnosis?
b. What is the cause of the disorder?
c. Write the reference ranges for the above all parameters.
d. Which are the other consequences of increased level of cholesterol?
e. What is good and bad cholesterol?

■ MULTIPLE CHOICE QUESTIONS (MCQs)

1. Rate controlling step of cholesterol biosynthesis is:
   a. Lanosterol → Cholesterol.
   b. HMG-CoA → Mevalonic acid + CoA
   c. Acetoacetyl-CoA + Acetyl-CoA → HMG-CoA + CoA
   d. Squalene → Lanosterol

2. Which one of the following require for the transport of fatty acids from cytosol to mitochondria?
   a. Carnitine   b. Creatine
   c. Citrate   d. ACP

3. Endogenous triglycerides in plasma are maximally carried in:
   a. VLDL   b. Chylomicrons
   c. LDL   d. HDL

4. Which of the following fatty acid has maximum number of carbon atoms:
   a. Oleic acid
   b. Linolenic acid
   c. Arachidonic acid
   d. Cervonic acid

5. How many ATPs are produced when palmitoyl-CoA, a 16-carbon saturated fatty acid is oxidized completely to CO_2 and H_2O?
   a. 96   b. 108
   c. 106   d. 135

6. Which of the following intermediates in the oxidation of odd-chain fatty acids is likely to appear in the urine in vitamin B_{12} deficiency?
   a. Succinic acid   b. Methylmalonic acid
   c. Propionic acid   d. Butyric acid

7. Which of the following statements is correct for fatty acid synthesis?
   a. Occurs in mitochondria
   b. Requires NADPH as a cofactor
   c. Requires NADH as a cofactor
   d. Intermediates are linked to coenzyme A

8. The following are the features of the fatty acid synthase complex, *except*:
   a. It is a dimer
   b. It is found within cytosol
   c. It requires pantothenic acid as a constituent
   d. It requires biotin as a cofactor

9. Which of the following is not true for LDL?
   a. Transport cholesterol to cells
   b. Contains apoB-100
   c. Contains apoC-II
   d. Is a marker for cardiovascular risk

10. Free fatty acids are transported in plasma as a:
   a. Component of VLDL
   b. Component of chylomicrons remnants
   c. Part of LDL
   d. Ligand bound to albumin

11. The concentration of the following is inversely related to the risk of cardiovascular disease:
   a. HDL
   b. LDL
   c. VLDL
   d. IDL

12. Which of the following is an abnormal form of lipoprotein?
   a. LDL
   b. IDL
   c. Lp(a)
   d. Chylomicron remnant

13. Ketone bodies cannot be utilized by which of the following?
   a. Brain
   b. Skeletal muscle
   c. RBCs
   d. Renal cortex

14. A key intermediate in the biosynthesis of both glycerophospholipids and triacylglycerol is:
   a. Diacylglycerol
   b. CDP-choline
   c. Phosphatidyl choline
   d. Phosphatidic acid

15. NADPH, utilized for synthesis of fatty acid, can be generated from:
   a. Citrate lyase
   b. Mitochondrial malate dehydrogenase
   c. Malic enzyme
   d. Citrate synthase

16. Ethanol is converted in the liver to:
   a. Acetone
   b. Acetaldehyde
   c. Methanol
   d. Lactate

17. The risk of heart attack can be decreased by, *except*:
   a. Cessation of smoking
   b. Lowered level of HDL
   c. Control of plasma cholesterol
   d. Lowered level of LDL

18. The form in which dietary lipids are transported from intestinal mucosal cells is:
   a. VLDL
   b. HDL
   c. Chylomicrons
   d. LDL

19. All of the following are amphipathic lipids, *except*:
   a. Triacylglycerol
   b. Phospholipids
   c. Cholesterol
   d. Fatty acids

20. The triacylglycerol present in adipose tissue is hydrolyzed by:
   a. Lipoprotein lipase
   b. Pancreatic lipase
   c. Hormone-sensitive lipase
   d. Phospholipase

21. During electrophoretic separation, the fastest moving lipoprotein is:
   a. HDL
   b. LDL
   d. VLDL
   d. Chylomicrons

22. Ketosis occurs in all of the following conditions, *except*:
   a. Diabetes mellitus
   b. Marasmus
   c. Prolonged starvation
   d. High fat diet

23. Bile acids are derived from:
   a. Phospholipids
   b. Triacylglycerol
   c. Fatty acids
   d. Cholesterol

24. Acetyl-CoA acts as a substrate for all the enzymes, *except*:
   a. HMG-CoA synthetase
   b. Malic enzymes
   c. Malonyl CoA synthetase
   d. Fatty acid synthetase

25. The following are the ketone bodies, *except*:
   a. Acetoacetyl-CoA
   b. β-hydroxy butyrate
   c. Acetone
   d. Acetoacetate

26. Satiety value of fat is due to which of the following hormone?
   a. Insulin
   b. Glucagon
   c. Thyroxine
   d. Enterogastron

27. Which of the following ketone bodies cannot be metabolized in human body?
   a. Acetoacetate
   b. Acetone
   c. β-hydroxybutyrate
   d. None of the above

28. Dietary fats after absorption appear in the circulation as
   a. HDL
   b. VLDL
   c. LDL
   d. Chylomicron

29. An important feature of Zellweger's syndrome is:
   a. Hypoglycemia
   b. Accumulation of phytanic acid in tissues
   c. Skin eruptions
   d. Accumulation of C_{26}–C_{38} polyenoic acid in brain tissues

30. Gaucher's disease is due to deficiency of the enzyme:
   a. Sphingomyelinase
   b. Glucocerebrosidase
   c. Galactocerbrosidase
   d. β-Galactosidase

31. An enzyme required for the synthesis of ketone bodies as well as cholesterol is:
   a. Acetyl-CoA carboxylase
   b. HMG-CoA synthetase
   c. HMG-CoA reductase
   d. All of the above

32. Niemann-Pick disease results from deficiency of:
   a. Ceramidase
   b. Sphingomyelinase
   c. β-Galactosidase
   d. Hexosaminidase A

33. Chylomicron remnants are catabolized in:
   a. Intestine
   b. Adipose tissue
   c. Liver
   d. Liver and intestine

34. Free glycerol cannot be used for triglyceride synthesis in
   a. Liver
   b. Kidney
   c. Intestine
   d. Adipose tissue

35. Adipose tissue lacks:
   a. Hormone-sensitive lipase
   b. Glycerol kinase
   c. cAMP-dependent protein kinase
   d. Glycerol-3-phosphate dehydrogenase

36. Propionyl-CoA formed by oxidation of fatty acids having an odd number of carbon atoms is converted into:
    a. Acetyl-CoA
    b. Acetoacetyl-CoA
    c. D-Methylmalonyl CoA
    d. Butyryl CoA

37. Acetyl-CoA carboxylase is activated by
    a. Malonyl-CoA   b. Citrate
    c. Palmitoyl-CoA   d. Acetoacetate

38. Refsum's disease results from a defect in the following pathway, *except*:
    a. Alpha-oxidation of fatty acids
    b. Beta-oxidation of fatty acids
    c. Gamma-oxidation of fatty acids
    d. Omega-oxidation of fatty acids

39. Human desaturase enzyme system cannot introduce a double bond in a fatty acid beyond:
    a. Carbon 9   b. Carbon 6
    c. Carbon 5   d. Carbon 3

40. Lovastatin is a:
    a. Competitive inhibitor of acetyl-CoA carboxylase
    b. Competitive inhibitor of HMG-CoA synthetase
    c. Noncompetitive inhibitor of HMG-CoA reductase
    d. Competitive inhibitor of HMG-CoA reductase

41. Abetalipoproteinaemia occurs due to a block in the synthesis of:
    a. Apoprotein A   b. Apoprotein B-48
    c. Apoprotein C   d. Apoprotein B-100

42. Mental retardation occurs in:
    a. Tay-Sachs disease
    b. Gaucher's disease
    c. Niemann-Pick disease
    d. All of these

43. Cholesterol is present in all of the following except:
    a. Egg   b. Fish
    c. Milk   d. Pulses

44. Which of the following is best described for the lipoprotein synthesized in the intestinal mucosa, containing a high concentration of triacylglycerol and mainly cleared from the circulation by adipose tissue and muscle:
    a. Chylomicron
    b. Low density lipoprotein
    c. Very low density lipoprotein
    d. High density lipoprotein

45. Which of the following is best described for the lipoprotein synthesized in the liver, contains high concentration of triacylglycerol and mainly cleared from the circulation by adipose tissue and muscle:
    a. Chylomicron
    b. Very low density lipoprotein
    c. High density lipoprotein
    d. Low density lipoprotein

46. Which of the following is not a part of fatty acid synthase
    a. Ketoacyl reductase
    b. Enoyl reductase
    c. Acetyl-CoA carboxylase
    d. Ketoacyl synthase

47. Which of the following is the major product of fatty acid synthase?
    a. Acetyl-CoA
    b. Acetoacetate
    c. Palmitoyl CoA
    d. Palmitate

48. The class of drugs called statins reduced blood cholesterol levels by:
    a. Preventing absorption of cholesterol from the intestine
    b. Inhibiting the conversion of 3-Hydroxy-3 methylglutaryl-CoA to mevalonate in the cholesterol biosynthesis
    c. Increasing the excretion of cholesterol via bile acids
    d. Stimulating the activity of LDL receptor

49. Which one of following statements is correct concerning the biosynthesis of cholesterol?
    a. Synthesis occurs in the cytosol of the cell.
    b. All carbon atoms in the cholesterol synthesis originates from acetyl-CoA
    c. The initial precursor is mevalonate
    d. Rate limiting enzyme is HMG-CoA synthase

50. HDL has the highest content of
    a. Saturated fatty acid
    b. Triglycerol
    c. Cholesterol
    d. Apolipoproteins

51. Which of the following will be elevated in the bloodstream about 2 hours after eating a high fat meal?
    a. HDL   b. Ketone bodies
    c. Chylomicrons   d. VLDL

52. Which of the following will be elevated in the bloodstream about 4 hours after eating a high fat meal?
    a. Chylomicrons
    b. High density lipoprotein
    c. Very low density lipoprotein
    d. Ketone bodies

53. Which of the following is best described for lipoproteins formed in the circulation by removal of triacylglycerol from very low density lipoprotein and containing cholesterol taken up from high density lipoprotein, cleared by the liver.
    a. Chylomicron
    b. High density lipoprotein
    c. Low density lipoprotein
    d. Very low density lipoprotein

54. What is the enzyme responsible for the breakdown of triglycerides into fatty acids and mono-acylglycerol in the intestine?
    a. Pancreatic lipase
    b. Lipoprotein lipase
    c. Hormone-sensitive lipase
    d. Phospholipase

55. What is the function of bile salt in the intestine?
    a. Activator of lipase
    b. Emulsifier
    c. Co-factor for cholesteryl esterase
    d. Inhibitor of lipid absorption

56. What is the precursor for bile salt synthesis?
    a. Fatty acid
    b. Glucose
    c. Cholesterol
    d. Glycerol

57. Which of the following class of fatty acids can be directly absorbed from the intestine?
    a. Very long-chain fatty acid
    b. Long-chain fatty acid
    c. Short-chain fatty acid
    d. Cholesterol esters

58. The lipid digestion process is regulated by different local hormones. The cholecystokinin hormone released from
    a. Mucosal cells
    b. Pancreatic delta cells
    c. Gastric parietal cells
    d. Pancreatic alpha cells

59. Lack of appropriate lipid absorption leads to a condition known as
    a. Metabolic syndrome
    b. Obesity
    c. Fatty liver
    d. Steatorrhea

60. A child was brought to the hospital with the clinical presentation of mental retardation, blindness, and muscular weakness. The biochemical examination showed the accumulation of GM2 gangliosides in the tissues. What is the possible cause of the disease?
    a. Tay-Sachs disease caused by hexosaminidase A deficiency
    b. Fabry disease caused by alpha-galactosidase deficiency
    c Krabbe disease caused by beta-galactosidase deficiency
    d. Gaucher disease caused by beta-glucosidase deficiency

61. All of the following are progressive stages of atherosclerosis, *except*:
    a. Plaque formation
    b. Plaque disruption
    c. Fatty streak formation
    d. High-density lipoprotein

62. Which of the following statements regarding HDLs is TRUE?
    a. HDLs are the largest lipoproteins.
    b. The protein content of HDLs is 10%.
    c. HDL removes cholesterol from the periphery and transports it to the kidneys.
    d. HDL removes cholesterol from the periphery and transports it to the liver.

63. Which of the following statements regarding ezetimibe is TRUE?
    a. Prevent uptake of cholesterol across the intestinal lumen
    b. Inhibit HMG-CoA reductase
    c. Used to lower blood sugar level
    d. Used to lower blood cholesterol level

64. Which of these statements regarding atherosclerosis is TRUE?
    a. Atherosclerosis is due to dysregulation of cholesterol
    b. Atherosclerosis is a process that targets arteries.
    c. Atherosclerosis is rapidly accelerated by genetic and environmental factors.
    d. All of the above

65. Which of the following is NOT considered a biomarker for atherosclerosis?
    a. HDL
    b. Lipoprotein(a)
    c. LDL
    d. Hyperhomocysteinemia

66. Ketogenesis occurs primarily in _____ of liver cells
    a. Mitochondria
    b. Cytosol
    c. Endoplasmic reticulum
    d. Golgi apparatus

67. Organ that can utilize energy formed in ketogenesis during prolong starvation are:
    a. Brain
    b. Skeletal muscle
    c. Heart
    d. All of the above

68. Isozymes primarily responsible for prostaglandin production by cells involves an inflammation:
    a. COX-I
    b. COX-II
    c. CPS I
    d. CPS II

69. Analgesic effects of aspirin is due to inhibition of
    a. Cyclooxygenase
    b. Catalase
    c. Peroxidase
    d. All of the above

70. The rate limiting step in prostaglandin synthesis is catalyzed by
    a. Arachidonic acid
    b. Phospholipase A_2
    c. Calcium
    d. Cyclooxygenase

71. A person on a fat free carbohydrate rich diet continues to grow obese. Which of the following lipoproteins is likely to be elevated in his blood?
    a. Chylomicrons
    b. VLDL
    c. LDL
    d. HDL

72. In uncontrolled diabetes mellitus, what is the cause of high level of VLDL and TAG:
    a. Increased hepatic lipase
    b. Increased LDL receptors
    c. Increased activity of lipoprotein lipase and decreased activity of hormone sensitive lipase
    d. Increased activity of hormone sensitive lipase and decreased lipoprotein lipase activity

73. A patient with eruptive xanthomas, drawn blood milky in appearance. Which lipoprotein is elevated in the plasma?
    a. Chylomicron
    b. Chylomicron remnants
    C. LDL
    d. HDL

74. Very high total cholesterol, elevated LDL, normal level of LDL receptors. What is the probable cause?
    a. Apo B100 mutation
    b. Complete deficiency of lipoprotein lipase
    c. Cholesterol acyltransferase deficiency
    d. Apo E defect

75. A patient was diagnosed with isolated increase in LDL. His father and brother had the same disease with increased cholesterol. The likely diagnosis is:
    a. Familial type III hyperlipoproteinemia
    b. Abetalipoproteinemia
    c. Familial LPL deficiency (type1)
    d. LDL receptor mutation

76. Absence of which apolipoprotein is responsible for the genetic disorder, familial type III hyperlipoproteinemia:
    a. Apo B100   b. Apo B48
    c. Apo E   d. Apo CII

77. Patient with abetalipoproteinemia frequently manifests with delayed blood clotting. This is due to inability to:
    a. Produce chylomicrons
    b. Produce VLDL
    c. Synthesize clotting factors
    d. Synthesize fatty acids

78. In prolonged fasting glycerol formed from triglyceride. Which of the following statements is true regarding glycerol?
    a. Used in synthesis of chylomicron
    b. It is directly used by tissues for energy needs
    c. It is formed due to increased activity of hormone sensitive lipase
    d. Glycerol acts as a substrate for gluconeogenesis
    e. It is formed by increased activity of lipoprotein lipase

ANSWERS FOR MCQs

1. b	2. a	3. c	4. c	5. c
6. b	7. b	8. d	9. c	10. d
11. a	12. c	13. c	14. d	15. c
16. b	17. b	18. c	19. a	20. c
21. a	22. b	23. d	24. b	25. a
26. d	27. b	28. d	29. d	30. b
31. b	32. b	33. c	34. d	35. b
36. c	37. b	38. a	39. a	40. d
41. b	42. d	43. d	44. a	45. b
46. c	47. d	48. b	49. b	50. d
51. c	52. c	53. c	54. a	55. b
56. c	57. c	58. a	59. d	60. a
61. d	62. d	63. a,d	64. d	65. a
66. a	67. d	68. d	69. a	70. b
71. b	72. d	73. a	74. a	75. d
76. c	77. a	78. c and d		

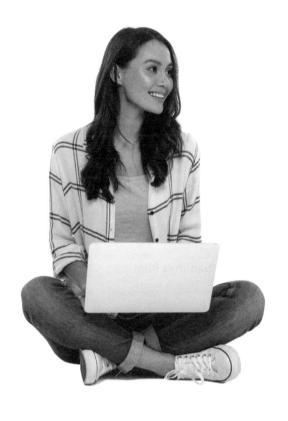

YOUR GUIDE AT EVERY STEP

Expert Knowledge Anytime, Anywhere

SCAN QR CODE
FOR MORE DETAILS

WHY CHOOSE US

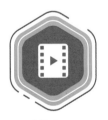

**Video
Lectures**

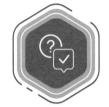

**Self-Assessment
Questions**

**Top
Faculty**

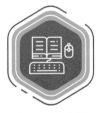

**New CBME
Curriculum**

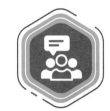

**Clinical Case
Based Approach**

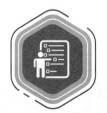

**NEET
Preparation**

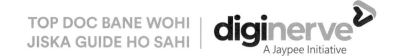

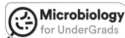
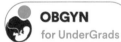

12 CHAPTER

Protein Metabolism

Competency	Learning Objectives
BI 5.3: Describe the digestion and absorption of dietary proteins. **BI 5.4:** Describe common disorders associated with protein metabolism. **BI 5.5:** Interpret laboratory results of analytes associated with metabolism of proteins.	1. Describe the digestion, absorption and transport of dietary proteins with associated disorders. 2. Describe amino acid pool. 3. Describe different stages of catabolism of amino acids. 4. Describe formation and transport of ammonia. 5. Describe urea cycle—pathway, significance, regulation and associated inborn disorders. 6. Describe the metabolism of amino acids—their role in biosynthesis of variety of specialized products and associated inborn disorders. 7. Describe biogenic amines and polyamines.

OVERVIEW

Proteins, the primary constituents of the body, may be structural or functional. A regular and adequate supply of protein in diet is essential for cell integrity and function. Dietary proteins are the primary sources of the nitrogen that is metabolized by the body. Adult man requires **70–100 g** protein per day.

The focus of this chapter is on the process of degradation of various amino acids and their related metabolic disorders.

We begin with a discussion of the breakdown of dietary proteins, and then proceed to a general description of the metabolic fates of amino groups and carbon skeletons.

DIGESTION AND ABSORPTION OF PROTEINS

Proteolytic enzymes (also called proteases) break down dietary proteins into their constituent amino acids. These enzymes are produced by three different organs; **the stomach, the pancreas** and **the small intestine.** The proteolytic enzymes include **endopeptidases** and **exopeptidases.**

- **Endopeptidases,** act on peptide bonds inside the protein molecule. Pepsin, trypsin chymotrypsin and elastase are endopeptidase.

- **Exopeptidases**, act at a peptide bond only at the end region of the chain. For example:
  - **Carboxypeptidase**, acts on the peptide bond only at the carboxyl terminal end on the chain.
  - **Aminopeptidase**, acts on the peptide bond only at the amino terminal end on the chain.

Digestion in Stomach

There is no digestion of protein in mouth. It starts in stomach. When protein enters the stomach, it stimulates the secretion of the hormone gastrin, which in turn, stimulates the release of **hydrochloric acid** by the parietal cells and (proenzyme or zymogen) **pepsinogen** by chief cells of gastric glands.

- **Hydrochloric acid:** Denatures proteins making their internal peptide bonds more accessible to subsequent hydrolysis by proteoses and provides an acid environment for the action of pepsin. As well as it acts as an antiseptic, kill most bacteria and other foreign cells.

- **Pepsinogen:** It is an inactive **proenzyme**, or **zymogen.** It is converted into active pepsin in the gastric juice by hydrochloric acid (HCl). Pepsin catalyzes the hydrolysis of peptide linkages within protein molecules. It has a fairly broad specificity but acts preferentially on linkages involving the **aromatic amino acids** tryptophan, tyrosine, and phenylalanine, as well as methionine and leucine. Action of pepsin results only partial degradation of proteins into a mixture of smaller units called peptides which then broken down further by pancreatic enzymes.

- **Rennin** is important in the digestive processes of infants. It is absent in adults. Rennin is also called **chymosin** or **rennet**.

Action of rennin is to clot milk. This is accomplished by the slight hydrolysis of the casein of milk to produce **paracasein**, which coagulates in the presence of calcium ions, resulting in an insoluble **calcium-paracaseinate** curd. Calcium paracaseinate is then acted on by **pepsin**.

$$\text{Casein} \xrightarrow{\text{Rennin}} \text{Paracasein} \xrightarrow{\text{Ca}^{++}} \underset{\substack{\text{(insoluble curd)}}}{\text{Ca paracaseinate}}$$

The purpose of this reaction is to convert milk into a more solid form to prevent the rapid passage of milk from the stomach of infants.

- ❖ Rennin and renin are different.
- ❖ **Rennin** is a proteolytic enzyme present in stomach and is involved in digestion of protein casein of milk.
- ❖ **Renin** also known as an angiotensinogenase, is a proteolytic enzyme, secreted by the kidneys and is involved in regulation of water and electrolyte balance and blood pressure.

Digestion in Intestine

Protein digestion is completed in the small intestine. As the acidic stomach contents pass into the small intestine, the low pH triggers secretion of the hormone **cholecystokinin** and **secretin**.

- **Cholecystokinin** stimulates secretion of pancreatic juice which contains inactive endopeptidases, trypsinogen, chymotrypsinogen, and procarboxypeptidase. These endopeptidases are active at pH 8.
- **Secretin** stimulates the pancreas to secrete **bicarbonate** into the small intestine to neutralize the gastric HCl.
  - **Trypsinogen, chymotrypsinogen,** and **pro-carboxypeptidase A** and **B** the zymogens of **trypsin, chymotrypsin,** and **carboxypeptidase** are synthesized and secreted by pancreas. Activation of the pancreatic inactive (proenzymes), **trypsinogen, chymotrypsinogen,** and **procarboxypeptidase** occurs by the action of **enteropeptidase (enterokinase)**, secreted by duodenal epithelial cells.
  - Enteropeptidase activates trypsinogen to trypsin and the activated trypsin in turn activates more trypsinogen. Trypsin also activates the chymotrypsinogen and procarboxypeptidase **(Figure 12.1)**.
  - The digestion of proteins now continues in the small intestine. **Trypsin,** and **chymotrypsin,** further hydrolyses the peptides that were produced by the action of pepsin in the stomach into smaller peptides.

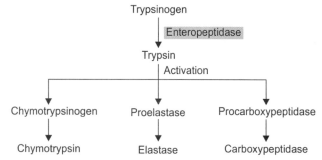

Figure 12.1: Activation of pancreatic proenzymes.

TABLE 12.1: Specificity of proteolytic enzymes.		
Enzyme	*Site of action*	*Cleavage points of peptide bond*
Pepsin	Stomach	Phe, Trp, Tyr, Leu (N)
Trypsin	Intestine	Lys, Arg (C)
Chymotrypsin	Intestine	Phe, Trp, Tyr (C)
Elastase	Intestine	Small nonpolar amino acids alanine, serine and glycine
Carboxypeptidase	Intestine	Successive C-terminal amino acids
Aminopeptidase	Intestinal mucosa	Successive N-terminal amino acids
Peptide bond cleavage occurs on either the carbonyl (C) or the amino (N) side of the indicated amino acid residues.		

This stage of protein digestion is accomplished very effectively, because pepsin trypsin, and chymotrypsin have different amino acid specificities **(Table 12.1)**.

- Chymotrypsin preferentially attacks peptide bonds involving the carboxyl groups of the aromatic amino acids (phenylalanine, tryptophan, and tyrosine).
- Trypsin attacks peptide bonds involving the carboxyl groups of the basic amino acids (lysine and arginine).
- Degradation of short peptides formed in the small intestine by the action of trypsin and chymotrypsin is then completed by **carboxypeptidase** (zinc-containing enzyme), and **aminopeptidases**
- **Carboxypeptidase** cleaves single amino acids from the carboxyl terminus of the peptides resulting in the liberation of free amino acids sequentially from the carboxyl end of the peptides.
- **Aminopeptidases** located on the brush border, cleave one amino acid at a time from the amino end of peptides.
  - The **dipeptidases** complete digestion of dipeptides to free amino acids. Dipeptidases are enzymes secreted by the small intestine. They are **exopeptidases.** They cleave dipeptides into 2 amino acids prior to absorption. These dipeptidases can then finally convert all ingested protein into free amino acids. Dipeptidases require **cobalt** or **manganese ions** for their activity. The hydrolysis of most proteins is thus completed to their constituent amino acids which are then ready for absorption into the blood.

■ The amino acids that are released by protein digestion are absorbed across the intestinal wall into the circulatory system, where they can be used for protein synthesis.

> Synthesis of enzymes as inactive precursors protects the exocrine cells from destructive proteolytic attack. The pancreas further protects itself against self-digestion by making a specific inhibitor, called **pancreatic trypsin inhibitor**. As trypsin is an activator of proteolytic enzymes, inhibition of trypsin effectively prevents premature production of active proteolytic enzymes within pancreatic cells.

Absorption of Amino Acids

The resulting mixture of free amino acids is transported into the epithelial cells lining the small intestine, through which the amino acids enter the blood capillaries in the villi and travel to the liver.

● The absorption of most amino acids involves an active **transport mechanism**, requiring ATP and specific transport proteins in the intestinal mucosal cells. Many transporters have **Na⁺-dependent mechanisms**, coupled with Na⁺ K⁺ pump, similar to those described for glucose absorption **(Figure 12.2)**.

● Several Na⁺-independent transport proteins are found in the brush-border membrane that is not specific for each amino acid but rather for the groups of structurally similar amino acids. All are specific for only **L-amino acid**. D-amino acids are transported by passive diffusion.

● There are 4 different carriers for amino acids:
1. Carrier for neutral amino acids (Ala, Val, Leu, Met, Phe, Tyr, Isoleucine)
2. Carrier for basic amino acids (Lys, Arg, and cysteine)
3. Carrier for acidic amino acids (Aspartic acid, Glutamic acid)

4. Carrier for imino amino acid (Proline) and glycine
● Alton Meister proposed that **glutathione (γ-glutamyl cysteinylglycine)** participates in absorption of amino acids in **intestine**, **kidneys** and **brain** and the cycle is called **gamma-glutamyl cycle** or **Meister cycle**.
● The amino acids, released by digestion, pass from the gut through hepatic portal vein to the liver.

> **Acute pancreatitis** is a disease caused by obstruction of the normal pathway by which pancreatic secretions enter the intestine. The zymogens of the proteolytic enzymes are converted to their catalytically active forms prematurely, inside the pancreatic cells, and attack pancreatic tissue itself. This causes unbearable pain and damage to the organ that can be fatal.

> ### Absorption of Intact Protein
>
> ❖ Small intestinal cells of fetal and newborn infants are able to absorb intact proteins, e.g., **immunoglobulin** IgA from **colostrum** of maternal milk are absorbed intact without loss of biologic activity, so that they provide passive immunity to the infant.
> ❖ The intact proteins are not absorbed by the adult intestine. However, in some adult individuals, small amount of intact proteins may be absorbed through the intestinal mucosa. These proteins often cause formation of antibodies against the foreign protein and are responsible for the symptoms of food allergies.

Disorders Associated with Amino Acid Transport

Genetic diseases arising from defects in amino acid transporters have been reported **(Table 12.2)**. Both the absorption of amino acids from the intestine and reabsorption from the glomerular filtrate are impaired. These disorders are discussed in details while discussing metabolism of individual amino acids.

▌ AMINO ACID POOL

Most proteins in the body are constantly being synthesized and then degraded. In healthy adults, the total amount of protein in the body remains constant because the rate of

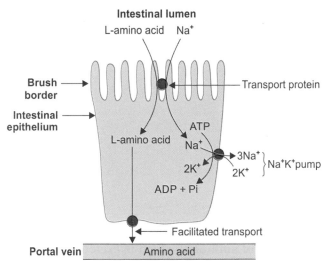

Figure 12.2: Stereospecific transport of L-amino acid across the intestinal epithelium.

TABLE 12.2: Amino acid transport system and disorder.

Transport system	Amino acid transported	Disorder associated with defective transport
Small neutral amino acids	Alanine, serine and threonine	Hartnup disease
Large neutral amino acids	Isoleucine, leucine, valine, tyrosine, tryptophan, phenylalanine	
Basic amino acids and cystine	Arginine, lysine and cystine	Cystinuria
Acidic amino acid	Glutamic acid and aspartic acid	
Imino acid and glycine	Proline, hydroxyproline and glycine	Glycinuria

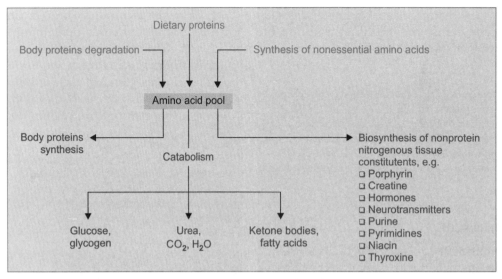

Figure 12.3: Amino acid pool.

protein synthesis is just sufficient to replace the protein that is degraded. This process is called **protein turnover**, which leads to the hydrolysis and resynthesis of **300–400 g of body proteins each day.** The turnover is high in infancy and decreases with age advance.

In contrast to carbohydrates and fat whose major function is to provide energy, the primary role of amino acids is to serve as building blocks of synthesis of tissue protein and other nitrogen-containing compounds. Amino acids, released by hydrolysis of dietary protein, and tissue proteins together constitute the **amino acid pool (Figure 12.3)**.

- Muscle and liver play major roles in maintaining circulating amino acids. Muscle generates over half of the total body pool of free amino acids, and liver is the site of disposal of excess nitrogen in the form of urea.
- After meal free amino acids, particularly **alanine** and **glutamine** are released from muscle into the circulation. Alanine is removed primarily by the liver, and glutamine is removed by the kidney. Glutamine also serves as a source of ammonia for excretion by the kidney.
- Branched-chain amino acids, particularly **valine**, are released by muscle and taken up predominantly by the brain **(Figure 12.4)**.
- In fasting state, branched-chain amino acids provided to the brain as an energy source. Alanine is a key glucogenic amino acid. The rate of hepatic gluconeogenesis from alanine is far higher than from all other amino acids.

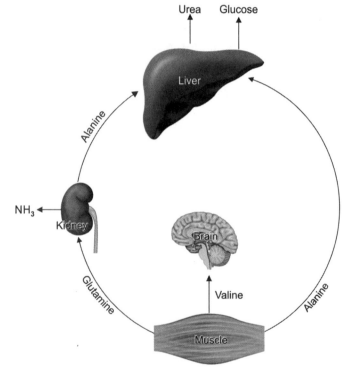

Figure 12.4: Amino acid exchanges between organs.

Contd...

- ❖ Interestingly, the liver cannot remove nitrogen from the branched-chain amino acids (leucine, isoleucine, and valine). Transamination of these amino acids takes place in muscle. Insulin promotes the uptake of branched-chain amino acids by muscle.

■ STAGES OF CATABOLISM OF AMINO ACIDS

In the catabolism, amino acids lose their **amino groups** in the form of **ammonia** which is excreted in the form of **urea** in the live by reactions of the **urea cycle. The remaining** carbon skeleton of amino acids, the α-keto acids

---

Why does the Muscle Release Alanine?

- ❖ Muscle can absorb and transaminate branch chain amino acids in order to use the carbon skeleton as fuel, however it cannot form urea. Consequently, the amino group is released into the blood as alanine **(Figure 12.12)**.

Contd...

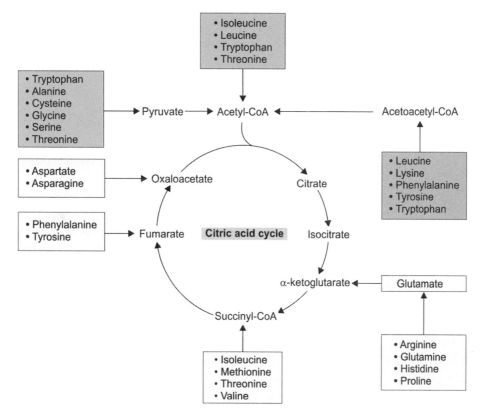

Figure 12.5: Metabolic fate of carbon skeleton of amino acids. **Yellow shade:** Glucogenic amino acids; **Red shade:** Ketogenic amino acid. Several amino acids are both glucogenic and ketogenic. Only two amino acids, leucine and lysine, are exclusively ketogenic.

undergo oxidation to carbon dioxide and water by reactions of **citric acid cycle**. The complete catabolism of amino acids includes following stages:

1. Removal of α-amino group in the form of **ammonia** by following reactions.
   - **Transamination** by the enzyme aminotransferase also called transaminase
   - **Deamination** may be **oxidative** or **non-oxidative**. Oxidative deamination is by glutamate dehydrogenase or amino acid oxidase. Non-oxidative deamination by amino acid dehydratase.
2. Transport of ammonia in the form of glutamine or alanine.
3. Disposal of ammonia in the form of **urea** in the liver.
4. Disposal (catabolism) of carbon skeleton of amino acids after the removal of α-amino group. The carbon skeletons of 20 amino acids converted to seven major products. All these products enter citric acid cycle **(Figure 12.5)** and are diverted to gluconeogenesis or ketogenesis or are completely oxidized to CO_2 and H_2O. The seven major products are:
   - Pyruvate
   - Acetyl-CoA
   - Acetoacetyl-CoA
   - α-ketoglutarate
   - Succinyl-CoA
   - Fumarate
   - Oxaloacetate

- Amino acids that are degraded to **acetyl-CoA** or **aceto-acetyl-CoA** are termed **ketogenic**, because they give rise to ketone bodies. Among 20 amino acids, only **leucine** and **lysine** are purely ketogenic.
- Amino acids that are degraded to **pyruvate**, **α-keto-glutarate**, **succinyl-CoA**, **fumarate** or **oxaloacetate**, are termed **glucogenic** because synthesis of glucose from these amino acids is possible.
- **Isoleucine, phenylalanine, tryptophan** and **tyrosine** are both **glucogenic** and **ketogenic**.
- The other fourteen amino acids are classed as purely glucogenic.

Figure 12.6 provides an overview of amino acid catabolism.

FORMATION AND TRANSPORT OF AMMONIA

Formation of Ammonia

Role of Transamination and Deamination Reaction in the Formation of Ammonia

Transamination Reactions

The first step in the catabolism of most L-amino acids is transfer of the α-amino groups, catalyzed by enzymes called **aminotransferase** or **transaminase**. In these transamination reactions, the α-amino group is transferred to the α-carbon atom of α-**ketoglutarate**, leaving behind the corresponding α-**keto acid** of the amino acid.

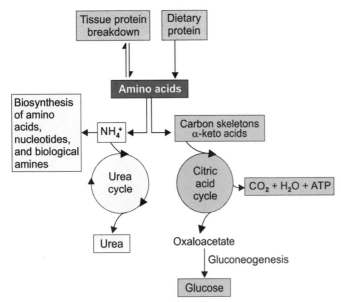

Figure 12.6: Amino acid catabolism overview.

- There is no net deamination (loss of amino groups) in these reactions, because the α-ketoglutarate becomes aminated as α-amino acid is deaminated **(Figure 12.7)**.
- The purpose of transamination reactions is to collect the amino groups from many different amino acids in the form **of L-glutamate**.
- The glutamate then functions as an amino group donor for biosynthetic pathways or for excretion pathways that lead to elimination of amino group in the form of ammonia.
- Cells contain various types of aminotransferases. Many are specific for **α-ketoglutarate** as an amino group acceptor but differ in their specificity for the L-amino acid. The enzymes are named for the amino group donor, e.g., **(Figure 12.8)**:
  - **Alanine transaminase (ALT):** It is also called **glutamate pyruvate transaminase (GPT)**, catalyzes the transfer of amino group of alanine to α-ketoglutarate resulting in the formation of pyruvate and L-glutamate and
  - **Aspartate transaminase (AST):** It is also called **glutamate oxaloacetate transaminase (GOT)**, catalyzes the transfer of the amino group of aspartate to α-ketoglutarate, resulting in the formation of oxaloacetate and L-glutamate.

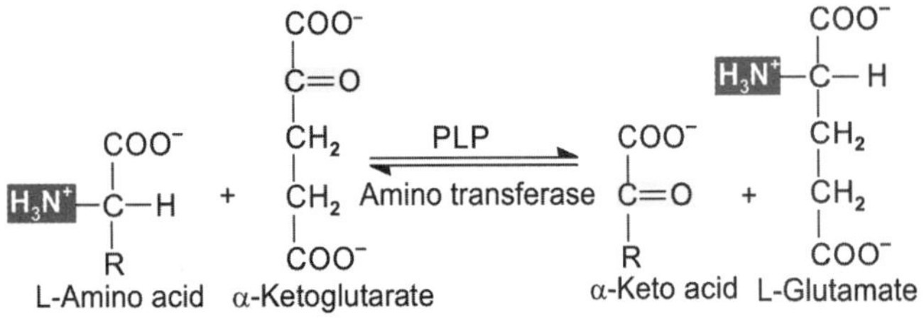

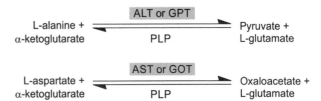

Figure 12.8: Reactions catalyzed by alanine transaminase and aspartate transaminase.

(ALT: alanine transaminase; AST: aspartate transaminase; GPT: glutamate pyruvate transaminase; GOT: glutamate oxaloacetate transaminase)

- The reactions catalyzed by aminotransferases are freely **reversible**.
- All amino transferases require **Pyridoxal phosphate (PLP)**, the coenzyme form of pyridoxine (vitamin B_6). Pyridoxal phosphate functions as an intermediate carrier of amino acid groups at the active site of aminotransferase.
- Most amino acids undergo transamination reaction except **lysine**, **threonine** and **proline**.

Metabolic Significance of Transamination Reactions

- To collect the amino groups from many various amino acids in the form of **L-glutamate**. The glutamate then functions as an amino group donor for biosynthetic pathways.
- Since transamination reactions are readily reversible, this permits transaminases to function both in amino acid catabolism and biosynthesis. L-glutamate, produced by transamination, can be used as an amino group donor in the synthesis of nonessential amino acids.

Clinical Significance of Aminotransferase or Transaminase

- Serum levels of some transaminases are elevated in some disease state and measurement of these are useful in medical diagnosis, e.g., ALT (GPT) and AST (GOT) are important in the diagnosis of liver and heart damage (*refer* Chapter: 5 Enzyme)
- It is also used to detect the toxic effects of some industrial chemicals like carbon tetrachloride, chloroform or other solvents.

Deamination Reaction

Deamination may be **oxidative** or **non-oxidative**. Oxidative deamination is by **glutamate dehydrogenase** or **amino acid oxidase**. Non-oxidative deamination by **amino acid dehydratase**.

Oxidative Deamination by Glutamate Dehydrogenase

As we have seen, the amino groups from many of the α-amino acids are collected in the liver in the form of the amino group of **L-glutamate** molecules. These amino groups are removed from glutamate in the form of **ammonia** by **glutamate dehydrogenase (GDH)**

In hepatocytes, glutamate is transported from the cytosol into mitochondria, where it undergoes oxidative

Figure 12.7: Transamination reaction.

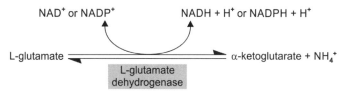

Figure 12.9: Oxidative deamination by L-glutamate dehydrogenase.

deamination, catalyzed by **L-glutamate dehydrogenase**. This enzyme is present in mitochondrial matrix. It is the only enzyme that can use **NAD⁺** or **NADP⁺** as the acceptor of reducing equivalents **(Figure 12.9)**.

Thus the net removal of α-amino groups to ammonia requires the combined action of glutamate transaminase and glutamate dehydrogenase. The combined action of an aminotransferase and glutamate dehydrogenase is referred to as **transdeamination**.

Glutamate dehydrogenase is inhibited allosterically by **GTP** and **ATP** and **NADH**; whereas GDP and ADP are allosteric activators. Thus decreased level of cellular energy accelerates the oxidation of amino acids to α-ketoglutarate which is oxidized by TCA cycle to liberate energy.

Metabolic Significance
- Glutamate dehydrogenase is located in mitochondria, as some of the other enzymes of urea cycle. This compart-mentalization of enzymes isolates free ammonia which is toxic.
- This freely reversible reaction functions both in amino acid catabolism and biosynthesis. Catabolically it channels nitrogen from glutamate to urea and anabolically it catalyzes amination of α-ketoglutarate by free ammonia to form glutamate.

Clinical Significance of Glutamate Dehydrogenase
GDH is present in normal serum in trace amount only, but increased activities are observed in cases of liver disease in which **hepatocellular damage** is present.

Oxidative Deamination by Amino Acid Oxidases

Both L and D amino acid oxidases occur in the **kidneys** and the **liver**. However, their activities are low. Amino acid oxidases convert α-amino acid to α-**imino acid** that decomposes to the corresponding α-**keto acid** with release of **ammonium ion (Figure 12.10)**. Amino acid oxidases use auto-oxidizable flavins (FMN or FAD) as coenzyme. The reduced flavin is reoxidized by molecular oxygen, forming hydrogen peroxide (H_2O_2) which is then split to O_2 and H_2O by **catalase.**

- D-amino acids present in the diet are metabolized by D amino acid oxidases in the liver.
- The function of D-amino acid oxidase present at high levels in the kidney is thought to be the detoxification of ingested D-amino acids derived from bacterial cell walls and from grilled foodstuffs. High heat causes some spontaneous racemization of the L-amino acids in proteins.

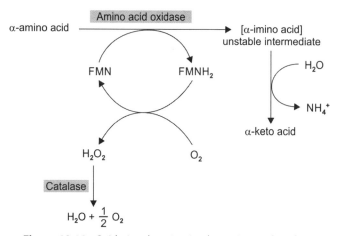

Figure 12.10: Oxidative deamination by amino acid oxidase.

Nonoxidative Deamination by Amino Acid Dehydratase

The α-amino groups of **serine** and **threonine** can be directly deaminated into NH_4^+ ion, without first being transferred to α-ketoglutarate. The presence of hydroxyl group attached to the α-carbon atom in each of these amino acids permits the deamination.

This direct deamination is catalyzed by **serine dehy-dratase** and **threonine dehydratase**, in which pyridoxal phosphate (PLP) is the coenzyme **(Figure 12.11)**. These enzymes are called dehydratase because dehydration precedes deamination.

Transport of Ammonia

In many tissues, including the brain, some processes such as nucleotide degradation also generate free ammonia. Since ammonia is extremely toxic, much of the free ammonia is immediately converted to nontoxic metabolites before export from the extrahepatic tissues into the blood and transport to the liver or kidneys. From extrahepatic tissues and muscles free ammonia is transported to the liver in two principal transport forms:
1. **Glutamine**
2. **Alanine**.

Transport of Ammonia in the Form of Glutamine

In many tissues (liver, kidney and brain), free ammonia is combined with **glutamate** to yield **glutamine** by the action of **glutamine synthetase (Figure 12.12)**. The glutamine, so formed, is a neutral nontoxic compound, which can readily

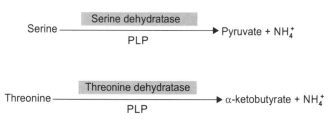

Figure 12.11: Nonoxidative deamination by amino acid dehydratase.

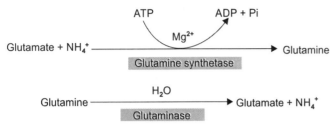

Figure 12.12: Formation and breakdown of glutamine.

pass through cell membrane, whereas **glutamate cannot**. Glutamine is normally present in blood in much higher concentrations than other amino acids. Glutamine also serves as a source of amino groups in a variety of biosynthetic reactions.

- The glutamine is carried via blood to the liver, where it can be acted upon by **glutaminase** to yield **glutamate** and **ammonia (Figure 12.12)**. The ammonia so formed is converted by the liver into **urea**.
- Some of the glutamate produced in the glutaminase reaction may be further processed in the liver by **glutamate dehydrogenase** (*see* **Figure 12.9**) releasing more ammonia and producing α-**ketoglutarate** (carbon skeletons) for metabolic fuel. However, most glutamate enters the transamination reactions required for amino acid biosynthesis and other processes.
- **Glutamine** is a major **transport** and temporary **storage** form of ammonia in the body.

> ❖ There are two human isoenzymes of mitochondrial glutaminase, termed **hepatic glutaminase** and **renal glutaminase**. Hepatic glutaminase level rise in response to high protein intake while renal glutaminase increases in **metabolic acidosis**.
> ❖ Excretion of ammonia into urine produced by the action of renal glutaminase in renal tubular cells regulates **acid-base balance**.
> ❖ In metabolic acidosis, there is an increase in glutamine processing and increase in ammonia formation by the kidneys.
> ❖ Not all the ammonia (NH_4^+) produced is converted to urea; some is excreted directly into the urine. In the kidney, the NH_4^+ forms salt with metabolic acids, facilitating their removal in the urine and serve as **buffer** in blood plasma.
> ❖ Production of ammonia from glutamine increases in metabolic acidosis and decreases in metabolic alkalosis.

Transport of Ammonia in the Form of Alanine

Alanine plays a special role in transporting ammonia to the liver in nontoxic form via a pathway called the **glucose-alanine cycle (Figure 12.13)**.

- In muscle amino groups from amino acids are collected in the form of **glutamate** by transamination.
- Glutamate can be converted to **glutamine** as described above, or glutamate can transfer its α-amino group to **pyruvate** by the action of **alanine amino transferase (ALT)** to form **alanine**. Alanine so formed passes into the blood and travels to the liver.

- In the liver by reverse reaction ALT transfers the amino group from alanine to α-ketoglutarate, forming pyruvate and glutamate. Glutamate can then enter mitochondria where **glutamate dehydrogenase** reaction release **ammonia**, or can undergo transamination with oxaloacetate to form **aspartate**, another nitrogen donor in urea synthesis, as we shall see. The overview of catabolism of amino groups is shown in **Figure 12.14**.

> Interestingly, the liver cannot remove nitrogen from the branched-chain amino acids (leucine, isoleucine, and valine). Transamination of these amino acids takes place in muscle. Insulin promotes the uptake of branched-chain amino acids by muscle.

UREA CYCLE: PATHWAY, SIGNIFICANCE, REGULATION AND ASSOCIATED INBORN DISORDERS

The ammonia formed in the breakdown of amino acids if not reused for the synthesis of new amino acids or other nitrogenous compounds, the excess ammonia is converted into **urea** in the urea cycle and excreted into the urine. This pathway was discovered in 1932 by **Hans Krebs** (who later also discovered the citric acid cycle) and a medical student associate, Kurt Henseleit.

Kreb's Henseleit urea cycle, is a major route for the metabolic disposal of ammonia. The series of reactions of urea cycle of occurs **exclusively in the liver**. Urea is formed from **ammonia**, **carbon dioxide** and α-**amino nitrogen** of **aspartate**, which requires **ATP**.

Enzymes catalyzing the urea cycle reactions are distributed between the **mitochondria** and the **cytosol** of the liver **(Figure 12.15)**. The first two reactions of urea cycle occur in the mitochondria, whereas the remaining three of the subsequent reactions take place in cytosol.

Sequence of Reactions

The sequence of reactions involved in the biosynthesis of urea, summarized in five steps as follows:

- I. **Formation of carbamoyl phosphate:** The biosynthesis of urea begins with the condensation of **carbon dioxide**, **ammonia** and **ATP** to form **carbamoyl phosphate**, a reaction catalyzed by mitochondrial **carbamoyl phosphate synthetase-I (CPS-I)**, a **key regulatory enzyme** for urea synthesis. Formation of carbamoyl phosphate requires two molecules of ATP. One ATP serves as a source of phosphate and second ATP is converted to AMP and PPi.

> ❖ **Carbamoyl phosphate synthetase-I** (CPS-I) is a hepatic mitochondrial enzyme functional in **urea synthesis.**
> ❖ **Carbamoyl phosphate synthetase-II** (CPS-II) is a cytosolic enzyme that uses **glutamine** rather than ammonia as a nitrogen source and functions in **pyrimidine** nucleotide biosynthesis (*see* **Chapter 18**).

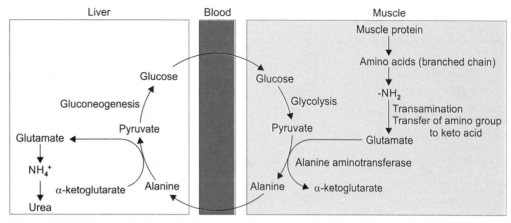

Figure 12.13: Glucose alanine cycle: Transport of ammonia in the form of alanine from muscle to liver.

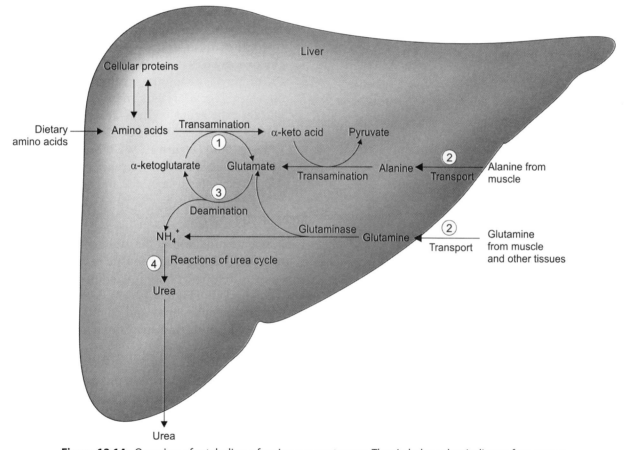

Figure 12.14: Overview of catabolism of amino groups to urea. The circled number indicates four stages.

II. **Formation of citrulline**: Carbamoyl phosphate donates its carbamoyl group to ornithine to form **citrulline** and release phosphate, in a reaction catalyzed by **ornithine transcarbamoylase**, Mg^{2+} requiring mitochondrial enzyme. The citrulline so formed now leaves the mitochondria and passes into the cytosol of the liver cell. Ornithine and citrulline are amino acids but are not found proteins. The next three reactions of the urea cycle take place in cytoplasm.

III. **Formation of argininosuccinate:** Citrulline is transported to cytoplasm, where it condenses with **aspartate**, a donor of the second amino group of urea. This reaction

is catalyzed by **argininosuccinate synthetase** which requires ATP. ATP is cleaved into AMP and pyrophosphate.

IV. **Formation of arginine and fumarate:** Argininosuccinate is cleaved by **argininosuccinase** (also called **argininosuccinate lyase**) to form free **arginine** and **fumarate**. The fumarate so formed returns to the pool of citric acid cycle intermediates. Thus, the carbon skeleton of aspartate is preserved in the form of fumarate.

Through fumarate urea cycle is linked with the citric acid cycle, the two **Krebs** cycles together have been referred to as the **Krebs bicycle (discussed onward)**.

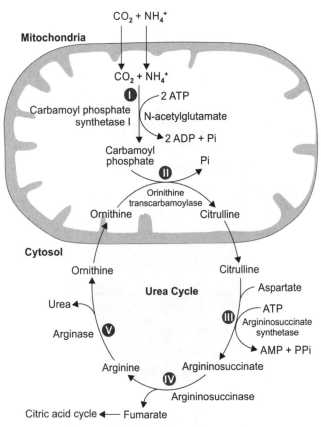

Figure 12.15: Reactions of urea cycle.

V. **Formation of urea and ornithine:** In the last reaction of urea cycle the liver hydrolytic enzyme **arginase**, cleaves arginine to yield urea and ornithine. Ornithine is thus regenerated and can enter mitochondria again to initiate another round of the urea cycle.

> The urea is excreted in the urine. Human beings excrete about 10 kg of urea per year.

Energy Cost of Urea Cycle

Four ATPs are consumed in the synthesis of each molecule of urea as follows:

- Two ATP are needed to make carbamoyl phosphate.
  - One ATP serves as a source of phosphate
  - Second ATP is converted to AMP + PPi
- One is required to make argininosuccinate
- One is required to restore AMP to ADP.

> The fumarate generated by the urea cycle is converted to malate and the malate is transported into the mitochondria (**Figure 12.17**). Inside the mitochondrial matrix **NADH** is generated in the malate dehydrogenase reaction. Each **NADH** molecule can generate **2.5 ATP** during mitochondrial respiration and reduces overall energetic cost of urea cycle. Net energy expenditure is only (4–2.5 = 1.5) 1.5 ATP.

Significance of Urea Cycle

- The toxic ammonia is converted into the harmless non-toxic urea.

- It disposes off two waste products, **ammonia** and **carbon dioxide**.
- It participates in the regulation of blood pH, which depends upon the ratio of dissolved CO_2, i.e., H_2CO_3 to HCO_3^-
- It forms semiessential amino acid, **arginine**. Arginine also serves as the precursor of the potent muscle relaxants nitric oxide (NO).

Regulation of Urea Cycle

- Urea cycle is regulated by **substrate availability**, higher the rate of ammonia formation higher the urea formation. This is the type of **feed forward** regulation for nonfunctional end product, in contrast to the feedback regulation for functional end product. Induction of urea cycle enzymes occurs in response to high protein diet or prolonged fasting when gluconeogenesis from amino acids is high.
- **Carbamoyl phosphate synthetase-I (CPS-I)** is an allosteric regulatory enzyme of urea cycle, which is allosterically activated by **N-acetylglutamate (NAG)**. NAG is synthesized from acetyl-CoA and glutamate to activate CPS-I (**Figure 12.16**). It has no other function. The synthesis of NAG increases after ingestion of protein-rich diet, by arginine and during starvation.

Krebs Bicycle

The fumarate produced in the argininosuccinase reaction of urea cycle is also an intermediate of the citric acid cycle. These two Krebs cycles are interconnected and referred to **Krebs bicycle (Figure 12.17)**. However, each cycle can operate independently and communication between them depends on the transport of intermediates between mitochondria and cytosol.

Enzymes of citric acid cycle, **fumarase** and **malate dehydrogenase** (MDH) are also present as **isoenzymes** in the cytosol. Fumarate formed in urea cycle can be converted to malate in the cytosol by **cytosolic MDH enzyme**. Then malate can be transported into mitochondria for use in

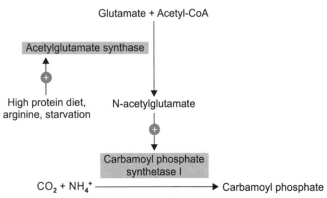

Figure 12.16: Activation of N-acetylglutamate.

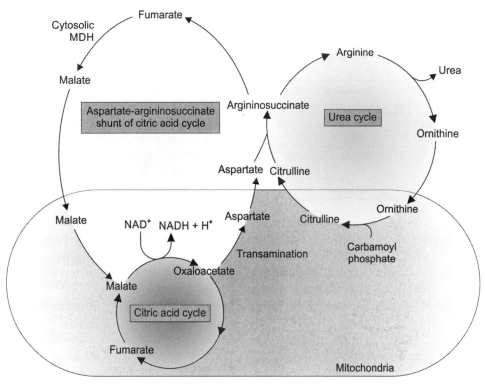

Figure 12.17: Krebs bicycle linking urea cycle and citric acid cycle.

the citric acid cycle. Malate in mitochondria oxidized to **oxaloacetate**. Oxaloacetate is transaminated to aspartate. Aspartate can be transported to cytosol where it serves as nitrogen donor in the urea cycle reaction catalyzed by argininosuccinate synthetase. The reactions linking citric acid cycle and urea cycle are known as the **"aspartate argininosuccinate shunt"** of citric acid cycle.

Significance of Krebs Bicycle

- It is involved in metabolic integration of nitrogen metabolism. The fumarate synthesized by urea cycle, links the **urea cycle**, **citric acid cycle** and **transamination** reactions **(Figure 12.15)**.
- Oxaloacetate which is formed from fumarate of urea cycle has also several other possible fates **(Figure 12.18)**.

Metabolic Inborn Disorders of Urea Cycle

Genetic defects have been documented for each of the urea enzymes. The metabolic disorders of urea biosynthesis are extremely rare. Since urea synthesis converts toxic

ammonia to nontoxic urea, all defects in urea synthesis result in **ammonia intoxication**. This intoxication is more severe when the metabolic block occurs at reaction I or II, since it accumulates ammonia itself. Deficiency of later enzymes result in the accumulation of other intermediates of the urea cycle, which are less toxic and therefore severity of symptoms is less (since some covalent linking of ammonia to carbon has already occurred if citrulline can be synthesized).

Disorders caused by genetic defects of urea cycle enzymes are given in **Table 12.3**. The clinical features and treatment of all five disorders are similar.

Urea cycle Disorder due to Transporter Defect

Hyperornithinemia-hyperammonemia-homocitrullinuria syndrome (HHH syndrome)

- ❖ **HHH syndrome** results from mutation of the **ORNT1 gene** that encodes the mitochondrial membrane **ornithine permease**.
- ❖ The failure to transport cytosolic ornithine into the mitochondria makes the urea cycle inoperable, with consequent hyperammonemia and hyperornithinemia.
- ❖ In absence of ornithine, mitochondrial carbamoyl phosphate, carbamoylates **lysine** to **homocitrulline**, results in homocitrullinuria.

Symptoms of Urea Cycle Disorders

Clinical symptoms, common to all urea cycle, disorders include:

- *Ammonia intoxication:* Ammonia toxicity causes cerebral impairment, ataxia, and epileptic seizures. In

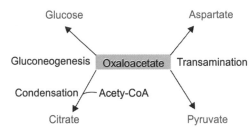

Figure 12.18: Fates of oxaloacetate.

TABLE 12.3: Disorders caused by genetic defects of urea cycle enzymes.

Disorders	Defective enzyme	Products accumulated
Hyperammonemia type-I	Carbamoyl phosphate synthetase-I	Ammonia
Hyperammonemia type-II	Ornithine transcarbamoylase	Ammonia
Citrullinemia	Argininosuccinate synthetase	Citrulline
Argininosuccinic aciduria	Argininosuccinase	Argininosuccinate
Argininemia	Arginase	Arginine

extreme cases there is swelling of the brain leading to death.

- Protein-induced vomiting
- Intermittent ataxia
- Irritability
- Lethargy
- Mental retardation.

Orotic Aciduria in Hyperammonemia Type II

The X-chromosome-linked deficiency termed hyperammonemia type II due to defect in **ornithine transcarbamoylase**. Hence carbamoyl phosphate accumulates in the mitochondria which reaches the cytoplasm and used for the synthesis of **pyrimidine** bases. Orotic acid, an intermediate in the pyrimidine synthesis accumulates which leads to orotic aciduria.

Why Ammonia is Toxic?

❖ In the body, about 98% of ammonia is in the protonated form (NH_4^+), which does not cross the plasma membrane. The small amount of NH_3 present readily crosses all membranes, including the blood-brain barrier, allowing it to enter cells, where much of it becomes protonated and can accumulate inside cells as NH_4^+.

❖ The accumulation of ammonia creates a serious biochemical problem because ammonia is very toxic. The damage from ammonia toxicity causes **cerebral (cognitive) impairment**, **ataxia**, and **epileptic seizures.** In extreme cases, there is **swelling of the brain** leading to **death.**

❖ Removal of cytosolic ammonia requires amination of α-ketoglutarate to **glutamate** by glutamate dehydrogenase **(Figure 12.9).** Then glutamate converted to **glutamine** by glutamine synthetase; (*see* **Figure 12.12).**

❖ In the brain, only **astrocytes**; star-shaped cells of the nervous system contains **glutamine synthetase**.

❖ For removal of ammonia in the brain more glutamate is diverted to the formation glutamine, which leads to depletion of glutamate in the brain. Depletion of glutamate affects the formation of gamma-aminobutyrate (GABA)

❖ Glutamate and gamma-aminobutyrate (GABA) are important **neurotransmitters;** the increased level of ammonia in the brain may reflect depletion of these neurotransmitters. Moreover, glutamine synthetase activity is insufficient to deal with excess NH_4^+.

❖ If extracellular concentration of NH_4^+ remains elevated, it disrupts the osmotic balance of nerve cell, causing swelling, resulting in brain edema.

Treatment

A protein-free diet is not the treatment option, because humans are incapable of synthesizing half of the 20 amino acids, and these essential amino acids must be provided in the diet. A variety of treatments are available for individuals with urea cycle defects. Many of these treatments must be accompanied by strict dietary control and supplements of essential amino acids. The treatment is as follows:

- Administration of benzoate and phenylacetate: In hyperammonemia type-I and hyperammonemia type-II, formation of citrulline and argininosuccinate is impaired. Citrulline and argininosuccinate cannot dispose of nitrogen atoms. Under these conditions, excess nitrogen accumulates in **glycine** and **glutamine** (**Figure 12.19**). By supplementing **benzoate** and **phenylacetate** the accumulated nitrogen is cleared from the body.
  - Benzoate reacts with glycine to form hippurate, which is excreted
  - Likewise, phenylacetate reacts with glutamine to form phenylacetylglutamine, which is also excreted.
- **Administration of carbamoyl glutamate an analog of N-acetylglutamate:** Deficiency of N-acetylglutamate synthase results in the absence of the normal activator (N-acetylglutamate) of carbamoyl phosphate synthetase I. This condition can be treated by administering **carbamoyl glutamate**, an analog of N-acetylglutamate to activate carbamoyl phosphate synthetase I.
- **Administration of arginine:** Supplementing the diet with arginine is useful in treating deficiencies of **ornithine transcarbamoylase**, argininosuccinate synthetase and argininosuccinase.

Laboratory Diagnostic Test for Urea Cycle Disorders

The most important step in diagnosing urea cycle disorders (UCDs) is clinical suspicion of **hyperammonemia.** Main clinical features include poor feeding, vomiting, lethargy, respiratory distress, seizures, if not detected and treated, early death may ensure. The basic tests used to help diagnose urea cycle disorders are:

- Blood ammonia
- Blood pH, CO_2, the anion gap

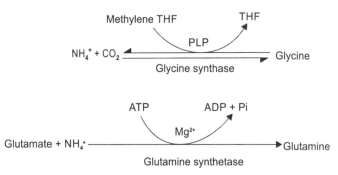

Figure 12.19: Synthesis of glycine and glutamine from ammonia.

- Plasma amino acids
- Urine organic acids
- Enzymatic diagnosis
- Genetic diagnosis
- **Blood ammonia:** A blood ammonia level is the first laboratory test in evaluating a patient with a suspected urea cycle defect. An elevated plasma ammonia level of 150 µmol/L or higher in neonates and >100 µmol/L in older children and adults, (with a normal anion gap and a normal blood glucose level) is a strong indication for the presence of a urea cycle defect. In neonates, it should be remembered that the basal ammonia level is elevated (less than 110 µmol/L) over that of adults, which typically is less than 35 µmol/L.
- **Blood pH, and CO$_2$, the anion gap:** The pH and CO$_2$ can vary with the degree of cerebral edema and hyper- or hypoventilation.
  - Hyperventilation secondary to the effect of hyper-ammonemia on the brain is a common early finding in hyperammonemic attacks, results in **respiratory alkalosis**.
  - Respiratory alkalosis can progress to acidosis, mostly if UCDs are diagnosed and treated late.
  - A blood gas analysis is, therefore, useful to guide the diagnosis of this type of metabolic disorders.
- **Plasma amino acids:** Certain amino acids are elevated in some urea cycle disorders and decreased in others, depending on where the block lies. Elevations or depressions of the intermediate molecules **arginine**, **citrulline**, and **argininosuccinate** will give clues to the point of defect in the cycle
- **Urine organic acids:** Urine organic acid analysis including the specific determination of **orotic acid**. Orotic acid is produced when there is an excess of **carbamoyl phosphate**. Excess carbamoyl phosphate used for the pyrimidine biosynthesis. Orotic acid is a catabolic product of pyrimidine.
  - Urinary orotic acid is measured to distinguish CPS1 deficiency or N-acetylglutamate synthase (NAGS) deficiency from ornithine transcarbamoylase (OTC) deficiency.
  - It is normal or low in CPS1 deficiency and NAGS deficiency and significantly elevated in OTC deficiency.
  - Urinary orotic acid excretion can also be increased in argininemia and citrullinemia.
- **Enzymatic diagnosis**: For enzymes, carbamoyl phosphate synthetase-I (CPSI), ornithine transcarbamoylase (OTC), and N-acetylglutamate synthase (NAGS) diagnosis is made on a liver biopsy specimen. Enzymatic testing for argininosuccinate synthetase (ASS), argininosuc-

TABLE 12.4: Causes of an abnormal levels of urea concentration.

Types	Causes
Prerenal uremia	• High protein diet • Any cause of increased protein catabolism, e.g., trauma, surgery, extreme starvation, diabetes mellitus, hemorrhage into gastrointestinal tract • Any cause of impaired renal perfusion, e.g., cardiac failure, ECF loses
Renal uremia	Any cause that leads to reduced GFR and leads to urea retention
Postrenal uremia	Any cause of obstruction to urine outflow, e.g., benign prostatic hypertrophy, malignant stricture or obstruction, stone
Reduced plasma urea concentration	Low protein diet, severe liver disease (decrease synthesis), water retention

cinase can be done on fibroblast samples and arginase can be tested on red blood cells.
- **Molecular genetic testing:** Molecular genetic testing is the primary method of diagnostic confirmation for all UCDs. Molecular testing of enzyme activity is the definitive diagnostic test.

Blood Urea

Normal range of blood urea for a healthy adult is **20–40 mg/dL**. High protein diet shows increase in level of blood urea concentration. In clinical practice, blood urea level is taken as an indicator of **renal function**. The term **uremia** is used to indicate increased blood urea levels. The causes of high blood urea are specified in **Table 12.4**.

METABOLISM OF AMINO ACIDS: THEIR ROLE IN BIOSYNTHESIS OF VARIETY OF SPECIALIZED PRODUCTS AND ASSOCIATED INBORN DISORDERS

Metabolism of Aliphatic Amino Acids

An aliphatic amino acid is an amino acid containing an aliphatic side chain. Glycine, alanine, valine, isoleucine and leucine are the aliphatic amino acids.

Metabolism of Glycine

Glycine is a nonessential or dispensable amino acid.

Synthesis of Glycine

It is synthesized from **serine** by removal of **hydroxymethyl** group from the side chain of serine. The methylene carbon group of hydroxymethyl is transferred to tetrahydrofolate and the hydroxy group is released as water **(Figure 12.20)**. This reaction is reversible, allowing glycine and serine to be interconverted.

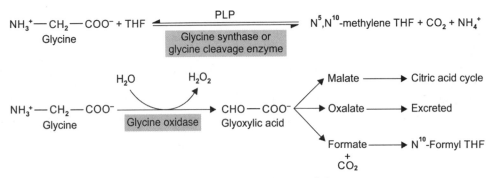

Figure 12.20: Synthesis of glycine from serine.
(THF = Tetrahydrofolate)

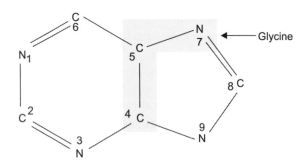

Figure 12.21: Catabolic pathways of glycine.

Catabolism of Glycine

Glycine is catabolized by following two ways:

1. The major pathway of glycine degradation is oxidative cleavage of glycine into CO_2 and NH_4^+ and a **methylene group (CH_2)** which is accepted by THF (**Figure 12.21**). This reversible reaction is catalyzed by **glycine synthase** also called **glycine cleavage enzyme** which is present in liver mitochondria. N^5,N^{10}-**methylene THF** formed in this reaction is used in certain biosynthetic pathways.

2. Glycine may be oxidatively deaminated by glycine oxidase to glyoxylic acid (**Figure 12.21**) which may be:
   - Decarboxylated to yield formaldehyde (formate) and CO_2
   - Converted to malate and then metabolized by the citric acid cycle
   - Oxidized to oxalate and excreted.

Metabolic defect of glyoxylate metabolism, associated with failure to convert glyoxylate to formate, as a result excess of glyoxylate is oxidized to oxalate.

Metabolic Importance of Glycine

Glycine is necessary for the formation of following products (**Figure 12.22**).

- **Synthesis of heme:** Glycine along with succinyl-CoA serves as a precursor for heme synthesis (*see* **Figure 14.2**).
- **Synthesis of glutathione:** Glycine is required for the formation of biologically important peptide, glutathione (γ-glutamyl-cysteinyl-glycine).
- **Formation of purine ring:** Glycine is required for the formation of purine ring. It provides C_4, C_5 and N_7 of the purine ring.

- **Formation of bile acids:** The water-insoluble bile acids; **cholic acid** and **chenodeoxycholic acid** are conjugated with glycine to form water-soluble **glycocholic acid** and **glycochenodeoxycholic acid** respectively. Conjugation lowers the pK of the bile salts, making them better detergents.
- Glycine is involved in **detoxification reactions**, e.g., benzoic acid is detoxicated by conjugating with glycine to hippuric acid.

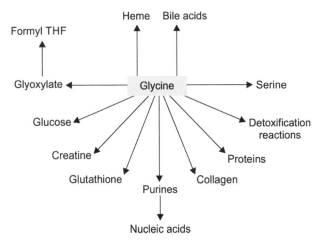

Figure 12.22: Metabolic importance of glycine.

- **Synthesis of creatine:** Glycine is necessary for the formation of creatine. It is synthesized from 3 amino acids, **glycine**, **arginine** and **methionine**. Creatine is present in muscle and brain tissue as the high energy compound **creatine phosphate**. Creatine phosphate functions as a **store of high energy phosphate** in muscle.
- **Collagen formation:** In collagen glycine occurs at every third position of a chain of the triple helix.
- Glycine is **glucogenic** amino acid, thus involved in the synthesis of glucose.
- Glycine is constituent of various tissue proteins, hormones and enzymes.
- By way of glyoxylate, it may form formate, which by THF may be incorporated into wide variety of biologically active compounds.

Metabolic Disorders of Glycine

Nonketotic Hyperglycinemia

- Nonketotic hyperglycinemia is due to defects in glycine cleavage enzyme, **glycine synthase** of catabolic pathway of glycine **(Figure 12.21)**.
- Nonketotic hyperglycinemia is characterized by elevated serum levels of glycine leading to severe mental deficiencies and death in very early childhood.
- At high levels, glycine is an inhibitory neurotransmitters leading to neurological defects.

Primary Hyperoxaluria

- It is an inborn error, characterized by high urinary **excretion of oxalate**. The metabolic defect involves a failure to catabolize glyoxylate, which therefore gets oxidized to **oxalate**.
- Increased level of oxalate results in **urolithiasis** (stone in urinary tract), **nephrocalcinosis** (presence of Ca deposits in kidneys) and **recurrent infections** of urinary tract.
- Death occurs in childhood or early adult life from renal failure or hypertension.

Glycinuria

- It is an inborn error characterized by increased excretion of **glycine** through urine, despite plasma concentration of glycine is normal.
- Since plasma levels are normal, glycinuria occurs probably due to a defect in renal tubular **reabsorption of glycine**.
- Glycinuria is characterized by increased tendency for the formation of oxalate renal stones.

Metabolism of Alanine

Alanine is a nonessential amino acid.

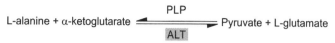

$$\text{L-alanine} + \alpha\text{-ketoglutarate} \underset{\text{ALT}}{\overset{\text{PLP}}{\rightleftharpoons}} \text{Pyruvate} + \text{L-glutamate}$$

Figure 12.23: Synthesis and catabolism of alanine.

Synthesis and catabolism of alanine: It is produced from pyruvate by a transamination reaction catalyzed by alanine transaminase (ALT) and may be metabolized back to pyruvate by a reversal of the same reaction **(Figure 12.23)**. Alanine is a major glucogenic amino acid.

Role of Alanine in Regulation of Blood Glucose
❖ In fasting, alanine plays a key role in maintaining the blood glucose level by gluconeogenesis.   ❖ Alanine is generated in muscle when the carbon skeleton of some amino acids is used as fuels. The nitrogen from these amino acids are transferred to pyruvate to form alanine by transamination reaction and transported to the liver, in the liver alanine undergoes reverse transamination reaction to form pyruvate.   ❖ The pyruvate is then converted to glucose by the gluconeogenesis. This process also helps maintain nitrogen balance.

Metabolism of Branched-chain Amino Acids

Valine, isoleucine and leucine are branched essential amino acids.

Catabolism of Branched-chain Amino Acids

The first three metabolic reactions for these branched-chain amino acids are similar and are catalyzed by common enzymes **(Figure 12.24)**. Therefore, the metabolism of three branched-chain amino acids is considered together. The common three reactions are as follows:

1. **Transamination:** The initial step in the degradation of the branched-chain amino acids is a transamination reaction to yield corresponding α-keto acids.
2. **Oxidative decarboxylation:** In the second step, the α-keto acids are oxidatively decarboxylated to the corresponding **acyl-CoA thioesters** by branched-chain **α-keto acid dehydrogenase complex**. TPP, FAD, lipoic acid, NAD$^+$ and CoA are required as coenzymes in this reaction.
3. **Dehydrogenation:** The third reaction is a FAD-dependent dehydrogenation, a reaction that resembles the first step of β-oxidation.

The subsequent reactions of all the three branched-chain amino acids differ and are catabolized as follows:

- **Valine** is converted to **succinyl-CoA** accounting for the **glucogenic** nature of the valine.
- **Isoleucine** is converted to **succinyl-CoA** and **acetyl-CoA**, accounting for the **ketogenic** and **glucogenic** nature of the isoleucine.
- **Leucine** forms **acetoacetate** and **acetyl-CoA** but does not produce succinyl-CoA, which accounts

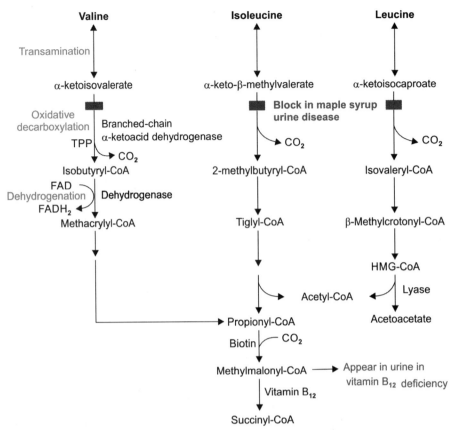

Figure 12.24: Degradation of the branched-chain amino acids (Valine, leucine and isoleucine).
(HMG-CoA: Hydroxymethylglutaryl-CoA)

for **exclusively the ketogenic** nature of the leucine. Leucine produces hydroxymethylglutaryl-CoA (HMG-CoA) intermediate product which is a precursor of cholesterol biosynthesis and ketone body formation.

Metabolic Disorders of Branched-chain Amino Acids

Maple Syrup Urine Disease (MSUD) or Branched-chain Keto Aciduria

It is an inborn error or branched-chain amino acids namely leucine, isoleucine and valine catabolism **(Figure 12.24)**.

Biochemical Cause

Maple syrup urine disease is due to inherited defect in the **branched-chain α-keto acid dehydrogenase**. Due to this defect α-keto acids of leucine, isoleucine and valine cannot be further metabolized. As a result, the branched-chain amino acids, leucine, isoleucine and valine, and their α-keto acids accumulate in blood, urine and CSF. Alpha keto acids impart a characteristic **sweet odor to the urine** of the affected individuals which resembles with **maple syrup** or **burnt sugar** hence the name.

Symptoms

Maple syrup urine disease is characterized by:
- Lethargy

- Failure to thrive
- Metabolic acidosis (ketoacidosis)
- Neurologic signs (mental retardation)
- Odor of maple syrup, in earwax, sweat or urine
- If untreated, it leads to coma and even death within one year after birth.

Laboratory Diagnostic Test for MSUD

Many infants with MSUD are identified through newborn screening programs. **Tandem mass spectrometry**, an advanced newborn screening test that screens for more than 30 different disorders through one blood sample, has aided in the diagnosis of MSUD.

- Infants with mild or intermittent forms of the disorder may have totally normal blood amino acids after birth and thus can be missed by newborn screening.
- In places where testing for MSUD is unavailable or where newborn screening fails to detect MSUD, a diagnosis may be suspected based upon symptomatic findings like lethargy, failure to thrive, neurologic signs or **odor of maple syrup** in earwax, sweat or urine.
- Tests to diagnose MSUD may include:
  - Urine analysis to detect high levels of branched-chain keto acids (ketoaciduria)
  - Blood analysis to detect abnormally high levels of branched-chain amino acids (BCAAs)

- Molecular genetic testing for mutations in the BCKDHA (Branched-chain keto acid dehydrogenase, alpha), BCKDHB and DBT (dihydrolipoamide branched-chain transacylase) genes are also available to confirm the diagnosis and is necessary for purposes of carrier testing for at-risk relatives and prenatal diagnosis for at-risk pregnancies.

Treatment

- Replacement dietary protein by mixture of amino acids that contain low or no leucine, isoleucine and valine.
- To monitor the effectiveness of the dietary treatment, plasma and urinary levels of branched-chain amino acids with dinitrophenylhydrazine (DNPH) should be measured constantly.

Metabolism of Aromatic Amino Acids

Phenylalanine, **tyrosine** and **tryptophan** are the aromatic amino acids. Phenylalanine and tryptophan are nutritionally essential amino acids but tyrosine is not as it can be synthesized from phenylalanine.

Metabolism of Phenylalanine and Tyrosine

Catabolism of Phenylalanine and Tyrosine

Phenylalanine metabolism is initiated by its oxidation to tyrosine which then undergoes oxidative degradation. Thus, catabolic pathway for phenylalanine and tyrosine is same as follows **(Figure 12.25)**:

- The first step is the hydroxylation of phenylalanine to tyrosine, a reaction catalyzed by **phenylalanine hydroxylase**. This enzyme is called monooxygenase (or mixed function oxygenase) because one atom of O_2 appears in the product and the other in H_2O. This enzyme requires tetrahydrobiopterin (H_4-biopterin) as a cofactor. The cofactor is oxidized to dihydrobiopterin (H_2-biopterin) during this reaction. The dihydrobiopterin produced is reduced back to tetrahydrobiopterin by dihydrobiopterin reductase which used NADPH as a reductant.
- The next step is transamination of tyrosine with ketoglutarate to P-hydroxyphenyl pyruvate, catalyzed by **tyrosine transaminase**.

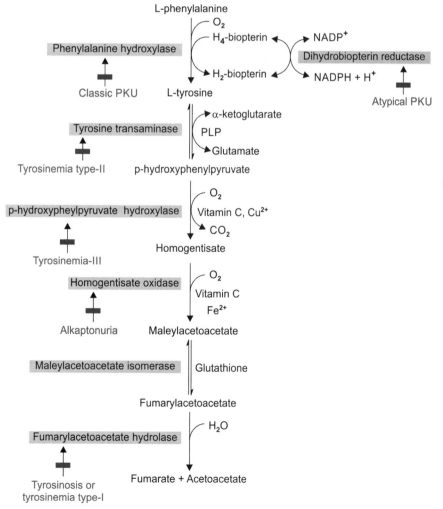

Figure 12.25: Catabolic pathway for phenylalanine and tyrosine showing metabolic disorders with respect to genetically defective enzymes.

- P-hydroxyphenyl pyruvate then reacts with O_2 to form **homogentisate**. This reaction is catalyzed by P-hydroxyphenylpyruvate **hydroxylase**, is called a dioxygenase because both atoms of O_2 become incorporated into product.
- Homogentisate is then cleaved by O_2 to yield 4-maleylacetoacetate. This reaction is catalyzed by another dioxygenase **homogentisate oxidase**.
- 4-maleylcetoacetate is then isomerized to 4-fumarylacetoacetate, by an enzyme maleylacetoacetate isomerase that uses glutathione as a cofactor.
- Finally, 4-fumarylacetoacetate is hydrolyzed by fumaryl acetoacetate hydrolase to fumarate, a glucogenic intermediate and **acetoacetate**, a ketogenic intermediate. Phenylalanine and tyrosine are therefore, both **glucogenic** and **ketogenic**.

Metabolic Disorders of Phenylalanine and Tyrosine

Phenylketonuria (PKU)

Phenylketonuria (PKU) is an inborn error of phenylalanine metabolism, associated with the inability to convert **phenylalanine** to **tyrosine**. The PKU is inherited in an autosomal recessive manner. The incidence of PKU is about 1 in 20,000 newborns.

Causes

- It is caused by a genetic defect in **phenylalanine hydroxylase**, the first enzyme in the catabolic pathway for phenylalanine.
- Phenylketonuria can also be caused a defect in the enzyme, **dihydrobiopterin reductase** that catalyzes the regeneration of tetrahydrobiopterin. Phenylalanine hydroxylase requires tetrahydrobiopterin as a cofactor. The cofactor is oxidized to dihydrobiopterin during the reaction. The dihydrobiopterin produced is reduced back to tetrahydrobiopterin by **dihydrobiopterin reductase**, which requires NADPH. PKU caused by deficiency of phenylalanine hydroxylase, is the most commonly encountered error.

Classification of PKU

PKU may be classified into three broad groups, given below. PKU caused by deficiency of phenylalanine hydroxylase, is the most commonly encountered error.

1. **Classic phenylketonuria** or hyperphenylalaninemia type-l, due to defect in **phenylalanine hydroxylase**
2. **Atypical phenylketonuria** or hyperphenylalaninemia type-II and III due to defect in **dihydrobiopterin reductase**
3. **Hyperphenylalaninemia type-IV and V** due to defect in **dihydrobiopterin** synthesis

Diagnostic Features of PKU

- In PKU, there is an **accumulation of phenylalanine** in tissues and blood and results in its increased excretion

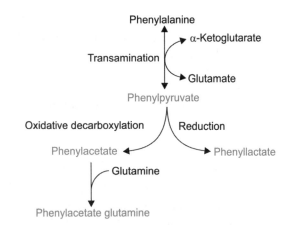

Figure 12.26: Alternative pathways of phenylalanine catabolism in phenylketonurics.

in urine, because it cannot be converted into tyrosine. Normally, three-quarters of phenylalanine molecules are converted into tyrosine, and the other quarter become incorporated into proteins. Since PKU patients cannot convert phenylalanine to tyrosine, by normal pathway, some minor pathway of phenylalanine becomes prominent in phenylketonurics **(Figure 12.26)**. In this pathway phenylalanine undergoes transamination with α-ketoglutarate to yield **phenylpyruvate**. Phenylalanine and phenylpyruvate (the keto acid) accumulate in blood and tissues and are excreted in the urine, hence the name **"phenylketonuria"**.

- Much of the **phenylpyruvate**, rather being excreted as such, is either decarboxylated to **phenylacetate**, or reduced to phenyllactate. Phenyllactate imparts a characteristic **mousy odor** to the urine, which have traditionally used to detect PKU in infants.
- Accumulation of phenylalanine or its metabolites in early life impairs normal development of the brain causing **mental retardation**. This may be caused by excess phenylalanine competing with the other amino acids for transport across the blood-brain barrier, resulting in a deficit of required metabolites. Untreated PKU is life-threatening, half die by age 20 years and three-quarters by age 30 years.
- **Hypopigmentation:** Phenylketonurics have a lighter skin color, fair hair and blue eyes due to deficiency of pigment melanin. The hydroxylation of tyrosine by tyrosinase is the first step in the formation of the pigment melanin is competitively inhibited by the high levels of phenylalanine in PKU (*see* **Figure 12.32**).

Treatment of PKU

Treatment of PKU Caused due to Defect in Phenylalanine Hydroxylase

- Low phenylalanine diet supplemented with tyrosine, because tyrosine is normally synthesized from phenylalanine. The aim is to provide just enough phenylalanine to meet the needs for growth and replacement.

- Proteins that have a low content of phenylalanine such as casein from milk are hydrolyzed and phenylalanine is removed by adsorption.
- A low phenylalanine diet must be started very soon after birth to prevent irreversible brain damage.

Treatment of PKU Caused due to Defect in Dihydrobiopterin Reductase

The treatment in this case is more complex than restricting the intake of phenylalanine and tyrosine. Tetrahydrobiopterin is also required for the formation of **L-3,4-dihydroxyphenylalanine (L-dopa)** and **5-hydroxytryptophan**, precursors of the **neurotransmitters**, **norepinephrine** and **serotonin**, respectively. In phenylketonuria of this type, these precursors must be supplied in the diet, along with tetrahydrobiopterin.

Diagnostic Tests for PKU

- In the past years, the urine of newborns was assayed by the addition of $FeCl_3$ which gives an olive color in the presence of phenylpyruvate.
- The phenylalanine level in blood is detected by screening by using Guthrie test a bacterial assay for phenylalanine is more reliable diagnostic test.
- The gene for human phenylalanine hydroxylase has been cloned, so that prenatal diagnosis of PKU is now possible with DNA probes.

Biochemical Basis for Mental Retardation in Phenylketonurics

The biochemical basis of retardation is not firmly established, but one hypothesis suggest that:

❖ The lack of hydroxylase reduces the amount of tyrosine, an important precursor to neurotransmitters such as dopamine.

❖ Moreover, high concentrations of phenylalanine prevent amino acid transport of any tyrosine present as well as tryptophan, a precursor to the neurotransmitter serotonin, into the brain. Because all three amino acids are transported by the same carrier, phenylalanine will saturate the carrier, preventing access to tyrosine and tryptophan.

❖ Finally, high blood levels of phenylalanine result in higher levels of phenylalanine in the brain, which disrupts myelination of nerve fibers and reduces the synthesis of several neurotransmitters.

Tyrosinemia

There are three types of tyrosinemia:
1. Tyrosinemia type-I (Tyrosinosis/Hepatorenal tyrosinemia)
2. Tyrosinemia type-II (Richner-Hanhart syndrome)
3. Tyrosinemia type-III (Neonatal tyrosinemia)

Tyrosinemia Type-I

- Tyrosinemia type-I, is also called **tyrosinosis** or **hepatorenal tyrosinemia**. It is caused by a genetic deficiency of **fumarylacetoacetate hydroxylase**.

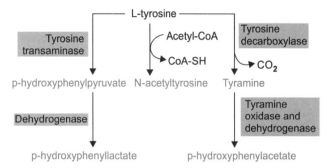

Figure 12.27: Alternative catabolic pathway for tyrosine in tyrosinemia.

- This defect results in accumulation and excretion of tyrosine and its metabolites such as P-hydroxyphenylpyruvate, P-hydroxyphenyllactate, P-hydroxyphenylacetate, N-acetyltyrosine and tyramine **(Figure 12.27)**.
- The deficiency of enzyme **fumarylacetoacetate hydroxylase** causes liver failure, kidney dysfunction, polyneuropathy and vitamin D resistant rickets.

Clinical Features

- In acute tyrosinosis, the infant exhibits diarrhea, vomiting and cabbage-like odor to skin and urine due to **succinyl-acetone** an abnormal metabolite, derived from fumaryl-acetoacetate. Death may occur in infancy due to acute liver failure (within first year of life).
- Whereas in chronic tyrosinosis in later life it develops liver cirrhosis and death occurs by age 10 years.

Diagnostic Test for Tyrosinemia Type-I

A diagnosis of tyrosinemia type I may be suspected in infants who display failure to thrive and an enlarged liver (hepatomegaly) during the first three months of life.

- The diagnosis is expected when tyrosine metabolites and succinylacetone are detected in the urine.
- It is also possible to make the diagnosis based on decreased activity of **fumarylacetoacetate hydroxylase** (FAH) in liver tissue but this test is not readily available.
- Molecular genetic testing for FAH gene mutations is available to confirm the diagnosis.
- Tyrosinemia type I may also be diagnosed through newborn screening programs. Succinylacetone can be measured on the newborn blood spot by tandem mass spectroscopy
- Carrier testing and prenatal diagnosis by DNA analysis are available if the specific gene-causing mutation has been identified in the family. Prenatal diagnosis is also possible by detection of succinylacetone in amniotic fluid.
- **Carrier testing** is a type of **genetic testing** to understand their risk of having a child with a genetic disorder.

Treatment

The patient should be kept on diet low in phenylalanine and tyrosine.

Tyrosinemia Type-II (Richner-Hanhart Syndrome)

Tyrosinemia type-II is caused by genetic deficiency of hepatic enzyme **tyrosine aminotransferase** (tyrosine transaminase).

Clinical Features

- Due to deficiency of hepatic enzyme tyrosine aminotransferase, the tyrosine cannot be metabolized by its routine pathway and is converted to p-hydroxyphenylacetate, N-acetyltyrosin and tyramine **(Figure 12.27)**. As a result, the tyrosine and its toxic metabolites accumulate in blood and tissues and appear in urine.
- The accumulation of tyrosine produces lesions in eye and skin and causes mild to moderate mental retardation.

Treatment

Diet low in tyrosine and phenylalanine is recommended. Diet with vitamin C may benefit the corneal and skin lesions of tyrosine aminotransferase deficiency, but not the mental retardation.

Tyrosinemia Type-III (Neonatal Tyrosinemia)

It is caused by absence of the enzyme **P-hydroxyphenylpyruvate hydroxylase** (dioxygenase). In neonatal tyrosinemia, serum tyrosine levels are high in premature infants resulting from an immature liver and its limited ability to synthesize the enzyme, **p-hydroxyphenylpyruvate hydroxylase**. As the liver matures, the accumulated tyrosine is metabolized and serum levels decrease to adult levels within 4–8 weeks of age. It is benign condition and responds well to ascorbic acid.

Alkaptonuria

This inherited metabolic disorder is due to defect in the enzyme **homogentisate oxidase**, which catalyzes oxidation of homogentisate to maleylacetoacetate **(Figure 12.25)**. As a result, the homogentisate accumulates in blood and body tissues and is excreted in large amounts in urine.

Clinical Features

- The urine of alkaptonuric patients becomes dark after being exposed to air. In presence of oxygen, the colorless homogentisate present in urine undergoes spontaneous oxidation to yield benzoquinone acetate, which polymerizes to form black brown pigment alkapton **(Figure 12.28)**. The alkapton imparts a characteristic black-brown color to urine **(Figure 12.29)**.
- Alkaptonuria is a harmless condition. Later in life patients may suffer from deposition of dark-colored alkapton pigments in connective tissues and bones. This results in black pigmentation of the sclera, ear, nose and cheeks and the clinical condition is known as ochronosis (because ochre color of the deposit).

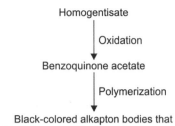

Homogentisate

↓ Oxidation

Benzoquinone acetate

↓ Polymerization

Black-colored alkapton bodies that binds to connective tissue (ochronosis)

Figure 12.28: Formation of alkapton bodies.

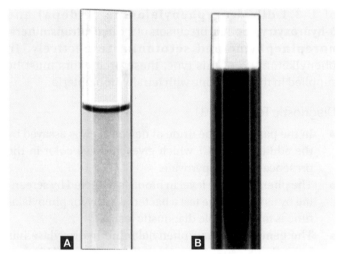

Figure 12.29: Urine samples from AKU patient. (A) Alkaptonuric urine normal color on excretion; (B) Darkens after standing.

Ochronosis leads to tissue damage and may develop joint pain, arthritis and backache.

Treatment

Since alkaptonuria is not considered life-threatening, this condition is not treated. Later in life, the symptoms of arthritis may be treated but the condition itself is not.

Diagnosis

The urine sample of patients of alkaptonuria turns dark on standing in air. The urine gives positive test with **ferric chloride** and **silver nitrate** due to reducing activity of homogentisate.

Albinism

It is an inborn error of tyrosine catabolism. It is due to inherited deficiency of enzyme **tyrosinase**. The inherited deficiency of tyrosinase impairs the synthesis of melanin from tyrosine (*see* **Figure 12.32**). Melanin is dark pigment of skin, hair, iris, and retinal epithelial cells. Melanin protects the body from harmful radiation of sunlight.

Clinical Features

- Impaired synthesis of melanin results in either hypopigmentation or no pigmentation of hair, skin and eyes and leads to white hair and skin.

- Albinos are highly sensitive to sunlight and can lead to skin cancer.
- The lack of melanin pigment in eyes is responsible for photophobia (intolerance to light) and nystagmus.

Biologically Important Compounds Derived from Tyrosine

Tyrosine serves as a precursor for following several biologically important compounds (**Figure 12.30**).

- Catecholamines
  - Dopamine
  - Norepinephrine
  - Epinephrine
- Melanin pigment
- Thyroxine.

Biosynthesis of Catecholamines

- Epinephrine (adrenaline), norepinephrine (noradrenaline) and dopamine are collectively called catecholamines. They are synthesized from tyrosine (**Figure 12.31**).
- Epinephrine and norepinephrine are produced by adrenal medulla and serve as **hormones**, whereas dopamine and norepinephrine produced in the CNS and postganglionic sympathetic nerves act as **neurotransmitter**.

> In Parkinson's disease, dopamine levels in the CNS are decreased because of a deficiency of cells that produce dopamine and depression is associated with low levels of serotonin.

Biosynthesis of Melanin Pigment

Melanin is a pigment. The synthesis of melanin occurs only in pigment producing cells called **melanocytes** (**Figure 12.32**).

- The first step is the conversion of tyrosine to **dihydroxyphenylalanine (dopa)**. In melanocyte, **tyrosinase** catalyzes this reaction.

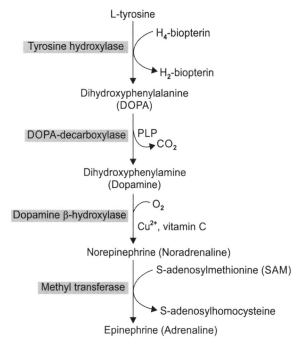

Figure 12.31: Synthesis of catecholamines.

- Tyrosinase also catalyzes the subsequent oxidation of dopa to dopaquinone.
- Dopaquinone is then converted to melanin. Tyrosinase does not require tetrahydrobiopterin but it utilizes copper as a cofactor

Biosynthesis of Thyroxine and Tri-iodothyroxine

The hormones thyroxine (T_4) and tri-iodothyroxine (T_3) are formed in the follicle cells of the thyroid gland by iodination of tyrosine residues of protein **thyroglobulin**. Monoiodo and diiodotyrosine residues are first formed and these then react to form T_3 and T_4 (**Figure 12.33**).

Metabolism of Tryptophan

Tryptophan is an **essential amino acid**, containing indol ring. Tryptophan is oxidized to produce alanine, which is glucogenic and acetyl-CoA, which is ketogenic. Thus, tryptophan is both glucogenic and ketogenic. Tryptophan is metabolized by **kynurenine pathway.**

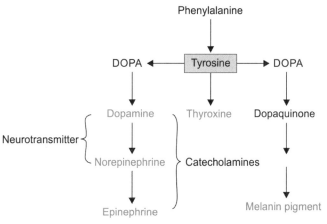

Figure 12.30: Biosynthesis of biologically important compounds from tyrosine.

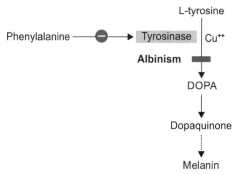

Figure 12.32: Biosynthesis of melanin.

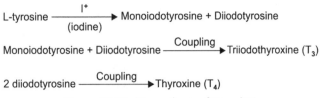

Figure 12.33: Biosynthesis of T3 and T4.

Kynurenine Pathway

In this pathway tryptophan is oxidized to kynurenine and alanine. Kynurenine is then converted to either **vitamin niacin** or **acetyl-CoA (Figure 12.34).**

- The initial reaction is an oxidation of tryptophan to formylkynurenine, catalyzed by the enzyme **tryptophan oxygenase** also called **tryptophan pyrrolase**, which is feedback inhibited by nicotinic acid derivatives, e.g., NADH or NADPH.
- Formylkynurenine is converted to kynurenine by removal of formyl group with the enzyme kynurenine formylase.
- Kynurenine is then metabolized to 3-hydroxy kynurenine by **kynurenine hydroxylase.**
- Next 3-hydroxykynurenine is converted to 3-hydroxyanthranilate and alanine by **kynureninase**, a PLP-dependent enzyme. A deficiency of **vitamin B$_6$ (pyridoxine)**

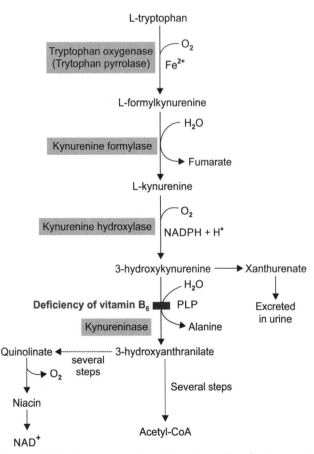

Figure 12.34: Kynurenine catabolic pathway of tryptophan and biosynthesis of vitamin niacin.

results in failure to catabolize the hydroxykynurenine, forming **xanthurenate (Figure 12.34)** and excreted in urine in vitamin B$_6$ deficiency.

- Next 3-hydroxyanthranilate undergoes decarboxylation forming vitamin niacin which can be converted to **NAD$^+$** and **NADP$^+$** or 3-hydroxyanthranilate can also be converted through a number of steps to acetyl-CoA.

> For every 60 mg of tryptophan, 1 mg equivalent of niacin can be generated.

Biologically Important Compounds Derived from Tryptophan

Tryptophan is a precursor for the synthesis of:
- Neurotransmitter serotonin
- Hormone melatonin
- Vitamin niacin (vitamin B$_3$)

Serotonin

Serotonin a **neurotransmitter** is synthesized by **neurons, pineal gland** and by the **argentaffin tissue** of the abdominal cavity. Normally, about 1–3% tryptophan is channeled to serotonin synthesis.

- Tryptophan is first oxidized to 5-hydroxytryptophan by **tryptophan hydroxylase**, which requires, **tetrahydrobiopterin** as a cofactor.
- 5-hydroxytryptophan undergoes decarboxylation to yield **serotonin** (5-hydroxytryptamine)
- Acetylation of serotonin followed by methylation in the pineal gland forms a **hormone melatonin (Figure 12.35).**
- The oxidative deamination of serotonin by the enzyme **monoamine oxidase (MAO)** leads the formation 5-hydroxyindoleacetic acid (5-HIAA), which is excreted.

Importance of Serotonin

- The most important physiological role of serotonin is that of a **neurotransmitter in serotonergic neurons** within the brain. In humans, serotonin is involved in a variety of behavioral patterns including.
  - Sleep
  - Perception of pain
  - Social behavior
  - Schizophrenia
  - Mental depression.
- Serotonin regulates mood, happiness, and anxiety. Low levels of serotonin leads to depression, anxiety, and suicidal behavior.
- Serotonin is responsible for stimulating the parts of the brain that control sleep and waking.
- It has been shown that alterations in serotonergic neuronal function in the CNS occur in severe depression which is due to reduced concentration of serotonin.

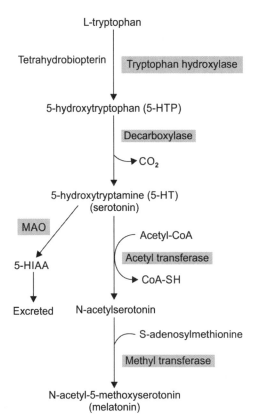

Figure 12.35: Formation of serotonin and melatonin from tryptophan.

(MAO: monoamine oxidase; 5-HIAA: 5-hydroxyindoleacetic acid)

- Serotonin in addition serving as **neurotransmitter** is a potent **vasoconstrictor** and stimulator of smooth muscle contraction.
- Clinically serotonin plays a role in **depression** and **carcinoid tumors**.

> Serotonin-deficient individuals treated with **antidepressant** drugs, such as, **amitriptyline** and **trazodone**. These drugs inhibit the reuptake of serotonin by the presynaptic neurons thereby increasing the concentration of serotonin at serotonergic synapses.

Carcinoid Syndrome or Argentaffinomas

A carcinoid syndrome is a serotonin secreting neoplasm. A carcinoid tumors develop from enterochromaffin cells, which are distributed widely throughout the gastrointestinal tract, biliary tract and gallbladder, pancreatic ducts, and bronchial tree.

Carcinoid tumors occur in any of these sites that overproduce serotonin, up to 60% of tryptophan (normal 1–3%) is diverted to serotonin formation. Therefore, niacin deficiency (pellagra) may also be seen in this carcinoid syndrome.

Clinical symptoms of carcinoid syndrome

Clinical symptoms of carcinoid syndrome includes:
- Prominent flushing
- Bronchial constriction
- Diarrhea

- Cardiac lesions and often is associated with heart failure.
- Individuals have large increases in urinary excretion of 5-HIAA.

Diagnostic test

- Measurement of urinary 5-HIAA (5-hydroxyindoleacetic acid) concentration. Carcinoid syndromes usually have large increase in urinary excretion of 5-HIAA, more than 25 mg/day compared with normal levels of less than 6 mg/day
- When an individual strongly suspect for carcinoid syndrome shows normal or borderline increases of 5-HIAA because:
  - Large amounts of serotonin produced are not being metabolized, in which case measurement of 5-HTP or serotonin is necessary for the diagnosis.
  - Secondly, secretion of 5-HIAA by the tumor is intermittent, in which case repeat specimen collections and serial measurements are needed to find out the abnormality.

Melatonin

- Melatonin is a hormone produced from serotonin by the pineal gland **(Figure 12.35)**.
- Synthesis of melatonin is regulated by **light dark cycle**. It is synthesized mostly at night.
- It is an inhibitor of **melanocyte-stimulating hormone (MSH)** and **adrenocorticotropic hormone (ACTH)**.
- Melatonin is a sleep-inducing substance and is involved in regulation of circadian rhythm of body. It may also be involved in regulating **reproductive functions**.

Metabolic Disorder of Tryptophan

Hartnup's Disease

- Hartnup's disease is an inherited disorder of tryptophan metabolism. This disorder was first of all reported in the family of **Hartnup**, therefore, named Hartnup's disease.
- It is due to defect in the intestinal and renal **transport of tryptophan** and other neutral amino acids and leads to tryptophan deficiency. Tryptophan deficiency ultimately leads to decreased synthesis of **vitamin niacin** and **serotonin**.
- Decreased synthesis of niacin leads to **pellagra**-like symptoms and decreased serotonin synthesis is responsible for **neurological symptoms** observed in Hartnup's disease.
- In addition to the neurological and pellagra like symptoms, there is **amino aciduria** due to failure of transport of amino acids from kidney. This causes increased urinary loss of alanine, serine, threonine, asparagine, glutamine, leucine, isoleucine, phenylalanine, tyrosine, tryptophan histidine glycine and citrulline.

- As well, any unabsorbed tryptophan remaining in the intestine is metabolized by intestinal bacteria to **indole acetic acid** and **indolepyruvic acid** which are subsequently excreted in urine.

Clinical Features

Hartnup disease causes:
- An intermittent photosensitive red scaly rash resembling the rash of pellagra
- Severe but reversible cerebellar ataxia
- Headache
- Muscle discomfort and
- Occasionally psychological disturbances
- Generalized neutral aminoaciduria.

Diagnosis

- Due to the variability of symptoms, unambiguous diagnosis can only be made through urine analysis. The test is based on the detection of elevated amino acids in the urine by chromatography.
- There is increased urinary excretion of **indole acetic acid** and **indolepyruvic acid** and other indole derivatives.
- Molecular genetic testing can confirm a diagnosis of Hartnup disease in some cases. Molecular genetic testing can detect genetic alterations in the *SLC19A6* gene known to cause the disorder, but usually is not necessary to obtain a diagnosis.

Therapy

Oral nicotinic acid supplementation will permit adequate synthesis of NAD$^+$ in patients with Hartnup disease. This corrects pellagra-like symptoms of the disorder. The aminoaciduria remains unaltered.

Metabolism of Sulfur-containing Amino Acids

The three sulfur-containing amino acids are **cystine**, **cysteine**, and **methionine**. Among these methionine is an essential amino acid whereas cysteine and cystine are nonessential amino acids. Cysteine and cystine are synthesized from two amino acids, **methionine**, which is nutritionally essential and **serine** is nonessential. **Cystine** and **cysteine** are readily interconvertible in the body.

Metabolism of Methionine

Methionine is metabolized by:
- Transfer of methyl group of methionine by **transmethylation** reactions.
- Conversion of demethylated portion of the methionine to **cysteine** and **cystine**.

Transfer of Methyl Group of Methionine by Transmethylation Reactions

Transfer of methyl group ($-CH_3$) from methionine to an acceptor molecule is termed as **transmethylation**. The methyl group of methionine becomes available for transmethylation only in an active form of methionine, **S-adenosylmethionine (SAM)**.
- ATP and an enzyme **methionine adenosyltransferase** are required for the activation of methionine to S-adenosylmethionine (**Figure 12.36**).
- The methyl group of active methionine (SAM) is very reactive and can be enzymatically transferred in the synthesis of many compounds. Some important transmethylation reactions are given below:
  - Norepinephrine to epinephrine
  - Phosphatidylethanolamine to phosphatidylcholine
  - Gunaidoacetoacetate to creatine
  - Ethanolamine to choline
  - Acetylserotonin to melatonin
  - Nucleotides to methylated nucleotides.

Conversion of Demethylated Portion of the Methionine to Cysteine and Cystine

- Removal of the methyl group from SAM forms **S-adenosyl homocysteine**. Hydrolytic cleavage of S-adenosyl homocysteine occurs to **homocysteine** and **adenosine**.

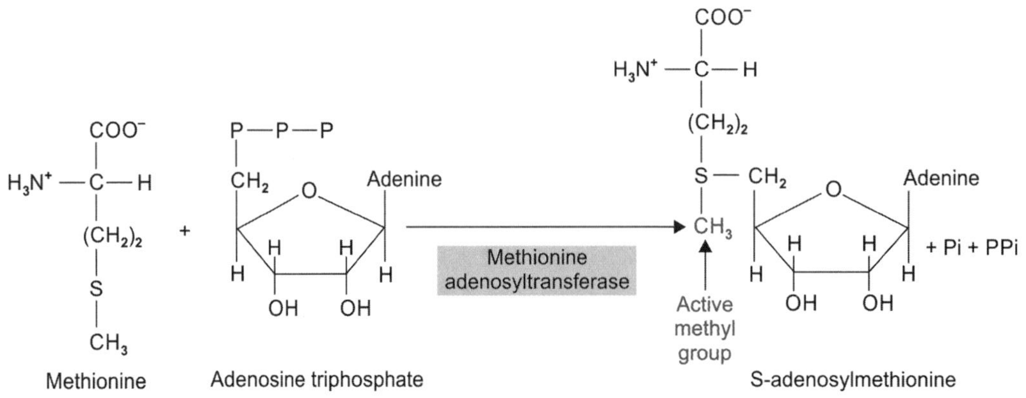

Figure 12.36: Formation of active methionine.

- Homocysteine then condenses with serine forming **cystathionine** by the enzyme cystathionine synthase.
- Hydrolytic cleavage of cystathionine forms **homoserine** plus **cysteine** by the enzyme cystathionine lyase, which requires cofactor pyridoxal phosphate (PLP). The cysteine then may be oxidized to cystine. Next homoserine is converted to α-ketobutyrate by homoserine deaminase. Then α-ketobutyrate undergoes oxidative decarboxylation to form propionyl-CoA which is catabolized by way of methylmalonyl-CoA and succinyl-CoA **(Figure 12.37)**.

> It should be noted that cysteine is synthesized from two amino acids, **methionine** and **serine**. Methionine furnishes the sulfur atom and serine furnishes the carbon skeleton.

Synthesis of Methionine from Homocysteine

Methionine can be regenerated by re-methylation of homocysteine, which requires both **tetrahydrofolate (THF)** and **vitamin B$_{12}$**. In this reaction, methyl group of **N^5-methyl THF** is transferred to vitamin B$_{12}$ forming **methyl B$_{12}$**. Then methyl B$_{12}$ transfers the methyl group to homocysteine which is converted to methionine. It should be noted that there is no net synthesis of methionine because homocysteine which serves as precursor for methionine has to be derived from methionine **(Figure 12.37)**.

Metabolism of Cysteine and Cystine

Synthesis of Cysteine and Cystine

Cysteine is a nutritionally nonessential, glucogenic amino acid. As discussed above, it is synthesized from two amino acids, methionine, which is nutritionally essential and serine, which is not. Methionine furnishes sulfur atom and serine furnishes the carbon skeleton **(Figure 12.37)**. Cystine is formed by oxidation of cysteine.

Catabolism of Cystine and Cysteine

The major catabolic fate of cystine is conversion of cystine to cysteine **(Figure 12.38)** a reaction catalyzed by **cystine reductase**. Catabolism of cystine then occurs simultaneously with that of cysteine. Cysteine can be catabolized by trans-amination pathway as follows:

- Cystine undergoes transamination reaction in the presence of α-ketoglutarate by the enzyme *cysteine transaminase* to form β-mercaptopyruvate and glutamate.
- β-mercaptopyruvate then undergoes desulfuration with **sulfur transferase** to form pyruvate and H$_2$S, which is converted to sulfide by reduced glutathione.
- The sulfide formed in the reaction is converted to sulfite and then to sulfate (SO$_4^{--}$).
- The sulfate thus formed is either excreted in the urine or converted to active sulfate, **phosphoadenosyl phosphosulfate (PAPS)** by using ATP.
- PAPS is used as a source of sulfur in the synthesis of **polysaccharides**, **glycolipids** and **sulpholipids** or used for **detoxification** reactions **(Figure 12.39)**.

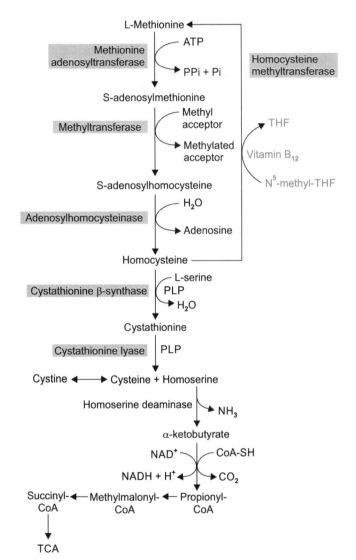

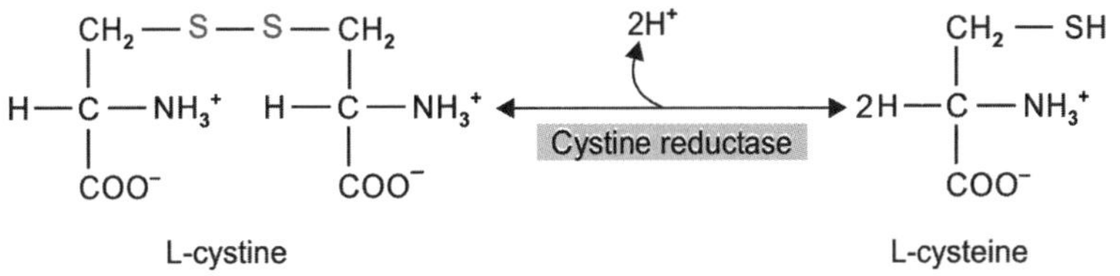

Figure 12.37: Catabolic pathway of methionine or biosynthetic pathway of cysteine.
(THF: Tetrahydrofolate)

Figure 12.38: Conversion of cystine to cysteine.

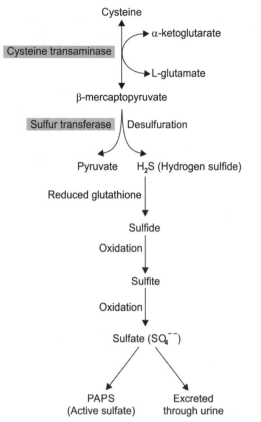

Figure 12.39: Transamination pathway for the catabolism of cysteine.
(PAPS = Phosphoadenosyl phosphosulfate)

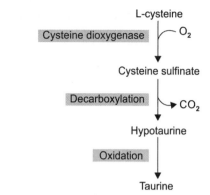

Figure 12.40: Formation of taurine from cysteine.

Importance of Cysteine

- The conversion of cysteine to pyruvate accounts for glucogenic nature and involved in formation of glucose.
- Cysteine is most important dietary source of sulfur.
- **Taurine** (an inhibitory neurotransmitter) is derived from cysteine **(Figure 12.40)**. Taurine conjugates with cholic acid (bile acid) to form taurocholic acid.
- Besides taurine, other physiologically important sulfur-containing compounds such as **insulin**, **coenzyme-A**, **glutathione** and **vasopressin** are derived from cysteine.
- It is also involved in detoxification mechanisms.

Metabolic Disorders of Sulfur-containing Amino Acids

Cystinuria (Cystinlysinuria)

Cystinuria is the most common inborn error of amino acid transport. Cystinuria is an inherited disorder in which kidney tubules fail to reabsorb the amino acids **cystine**, **ornithine**, **arginine** and **lysine** (the mnemonic is **COAL**). This is characterized by massive urinary excretion of cystine, ornithine, arginine and lysine.

Cause
Normally, these amino acids are filtered by the glomerulus and reabsorbed in the proximal renal tubule by specific

carrier proteins. In cystinuria defect in the carrier proteins leads to the excretion of all these four amino acids.

Clinical Features
Since cystine is the least soluble it's over excretion often leads to precipitation and formation of **cystine calculi** (stones) in the renal tubules and leads to obstruction, infection and renal insufficiency in cystinuric patient. The amino acids **lysine**, **arginine**, and **ornithine** are also excreted in massive amounts in this disorder. However, these amino acids dissolve more readily in the urine (more soluble) and are not associated with any particular symptoms.

The initial symptom of cystinuria is usually sharp pain in the lower back or side of the abdomen (renal colic). Other symptoms may include blood in the urine (hematuria), obstruction of the urinary tract (ureters), and/or infections of the urinary tract. Frequent recurrences ultimately may lead to kidney damage.

Treatment
Treatment involves ingestion of large amounts of water, which increases cystine solubility through maintenance of alkaline urine.

Cystinosis (Cystine Storage Disease)

Cystinosis is a rare but serious lysosomal disorder.

Cause
It is caused by a defective carrier that transports cystine across the lysosomal membrane from lysosomal vesicles to the cytosol.

Clinical Features
Cystine accumulates in the lysosomes in many tissues and forms crystals impairing their function. Cystinosis is usually accompanied by a generalized aminoaciduria. Patients usually die within 10 years due to acute renal failure.

Homocystinuria

Homocystinurias are a group of disorder of methionine metabolism. It is characterized by high blood and urinary levels of **homocysteine** and **methionine**. Four metabolic

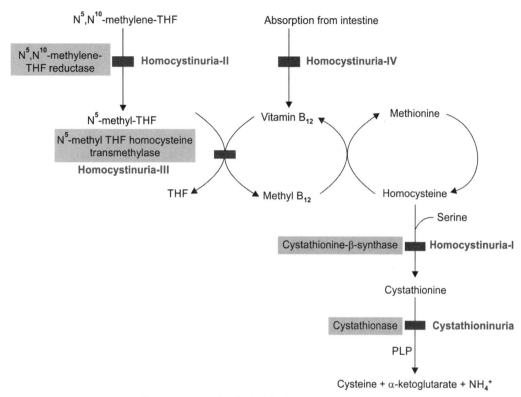

Figure 12.41: Metabolic blocks in homocystinuria.

TABLE 12.5: Different types of homocystinuria with their defects.

Types	Defects
Homocystinuria-I	Cystathionine-β-synthase
Homocystinuria-II	Synthesis of N^5-methyl tetrahydrofolate
Homocystinuria-III	Deficiency of methyl B_{12}
Homocystinuria-IV	Defective intestinal absorption of vitamin B_{12}

defects cause four types of homocystinuria **(Figure 12.41 and Table 12.5)**.

Homocystinuria type-I: It is due to defect in the enzyme **cystathionine synthase**, which converts homocysteine to cystathionine **(Figure 12.41)**. As a result, homocysteine accumulates in blood and appears in urine.

● The accumulation of homocysteine causes skeletal abnormalities, ectopia lentis (dislocation of the lenses in the eyes), osteoporosis, mental retardation and thrombosis. Thrombosis may result in myocardial infarction, pulmonary embolism or stroke.

● A deficiency of cystathionine synthase is the most common cause of homocystinuria. Other types of homocystinuria are due to defects in the remethylation of homocysteine to form methionine.

Homocystinuria type-II and III: In type-II and III, there is deficiency in synthesis of N^5-**methyltetrahydrofolate** and **methyl B_{12}** respectively. Both N^5-methyl THF and methyl B_{12} are required for the remethylation of homocysteine to form methionine.

Homocystinuria type-IV: It is due to defective intestinal absorption of vitamin B_{12}.

Diagnosis

Homocystinuria is due to **cystathionine beta-synthase (CBS)** deficiency.

● Tests are performed to determine the levels of the enzyme cystathionine beta-synthase in certain cells or tissues of the body.

● A diagnosis may be confirmed by a variety of specialized tests. Tests that can detect elevated levels of homocystine, methionine, or homocysteine in the plasma or urine may be used to help confirm a diagnosis of homocystinuria.

● Homocystinuria due to CBS deficiency may also be diagnosed through newborn screening programs. Newborn screening for homocystinuria due to CBS deficiency specifically tests for methionine levels.

Treatment

● The biochemical defect in cystathionine β synthase can be corrected in some cases by providing pyridoxine (vitamin B_6). Pyridoxine is needed to activate the enzyme cystathionine β synthase.

● Those with complete enzyme deficiency should be treated with a diet low in methionine and supplemented with cysteine.

● Vitamin B_{12} may be given in instances of vitamin B_{12} deficiency.

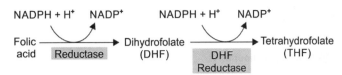

Figure 12.42: Formation of tetrahydrofolate from folic acid.

One-carbon Metabolism

Groups, containing single carbon atoms are called one-carbon groups. One-carbon groups are formed from several amino acids like, **serine**, **glycine**, **histidine** and **tryptophan** during their metabolism. One-carbon groups formed during this amino acid metabolism are:

- Methyl (CH_3)
- Methylene (CH_2)
- Methenyl (CH)
- Formyl (CHO)
- Formimino $(CH=NH)$

These one-carbon groups are transferred through **tetrahydrofolate (THF)**. Tetrahydrofolate is formed from vitamin folic acid **(Figure 12.42)**. One-carbon groups carried by THF are attached either to nitrogen N^5 or N^{10} or to both N^5 and N^{10} **(Figure 12.43)**. The different one-carbon derivatives of THF are as follows:

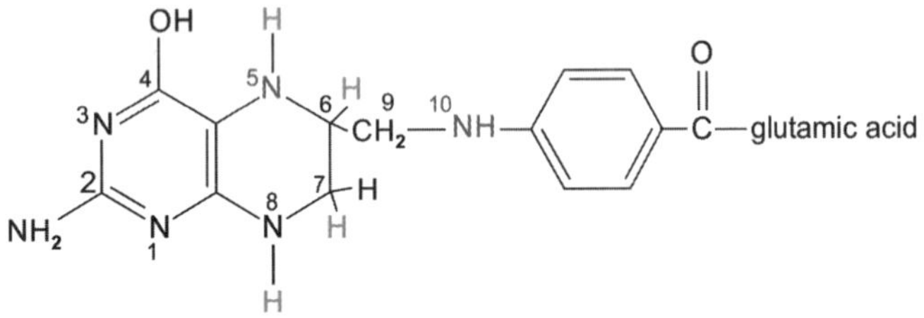

Figure 12.43: Structure of tetrahydrofolate.

- N^5-methyl THF
- N^5, N^{10}-methylene THF
- N^5, N^{10}-methenyl THF
- N^5-formyl-THF
- N^5-formimino-THF.

These different derivatives of THF are interconvertible. **Figure 12.44** shows sources of one-carbon groups and their utilization.

> It should be noted that CO_2 is also a one-carbon group, is carried by vitamin biotin. However, biotin is not considered as a member of one-carbon pool.

Sources of One-carbon Groups

- **Formate** produced in the degradation of **glycine** and **tryptophan** reacts with THF to form N^{10}-**formyl TH** **(Figure 12.44)**.
- Histidine during its degradation produces **formimino glutamate (FIGLU)**, which reacts with THF forming N^5-**formimino-THF** which on releasing ammonia generates N^5, N^{10}-**methenyl THF**.
- Serine is the major one-carbon source. When serine is converted to glycine N^5, N^{10}-**methylene THF** is formed.
- Methyl groups of choline and betaine reacts with THF to form N^5-**methyl THF**.
- Active form of methionine, **S-adenosylmethionine (SAM)** carries methyl groups and acts as a methyl group donor.

Utilization of One-carbon Groups

One-carbon groups carried by THF are used for the synthesis of other biologically important compounds, e.g., **(Figure 12.44)**.

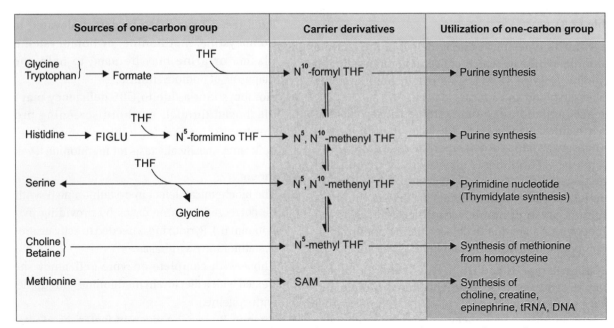

Figure 12.44: One-carbon metabolism showing source of carrier derivative and recipients of one-carbon groups.

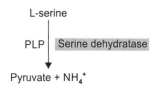

L-serine

PLP | Serine dehydratase

Pyruvate + NH$_4^+$

Figure 12.45: Degradation of serine.

- Synthesis of serine from glycine.
- Synthesis of pyrimidine nucleotide thymidylate (TMP).
- Synthesis of purine bases.
- Synthesis of methionine from homocysteine.
- Methyl group carried by SAM is used for the synthesis of choline, creatine, epinephrine, carnitine, t-RNA, DNA, etc.

Importance of One-carbon Group Metabolism

One-carbon groups at different levels of oxidation are transferred and made available by way of the tetrahydrofolate and vitamin B$_{12}$ coenzymes for use in a wide variety of vital anabolic processes.

Metabolism of Hydroxy Group-containing Amino Acids

Serine, threonine and **tyrosine** are the hydroxy group containing amino acids. Tyrosine is discussed already under aromatic amino acids.

Metabolism of Serine

Serine is a nonessential amino acid.

Synthesis of Serine

Serine is synthesized from glycine by transfer of hydroxymethyl group from N^{5}N^{10}-methylene THF (*see* **Figure 12.20**).

Catabolism of Serine

- In humans, serine is catabolized via glycine and N^5,N^{10}-methylene tetrahydrofolate. The reaction is catalyzed by **serine hydroxy methyl transferase (Figure 12.20)**. Further catabolism of serine merges with that of glycine.
- In many mammals, serine is degraded by serine dehydratase, an enzyme that requires pyridoxal phosphate (PLP) and produces NH$^+$ and pyruvate **(Figure 12.45)**. This pathway appears to be a minor one in humans.

Importance of Serine

- Serine is a constituent of phospholipid, **phosphatidylserine**, found in brain.
- After decarboxylation serine gives rise to **ethanolamine** which is the constituent of another phospholipid, **phosphatidylethanolamine** (cephalin).
- Serine also takes part in the synthesis of cysteine **(Figure 12.37)**.

Metabolism of Threonine

Threonine is an essential and **glucogenic amino acid**.

Catabolism of Threonine

Threonine is degraded by two pathways:
1. Threonine is cleaved to acetaldehyde and glycine by threonine aldolase. Acetaldehyde is then oxidized to acetate, which then is converted to acetyl-CoA **(Figures 12.46A and B)**.
2. Threonine dehydratase produces α-ketobutyrate. Subsequently, α-ketobutyrate is oxidatively decarboxylated to yield propionyl-CoA, which is then carboxylated to methylmalonyl-CoA, which, in turn, is

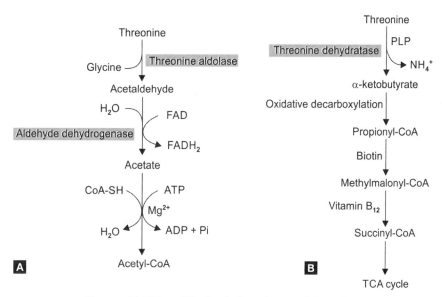

Figures 12.46A and B: Catabolic pathways of threonine.

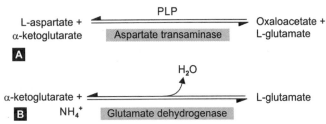

Figures 12.47A and B: Synthesis and degradation of L-glutamate.

isomerized to succinyl-CoA. Succinyl-CoA enters the Kreb's cycle, and gives rise to pyruvate **(Figure 12.46B)**. Threonine is thus glucogenic amino acid.

Metabolism of Acidic Amino Acids

Metabolism of Glutamic Acid

Glutamic acid is a **nonessential**, **glucogenic** amino acid.

Synthesis of Glutamic Acid

It is synthesized from α-ketoglutarate an intermediate of citric acid cycle by:
- Transamination **(Figure 12.47A)**.
- By reductive amination of a ketoglutarate catalyzed by glutamate dehydrogenase **(Figure 12.47B)**.

Catabolism of Glutamic Acid

When glutamate is degraded, it is converted back to α-ketoglutarate either by transamination or by glutamate dehydrogenase reaction **(Figures 12.47A and B)**.

Importance of Glutamic Acid

- A number of other amino acids like glutamine, proline and arginine are derived from glutamate.
- Glutamate involved in the synthesis of glutathione, (α-glutamyl-cysteinyl glycine) which is involved in the reduction of H_2O_2 to H_2O and transport of amino acids into cells of kidney and intestine.
- Glutamate is decarboxylated at C-1 to form amine **gamma-aminobutyric acid (GABA)**, which serves as a **neurotransmitter.**

Metabolism of Glutamine

Glutamine is an amide of glutamate.

Synthesis and Degradation of Glutamine

It is produced from glutamate by glutamine synthetase, which adds NH^+ to the carboxyl group of the side chain, forming an amide. Glutamine is reconverted to glutamate by a different enzyme, glutaminase, which is particularly important in the kidney **(Figure 12.48)**.

Importance of Glutamine

- **Glutamine is the major transport form of ammonia.**

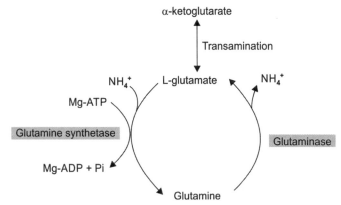

Figure 12.48: Synthesis and degradation of glutamine.

- Glutamine is the principal source of ammonia in the kidney and plays an important role in the maintenance of acid-base balance.
- Glutamine participates in a number of biosynthetic reactions, usually by supplying amino or ammonia nitrogen, e.g., in the formation of arginine, carbamoyl phosphate, purines, etc.

Metabolism of Aspartic Acid

Aspartic acid is a nonessential, glucogenic amino acid.

Synthesis and Degradation of Aspartic Acid

Aspartate is synthesized from Krebs citric acid cycle intermediate, oxaloacetate by transamination reaction. Because the transamination reaction is readily reversible, aspartate can be converted to oxaloacetate, an intermediate of citric acid cycle **(Figure 12.47A)**.

Importance of Aspartic Acid

- In the urea cycle, aspartate reacts with citrulline to form argininosuccinate, which is cleaved, forming an essential amino acid arginine and fumarate.
- Aspartate reacts with inosine monophosphate (IMP) to form AMP.

Metabolism of Asparagine

Asparagine is an amide of aspartate.

Synthesis and Degradation of Asparagine

Asparagine is formed from aspartate by a reaction in which glutamine provides the nitrogen for formation of the amide group. Hydrolytic release of the amide nitrogen of asparagine as ammonia and aspartate is catalyzed by **asparaginase (Figure 12.49)**.

Certain types of tumor cells, particularly leukemic cells, require asparagine. Therefore, asparaginase has been used as an antitumor agent. It acts by converting asparagine to aspartate, decreasing the amount of asparagine available for tumor cell growth.

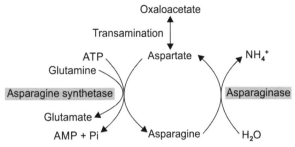

Figure 12.49: Synthesis and degradation of aspartate and asparagine.

Metabolism of Imino Acid

Metabolism of Proline

Proline is a nonessential, glucogenic amino acid.

Synthesis of Proline

Proline is formed from glutamate by reversal of the reactions of proline catabolism (**Figure 12.50**).

Glutamate is first phosphorylated and then converted to glutamate γ-semialdehyde by reduction.

This semialdehyde spontaneously cyclizes and reduction of this cyclic compound yields proline.

Degradation of Proline

Proline rather than undergoing direct transamination is oxidized to dehydroproline, which adds water, forming glutamate γ-semialdehyde. This is further oxidized to glutamate and transaminated to α-ketoglutarate (**Figure 12.51**).

Importance of Proline

- Proline serves as a precursor of hydroxyproline. Hydroxyproline is an important constituent of **collagen** which stabilizes the collagen triple helix. Collagen contains about one-third glycine and one-third proline plus hydroxyproline.
- Proline and ornithine are readily interconverted in the body. Thus, proline may yield ornithine for urea synthesis or ornithine may be broken down via proline (**Figure 12.50**).

Metabolic Disorders of Proline

Two autosomal recessive hyperprolinemias have been reported. Mental retardation occurs in half of the known cases but neither type is life-threatening. Two types of hyperprolinemia, called type-I and type-II, resulting in increase in blood and urine levels of proline are as follows:

Hyperprolinemia type-I: The metabolic block in type-I is at proline dehydrogenase (**Figure 12.51**). There is no associated impairment of hydroxyproline catabolism.

Hyperprolinemia type-II: The metabolic block occurs at glutamate γ-semialdehyde dehydrogenase (**Figure 12.51**). Since, the same dehydrogenase functions in hydroxypro-

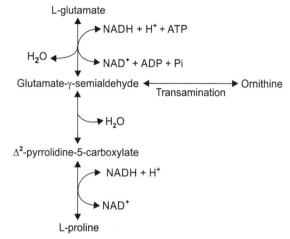

Figure 12.50: Synthesis of proline from glutamate.

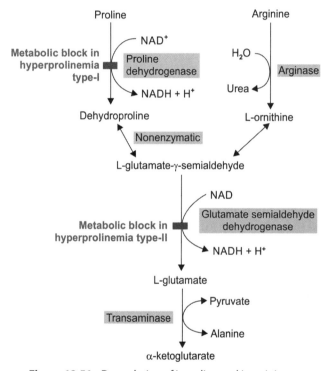

Figure 12.51: Degradation of L-proline and L-arginine to α-ketoglutarate.

line catabolism, both proline and hydroxyproline catabolism are affected. The urine contains the hydroxyproline catabolites.

Metabolism of Basic Amino Acids

Metabolism of Arginine

Arginine is considered to be a semiessential amino acid. It can be synthesized in the body but not in quantities sufficient to permit normal growth. It is thus an amino acid, which is essential for growth but not for maintenance.

Synthesis and Degradation of Arginine

- Arginine is synthesized from glutamate. Glutamate is reduced to glutamate-γ-semialdehyde, which is then

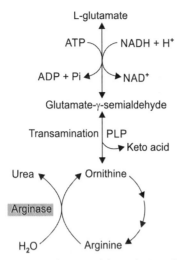

Figure 12.52: Synthesis and degradation of arginine.

transaminated to yield ornithine, an intermediate of urea cycle. The reactions of the urea cycle convert ornithine to arginine.

- Arginine is cleaved by arginase to form urea and ornithine. If ornithine is present in amounts in excess of those required for the urea cycle, it is transaminated to glutamate semialdehyde which is reduced to glutamate **(Figure 12.52)**.

Importance of Arginine

- Arginine takes part in the formation of urea.
- Arginine is involved in the synthesis of creatine, an important constituent of muscle. In the formation of creatine, the guanidinium group of arginine is transferred to glycine.
- Nitric oxide is synthesized from arginine **(Figure 12.53)**. Nitric oxide is a biological messenger in a variety of physiological responses including vasodilation, neurotransmission and the ability to kill tumor cells and parasites.

Metabolism of Histidine

Histidine like arginine is a nutritionally semiessential amino acid and is glucogenic.

Degradation of Histidine

Degradation of histidine occurs mainly in the liver. The major pathway and principal intermediates are shown in **Figure 12.54**

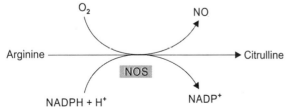

Figure 12.53: Synthesis of nitric oxide.
(NOS: nitric oxide synthase; NO: nitric oxide)

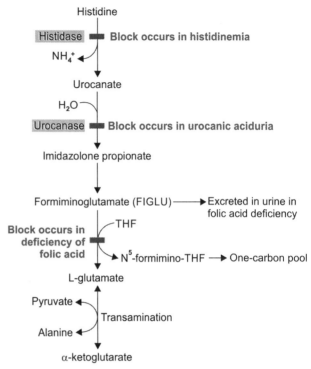

Figure 12.54: Degradation of histidine.

- In a series of steps, histidine is converted to formimino-glutamate (FIGLU).
- The subsequent reactions transfer one-carbon group, i.e., formimino group of FIGLU to the tetrahydrofolate (THF) to form N^5-formimino-THF leaving L-glutamate.
- N^5-formimino-THF may be used in one-carbon metabolism **(Figure 12.44)**.

In folic acid deficiency, transfer of formimino group of FIGLU to THF reaction is partially or totally blocked, and FIGLU is excreted in the urine. Excretion of FIGLU, therefore, provides a diagnostic test for folic acid deficiency.

Importance of Histidine

Histidine has several other important functions in addition to the general role of amino acids in tissue protein formation as follows:

- Upon decarboxylation, it forms **histamine**, which reduces blood pressure, is a vasodilator and increases the secretion of gastric juice. Allergic reactions stimulate an excessive liberation of histamine.
- Histidine is involved in the formation of biologically important peptides like **carnosine** and **anserine** present in muscle, **ergothioneine** present in erythrocytes, liver and brain.

Metabolic Disorders of Histidine

Two benign hereditary disorders of histidine catabolism are **(Figure 12.54)**:

1. **Histidinemia:** Histidinemia is characterized by elevated blood and urine histidine. The defective enzyme is

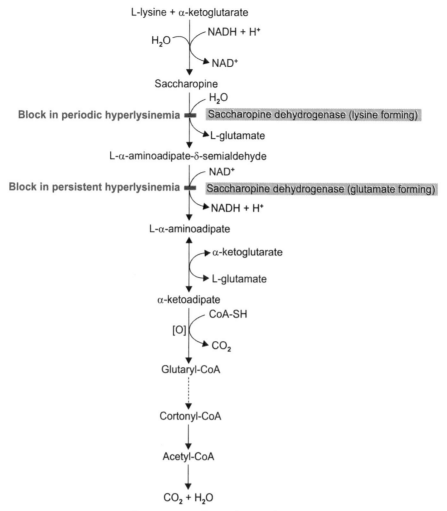

L-lysine + α-ketoglutarate

H₂O — NADH + H⁺

NAD⁺

Saccharopine

H₂O

Block in periodic hyperlysinemia ━ Saccharopine dehydrogenase (lysine forming)

L-glutamate

L-α-aminoadipate-δ-semialdehyde

NAD⁺

Block in persistent hyperlysinemia ━ Saccharopine dehydrogenase (glutamate forming)

NADH + H⁺

L-α-aminoadipate

α-ketoglutarate

L-glutamate

α-ketoadipate

CoA-SH

[O]

CO_2

Glutaryl-CoA

Cortonyl-CoA

Acetyl-CoA

CO_2 + H_2O

Figure 12.55: Degradation of L-lysine.

histidase, resulting in impaired conversion of histidine to urocanate.

2. **Urocanic aciduria:** It is characterized by elevated excretion of urocanate; it results from a defective urocanase enzyme.

Metabolism of Lysine

Lysine is a nutritionally essential amino acid. Lysine is both glucogenic and ketogenic amino acid. It contains two amino groups, neither of which can undergo direct transamination. Lysine is involved in the synthesis of carnitine, which serves to shuttle fatty acyl groups across mitochondrial membrane.

Catabolism of Lysine

Lysine is degraded by a complex pathway in which saccharopine, α-ketoadipate and crotonyl-CoA are intermediates **(Figure 12.55)**. Ultimately, lysine generates acetyl-CoA.

Metabolic Disorders of Lysine

Two inherited disorders of lysine metabolism have been reported:

1. Periodic hyperlysinemia
2. Persistent hyperlysinemia.

- **Periodic hyperlysinemia:** It is characterized by hyperammonemia and elevated plasma lysine. Elevated liver lysine levels competitively inhibit liver arginase, causing hyperammonemia and show the clinical symptoms of ammonia intoxication. The biochemical cause of hyperlysinemia is uncertain.

- **Persistent hyperlysinemia:** Persistent hyperlysinemia is believed to be inherited as an autosomal recessive trait. In addition to impaired conversion of lysine and α-ketoglutarate to saccharopine, some patients cannot cleave saccharopine. Persistent hyperlysinemia is not associated with hyperammonemia. Some patients are mentally retarded.

BIOGENIC AMINES AND POLYAMINES

Biogenic Amines

Decarboxylation of amino acids results in the formation of **amines**. These amines are called **biogenic amines**. They

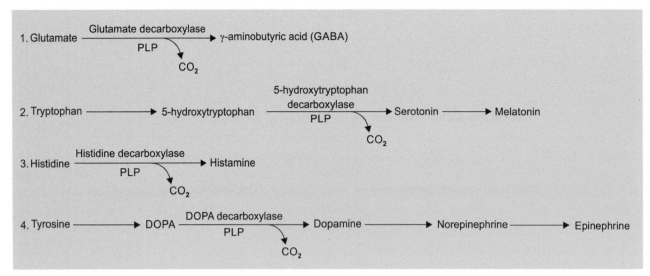

Figure 12.56: Synthesis of biogenic amines by PLP-dependent decarboxylation of amino acids.

have diverse biological function. Decarboxylation reactions are catalyzed by **PLP-dependent decarboxylases**. The important biogenic amines formed by decarboxylation of amino acids are given below **(Figure 12.56)**.

- **γ-aminobutyric acid (GABA):** It is an inhibitory neurotransmitter derived from glutamate on decarboxylation. In vitamin B$_6$ deficiency, under production of GABA leads to convulsions (epileptic seizures) in infants and children.
- **Serotonin and melatonin:** These are produced from tryptophan. Serotonin is a neurotransmitter and stimulates the cerebral activity. Melatonin is a sleep-inducing substance and is involved in regulation of circadian rhythm of body.
- **Histamine:** It is produced by decarboxylation of histidine. It is a vasodilator and lowers blood pressure. It is involved in allergic reactions.
- **Catecholamines (dopamine, norepinephrine and epinephrine):** Synthesis of catecholamines from tyrosine requires PLP-dependent DOPA decarboxylase. Catecholamines are neurotransmitters and involved in metabolic and nervous regulation. Some of the most important biogenic amines and their functions are given in **Table 12.6**.

Polyamines

Biological amines made up of multiple amino acids called polyamines, e.g., putrescine, spermidine, spermine. Polyamines are positively charged at physiological pH and associate with negatively-charged nuclear DNA. These are present in high concentration in semen. The concentration of polyamines in brain is about 2 mM.

Functions of Polyamines

- Polyamines are involved in regulation of **transcription** and **translation**.

TABLE 12.6: Some important biogenic amines and their function.

Amines	Amino acid precursors	Functions
Dopamine	Tyrosine	Neurotransmitter
Norepinephrine	Tyrosine	Neurotransmitter
Epinephrine	Tyrosine	Hormone
Tyramine	Tyrosine	Vasoconstrictor
Serotonin	Tryptophan	Vasoconstrictor
Melatonin	Tryptophan	Vasoconstrictor
GABA	Glutamate	Neurotransmitter
Histamine	Histidine	Vasodilator
Taurine	Cysteine	Neurotransmitter
Spermine	Ornithine and methionine	Growth factor, regulator of transcription and translation

- They act as a growth factor and function in cell proliferation and growth.
- Polyamines are involved in stabilization of intact cells, subcellular organelles and membranes.

Biosynthesis of Polyamines

- **Putrescine**, **spermidine** and **spermine** are derived from **ornithine** and **methionine**.
- Ornithine is derived from arginine. Arginine undergoes a decarboxylation to form putrescine and carbon dioxide **(Figure 12.57)** by an enzyme **ornithine decarboxylase**.
- **S-Adenosylmethionine** undergoes a **decarboxylation** to form **5-adenosylmethiopropylamine**, by an enzyme S-adenosylmethionine decarboxylase.

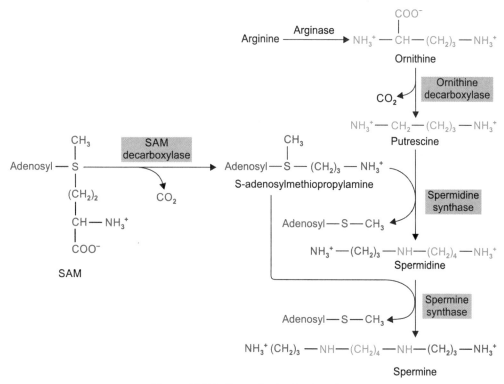

Figure 12.57: Biosynthesis of polyamines.
(SAM = S-Adenosylmethionine)

- S-Adenosylmethiopropylamine donates aminopropyl group to putrescine and then to spermidine to form spermine.
- It is presumed that the 15% of methionine which cannot be used for cysteine synthesis in minimal diets is used for polyamine synthesis.

Catabolism and Excretion of Polyamines

- The enzyme polyamine oxidase present in liver peroxisomes oxidizes spermine to spremidine and spermidine to putrescine.
- Putrescine is then oxidized by a copper-containing diamine oxidase to CO_2 and NH_3.

- Major portions of putrescine and spermidine are excreted in urine after conjugation with acetyl-CoA as acetylated derivatives.

Clinical Significance of Polyamines

- Polyamines and their derivatives have application in diagnosis and treatment of cancer.
- Their levels have been shown to increase in response to cell growth and differentiation.
- Their concentration is elevated in body fluids of cancer patients.
- Assays of urinary and blood polyamines have been used to detect cancer and to determine the success of therapy (diagnostic indicator).

ASSESSMENT QUESTIONS

▌ STRUCTURED LONG ESSAY QUESTIONS (SLEQs)

1. Describe the metabolism of tryptophan under the following headings:
   i. Catabolic pathway
   ii. Biologically important compounds derived
   iii. Metabolic disorder
2. Describe the metabolism of methionine under the following headings:

   i. Active form of methionine
   ii. Catabolic pathway
   iii. Importance of active form of methionine
   iv. Name the metabolic disorders with defective enzymes
3. Describe the metabolism of ammonia under the following headings:
   i. Formation of ammonia
   ii. Transport of ammonia
   iii. Disposal of ammonia in the form of urea with pathway

4. Describe the metabolism of phenylalanine and tyrosine under the following headings:
   i. Catabolism with pathway
   ii. Name the metabolic disorders with defective enzymes
   iii. Biologically important compounds derived
5. Describe urea cycle under the following headings:
   i. Pathway
   ii. Energy cost
   iii. Significance
   iv. Metabolic inborn errors
6. Describe the metabolism of glycine under the following headings:
   i. Synthesis
   ii. Catabolism
   iii. Metabolic importance
   iv. Name the metabolic disorders with defective enzymes
7. Describe the metabolism of branched-chain amino acids under the following headings:
   i. Catabolism
   ii. Metabolic disorders
8. Describe the metabolism of cysteine under the following headings:
   i. Synthesis
   ii. Catabolic pathway
   iii. Biologically important compounds derived
   iv. Metabolic disorder

SHORT ESSAY QUESTIONS (SEQs)

1. What is transamination reaction? Give its metabolic and clinical significance.
2. What is deamination reaction? Give its metabolic and clinical significance.
3. Write metabolic disorders of urea cycle with defective enzyme.
4. What is phenylketonuria? Give its causes, types, and clinical manifestations.
5. What is alkaptonuria? Give its causes and clinical manifestations.
6. What is homocystinuria? Give its causes, types, and clinical manifestations.
7. What is Hartnup disease? Give its causes, clinical manifestations and diagnostic tests.
8. Write biologically important compound derived from tyrosine and its importance.
9. Write biologically important compound derived from tryptophan and its importance.
10. What is maple syrup urine disease? Give its causes, clinical manifestations and diagnostic tests.
11. Give an account of the formation of specialized products from glycine.
12. Describe the digestion and absorption of proteins
13. What is biogenic amine and polyamines? Give its examples and importance
14. What is one-carbon pool? Give its importance.

SHORT ANSWER QUESTIONS (SAQs)

1. Write name of two endopeptidases with their specifications.
2. Give clinical significance of transamination reaction.
3. Write name of enzymes, which are deficient in phenylketonuria and alkaptonuria.
4. Name four proteolytic enzymes and their site of action.
5. Give four significances of urea cycle.
6. Give biologically important compound derived from tyrosine and tryptophan.
7. Write name of different types of homocystinuria with their defects.
8. Why ammonia is toxic? Justify.
9. Write name of amino acids required for formation of creatine and give the importance of creatine.
10. Active form of methionine and its function.
11. Write name of urea cycle disorders.
12. Why hyperammonemia type II (urea cycle disorders) cause orotic aciduria.
13. Write differences between CPSI and CPS II.
14. Enumerate compounds formed from plycine.
15. Write laboratory diagnosis of phenylketonuria.
16. How epinephrine is synthesized in the body?
17. What is carcinoid syndrome? Give its clinical symptoms.
18. Which enzyme is deficient in albinism? Mention two clinical features of albinism.
19. What is the role of γ-aminobutyric acid in the body? Name the amino acid from which it is derived.
20. Mention the amino acids which take part in one-carbon pool.
21. What is transmethylation reaction? Mention two transmethylation reactions.
22. Maple syrup urine disease (MSUD) is inborn error of which amino acids? Name the defective enzyme.
23. What are biogenic amines? Give four examples.
24. Write functions and products of histidine and serine.
25. Write functions and products of aspartate and asparagine.
26. Write functions and products of glutamate and glutamine.

CASE VIGNETTE-BASED QUESTIONS (CVBQs)

Case Study

1. **A 3-year-old boy was admitted to hospital with the symptoms of pellagra, accompanied by mental retardation and excessive excretion of neutral amino acids. He was diagnosed as having Hartnup disease.**
   Questions
   a. What is the cause of Hartnup disease?
   b. Why does it show mental retardation and pellagra-like symptoms?
   c. How will you treat pellagra like symptoms?
   d. Can aminoaciduria be treated?

2. **A 5-month-old female infant was admitted to hospital with a complaint of vomiting and a failure to gain weight. The mother also reported that the child would**

oscillate between periods of irritability and lethargy, biochemical investigations of the patient indicated markedly increased concentration of plasma ammonia (550 µg/dL).

Questions

a. Name the probable disorder.
b. What is the cause of the disorder?
c. Name the transport form of ammonia.
d. What will be the nutritional therapy for the patient?

3. **A full term infant was observed to have a lack of pigmentation, blue eyes, white hair and confirmed as a case of albinism.**

Questions

a. Name the deficient pigment.
b. Name the enzyme responsible for the defect.
c. Write biochemical reaction catalyzed by the enzyme.
d. Name the amino acid, from which the pigment is synthesized.

4. **A 20-year-old man came to the emergency room with severe pain in his right side and back. Subsequent examination and evaluation indicated a kidney stone and increased excretion of cystine, arginine and lysine in the urine and diagnosed as a case of cystinuria.**

Questions

a. What is the cause of cystinuria?
b. Why is there formation of kidney stone?
c. How is the condition to be treated?
d. Name the biosynthetic precursor of cysteine.

5. **A 5-month-old female infant was hospitalized. A diagnosis of classic phenylketonuria (PKU) was made.**

Questions

a. Name the defective enzyme of classic phenylketonuria.
b. Name the other types of PKU with their defective enzymes.
c. What are the characteristics of PKU?
d. Name diagnostic test for PKU.

6. **A patient was diagnosed as having alkaptonuria.**

Questions

a. Outline the biochemical pathway and point out metabolic defect which leads to this condition.
b. State the changes in urine, on standing, in such patients. Why?
c. What is ochronosis?
d. What is the treatment?

7. **A 40-year-old woman presented with progressive skin pigmentation. X-ray spine shows calcification of intervertebral discs. On adding Benedict's reagent to urine, it gives greenish brown precipitate and blue-black supernatant fluid.**

Questions

a. What is the diagnosis?
b. Disorder concern with which biomolecule.
c. Why Benedict test gives greenish brown precipitate.
d. Name the defective enzyme.

MULTIPLE CHOICE QUESTIONS (MCQs)

1. **Histidine is converted to histamine by:**
   a. Transamination
   b. Decarboxylation
   c. Hydroxylation
   d. Reduction

2. **In Maple-syrup urine disease, which of the following compound is accumulated?**
   a. Homogentisate
   b. Methylmalonyl-CoA
   c. Branched-chain α-keto acids
   d. Homocysteine

3. **The methylene group, transferred to glycine in converting it to serine, comes from:**
   a. S-Adenosylmethionine
   b. Methylene-B_{12}
   c. Carboxybiotin
   d. N^5,N^{10}-methylene-THF

4. **If urine sample darkens on standing: The most likely condition is:**
   a. Phenylketonuria   b. Alkaptonuria
   c. Maple syrup disease   d. Tyrosinemia

5. **Which type of reaction is conversion of norepinephrine to epinephrine?**
   a. Transamination   b. Decarboxylation
   c. Transmethylation   d. Phosphorylation

6. **Phenylketonuria results due to the absence of the enzyme:**
   a. Phenylalanine oxidase
   b. Phenylalanine hydroxylase
   c. Phenylalanine transaminase
   d. Phenylalanine oxygenase

7. **Which of the following amino acid cannot undergo transamination?**
   a. Lysine   b. Alanine
   c. Aspartic acid   d. Glutamic acid

8. **The amino acid required for synthesis of heme is:**
   a. Glutamine   b. Glutamic acid
   c. Glycine   d. Lysine

9. **All of the following are synthesized from tyrosine, *except*:**
   a. Melanin   b. Serotonin
   c. Dopamine   d. Epinephrine

10. **The fate of ammonia in brain is:**
    a. Conversion to urea
    b. Conversion to glutamate
    c. Conversion to aspartate
    d. Remains as such

11. **Which of the following amino acid can undergo deamination by dehydration?**
    a. Threonine   b. Alanine
    c. Tryptophan   d. Glycine

12. **Transamination of oxaloacetate results in the formation of:**
    a. Aspartic acid   b. Valine
    c. Alanine   d. Serine

13. All of the following are intermediates formed by amino acid degradation, *except*:
    a. α-ketoglutarate
    b. Oxaloacetate
    c. Fumarate
    d. Citrate

14. In alkaptonuria, which of the following accumulates abnormally in the urine?
    a. Phenylalanine
    b. Acetoacetate
    c. Homogentisate
    d. Fumarate

15. The reactions of urea cycle occur in:
    a. The cytosol
    b. The mitochondria
    c. The mitochondrial matrix and the cytosol
    d. Lysosomes

16. All of the following statements are true in the transamination of amino acids, *except*:
    a. Ammonia is neither consumed nor produced
    b. Requires pyridoxal phosphate
    c. The amino group acceptor is α-keto acid
    d. All amino acids can undergo transamination

17. Tetrahydrobiopterine is used as a coenzyme in the metabolism of:
    a. Folic acid
    b. Phenylalanine
    c. Glycine
    d. Asparagine

18. Which of the following pathways occurs in the mitochondria and cytoplasm?
    a. Urea cycle
    b. TCA cycle
    c. Glycolysis
    d. Oxidative phosphorylation

19. Which of the following amino acid is involved in the synthesis of carnitine?
    a. Lysine
    b. Phenylalanine
    c. Tryptophan
    d. Threonine

20. The following enzymes are involved in digestion and absorption of protein, *except*:
    a. Trypsinogen
    b. Amylase
    c. Pepsin
    d. Chymotrypsin

21. Norepinephrine is converted to epinephrine by:
    a. Transamination
    b. Transmethylation
    c. Transcarboxylation
    d. Decarboxylation

22. Following enzymes are endopeptidase, *except*:
    a. Pepsin
    b. Trypsin
    c. Chymotrypsin
    d. Aminopeptidase

23. Which amino acid does not take part in one-carbon transfer reactions?
    a. Glycine
    b. Serine
    c. Alanine
    d. Histidine

24. Carboxypeptidase contains which of the following mineral?
    a. Fe
    b. Cu
    c. Ca
    d. Zn

25. For metabolic disorder of urea cycle which statement is not correct?
    a. Ammonia intoxication is most severe when the metabolic block occurs prior to reactions 3 of the urea cycle
    b. Clinical symptoms include mental retardation
    c. Clinical signs include hyperammonemia
    d. Glutamate provides the second nitrogen of argininosuccinate

26. Select incorrect statement of the following:
    a. Threonine contribute to biosynthesis of coenzyme A
    b. Histamine arises by decarboxylation of histidine
    c. Serotonin and melatonin are metabolites of tryptophan
    d. Glycine, arginine and methionine each contribute atoms for biosynthesis of creatine

27. In the formation of urea from ammonia all of the following are true, *except*:
    a. Ornithine transcarbamoylase catalyzes the rate limiting step
    b. Aspartate supplies one of the nitrogen found in urea.
    c. This is an energy required process
    d. Fumarate is produced

28. Following components are required for the urea formation, *except*:
    a. Ammonia
    b. α-amino group of aspartate
    c. CO_2
    d. NADPH

29. Which of the following is true for aminotransferase?
    a. Catalyze irreversible reaction
    b. Require pyridoxal phosphate as a cofactor
    c. Catalyze reaction that result in net loss of amino group in the form of ammonia
    d. Usually require glutamine as one of the reacting pair

30. Which of the following statements are true for the reaction catalyzed by glutamate dehydrogenase? *Except*:
    a. It catalyzes oxidative deamination
    b. Requires NADH or NADPH
    c. Net removal of α-amino group of amino acid to ammonia
    d. Is an irreversible reaction

31. The number of ATP required for urea synthesis is:
    a. 0
    b. 1
    c. 2
    d. 4

32. A compound that link citric acid cycle and urea cycle is:
    a. Malate
    b. Citrate
    c. Succinate
    d. Fumarate

33. The two nitrogen atoms in urea are contributed by:
    a. Ammonia and glutamate
    b. Glutamine and glutamate
    c. Ammonia and aspartate
    d. Ammonia and alanine

34. A coenzyme required for the synthesis of glycine from serine is:
    a. ATP
    b. Pyridoxal phosphate
    c. TPP
    d. NAD

35. Cysteine is synthesized from methionine and
    a. Serine
    b. Homoserine
    c. Homocysteine
    d. Threonine

36. Methionine is synthesized in human body from:
    a. Cysteine and homoserine
    b. Homocysteine and serine
    c. Cysteine and serine
    d. None of these

37. Free ammonia is released during:
    a. Oxidative deamination of glutamate
    b. Catabolism of purines
    c. Catabolism of pyrimidines
    d. All of these

38. Ammonia is transported from muscles to liver mainly in the form of:
    a. Free ammonia
    b. Glutamine
    c. Asparagine
    c. Alanine

39. Maple syrup urine disease is an inborn error of metabolism of:
    a. Sulfur-containing amino acids
    b. Aromatic amino acids
    c. Branched-chain amino acids
    d. Dicarboxylic amino acids

40. FIGLU is an intermediate product of:
    a. Histidine
    b. Arginine
    c. Cystine
    d. Methionine

41. Normal range of serum urea is:
    a. 0.6–1.5 mg/dL
    b. 9–11 mg/dL
    c. 20–40 mg/dL
    d. 60–100 mg/dL

42. The symptom of ammonia intoxication includes:
    a. Blurring of vision
    b. Constipation
    c. Skin lesion
    d. Diarrhea

43. The milk protein in the stomach of the infants is digested by:
    a. Pepsin
    b. Trypsin
    c. Chymotrypsin
    d. Rennin

44. Rennin acts on casein of milk in infants in presence of:
    a. Mg^{++}
    b. Zn^{++}
    c. Co^{++}
    d. Ca^{++}

45. Neonatal tyrosinemia improves on administration of:
    a. Thiamine
    b. Riboflavin
    c. Pyridoxine
    d. Ascorbic acid

46. Absence of phenylalanine hydroxylase causes:
    a. Neonatal tyrosinemia
    b. Classic phenylketonuria
    c. Primary hyperoxaluria
    d. Albinism

47. Richner-Hanhart syndrome is due to defect in:
    a. Tyrosinase
    b. Phenylalanine hydroxylase
    c. Hepatic tyrosine transaminase
    d. Fumaryloacetoacetate hydrolase

48. Tyrosinosis is due to defect in the enzyme:
    a. Fumarylacetoacetate hydrolase
    b. P-hydroxyphenylpyruvate hydroxylase
    c. Tyrosine transaminase
    d. Tyrosine hydroxylase

49. Cabbage odor/rancid butter smell is a feature seen usually in:
    a. Phenylketonuria
    b. Tyrosinemia
    c. Isovaleric academia
    d. Multiple carboxylase deficiency

50. Increased urinary indole acetic acid is diagnostic of:
    a. Maple syrup urine disease
    b. Hartnup disease
    c. Homocystinuria
    d. Phenylketonuria

51. An inborn error, maple syrup urine disease is due to deficiency of the enzyme:
    a. Glycinase
    b. Phenylalanine hydroxylase
    c. Fumarylacetoacetate hydrolase
    d. α-ketoacid dehydrogenase

52. Alkaptonuria occurs due to deficiency of the enzyme:
    a. Maleylacetoacetate isomerase
    b. Homogentisate oxidase
    c. P-hydroxyphenylpyruvate hydroxylase
    d. Fumarylacetoacetate hydrolase

53. Ochronosis occurs in:
    a. Tyrosinemia
    b. Tyrosinosis
    c. Alkaptonuria
    d. Richner-Hanhart syndrome

54. Hormone synthesized from tyrosine is:
    a. Calcitriol
    b. Calcitonin
    c. Thyroxine
    d. Cortisol

55. The amino acid producing (major source of) ammonia in kidney is:
    a. Glutamine
    b. Alanine
    c. Aspartate
    d. Glutamate

56. Maple syrup urine disease is due to deficiency of?
    a. Decarboxylation
    b. Dehydroxylation
    c. Transamination
    d. Deamination

57. Transfer of an amino group from an amino acid to an alpha keto acid is done by?
    a. Transaminases
    b. Amnases
    c. Transketolase
    d. Decarboxylase

58. The amino acid which serves as a carrier of ammonia from skeletal muscle to liver is:
    a. Alanine
    b. Methionine
    c. Arginine
    d. Glycine

59. Which end product of citric acid cycle is used in detoxification of ammonia in brain:
    a. Oxaloacetate
    b. Alpha ketoglutarate
    c. Succinate
    d. Citrate

60. Urea is end product of:
    a. Amino acid-nitrogen metabolism
    b. HMP pathway
    c. Fatty acid-oxidation
    d. Glycogenolysis

61. Amino acids secreted in cystinuria are all, *except*:
    - a. Ornithine
    - b. Histidine
    - c. Arginine
    - d. Lysine

62. Tryptophan is a precursor for synthesis of which of the following:
    - a. Vitamin B_3 (niacin)
    - b. Serotonin
    - b. Melatonin
    - d. All of the above

63. Tryptophan acts as a precursor for the synthesis which vitamin?
    - a. Vitamin K
    - b. Vitamin B_{12}
    - c. Vitamin D
    - d. Vitamin B_3

64. Serotonin is synthesized in which cell?
    - a. Liver cell
    - b. Muscle cell
    - c. Neuron cell
    - d. Both a and b

65. Melatonin acts as an inhibitor for which hormone?
    - a. Insulin
    - b. ACTH
    - c. Glucagon
    - d. All of the above

66. Which enzyme degrades serotonin to 5-hydroxyindoleacetate?
    - a. Monoamine oxidase
    - b. Diamine oxidase
    - c. Triamine oxidase
    - d. Tetraamine oxidase

67. Which of the following statement is not true?
    - a. Melatonin is a hormone
    - b. Serotonin is also called as 5-hydroxytryptamine
    - c. Xanthurenate is toxic and cannot be excreted in urine
    - d. Vitamin B_3 is also known as niacin

68. Which organ is affected due to the deficiency of serotonin?
    - a. Brain
    - b. Heart
    - c. Lungs
    - d. Kidney

69. Which of the following act as precursor for the synthesis of melatonin?
    - a. Pyruvate
    - b. Acetyl-CoA
    - c. Serotonin
    - d. Lactate

70. Homocysteine, a precursor for production of cysteine is formed from:
    - a. Serine
    - b. Methionine
    - c. Glycine
    - d. Alanine

71. All of the following substances formed from cysteine, *except*:
    - a. Aurine
    - b. Insulin
    - c. Glutathione
    - d. Serotonine

ANSWERS FOR MCQs

1. b	2. c	3. d	4. b	5. c
6. b	7. a	8. c	9. b	10. b
11. a	12. a	13. d	14. c	15. c
16. d	17. b	18. a	19. a	20. b
21. b	22. d	23. c	24. d	25. d
26. a	27. a	28. d	29. b	30. d
31. d	32. d	33. c	34. b	35. a
36. d	37. a	38. c	39. c	40. a
41. c	42. a	43. d	44. d	45. d
46. b	47. c	48. a	49. b	50. b
51. d	52. b	53. c	54. c	55. a
56. a	57. a	58. a	59. b	60. a
61. b	62. d	63. d	64. c	65. b
66. a	67. c	68. a	69. c	70. b
71. d				

13 CHAPTER

Integration of Metabolism and Metabolic Processes in Fed, Fasting, and Starvation States

Competency	Learning Objectives
BI 6.1: Discuss the metabolic processes that take place in specific organs in the body in the fed and fasting states.	1. Describe integration of metabolic processes of carbohydrate, protein and lipid at cellular and at tissue or organ level and significance. 2. Describe the metabolic processes and role of specific organs in fed, fasting, and starvation states.

OVERVIEW

We have studied the biochemistry of metabolism of carbohydrate, lipid, and protein, one pathway at a time. We have seen how useful energy is extracted from fuels and used to power biosynthetic reactions. Not all the major metabolic pathways operate in every tissue at any given time. However, cells and organs cooperate for the common good of the body. Together they control the everyday challenges of overeating, fasting, and muscular activity.

The metabolism of carbohydrate, lipids, and proteins are interrelated, and occur simultaneously. All products of digestion are metabolized to a common product, acetyl-CoA, which is then oxidized by citric acid cycle to yield ATP **(Figure 13.1)**. The best way to understand the inter-relationships of the pathways is to learn the changes in metabolism during the starvation and feed state. Feed refers to the intake of meals after which the fuel is stored as glycogen and triacylglycerol to meet metabolic needs of fasting. Cells of the body die without the provision of continuous supply of energy for ATP synthesis to meet their needs.

This chapter focuses on the integration of the major metabolic processes of **carbohydrate, protein**, and **lipids**. The chapter begins with the discussion on **integration of metabolism** at **cellular level** followed by integration of metabolism at **tissue** or **organ level**. This chapter also

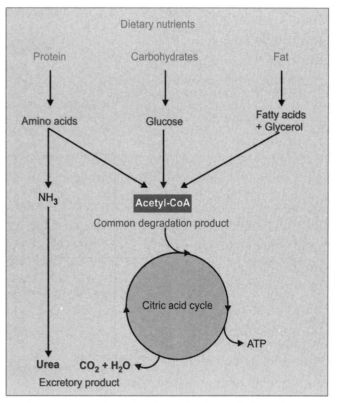

Figure 13.1: Outline of pathways for the catabolism of three principal nutrients, carbohydrate, protein, and fat.

describes metabolic changes occur in **fed, fasting**, and **starvation**.

INTEGRATION OF METABOLISM: AT CELLULAR AND AT TISSUE OR ORGAN LEVEL AND ITS SIGNIFICANCE

The coordination of various anabolic and catabolic pathways of **carbohydrates**, **lipids**, and **proteins** to supply; energy, or precursors for the biosynthesis of compounds which are required by the cells for maintenance or growth is called integration of metabolism. This integration of metabolism must be considered at two levels:

1. Cellular level
2. Tissue or organ level.

Integration of Metabolism at Cellular Level

Integration of metabolism at cellular level includes the flow of key metabolites, e.g., glucose, fatty acids, glycerol, and amino acids, between different metabolic pathways in the cell **(Figure 13.2)**, for the conversion of:

- Carbohydrates into fats and fats into carbohydrates.
- Carbohydrates into proteins and proteins into carbohydrates.
- Proteins into fats.

Conversion of Carbohydrates into Fats and Fats into Carbohydrates

- Carbohydrates (glucose) are metabolized via glycolytic pathway to pyruvate and then pyruvate to acetyl-CoA by pyruvate dehydrogenase reaction. Acetyl-CoA is the precursor for synthesis of **fatty acids**. Fatty acids, that are produced, combine with glycerol to form **triacylglycerol**. Glycerol may also be supplied from the glycolysis as glycerol-3-phosphate, particularly in tissues having no glycerol kinase. Thus, carbohydrates can easily form fat.

- Only a fatty acid having an odd number of carbon atoms is glucogenic as it forms a molecule of **propionyl-CoA** upon β-oxidation. Propionyl-CoA can be converted to **succinyl-CoA**, (*see* **Figure 10.23**) an intermediate of citric acid cycle, which can be converted to glucose by gluconeogenesis. There cannot be a net conversion of fatty acids having an even number of carbon atoms (which form acetyl-CoA) to glucose or glycogen. Conversion of acetyl-CoA to glucose is not possible because:

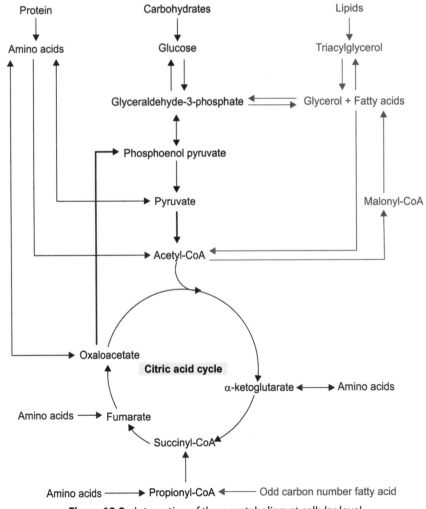

Figure 13.2: Integration of three metabolism at cellular level.

- The pyruvate dehydrogenase reaction is essentially nonreversible which prevents the direct conversion of acetyl-CoA to pyruvate.
- Secondly, there cannot be a net gain of oxaloacetate via citric acid cycle, since one molecule of oxaloacetate is consumed to condense with acetyl-CoA and only one molecule of oxaloacetate is regenerated **(Figure 10.15)**. It is not formed denova when acetyl-CoA is oxidized by citric acid cycle.
- The glycerol moiety of triacylglycerol will form glucose after activation to glycerol-3-phosphate and this is an important source of glucose in starvation.

Conversion of Carbohydrates into Proteins and Proteins into Carbohydrates

- Many carbon skeletons of the **nonessential amino acids** can be produced from carbohydrate via the intermediates of citric acid cycle (*see* **Figure 12.5**) and transamination.
- By reversal of transamination glucogenic amino acids yield carbon skeletons that are either members or precursors of the citric acid cycle. They are therefore readily converted by gluconeogenesis to glucose and glycogen.

Conversion of Proteins to Fats

- Conversion of carbon skeletons of glucogenic amino acids to fatty acids is possible either by formation of pyruvate and acetyl-CoA. Generally, however, the net conversion of amino acids to fat is not a significant process.
- It is not possible for a net conversion of fatty acids to amino acids to take place.

Integration of Metabolism at Tissue or Organ Level

Integration of metabolism at tissue or organ level includes the inter-relationship of different tissues and organs in maintaining an appropriate metabolic state for the whole body. All metabolic pathways are not present in all cells and tissues, and their distribution varies among the major tissues.

The types of fuels that are **imported**, **exported**, and **stored** also vary, depending on the tissues **(Figure 13.3)**. The major organs along with their most important metabolic functions are discussed here.

Role of Liver

Major roles of the liver include the following:
- Liver maintains blood glucose levels. During the fed state, the liver takes up excess glucose and stores it as

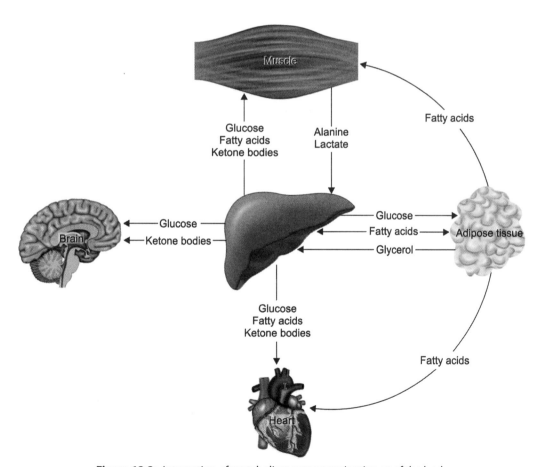

Figure 13.3: Integration of metabolism among major tissues of the body.

glycogen or converts it to fatty acids. During the fasting state, the **glycogenolysis** and **gluconeogenesis** by the liver are the major sources of glucose for the rest of the body.

- The liver serves as the major site of fatty acid synthesis.
- The liver synthesizes ketone bodies during starvation.

Role of Skeletal Muscle

- Skeletal muscle maintains large stores of **glycogen**, which provide a source of glucose for energy during physical exertion.
- In resting muscle, the preferred fuel is **fatty acids**. During starvation, free fatty acids and ketone bodies are oxidized in preference to glucose in muscle by inhibiting its entry into the cell.
- The **protein** contained in muscle may be mobilized as a fuel source in the form of **amino acids**, if no other fuel is available.
- **Pyruvate**, the product of glycolysis in the skeletal muscle, may be converted to either **lactate** (by anaerobic glycolysis by Cori cycle, **See Figure 10.20**) or **alanine** (by transamination) and exported to the liver (by Glucose alanine cycle, **See Figure 10.22**) where it is used to regenerate glucose via gluconeogenesis.

Role of Adipose Tissue

The primary function of the adipose tissue is the storage of metabolic fuel in the form of **triacylglycerols**.

- During the fed state, the adipose tissues synthesize **triacylglycerols** from glucose and free fatty acids.
- During the fasting state, triacylglycerols are converted to **glycerol** and **fatty acids**. Fatty acids are exported to the liver and other tissues as a fuel.
- In adipose tissue, glycerol liberated cannot be reused in the synthesis of triacylglycerols, because adipocytes lack glycerol kinase. Therefore, the glycerol, which is released transported to the liver, and kidney which contain glycerol kinase, which can phosphorylate it. The resulting glycerol phosphate can be used to form triacylglycerol in the liver or to be converted to DHAP.

Role of Brain

Brain tissue normally uses **glucose** as an exclusive fuel, except during starvation, when it can adapt to use ketone bodies as an energy source. The brain contains essentially no fuel reserves and must be continuously supplied with fuel from the **liver (Figure 13.3)**.

Role of Heart Muscle

Heart muscle contains essentially no fuel reserves and must be continuously, supplied with fuel from liver and adipose tissue **(Figure 13.3)**.

Significance of Integration of Metabolism

- Integration of metabolism ensures a supply of suitable fuel for all tissues, at all times from the **fully fed state** to the totally **starved state**.
- Under positive caloric balance, i.e., in well fed state a significant proportion of the food energy intake is stored as either **glycogen** or **fat**.
- Under negative caloric balance, i.e., in starvation, fatty acids are oxidized in preference to glucose, to spare glucose for those tissues, (e.g., brain and erythrocytes) that require it under all conditions.
- Under conditions of carbohydrate shortage, available fuels are oxidized in the following order of preference:
  - Ketone bodies
  - Free fatty acids
  - Glucose.

THE METABOLIC PROCESSES AND ROLE OF SPECIFIC ORGANS IN FED, FASTING, AND STARVATION STATES

Starvation is the deprivation of the food and thereby deprivation of exogenous supply of calories to meet the energy demands of the body for basal metabolism and other activities. Starvation, in a strict biochemical sense, begins immediately after the absorption of a meal is complete.

Starvation is not always the result of unavailability or scarcity of food. Any medical condition, which prevents consumption or utilization of available food will effectively lead to starvation, e.g., trauma, surgery, cancer cachexia, infections, malabsorption, etc.

We begin with a physiological condition the **starved-fed cycle** or **fast-fed cycle**, which occurs after an evening meal and through the 12 hours overnight fast.

- This nightly starved fed cycle has three stages: **the well fed state after meal** the **early fasting phase during night** and **the refed state after breakfast**.
- The starved-fed cycle is the physiological response to a fast. Here we discuss metabolic changes in the context of four normal metabolic states:
  1. The well fed state after meal or postprandial state.
  2. The early fasting phase during night or postabsorptive phase, which covers the 12 hours overnight fast.
  3. The refed state after breakfast.
  4. Prolonged starvation, which lasts longer than 24 hours and can extend into several days or weeks.
- The changes in metabolism from one stage into the next are not abrupt but gradual.
- The main purpose of the many biochemical changes in these metabolic phases is to maintain constant **blood glucose** level, which is maintained by the combined action of **insulin** and **glucagon**.
  - Insulin signals body tissues, especially liver, muscle, and adipose tissue that blood glucose is higher than

necessary, as a result, cells take up excess glucose from the blood and convert it to **glycogen** and **triacylglycerols** for storage.

- Glucagon signals that blood glucose is too low, and tissues respond by producing glucose through **glycogen breakdown** and **gluconeogenesis** in the liver and by oxidizing fats to reduce the need for glucose.

Metabolic Changes in Well-fed State after Meal or Postprandial State

Figure 13.4 illustrates the role of specific organs in the metabolism in well-fed state.

After consumption and digestion of an evening meal, **glucose** and **amino acids** are transported from intestine to the blood. The dietary lipids are packaged into **chylomicrons** and transported to the blood by lymphatic system. This fed condition leads to the **increase in blood glucose** level. The high blood glucose concentration leads to secretion of **insulin**.

- Insulin **stimulates** the **glycogen synthesis** in both **muscle** and **liver** and **suppresses gluconeogenesis** in the liver, and stimulates **protein synthesis**.
- Insulin also accelerates **glycolysis** in the liver, which in turn increases the **synthesis of fatty acids**.

- The high insulin level in the fed state promotes the entry of **glucose** into **muscle** and **adipose tissue**. Insulin stimulates the synthesis of glycogen by muscle as well as by the liver. When there is plenty of glucose in blood, it is stored as a **glycogen**, so as to be able to release glucose in times of scarcity.
- **Figure 13.5** show the various metabolic effects of insulin on blood glucose.
  - Liver possesses an isoenzyme of hexokinase called **glucokinase**, which converts glucose into glucose 6-phosphate. Glucokinase has **high K_m** value and is thus active only when blood glucose level is high. Moreover, glucokinase is **not inhibited** by **glucose 6-phosphate** as hexokinase is. Consequently, the liver forms glucose 6-phosphate more rapidly, as blood glucose level rises. The increased level of glucose 6-phosphate, leads to the formation of glycogen.
  - In the liver insulin accelerates glycolysis and oxidation of pyruvate to acetyl-CoA. Excess acetyl-CoA not needed for energy production is used for **fatty acid synthesis**, and fatty acids are exported from the liver to adipose tissue as the **triacylglycerol** of VLDL.
  - Insulin stimulates the synthesis of triacylglycerol in adipose tissue, from fatty acids released from the triacylglycerol of VLDL. These fatty acids are

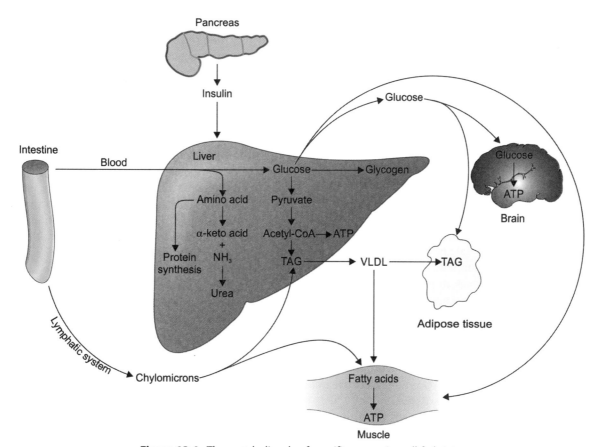

Figure 13.4: The metabolic role of specific organs in well-fed state.
(TG: triacylglycerol)

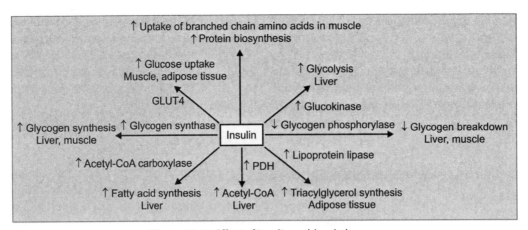

Figure 13.5: Effect of insulin on blood glucose.
(GLUT4: glucose transporter-4; PDH: pyruvate dehydrogenase)

ultimately derived from the excess glucose taken from blood by the liver.

- The action of insulin also affects protein metabolism. Insulin promotes the uptake of **branched chain amino acids** (valine, leucine, and isoleucine) by muscle.
- Insulin stimulates protein synthesis, which favors building up of muscle protein. In addition it inhibits the intracellular degradation of proteins.

> The lack of insulin activity in **diabetes mellitus** results in failure of transfer of glucose from the blood into cells and leads to hyperglycemia. The body responds as it were in the fasting state.

Metabolic Changes in Early Fasting Phase During Night

If we eat another meal within a few hours, we return to the fed state. However, if we continue to fast over a 12 hours period, we enter the basal state also known as the **postabsorptive state. Figure 13.6** illustrates the main features of the metabolic changes occur during early fasting.

Blood glucose level is highest approximately 1 hour after meal and then decrease as tissues oxidize glucose or convert it to storage forms of fuel. Within about 1 hour after a meal, blood glucose levels begin to fall and by 2 hours the level returns to the fasting range (70–100 mg/dL).

- For the brain, the erythrocytes, the bone marrow, the renal medulla and peripheral nerves glucose is the major fuel and which has to be supplied for their energy needs. Most neurons lack enzymes required for oxidation of fatty acids but they can use ketone bodies to a limited extent. Red blood cells lack mitochondria, which contain enzymes of fatty acid and ketone body oxidation, and can use only glucose as a fuel. Therefore, it is essential to maintain the blood glucose level within normal range.
- However, the tissues such as muscle can readily use free fatty acids, released from adipose tissue.
- The blood glucose level is maintained within normal level (at or above 70 mg/dL) by the following ways:
  1. The decrease in blood glucose causes decrease in **insulin** secretion and stimulates secretion of

glucagon (**Figure 13.7**). Just as insulin signals the fed state, **glucagon** signals the **starved state**. Glucagon is secreted by α-cells of the pancreas in response to low blood sugar level in the fasting state.

2. The main target organ of glucagon is the liver. Glucagon causes an increase in blood glucose concentration in several ways (**Figure 13.8**).
   - Glucagon stimulates **glycogen breakdown** and inhibits glycogen synthesis by triggering cAMP (**Figure 10.30**) leading to the phosphorylation and activation of **phosphorylase** and the inhibition of **glycogen synthase**.
   - The glucose formed by breakdown of liver glycogen is then released from the liver into the blood. The liver glycogen is capable of maintaining the blood glucose concentration at normal values for **8 to 12 hours (Figure 13.7)**. Thus, hepatic glycogenolysis is a transient response to starvation.

3. In response to low insulin level the entry of glucose into the muscle and adipose tissue decreases. The diminished utilization of glucose by muscle and adipose tissue also contributes to maintain the blood glucose level. By stimulating glycogen breakdown glucagon facilitates the liver to provide glucose for brain (which is exclusively dependent on glucose as fuel), and restoring blood glucose to its normal level.

4. As the liver glycogen store begins to be depleted, another mechanism, **gluconeogenesis** is used to maintain blood glucose levels. In gluconeogenesis, **lactate**, **glycerol**, and **amino acids** are used as precursors to glucose.
   - Gluconeogenesis initially occurs from **lactate** (obtained from glycolysis in red blood cell) and **alanine** (coming from muscle, a key glucogenic amino acid). The rate of hepatic gluconeogenesis from alanine is far higher than from all other amino acids. But it should be noted that there is no net synthesis or gain of glucose by this process using lactate and alanine as the precursors. It simply replaces glucose that had already been converted

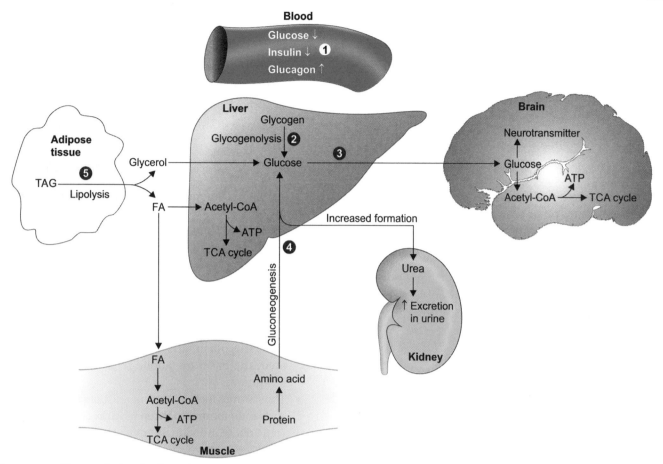

Figure 13.6: The metabolic role of specific organs during early fasting. The circled number indicates the approximate order in which processes begin to occur.

(TG: triacylglycerol; FA: fatty acid; AA: amino acid)

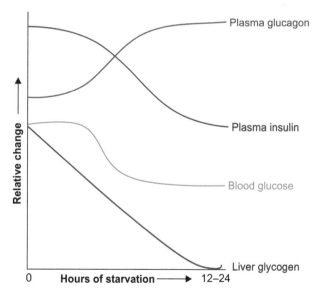

Figure 13.7: Release of fuel from the body stores due to changes in hormone level during the onset of starvation.

glucose, but only a limited amount is available as well as there is no net synthesis or gain of glucose by this process.

♦ Thus, for the net synthesis of glucose to take place, another source of carbon is required. The only potential source of glucose is the **carbon skeletons** of amino acids derived from the **breakdown of muscle proteins**.

Why does the Muscle Release Alanine?

❖ Muscle can absorb and transaminate branch chain amino acids in order to use the carbon skeleton as fuel, however it cannot form urea. Consequently, the amino group is released into the blood as **alanine (Figure 12.13)**.

❖ Interestingly, the liver cannot remove nitrogen from the branched chain amino acids (leucine, isoleucine, and valine). Transamination of these amino acids takes place in muscle. Insulin promotes the uptake of branched chain amino acids by muscle.

into lactate and alanine by tissues such as muscle and RBC.

♦ The glycerol released from adipose tissue by lipolysis of triacylglycerol can be converted into

5. Glucagon like epinephrine affects **adipose tissue**, activating triacylglycerol breakdown by triggering cAMP-dependent phosphorylation of **perilipin** and **hormone sensitive lipase**.

♦ The activated **hormone sensitive lipase** hydrolyses triacylglycerol to free fatty acids and glycerol.

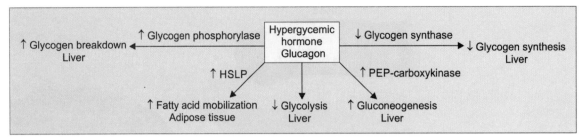

Figure 13.8: Effect of glucagon on blood glucose.

(PFK-1: phosphofructokinase-1; HSLP: hormone sensitive lipoprotein lipase; PEP carboxykinase: phosphoenol pyruvate carboxykinase)

Liberated free fatty acids are transported to the liver and other tissues as fuel. Both muscle and liver use fatty acids as fuel when the blood glucose level drops, sparing glucose for the brain.

- Increased amount of glycerol is transported to the liver, which is a substrate for gluconeogenesis.
- Glucagon also inhibits **fatty acid synthesis** by diminishing the production of pyruvate and by lowering the activity of **acetyl-CoA carboxylase**, (regulatory enzyme in fatty acid synthesis) by maintaining it in the inactive phosphorylated state.

- The net effect of glucagon is therefore to stimulate glucose synthesis and release by the liver and to mobilize fatty acids from adipose tissue, to be used instead of glucose by tissues other than the brain.

The Refed State after Breakfast

Earlier, we considered the **metabolic changes** occur during **overnight** or **early fasting**. After overnight fast when individual having breakfast, the body returns to the fed state.

- Fat is processed exactly as it is processed in the normal fed state.
- However, glucose is not processed as it is processed in the normal fed state. The liver does not initially absorb glucose from the blood, but instead, spares it for the other tissues.
- Furthermore, the liver remains in a **gluconeogenic mode** for 2 to 3 hours after feeding. The newly synthesized glucose by gluconeogenesis is used to replenish the liver's glycogen stores. As the blood glucose concentration continues to rise, the liver completes the replenishment of its glycogen stores with end of gluconeogenic mode of the liver and start synthesizing glycogen from fresh blood glucose.
- After complete replenishment of liver glycogen stores, the remaining excess glucose is processed for fatty acid synthesis.

Metabolic Changes Occur During Prolonged Starvation

When fasting state is prolonged, the condition is called **starvation**. Let us now examine what are the adaptations if fasting is prolonged to the point of starvation. **Figure 13.9** illustrates the metabolic role of specific organs during **prolonged starvation**.

- In starvation, energy has to be derived from the body's own stores.
    - A typical well-nourished 70 kg man has fuel reserves totaling about **165,000 kcal (Table 13.1)**.
    - The energy, needed for 24-hour period, ranges from about 1,600 kcal in the basal state to 6,000 kcal depending on the extent of activity.
    - However, the carbohydrate reserves are exhausted in only a day. The total energy, immediately available from the plasma, is very small, and would only meet the basal metabolic requirements for about 80 minutes.
    - Thus, stored fuels are enough to meet caloric needs in starvation for **one to three months** and in the case of some obese individuals, much longer.

Metabolic Changes on the First Day of Starvation

The metabolic changes on the first day of starvation are like those after overnight fast.

- The low blood glucose level leads to decreased secretion of insulin and increased secretion of glucagon.
- The **lipolysis**, breakdown of triacylglycerol in adipose tissue and **gluconeogenesis** in liver are the predominant metabolic processes.
- The concentration of **acetyl-CoA** and **citrate** increase due to increased breakdown of triacylglycerol.
- Acetyl-CoA and citrate inhibits glycolysis.
- The uptake of glucose by muscle is markedly diminished because of the low insulin level, whereas fatty acids enter freely. Now muscle uses no glucose and depends exclusively on fatty acids for fuel.
- The β-oxidation of fatty acids by muscle stops the conversion of pyruvate into acetyl-CoA, because acetyl-CoA stimulates the **phosphorylation** of the **pyruvate dehydrogenase complex**, which makes it inactive.
- Hence, pyruvate, lactate, and alanine are exported to the liver for conversion to glucose by gluconeogenesis.
- Glycerol derived from the degradation of triacylglycerols is also a precursor for the synthesis of glucose by the liver.
- **Proteolysis** also provides **carbon skeletons** for gluconeogenesis. During starvation, degraded proteins are not replenished and serve as carbon sources for glucose synthesis.

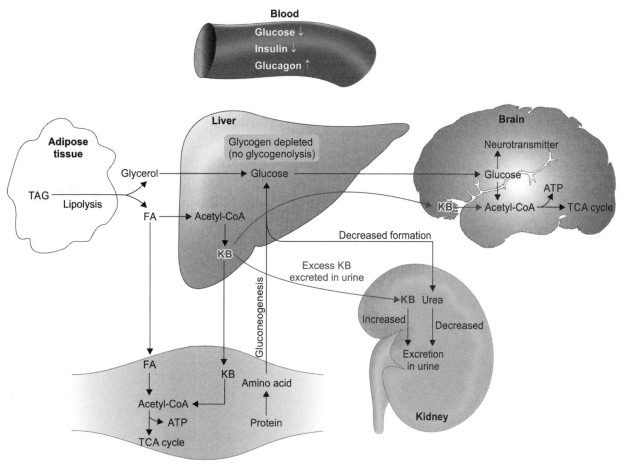

Figure 13.9: The metabolic role of specific organs during prolonged starvation.
(TG: triacylglycerol; FA: fatty acid; KB: ketone bodies; AA: amino acid)

Type of fuel	Weight (kg)	Caloric equivalent (thousands of kcal)	Estimated survival
TABLE: 13.1: Fuel reserved in well-nourished 70 kg man.			
Triacylglycerol (adipose tissue)	15	140	3 months
Proteins (mainly muscle)	6	24	
Glycogen (muscle, liver)	0.23	0.90	
Circulating fuels (glucose, fatty acids, triacylglycerols)	0.023	0.10	
Total		165	

- Initial sources of protein are those that turn over rapidly, such as proteins of the intestinal epithelium (digestive enzymes) and the secretions of the pancreas, as these enzymes are no longer needed. These are so-called **labile proteins**, the loss of which does not affect the integrity of the tissues.
- Then there is a rapid breakdown of muscle protein, providing amino acids that are used by the liver for gluconeogenesis. The major gluconeogenic amino acids, coming from muscle, are **alanine** and **glutamine**.
- Glucagon increases the uptake of alanine by the liver.

- The processes, which take place in early fasting cannot go on indefinitely, because, although they provide efficiently for the body's energy requirements, they will soon deplete the substantial proportion of body protein. However, breakdown of proteins will carry out a loss of function. It is known that death results when 30 to 50% of the body protein is lost. Adjustments to metabolism are made after 24 to 48 hours, which conserve body protein.

> Protein undergoes three phases of depletion, **rapid depletion at first** then the **greatly slowed depletion**, and **finally rapid depletion again** shortly before death.

Metabolic Changes after Three Days of Starvation

Now we will see how is the loss of muscle protein reduced?

- After about 3 days of starvation, the liver forms large amounts of **ketone bodies**, **acetoacetate** and β-**hydroxybutyrate**. The synthesis of ketone bodies from acetyl-CoA increases markedly (producing the state of **ketosis**) because:
  - Citric acid cycle is unable to oxidize all of the acetyl-CoA generated by the degradation of fatty acids.

- Gluconeogenesis depletes the supply of oxaloacetate, which is essential for the entry of acetyl-CoA into the citric acid cycle. Consequently, liver produces large quantities of ketone bodies and released into the blood.
- At this time, the brain begins to consume significant amounts of acetoacetate in place of glucose.
- After 3 days of starvation about a quarter of the energy needs of the brain are met by ketone bodies.
- The heart also uses ketone bodies as fuel.

Metabolic Changes after Several Weeks of Starvation

- After several weeks of starvation, **ketone bodies** become the major fuel of the brain. As the supply of ketone bodies increases and the supply of glucose diminish, the brain reduces its utilization of glucose and begins to consume appreciable amounts of ketone bodies in place of glucose.
- The increased use of ketone bodies by the brain is a simple mass action effect of the increased availability of the ketone bodies, which like glucose, now can cross the blood-brain barrier.

> ❖ Up to half the energy requirement of the brain can be met by ketone bodies. They can cross the blood brain barrier and diffuse into brain cells where they are reconverted to acetyl-CoA in the mitochondria.
> ❖ The brain does not use amino acids in significant amounts as such but can use glucose derived from glucogenic amino acids in the liver.
> ❖ It does not use fatty acids in significant amounts as they do not cross the blood brain barrier **(Figure 13.10)**.

- After several weeks of starvation, ketone bodies become the major fuel of the brain. Although the brain still has a residual glucose requirement, not only for provision of energy, but also for synthesis of **neurotransmitters**. Only 40 g. of glucose is needed per day for the brain as compared with about 120 g in the first day of starvation.
- Therefore, less muscle is degraded than in the first days of starvation. The breakdown of **20 g of muscle** compared with **75 g** early in starvation is most important for survival. This sequence of events leads to at least partial preservation of the protein stores of the body.
- During the conversion of amino acid to glucose by gluconeogenesis, the nitrogen of the amino acid is converted to urea and so production of urea decreases during prolonged starvation, as compared to its production in short-term starvation. Decrease in nitrogen excretion occurs from around 12 to 15 g/day to 3 to 4 g/day, following 4 to 6 weeks of starvation **(Figure 13.11)**. Urea nitrogen diminishes markedly, suggesting that fewer amino acids undergo gluconeogenesis in the liver.

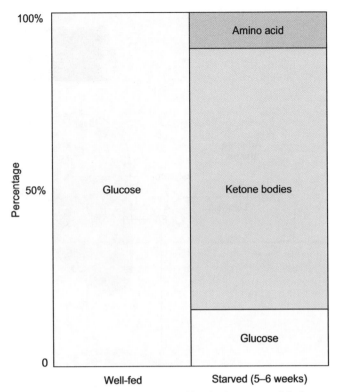

Figure 13.10: Fuel source used by the brain in well-fed and starved state.

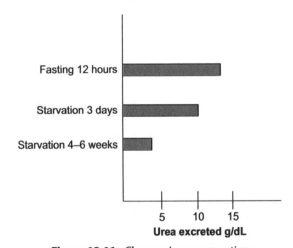

Figure 13.11: Changes in urea excretion during prolonged fasting.

- Because of these adaptive mechanisms the person's survival time is mainly determined by the size of the **triacylglycerol depot**. When the triacylglycerol stores are completely exhausted, the only source of fuel remains is **protein**. So degradation of proteins accelerates, and thus, muscle proteins heavily drained as a source of energy. At that time, the protein stores once again enter a stage of **rapid depletion**. Because proteins are also essential for the maintenance of cellular function, death ordinarily ensues when the proteins of the body have been depleted to about half their normal level. The death invariably results from a loss of heart, liver, or kidney function.

STRIKE A NOTE

❖ Circulating glucose concentrations do not drop below 70 mg/dL even in prolonged starvation.
❖ Carbohydrate reserves (glycogen) are depleted after 8 to 12 h of starvation.
❖ The first priority of metabolism in starvation is to provide sufficient glucose to the brain and other tissues that are absolutely dependent on glucose.
❖ Gluconeogenesis plays an essential role in maintaining blood glucose during both the **early fasting phase** and **prolonged starvation**.
❖ During starvation, the kidney becomes an important site of gluconeogenesis and may contribute as much as half of the blood glucose.
❖ The major substrates for gluconeogenesis are amino acids derived from skeletal muscle protein breakdown.
❖ The major glucogenic amino acid coming from muscle to liver for gluconeogenesis during starvation is alanine.
❖ The second priority of metabolism in starvation is to preserve protein. This is accomplished by using fatty acids and ketone bodies in place of glucose as a fuel.
❖ During starvation, most tissues utilize fatty acids and/or ketone bodies to spare glucose for the brain.
❖ Glucose utilization by the brain is decreased during prolonged starvation as the brain start utilizing ketone bodies as the major fuel.
❖ Ketosis is a metabolic adaptation to starvation, arises as a result of deficiency in available carbohydrate.
❖ Protein undergoes three phases of depletion, rapid depletion at first then the greatly slowed depletion, and finally rapid depletion again shortly before death.

ASSESSMENT QUESTIONS

STRUCTURED LONG ESSAY QUESTIONS (SLEQs)

1. Describe the integration metabolism under the following headings:
   i. Definition
   ii. At cellular level
   iii. At tissue/organ level
   iv. Significance
2. Describe the metabolic changes that occur during:
   i. Well-fed state
   ii. Fasting state during night
   iii. Starvation state
3. Metabolic changes occur during fed fasting and starvation states with a role of specific organs.

SHORT ESSAY QUESTIONS (SEQs)

1. Define integration metabolism. Write integration metabolism at cellular level.
2. Define integration metabolism. Write integration metabolism at tissue or organ level.
3. Write metabolic changes in fed state.
4. Write metabolic changes in fasting state during night.
5. What is integration of metabolism? Write role of liver in integration of metabolism.
6. What is integration of metabolism? Write role of adipose tissue in integration of metabolism.

SHORT ANSWER QUESTIONS (SAQs)

1. There is no net gain of glucose from lactate and alanine by gluconeogenesis. Justify?
2. During starvation protein undergoes three phases of depletion. Justify?

3. Write metabolic priority during starvation.
4. Which pathway occurs during all phases of starvation? Why?
5. Metabolic processes which take place in early fasting cannot continue with prolonged fasting. Justify?

CASE VIGNETTE-BASED QUESTIONS (CVBQs)

Case Study

1. **A patient attending an obesity clinic is found to have ketonuria. The patient is on a low carbohydrate diet in order to lose weight. There is no glycosuria. Blood glucose level was, found 80 mg/100 mL:**
   a. Explain the cause of ketonuria.
   b. How blood glucose level is maintained in this patient?
   c. Name the test to confirm ketonuria.
   d. What is ketosis?

MULTIPLE CHOICE QUESTIONS (MCQs)

1. **The first priority of metabolism in starvation is to provide which of the following substances to the brain and other tissue?**
   a. Fatty acids   b. Ketone bodies
   c. Glucose   d. Cholesterol

2. **During starvation, blood or tissue levels of all of the following are elevated, *except*:**
   a. Free fatty acids   b. Ketone bodies
   c. Glucagon   d. Insulin

3. **Which of the following processes plays an essential role in maintaining blood glucose during early and prolonged starvation?**
   a. Glycolysis   b. Gluconeogenesis
   c. Ketogenesis   d. Glycogenolysis

4. In starvation, muscle protein is spared by:
   a. Using fatty acids and ketone bodies
   b. By increasing rate of gluconeogenesis
   c. By inhibiting glucose utilization
   d. By stimulating protein synthesis

5. In prolonged starvation, the main energy source of brain is:
   a. Glucose
   b. Ketone bodies
   c. Fructose
   d. Fatty acids

6. The major glucogenic amino acid coming from muscle to liver for gluconeogenesis during starvation is:
   a. Threonine
   b. Methionine
   c. Alanine
   d. Glycine

7. During early fasting glucose is derived from:
   a. Glycogen
   b. Amino acids
   c. Fatty acids
   d. Ketone bodies

8. Fatty acid or ketone bodies are used as energy source in:
   a. Intraprandial phase
   b. Postabsorptive phase
   c. Prolonged starvation
   d. Fully fed state

9. During starvation free fatty acids and ketone bodies are oxidized in preference to glucose in muscle by impairing, *except*:
   a. Uptake of glucose by the cell
   b. Phosphorylation by hexokinase and phosphofructokinase
   c. Pyruvate dehydrogenase activity
   d. Lactate dehydrogenase activity

10. During starvation, the first reserve nutrient to be depleted is:
    a. Glycogen
    b. Proteins
    c. Triglycerides
    d. Cholesterol

11. Synthesis of the following enzymes is increased during starvation.
    a. Digestive enzymes
    b. Gluconeogenic enzymes
    c. Glycolysis enzymes
    d. Glycogenesis enzymes

12. In fasting which of the following metabolites will be elevated in blood after 24 hours?
    a. Triacylglycerol   b. Glucose
    c. Free fatty acid   d. Glycogen

13. On prolonged fasting which of the following metabolites will be elevated in blood after 3 days?
    a. Ketone bodies
    b. Glycogen
    c. Triacylglycerol
    d. Glucose

14. After overnight fast one would expect increased activity of what?
    a. Hepatic glycogen synthase
    b. Pyruvate dehydrogenase
    c. Hormone sensitive lipase
    d. Pancreatic lipase

15. After overnight fast one would expect glucose transporter activity to be what?
    a. Decreased in brain cell
    b. Enhanced in adipocytes
    c. Decreased in red blood cells
    d. Decreased in muscle cells

16. Which one of the following statements is correct for metabolism during prolonged starvation compared to early or short term starvation?
    a. The degradation of proteins is increased
    b. The rate of gluconeogenesis in liver is decreased
    c. The formation of ketone bodies is decreased
    d. Heart generates more of its energy from glucose

17. Which of the following statements are correct for amino acid metabolism during the fasting state compared with the fed state? *Except.*
    a. Glutamine and alanine are released in increased amounts
    b. Glucose is preserved for the brain
    c. Alanine is utilized for glucose synthesis
    d. Alanine is utilized for protein synthesis

18. Which of the following occurs in cardiac muscle but not in the brain, even in the fasted state?
    a. Fatty acid oxidation
    b. Glycolysis
    c. TCA cycle
    d. Glucose uptake via a glucose transporter

19. During starvation, ketone bodies are used as a fuel by:
    a. Erythrocytes
    b. Brain
    c. Liver
    d. All of these

20. Which type of metabolic fuel is utilized for generating glucose under conditions of severe starvation?
    a. Glycogen
    b. Fats
    c. Starch
    d. Amino acids

21. Liver glycogen is used in fasting to provide glucose. Muscle glycogen is not. What is the explanation for this?
    a. Muscle does not have a debranching enzyme
    b. Muscle cannot degrade glycogen further than glucose-1-phosphate
    c. Muscle lacks glucose-6-phosphatase
    d. The liver provides all the glucose necessary for metabolism and there is no need for muscle to do the same

22. Which of the following organs utilizes glucose, fatty acid, and ketone bodies as fuel?
    a. Heart
    b. Liver
    c. RBC
    d. Brain

23. **In fasting state which of the following is false?**
    a. Insulin level falls
    b. Level of cAMP is high
    c. Glycogenesis is active
    d. Lipolysis active

24. **Which of the following pathway is active in high insulin glucagon ratio?**
    a. Glycogenolysis
    b. Lipolysis
    c. Pyruvate dehydrogenase
    d. Gluconeogenesis

25. **After 48 hours of fasting which of the following do not be active?**
    a. Lipolysis
    b. Ketone body synthesis
    c. Gluconeogenic substrates are depleted
    d. Glycogenolysis

26. **Which of the following enzyme activity decrease in fasting?**
    a. Hormone sensitive lipase
    b. Glycogen Phosphorylase
    c. Acetyl-CoA carboxylase
    d. CPS I

ANSWERS FOR MCQs

1. c	2. d	3. b	4. a	5. b
6. c	7. a	8. c	9. a	10. a
11. b	12. c	13. a	14. c	15. d
16. b	17. d	18. a	19. b	20. d
21. c	22. a	23. c	24. c	25. d
26. c				

Hemoglobin Metabolism

Competency	Learning Objectives
BI 6.11: Describe the functions of heme in the body and describe the processes involved in its metabolism and describe porphyrin metabolism.	1. Describe biosynthesis of heme: Pathway, regulation, significance and associated disorder. 2. Describe catabolism of heme: Formation, transport, conjugation, secretion and excretion of bilirubin. 3. Describe disorders of bilirubin metabolism: Hyperbilirubinemia. 4. Describe laboratory tests done to differentiate jaundice.

OVERVIEW

Heme is the prosthetic group of several proteins and enzymes including **hemoglobin, myoglobin, cytochrome, cytochrome P450, enzymes** like **catalase**, certain **peroxidase**, and **tryptophan pyrrolase**. Heme is synthesized from **porphyrin** and **iron**. Porphyrin ring is coordinated with an atom of iron to form heme **(Figure 14.1)**.

Porphyrins are cyclic molecule formed by the linkage of 4-pyrrol rings through methenyl bridges. Eight side chains serve as substituents on the porphyrin ring, two on each pyrrol. These side chains may be acetyl (A), propionyl (P), methyl (M) or vinyl (V) groups. Different porphyrins vary in nature of the side chains that are attached to each of the four pyrrol rings. The side chains of the porphyrin can be arranged in four different ways designated by roman numerals I to IV. **Only type III isomer is physiologically important in humans**.

Heme and its immediate precursor, **protoporphyrin IX** are both of **type III porphyrins**. However, they are sometimes identified as belonging to series IX, because they were designated ninth in a series of isomer postulated by **Hans Fischer**, the pioneer worker of porphyrin chemistry.

BIOSYNTHESIS OF HEME: PATHWAY, REGULATION, SIGNIFICANCE AND ASSOCIATED DISORDER

Biosynthesis of Heme

Heme synthesis takes place in all cells (except in mature erythrocytes), but occurs to the greatest extent in the **bone marrow** and **liver**, where the requirements for incorporation of heme into hemoglobin and cytochromes are high. Biosynthesis of heme may be divided into three stages **(Figure 14.2)**:

1. Biosynthesis of δ-**aminolevulinate (ALA)** from the precursor **glycine** and **succinyl-CoA**
2. Formation of **porphobilinogen (PBG)** from two molecules of δ-**aminolevulinate**
3. Conversion of the porphobilinogen to the cyclic **tetrapyrrol porphyrin ring** and **heme**.

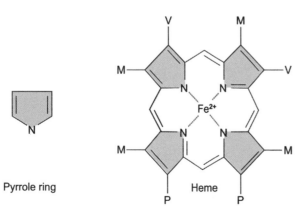

Pyrrole ring Heme

Figure 14.1: A heme molecule showing a pyrrol molecule and an atom of iron (Fe^{2+}) in the center of the porphyrin ring, which is tetrapyrrol structure.
(M: methyl; V: vinyl; P: propionyl)

It is to be noted that the first and last three enzymatic steps are catalyzed by enzymes that are in the **mitochondrion**, whereas the intermediate steps take place in the **cytosol**.

- The first step in the biosynthesis of porphyrins is the condensation of **glycine** and **succinyl-CoA** to form δ-aminolevulinate **(ALA)**, which occurs in mitochondria. This reaction is catalyzed by **δ-aminolevulinate synthase (δ-ALAS)** and **PLP** (pyridoxal phosphate) is also necessary in this reaction to activate glycine. **This is the rate controlling step in heme synthesis**.

In human, there are two isoenzymes of ALA synthase present. ALAS-1 is present throughout the body, whereas ALAS-2 is expressed in erythrocyte precursor cells.

- In the cytosol two molecules of δ-ALA condense to form 2 molecules of water and one of **porphobilinogen (PBG)**. This dehydration reaction is catalyzed by **δ-aminolevulinate dehydratase**, also called **porphobilinogen synthase (PBGS)**, which is a **zinc** containing enzyme.

- ❖ δ-aminolevulinate dehydratase enzyme is inhibited by relatively low concentrations of **lead (Pb)**. ALA dehydratase and Ferrochelatase are Zn^{2+} dependent metalloenzymes. Pb^{2+} replaces the Zn^{2+} at the active site and inhibits them.
- ❖ This accounts for the large excretion of ALA in the urine of a person who is affected with lead poisoning.
- ❖ The quantitative determination of ALA in urine is one of the better analytical means of monitoring the severity and control of lead poisoning in human subjects.

- Four porphobilinogen molecules condense to form a **linear tetrapyrrol (hydroxmethylbilane, HMB)**. The reaction is catalyzed by **PBG deaminase**, also known as **uroporphyrinogen-I synthase (or HMB synthase)**. Linear tetrapyrrol cyclizes to **uroporphyrinogen III** by **uroporphyrinogen III cosynthase**. At this point basic ring structure (porphyrin skeleton) is formed.

Under normal conditions, the uroporphyrinogen formed is almost exclusively the type III isomer but in certain of the porphyrias (discussed later), the type I isomers of porphyrinogens are formed in excess.

- Subsequent reactions alter the side chains and the degree of saturation of the porphyrin ring as follows:
  - Uroporphyrinogen III is converted to **coproporphyrinogen III** by **decarboxylation** of all of the acetate side chain groups, to methyl (M) substituents. The reaction is catalyzed by **uroporphyrinogen decarboxylase**.
  - Coproporphyrinogen III then enters the mitochondria, where it is converted to **protoporphyrinogen-IX**

by the mitochondrial enzyme **coproporphyrinogen oxidase**. This enzyme catalyzes the conversion of two of the propionate side chains into vinyl groups by oxidative decarboxylation. This enzyme is able to act only on type-III coproporphyrinogen; that is why type-I protoporphyrins do not generally occur in nature.

- The oxidation of protoporphyrinogen-IX to **protoporphyrin** is catalyzed by another mitochondrial enzyme, **protoporphyrinogen oxidase**.
- The final step in heme synthesis involves the incorporation of **ferrous ion (Fe^{2+})** into protoporphyrin in a reaction catalyzed by mitochondrial **heme synthase** or **ferrochelatase**.

Many porphyrin-containing metalloproteins have heme as their prosthetic group; these are known as **hemoproteins**. Hemes are most commonly recognized as components of hemoglobin, but are also found in a number of other biologically important hemoproteins such as **myoglobin, cytochromes, catalases, heme peroxidase**, and **endothelial nitric oxide synthase**.

Regulation of Heme Synthesis

Several factors regulate heme biosynthesis:

- δ-**aminolevulinic acid synthase (ALAS)**, a **mitochondrial allosteric enzyme** that catalyzes rate controlling step of heme biosynthetic pathway, is feedback inhibited by heme **(Figure 14.2)**.
- Regulation also occurs at the level of enzyme synthesis. Increased level of heme represses the synthesis of δ-aminolevulinic acid synthase and decreased level of heme induces the synthesis of δ-aminolevulinic acid synthase.
- The iron atom itself activates heme synthesis.

Factors that Affect Heme Synthesis

- Several drugs induce the synthesis of hepatic ALAS, e.g., steroid hormone metabolites, ethanol, barbiturates, griseofulvin etc. Most of the drugs are metabolized in the liver by utilizing **cytochrome P450**. Maximum amount of heme is consumed for the formation of cytochrome P450, which in turn reduces the intracellular heme concentration. Reduced heme concentration increases rate of heme synthesis to meet the needs of the cells by inducing ALA synthase.
- **Lead** can inactivate δ-**ALA dehydratase** and **ferrochelatase** by combing with essential thiol groups of these enzymes. Signs of lead poisoning include:
  - Elevated levels of **protoporphyrin in erythrocytes**
  - Elevated urinary levels of **ALA** and **coproporphyrin III**.
  - Production of **heme** is decreased.

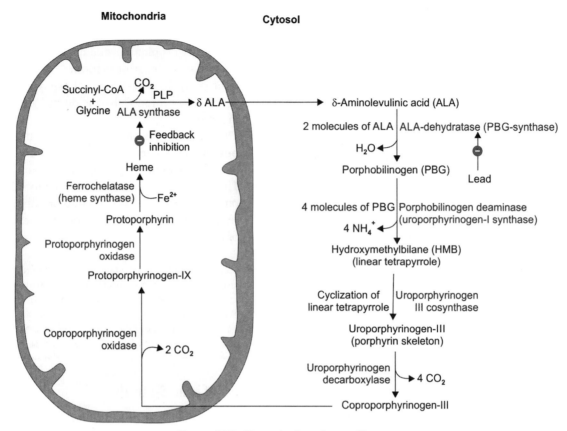

Figure 14.2: Biosynthetic pathway of heme.

- **Anemia** results from lack of hemoglobin and
- Energy production decreases due to lack of cyto-chromes for the electron transport chain.
- **Isonicotinic acid hydrazide (isoniazid, INH), an anti-tuberculosis agent,** inhibits heme synthesis **by limiting PLP availability to ALAS. INH reacts with pyridoxal to form pyridoxal isonicotinoyl hydrazone** which can cause sideroblastic anemia as a side-effect.

Significance of Heme

Heme plays multiple roles in cellular processes as follows:

- Heme exists as a prosthetic group in numerous proteins and enzymes including hemoglobin, myoglobin, cytochrome, cytochrome P450, enzymes like catalase, certain peroxidase, and tryptophan pyrrolase.
- The strong affinity of heme toward oxygen makes it possible for hemoglobin and myoglobin (heme-containing proteins), to function in oxygen transport and storage.
- Heme also participates in electron transfer reactions, detoxification of xenobiotics, signal transduction, and regulation of transcription, translation, microRNA processing, mitochondrial protein import, protein stability, and differentiation.
- Malfunction of heme synthesis can lead to disorders such as anemia and porphyrias.

Disorders of Heme Biosynthesis

Porphyrias

The porphyrias are rare group of genetic disorders resulting from deficiencies of enzymes in the biosynthetic pathway for heme, and leads to accumulation and increased excretion of **porphyrins** or **porphyrin precursors** (ALA and PBG). Porphyria is named from the ancient Greek word *porphura*, meaning purple. Purple color caused by pigment like porphyrins in the urine of some patients with defects in heme synthesis. **Six** types of porphyrias reported worldwide.

Most of the porphyrias are inherited **autosomal dominant** except **congenital erythropoietic porphyria** which is genetically **autosomal recessive** disease.

Classification of Porphyria

Porphyrias are classified on the basis of the tissue where the enzyme deficiency occurs. These are **(Table 14.1)**:

1. **Erythropoietic** porphyria (enzyme deficiency occurs in erythropoietic cells of bone marrow). For example:
   - Congenital erythropoietic porphyria
   - Protoporphyria
2. **Hepatic** porphyria (enzyme deficiency occurs in liver). For example:
   - Acute intermittent porphyria
   - Porphyria cutanea tarda

TABLE 14.1: Types of porphyrias and their major findings.

Type	Class	Enzyme involved	Major signs and symptoms
Acute intermittent porphyria	Hepatic	Uroporphyrinogen I Synthase (PBG deaminase or hydroxymethylbilane synthase)	Abdominal pain, neuropsychiatric symptoms
Congenital erythropoietic	Erythropoietic	Uroporphyrinogen III synthase	Photosensitivity
Porphyria cutanea tarda	Hepatic	Uroporphyrinogen decarboxylase	Photosensitivity
Hereditary coproporphyria	Hepatic	Coproporphyrinogen oxidase	Photosensitivity, abdominal pain, neuropsychiatric symptoms
Variegate porphyria	Hepatic	Protoporphyrinogen oxidase	Photosensitivity, abdominal pain, neuropsychiatric symptoms
Protoporphyria	Erythropoietic	Ferrochelatase	Photosensitivity

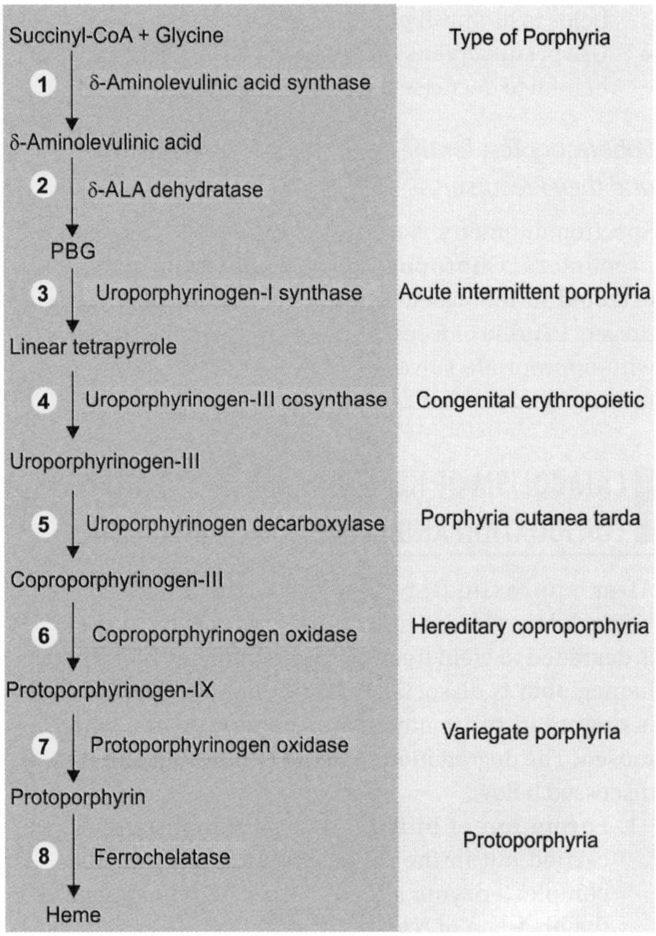

Succinyl-CoA + Glycine   Type of Porphyria

1 δ-Aminolevulinic acid synthase

δ-Aminolevulinic acid

2 δ-ALA dehydratase

PBG

3 Uroporphyrinogen-I synthase   Acute intermittent porphyria

Linear tetrapyrrole

4 Uroporphyrinogen-III cosynthase   Congenital erythropoietic

Uroporphyrinogen-III

5 Uroporphyrinogen decarboxylase   Porphyria cutanea tarda

Coproporphyrinogen-III

6 Coproporphyrinogen oxidase   Hereditary coproporphyria

Protoporphyrinogen-IX

7 Protoporphyrinogen oxidase   Variegate porphyria

Protoporphyrin

8 Ferrochelatase   Protoporphyria

Heme

Figure 14.3: Porphyrias caused by mutations of enzymes.

- Hereditary coproporphyria
- Variegate porphyria

Major types of porphyria and deficient of enzymes are shown in **Figure 14.3**.

Mnemonic

All congenital porphyria comprise variable presentation (ACPCVP)

- **A:** Acute intermittent porphyria (Deficient of enzyme: porphobilinogen deaminase or hydroxymethylbilane synthase).
- **C:** Congenital erythropoietic porphyria (Deficient of enzyme: uroporphyrinogen III synthase).

- **P:** Porphyria cutanea tarda (Deficient of enzyme: uroporphyrinogen decarboxylase).
- **C:** Coproporphyria (Deficient of enzyme: coproporphyrinogen oxidase).
- **V:** Variegate porphyria (Deficient of enzyme: protoporphyrinogen oxidase).
- **P:** Protoporphyria (Deficient of enzyme: ferrochelatase).

Clinical Features

Clinical features depend upon the accumulated products **(Figure 14.4)**. Major signs and symptoms of porphyria are:

1. Photosensitivity
2. Abdominal pain
3. Neuropsychiatric symptoms

- Where the enzyme block occurs early in the pathway prior to the formation of porphyrinogens, **ALA** and **PBG** will accumulate in the body tissues and fluids. These compounds can impair the function of abdominal nerve and central nervous system, resulting in **abdominal pain** and **neuropsychiatric symptoms**.
- On the other hand, enzyme blocks later in the pathway, result in the accumulation of the **porphyrinogens** which on exposure to light auto-oxidized to corresponding **porphyrin** derivatives, causes **photosensitivity** to

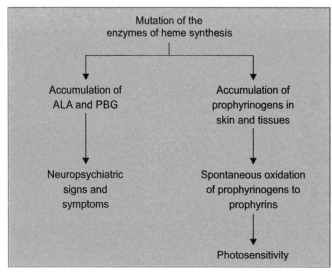

Figure 14.4: Biochemical basis of the major signs and symptoms of porphyrias.

visible light and **skin injuries (Figure 14.5)**. The injuries occur in the exposed areas where sunlight activates porphyrins, which reacts with molecular oxygen to form **oxygen radicals** in the skin. These oxygen radicals injure lysosomes and other organelles. Damaged lysosomes release their degradative enzymes causing skin damage.

- **Hydroxymethylbilane** is the 1st porphyrin of the pathway which is able to absorb light and cause photosensitivity. Hence, defects above will have no **photosensitivity** and defects below will have **photosensitivity**.

- One of the rare porphyrias, **congenital erythropoietic porphyria**, results in an accumulation of uroporphyrinogen I, an abnormal isomer. Uroporphyrin I, coproporphyrin I, also accumulate. The urine of patients having this disease is red because of excretion of large amounts of uroporphyrinogen I. Their teeth exhibit a strong red fluorescence under ultraviolet light (**Figure 14.6**) because of the deposition of porphyrins.

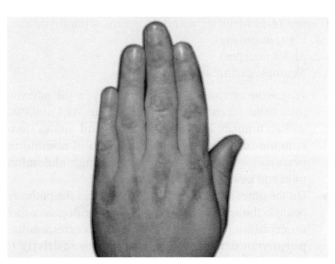

Figure 14.5: Skin lesion in a patient with porphyria cutanea tarda.

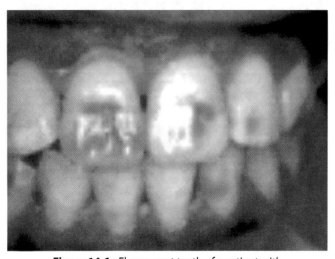

Figure 14.6: Fluorescent teeth of a patient with porphyria cutanea tarda.

Treatment of Porphyria

Present treatment of porphyria is basically symptomatic. The symptoms of most porphyrias are now readily controlled with dietary changes or administration of heme or heme derivatives. This includes:

- Ingestion of large amounts of **carbohydrate**, and administration of **hematin** to repress synthesis of ALA synthase. ALA synthase diminish production of harmful heme precursors.
- Avoid drugs that cause production of **Cytochrome P450**.
- β-carotene decreases the production of free radicals and helps to diminish photosensitivity.
- Use of **sunscreens** that filter out visible light can also be helpful to decrease the photosensitivity.

Laboratory Test for the Detection of Porphyrins and their Precursors

Spectrophotometry is used to detect porphyrins and their precursors. Coproporphyrins and uroporphyrins are excreted in increased amounts in the porphyrias. When present in urine or feces, they can be separated by extraction with appropriate solvents, then identified and quantified using spectrophotometric methods.

CATABOLISM OF HEME: FORMATION, TRANSPORT, CONJUGATION AND EXCRETION OF BILIRUBIN

After approximately 120 days, the heme group of hemoglobin released from dying erythrocytes in the spleen is degraded to yield free Fe^{2+} and, ultimately bilirubin. First hemoglobin is dissociated into **heme** and **globin**. Globin is degraded to its constituent amino acids, which are reused. The degradation of heme to bilirubin and its fate is discussed below.

1. **Formation of bilirubin:** The catabolism of heme is carried out in the microsomal fractions of cells by a complex enzyme system called **heme oxygenase**, in the presence of **NADPH** and **O$_2$**. Ferric ion and carbon monoxide (CO) are released with production of the green pigment **biliverdin**. Biliverdin is reduced to red yellow colored **bilirubin (Figure 14.7)**. Bilirubin and its derivatives are collectively termed **bile pigments**.
   - One gram of hemoglobin yields 35 mg of bilirubin.
   - The daily bilirubin formation in human adults is approximately **250 to 350** mg deriving mainly not only from hemoglobin but from ineffective erythropoiesis and from various other heme proteins such as cytochrome P450.
   - The further metabolism and excretion of bilirubin occurs in the **liver** and **intestine**.
   - The catabolism of heme is regulated at the first step, catalyzed by **heme oxygenase**.
2. **Transport and uptake of bilirubin by the liver:**

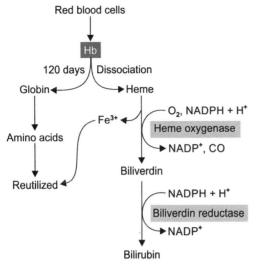

Figure 14.7: Degradation of hemoglobin to bilirubin.

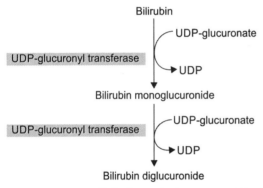

Figure 14.8: Conjugation of bilirubin with glucuronic acid in the liver.

- Bilirubin is only sparingly water-soluble. Bilirubin formed in peripheral tissues is transported to the **liver** by binding to **serum albumin**.
- In the liver the bilirubin is removed from albumin and taken up by hepatocyte. Once internalized, bilirubin binds to cytosolic proteins, such as glutathione S-transferase, previously known as ligandin to prevent bilirubin from re-entering the blood stream.

> Antibiotics and certain other drugs compete with bilirubin for binding to albumin. Thus, antibiotics can displace bilirubin from albumin and diffuse into tissues.

3. **Conjugation and secretion of bilirubin:**
   - Hepatocytes convert sparingly soluble, nonpolar bilirubin to a more soluble, polar form, by conjugation with two molecules of glucuronic acid.
   - This reaction is catalyzed by **UDP-glucuronyl transferase** using UDP-glucuronate as a source of glucuronate. Bilirubin monoglucuronide is formed first then it is subsequently converted to the **bilirubin diglucuronide (Figure 14.8)**.

- Most of the bilirubin secreted in the bile is in the form of bilirubin diglucuronide, (conjugated form of bilirubin) which occurs by an active transport mechanism and is a **rate limiting step for the entire process of hepatic bilirubin metabolism**.
- Unconjugated bilirubin is not secreted into bile.

4. **Excretion of bilirubin:**
   - Bilirubin is excreted in the form of **stercobilin** and **urobilinogen** through feces and urine, respectively.
   - Following secretion into bile, conjugated bilirubin passes through the hepatic and common bile ducts into the intestinal lumen.
   - Bilirubin diglucuronide is hydrolyzed in the intestine by **bacterial enzymes β-glucuronidase** to liberate **free bilirubin**.
   - The free bilirubin so formed is further reduced to a colorless **urobilinogen**, a part of which absorbed from the gut into the portal circulation **(Figure 14.9)**. The urobilinogen which is absorbed into portal circulation can take two alternative routes.
     - A part of it enters the systemic circulation and transported to the kidneys, where it is oxidized to **urobilin** (orange yellow pigment) and excreted in urine. The normal umber yellow color of urine is due to urobilin.
     - A part of the urobilinogen is returned to the liver and re-excreted through liver to the intestine, known as **enterohepatic urobilinogen cycle**.
   - The major portion of urobilinogen which remains within intestinal lumen is reduced further in the intestine to **stercobilinogen**, which is excreted as an oxidized brown pigment **stercobilin** in the faeces. The characteristic brown color of stool is due to stercobilin. **Figure 14.8** shows the five major processes involved in the metabolism of hemoglobin.

STRIKE A NOTE

- ❖ Heme breakdown pathway is the only **endogenous source of carbon monoxide (CO) in humans**. A fraction of the carbon monoxide is released via the respiratory tract. Thus, the measurement of carbon monoxide in an exhaled breath provides an index of the quantity of heme that is degraded in an individual.
- ❖ The CO produced by heme oxygenase is toxic at high concentrations, but very low concentrations generated during heme degradation have some regulatory and/or signaling functions.
- ❖ Bilirubin is much less soluble in aqueous media than is biliverdin.
- ❖ Bilirubin is a very effective and most abundant antioxidant; whereas biliverdin is not.

DISORDERS OF BILIRUBIN METABOLISM: JAUNDICE AND CONGENITAL HYPERBILIRUBINEMIA

- The normal concentration of serum bilirubin is:
  - *Total bilirubin:* 0.1 to 1.0 mg/dL

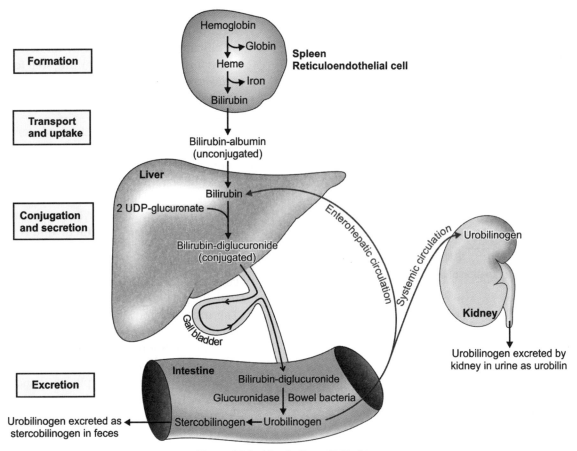

Figure 14.9: Metabolism of bilirubin.

- *Conjugated (direct) bilirubin:* 0.1 to 0.4 mg/dL
- *Unconjugated (indirect) bilirubin:* 0.2 to 0.7 mg/dL.
- Diseases or conditions that interfere with bilirubin metabolism may cause a rise in its serum concentration. When **bilirubin in the blood** (unconjugated or conjugated) **exceeds 1 mg/dL**, **hyperbilirubinemia** exists.
- Hyperbilirubinemia may be due to:
  - Increased bilirubin production
  - Decreased hepatic uptake
  - Decreased hepatic conjugation
  - Decreased excretion of bilirubin into bile.
- In all these situations bilirubin accumulates in the blood, and when it reaches a certain concentration, approximately **2.2–5 mg/dL**, it diffuses into the tissues. The skin and sclera (whites of the eyes) appear yellowish due to deposition of bilirubin in the tissues. The condition is called **jaundice** or **icterus**. The cell toxicity associated with jaundice may be due to bilirubin levels in excess of the serum albumin needed to solubilize it. Hyperbilirubinemia may be **acquired** or **inherited** (Table 14.2).

Acquired hyperbilirubinemia are:
- Hemolytic jaundice (prehepatic jaundice)
- Hepatic jaundice (hepatocellular jaundice)
- Obstructive jaundice (posthepatic jaundice)
- Neonatal jaundice (physiological jaundice)

Type	Conjugated hyperbilirubinemia	Unconjugated hyperbilirubinemia
Acquired	• Obstructive jaundice • Hepatic jaundice	• Hemolytic jaundice • Hepatic jaundice • Neonatal jaundice
Inherited	• Dubin-Johnson syndrome • Rotor syndrome	• Crigler-Najjar syndrome • Gilbert's syndrome

TABLE 14.2: Conjugated and unconjugated hyperbilirubinemia.

Inherited hyperbilirubinemia are:
- Gilbert's syndrome
- Crigler-Najjar syndrome
- Dubin-Johnson syndrome
- Rotor syndrome.

Acquired Hyperbilirubinemia

Prehepatic or Hemolytic Jaundice

In prehepatic or hemolytic jaundice, there is increased breakdown of hemoglobin to bilirubin at a rate in excess of the ability of the liver cell to conjugate and excrete it. Excess hemolysis may be due to:
- Sickle hemoglobin
- Deficiency of enzyme **glucose-6-phosphate dehydrogenase**
- Incompatible blood transfusion.

Since the excess bilirubin is **unconjugated**, it cannot be excreted in the urine. The urine color is normal; therefore it is also called **"acholuric jaundice"**. More than normal amounts of bilirubin are excreted into the intestine, resulting in an increased amount of urobilinogen in feces and urine. The main biochemical features of the hemolytic jaundice are:

- Increased plasma concentration of unconjugated bilirubin
- Increased amount of urobilinogen in urine and feces
- Absence of bilirubin in the urine.

Hepatocellular or Hepatic Jaundice

In this kind of jaundice, there is some disorder of the liver cells or the bile passage within the liver. Hepatic parenchymal cell damage impairs conjugation of bilirubin and results in **unconjugated hyperbilirubinemia**. Patients with jaundice due to hepatocellular damage commonly have obstruction of the biliary tree with the liver that results in the **presence of some conjugated hyperbilirubinemia** also. Hepatocellular damage is usually caused by:

- Infections (viral hepatitis)
- Toxic chemicals (such as alcohol, chloroform, carbon tetrachloride, etc.)
- Drugs
- Cirrhosis.

The main biochemical features are:

- Increased serum concentration of conjugated and unconjugated bilirubin
- Decreased amount of urobilinogen in urine and feces
- Presence of bilirubin in the urine
- Raised level of alanine transaminase (ALT) and aspartate transaminase (AST) enzymes (hepatic cell damage allows intracellular enzymes to leak into the blood).

Post hepatic or Obstructive Jaundice

This occurs when there is an obstruction in the passage of conjugated bilirubin from the liver cells to the intestine. The condition is also called **cholestasis**, (the obstruction of biliary flow). The obstruction may be intrahepatic or extrahepatic. Extrahepatic cholestasis occurs due to:

- Blockage of the common bile duct by gallstones
- Carcinoma of the head of the pancreas
- Carcinoma of the duct itself.

The main biochemical manifestations of obstructive jaundice are:

- Increased plasma concentration of conjugated bilirubin
- Absence of urobilinogen in feces and urine
- The presence of bilirubin and bile salts in the urine
- Raised level of plasma alkaline phosphatase (ALP). ALP is normally excreted through bile. Obstruction to the flow of bile causes regurgitation of enzyme into the blood resulting in increased serum concentration.

Neonatal Jaundice (Physiologic Jaundice)

Newborn infants sometime develop jaundice because; the liver of the newborn is deficient in enzyme **UDP-glucuronyl transferase**, necessary for conjugation. Mild jaundice in the first few days after birth is common and physiological. It results from an accelerated **hemolysis** and **immature liver enzyme system** for conjugation of bilirubin in the newborn. The enzyme deficiency is more serious with increasing degrees of prematurity.

Since the increased bilirubin is unconjugated, it is capable of penetrating the blood brain barrier when its concentration in plasma exceeds 20–25 mg/dL. This results in a **hyperbilirubinemia toxic encephalopathy** or **kernicterus**, which can cause mental retardation

A traditional treatment to reduce excess bilirubin, exposure to fluorescent lamp, causes a photochemical conversion of bilirubin to compounds that are more soluble and easily excreted.

Inherited Hyperbilirubinemias

There is a group of inherited disorders of bilirubin metabolism, in which either **unconjugated** or **conjugated hyperbilirubinemia** is the only detectable abnormality. Most of these disorders occur due to mutations in the gene encoding for certain enzymes of bilirubin metabolism.

Gilbert's Syndrome

Gilbert's syndrome is an inherited disease characterized by mild benign (harmless) unconjugated hyperbilirubinemia due to:

- Impaired hepatic uptake of bilirubin
- Partial conjugation defect due to reduced activity of **UDP-glucuronyl transferase**.

Crigler-Najjar Syndrome

This is a rare autosomal recessive disorder due to total absence of **hepatic glucuronyl transferase** enzyme. As a result conjugation does not take place. There are two forms of this condition:

- **Type-I** is characterized by complete absence of the conjugating enzyme **glucuronyl transferase** and therefore no conjugated bilirubin is formed and unconjugated bilirubin accumulates in serum, above 20 mg/dL. It causes severe jaundice, brain damage with kernicterus and early death. Phototherapy reduces plasma bilirubin levels to some extent, but phenobarbital has no beneficial effect. The disease is often fatal within the first 15 months of life.
- **Type-II** is a less severe form in which the enzyme deficiency is partial and serum bilirubin tends not to exceed 20 mg/dL of serum. A patient responds to treatment with large dose of phenobarbital and is compatible with more prolonged survival.

TABLE 14.3: Laboratory findings in the differential diagnosis of jaundice.

Condition	Serum bilirubin		Urine	Urine	Fecal
	Conjugated (direct)	**Unconjugated (indirect)**	**Urobilinogen**	**Bilirubin**	**Urobilinogen**
Normal	0.1–0.4 mg/dL	0.2–0.7 mg/dL	0.4 mg/24 h	Absent	40–280 mg/24 h
Hemolytic	Normal	Increased	Increased	Absent	Increased
Hepatocellular	Increased	Increased	Decreased (if micro-obstruction is present)	Present (if micro-obstruction is present)	Decreased
Obstructive	Increased	Normal	Absent	Present	Trace to absent

Dubin-Johnson Syndrome

This is harmless autosomal recessive disorder and is due to defective hepatic secretion of **conjugated bilirubin** into the bile and is characterized by slightly raised plasma **conjugated bilirubin** level in childhood or during adult life.

The conjugated hyperbilirubinemia is caused by mutations in the gene encoding the protein involved in the secretion of conjugated bilirubin into bile. It is also characterized by abnormal black pigment in the hepatocytes, imparting a dark brown to black color to the liver.

Rotor Syndrome

It is similar in most respects to the Dubin-Johnson syndrome but liver cells are not pigmented.

LABORATORY TESTS DONE TO DIFFERENTIATE JAUNDICE

1. **Serum bilirubin: Van den Bergh test** is a chemical method to estimate bilirubin in serum.
   - Bilirubin + Ehrlich's Diazo reagent (diazotized sulfanilic acid)

- Radish purple azo-pigment is formed.
- They are analyzed by photometry at 540 nm.

The two types of reactions of Van den Bergh test are: **Direct and indirect**

- For conjugated bilirubin direct Van den Bergh test is positive, so **conjugated bilirubin** is called **direct bilirubin**
- For unconjugated bilirubin indirect Van den Bergh test is positive, so **unconjugated bilirubin** is called **indirect bilirubin**

2. **Test in urine:** Urine is tested for presence of **bilirubin**, **urobilinogen** and **bile salts**
   - Urine bilirubin is tested by modified **Fouchet's test**
   - Urine and fecal urobilinogen is tested by **Ehrlich's test**
   - Urine bile salts tested by Hay's test, and Pettenkofer test

3. **Liver enzyme assay**
   - Transaminases (AST and ALT) elevated in hepatitis
   - Alkaline phosphatase elevated in obstructive jaundice
   - 5' Nucleotidase in obstructive jaundice

Table 14.3 summarizes laboratory findings in the differential diagnosis of jaundice.

ASSESSMENT QUESTIONS

STRUCTURED LONG ESSAY QUESTIONS (SLEQs)

1. Describe heme biosynthesis under following headings:
   i. Pathway
   ii. Regulation
   iii. Different types of porphyria with defective enzymes
2. Describe the catabolism of heme under following headings:
   i. Formation of bilirubin
   ii. Fate of bilirubin
   iii. Acquired disorder of bilirubin metabolism

SHORT ESSAY QUESTIONS (SEQs)

1. What are porphyrias? Describe any three porphyrias.
2. What are the signs and symptoms of porphyria? Give biochemical basis of the same.

3. Write laboratory investigations in different types of Jaundice.
4. What is hyperbilirubinemia? Write congenital hyperbilirubinemias.
5. Write differential diagnosis of jaundice.

SHORT ANSWER QUESTIONS (SAQs)

1. Name any two congenital hyperbilirubinemias and their defective enzyme.
2. Write regulation of heme synthesis.
3. Name defective enzyme, in acute intermittent porphyria and congenital erythropoietic porphyria.
4. Write significance of Van den Berg test.
5. Write urinary findings in jaundice.

CASE VIGNETTE-BASED QUESTIONS (CVBQs)

Case Study

1. **A 53-year-old woman developed a hyperpigmentation and rash on her neck and photosensitive nature, a diagnosis of porphyria cutanea tarda was considered.**

   Questions
   a. What is porphyria?
   b. What are the types of porphyria?
   c. Which enzyme is defective in porphyria cutanea tarda?

2. **A 45-year-old woman complains of acute abdominal pain and vomiting following fatty food. The biochemical investigations are:**
   a. **Raised serum conjugated bilirubin.**
   b. **Significantly raised serum alkaline phosphatase.**
   c. **Excretion of dark yellow colored urine.**
   d. **Fouchet's test on fresh urine shows green color.**

   Questions
   a. Name the disease.
   b. Give differential diagnosis of the condition.

3. **A 50-year-old woman visited hospital with history of anorexia, nausea, and flu like symptoms. She had noticed that her urine had been dark in color over the past 2 days. Her LFTs were as follows:**
   i. Total bilirubin (direct and indirect): Increased
   ii. AST and ALT: Marked increased activity
   iii. Alkaline phosphatase: Increased

   Questions
   a. Comment on these results.
   b. What is the differential diagnosis?

4. **A 30-year-old male presented at clinical with history of intermittent abdominal pain and episodes of confusion and psychiatric problems. Laboratory tests revealed increase of urinary δ-aminolevulinate and porphobilinogen. Mutational analysis revealed a mutation in the gene for uroporphyrinogen synthase (porphobilinogen deaminase).**

   Questions
   a. What is the probable diagnosis?
   b. What is the cause of abdominal pain and psychiatric problem?
   c. The disorder concern with which metabolic pathway.
   d. Name some other disorders related to same pathway.

5. **A 62-year-old female presented at clinic with intense jaundice she had noted that her stools had been very pale. Lab test revealed a very high level of direct bilirubin. The level of alkaline phosphates was markedly elevated.**

   Questions
   a. What is the probable diagnosis?
   b. Why color of stool is very pale?
   c. What is the status of urine bilirubin?
   d. What is direct and indirect bilirubin?

6. **A 58-year-old man complained of increased skin lesion formation on his hands, forehead, neck, and ears on exposure to the sun. Laboratory findings showed an increase in urinary uroporphyrin with normal levels of ALA and porphobilinogen. Mutational analysis showed mutation in the gene for uroporphyrinogen decarboxylase.**

   Questions
   a. What is the probable type of porphyria?
   b. Which are the other types of porphyria?
   c. What is the cause of skin lesion?
   d. What is porphyria?

7. **A boy presented at clinic with staining of teeth and raised coproporphyrinogen I levels, and increased photosensitivity:**

   Questions
   a. What is the probable type of porphyria?
   b. Which enzyme is deficient?
   c. What is the cause of photosensitivity?
   d. Name other types of porphyria

8. **A 14-year-old girl was admitted to the medical ward after she developed yellowish discoloration of the eye, marked loss of appetite, low grated fever (100–101°F) nausea and occasional vomiting in the last one week. She had pain in the right hypochondrium and urine was high colored. She looked weak and malnourished also:**

   Serum LFT was done and following were the results:
   – Total Bilirubin   –8 mg%
   – Direct Bilirubin   –4.8 mg%
   – Serum AST   –980 IU/L
   – Serum ALT   –1210 IU/L
   – Serum ALP   –20 KA units

   Questions
   a. What is the probable diagnosis? Justify.
   b. What are the common causes of the above diagnosed case?
   c. Which metabolism is mainly affected in the above case?
   d. What is the reference ranges of the above parameters?
   e. What test would you do to detect the bile pigments in the urine sample of this patient? Explain the likely results of these tests.

MULTIPLE CHOICE QUESTIONS (MCQs)

1. Acute intermittent porphyria is accompanied by increased urinary excretion of:
   a. Porphobilinogen   b. Heme
   c. Bilirubin   d. Biliverdin

2. The normal brown red color of feces results from the presence of:
   a. Stercobilin   b. Bilirubin
   c. Biliverdin   d. Bilirubin diglucuronide

3. The end product of catabolism of heme is:
   a. Bile acids   b. Bile salts
   c. Bile pigment   d. Uric acid

4. Unconjugated bilirubin is raised mostly in:
   a. Hemolytic jaundice
   b. Obstructive jaundice
   c. Carcinoma of pancreas
   d. Stone in gallbladder

5. The rate limiting reaction in heme synthesis is catalyzed by:
   a. δ-ALA dehydratase
   b. δ-ALA synthase
   c. Ferrochelatase
   d. Uroporphyrinogen decarboxylase

6. Which of the following statements is not applicable to bilirubin?
   a. Bilirubin is carried in the plasma to the liver bound to albumin
   b. High levels of bilirubin can cause damage to brain of newborn infants.
   c. Bilirubin is water soluble
   d. Bilirubin does not contain iron

7. The biosynthesis of heme requires all of the following, *except*:
   a. Succinyl CoA
   b. Glycine
   c. Ferrous ion
   d. Glutamine

8. Lead poisoning leads to increased level of:
   a. Bilirubin
   b. δ-aminolevulinic acid
   c. Porphobilinogen
   d. Coproporphyrin

9. Increased level of conjugated bilirubin in blood occurs in the following condition, *except*:
   a. Hemolytic jaundice
   b. Hepatocellular jaundice
   c. Obstructive jaundice
   d. Dubin-Johnson syndrome

10. In lead poisoning which of the following is seen in urine:
    a. δ-aminolevulinic acid
    b. Uroporphyrin
    c. Coproporphyrin
    d. Protoporphyrin

11. Acute intermittent porphyria is caused by:
    a. Protoporphyrinogen oxidase
    b. Coproporphyrinogen oxidase
    c. Ferrochelatase
    d. HMB synthase

12. The porphyria which does not show photosensitivity is:
    a. Acute intermittent porphyria
    b. Erythropoietic porphyria
    c. Hereditary coproporphyria
    d. Porphyria cutanea tarda

13. Hepatic glucuronyl transferase deficiency occurs in which of the following condition:
    a. Dubin-Johnson syndrome
    b. Crigler-Najjar syndrome
    c. Lesch-Nyhan syndrome
    d. None of the above.

14. Protoporphyria is due to deficiency of:
    a. Protoporphyrinogen oxidase
    b. Coproporphyrinogen oxidase
    c. Ferrochelatase
    d. Uroporphyrinogen decarboxylase

15. Porphyrias is a inherited disorder of which of the following synthetic pathway:
    a. Glycogen
    b. Heme
    c. Purine nucleoids
    d. Cholesterol

16. Heme biosynthesis does not occur in:
    a. Osteocytes
    b. Liver
    c. RBC
    d. Erythroid cells of bone marrow

17. In variegate porphyria the defective enzyme is:
    a. Protoporphyrinogen oxidase
    b. Coproporphyrinogen oxidase
    c. Ferrochelatase
    d. Uroporphyrinogen decarboxylase

18. A 10-year-boy presents with increase bilirubin in urine and no urobilinogen. Diagnosis is:
    a. Gilbert syndrome
    b. Hemolytic jaundice
    c. Viral hepatitis
    d. Obstructive jaundice

19. All of the following types of porphyrias are autosomal dominant, *except:*
    a. Acute intermittent porphyria
    b. Congenital erythropoietic porphyria
    c. Hereditary coproporphyria
    d. Porphyria cutanea tarda

20. What is expected out of Van den Bergh reaction in hepatic jaundice?
    a. Direct positive
    b. Indirect positive
    c. Biphasic
    d. None of the above

21. A girl licks paint that is peeled off from the toys, develop acute abdominal pain, tingling sensation of hands and legs and weakness. Which enzyme is inhibited in this child?
    a. ALA synthase
    b. Heme oxygenase
    c. Coproporphyrinogen oxidase
    d. ALA dehydratase

22. A boy with staining of teeth and raised coproporphyrin-I levels and increased risk of photosensitivity, the enzyme deficient is:
    a. Uroporphyrinogen synthase
    b. Uroporphyrinogen III synthase
    c. Uroporphyrinogen decarboxylase
    d. Coproporphyrinogen oxidase

ANSWERS FOR MCQs

1. a	2. a	3. c	4. a	5. b
6. c	7. d	8. b	9. a	10. a
11. d	12. a	13. b	14. c	15. b
16. c	17. a	18. d	19. b	20. c
21. d	22. b			

15 CHAPTER

Minerals

Competency	Learning Objectives
BI 6.9: Describe the functions of various minerals in the body, their metabolism and homeostasis. **BI 6.10:** Enumerate and describe the disorders associated with mineral metabolism.	1. Describe metabolism of sodium and potassium: Sources, RDA, absorption and transport, functions, reference range, homeostasis, and associated disorders. 2. Describe metabolism of calcium, phosphorus, and magnesium: Sources, RDA, absorption and transport, functions, reference range, homeostasis, and associated disorders. 3. Describe metabolism of trace elements: Sources, RDA, absorption and transport, functions, and associated disorders.

OVERVIEW

Minerals are inorganic elements, required for a variety of functions. The minerals required in human nutrition can be grouped into **macrominerals** and **microminerals (trace elements)**. The macrominerals are required in excess of **100 mg/day**. The microminerals or trace elements are required in amounts **less than 100 mg/day**.

The major minerals required in human nutrition are given in **Table 15.1**. The principal functions and deficiency manifestations of each of the macro and microminerals are summarized in **Table 15.2**.

METABOLISM OF SODIUM AND POTASSIUM

Sodium and potassium are grouped together because they have an important role in maintaining:
- Electrical neutrality
- Osmotic pressure
- Water and acid-base balance.

Na⁺ is the major cation of **extracellular fluids**, while **potassium (K⁺)** is of **intracellular fluids**. Plasma concentrations of these ions are:
- **Sodium:** 135 to 145 mEq/L
- **Potassium:** 3.5 to 5 mEq/L.

TABLE 15.1: Major minerals required in human nutrition.

Macrominerals	Microminerals or trace elements
Sodium	Copper
Potassium	Fluoride
Calcium	Iodine
Phosphorus	Iron
Magnesium	Molybdenum
Sulfur	Selenium
	Zinc

Sodium

The total body sodium of the average 70 kg man is approximately 3,700 mmol or 1.8 g/kg, of which approximately 75% is exchangeable and 25% is nonexchangeable, which is incorporated into tissues such as bone. Most of the exchangeable sodium is in the extracellular fluid. In the extracellular fluid the sodium concentration is tightly regulated at **140 mEq/L**.

Dietary Food Sources

Table salt (NaCl), salty foods, animal foods, milk, baking soda, baking powder, some vegetables.

TABLE 15.2: Principal functions and deficiency manifestations of macrominerals and microminerals.

Element	Metabolic function	Deficiency manifestation
Macrominerals		
Sodium	Principal extracellular cation, buffer constituent, water and acid-base balance, cell membrane permeability	Dehydration, acidosis, excess leads to edema, and hypertension
Potassium	Principal intracellular cation, buffer constituent, water and acid-base balance, neuromuscular irritability	Muscle weakness, paralysis and mental confusion, acidosis
Calcium	Constituent of bone and teeth, blood clotting, regulation of nerve, muscle and hormone function	Tetany, muscle cramps, convulsions, osteoporosis, rickets
Phosphorus	Constituent of bone and teeth, nucleic acids, and NAD, FAD, ATP, etc. Required for energy metabolism	Growth retardation, skeletal deformities, muscle weakness, cardiac arrhythmia
Magnesium	Cofactor for phosphate transferring enzymes, constituent of bones and teeth, muscle contraction, nerve transmission	Muscle spasms, tetany, confusions, seizures
Microminerals or trace elements		
Copper	Constituent of oxidase enzymes, e.g., tyrosinase, cytochrome oxidase, ferroxidase and ceruloplasmin, iron absorption and mobilization	Microcytic hypochromic anemia, depigmentation of skin, hair. Excessive deposition in liver in Wilson's disease
Fluoride	Constituent of bone and teeth, strengthens bone and teeth	Dental caries
Iodine	Constituent of thyroid hormones (T_3 and T_4)	Cretinism in children and goiter in adults
Iron	Constituent of heme and nonheme compounds and transport, storage of O_2	Microcytic anemia
Molybdenum	Constituent of xanthine oxidase, sulfite oxidase, and aldehyde oxidase	Xanthinuria
Selenium	Antioxidant, cofactor for glutathione peroxidase, protects cell against membrane lipid peroxidation	Cardiomyopathy
Zinc	Cofactor for enzymes in DNA, RNA and protein synthesis, constituent of insulin, carbonic anhydrase, carboxypeptidase, LDH, alcohol dehydrogenase, alkaline phosphatase, etc	Growth failure, impaired wound healing, defects in taste and smell, loss of appetite

Recommended Dietary Allowance (RDA) per Day

- 1 to 5 g
- 5 g NaCl per day is recommended for adults without history of hypertension
- 1 g NaCl per day is recommended with history of hypertension.

Homeostasis of Sodium

Sodium readily absorbed in the bloodstream via the epithelial cell by an active transport. Dietary intakes of Na⁺ are very variable worldwide but are usually matched by their corresponding urinary losses. There is normally little loss of these ions through the skin (sweat) and in the feces. Urinary sodium output is regulated by four mechanisms:

1. **The renin-angiotensin-aldosterone system (RAAS)** (For discussion of mechanisms refer, **Water and Electrolyte Balance; Chapter 16**).
2. **Atrial natriuretic peptide** (For discussion of mechanisms refer, **Water and Electrolyte Balance; Chapter 16**).
3. **The glomerular filtration rate (GFR):** The rate of Na⁺ excretion is related to the GFR. When the GFR falls actually, less Na⁺ is excreted and vice-versa.

4. **Dopamine:** An increase in filtered sodium load causes increased dopamine synthesis by proximal tubule cells. The dopamine then acts on the distal tubule to stimulate Na⁺ excretion.

Metabolic Functions

- It maintains the **osmotic pressure** and **water balance**
- It is a constituent of **buffer** and involved in the maintenance of **acid-base balance**
- It maintains **muscle** and nerve **irritability** at the proper level
- Sodium is involved in **cell membrane permeability**.

Clinical Conditions Related to Plasma Sodium Level Alterations

For discussion of clinical conditions related to plasma sodium level alterations refer, **Water and Electrolyte Balance; Chapter 16.**

Potassium

Potassium is the main **intracellular cation**. About 98% of total body potassium is in cells (150–160 mEq/L), only 2%

in the ECF (3.5–5 mEq/L). Total body potassium in an adult male is about 50 mEq/kg of body weight and is influenced by age, sex, and muscle mass, since most of the body's potassium is found in muscles.

Dietary Food Sources

Vegetables, fruits, whole grain, meat, milk, legumes, and tender coconut water.

Recommended Dietary Allowance per Day

2 to 5 g.

Serum Potassium

Normal range of serum potassium is **3.5** to **5 mEq/L**.

Body Potassium Homeostasis

Potassium is absorbed readily by passive diffusion from gastrointestinal tract. The amount of potassium in the body depends on the balance between potassium intake and output. Potassium output occurs through three primary routes, the **gastrointestinal tract**, the **skin**, and the **urine**.

- Under normal conditions loss of potassium through gastrointestinal tract and skin is very small. The major means of K^+ excretion is by the kidney.
- The kidney is capable of regulating the excretion of potassium to maintain the body potassium homeostasis. Intake is normally closely matched by the urinary excretion.
- Nearly all the potassium filtered at the glomerulus is reabsorbed in the proximal tubule. Less than 10% reaches the distal tubule, where the main regulation of potassium excretion occurs. Secretion of potassium in response to alterations in dietary intake occurs in the distal tubules.
- The **distal tubule** is an important site of **sodium reabsorption**. When sodium is reabsorbed, the tubular lumen becomes electronegative in relation to the adjacent cell and cations in the cell (e.g., K^+ or H^+) move into the lumen to balance the charge.
- **Thus during the sodium reabsorption there is an obligatory loss of potassium.** The rate of excretion of potassium depends on the rate of reabsorption of sodium by the distal tubule and on the concentration of potassium in the tubular cells.

Metabolic Functions

- Potassium maintains the intracellular **osmotic pressure, water balance, and acid-base balance**.
- It influences neuromuscular activity of cardiac and skeletal muscle
- Several glycolytic enzymes need potassium for their function
- Potassium is required for **transmission of nerve impulses**

- Nuclear activity and protein synthesis are dependent on potassium.

METABOLISM OF CALCIUM, PHOSPHORUS, AND MAGNESIUM

Calcium

Calcium is the most abundant mineral in the body. The adult human body contains about 1 kg of calcium. About 99% the body's calcium is present in bone together with phosphate as the mineral **hydroxyapatite [Ca$_{10}$ (PO$_4$)$_6$ (OH)$_2$]**, with small amounts in soft tissue and extracellular fluid **(Table 15.3)**.

Calcium is present in plasma in three forms:

1. **Free** or **unbound** or **ionic calcium, Ca^{2+}:** In blood 50% of the plasma calcium is free, unbound, ionic form which is functionally most active.
2. **Bound calcium:** 40% of the plasma calcium is bound to protein mostly to albumin.
3. **Complex calcium:** 10% of the plasma calcium is in complex with anions including bicarbonate HCO$_3^-$), phosphate (H$_2$PO$_4^-$), lactate and citrate.

All these three forms are in equilibrium with one another **(Figure 15.1). Unbound calcium (Ca^{2+}) is biologically active fraction of the total calcium in plasma** and maintenance of its concentration, within tight limits is required for nerve function, membrane permeability, muscle contraction, and hormone secretion.

TABLE 15.3: Distribution of calcium, phosphorus, and magnesium in the body.

Tissue	Relative distribution (%)		
	Calcium	Phosphorus	Magnesium
	1,000 g (Total)	600 g (Total)	25 g (Total)
Skeleton (bone)	99%	85%	55%
Soft tissue	1%	15%	45%
Extracellular fluid	<0.2%	<0.1%	1%

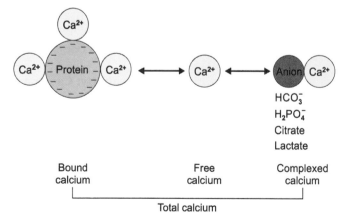

Figure 15.1: Equilibrium between physiochemical states of calcium in plasma.

Functions

- **Formation of bone and teeth:** 99% of the body's calcium is located in bone in the form of **hydroxyapatite crystal [3Ca$_3$ (PO$_4$)$_2$ Ca (OH)$_2$].** The hardness and rigidity of bone and teeth are due to hydroxyapatite. About 1 kg calcium is found in the skeleton of average adult man.
- **Blood coagulations:** Calcium present in platelets involved in blood coagulation, the conversion of an inactive protein prothrombin into an active thrombin requires calcium ions.
- **Muscle contraction:** Muscle contraction is initiated by the binding of calcium to troponin.
- **Release of hormones:** The release of certain hormones like parathyroid hormone, calcitonin, etc., requires calcium ions.
- **Release of neurotransmitters:** Influx (entry) of Ca^{2+} from extracellular space into neurons causes release of neurotransmitter.
- **Regulation of enzyme activity:** Activation of number of enzymes or binding proteins requires Ca^{2+} as a specific cofactor; calcium ions stabilize the active conformation of the enzyme, for example:
  - Allosteric activation of enzyme glycogen phosphorylase of glycogenolysis.
  - Activation of salivary and pancreatic α-amylase.
  - Three enzymes of TCA cycle: Pyruvate dehydrogenase, isocitrate dehydrogenase, and α-ketoglutarate dehydrogenase are activated by Ca^{2+}.
  - Pyruvate kinase, a rate limiting enzyme of glycolytic pathway is inhibited by calcium.
  - Calcium binds trypsin near its active site to prevent auto-digestion of trypsin.
- **Second messenger:** Calcium acts as a second messenger for hormone action. For example, it acts as a second messenger for **epinephrine** and **glucagon**. Ca also functions as a **third messenger** for some hormones such as **antidiuretic hormone (ADH).**
- **Cardiac activity:** Cardiac muscle depends on extracellular Ca^{2+} for contraction. Myocardial contractility increases with increased Ca^{2+} concentration and decreases with decreased calcium concentration. If cardiac muscle is deprived of Ca^{2+} ions, it ceases to beat within approximately 1 minute.
- **Membrane integrity and permeability:** Calcium is required for maintenance of integrity and permeability of the membrane.

Dietary Sources

The main dietary sources of calcium are:
- Milk and dairy products (half a liter of milk contains approximately 1,000 mg of calcium)
- Cheese
- Cereal grains
- Legumes
- Nuts
- Vegetables.

Recommended Dietary Allowance Per Day

- **Adults:** 800 mg/day
- **Women during pregnancy and lactation and for teenagers:** 1,200 mg/day
- **Infants:** 300–500 mg/day.

Absorption

Calcium is absorbed from small intestine and the degree of absorption is affected by different factors. Some of these are discussed below:

Factors that Stimulate Calcium Absorption

- **Vitamin D** stimulates absorption of calcium from intestine by inducing the synthesis of calcium binding protein, necessary for the absorption of calcium from intestine.
- **Parathyroid hormone** (PTH) stimulates calcium absorption indirectly via activating vitamin D.
- **Acidic pH:** Since, calcium salts are more soluble in acidic pH, the acidic foods and organic acids (citric acid, lactic acid, pyruvic acid, etc.) favor the absorption of calcium from intestine.
- **High protein diet** favors the absorption of calcium. Basic amino acids, lysine, and arginine derived from hydrolysis of the dietary proteins increase calcium absorption.
- **Lactose** is known to increase the absorption of calcium, by forming soluble complexes with the calcium ion.

Factors that Inhibit Calcium Absorption

- **Phytates** and **oxalates** bind dietary calcium forming insoluble salts which cannot be absorbed from the intestine. Phytates present in many cereals and oxalates present in green leafy vegetables.
- **High fat diet** decreases the absorption of calcium. High amounts of fatty acids derived from hydrolysis of dietary fats react with calcium to form insoluble calcium soaps which cannot be absorbed.
- **High phosphate content** in diet causes precipitation of calcium as calcium phosphate and thereby lowers the ratio of Ca:P in the intestine. The Ca:P ratio should be 1:2–2:1 for optimum absorption of calcium. When food contains almost equal amounts of calcium and phosphorus there is maximum absorption of calcium.
- **High fiber diet** decreases the absorption of calcium from intestine.

Excretion

The excretion of calcium is partly through the **kidneys** but mostly by way of the small intestine through feces. Small amount of calcium may also be lost in sweat.

Homeostasis of Plasma Calcium

The plasma calcium concentration in normal individual is approximately **9–11 mg%** (2–3 mEq/L). Homeostasis of plasma calcium is dependent on the:

- Functions of three main organs:
  1. Bone
  2. Kidney
  3. Intestine.
- Functions of three main hormones:
  1. Parathyroid hormone (PTH)
  2. Vitamin D or cholecalciferol or calcitriol
  3. Calcitonin.
- The four major regulating processes are:
  1. Absorption of calcium from the intestine, mainly through the action of vitamin D.
  2. Reabsorption of calcium from the kidney, mainly through the action of parathyroid hormone and vitamin D.
  3. Demineralization of bone mainly through the action of parathyroid hormone, but facilitated by vitamin D.
  4. Mineralization (calcification) of bone through the action of calcitonin.

Mechanism (Figure 15.2)

- In response to drop in the blood calcium level parathyroid hormone is secreted by the parathyroid gland. It acts on **intestine**, bone and **kidney** to increase the plasma calcium concentration.
- Action of PTH on intestine is indirect via the formation of calcitriol; active form of vitamin D. PTH stimulates the production of **calcitriol**; an active form of **vitamin D**. Calcitriol then increases **absorption of calcium** and **phosphate** from **intestine** by stimulating the following processes:
  - Absorption of calcium and phosphorus from intestine by inducing synthesis of calcium binding protein necessary for the absorption of calcium from intestine.
  - Reabsorption of calcium and phosphorus from the kidney.
  - Mobilization of calcium and phosphorus from the bone.

  PTH stimulates mobilization of **calcium** and **phosphate** from bones by stimulating **osteoclast activity**.
  - Osteoclast activity results in **demineralization of the bone**.
  - Uptake of calcium and phosphate by bone is also decreased by PTH resulting in an increase in blood calcium and phosphate level.
- In **kidney** PTH increases the **tubular reabsorption** of **calcium** and decreases renal excretion of calcium.
- PTH increases **excretion** of **phosphate** by **inhibiting its renal reabsorption**.
- Thus, overall effects of PTH and calcitriol elevate **plasma calcium** level. In response to rise in the blood calcium

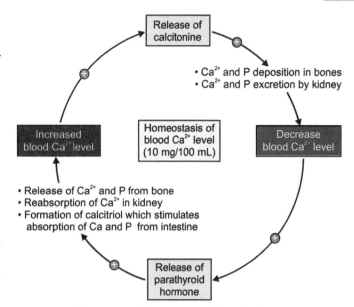

Figure 15.2: Homeostasis of blood calcium.

level **calcitonin** hormone is secreted by the thyroid gland. Action of calcitonin on the bones is opposite to that of the PTH.
- It inhibits calcium mobilization from bone and increases bone calcification (mineralization) by increasing the **osteoblasts** activity.
- In the kidney, it stimulates the excretion of calcium and phosphorus, thereby decreasing the blood calcium level.

STRIKE A NOTE

- In kidney, PTH **increases** the tubular **reabsorption of calcium** and decreases renal excretion of calcium.
- In kidney, PTH **decreases** the tubular **reabsorption of phosphate** and increases renal excretion of phosphate.
- The phosphate, which is not reabsorbed in the renal tubule acts as an important **urinary buffer**.
- Calcium is excreted more in the stool (850 mg/day) and less in urine (150 mg/day), whereas phosphate is excreted more in urine (1000 mg/day) and less in stool (400 mg/day).

Clinical Conditions Related to Plasma Calcium Level Alterations

Hypocalcemia

Hypocalcemia is characterized by lowered levels of plasma calcium. The causes of hypocalcemia include:
- **Hypoparathyroidism:** The most common cause of hypoparathyroidism is neck surgery, or due to magnesium deficiency. Magnesium stimulates the secretion of PTH by the parathyroid glands.
- **Vitamin D deficiency:** This may be due to dietary deficiency, malabsorption or little exposure to sunlight. It may lead to bone disorders, osteomalacia in adults, and rickets in children.

- **Renal disease:** The diseased kidneys fail to synthesize calcitriol due to impaired hydroxylation.

Clinical Features of Hypocalcemia

The clinical features of hypocalcemia include:
- Neuromuscular irritability
- Neurologic features such as tingling, tetany, numbness (fingers and toes)
- Muscle cramps
- Cardiovascular signs such as an abnormal ECG
- Cataracts.

Hypercalcemia

Hypercalcemia is characterized by **increased plasma calcium** level. The most common causes of hypercalcemia are:
- Hyperparathyroidism
- Malignant disease:
  - The cancer can metastasize to bone and make calcium leak out into the bloodstream from bones, so the level in the blood increases.
  - The second cause is by tumors that secrete **parathyroid hormone related peptide (PTHrP)**, a protein that has similar action to parathyroid hormone (PTH) stimulate bone resorption.
  - The types of cancers that are most commonly associated with hypercalcemia are:
    - Multiple myeloma
    - Breast cancer
    - Lung cancer
    - Kidney cancer
    - Prostate cancer.

Clinical Features of Hypercalcemia

- Neurological symptoms such as depression, confusion, inability to concentrate
- Muscle weakness
- Gastrointestinal problems such as anorexia, abdominal pain, nausea and vomiting, and constipation
- Renal features such as polyuria and polydipsia
- Cardiac arrhythmias.

Rickets

- Rickets is characterized by defective calcification of bones.
- This is may be due to deficiency of vitamin D or due to dietary deficiency of calcium and phosphorus or both.

Osteoporosis

- Osteoporosis means porous bones; due to lowered bone density.
- Dietary deficiency of calcium and phosphorus, as well as **low estrogen in elderly women, low testosterone**

in men, lack of vitamin D causes demineralization of the bone resulting in lowered bone density.

Phosphorus

Phosphorus is a widely distributed important element in the human body (*see* **Table 15.3**). Adults contain about 400 to 700 g of phosphorus, about 80% of which is combined with calcium in bones and teeth. It is present in the form of organic and inorganic phosphate.
- In the soft tissues most phosphate is organic, as a component of **phospholipids**, **phosphoproteins**, **nucleic acids**, and **nucleotides**.
- In the ECF phosphorus is mostly present in the inorganic form, where it exists as a mixture of HPO_4^{--} and $H_2PO_4^{-}$ at physiological pH. The ratio of $HPO_4^{--}/H_2PO_4^{-}$ is pH dependent.

Functions

- **Constituent of bone and teeth:** Inorganic phosphate is a major constituent of **hydroxyapatite** in bone, thereby playing an important role in structural support of the body.
- **Acid-base regulation:** Mixture of HPO_4^{--} and $H_2PO_4^{-}$ constitutes the **phosphate buffer** which plays a role in maintaining the pH of body fluid.
- **Energy storage and transfer reactions:** High energy compounds, e.g., ATP, ADP, creatine phosphate, etc. which play a role of storage and transport of energy, contain phosphorus.
- **Essential constituent:** Phosphate is an essential element in phospholipid of cell membrane, nucleic acids (RNA and DNA), nucleotides (NAD, NADP, cAMP, cGMP, etc.)
- **Regulation of enzyme activity:** Phosphorylation and dephosphorylation of enzymes modify the activity of many enzymes.

Dietary Sources

The foods rich in calcium are also rich in phosphorus, i.e., milk, cheese, beans, eggs, cereals, fish, and meat.

Recommended Dietary Allowance per Day

- The recommended dietary allowance for both men and women is **800 mg/day**.
- The amount during pregnancy and lactation is **1200 mg/day**.

Absorption

- Like calcium, phosphorus is absorbed from small intestine and the degree of absorption is similarly affected by different factors as that of calcium.
- Vitamin D stimulates the absorption of phosphate along with calcium.

- Acidic pH favors the absorption of phosphorus.
- Phytates and oxalates decrease absorption of phosphate from intestine.
- Optimum absorption of calcium and phosphate occurs when dietary Ca:P ratio is 1:2 to 2:1.

Excretion

Phosphates are mainly excreted by the kidneys as NaH_2PO_4 through urine (unlike calcium). PTH decreases the reabsorption of phosphorus from the tubules and cause increased excretion of phosphorus in urine.

Plasma Phosphorus

Plasma contains **2.5 to 4.5 mg/dL** of inorganic phosphate. Plasma phosphate concentration is controlled by the kidney, where tubular reabsorption is reduced by PTH. **The phosphate which is not reabsorbed in the renal tubule acts as urinary buffer.**

Clinical Conditions Related to Plasma Phosphorus Concentration Alterations

Hypophosphatemia

In hypophosphatemia serum inorganic phosphate concentration is less than 2.5 mg/dL.

Causes of Hypophosphatemia

- **Hyperparathyroidism:** High PTH increases phosphate excretion by the kidneys and this leads to low serum concentration of phosphate.
- **Congenital defects** of tubular phosphate reabsorption, e.g., **Fanconi's syndrome**, in which phosphate is lost from body.

Clinical Symptoms of Hypophosphatemia

- As phosphate is an important component of ATP, cellular function is impaired with hypophosphatemia and leads to muscle pain and weakness and decreased myocardial output.
- If hypophosphatemia is chronic; rickets in children or osteomalacia in adults may develop.

Hyperphosphatemia

Causes of Hyperphosphatemia

- **Renal failure:** This is the most common cause in which phosphate excretion is impaired.
- **Hypoparathyroidism:** Low PTH decreases phosphate excretion by the kidney and leads to high serum concentration.

Clinical Symptoms of Hyperphosphatemia

Elevated serum phosphate may cause a decrease in serum calcium concentration; therefore **tetany** and **seizures** may be the presenting symptoms.

Magnesium

The body contains about **25 g** of magnesium, most of which (55%) is present in the bones in association with calcium and phosphorus, a small proportion of the body's content is in the ECF (*see* **Table 15.3**).

Functions

- Magnesium is essential for the activity of many enzymes. Magnesium is a cofactor for more than 300 enzymes in the body; in addition, magnesium is allosteric activators of many enzyme systems. It plays an important role in oxidative phosphorylation, glycolysis, cell replication, nucleotide metabolism, protein synthesis, and many ATP dependent reactions.
- Magnesium influences the secretion of PTH by the parathyroid glands.
- Hypomagnesemia may cause hypoparathyroidism.
- Magnesium along with sodium, potassium, and calcium controls the neuromuscular irritability.
- It is an important constituent of bone and teeth.

Dietary Sources

Although most foods contain considerable magnesium it is especially abundant in the **chlorophyll of green leafy vegetables**. As magnesium is an essential part of chlorophyll, green vegetables are an important dietary source, as are cereals, pulses, nuts, meat, eggs, and milk.

Recommended Dietary Allowance per Day

- RDA of the adult man is **350 mg/day** and for women **300 mg/day**.
- More magnesium is required during pregnancy and lactation (450 mg/day).

Absorption

About 30 to 40% of the dietary magnesium is absorbed from the small intestine. Vitamin D and PTH increase the absorption of magnesium from intestine. Large amounts of calcium and phosphate in diet reduce the absorption of magnesium from intestine.

Excretion

Magnesium is excreted mainly by way of intestine. All unabsorbed magnesium as well as that in biliary excretion and intestinal secretion are excreted through feces. A fraction of absorbed magnesium is excreted by the kidneys through urine.

Serum Magnesium

Human blood serum magnesium concentration is **1 to 3.5 mg/dL**. The mechanism of control is poorly understood. Renal conservation of magnesium is partly controlled by

PTH and aldosterone. PTH increases tubular reabsorption of magnesium similar to that of calcium. Aldosterone increases its renal excretion as it does for potassium.

Clinical Conditions Related to Plasma Magnesium Concentration Alterations

Hypomagnesemia

Hypomagnesemia is an abnormally low serum magnesium level. It is usually associated with magnesium deficiency. Since magnesium is present in most common foodstuffs, low dietary intakes of magnesium are associated with general nutritional insufficiency, accompanied by intestinal malabsorption, severe vomiting, diarrhea or other causes of intestinal loss.

The symptoms of hypomagnesemia are very similar to those of hypocalcemia, impaired neuromuscular function such as tetany, hyperirritability, tremor, convulsions, and muscle weakness.

Hypermagnesemia

Hypermagnesemia is uncommon but is occasionally seen in renal failure. Depression of the neuromuscular system is the most common manifestation of hypermagnesemia.

■ METABOLISM OF TRACE ELEMENTS

Microminerals or trace elements are present in the body in very small amounts (micrograms to milligrams) that are essential for certain biochemical processes. Trace elements required by humans are:
- Copper
- Fluoride
- Iodine
- Iron
- Manganese
- Molybdenum
- Selenium
- Zinc.

Copper (Cu)

A 70 kg human adult body contains approximately 80 mg of copper. It is present in all tissues. The highest concentrations are found in liver and kidney, with significant amount in cardiac and skeletal muscle and in bone.

Dietary Food Sources

Shellfish, liver, kidneys, egg yolk, and some legumes are rich in copper.

Recommended Dietary Allowance Per Day

2 to 3 mg.

Functions

- Copper is an essential constituent of many enzymes which involve oxidation-reduction reactions.
  - Cytochrome oxidase
  - Superoxide dismutase
  - Dopamine β-hydroxylase
  - Tyrosinase
  - Tryptophan dioxygenase
  - Lysyl oxidase.
- Copper is required for:
  - **Iron absorption: Ceruloplasmin**, the major copper containing protein in plasma has **ferroxidase** activity that oxidizes ferrous ion to ferric state before its binding to transferrin (transport form of iron).
  - **Synthesis of hemoglobin:** Copper is a constituent of **ALA synthase** enzyme required for heme synthesis
  - **Synthesis of melanin pigment:** Copper is constituent of enzyme tyrosinase
  - **Synthesis of collagen and elastin:** Lysyl oxidase, a copper containing enzyme converts certain lysine residues to allysine needed in the formation of collagen and elastin.

Absorption and Excretion

About 10% of the average daily dietary copper is absorbed mainly from the duodenum. Absorbed copper is transported to the liver bound to albumin and exported to peripheral tissues mainly (about 90%) bound to ceruloplasmin and to a lesser extent (10%) to albumin. The main route of excretion of copper is in the bile into the gut.

Plasma Copper

Normal plasma concentrations are usually between **100** and **200 µg/dL** of which 90% is bound to ceruloplasmin and 10% to albumin.

Deficiency Manifestation

Both children and adults can develop symptomatic deficiency. Premature infants are the most susceptible since the copper stores in the liver are start in the third trimester of pregnancy. Signs of copper deficiency include:
- **Neutropenia** (decreased number of neutrophils) and **hypochromic anemia** in the early stages.
- **Osteoporosis** and various bone and joint abnormalities, due to impairment in copper-dependent cross-linking of bone collagen and connective tissue.
- **Decreased pigmentation of skin** due to depressed copper dependent tyrosinase activity, which is required in the biosynthesis of skin pigment melanin.
- In the later stages **neurological abnormalities** (such as spasticity or neuropathy) probably caused by depressed **cytochrome oxidase** activity.

Inborn Errors of Copper Metabolism

There are two inborn errors of copper metabolism:
1. Menke's syndrome
2. Wilson's disease.

Menke's Syndrome or Kinky-hair Disease

- It is very rare, fatal, **X-linked recessive** disorder.
- The genetic defect is in **absorption of copper** from intestine.
- Both serum copper and ceruloplasmin and liver copper content are low.
- Clinical manifestations occur early in life and include:
  - Kinky or twisted brittle hair (steely) due to loss of copper catalyzed disulfide bond formation
  - Depigmentation of the skin and hair
  - Seizures
  - Mental retardation and
  - Vascular defects (lesions of the blood vessels).

Wilson's Disease

- Wilson's disease is an inborn error of copper metabolism.
- It is an autosomal recessively inherited disorder caused by a mutation in the **gene ATP7B** that codes for a cation transporting enzyme involved in copper transport which leads to impaired:
  - Copper excretion into bile
  - Reabsorption of copper in the kidney
  - Hepatic incorporation of copper into ceruloplasmin.

Clinical Manifestations

- **Copper toxicity** occurs due to copper deposition in liver, brain, and kidney.
- Copper deposits in the eye can sometimes be seen as a **yellow** or **brown pigment** around the iris, **Kayser-Fleischer (KF) rings**.
- Excessive deposition of copper in:
  - Brain leads to neurological symptoms
  - Liver leads to cirrhosis and
  - Kidney leads to renal tubular damage
- The disease is also characterized by increased excretion of copper in urine and low levels of copper and ceruloplasmin in plasma.

Treatment

- Treatment is by administration of a chelating agent, **penicillamine** to promote urinary copper excretion.
- Patients are maintained on oral penicillamine for life.
- **Liver transplantation** may also be considered, particularly in young patients with severe disease.

Fluorine (F)

In the form of fluoride, fluorine is incorporated into the structure of teeth and bone.

Dietary Food Sources

The body receives fluorine mainly from drinking water. Some sea fish and tea also contain small amount of fluoride.

Recommended Dietary Allowance per Day

1.5 to 4 mg per day or **1 to 2 ppm** (since it is present in water it is expressed as ppm).

Absorption and Excretion

Inorganic fluoride is absorbed readily in the stomach and small intestine and distributed almost entirely to bone and teeth. About 50% of the daily intake is excreted through urine.

Functions

- Fluoride is required for the proper formation of **bone** and **teeth**.
- Fluoride becomes incorporated into **hydroxyapatite**, the crystalline mineral of bones and teeth to form **fluoroapatite**.
- Fluoroapatite increases **hardness** of **bone** and **teeth**.
- It provides protection against **dental caries** and attack by acids.

Deficiency Symptoms

Deficiency of fluoride leads to **dental caries** and **osteoporosis**.

Toxicity

- Excessive amounts of fluoride can result in dental fluorosis. This condition results in teeth with a patch, dull white, even chalk looking appearance. A brown mottled appearance can also occur **(Figure 15.3)**.
- It is known to **inhibit** several enzymes especially **enolase** of glycolysis.

Iodine (I$_2$)

The adult human body contains about **50 mg** of iodine. The blood plasma contains **4 to 8 µg** of protein bound iodine (PBI) per 100 mL.

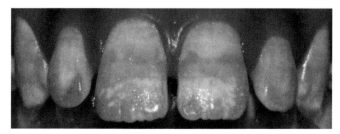

Figure 15.3: Formation of dull white patch with a chalk looking appearance on teeth due to fluorosis.

Dietary Food Sources

Seafood, drinking water, iodized table salt, onions, vegetables, etc.

Recommended Dietary Allowance Per Day

100 to 150 µg for adults.

Functions

The most important role of iodine in the body is in the synthesis of thyroid hormones, **triiodothyronine (T_3)** and **tetraiodothyronine (T_4)**, which influence a large number of metabolic functions.

Absorption and Excretion

Iodine in the diet absorbed rapidly in the form of iodide from small intestine. Normally, about 1/3rd of dietary iodide is taken up by the thyroid gland, a little by the mammary and salivary glands. The rest is excreted by the kidneys.

Nearly 70 to 80% of iodine is excreted by the kidneys; small amounts are excreted through bile, skin, and saliva. Milk of lactating women also contains some iodine.

Deficiency Manifestation

Deficiency of iodine occurs in several regions of the world, where the iodine content of soil and therefore of plants is low. A deficiency of iodine in children leads to **cretinism** and in adult endemic **goiter**.

- **Cretinism:** Severe iodine deficiency in mothers leads to intrauterine or neonatal hypothyroidism results in cretinism in their children. Cretinism is characterized by mental retardation, slow body development, dwarfism, and characteristic facial structure.
- **Goiter:** A goiter is an **enlarged thyroid** with decreased thyroid hormone production. An iodine deficiency in adults stimulates the proliferation of thyroid epithelial cells, resulting in enlargement of the thyroid gland. The thyroid gland collects iodine from the blood and uses it to make thyroid hormones. In iodine deficiency, the thyroid gland undergoes compensatory enlargement in order to extract iodine from blood more efficiently.

Iron (Fe)

A normal adult possesses **3 to 5 g** of iron. This small amount is used again and again in the body. Iron is called a **one way substance**, because very little of it is excreted. Iron is not like vitamins or most other organic or even inorganic substances, which are either inactivated or excreted in course of their physiological function.

Dietary Food Sources

The best sources of food iron include liver, meat, egg yolk, green leafy vegetables, whole grains, and cereals. There are two types of food iron:

- In animal foods, iron is often attached to proteins called **heme proteins** and referred to as **heme iron** and is found in meat, poultry, and fish.
- In plant foods, iron is not attached to heme proteins and is classified as **nonheme iron**, found in green leafy vegetables.

Recommended Dietary Allowance Per Day

- **Adult men and postmenopausal women:** 10 mg
- **Premenopausal women:** 15–20 mg
- **Pregnant women:** 30–60 mg.

Women require greater amount than men due to the physiological loss during menstruation.

Functions

Iron is required for:

- Synthesis of heme compound like hemoglobin, myoglobin, cytochromes, catalase, and peroxidase.
- Synthesis of nonheme iron (NHI) compounds, e.g., iron-sulfur proteins of flavoprotein, succinate dehydrogenase, and NADH dehydrogenase.
- Thus iron helps mainly in the **transport, storage**, and **utilization of oxygen**.

Absorption Transport, Storage, and Excretion of Iron

The normal intake of iron is about 10 to 20 mg/day. Normally, about 5 to 10% of dietary iron is absorbed. Most absorption occurs in the duodenum.

- **Nonheme iron** bound to organic acids or proteins is absorbed in the ferrous (Fe^{2+}) state into the mucosal cell as follows:
  - The gastric acid, HCl and organic acids in the diet convert bound nonheme compound of the diet into **free ferric (Fe^{3+}) ions**.
  - These free ferric ions are reduced with ascorbic acid and glutathione of food to more soluble ferrous (Fe^{2+}) form which is transported into mucosal cell by a **divalent metal ion transporter (DMT)**.
  - After absorption Fe^{2+} is oxidized in mucosal cells to Fe^{3+} by the enzyme **Ferroxidase**, which then combines with **apoferritin** to form **ferritin**. Ferritin is a temporary storage form of iron **(Figure 15.4)**.
- Heme iron of food is absorbed as such separately through **heme transporter (HT)** by the intestinal mucosal cells. It is subsequently broken down by **heme oxygenase** with the release of **iron** in the cells.

Factors Affecting Iron Absorption

- **State of iron stores in the body:** Absorption is increased in **iron deficiency** and decreased when there is iron overload.
- **Ferroportin** and **divalent metal ion transporter** are inhibited by **hepcidin**, a peptide secreted by the liver

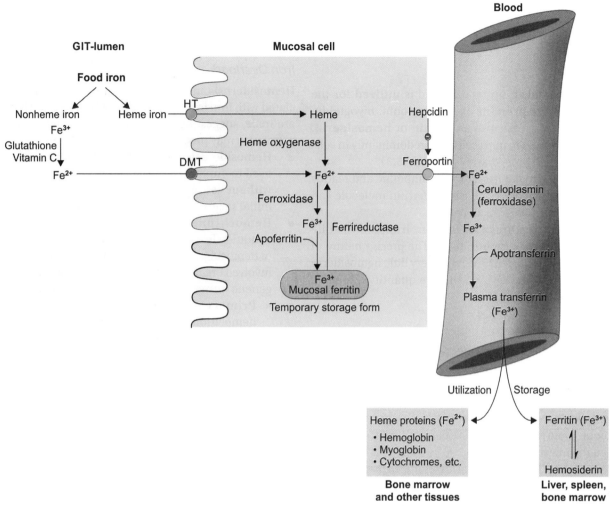

Figure 15.4: Absorption, storage, and utilization of food iron.
(HT: heme transporter; DMT: divalent metal transporter)

when body iron reserves are adequate. In response to hypoxia, anemia, or hemorrhages, the synthesis of hepcidine is reduced, leading to increased synthesis of ferroportin and increased iron absorption.

- **Rate of erythropoiesis** (the process of red blood cell production). When rate of erythropoiesis is increased, absorption may be increased even though the iron stores are adequate or overloaded.
- **The contents of the diet:** Substances that form soluble complexes with iron, e.g., ascorbic acid (vitamin C) facilitates absorption. Substances that form insoluble complexes, e.g., phosphate, phytates and oxalates inhibit absorption. Alcohol and fructose also enhance iron absorption. Absorption of iron is impaired by calcium. A glass of milk with a meal significantly reduces iron absorption.
- **Nature of gastrointestinal secretions and the chemical state of the iron:** Iron in the diet does not usually become available for absorption unless released in free form during digestion. This depends partly on gastric acid (HCl) production. Ferrous (Fe^{2+}) is more readily

absorbed than ferric form (Fe^{3+}) and the presence of HCl, helps to keep iron in the Fe^{2+} form.

Transport

- The transfer of iron from the storage ferritin (Fe^{3+} form) to plasma involves reduction of Fe^{3+} to Fe^{2+} in the mucosal cell with the help of ferroreductase **(Figure 15.3)**.
- Fe^{2+} then enters the plasma via a transport protein **ferroportin**, where it is reoxidized to Fe^{3+} by a copper protein, **ceruloplasmin** (ferroxidase).
- Fe^{3+} is then incorporated into **transferrin** by combining with **apotransferrin**. Apotransferrin is a specific iron binding protein. Each apotransferrin can bind with two Fe^{3+} ions. Once transferrin is saturated with iron, any that has accumulated in the mucosal cells is lost when the cells are shed.
- Ferroportin and divalent metal ion transporter are inhibited by **hepcidin**, a peptide secreted by the liver when body iron reserves are adequate. In response to hypoxia, anemia, or hemorrhage, the synthesis of hepcidine is reduced, leading to increased synthesis of

ferroportin and increased iron absorption. As a result of this mucosal barrier, only ~10% of dietary iron is absorbed.

Storage

Iron in blood is taken up by cells and is **utilized** for the formation of **heme proteins** like hemoglobin, myoglobin, cytochromes, etc., or **stored** as **ferritin** or **hemosiderin**. Storage of iron occurs in most cells but predominantly in cells of liver, spleen, and bone marrow **(Figure 15.3)**.

- **Ferritin** is the major iron storage compound and readily available source of iron. Each apoferritin molecule can take up about 4500 iron atoms.
- In addition to storage as ferritin, iron can also be found in a form of **hemosiderin**. The precise nature of hemosiderin is unclear. Normally very little hemosiderin is to be found in the liver, but the quantity increases during iron overload.

Excretion

Iron is not excreted in the urine, but is lost from the body via the **bile**, **feces**, and in **menstrual blood**. Iron excreted in the feces is exogenous, i.e., dietary iron that has not been absorbed by the mucosal cells is excreted in the feces.

- In male, there is an average loss of endogenous iron of about 1 mg/day through desquamated cells of the skin and the intestinal mucosa.
- Females may have additional losses due to menstruation or pregnancy.

Disorders of Iron Metabolism

The major disorders of iron metabolism is **iron deficiency anemia** and **iron overload**.

Iron Deficiency Anemia

- A deficiency of iron causes a reduction in the rate of hemoglobin synthesis and erythropoiesis, and can result in **iron deficiency anemia**.
- Iron deficiency causes low hemoglobin resulting in **hypochromic microcytic anemia** in which the size of the red blood cells are much smaller than normal and have much reduced hemoglobin content.
- Iron deficiency anemia is the commonest of all single nutrient deficiencies. The main causes are:
  - **Deficient intake:** Including reduced bioavailability of iron due to dietary fiber, phytates, oxalates, etc.
  - **Impaired absorption:** For example, intestinal malabsorptive disease, and abdominal surgery.
  - **Excessive loss:** For example, menstrual blood loss in women and in men from gastrointestinal bleeding (in peptic ulcer, diverticulosis or malignancy).

Clinical features of anemia: Weakness, fatigue, dizziness, and palpitation. Nonspecific symptoms are nausea, anorexia, constipation, and menstrual irregularities. Some individuals develop pica, a craving for unnatural articles of food such as clay or chalk.

Iron Overload

Hemosiderosis and **hemochromatosis** are conditions associated with iron overload. At least 90% of affected individuals are male, suggesting that iron losses in menstruation and pregnancy may protect females.

- **Hemosiderosis:** Hemosiderosis is a term that has been used to imply an increase in iron stores as hemosiderin **without associated tissue injury**. Hemosiderosis is an initial stage of iron overload.
- **Hemochromatosis:** Hemochromatosis is a clinical condition in which excessive deposits of iron in the form of hemosiderin are present in the tissues, **with injury** to involved organs. The causes of hemochromatosis may be genetic (primary) or acquired (secondary).
  - **Primary or genetic hemochromatosis:** Primary hemochromatosis is a hereditary disorder, due to an unregulated increase in the intestinal absorption of iron from normal diet. Patients with hemochromatosis absorb about 4 mg of iron per day rather than 1 mg from gastrointestinal tract. Iron is deposited as hemosiderin in liver, pancreas, heart, and other organs. After accumulating for years, the excessive amounts of intracellular iron lead to tissue injury and ultimately organ failure. At this stage the amount of storage iron may exceed **20 rather than the normal 3 to 4 g**.
  - **Secondary or acquired hemochromatosis:** The main causes of acquired hemochromatosis are:
    - Chronic overload: This occurs when the diet contains excess absorbable iron, e.g., acid containing food cooked in iron pot.
    - Parenteral administration of iron or chronic blood transfusion for blood disorders, e.g., thalassemia.
    - Alcohol abuse due to an ethanol induced increase in iron absorption.

Clinical Symptoms of Hemochromatosis

Clinical symptoms of hemochromatosis are related to the involved organ systems as follows:

- **Liver:** Leading to cirrhosis
- **Pancreas:** Leading to fibrotic damage to pancreas with diabetes mellitus
- **Skin:** Skin pigmentation, bronzed diabetes
- **Endocrine organ:** Leading to hypothyroidism, testicular atrophy
- **Joints:** Leading to arthritis
- **Heart:** Leading to arrhythmia and heart failure.

Iron Toxicity

- Acute overdose, mainly occurring in children may cause severe or even fatal symptoms due to toxic effect of free iron in plasma which may be life-threatening. Symptoms include:

- Nausea
- Vomiting
- Abdominal pain
- Diarrhea and
- Hematemesis
- In severe cases, hypotension, liver damage, and coma can result.

Molybdenum (Mo)

Dietary Food Sources

Liver and kidney are good meat sources, whole grains, legumes, and leafy vegetables serve as vegetable sources.

Recommended Dietary Allowance Per Day

0.15 to 0.5 mg.

Functions

Molybdenum is a constituent of the following enzymes:
- Xanthine oxidase
- Aldehyde oxidase
- Sulfite oxidase.

Absorption and Excretion

Dietary molybdenum is readily absorbed by the intestine and is excreted in urine and bile.

Deficiency Manifestation

Deficiency of molybdenum has been reported to cause **xanthinuria** with low plasma and urinary uric acid concentration.

Selenium (Se)

Dietary Food Sources

Liver, kidney, seafood, and meat are good sources of selenium. Grains have a variable content depending on the region where they are grown.

Recommended Dietary Allowance Per Day

50 to 200 µg for normal adults.

Functions

- Selenium is an antioxidant functions as an **antioxidant** along with vitamin E.
- Selenium in the form of **selenocysteine** is a constituent of enzyme **glutathione peroxidase**. Glutathione peroxidase has a cellular **antioxidant** function that protects cell proteins, cell membranes, lipids, and nucleic acids from oxidative damage by H_2O_2 and a variety of hydroperoxides.

- Selenium, as a constituent of glutathione peroxidase is important in preventing lipid peroxidation and protecting cells against superoxide (O_2^-) and some other free radicals.
- Selenocysteine is also a constituent of **iodothyronine deiodinase**, the enzyme that converts thyroxine to triiodothyronine.

Absorption and Excretion

The principal dietary forms of selenium **selenocysteine** and **selenomethionine** are absorbed from gastrointestinal tract. Selenium homeostasis is achieved by regulation of its excretion via urine.

Deficiency Manifestations

- **Keshan disease**, a cardiomyopathy found in children and young women living in regions of China where dietary intake of selenium is low (<20 µg/d).
- Its most common symptoms include **dizziness, loss of appetite, nausea, abnormal electrocardiograms**, and **congestive heart failure**.

Selenium Toxicity (Selenosis)

Chronic ingestion of high amounts of selenium leads to **selenosis**, characterized by hair and nail brittleness and loss, garlic breath odor, skin rash, myopathy, irritability, and other abnormalities of the nervous system.

Zinc (Zn)

Total zinc content of the adult body is about 2 g. In blood, RBCs contain very high concentration of zinc as compared to plasma. Most of the zinc in the body is found in the liver, bone, blood (75% in erythrocytes), testes, pancreas, and epidermal tissues. It is excreted mainly through feces.

Dietary Food Sources

- Meat, liver, seafood, and eggs are good sources.
- Other sources of zinc are wheat, cereals, peas, beans, and nuts.
- Milk including breast milk also is a good source of zinc. **The colostrum is an especially rich source.**
- Zinc is more readily absorbed from vegetables than animal sources.

Recommended Dietary Allowance Per Day

The requirement for adults is **15–20 mg/day**. It is more during the period of growth pregnancy and lactation.

Functions

- Zinc is essential for the function and structure of several enzymes. Zinc is a component of many metalloenzymes in the body. More than 70 metalloenzymes are known to be associated with zinc. A few important ones are:

- Dehydrogenases
- Peptidases
- Phosphatases
- Isomerase
- Transcarbamylase
- Carbonic anhydrase
- DNA polymerases and RNA-polymerases required for DNA and RMA synthesis
- Porphobilinogen (PBG) synthase required for heme synthesis.

- **Zinc is necessary for the growth and division of cells**. Zinc is involved in the synthesis and stabilization of proteins, DNA, and RNA.
- Zinc is an important element in wound healing as it is a necessary factor in the biosynthesis and integrity of connective tissue.
- Zinc is required for the secretion and storage of insulin from the β-cells of pancreas.
- Zinc is necessary for the binding of steroid hormone receptors and several other transcription factors to DNA.
- Zinc is required for normal spermatogenesis, fetal growth, and embryonic development.
- **Gustine**, a Zn containing protein present in saliva is required for the development and functioning of taste buds. Therefore, zinc deficiency leads to loss of taste acuity.

Absorption and Excretion

Approximately 20 to 30% of ingested dietary zinc is absorbed in small intestine. It is transported in blood plasma mostly by albumin and α_2-macroglobulin. Zinc is excreted in urine, bile, in pancreatic fluid and in milk in lactating mothers.

Deficiency Manifestation

Zinc deficiency has many causes, but malnutrition and malabsorption are the most common. Clinical symptoms of zinc deficiency include:

- Growth failure
- Hair loss
- Anemia
- Reduced taste acuity (Loss of taste sensation)
- Hypogonadism (impaired spermatogenesis)
- Neuropsychiatric symptoms
- Delayed wound healing.

Acrodermatitis enteropathica: A rare inherited disorder of zinc metabolism is due to an inherited defect in zinc absorption that causes low plasma zinc concentration and reduced total body content of zinc; it is manifested in infancy as skin rash.

ASSESSMENT QUESTIONS

■ STRUCTURED LONG ESSAY QUESTIONS (SLEQs)

1. Describe metabolism of calcium under the following headings:
   i. Functions
   ii. Sources and nutritional requirements
   iii. Factors affecting absorption
   iv. Regulation of plasma calcium level
   v. Clinical conditions related to plasma calcium level alterations
2. Describe metabolism of phosphorus under the following headings:
   i. Functions
   ii. Sources and nutritional requirements
   iii. Factors affecting absorption
   iv. Regulation of plasma phosphorus level
   v. Clinical conditions related to plasma phosphorus level alterations
3. Describe metabolism of iron under the following headings:
   i. Functions
   ii. Sources and nutritional requirements
   iii. Absorption, transport, storage, and excretion with diagram
   iv. Disorders of metabolism

■ SHORT ESSAY QUESTIONS (SEQs)

1. Write factors affecting calcium absorption.
2. Write regulation of serum calcium level.
3. Write disorders of iron overload.
4. Write cause and symptoms of Wilson's disease.
5. Write cause and symptoms of Menke's syndrome.
6. Write causes and manifestations of iron deficiency.
7. What are good dietary sources of iron? Explain how iron is absorbed from the gastrointestinal tract.

■ SHORT ANSWER QUESTIONS (SAQs)

1. Factors that inhibit calcium absorption.
2. State factors affecting iron absorption.
3. What are the richest sources of iron?
4. What is the cause of Wilson's disease?
5. Name trace elements giving biochemical role of any two trace elements.
6. Name four enzymes having copper as an integral component.
7. What is the cause of Menke's syndrome?
8. Deficiency manifestation of iodine.

9. What is hemosiderin?
10. Name two enzymes having molybdenum as a constituent.
11. Name two enzymes containing zinc.
12. Write functions of selenium.
13. Write any four functions of calcium.
14. Name the hormones that regulate blood calcium level.
15. Write any four functions of phosphate.
16. Write any four biochemical functions of iron.
17. What are the transport and storage forms of iron?
18. Write functions of iodine
19. What is fluorosis and write its cause.
20. Write four functions of copper.

CASE VIGNETTE-BASED QUESTIONS (CVBQs)

Case Study

1. A 15-year-old girl presented with abdominal pain. She became jaundiced and she subsequently died of liver failure. At postmortem of her liver copper concentration was found to be grossly increased.

   Questions
   a. What is the diagnosis?
   b. What is the cause of liver failure?
   c. What is the cause of increased copper concentration in liver?
   d. What is the normal plasma concentration of copper?

2. A patient in the hospital had seizures and usually appeared weak and tired. Physical finding was deposition of copper in the eyes as brown pigment (the Kayser-Fleischer ring) and hepatomegaly. A diagnosis of Wilson's disease was made.

   Questions
   a. What is the biochemical problem in Wilson's disease?
   b. Name two copper containing enzymes.
   c. Give functions and sources of copper.

3. A 35-year-old man, who required total intravenous feeding (with no assessment of his trace metal status), for four months, developed a skin rash, with accompanying hair loss, reduced taste acuity, and delayed wound healing. He was clearly diagnosed zinc deficient.

   Questions
   a. Give food sources of zinc.
   b. RDA for zinc.
   c. Functions of zinc.
   d. Name two enzymes having zinc as a constituent.

4. A 40-year-old woman complains of tiredness and appears pale. She is experiencing a heavy and prolonged monthly menstrual flow and her hemoglobin concentration is 90 g/L (normal range 120–160 g/L).

   Questions
   a. What is your probable diagnosis?
   b. How can the complaints be relieved?
   c. Give RDA and factors affecting absorption of the deficient biochemical substance.

5. A 18-year-old female comes to her physician complaining about feeling tired and her physician performs a physical examination and diagnosis of anemia was made. Her blood investigations showed decreased level of ceruloplasmin.

   Questions
   a. What is the cause of anemia.
   b. What type of anemia does this patient exhibit?
   c. What is ceruloplasmin.
   d. What are the functions of ceruloplasmin?

6. A 57-year-old man was admitted to clinic who exhibits a brown pigment ring (KF ring) around his cornea and also some signs of neurological impairment.

   Questions
   a. What is the probable diagnosis?
   b. Cause of disorder.
   c. Suggest treatment for the disorder.
   d. Name supportive investigations.

7. A 50-year-old woman presented at clinic, who is pale and tired she has iron deficiency anemia.

   Questions
   a. What is the normal reference plasma level of iron?
   b. Write RDA for iron.
   c. What is the transport form of iron?
   d. Write storage form of iron.

MULTIPLE CHOICE QUESTIONS (MCQs)

1. Normal serum sodium level is:
   a. 135–145 mEq/L   b. 150–160 mEq/L
   c. 120–130 mEq/L   d. 170–180 mEq/L

2. In wound healing the following trace element is involved:
   a. Iron   b. Copper
   c. Zinc   d. Selenium

3. The mineral having sparing action of vitamin E:
   a. Chromium   b. Iron
   c. Iodine   d. Selenium

4. Wilson's disease is characterized by impaired:
   a. Copper excretion into bile
   b. Reabsorption of copper in the kidney
   c. Hepatic incorporation of copper into ceruloplasmin
   d. All of the above

5. Glutathione peroxidase contains:
   a. Calcium   b. Iron
   c. Selenium   d. Chromium

6. Hemochromatosis is due to excessive deposition of:
   a. Iron in the form of hemosiderin
   b. Copper
   c. Zinc
   d. Iodine

7. Transferrin is involved in:
   a. Hormone metabolism
   b. Diagnosis of Wilson's disease
   c. Transport of iron
   d. Transport of bilirubin

8. **The major storage form of iron is:**
   a. Transferrin
   b. Ceruloplasmin
   c. Ferritin
   d. Hemosiderin

9. **The element that prevents the development of dental caries:**
   a. Fluorine
   b. Calcium
   c. Phosphorus
   d. Selenium

10. **Carbonic anhydrase contains mineral:**
    a. Copper
    b. Iodine
    c. Zinc
    d. Iron

11. **Molybdenum is a constituent of all of the following, *except*:**
    a. Xanthine oxidase
    b. Aldehyde oxidase
    c. Sulfite oxidase
    d. Cytochrome oxidase

12. **Transport form of iron is:**
    a. Transferrin
    b. Ferritin
    c. Hemosiderin
    d. Ceruloplasmin

13. **Iodine is required for the formation of:**
    a. Vitamin B_{12}
    b. Thyroxine
    c. Insulin
    d. Calcitonin

14. **Which of the following minerals is known as glucose tolerance factor (GTF)?**
    a. Chromium
    b. Cobalt
    c. Calcium
    d. Copper

15. **Intestinal absorption of iron is enhanced by:**
    a. Phytic acid
    b. Ascorbic acid
    c. Oxalic acid
    d. Alkaline pH

16. **Element called "one way substance" is:**
    a. Iodine
    b. Iron
    c. Copper
    d. Calcium

17. **Which of the following minerals stimulates secretion of PTH?**
    a. Iodine
    b. Magnesium
    c. Copper
    d. Sodium

18. **Iron is a component of:**
    a. Hemoglobin
    b. Ceruloplasmin
    c. Transferase
    d. Transaminase

19. **Daily requirement of iron for normal adult male is about:**
    a. 5 mg
    b. 10 mg
    c. 15 mg
    d. 20 mg

20. **The total iron content of the human body is:**
    a. 400–500 mg
    b. 1–2 g
    c. 2–3 g
    d. 4–5 g

21. **A good source of iron is:**
    a. Spinach
    b. Milk
    c. Tomato
    d. Potato

22. **The deficiency of copper decreases the activity of the enzyme:**
    a. Lysyl oxidase
    b. Lysine hydroxylase
    c. Tyrosine oxidase
    d. Proline hydroxylase

23. **Wilson's disease is a condition of toxicosis of:**
    a. Iron
    b. Copper
    c. Chromium
    d. Molybdenum

24. **In Wilson's disease:**
    a. Copper fails to be excreted in the bile
    b. Copper level in plasma is decreased
    c. Ceruloplasmin level is increased
    d. Intestinal absorption of copper is decreased

25. **Menke's disease is due to an abnormality in the metabolism of:**
    a. Iron
    b. Manganese
    c. Magnesium
    d. Copper

26. **Menke's disease (Kinky or steel hair disease) is a X-linked disease characterized by:**
    a. High levels of plasma copper
    b. High levels of ceruloplasmin
    c. Low levels of plasma copper and of ceruloplasmin
    d. High level of hepatic copper

27. **Mitochondrial superoxide dismutase contains:**
    a. Zinc
    b. Copper
    c. Magnesium
    d. Manganese

28. **Mitochondrial pyruvate carboxylase contains:**
    a. Zinc
    b. Copper
    c. Manganese
    d. Magnesium

29. **Molybdenum is a constituent of:**
    a. Hydroxylases
    b. Oxidases
    c. Transaminases
    d. Transferases

30. **Metallic constituent of "Glucose tolerance factor" is:**
    a. Sulfur
    b. Cobalt
    c. Chromium
    d. Selenium

31. **Selenium is a constituent of the enzyme:**
    a. Glutathione peroxidase
    b. Homogentisate oxidase
    c. Tyrosine hydroxylase
    d. Phenylalanine hydroxylase

32. **Excess intake of cobalt for longer periods leads to:**
    a. Polycythemia
    b. Megaloblastic anemia
    c. Pernicious anemia
    d. Microcytic anemia

33. **Fluorosis occurs due to:**
    a. Drinking water containing less fluorine
    b. Drinking water containing high calcium
    c. Drinking water containing high fluorine
    d. Drinking water containing heavy metals

34. **An important zinc containing enzyme is:**
    a. Carbonic anhydrase
    b. Isocitrate dehydrogenase
    c. Cholinesterase
    d. Lipoprotein lipase

35. **Acrodermatitis enteropathica is due to defective absorption of:**
    a. Manganese
    b. Molybdenum
    c. Iodine
    d. Zinc

36. **Intestinal absorption of calcium is hampered by:**
    a. Phosphate
    b. Phytates
    c. Proteins
    d. Lactose

37. **What are the functions of potassium?**
    a. In muscle contraction
    b. Cell membrane function
    c. Enzyme action
    d. All of these

38. **Hypocalcemia can occur in all the following, *except*:**
    a. Rickets
    b. Osteomalacia
    c. Hyperparathyroidism
    d. Intestinal malabsorption

39. **Normal range of serum potassium is:**
    a. 2.1–3.4 mEq/L b. 3.5–5.3 mEq/L
    c. 5.4–7.4 mEq/L d. 7.5–9.5 mEq/L

40. **Iron is stored in the form of:**
    a. Ferritin and transferrin
    b. Transferrin and hemosiderin
    c. Hemoglobin and myoglobin
    d. Ferritin and hemosiderin

41. **Iron is transported in blood in the form of:**
    a. Ferritin b. Hemosiderin
    c. Transferrin d. Hemoglobin

42. **Zinc is involved in storage and release of:**
    a. Histamine b. Acetylcholine
    c. Epinephrine d. Insulin

43. **Molybdenum is a cofactor for:**
    a. Xanthine oxidase b. Aldehyde oxidase
    c. Sulfite oxidase d. All of these

44. **A trace element having antioxidant function is:**
    a. Selenium b. Tocopherol
    c. Chromium d. Molybdenum

45. **Selenium is a constituent of:**
    a. Glutathione reductase
    b. Glutathione peroxidase
    c. Catalase
    d. Superoxide dismutase

46. **Selenium decreases the requirement of:**
    a. Copper b. Zinc
    c. Vitamin D d. Vitamin E

47. **The general functions of minerals are:**
    a. The structural components of body tissues
    b. In the regulation of body fluids
    c. In acid-base balance
    d. All of these

48. **Hyponatremia caused by each of the following, *except*:**
    a. Prolonged vomiting or diarrhea
    b. Aldosterone deficiency
    c. Renal failure
    d. Excessive aldosterone secretion

49. **A hemolytic sample will cause falsely increased levels of each of the following, *except*:**
    a. Potassium
    b. Sodium
    c. Phosphate
    d. Magnesium

50. **PTH (parathyroid hormone) increases:**
    a. Osteoblast activity
    b. Reabsorption of Ca^{++} in the distal tubules
    c. Reabsorption of phosphate in the distal tubules
    d. Excretion of Ca^{++} in the distal tubules

51. **A patient with chronic kidney disease is noted to have hyperphosphatemia. The regulators of serum phosphate concentration include all of the following, *except*:**
    a. PTH
    b. Calcitriol
    c. Calcitonin
    d. 1,25 vitamin D

52. **A 34-year-old man with normal kidney function is noted to have an elevated phosphorus level, the cause of hyperphosphatemia is:**
    a. Fanconi's syndrome
    b. Hypoparathyroidism
    c. Multiple myeloma
    d. Hyperparathyroidism

ANSWERS FOR MCQs

1. a	2. c	3. d	4. d	5. c
6. a	7. c	8. c	9. a	10. c
11. d	12. a	13. b	14. a	15. b
16. b	17. b	18. a	19. b	20. d
21. a	22. a	23. b	24. a	25. d
26. c	27. c	28. c	29. b	30. c
31. a	32. a	33. c	34. a	35. d
36. b	37. d	38. c	39. b	40. d
41. c	42. d	43. d	44. a	45. b
46. d	47. d	48. d	49. b	50. b
51. c	52. b			

16 CHAPTER

Water and Electrolyte Balance

Competency	Learning Objectives
BI 6.7: Describe the processes involved in maintenance of normal pH, water and electrolyte balance of body fluids and the derangements associated with these.	1. Describe total body water and its distribution. 2. Describe electrolytes and their distribution in ICF and ECF. 3. Describe regulation of water and electrolyte balance. 4. Describe disorders associated with water and electrolyte imbalances.

■ OVERVIEW

Water is the most abundant constituent of the human body accounting approximately 60–70% of the body mass in a normal adult. Water content of the body changes with age. It is about 75% in the newborn and decreases to less than 50% in older individuals. Water content is **greatest** in **brain** tissue and **least** in **adipose tissue**.

Water is a medium in which body solutes, both organic and inorganic, are dissolved and metabolic reactions take place. It acts as a vehicle for transport of solutes. Water itself participates as a substrate and a product in many chemical reactions, e.g., in glycolysis, citric acid cycle and mitochondrial respiratory chain. The stability of subcellular structures and activities of numerous enzymes are dependent on adequate cell hydration.

Water is involved in the regulation of **body temperature** because of its highest **latent heat of evaporation**. Water also acts as a **lubricant** in the body so as to prevent friction in joints, pleura, peritoneum and conjunctiva. A relative deficiency and an excess of water impair the function of tissues and organs. This chapter focuses on:

- Compartmentalization of body fluid and its inorganic solutes (electrolytes).
- Physiological mechanisms involved in maintenance of this compartmentalization.
- Pathophysiological events that occur due to alter composition of body fluid.

■ TOTAL BODY WATER AND ITS DISTRIBUTION

Total body water (TBW), includes water both inside and outside of cells and water normally present in the gastrointestinal and genitourinary systems. Total body water can be theoretically divided into two main compartments **extracellular water (ECW)** and **intracellular water (ICW)** **(Figure 16.1)**.

- The **ECW** includes all water external to cell membranes and constitutes the medium through which all metabolic exchange occurs. The ECW can be further subdivided into, **intravascular water**, i.e., **plasma** and **extravascular water**, i.e., **interstitial fluid**.

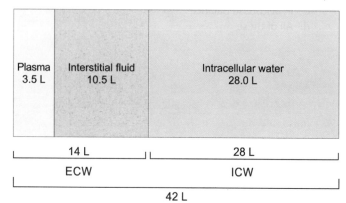

Figure 16.1: Body water compartments.

- The **ICW** includes all water within cell membranes and constitutes the medium in which chemical reactions of cell metabolism occur.

Distribution of Body Water

- In a 70 kg adult, the total body water is about **42 L**. About **28 L** of water is as intracellular water **(ICW)** and 14 L of extracellular water **(ECW)**.
- The ECW is distributed as **3.5 L plasma water** (intravascular water) and **10.5 L interstitial water** (extravascular) **(Table 16.1)**.
- Distribution of water between intracellular and extracellular compartments is affected by **colloidal osmotic pressure** and **osmolality**.
- Osmolality depends on the amount of osmotically active substances in these compartments. Electrolyte and water balance are dependent on each other and cannot be considered separately.
- The body water is maintained within the fairly constant limits by a regulation between the **intake** and **output** as shown in **Table 16.2**.
- Under normal conditions water intake include:
  - Approximately, one-half to two-thirds of water intake is in the form of **oral fluid intake**
  - Approximately, one-half to one-third is in the form of oral intake of **water in food**
  - In addition, a small amount of water (150–350 mL/day) is produced during metabolism of food called **metabolic water** or **water of oxidation**

Oral fluid intake is the only source of water that is regulated in response to changes in ECW volume and osmolarity.

- Routes of water excretion (water output) include:
  - Urinary water loss
  - Insensible water loss through skin and lung
  - Sensible perspiration through sweat
  - Gastrointestinal water loss through stool
- The kidney is the principal organ regulating the volume and composition of the body fluids. Urine volume varies over a wide range in response to changes in ECW volume and osmolarity.
- Loss of water by diffusion through the skin and through the respiratory tract is known as **insensible water** loss because it is not visible. It is the only route by which water is lost without solute. Normally, half of insensible water loss occurs through the skin and half through the respiratory tract. Insensible water loss varies directly with surrounding temperature, body temperature and activity and inversely with surrounding humidity.
- **Sensible perspiration** is negligible in cool environment but increases with surrounding temperature, body temperature or physical activity. Sodium and chloride are the major ionic components of sweat. An increase in ECW osmolarity causes a decrease in the rate of sensible perspiration. Water loss from the gastrointestinal tract through stool is approximately 200 mL/day.
- As a result of the balance between water intake and water excretion, extracellular water osmolarity is maintained constant at **285–298 mOsm/L**.
- Average daily water turnover in the adult, is approximately **2500 mL**. However, the range of water turnover depends on **intake**, **environment** and **activity** (Table 16.2).

❖ The osmolality is the number of solute particles per unit weight of water, irrespective of the size, or nature of the particles. Therefore, on a weight basis low molecular weight solutes contribute much more to the osmolality than high molecular weight solutes.

❖ The units of osmolality are **mmol/1 kg** of water. This determines osmotic pressures exerted by a solution across a membrane, when the concentration is expressed as **osmoles per liter** of solution, it is called osmolarity. Adding material to a liter of water is molality and adding water to material to make a liter of solution is **molarity**.

❖ Osmolality affects the movement of water across cell membranes.

TABLE 16.1: Distribution of water.

Compartment	Percentage of TBW	Volume in 70 kg man
Total body water (TBW)	–	42 L
Extracellular water (ECW)	33%	14 L
a. Plasma	8%	3.5 L
b. Interstitial water	25%	10.5 L
Intracellular water (ICW)	67%	28.0 L

TABLE 16.2: Daily intake and output of body water in normal adult.

	Daily intake of water (mL/day)				Daily output of water (mL/day)		
Source	Normal	Hot environment	Strenuous work	Source	Normal	Hot environment	Strenuous work
Drinking water	1200	2200	3400	Urine	1400	1200	500
Water from food	1000	1000	1150	Insensible water loss Skin Lung	400 400	400 300	400 600
Water of oxidation/ Metabolic water	300	300	450	Sensible water loss Sweat	100	1400	3300
				Gastrointestinal water loss Stool	200	200	200
Total	**2500**	**3500**	**5000**	**Total**	**2500**	**3500**	**5000**

ELECTROLYTES AND THEIR DISTRIBUTION IN ICF AND ECF

Electrolytes are the inorganic minerals which are readily dissociated into **positively charged (cations)** and **negatively charged (anions)** ions.

- In physiology, the primary electrolytes are sodium (Na^+), potassium (K^+), calcium (Ca^{2+}), magnesium (Mg^{2+}), chloride (Cl^-), phosphate (HPO_4^{2-}), and bicarbonate (HCO_3^-).
- The term electrolytes applied in medicine to the four ions in plasma, (Na^+, K^+, Cl^- and HCO_3^-) that exert the greatest influence on **water balance** and **acid-base balance**.
- In the assessment of acid-base disorders, commonly measured electrolytes are serum Na^+, K^+, H^+ (as pH), Cl^-, and HCO_3^-. Other anions (e.g., sulfates, phosphates, proteins) and cations (e.g., calcium, magnesium, and proteins) are not measured routinely but can be estimated indirectly, since (to maintain electrical neutrality) the sum of the cations must equal that of the anions.
- Normal cellular functions and survival requires electrolytes which are maintained within narrow limits. The concentration of electrolytes is expressed as **milliequivalent per liter (mEq/L) rather than milligrams**.
- Electrolytes produce osmotic pressure. This osmotic pressure helps in maintaining water balance.

Distribution of Electrolytes

The electrolytes are well distributed in ECF and ICF and play an important role in distribution and retention of body water by regulating the osmotic equilibrium. Total concentration of cations and anions in each compartment (ECF and ICF) is equal to maintain electrical neutrality. The concentration of electrolytes in extracellular and intracellular fluid is shown in **Table 16.3**. There are striking differences in composition between the two fluids.

- **Sodium** is the principal cation of the **extracellular fluid** and comprises over 90% of the total cations, but has a low concentration in intracellular fluid and constitutes only 8% of the total cations
- **Potassium** by contrast, is the principal cation of **intracellular fluid** and has a low concentration in extracellular fluid. About 98% of total body potassium is in cells (150–160 mEq/L), only 2% in the ECF (3.5–5 mEq/L).
- Similar differences exist with the anions. **Chloride (Cl^-)** and **bicarbonate (HCO_3^-)** which predominate in the **extracellular fluid**, while **phosphate** is the principal anion within the cells.
- The body water balance is closely linked to the balance of dissolved electrolytes, the most important of which are Na^+ and K^+.

TABLE 16.3: Electrolyte content of ECF and ICF and their concentration.

Ions	Extracellular fluid mEq/L	Intracellular fluid mEq/L
Cations		
Na^+	142	10
K^+	5	150
Ca^{++}	5	2
Mg^{++}	3	40
Total	**155**	**202**
Anions		
Cl^-	103	2
HCO_3^-	27	10
HPO_4^-	2	140
SO_4^{--}	1	5
Organic acids	6	5
Protein	16	40
Total	**155**	**202**

- The osmotic pressure of **extracellular fluids** is determined by the concentration of Na^+ and its associated anions (Cl^-), it accounts for over 90% of the osmolality and thus Na^+ concentration determines the extracellular fluid volume.
- K^+ similarly determines **intracellular osmolality** to a large extent. Serum potassium concentration does not vary appreciably in response to water loss or retention. But even a small change in intracellular potassium concentration will cause a big change in the serum potassium content.

REGULATION OF WATER AND ELECTROLYTE BALANCE

Distribution of water between intracellular and extracellular compartments is affected by **colloidal osmotic pressure** and **osmolality**.

- Since **osmolality** is dependent on the number of **electrolytes** (solute particles), electrolyte and water balance are dependent on each other and cannot be considered separately.
- Water content of ECF and ICF depends on the **concentration of electrolytes** (osmotically active ions) in it. The major determinant factor is the **sodium (Table 16.4)**.

TABLE 16.4: Osmolality exerted by various electrolytes of plasma.

Electrolytes	Osmolality mOsm/kg	Percentage of total
Sodium	270	92
Potassium	7	
Calcium	3	
Magnesium	1	
Urea	5	8
Glucose	5	
Proteins	1	
Total	**292**	

- If the electrolyte concentration is high, fluid moves into that compartment by **osmotic pressure** exerted by electrolytes.
- Change in concentration of osmotically active ions (electrolytes) in either of water compartments creates a **gradient of osmotic pressure**. As a result, movement of water between compartments occurs.
- Water diffuses from a compartment of **low osmolality to one of high osmolality** until osmotic pressures are identical in both of them. The normal osmolality of plasma varies from, **285–295 mOsm/kg**. It is maintained by the **kidney** which excretes either water or solute as the case may be.
- Kidneys regulate water and electrolyte balance and maintain osmolality of plasma **(285–295 mOsm/kg)** by:
  1. Hypothalamic mechanisms controlling thirst
  2. Antidiuretic hormone or vasopressin
  3. Renin-angiotensin-aldosterone system (RAAS)
  4. Atrial natriuretic factor (ANF)

- ❖ **Osmotic pressure** is an important factor that determines the distribution of water among body water compartments. Osmotic pressure is the force that tends to move water from dilute solutions to concentrated solutions. The effective osmotic pressure of a solution depends on the **total number of solute particles** in solution and the **permeability characteristics** of the particular membrane.
- ❖ Crystalloids and water can easily diffuse across membranes, but an osmotic gradient is provided by the nondiffusible colloidal protein particles. The **colloidal osmotic pressure** exerted by **proteins** maintains the intracellular and intravascular fluid compartments. If this gradient is reduced, the fluid will drive out and accumulate in the interstitial space leading to **edema**.

Hypothalamic mechanism and role of antidiuretic hormones:

- It regulates **water intake** and **water output**. The regulatory areas of **water intake** and **water output** are located in separate areas of the hypothalamus in the brain.
  - **Water intake** is normally controlled by the sensation of **thirst**
  - **Water output** by the action of **antidiuretic hormone (ADH)**.
- An increase in plasma **osmolarity** (due to deficiency of water) causes **sensation of thirst** and stimulates hypothalamic thirst center, which results in an increase in water intake.
- An increase in plasma **osmolarity** also stimulates hypothalamus to release **ADH**. ADH then increases water reabsorption by the kidney. All these events ultimately help to restore the plasma osmolality.
- Conversely, a large intake of water causes fall in osmolarity suppresses thirst as well as reduces ADH secretion, leading to a diuresis, excreting large volume of dilute urine **(Figure 16.2)**.

Renin-angiotensin-aldosterone system (RAAS):

- A fall in ECF volume results in decrease in renal plasma flow with reduction in Na in the fluid of the distal tubule
- **Renin** is secreted in response to a reduction in Na^+ in the fluid of the distal tubule which results in retention of ECF volume.
- Renin converts **angiotensinogen** in plasma to **angiotensin I**, which in turn is converted to **angiotensin-II**

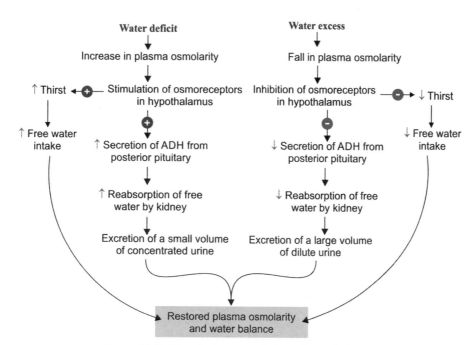

Figure 16.2: Hypothalamic regulation of water balance.

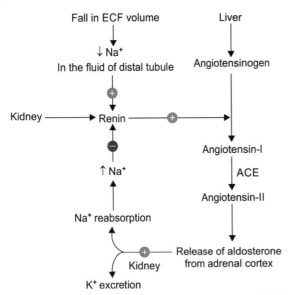

Figure 16.3: Renin-angiotensin-aldosterone system (RAAS).

by **angiotensin-converting enzyme (ACE)**, which stimulates:

- Aldosterone secretion by the adrenal cortex
- Thirsting behavior
- ADH secretion **(Figure 16.3)**.
- Aldosterone stimulates Na^+ reabsorption in the renal tubules in the exchange of H^+ and K^+. As a result of Na^+ reabsorption, water is retained by the body and **ECW restored to normal**.

Atrial Natriuretic Factors

Atrial natriuretic factor (ANF) is a **polypeptide hormone** secreted by the right atrium of the heart.

- It increases Na^+ and water excretion by the kidney.
- In negative sodium and water balance ANF is inhibited and sodium balance become positive and ECW is restored to normal.

◼ DISORDERS OF WATER AND ELECTROLYTE BALANCE

Under most conditions, disturbances of **free water** and **electrolyte balance** occur simultaneously. In most cases, it is a combination of **dehydration** together with an **electrolyte deficit**. Fluid and electrolyte disorders are caused by a temporary disturbance in the body's levels of fluids and electrolytes.

- A disturbance of body water balance in which more fluid is lost from the body than is absorbed results in **dehydration** of the tissues. In contrast, the rapid ingestion of large quantities of water can lead to **overhydration (water intoxication)**.
- **Electrolyte imbalances** occur commonly as a result of:
  - Loss of electrolytes
  - Shifts of certain electrolytes, or
  - Relative changes in concentrations caused by loss of water.

- Common electrolyte imbalances include **hyponatremia, hypernatremia, hypokalemia** and **hyperkalemia**.

Dehydration

Dehydration is the disorders of **water** and **electrolyte balance**, which is due to:

1. Imbalance of water intake and output or
2. Sodium intake and output

- Dehydration may be defined as a state in which loss of water exceeds that of intake, as a result of which body's water content gets reduced and the body is in negative water balance.
- Dehydration may be of two types:
  1. Due to pure water deficiency, without loss of electrolytes, called **simple dehydration**
  2. Due to combine deficiency of water and electrolyte, sodium.

Simple Dehydration (Deficit of Water)

- Simple dehydration, defined as decrease in total body water with relatively normal total body sodium.
- It may result from:
  - Failure to replace obligatory water losses or
  - Failure of the regulatory mechanisms that promotes conservation of the water by the kidney.
- Simple dehydration is associated with:
  - **hypernatremia**, i.e. increased level of sodium
  - **Increase in ECW osmolarity** because water balance is negative and sodium balance is normal.
- The increase in ECW osmolarity (as water is lost from the body) results in movement of water out of the ICW compartment and results in **contraction of both the ECW** and **ICW** compartments.

Dehydration due to Combined Water and Sodium Deficiency

- Dehydration due to combined water and sodium deficiency is more common than simple dehydration.
- Thus, dehydration results from a net negative balance of water and sodium.
- In this case water balance may be:
  - More negative than sodium balance; **called hypernatremic** or **hyperosmolar** dehydration.
  - Equal to sodium balance called; **normonatremic** or **isomolar** dehydration
  - Less negative than sodium balance called; **hyponatremic** or **hyposmolar dehydration**
- Hypernatremic dehydration is the most common type of dehydration.

In Hypernatremic or Hyperosmolar Dehydration

- Water balance is more negative than sodium balance
- Increase in ECW osmolarity causes water to move out of the cell and **contraction of ICW volume occurs**.

Causes of hypernatremic dehydration
- Excessive sweating if free water intake is inadequate.
- Water and food deprivation.
- Diuretic therapy if free water intake is inadequate.
- Osmotic diuresis with glycosuria.

In Normonatremic Dehydration or Isomolar

- Water balance is equally negative to sodium balance.
- No changes occur in ECW and ICW osmolarity.
- Water does not move out of or into cells.

Causes of normonatremic dehydration are:
- Vomiting
- Diarrhea

In Hyponatremic or Hyposmolar Dehydration

- Water balance is less negative to sodium balance.
- Decrease in ECW osmolarity causes water to move into cells and results in increased ICW volume and decreased ECW volume.

Causes of hyponatremic/hyposmolar dehydration
- Salt-wasting renal disease.
- Adrenocortical insufficiency, Addison's disease.
- Diuretic therapy if free water intake is excessive.
- Excessive sweating.

Clinical Findings

- The signs and symptoms of dehydration include:
  - Thirst
  - Wrinkled skin
  - Dry mucous membranes
  - Muscle cramps
  - Oliguria (decreased urine output)
  - Sunken eyeballs
  - Increased blood urea nitrogen, and increased haematocrit.
  - With increasing severity, weakness, hypotension and shock may occur.
- The first and most important clinical finding in dehydration is **dryness** and **wrinkling of the skin**, which gives the body and face a shrunken appearance. The eyes recede into the sockets, sunken eyes is the remarkable clinical findings of dehydration.

Overhydration or Water Intoxication

- **Overhydration** or **water intoxication** is defined as increase in total body water (TBW) with normal total body sodium.
- It rarely results from excessive water consumption (polydipsia). A normal healthy individual can consume a large volume of water without producing any deleterious effects, as the normal individual has the capacity to excrete large volume of dilute urine, when excess of free water (without electrolyte) is given.

- More often water intoxication results due to the retention of excess water in the body, which can occur due to:
  - Renal failure
  - Excessive administration of fluids parenteral
  - Hypersecretion of ADH (syndrome of inappropriate ADH secretion, SIADH).
- This results in hyponatremia and hyposmolarity of the ECW with expansion of the ECW and ICW compartments.

Clinical Findings

Acute fall in serum sodium results in nausea, vomiting, headache, muscular weakness, confusion, seizures and in severe cases convulsions, coma and even death can occur.

Hypernatremia

- Hypernatremia is an increase in serum sodium concentration above the normal range of 135–145 mEq/L. The causes of hypernatremia are:
  - **Water depletion**, may arise from a decreased intake or excessive loss of water with normal sodium content, which occur in diabetes insipidus.
  - **Water and sodium depletion**, if more water than sodium is lost, e.g., diabetes mellitus (osmotic diuresis) and excessive sweating or diarrhea in children.
  - **Excessive sodium intake or retention** in the ECF due to excessive aldosterone secretion, e.g., **Cohn's syndrome** and in **Cushing's syndrome**, where there is excess cortisol production due to hyperactivity of adrenal cortex. Cortisol has mineralocorticoid activity.
- If hypernatremia is due to water loss, then the symptoms are therefore those of dehydration and if it is due to excess salt gain, lead to **hypertension** and **edema**.

Hyponatremia

- Hyponatremia is a significant fall in serum sodium concentration below the normal range 135 to 145 mEq/L. The causes of hyponatremia are:
  - **Retention of water**: Retention of water dilutes the constituents of the extracellular space causing hyponatremia, which occur in heart failure, liver disease, nephrotic syndrome, renal failure, syndrome of inappropriate ADH secretion (SIADH).
  - **Loss of sodium**: This occurs only when there is pathological sodium loss. Such losses may be from gastrointestinal tract, e.g., vomiting, diarrhea, and fistula or in urine. Urinary loss may be due to aldosterone deficiency (Addison's disease).
- Symptoms of hyponatremia are: constant thirst, muscle cramps, nausea, vomiting, abdominal cramps, weakness and lethargy.

Hyperkalemia

Serum potassium concentration does not vary appreciably in response to water loss or retention. But even a small

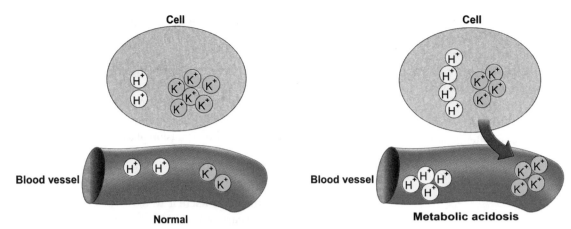

Figure 16.4: Hyperkalemia is associated with metabolic acidosis.

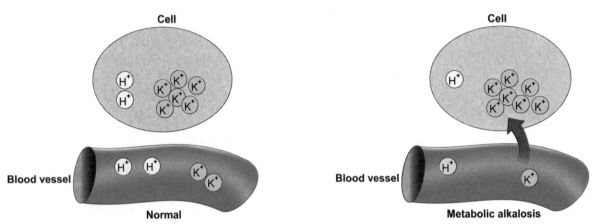

Figure 16.5: Hypokalemia is associated with metabolic alkalosis.

change in intracellular potassium concentration will cause a big change in the serum potassium content.

- Hyperkalemia is a clinical condition associated with elevated plasma potassium above the normal range (3.5 mEq/L–5 mEq/L).
- The causes of hyperkalemia:
  - **Renal failure:** The kidney may not be able to excrete a potassium load when GFR is very low.
  - **Metabolic acidosis:** Due to redistribution of potassium from the intracellular to extracellular fluid space. In acidosis, the concentration of H⁺ ions increases, so potassium ions inside cells are displaced from the cell by hydrogen ions in order to maintain electrochemical neutrality **(Figure 16.4)**.
  - **Cell damage:** Nearly all the total body potassium (98%) is inside the cells. If there is significant tissue damage, the contents of cells, including potassium, leak out the extracellular compartment causing increase in serum potassium. For example, in **rhabdomyolysis** (a condition in which skeletal muscle is broken down), trauma and malignancy.
  - **Insulin deficiency:** Insulin stimulates cellular uptake of potassium. In diabetes mellitus where there is insulin deficiency, hyperkalemia is an associated feature.

- First manifestation is cardiac arrest, changes in electro-cardiogram, cardiac arrhythmia, muscle weakness which may be preceded by paresthesia (abnormal tingling sensation).
- Sever hyperkalemia is immediately life-threatening, and death may occur with no clinical warning signs.

Hypokalemia

- Hypokalemia is a significant fall in serum potassium concentration below the normal range (3.5–5 mEq/L).
- The causes of low plasma concentration of potassium are:
  - **Gastrointestinal losses:** Potassium may be lost from the intestine due to vomiting, and diarrhea.
  - **Renal losses:** Due to renal disease, administration of diuretics,
  - **Increased aldosterone production:** Aldosterone increases sodium reabsorption in the renal tubules at the expense of potassium and hydrogen ions.
  - **Metabolic alkalosis:** An alkalosis may cause a shift of potassium from the ECF to the ICF. In alkalosis the concentration of H⁺ ions decreases, so potassium ions move inside cells in order to maintain electrochemical neutrality **(Figure 16.5)**.
- **Symptoms of hypokalemia:** Anorexia, nausea, vomiting, muscle cramps, or tenderness, lethargy and confusion.

ASSESSMENT QUESTIONS

▌STRUCTURED LONG ESSAY QUESTIONS (SLEQs)

1. Describe electrolyte metabolism under following headings:
   i. Distribution of electrolytes in ECF and ICF
   ii. Plasma concentrations of sodium and potassium
   iii. Disorders of electrolyte (sodium and potassium) imbalance
2. Describe the water and electrolyte balance under the following headings:
   i. Name the regulating factors
   ii. Mechanism of each regulating factor
   iii. Dehydration

▌SHORT ESSAY QUESTIONS (SEQs)

1. What is total body water? Write its distribution and factors that affect distribution of water in the body.
2. Define dehydration? Write its types, causes and clinical symptoms of dehydration.
3. Write regulation of water and electrolyte balance in the body.
4. Write causes and symptoms of hypernatremia and hyponatremia.
5. Write causes and symptoms of hyperkalemia and hypokalemia.

▌SHORT ANSWER QUESTIONS (SAQs)

1. Enumerate factors involved in the regulation of water and electrolyte balance.
2. Give causes and symptoms of dehydration.
3. What is total body water? Write its distribution in the body.
4. Define water intoxication. Write its causes and symptoms.
5. Name the major intracellular and extracellular anion and give its reference range.
6. Name the major intracellular and extracellular cation and give its reference range.
7. Write the normal serum sodium and potassium level.
8. Write two causes of hyponatremia and hyperkalemia.

▌CASE VIGNETTE-BASED QUESTION (CVBQ)

Case Study

1. **A 40-year-old female was brought to the hospital with complaints of persistent vomiting, loose motions, cramps and extreme weakness, sunken eyes and dry tongue.**
   Questions
   a. Name the condition arising due to the above symptoms.
   b. What are the causes for the condition?
   c. Which are the different types of the condition?
   d. Suggest the treatment.

▌MULTIPLE CHOICE QUESTIONS (MCQs)

1. **Chief anion of ECF is:**
   a. Cl^-
   b. HCO_3^-
   c. HPO_4^{--}
   d. Protein
2. **In ICF, main cation is:**
   a. Na^+
   b. K^+
   c. Ca^{++}
   d. Mg^{++}
3. **Which of the following is correct about intracellular water (ICW)?**
   a. Amount less than ECW
   b. Amount more than ECW
   c. Amount equal to ECW
   d. None of the above
4. **Which of the following hormones affects fluid and electrolyte balance?**
   a. Epinephrine
   b. Glucagon
   c. Thyroxine
   d. Aldosterone
5. **Distribution of water between intracellular and extracellular compartments depends on all of the following, *except*:**
   a. Osmolality
   b. Osmolarity
   c. Colloidal osmotic pressure
   d. Surface tension
6. **Source of daily output of water is:**
   a. Urine
   b. Insensible water (skin and lungs)
   c. Sensible water (sweats and stool)
   d. All of the above
7. **Metabolic water is:**
   a. Water from food
   b. Drinking water
   c. Water derived from metabolism
   d. Total body water
8. **Water and electrolyte balance is regulated by, *except*:**
   a. ADH
   b. Renin-angiotensin-aldosterone system (RAAS)
   c. Atrial natriuretic factor (ANF)
   d. Insulin
9. **Main anions of ICF is:**
   a. Cl^-
   b. HPO_4^{--}
   c. HCO_3^-
   d. SO_4^{--}
10. **Main cation of ECF is:**
    a. Na^+
    b. K^+
    c. Ca^{++}
    d. Mg^{++}
11. **Which of the following has greatest water content?**
    a. Liver
    b. Adipose tissue
    c. Brain
    d. Kidney
12. **Which of the following has least water content?**
    a. Pancreas
    b. Brain
    c. Liver
    d. Adipose tissue

13. **In a 70 kg adult, the total body water content is:**
    a. 42 L   b. 28 L
    c. 14 L   d. 3.5 L

14. **The largest portion of total body water is found in which of the tissue?**
    a. Intracellular fluid
    b. Extracellular fluid
    c. Interstitial fluid
    d. Plasma

15. **The daily water allowance for normal adult (60 kg) is about:**
    a. 200–600 mL   b. 500–800 mL
    c. 800–1500 mL   d. 1800–2500 mL

16. **Insensible loss of body water of normal adult is about:**
    a. 50–100 mL   b. 100–200 mL
    c. 300–500 mL   d. 600–1000 mL

17. **Vasopressin (ADH):**
    a. Enhance reabsorption of water from kidney
    b. Decreases reabsorption of water
    c. Increases excretion of calcium
    d. Decreases excretion of calcium

18. **In primary dehydration:**
    a. Intracellular fluid volume is reduced
    b. Intracellular fluid volume remains normal
    c. Extracellular fluid volume is much reduced
    d. Extracellular fluid volume is much increased

19. **Osmotically active substances in plasma are:**
    a. Sodium
    b. Chloride
    c. Proteins
    d. All of these

20. **Osmotic pressure of plasma is:**
    a. 80–100 milliosmole/liter
    b. 180–200 milliosmole/liter
    c. 280–300 milliosmole/liter
    d. 380–400 milliosmole/liter

21. **The water produced during metabolic reactions in an adult is about:**
    a. 100 mL/day
    b. 300 mL/day
    c. 500 mL/day
    d. 700 mL/day

22. **The daily water loss through gastrointestinal tract in an adult is about:**
    a. 500 mL/day   b. 200 mL/day
    c. 300 mL/day   d. 400 mL/day

23. **Body water is regulated by the hormone:**
    a. Oxytocin   b. ACTH
    c. FSH   d. Epinephrine

24. **Edema can occur when:**
    a. Plasma Na and Cl are decreased
    b. Plasma Na and Cl are increased
    c. Plasma proteins are decreased
    d. Plasma proteins are increased

ANSWERS FOR MCQs

1. a	2. b	3. b	4. d	5. d
6. d	7. c	8. d	9. b	10. a
11. c	12. d	13. a	14. a	15. d
16. d	17. a	18. a	19. d	20. c
21. b	22. b	23. a	24. c	

Acid-base Balance

Competency	Learning Objectives
BI 6.7: Describe the processes involved in maintenance of normal pH, water and electrolyte balance of body fluids and the derangements associated with these. **BI 6.8:** Discuss and interpret results of arterial blood gas (ABG) analysis in various disorders.	1. Describe acids, bases and buffers and normal pH of the body fluids. 2. Describe metabolic sources of acids and bases which tend to alter pH of the body fluids. 3. Describe maintenance of normal blood pH by buffers, respiratory and renal mechanism. 4. Describe disorders associated with acid-base balance: acidosis and alkalosis. 5. Discuss arterial blood gas (ABG) analysis in acidosis and alkalosis. 6. Describe anion gap and its significance.

OVERVIEW

The normal process of metabolism results in the net formation of **40** to **80 nmol of hydrogen ions per 24 hours**, principally from the oxidation of sulfur containing amino acids. Metabolism generates **carbon dioxide** which is dissolves in H_2O forming **carbonic acid**, which in turn dissociates, releasing hydrogen ion. In addition metabolism generates strong acids such as **sulphuric acid** and **organic acids** such as **uric acid**, **lactic acid**, and others, all become sources of hydrogen ion in the extracellular fluid.

● Changes in pH affect the **ionization of protein** molecules and consequently activity of many enzymes.

● Changes in pH together with the partial pressure of **carbon dioxide (pCO$_2$)** change the shape of the **hemoglobin**.

● A decrease in pH increases sympathetic tone and may lead to **cardiac dysrhythmias**.

The homeostatic mechanisms for hydrogen ions and carbon dioxide are very efficient. Temporary imbalances can be absorbed by buffering and as a result, the hydrogen ion concentration of the body is maintained within narrow limits of **pH 7.35 to 7.45 (35–45 nmol/L)** in extracellular

fluid (ECF). The intracellular hydrogen ion concentration is slightly higher, but is also strictly controlled.

In disease however, imbalances between the rates of acid formation and excretion can develop and may persist, resulting in **acidosis** and **alkalosis**. This chapter discusses the body's mechanisms to maintain acid-base balance and its disorders.

ACIDS, BASES, AND BUFFERS AND NORMAL pH OF THE BODY FLUIDS

An acid is defined as a substance that releases protons or hydrogen ions (H^+), e.g., hydrochloric acid (HCl), carbonic acid (H_2CO_3).

$$HCl \rightarrow H^+ + Cl^-$$
$$H_2CO_3 \rightarrow H^+ + HCO_3^-$$

A base is a substance that accepts protons or hydrogen ions, e.g., bicarbonate ion (HCO_3^-), and phosphate ion HPO_4^{--}

$$HCO_3^- + H^+ \rightarrow H_2CO_3$$
$$HPO_4^{--} + H^+ \rightarrow H_2PO_4^-$$

● Proteins in the body also function as bases, because some of the amino acids accept hydrogen ions, e.g., **hemoglobin** in red blood cells and plasma protein

TABLE 17.1: Normal pH of body fluids.

Body fluid	pH
Extracellular fluid • Arterial blood • Venous blood and interstitial fluid	 7.40 7.35
Intracellular fluid	6.0–7.4
Urine	4.5–8.0
Gastric HCl	0.8

especially **albumin** are the most important of the body's bases.

- **Buffer** is a solution of weak acid and its corresponding salt, which resists a change in pH when a small amount of acid or base is added to it. By buffering mechanism a strong acid (or base) is replaced by a weaker one.

Normal pH of the Body Fluids

The normal pH of **arterial blood is 7.4**, whereas the pH of venous blood and interstitial fluids is about **7.35** because of the extra amounts of carbon dioxide (CO_2), released from the tissues form H_2CO_3 in these fluids. **Thus, the pH of blood is maintained within a remarkable constant level of 7.35 to 7.45**. Normal pH of body fluids is shown in **Table 17.1**.

The maintenance of a constant pH is important because, the activities of almost all enzyme systems in the body are influenced by hydrogen ion concentration. Therefore, changes in hydrogen ion concentration alter virtually all cell and body functions, the conformation of biological structural components and uptake and release of oxygen.

Why Maintenance of a pH is Important?

- ❖ Changes in pH affect ionization and conformation of protein.
- ❖ Activities of almost all enzyme systems in the body are affected by hydrogen ion concentration which alters nearly all cell and body functions.
- ❖ A change in pH alters the conformation hemoglobin and hampers the uptake and release of oxygen.
- ❖ A decrease in pH increases sympathetic tone and may lead to **cardiac dysrhythmias**.

▮ METABOLIC SOURCES OF ACIDS AND BASES WHICH TEND TO ALTER pH OF THE BODY FLUIDS

Metabolic Sources of Acids

During metabolic processes two types of acids are produced:
1. **Fixed acids are nongaseous acids such as:**
   - Phosphoric and sulphuric acids, produced from the sulfur and phosphorus of proteins and lipoproteins.
   - Organic acids such as pyruvic acid, lactic acid, keto acids (acetoacetic and β-hydroxybutyric acid), and uric acid.

2. **Volatile acids:** The physiologically important volatile acid is **carbonic acid (H_2CO_3)**. In physiology, carbonic acid (H_2CO_3) is described as *volatile acid* or *respiratory acid*, because it is the only acid excreted as a gas by the lungs. It plays an important role in the bicarbonate buffer system to maintain acid-base homeostasis.

Metabolic Sources of Bases

Catabolism of few food materials produces bases. For example:
- Citrate salts of fruit juices may produce bicarbonate salt.
- Deamination of amino acids produces ammonia.
- Formation of biphosphate and acetate also contributes to alkalinizing effect.

▮ MAINTENANCE OF NORMAL BLOOD pH

To maintain the blood pH at **7.35** to **7.45**, there are three primary systems that regulate the hydrogen ion concentration in the body fluids. These are:
- **Buffer mechanism:** First line of defense.
- **The respiratory mechanism:** Second line of defense.
- **Renal mechanism:** Third line of defense.

The first two lines of defense keep the hydrogen ion concentration from changing too much until the more slowly responding third line of defense, the kidneys, can eliminate the excess acid or base from the body.

Buffer Systems and their Role in Acid-base Balance

A buffer is a mixture of a weak acid and a salt of its conjugate base (if one molecule differs from another by only a proton, the two are called as conjugate acid-base pair). A buffer can reversibly bind hydrogen ions. The general form of the buffering reaction is:

$$\text{Buffer} + H^+ \rightleftharpoons H \text{ buffer}$$

- Thus, a **free H^+** combines with the buffer to form a **weak acid (H buffer)**, that can either remain as an undissociated molecule or dissociates back to buffer and H^+.
- When the hydrogen ion concentration increases, the reaction is forced to the right and more hydrogen ions bind to the buffer, as long as the available buffer is present.
- Conversely, when the hydrogen ion concentration decreases, the reaction shifts towards the left and hydrogen ions are released from the buffer. In this way, changes in hydrogen ion concentration are minimized.

Buffering capacity depends on the concentration of the buffer, and relationship between the pKa of the buffer and the desired pH. The pKa is the pH at which a buffer exists in equal proportions with its acid and conjugate base. A buffer is considered most effective within ±2 pH units of its pKa; it has the maximum buffering capacity when its pKa equals the pH. For the maximum blood buffering, the pKa of the buffers should, therefore, be near physiologic pH, that is, pH 7.4.

- The buffer systems of the blood, tissue fluids, and cells; immediately combine with acid or base to prevent excessive changes in hydrogen ion concentration.
- When there is a change in hydrogen ion concentration, the buffer systems of the body fluids react within a fraction of a second to minimize these changes.
- Buffer systems do not eliminate hydrogen ions from the body or add them to the body but only keep them tied up until balance can be re-established. Various buffer systems present in human body are given below.

Blood Buffers

The most important physiological buffer systems of plasma (extracellular buffer) and erythrocytes (intracellular buffer) are **(Table 17.2)**:
- Buffers of **extracellular fluid** present in plasma.
  - Bicarbonate buffer ($NaHCO_3/H_2CO_3$).
  - Phosphate buffer (Na_2HPO_4/NaH_2PO_4).
  - Protein buffer (Na protein/H protein).
- Buffers of **intracellular fluid** present in RBCs
  - Bicarbonate buffer ($KHCO_3/H_2CO_3$).
  - Phosphate buffer (K_2HPO_4/KH_2PO_4).
  - Hemoglobin buffer (KHb/HHb), ($KHbO_2/H.HbO_2$).

The Bicarbonate Buffer System (HCO_3^-/H_2CO_3)

The bicarbonate buffer system is the most important **extracellular buffer**. Although bicarbonate buffer system has a relatively low buffering capacity with pKa 6.3 it plays an important role in maintaining blood pH, because of:
- Its **high concentration**, and
- The two elements of the buffer system, **HCO_3^-** and **H_2CO_3** are regulated by increasing or decreasing the rate of reabsorption of HCO_3^- by the kidneys, and by altering the rates of removal or retention of CO_2 and thereby H_2CO_3 by the lungs on a minute by minute basis.

> Under physiological conditions, with a plasma pH 7.4, the ratio of bicarbonate to carbonic acid (HCO_3^-/H_2CO_3) is **20:1**.

Mechanism of Action of Bicarbonate Buffer

- When a strong acid, such as HCl, is added to the bicarbonate buffer solution, the increased hydrogen ions are buffered by **HCO_3^{--}**. Thus, hydrogen ions from strong acid HCl react with HCO_3^- to form very weak acid H_2CO_3, which, in turn, forms CO_2 and H_2O. The net result therefore is that, the excess CO_2 greatly stimulates respiration, which eliminates the CO_2 from extracellular fluid.

$$HCO_3^- + H^+ \rightarrow H_2CO_3 \rightarrow CO_2 + H_2O$$

- The opposite reactions take place when a strong base such as sodium hydroxide (NaOH), is added to the bicarbonate buffer solution. In this case, the hydroxyl ions (OH-) from NaOH are buffered by H_2CO_3. NaOH combines with H_2CO_3 to form very weak base $NaHCO_3^-$ and H_2O. Thus, the $NaHCO_3$ replaces the strong base NaOH.

$$NaOH + H_2CO_3 \rightarrow NaHCO_3 + H_2O$$

The Phosphate Buffer System ($HPO_4^{--}/H_2PO_4^-$)

The phosphate buffer system is not important as a **blood buffer**; it plays a major role in buffering **renal tubular fluid** and **intracellular fluids**. The phosphate buffer is especially important in the tubular fluids of the kidneys for two reasons:
1. Phosphate usually becomes concentrated in the tubules, thereby increasing the buffering power of the system
2. The tubular fluid usually has a considerably lower pH than extracellular fluid, closer to the pKa 6.8 of the system.

Mechanism of Action of Phosphate Buffer

- The main elements of the phosphate buffer system are **HPO_4^{--}** and **$H_2PO_4^-$**.
- When a strong acid such as HCl is added to a mixture of these two substances, the H^+ is accepted by the base HPO_4^{--} and converted to $H_2PO_4^-$ and strong acid HCl is replaced by a weak acid NaH_2PO_4 and decrease in pH is minimized.

$$HCl + Na_2HPO_4 \rightarrow NaH_2PO_4 + NaCl$$

- When strong base, such as NaOH, is added to the buffer system, the OH- is buffered by the $H_2PO_4^-$ to form HPO_4^{--} and water. Thus strong base NaOH is replaced by weak base HPO_4^{--}, causing slight increase in the pH.

$$NaOH + NaH_2PO_4 \rightarrow Na_2HPO_4 + H_2O$$

> At a plasma pH of 7.4 the ratio HPO_4^- : $H_2PO_4^-$ is 4:1.

Protein Buffer

Plasma Protein Buffer (Na Protein/H Protein)

- In the blood, plasma proteins especially **albumin** acts as buffer because:
  - Proteins contain a large number of dissociable acidic (COOH) and basic (NH_2) groups in their structure.
  - In acid solution they act as a buffer in that, the basic amino group (NH_2) takes up excess H^+ ions forming (NH_3^+).

Buffer system	Plasma (extracellular) buffer	Erythrocyte (intracellular) buffer
Bicarbonate	$NaHCO_3/H_2CO_3$	$KHCO_3/H_2CO_3$
Phosphate	Na_2HPO_4/NaH_2PO_4	K_2HPO_4/KH_2PO_4
Protein	Na Protein/H. Protein	KHb/H.Hb $KHbO_2/H.HbO_2$

TABLE 17.2: The principal buffers of the blood.

- Whereas in basic solutions the acidic COOH groups give up hydrogen ion forming OH⁻ of alkali to water.
- Other important buffer groups of proteins in the physiological pH range are the **imidazole groups of histidine**. Each albumin molecule contains 16 **histidine** residues.

Hemoglobin Buffer (KHb/HHb and KHbO₂/HHbO₂)

Hemoglobin is the major **intracellular buffer** of the blood which is present in erythrocytes. High concentration and appropriate pKa makes hemoglobin the dominant buffering agent of blood at physiological pH. It buffers **carbonic acid (H₂CO₃)** and its **anhydride CO₂** from the tissues.

Mechanism of Action of Hemoglobin Buffer

Hemoglobin works effectively in cooperation with the bicarbonate buffer system. The various reactions occur in regulation of body pH by hemoglobin are given below **(Figure 17.1)**.

- **In the lungs** deoxyhemoglobin carried from tissue is oxygenated to oxyhemoglobin (HbO₂). The formation of oxyhemoglobin from reduced hemoglobin (HHb) releases **hydrogen** ions which are buffered by bicarbonate (HCO₃⁻) to form **carbonic acid (H₂CO₃)**. The carbonic acid formed is converted quickly in the presence of the **carbonic anhydrase (CA)** to **carbon dioxide** and **water**, which is eliminated by ventilation. This buffering effect reduces the pH change as a result of the oxygenation of HHb. The low CO₂ tension in the lung shifts the equilibrium towards the production of CO₂ which is continually eliminated in the expired air **(Figure 17.1)**.

$$H^+ + HCO_3^- \rightleftharpoons H_2CO_3 \rightleftharpoons H_2O + CO_2$$

As the concentration of HCO₃⁻ in the erythrocytes is dropped, (as these are used to buffer oxyhemoglobin), bicarbonate ions from the plasma where its concentration is higher enters into the erythrocyte. To preserve electroneutrality, some negative ion must enter the plasma. Since the cell is readily **permeable to chloride** ions, a shift of **chloride ions** in exchange for the **bicarbonate ions** occurs in the lungs. The chloride ions leave erythrocyte for each bicarbonate molecule that enters it. This change is called the **chloride shift**.

- **In the tissues**, the oxygen tension is reduced and hence oxyhemoglobin dissociates delivering O₂ to the cells and deoxyhemoglobin is formed. CO₂ produced by metabolism enters the blood, where it is hydrated to form H₂CO₃ by **carbonic anhydrase (CA)**. The H₂CO₃ thus formed ionizes to form H⁺ and HCO₃⁻ and results in decrease in blood pH.
- Deoxyhemoglobin acts as a **buffer** and accepts these H⁺ ions to form HHb (weak acid) and HCO₃⁻. The H⁺ ions produced from H₂CO₃ does not cause any change in pH

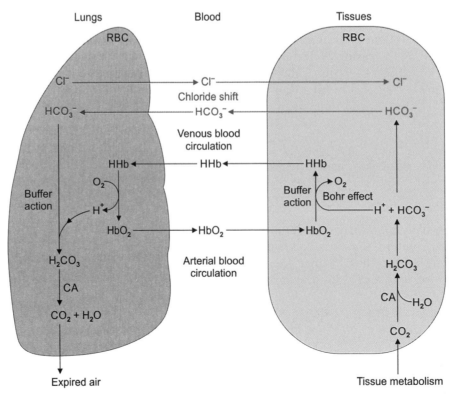

Figure 17.1: Buffering action of hemoglobin in coordination with bicarbonate buffer and role of respiration (lungs) in maintenance of normal blood pH.

(CA: carbonic anhydrase)

because of the buffering action of deoxyhemoglobin (**Figure 17.1**).

- Now, the increase in bicarbonate concentration in the erythrocyte leads to diffusion of these ions from the erythrocytes into the plasma where its concentration is low. Again a shift of chloride ions in exchange for the bicarbonate ions occurs in the tissues but this time chloride ions enter the erythrocyte for each bicarbonate ion that leaves it.

- When the blood returns to the lungs, these H$^+$ ions are released as a result of the formation of oxyhemoglobin. Since oxyhemoglobin is a stronger acid results in the release of H$^+$ and the newly released H$^+$ ion is promptly neutralized by HCO$_3^-$. This reaction is necessary for the liberation of CO$_2$ in the lungs.

> ❖ The transport of an appreciable quantity of the CO$_2$ released from the tissues without change in pH is called **isohydric transport of CO$_2$**.
> ❖ Most of the CO$_2$ is transported in the plasma as bicarbonate (HCO$_3^-$) (**Figure 17.1**).
> ❖ Because HCO$_3$ is much more soluble in blood plasma than is CO$_2$, this indirect route increases the blood's capacity to carry CO$_2$ from the tissues to the lungs.

STRIKE A NOTE

- ❖ Any nonvolatile acid stronger than carbonic acid can be buffered by bicarbonate (HCO$_3^-$).
- ❖ Plasma bicarbonate is a measure of the base that remains after all acids, stronger than carbonic acid has been neutralized. It represents the reserve of alkali available for the neutralization of such strong acids and it has been termed as the **alkali reserve**.
- ❖ The average normal ratio of the concentration of HCO$_3^-$ and H$_2$CO$_3$ in plasma is **25 mmol/L to 1.25 mmol/L = 20:1**.
- ❖ Subsequently any changes in the concentration of either bicarbonate (HCO$_3^-$) or carbonic acid (H$_2$CO$_3$) and therefore in the ratio HCO$_3^-$:H$_2$CO$_3$ accompanied by a change in pH.
- ❖ The phosphate buffer system has a **pKa of 6.8**, which is close to the normal pH of 7.4 in the body fluids and this allows the system maximum buffering power. However, its concentration in both plasma and erythrocytes is low, i.e., only 8% of the concentration of the bicarbonate buffer. Therefore, the total buffering power of the phosphate system in the blood is much less than that of the bicarbonate buffering system.
- ❖ Organic phosphate in the form of **2,3 bisphosphoglycerate (2,3 BPG)**, present in erythrocytes in a concentration of about 4.5 mmol/L, accounts for about 16% of the noncarbonate buffer value of erythrocyte fluid.
- ❖ Proteins, especially albumin, account for the greatest portion (95%) of the nonbicarbonate buffer value of the plasma. Each albumin molecule contains **16 histidine** residues.
- ❖ Each Hb molecule contains **38 molecules of histidine**.
- ❖ The **imidazole group** of histidine has a pKa of approximately 7.3, fairly close to 7.4 and has maximum buffering capacity at physiological pH range.
- ❖ Hb buffers carbonic acid (H$_2$CO$_3$).
- ❖ **Oxyhemoglobin** is a **stronger acid** results in the release of H$^+$, which is buffered by KHCO$_3^-$.

Respiratory Mechanism in Acid-base Balance

The second line of defense against acid-bases disturbances is by regulating the concentration of carbonic acid (H$_2$CO$_3$) in the blood and other body fluids by the lungs. The respiratory center regulates the removal or retention of CO$_2$ and thereby H$_2$CO$_3$ from the extracellular fluid by the lungs. Thus lungs, function by maintaining one component (H$_2$CO$_3$) of the bicarbonate buffer as follows:

- An increase in (H$^+$) or (H$_2$CO$_3$) stimulates the respiratory center to increase the rate of respiratory ventilation. When the ventilation rate increases, more CO$_2$ is released from the blood and pH increases.

- Similarly, an increase in (OH$^-$) or (HCO$_3^-$) depresses respiratory ventilation. A decrease in ventilation rate will cause a decrease in release of CO$_2$ from the blood. The increased blood CO$_2$ will result in the formation of more H$_2$CO$_3$. Thus, there will be decrease in pH.

- Thus, when the rate of ventilation is increased, excess acid (H$_2$CO$_3$) in the form of CO$_2$ is quickly removed. Similarly, when the rate of ventilation is decreased, acid (H$_2$CO$_3$) in the form of CO$_2$ is added to neutralize excess alkali (HCO$_3^-$).

> Respiratory system acts as a **controller** of H$^+$ concentration (**Figure 17.2**). Increased H$^+$ concentration stimulates respiratory center and alveolar ventilation. This decreases the concentration of CO$_2$ in extracellular fluid and reduces H$^+$ concentration back to normal. Conversely, decreased H$^+$ concentration below normal depresses respiratory center and alveolar ventilation and H$^+$ concentration increases back to normal.

Renal Mechanism in Acid-base Balance

Renal mechanism is the **third-line of defense** in acid-base balance. Long-term acid-base control is exerted by renal mechanisms. Kidney participates in the regulation of acid-

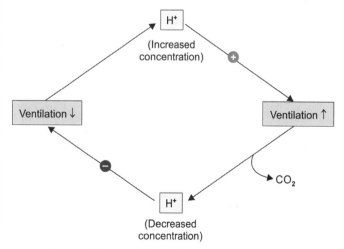

Figure 17.2: Regulation of H$_2$CO$_3^-$ concentration by respiratory system.

base balance primarily by **conservation of HCO$_3^-$ (alkali reserve)** and excretion of acid as the case may be.

- The pH of the initial glomerular filtrate is approximately 7.4 same as that of plasma, whereas the average urinary pH is approximately 6.0 due to the renal excretion of nonvolatile acids produced by metabolic processes. The pH of the urine may vary from 4.5 to 8.0 corresponding to the case of acidosis or alkalosis. In acidosis, excretion of acids is increased and base is conserved, in alkalosis, the opposite occurs. This ability to excrete variable amounts of acid or base makes the kidney, the final defense mechanism against change in body pH.

- Renal conservation of HCO$_3^-$ and excretion of acid occur through four key mechanisms
  1. Exchange of H$^+$ (formed in tubular cell) with Na$^+$ of tubular fluid. **(Figure 17.3)**
  2. Reabsorption (recovery) of bicarbonate from tubular fluid **(Figure 17.3)**
  3. Formation of ammonia and excretion of ammonium ion (NH$_4^+$) in the urine **(Figure 17.4)**
  4. Excretion of H$^+$ as H$_2$PO$_4^-$ in urine **(Figure 17.5)**.

Exchange of H$^+$ for Na$^+$ of Tubular Fluid

- In renal tubular cells, the carbonic anhydrase catalyzes the formation of carbonic acid (H$_2$CO$_3$) from CO$_2$ and water. The carbonic acid, thus formed dissociates to yield H$^+$ and HCO$_3^-$.

- The H$^+$ ions formed in tubular cells are secreted into the tubular fluid in exchange for Na$^+$ present in tubular fluid **(Figure 17.3)**. Na$^+$-H$^+$ exchange is enhanced in state of acidosis and inhibited in alkalosis states.

- The bicarbonate anion formed by the dissociation of H$_2$CO$_3$ in the tubular cell diffuses into the blood as the accompanying ion to Na$^+$ and HCO$_3^-$ is thus conserved and increases the **'alkali reserve'** of the body.

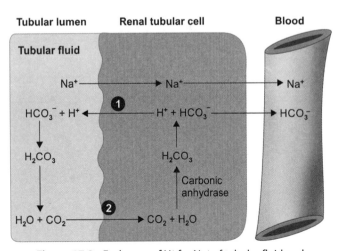

Figure 17.3: Exchange of H$^+$ for Na$^+$ of tubular fluid and reabsorption of bicarbonate from tubular fluid.

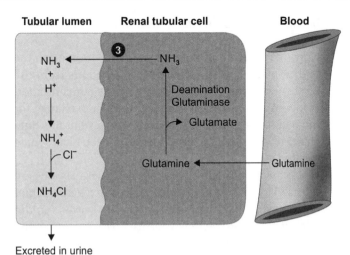

Figure 17.4: Formation of ammonia and excretion of ammonium ions in the urine.

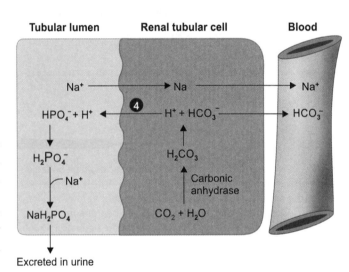

Figure 17.5: Excretion of H$^+$ as H$_2$PO$_4^-$ in urine.

Reabsorption (Recovery) of Bicarbonate from Tubular Fluid

- Some H$^+$ that are secreted into the tubular fluid in exchange of Na$^+$ react with HCO$_3^-$ in the tubular fluid to form H$_2$CO$_3$, which is dehydrated to CO$_2$ and H$_2$O by an enzyme carbonic anhydrase.

- The increase in CO$_2$ in tubular fluid causes carbon dioxide to diffuse into the tubular cell where it reacts with H$_2$O to form H$_2$CO$_3$ and subsequently, H$^+$ and HCO$_3^-$. Thus, reabsorption of bicarbonate is in terms of diffusion of CO$_2$ into tubular cells and its subsequent conversion to HCO$_3^-$ **(Figure 17.3)**.

- The process of bicarbonate reabsorption is enhanced in states of acidosis and decreased in alkalosis.

- The kidney reabsorbs almost all filtered bicarbonate at plasma bicarbonate concentration below 25 mEq/L. Only when bicarbonate levels become elevated above 25 mEq/L bicarbonate will be excreted into the urine.

Formation of Ammonia and Excretion of Ammonium Ions (NH$_4^+$) in the Urine

- Ammonia (the urinary buffer) is produced by **deamination of glutamine** in renal tubular cell. **Glutaminase** present in tubular cells catalyzes this reaction.
- Ammonia is a gas and diffuses readily across the cell membrane into the tubular lumen, where it buffers hydrogen ions to form ammonium (NH$_4^+$) ions **(Figure 17.4)**.
- The NH$_4^+$ ions formed in the tubular lumen cannot diffuse back into tubular cells and thus, is trapped in the tubular urine and excreted with anions, such as phosphate, chloride or sulphate.
- The rate of glutamine uptake from the blood and its utilization by the kidney depends on the amount of acid which must be excreted to maintain a normal blood pH. As the level of H$^+$ ions of the blood increases (pH decreases), glutamine uptake increases. During a metabolic acidosis, the excretion of NH$_4^+$ by the kidney increases several fold.

The removal of hydrogen ions as NH$_4^+$ decreases the requirement of bicarbonate to buffer the urine.

Excretion of H$^+$ Ions as H$_2$PO$_4^-$ in Urine

- The hydrogen ions secreted into the tubular fluid in exchange of Na$^+$ are buffered by HPO$_4^{--}$ of phosphate buffer. HPO$_4^{--}$ combines with the secreted H$^+$ and is converted to H$_2$PO$_4^-$ and is excreted in the urine as NaH$_2$PO$_4$ **(Figure 17.5)**.
- This process depends on the amount of phosphate filtered by the glomeruli and the pH of urine. Acidemia increases phosphate excretion and thus provides additional buffer for reaction with H$^+$.
- A decrease in the glomerular filtration rate (GFR) with renal disease may result in a decrease of H$_2$PO$_4^-$ excretion.

◼ DISORDERS ASSOCIATED WITH ACID-BASE BALANCE

Bicarbonate buffer (HCO$_3^-$/H$_2$CO$_3$) system is the most important buffering system of the body. Acid-base balance depends on the ratio **HCO$_3^-$/H$_2$CO$_3$**. At pH 7.4 the ratio of the concentration of HCO$_3^-$ and H$_2$CO$_3$ in plasma is **20:1**. Any changes in the concentration of either **bicarbonate (HCO$_3^-$)** or **carbonic acid (H$_2$CO$_3$)** is accompanied by a change in ratio and pH. The concentration of **carbonic acid (H$_2$CO$_3$)** is regulated by **lungs** and concentration of **bicarbonate**, is regulated by **kidneys**.

- The term **"acidemia"** describes the state of an arterial blood pH less than 7.35, while **acidosis** is used to describe the pathological conditions leading to these states
- The term **"alkalemia"** describes the state of an arterial blood pH greater than 7.45, while **alkalosis** is used to describe the pathological conditions leading to these states.

Acidosis and Alkalosis

- **Acidosis** may be defined as an abnormal condition caused by the accumulation of excess acid in the body or by the loss of alkali from the body.
- **Alkalosis** is an abnormal condition caused by the accumulation of excess alkali in the body or by the loss of acid from the body.
- More than one type of pathological process can occur simultaneously, giving rise to a **mixed acid-base disturbance**, in which the blood pH may be low, high or within the normal level.
- Unrecognized or untreated disturbances in acid-base balance can be fatal.
- Acid-base disorders are classified, in terms of their immediate cause, as follows **(Figure 17.6)**:
  1. **Metabolic acidosis:** Decrease in bicarbonate (HCO$_3^-$) concentration.

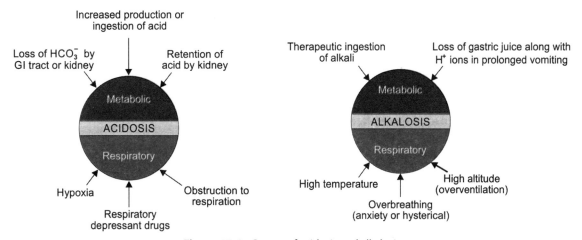

Figure 17.6: Causes of acidosis and alkalosis.

2. **Metabolic alkalosis:** Increase in bicarbonate (HCO_3^-) concentration.
3. **Respiratory acidosis:** Increase in pCO_2 or H_2CO_3 concentration.
4. **Respiratory alkalosis:** Decrease in pCO_2 or H_2CO_3 concentration.

Compensatory mechanism against acidosis and alkalosis

Any derangement of acid-base balance produces compensatory changes to restore homeostasis as follows:

- If acidosis is caused by an increase of H_2CO_3, increase in the HCO_3^- occurs to maintain the ratio of **HCO_3^-/H_2CO_3** (20:1).
- If acidosis is from loss of alkali (HCO_3^-), a simultaneous decrease in the H_2CO_3 occurs to maintain the ratio.
- If alkalosis arising from an increased amount of alkali (HCO_3^-) may be compensated by an increased retention of carbonic acid.
- If alkalosis is due to a decrease in H_2CO_3, simultaneously, a decrease in the HCO_3^- occurs.
- In all these four conditions, if the ratio HCO_3^-/H_2CO_3 remains within limits, i.e., about **16:1 to 25:1**, corresponding to pH 7.3 to 7.5, the condition is called **compensated acidosis** and **compensated alkalosis**.
- When the ratio actually changes and pH is outside of the normal range the term **uncompensated** is used.
  - In **uncompensated acidosis**, the pH falls to an abnormal level and the patient may go into coma.
  - In **uncompensated alkalosis**, the pH rises to an abnormal level and leads to neuromuscular irritability and tetany.

Metabolic Acidosis

A fall in blood pH due to a decrease in bicarbonate levels of plasma is called **metabolic acidosis**.

- Decrease in bicarbonate levels may be due to:
  - Increased production of acids. In uncontrolled diabetes mellitus and starvation there is an excessive production of acetoacetic acid and β-hydroxybutyric acid. These acids are buffered by utilizing base component (i.e., HCO_3^-) of the bicarbonate buffer. Consequently the concentration of bicarbonate ions fall giving rise to bicarbonate deficit and results in metabolic acidosis (ketoacidosis).
  - In lactic acidosis (increased level of lactic acid) occurs in vigorous exercise.
  - In nephritis (chronic renal failure), kidney may not be able to excrete acids in sufficient amounts that leads to retention of acids.
  - Excessive loss of bicarbonate occurs in the urine in renal tubular dysfunction and form GI tract in severe diarrhea.

Compensatory Mechanisms

Metabolic acidosis is compensated by:

- Increasing rate of respiration to wash out CO_2 (hence H_2CO_3) faster. Consequently, the ratio $HCO_3^-:H_2CO_3$ is elevated.
- Increasing excretion of H+ ions as NH_4^+ ions.
- Increasing elimination of acid ($H_2PO_4^-$) in the urine.

All these compensatory mechanisms tend to reduce carbonic acid to keep the pH in the normal range and a compensated acidosis results.

Respiratory Acidosis

It results from an increase in concentration of **carbonic acid (H_2CO_3)** in plasma. An increase in concentration of H_2CO_3 is due to decrease in alveolar ventilation, and that leads to retention of CO_2. Decreased alveolar ventilation may occur in following circumstances.

- **Obstruction to respiration:** This may occur in pneumonia, emphysema, asthma, etc.
- **Depression of respiration:** Administration of respiratory depressant toxic drugs, e.g., morphine depresses the respiratory center.

Compensatory Mechanisms

- Increase in renal reabsorption of bicarbonate.
- Rise in urinary acid ($H_2PO_4^-$) and ammonia.

Metabolic Alkalosis

A rise in blood pH due to rise in the bicarbonate levels of plasma is called **metabolic alkalosis**. This is seen in the following conditions:

- Loss of gastric juice along with H+ ions in prolonged and severe vomiting.
- Therapeutic administration of large dose of alkali (as in peptic ulcer) or chronic intake of excess antacids.

Compensatory Mechanisms

- Increased excretion of alkali (HCO_3^-) by the kidney
- Diminished formation of ammonia
- Respiration is depressed to conserve CO_2.

Respiratory Alkalosis

A rise in blood pH due to lowered concentration of CO_2 or H_2CO_3, due to hyperventilation. This occurs in the following conditions:

- Anxiety or hysteria
- Fever
- Hot baths
- At high altitude
- Working at high temperature, etc.

Compensatory Mechanisms

- Reduction of urinary ammonia formation
- Increased excretion of bicarbonate
- Decreased elimination of acid **$H_2PO_4^-$** in the urine.

TABLE 17.3: Acid-base disorders and their clinical causes.

Acid-base disorders	Clinical causes
Metabolic acidosis	• Diabetes mellitus (Ketoacidosis) • Lactic acidosis • Therapeutic administration of HCl • Renal failure • Severe diarrhea • Renal tabular acidosis due to loss of HCO_3^- ions
Respiratory acidosis	• Chronic obstructive airways disease, asthma, emphysema, and pneumonia • Cardiac arrest, severe hypoxia • Weakness of respiratory muscle, e.g., in poliomyelitis, multiple sclerosis • Chest deformities, thoracic trauma, pneumothorax myopathies • Administration of respiratory depressant toxic drugs, e.g., morphine
Metabolic alkalosis	• Loss of gastric juice along with H^+ ions • Nasogastric drainage (loss of H^+ ions) • Hypokalemia • Therapeutic administration of alkali
Respiratory alkalosis	• Hyperventilation (anxiety, fever) • Hot baths • High altitudes • Working at high temperature • Salicylate poisoning

Mixed Acid-base Disturbances

- More than one type of pathological condition can occur simultaneously, giving rise to a **mixed acid-base imbalance**, in which the blood pH may be low, high or within the normal level.
- Respiratory and metabolic disorders of acid-base balance can occur together. For example, some patients with chronic renal failure (which causes a primary metabolic acidosis) may also have chronic obstructive airways disease, which causes a primary respiratory acidosis.
- Plasma (H^+) will be increased in these patients, but the results for plasma CO_2 and concentration of (HCO_3^-) cannot be predicted. The history and clinical findings must be taken into account.

Table 17.3 summarizes the clinical causes of acid-base disorders.

Clinical Cases

1. A young man with a history of dyspepsia and excessive alcohol intake who gives a history of vomiting. Blood gas results are:
   - ➤ pH = 7.5 *(alkalosis)*
   - ➤ HCO_3^- = 47 mEq/L *(metabolic alkalosis due to loss of H^+ from gut)*
   - ➤ PCO_2 = 55 mm Hg *(respiratory acidosis, signifying compensation)*
2. A patient who has had an acute asthmatic attack. Blood gas results are:
   - ➤ pH = 7.6 *(alkalosis)*
   - ➤ pCO_2 = 20 mm Hg *(respiratory alkalosis)*
   - ➤ HCO_3^- = 22 mEq/L *(not low, hence uncompensated)*
   Therefore, uncompensated respiratory alkalosis.

Contd...

Contd...

3. A patient with chronic bronchitis. Blood gas results are:
   - ➤ pH = 7.356 (normal, so there is either no acid-base disturbance or a fully compensated one)
   - ➤ pCO_2 = 70 mm Hg (respiratory acidosis)
   - ➤ HCO_3^- = 40 mEq/L *(metabolic alkalosis)*

In view of the history, it will most likely be a fully compensated respiratory acidosis. The other possibility is a fully compensated metabolic alkalosis.

ARTERIAL BLOOD GAS ANALYSIS IN ACID-BASE IMBALANCE

Arterial blood gas analysis in acid-base imbalance is given in **Table 17.4**.

- The assessment of acid-base status is usually done by **arterial blood gas (ABG) analyser (Figure 17.7)** which measures **pH, pCO_2,** and **pO_2** directly by means of electrodes.

TABLE 17.4: Arterial blood gas analysis in acid-base imbalance.

Disorders	Primary responses		Compensatory responses
Metabolic acidosis	↑[H^+] ↓pH	↓ (HCO_3^-) Decrease in plasma bicarbonate concentration	↓ pCO_2 Hyperventilation
Metabolic alkalosis	↓[H^+] ↑pH	↑ (HCO_3^-) Increase in plasma bicarbonate concentration	↑ pCO_2 Hypoventilation
Respiratory acidosis	↑[H^+] ↓pH	↑ pCO_2 Increase in plasma carbonic acid	↑ (HCO_3^-) Increase renal bicarbonate reabsorption
Respiratory alkalosis	↓[H^+] ↑pH	↓ pCO_2 Decrease in plasma carbonic acid	↓ (HCO_3^-) Decrease renal bicarbonate reabsorption

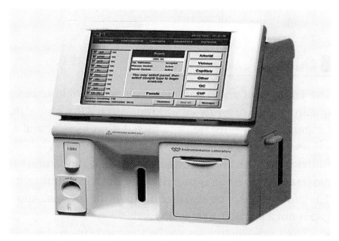

Figure 17.7: Arterial blood gas (ABG) analyzer.

TABLE 17.5: Normal range of arterial and venous blood gases.

Value	Arterial blood	Venous blood
pH	7.40 (7.35–7.45)	7.36 (7.31–7.41)
PO$_2$	80–100 mm Hg	35–40 mm Hg
O$_2$ saturation	95%	70–75%
PCO$_2$	35–45 mm Hg	41–51 mm Hg
HCO$_3^-$	22–26 mEq/L	22–26 mEq/L
BE	–2 to +2	–2 to +2

(O$_2$: oxygen; PO$_2$: partial pressure of oxygen; pH: acidity/alkalinity; PCO$_2$: partial pressure of carbondioxide; HCO$_3^-$: bicarbonate in blood; BE: base excess)

- The acid-base status of the body fluid is assessed by the measurement of **blood pH** and **pCO$_2$**.
- Arterial blood gas analysis is a common investigation in **emergency** departments and **intensive care** units for monitoring patients with **acute respiratory failure**.
- An ABG analysis can help in the assessment of a patient's **gas exchange**, **ventilatory control**, and **acid-base balance**. The normal range of arterial and venous blood gases, which are widely used parameters, are given in **Table 17.5**.
- Accurate results for ABG depend on proper manner of **collecting**, **handling**, and **analyzing** the specimen. The most common problems that are encountered are:
  - Collection of nonarterial samples
  - Air bubbles in the sample
  - Use of inadequate or excessive anticoagulant
  - Delayed analysis of a noncooled sample
- The ABG analysis becomes necessary because it:
  - Helps in confirming diagnosis
  - Guides treatment plan
  - Helps in ventilator management and improvement in acid/base management
- Interpretation of an arterial blood gas result should not be done without considering the clinical findings. The results change as the body compensates for the underlying problem.

ANION GAP

The concept of anion gap originally was developed as a quality control rule when it was found that if the sum of the Cl$^-$ and HCO$_3^-$ values was subtracted from the Na$^+$ and K$^+$ values the difference or 'gap' averaged 16 mmol/L in healthy individuals. The concentration of anions and cations in plasma must be equal to maintain electrical neutrality. Therefore, there is no real anion gap in the plasma. Anion gap is not a physiological reality.

- The term electrolytes applied in medicine to the four ions in plasma, (Na$^+$, K$^+$, Cl$^-$ and HCO$_3^-$) that exert the greatest influence on water balance and acid-base balance.
- In the assessment of acid-base disorders, commonly measured electrolytes are serum Na$^+$, K$^+$, H$^+$ (as pH), Cl$^-$, and HCO$_3^-$. Other anions (e.g., sulfates, phosphates, proteins) and cations (e.g., calcium, magnesium, and proteins) are not measured routinely.
- Serum Na+ and K+ content accounts for 95% of cations, and Cl$^-$ and HCO$_3^-$ for about 85% of anions. The unmeasured anion is commonly known as the **anion gap**, which is normally 12 ± 4 mEq/L.

Thus, **anion gap** is a measurement of the difference between the sums of "routinely measured" cations and the sum of the "routinely measured" anions in the blood. The anion gap = (Na$^+$ + K$^+$) – (Cl$^-$ + HCO$_3^-$) and is estimated as:

Anion gap (Unmeasured anions)
$$= ([Na^+] + [K^+]) - ([Cl^-] + [HCO_3^-])$$
$$= (142 + 4) - (103 + 27)$$
$$= 146 - 130$$
$$= 16 \text{ mEq/L}$$

Significance of Anion Gap

- Acid-base disorders are often associated with alterations in the anion gap.
- The **anion gap** value is useful in assessing the acid-base status of a patient and in diagnosing metabolic acidosis. In metabolic acidosis the anion gap can increase or remain normal depending on the cause of acidosis.
- Disorders that cause a high anion gap are metabolic acidosis, dehydration, therapy with sodium salts of strong acids, therapy with certain antibiotics and alkalosis.
- A decrease in the normal anion gap occurs in various plasma dilution states, hypercalcemia, hypermagnesemia, hypernatremia, and hypoalbuminemia.
- Evaluation of **mixed acid-base abnormalities** requires an understanding of the anion gap. Clinical findings and history are also necessary to define the factors that may contribute to the development of mixed acid-base disorders.

Metabolic Acidosis Associated with Increased Anion Gap

- In metabolic acidosis, the plasma HCO$_3^-$ is reduced. To keep electroneutrality, the concentration of anions (either Cl$^-$ or an unmeasured anion) must increase. If the decrease in plasma HCO$_3^-$ is not accompanied by increased Cl$^-$, the anion gap value will increase and referred to as **increased anion gap acidosis** or **normochloremic acidosis**.
- Metabolic acidosis caused by excess nonvolatile acids (besides HCl), such as lactic acid, or keto acids is

TABLE 17.6: Metabolic acidosis associated with normal and increased plasma anion gap.

Increased anion gap	Normal anion gap

• Diabetic ketoacidosis
• Renal failure
• Methanol toxicity
• Alcoholic ketoacidosis
• Paracetamol toxicity
• Lactic acidosis
• Ethylene glycol poisoning
• Salicylate toxicity (present in aspirin)
	• Gastrointestinal fluid loss
	  ❯ Diarrhea
	  ❯ Pancreatitis
	  ❯ Intestinal fistula
	• Renal tubular acidosis
	• Acetazolamide therapy (carbonic anhydrase inhibitor)

associated with an increased plasma anion gap because the fall in HCO_3^- is not compensated by an equal increase in Cl^-. A useful **mnemonic** help to remember some of the causes of an increase anion gap metabolic acidosis is **DR MAPLES (Table 17.6)**.

Metabolic Acidosis Associated with Normal Anion Gap

● In contrast to high anion gap acidosis, plasma Cl^- increases in proportion to the fall in plasma HCO_3^- and the anion gap is remained normal, this referred to as **hyperchloremic metabolic acidosis** or **normal anion gap acidosis**.

● The cause of normal anion gap acidosis is the loss of bicarbonate rich fluid from either the kidney (renal tubular acidosis or acetazolamide therapy) or gastrointestinal tract (diarrhea). As HCO_3^- is lost, Cl^- ions are reabsorbed with Na^+ or K^+ to maintain electroneutrality.

> Acetazolamide therapy is used to treat glaucoma. By inhibiting **carbonic anhydrase** activity in the eye, it reduces the formation of aqueous humor. Inhibition of the enzyme in renal tubular cells and erythrocytes impairs H^+ secretion and HCO_3^- formation.

ASSESSMENT QUESTIONS

STRUCTURED LONG ANSWER QUESTIONS (SLAQs)

1. Discuss the mechanisms for regulation of blood pH under following headings:
   i. Normal blood pH range
   ii. Buffer mechanism
   iii. Respiratory mechanism
   iv. Renal mechanism
2. Discuss the role of buffers in regulation of blood pH under following headings:
   i. Normal blood pH range
   ii. Name the buffer systems in the body
   iii. Buffer mechanism
   iv. Metabolic acidosis with its compensatory mechanisms
3. Discuss the mechanisms for regulation of blood pH under following headings:
   i. Normal blood pH range
   ii. Role of lungs
   iii. Role of kidney
   iv. Respiratory acidosis with its compensatory mechanisms
4. Discuss the role of kidney in regulation of acid-base balance under following headings:
   i. Normal blood pH range
   ii. Mechanisms with diagram
   iii. Metabolic and respiratory alkalosis
   iv. Compensatory mechanisms for metabolic and respiratory alkalosis
5. Discuss the disorders associated with derangement of acid-base balance under the following headings:
   i. Define acidemia and alkalemia
   ii. Metabolic acidosis with compensatory mechanisms
   iii. Metabolic alkalosis with compensatory mechanisms

   iv. Respiratory acidosis with compensatory mechanisms
   v. Respiratory alkalosis with compensatory mechanisms

SHORT ESSAY QUESTIONS (SEQs)

1. Name various blood buffers. Write the mechanism of action of bicarbonate buffer.
2. Write causes of metabolic acidosis and their compensatory mechanisms.
3. Write the role of kidney in regulation of blood pH.
4. Write mechanism of action of hemoglobin as a buffer.
5. What is anion gap? How it is measured? Write the status of anion gap in metabolic acidosis.
6. What is arterial blood gas analysis (ABG)? Write different parameters with their reference range. Give importance and common problem encountered in ABG analysis

SHORT ANSWER QUESTIONS (SAQs)

1. What is metabolic acidosis? Name any two pathological conditions which lead to metabolic acidosis.
2. Write the role of lungs in compensatory metabolic acidosis
3. Write the role of kidney in compensatory respiratory acidosis
4. What are buffers? Name important buffers of blood.
5. Name four renal mechanisms in acid-base balance.
6. What is respiratory acidosis? Name pathological conditions which lead to respiratory acidosis.
7. Write the role of phosphate buffer in acid-base balance.
8. Write definition and importance chloride shift.
9. Write definition and importance alkali reserve.
10. Write definition and clinical importance of anion gap.

11. Write causes and compensatory mechanisms for metabolic acidosis.
12. Write causes and compensatory mechanisms for metabolic alkalosis.
13. Write causes and compensatory mechanisms for respiratory acidosis.
14. Write causes and compensatory mechanisms for respiratory alkalosis.
15. Enumerate any four causes for high anion gap metabolic acidosis.
16. Write definition and importance isohydric transport of CO_2.

■ CASE VIGNETTE-BASED QUESTIONS (CVBQs)

Case Study

1. **A 38-year-old man reported in the emergency ward of a hospital emergency with complaints of persistent vomiting for one week. He had generalized muscular cramps. On examination, he appeared dehydrated and had shallow respiration. Blood sample was analyzed with the following results:**

pH	=	7.8
Bicarbonates	=	35 mEq/L
pCO_2	=	50 mm Hg
Na^+	=	145 mEq/L
K^+	=	2.9 mEq/L

   Questions
   a. Identify the nature of acid-base disorder.
   b. What could be the cause of this acid-base disorder?
   c. What is the cause of shallow respiration?
   d. Give reason for development of muscle cramps.

2. **A 50-year-old male was admitted with a history of chronic obstructive airways disease for many years. On examination, he was found cyanosed, and breathless. Blood sample was analyzed with the following results:**

Blood pH	=	below normal
pCO_2	=	markedly elevated
(HCO_3^-)	=	markedly elevated

   Questions
   a. Identify the nature of acid-base disorder.
   b. What could be the cause of elevated pCO_2?
   c. What could be the cause of elevated (HCO_3^-)?

3. **A person presents himself with untreated diabetes mellitus. He is treated for acidosis.**

   Questions
   a. What is the type of acidosis?
   b. What is the normal bicarbonate/carbonic acid ratio? What will happen to the ratio in this patient?
   c. How will compensation occur?
   d. What is the role of kidney in correcting acidosis?

4. **A 28-year-old man was admitted to hospital with a crushed chest. The biochemical results on arterial blood gases were found with high [H^+] and pCO_2.**

Questions
a. What is the acid-base disorder?
b. Write compensatory mechanism for the disorder
c. What is the normal blood pH?
d. What is the normal blood pCO_2?

5. **A 56-year-old woman was admitted seriously ill and confused. The patient had systemic edema. Diagnosis was that the patient had mixed acid-base disorder. On admission the following biochemical results were obtained:**

   i. Low [H^+] concentration (Increased blood pH)
   ii. Increased bicarbonate concentration
   iii. Increase in pCO_2 is too high.

   Questions
   a. What is the evidence for the disorder?
   b. Which are the other acid-base disorders?
   c. What is the normal blood pH?
   d. What is the normal blood pCO_2?

6. **In a patient, Blood gas analysis showed following findings:**

HCO_3^-	=	24 mEq/L
H_2CO_3	=	2.7 mEq/L
PCO_2	=	90 mm Hg
pH	=	7.05

   Questions
   a. What is your probable diagnosis? Justify.
   b. What are the causes for above condition?
   c. What is the compensatory mechanism of diagnosed condition?

7. **In a patient, ABG analysis showed:**

HCO_3^-	=	24 mEq/L
H_2CO_3	=	0.6 mEq/L
$HCO_3^- : H_2CO_3$	=	40 : 1
PCO2	=	20 mm Hg
pH	=	7.7

   Questions
   a. What is your probable diagnosis? Justify.
   b. What are the causes for above condition?
   c. What is the compensatory mechanism of diagnosed condition?

8. **In a patient, ABG analysis showed:**

HCO_3^-	=	15 mEq/L
H_2CO_3	=	1.2 mEq/L
$HCO_3^- : H_2CO_3$	=	12.5 : 1
PCO_2	=	40 mm Hg
pH	=	7.2

   Questions
   a. What is your probable diagnosis?
   b. What are the causes for above condition?
   c. What is the compensatory mechanism of diagnosed condition?

9. **In a patient, ABG analysis showed:**

HCO_3^-	=	38 mEq/L
H_2CO_3	=	1.2 mEq/L

$HCO_3^- : H_2CO_3$ = 31.7 : 1

PCO_2 = 40 mm Hg

pH = 7.6

Questions

a. What is your probable diagnosis?

b. What are the causes for above condition?

c. What is the compensatory mechanism of diagnosed condition?

MULTIPLE CHOICE QUESTIONS (MCQs)

1. **Metabolic acidosis is primarily due to:**
   a. Increase in carbonic acid
   b. Decrease in carbonic acid
   c. Decrease in bicarbonate
   d. Increase in bicarbonate

2. **In compensated metabolic acidosis plasma:**
   a. HCO_3^-/H_2CO_3 ratio is increased
   b. Total CO_2 content is decreased
   c. HCO_3^-/H_2CO_3 ratio is decreased
   d. None of the above

3. **Important buffer in extracellular fluid is:**
   a. Hemoglobin
   b. Bicarbonate
   c. Protein
   d. Phosphate

4. **All of the following are associated with metabolic alkalosis, except:**
   a. Rise in blood pH
   b. Rise in bicarbonate plasma levels
   c. Loss of H^+ ions
   d. Decrease in bicarbonate plasma levels

5. **Metabolic acidosis is associated with all of the following, except:**
   a. Increased elimination of acid in urine
   b. Increased formation of ammonia
   c. Increased respiration
   d. Diminished formation of ammonia

6. **The normal pH of plasma is maintained by all of the following, except:**
   a. Plasma buffer
   b. Lung's mechanism
   c. Heat mechanism
   d. Renal mechanism

7. **Normal pH of blood is:**
   a. 7.0
   b. 7.2
   c. 7.4
   d. 7.6

8. **At blood pH 7.4, the ratio of $NaHCO_3/H_2CO_3$ will be:**
   a. 5:1
   b. 10:1
   c. 20:1
   d. 4:1

9. **At blood pH 7.4, the ratio of $HPO_4^-/H_2PO_4^-$ will be:**
   a. 4:1
   b. 5:1
   c. 20:1
   d. 1:20

10. **Respiratory acidosis results from:**
    a. Obstruction to respiration
    b. Diabetes mellitus
    c. Starvation
    d. Hyperventilation

11. **Which of the following is volatile acid?**
    a. Phosphoric acid
    b. Carbonic acid
    c. Sulfuric acid
    d. Lactic acid

12. **Physiologically important carbonic acid (H_2CO_3) present in the body is equivalent to:**
    a. 36 liters of 0.1 N acid
    b. 56 liters of 1 N acid
    c. 36 liters of 1 N acid
    d. 36 liters of 0.01 N acid

13. **Carbonic acid (H_2CO_3) is buffered by:**
    a. Bicarbonate buffer
    b. Phosphate buffer
    c. Hemoglobin buffer
    d. None of the above

14. **Plasma bicarbonate is decreased in:**
    a. Respiratory alkalosis
    b. Respiratory acidosis
    c. Metabolic alkalosis
    d. Metabolic acidosis

15. **Plasma bicarbonate is increased in:**
    a. Respiratory alkalosis
    b. Metabolic alkalosis
    c. Respiratory acidosis
    d. Metabolic acidosis

16. **Total CO_2 is increased in:**
    a. Respiratory acidosis
    b. Metabolic acidosis
    c. Respiratory alkalosis
    d. All of the above

17. **Metabolic acidosis is caused in:**
    a. Pneumonia
    b. Prolonged starvation
    c. Depression of respiratory center
    d. Hysterical hyperventilation

18. **Respiratory alkalosis occurs in:**
    a. Hysterical hyperventilation
    b. Depression of respiratory center
    c. Renal diseases
    d. Loss of intestinal fluids

19. **Morphine poisoning causes:**
    a. Metabolic acidosis
    b. Respiratory acidosis
    c. Metabolic alkalosis
    d. Respiratory alkalosis

20. **Respiratory acidosis results from:**
    a. Retention of carbon dioxide
    b. Excessive elimination of carbon dioxide
    c. Retention of bicarbonate
    d. Excessive elimination of bicarbonate

21. **Respiratory acidosis can occur in all of the following** *except*:
    a. Administration of respiratory depressant toxic drugs
    b. Hysterical hyperventilation
    c. Pneumonia
    d. Emphysema

22. **Respiratory alkalosis can occur in:**
    a. Bronchial asthma
    b. Collapse of lungs
    c. Hysterical hyperventilation
    d. Bronchial obstruction

23. **Anion gap is the difference in the plasma concentrations of:**
    a. (Chloride) – (Bicarbonate)
    b. (Sodium) – (Chloride)
    c. (Sodium + Potassium) – (Chloride + Bicarbonate)
    d. (Sum of cations) – (Sum of anions)

24. **Normal anion gap in plasma is about:**
    a. 5 mEq/L   b. 15 mEq/L
    c. 25 mEq/L   d. 40 mEq/L

25. **Anion gap is normal in:**
    a. Hyperchloremic metabolic acidosis
    b. Diabetic ketoacidosis

    c. Lactic acidosis
    d. None of the above

26. **Anion gap is increased in:**
    a. Renal tubular acidosis
    b. Metabolic acidosis resulting from diarrhea
    c. Metabolic acidosis resulting from intestinal obstruction
    d. Diabetic ketoacidosis

27. **Which of the following true for anion gap in plasma:**
    a. There is no real anion gap in the plasma.
    b. Anion gap is not a physiological reality.
    c. The anion gap is the difference between unmeasured anions and unmeasured cations
    d. All of the above

28. **Metabolic alkalosis can occur in:**
    a. Severe diarrhea
    b. Renal failure
    c. Recurrent vomiting
    d. Excessive use of carbonic anhydrase inhibitors

▮ ANSWERS FOR MCQs

1. c	2. c	3. b	4. d	5. d
6. c	7. c	8. c	9. a	10. a
11. b	12. c	13. c	14. d	15. b
16. a	17. b	18. a	19. b	20. a
21. b	22. c	23. c	24. b	25. a
26. b	27. d	28. c		

Purine and Pyrimidine Nucleotide Metabolism

Competency	Learning Objectives
BI 6.2: Describe and discuss the metabolic processes in which nucleotides are involved. **BI 6.3:** Describe the common disorders associated with nucleotide metabolism. **BI 6.4:** Discuss the laboratory results of analytes associated with gout and Lesch-Nyhan syndrome.	1. Describe the de novo synthesis of purine nucleotides and its regulation. 2. Describe salvage pathway of purine nucleotides synthesis and its significance. 3. Describe catabolism of purine nucleotides and associated disorders. 4. Describe biochemical basis of clinical manifestations of gout and Lesch-Nyhan syndrome. 5. Describe de novo synthesis of pyrimidine nucleotides and its regulation. 6. Describe catabolism of pyrimidine nucleotides, and associated disorders.

OVERVIEW

Purine and pyrimidine nucleotides are required for the synthesis of the **nucleic acids**, DNA and RNA and many critical cellular functions. **Purine** and **pyrimidine** nucleotides are **dietary nonessential** components. Dietary nucleic acids and nucleotides do not provide essential constituents for the biosynthesis of endogenous nucleic acids. The dietary purines and pyrimidines are neither converted to nucleotides nor incorporated into nucleic acids.

Purine bases are oxidized to **uric acid** and **pyrimidines** bases are oxidized to **CO_2** and **ammonia**, which are subsequently excreted in the urine.

Nucleotide biosynthetic pathways are very important as intervention points for therapeutic agents. Many of the most widely used drugs in the treatment of cancer block steps in nucleotide biosynthesis, particularly steps in the synthesis of DNA precursor.

DE NOVO SYNTHESIS OF PURINE NUCLEOTIDES

In de novo pathway the purine ring is assembled on **ribose-5-phosphate**. The two parent purine nucleotides of nucleic acids are:

1. **Adenosine monophosphate, AMP** (contains adenine purine base) and
2. **Guanosine monophosphate, GMP** (contains guanine purine base).

Precursors for the De novo Synthesis of Purine

Purine ring is formed from a variety of precursors. **Figure 18.1** shows the sources of the **carbon**, and **nitrogen** atoms of the purine ring structure:

- Glycine provides C_4, C_5 and N_7
- Aspartate provides N_1
- Glutamine provides N_3 and N_9
- Tetrahydrofolate derivatives furnish C_2 and C_8
- Carbon dioxide provides C_6.

Major Steps of De Novo Synthesis of Purine Nucleotides

Purine synthesis is a **multi-step** process that requires **ribose-5-phosphate** derived from **pentose phosphate**. The precursors (**Figure 18.1**) forming the purine ring are successively added to ribose-5-phosphate. Thus, purines are directly synthesized as **nucleotide** by assembling the precursors that comprise the purine ring system directly on the ribose. Here we will discuss only the major steps.

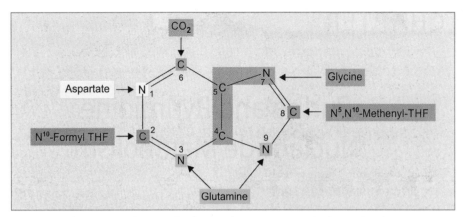

Figure 18.1: Source of carbon and nitrogen atoms in the purine ring.

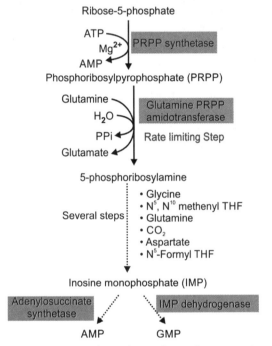

Figure 18.2: De novo pathway for synthesis of purine nucleotides.

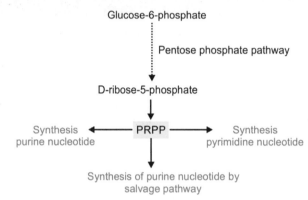

Figure 18.3: Formation and use of PRPP.

- IMP is formed by contributing; aspartic acid (N-1), glutamine (N-3 and N-9), glycine (C-4, C-5, and N-7), CO_2 (C-6), and THF one-carbon derivatives (C-2 and C-8) **(Figure 18.2)**.
- Inosine monophosphate (IMP) is the immediate precursor to GMP and AMP. Both **AMP** and **GMP** are produced from IMP.

❖ Deoxyribonucleotides, the building blocks of DNA, are not synthesized by de novo synthesis but are formed from their corresponding ribonucleotides. Deoxyribonucleotides are synthesized by reduction of ribonucleotide **(Figure 18.4)**.

❖ The 2'-hydroxyl group on the ribose moiety is replaced by a hydrogen atom. Reduction at 2'-carbon of purine and pyrimidine ribonucleotides, catalyzed by the **ribonucleotide reductase** forms the deoxyribonucleotides. The enzyme ribonucleotide reductase is responsible for the reduction reaction for all four ribonucleotides.

❖ The enzyme is active only when cells have actively synthesizing DNA, preparative to cell division.

❖ Reduction requires thioredoxin (a protein cofactor), thioredoxin reductase (a flavoprotein) and NADPH.

- The biosynthesis of purine begins with ribose-5-phosphate which is converted to **phosphoribosyl pyrophosphate, PRPP** by the transfer of pyrophosphate group from ATP to C-1 of the ribose-5-phosphate. This reaction is catalyzed by the enzyme **PRPP synthetase (Figure 18.2)**.
- PRPP is required for both pyrimidine and purine de novo synthesis. It is an intermediate in the purine salvage pathway **(Figure 18.3)**.
- PRPP is aminated by the addition of the amide group from **glutamine** to form amino sugar **5-phosphoribosylamine**. The enzyme that catalyzes the transfer of the amide nitrogen is called **glutamine PRPP amidotransferase**.
- The synthesis of phosphoribosylamine from PRPP is the **first committed (rate limiting) step** in the formation of inosine monophosphate (IMP).

Regulation of De Novo Synthesis of Purine Nucleotide

The de novo synthesis of purine nucleotides is regulated by feedback inhibition at three sites.

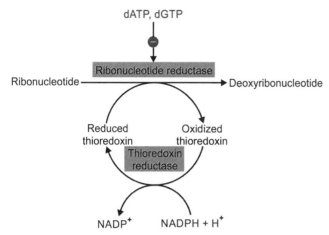

Figure 18.4: Synthesis of deoxyribonucleotide.

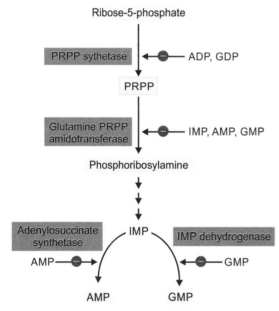

Figure 18.5: Three major feedback mechanism for the control of de novo purine biosynthesis.

1. The overall determinant of the rate of de novo purine nucleotide biosynthesis is the **concentration of PRPP**. The rate of PRPP synthesis depends on the availability of **ribose 5-phosphate** and on the activity of **PRPP synthetase**. PRPP synthetase enzyme is inhibited allosterically by **ADP** and **GDP**.

2. The synthesis of **phosphoribosylamine** from **PRPP** is the **committed (rate limiting) step** in the synthesis of purine nucleotides. This reaction is catalyzed by the allosteric enzyme **glutamine PRPP amidotransferase** which is feedback inhibited by the end products **IMP**, **AMP**, and **GMP**. Thus, whenever either AMP or GMP accumulates to excess, this reaction is inhibited **(Figure 18.5)**.

3. Third control mechanism, exerted at a later stage, in which AMP and GMP regulate their formation from IMP **(Figure 18.5)**.

SALVAGE PATHWAY OF PURINE NUCLEOTIDES SYNTHESIS AND ITS SIGNIFICANCE

Normally, the nucleotides are synthetized de novo from amino acids and other precursors. A small part of purine bases, however, is **'recycled to purine nucleotide'** from degraded DNA of broken-down cells. This is termed the **"salvage pathway"**.

Free purine and **pyrimidine bases** are constantly released in cells during the metabolic degradation of nucleic acids and nucleotides. However, free purines are in large part salvaged and reused to make purine nucleotides, in a pathway much simpler than the de novo synthesis of purine nucleotides described earlier. A similar salvage pathway exists for pyrimidine bases in microorganisms and possibly in mammals.

- In the de novo synthesis of purine nucleotides, purine ring is assembled step by step on ribose-5-phosphate in a long series of reactions. The salvage pathway is much simpler and requires far less energy than does de novo synthesis. It consists of a single reaction.

  - One of the primary salvage pathways consists of a single reaction catalyzed by **adenosine phosphoribosyl-transferase, (APRTase)** in which free **adenine** reacts with **PRPP** to yield the corresponding adenine nucleotide **(Figure 18.6)**.

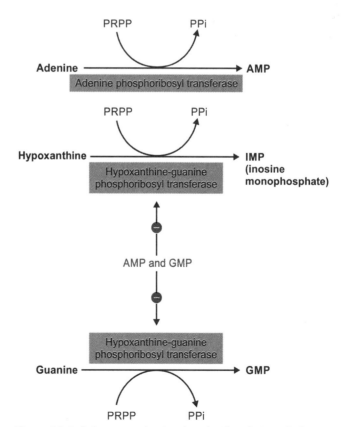

Figure 18.6: Salvage reaction by phosphoribosylation of adenine, hypoxanthine and guanine.

- Free **guanine** and **hypoxanthine** (the deamination product of adenine) are salvaged in the same way by **hypoxanthine-guanine phosphoribosyltransferase (HGPRTase)**, to yield GMP and IMP from guanine and hypoxanthine respectively **(Figure 18.6)**.

Significance of Salvage Pathway

- HGPRTase is the "salvage enzyme" for the purines—it channels **hypoxanthine** and **guanine** back into DNA synthesis.
- Salvage pathway provides purine nucleotides for tissues, incapable of their biosynthesis by de novo pathway.
- For example, human brain, erythrocytes and polymorphonuclear leukocytes cannot synthesize 5-phosphoribosylamine due to low level of **PRPP amidotransferase** and therefore depends in part on salvage pathways for purine nucleotides.
- Failure of HGPRTase enzyme results:
  - Increased **uric acid** formation as cell breakdown products cannot be reused, and are therefore degraded to uric acid.
  - Stimulation of de novo pathway due to an excess of PRPP.

CATABOLISM OF PURINE NUCLEOTIDES AND ASSOCIATED DISORDERS

The end product of purines (adenine and guanine) is **uric acid (Figure 18.7)**.

- Purine nucleotides (AMP and GMP) are degraded by a pathway, in which the phosphate group is removed by the action of **nucleotidase;** to yield the nucleoside, **adenosine** or **guanosine**.
- **Adenosine** is then **deaminated** to **inosine** by **adenosine deaminase**.
- Inosine is then hydrolyzed by **purine nucleoside phosphorylase** to yield its purine base **hypoxanthine** and ribose-1-phosphate.
- Hypoxanthine is oxidized successively to **xanthine** and then **uric acid**, by **xanthine oxidase, a molybdenum** and **iron-containing flavoprotein**. In this reaction molecular oxygen is reduced to H_2O_2, which is decomposed to H_2O and O_2, by catalase.
- **Guanosine** is cleaved to **guanine** and ribose-1-phosphate by **purine nucleoside phosphorylase** enzyme.
- Guanine undergoes hydrolytic removal of its amino group by **guanase** to yield **xanthine**, which is converted to **uric acid** by **xanthine oxidase**.
- A healthy adult human excretes **uric acid** at a rate of about **0.6 g/24 hour**

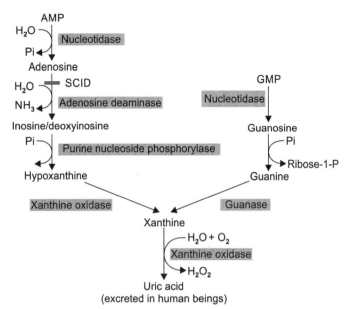

Figure 18.7: Catabolism of purine nucleotides.
(SCID: Severe combined immunodeficiency)

> ❖ The pathway for the degradation of AMP includes an extra step because adenosine is not a substrate for **nucleoside phosphorylase**. In the extra step, adenosine is deaminated to **inosine**, which is a substrate for nucleoside phosphorylase.
> ❖ Uric acid plays a beneficial role as a potent **antioxidant**. It is a very effective scavenger of free radicals. Indeed, urate is about as effective as ascorbate as an antioxidant.

Disorders of Purine Metabolism

The catabolism of the purines; adenine and guanine produces **uric acid**. At physiological pH, uric acid is mostly ionized and present in plasma as **sodium urate**. An elevated serum urate concentration is known as **hyperuricemia**. **Uric acid** and **urate** are relatively **insoluble** molecules which readily precipitate out of aqueous solutions such as urine or synovial fluid.

The average normal blood serum level of uric acid is **4 to 7 mg per 100 mL**. The majority of uric acid is **excreted** via the **kidney**. The upper normal range is 7 mg per 100 mL, which is above the solubility of sodium urate in water which is 6.4 mg per 100 mL. Elevated serum urate concentration is known as **hyperuricemia**.

- Formation of uric acid, depends on the rate of:
  - De novo synthesis of purines
  - The metabolism of endogenous DNA, RNA and other purine-containing molecule such as ATP
  - The breakdown of dietary nucleic acids
- Hyperuricemia may arise from:
  - **Increased uric acid formation**, which may be due to primary (genetic) or secondary cause or
  - **Decreased uric acid excretion** by the kidney.
- The common causes of hyperuricemia are summarized in **Figure 18.8**. Genetic causes of hyperuricemia are

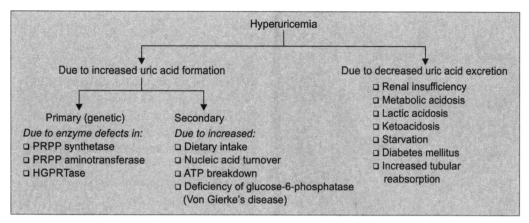

Figure 18.8: The causes of hyperuricemia.

known as **primary disorders**, and secondary hyperuricemia may be caused by a variety of other diseases.

- Hyperuricemia is aggravated by **alcohol**, as ethanol increases the turnover of **ATP** and **uric acid** production.
- Ethanol in excess may cause the accumulation of organic acids, which compete with the tubular secretion of uric acid.
- Disorders such as **ethanol intoxication**, **diabetic ketoacidosis** and **starvation** lead to elevations of lactic acid, β-hydroxybutyric acid and acetoacetic acid and will compete with the tubular secretion of uric acid and cause hyperuricemia.

The consequence of this leads to the condition, **gout**.

Gout

Gout is a clinical syndrome associated with **hyperuricemia** and recurrent **acute arthritis**. Hyperuricemia is not always associated with gout. Gout occurs predominantly in males. The increased serum uric acid is due to either increased formation of uric acid or its decreased renal excretion. Gout is classified into two broad types:

1. Primary gout
2. Secondary gout

Primary Gout

- In primary gout, increased level of uric acid is associated with increased synthesis of purine nucleotides.
- Increased synthesis of purine nucleotides is caused by defective enzymes of purine nucleotide biosynthesis, such as:
  - PRPP synthetase
  - Glutamine PRPP amidotransferase
  - HGPRTase
- In normal course, **PRPP synthetase** and **glutamine PRPP amidotransferase** are allosterically feedback regulated by its own product AMP and GMP **(Figure 18.5)**. But due to loss of allosteric feedback regulation,

abnormally high level of PRPP synthetase and glutamine PRPP amidotransferase results in excessive production of PRPP, which in turn accelerates the rate of de novo synthesis of purine nucleotides. Increased synthesis is associated with increased break down to uric acid.

- **HGPRTase deficiency:** The enzyme HGPRTase catalyzes the synthesis of GMP from guanine and IMP from hypoxanthine by salvage pathway **(Figure 18.6)**. Deficiency of HGPRTase leads to reduced synthesis of IMP and GMP by salvage pathway and increases the level of PRPP. Increased level of PRPP accelerates the purine nucleotide biosynthesis by de novo pathway.

Symptoms of Primary Gout

- Elevated concentration of **uric acid** in the blood and tissues. The joints become inflamed, painful, and arthritic due to abnormal deposition of sodium urate crystals.
- Patients with primary gout often show deposition of urate as tophi (clusters of urate crystals) in soft tissues **(Figure 18.9)** that affects the joints and leads to painful arthritis.

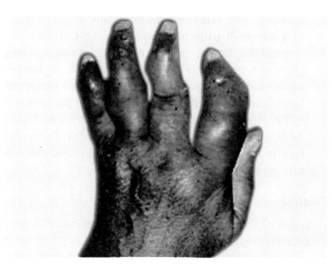

Figure 18.9: Deposition of urate as tophi in soft tissues.

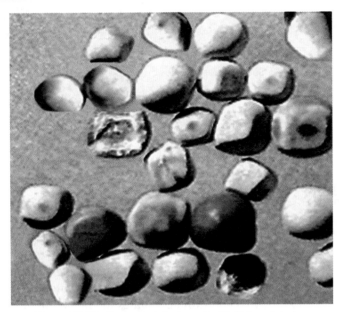

Figure 18.10: Urate crystals deposited in kidney tubules.

- The kidneys are also affected, since excess urate **(Figure 18.10)** is also deposited in the kidney tubules and leads to renal failure.

Secondary Gout

Secondary gout results from a variety of diseases that cause an **elevated destruction of cells** or **decreased elimination of uric acid** as follows:

- Elevated destruction of cells is accompanied by increased degradation of nucleic acids to uric acid, which occurs in **cancers** (leukemia, polycythemia), **psoriasis** and **hypercatabolic states** (starvation, trauma, etc.).
- Decreased elimination of uric acid occurs in chronic **renal disease** due to reduced glomerular filtrate rate.
- **Glucose-6-phosphatase deficiency:** Glucose-6-phosphatase enzyme is not directly involved in purine synthesis. It is involved indirectly with biosynthesis of purine nucleotide. In type-I glycogen storage disease, **Von Gierke's disease** due to deficiency of **glucose-6-phosphatase**, glucose-6-phosphate cannot be converted to glucose. Accumulated glucose-6-phosphate is then metabolized via **hexose monophosphate pathway**, which in turn generates large amounts of **ribose-5-phosphate**, a precursor of PRPP. The increased synthesis of PRPP then enhances de novo synthesis of purine nucleotides. Increased synthesis is associated with increased break down to uric acid.

Treatment of Gout

Gout can be treated by a combination of nutritional therapy and drug therapy.

- Foods especially rich in nucleotides and nucleic acids such as liver or coffee and tea, which contain the purines

caffeine and **theobromine**, are withheld from the diet. Restriction in intake of alcohol is also advised.

- Major improvement follows the use of the drug **allopurinol**, an analog of hypoxanthine which inhibits **xanthine oxidase competitively**, the enzyme responsible for converting purines into uric acid. This leads to reduced formation of uric acid and accumulation of xanthine and hypoxanthine, which are more soluble and thus easily excreted.

Lesch-Nyhan Syndrome (LNS)

Lesch-Nyhan syndrome is an inherited X-linked recessive disorder that affects only males. It is caused by a **complete lack of hypoxanthine-guanine phosphoribosyltransferase (HGPRTase)**, an enzyme which is involved in salvaging purine bases for resynthesis to purine nucleotides (*see* **Figure 18.6**).

- In the absence of HGPRTase, the salvage pathway is inoperative and purines cannot be reconverted to nucleotides; instead they are degraded to uric acid.
- The genetic lack of HGPRTase also leads to an overproduction of PRPP, which stimulates purine biosynthesis. Because of increased purine synthesis, the degradation product uric acid also increases. This results in increased concentration of uric acid in plasma and urine and gout like damage to tissue.

Symptoms

The symptoms include:

- Hyperuricemia
- Gout
- Urinary tract stones
- The neurological symptoms or mental retardation
- Spasticity (abnormal muscle tightness due to prolonged muscle contraction associated with damage to the brain, spinal cord or motor nerves) **(Figure 18.11A)**.
- Self-mutilation (painful, destructive biting of fingers and lips) **(Figures 18.11B and C)**
- Behave aggressively towards others

Children with this genetic disorder, which becomes manifest by the age of 2 years, are sometimes poorly coordinated and have intellectual deficits. In addition, they are extremely aggressive and show uncontrollable self-destructive tendencies; they mutilate themselves by biting off their fingers, toes, and lips. Elevated levels of urate in the serum lead to the formation of kidney stones early in life, followed by the symptoms of gout years later.

Biochemical Basis of Neurological Symptoms of Lesch-Nyhan Syndrome

- **Brain** is dependent on **salvage pathway** for supply of **purine nucleotides** because activity of **amidotransferase** that catalyzes the committed step in the de novo synthesis is low in the brain.

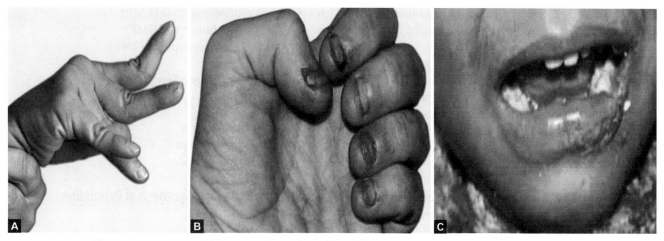

Figures 18.11A to C: (A) Spasticity; (B and C) Self-mutilation: Symptoms of Lesch-Nyhan syndrome.

- Brain cells normally have much higher levels of purine salvage enzyme (HGPRTase) than other cells and use salvage pathway for the synthesis of IMP and GMP.
- ATP formed by salvage pathway acts as a **neurotransmitter** in both peripheral and central nervous systems.
- Lack of HGPRTase results in imbalance of key neurotransmitters

Treatment

Allopurinol reduces uric acid formation but does not alleviate the neurologic symptoms. This syndrome is potential target for gene therapy.

Adenosine Deaminase Deficiency (ADA Deficiency)

- **Adenosine deaminase deficiency (ADA deficiency)** is an autosomal recessive metabolic disorder due to mutation in the *ADA gene*.
- Adenosine deaminase deficiency damages the **immune system** and causes **severe combined immunodeficiency (SCID)**.
- Adenosine deaminase (ADA) deficiency leads to accumulation of **adenosine**, **deoxyadenosine**, and **dATP**.
- As dATP level rises, **ribonucleotide reductase** is inhibited **(Figure 18.4)** and causes a reduction of other deoxyribonucleotides (e.g., dCTP) required for DNA synthesis; this leads to inhibition of cell division.
- ADA enzyme is found throughout the body but is most active in lymphocytes. Lymphocytes usually contain high quantity of ADA. Therefore ADA deficiency is mainly manifested as reduced lymphocytes. ADA deficiency hampers both T-lymphocyte and B-lymphocyte-mediated functions, namely, cellular and humoral immunity.

Symptoms

- Symptoms of SCID occur in infancy and include severe recurring or life-threatening **infections** especially viral infections, which may result in pneumonia and chronic diarrhea.
- The condition is fatal, often leading to death at an early age usually within the first year or two of life, unless infants receive immune-restoring treatments, such as transplants of blood-forming stem cells, gene therapy, or enzyme therapy.

Treatment

Individual with ADA deficiency lack an effective immune system and do not survive unless treated. Current therapies include:
- Bone marrow transplants from a matched donor to replace the hematopoietic stem cells those mature into B and T lymphocytes.
- Enzyme replacement therapy, requiring once or twice per week intramuscular injection of active ADA, is effective, but the therapeutic benefit declines after 8–10 years and complication arise, including malignancies.
- Permanent cure requires replacing the defective gene with a functional one in bone marrow cells.
- Adenosine deaminase deficiency was one of the first targets of human **gene therapy** trials in 1990. Gene therapy is rapidly becoming a viable path for long-term restoration of immune function for these patients.

BIOCHEMICAL BASIS OF CLINICAL MANIFESTATIONS OF GOUT AND LESCH-NYHAN SYNDROME

Use of Biochemical Testing for the Detection of Gout

- **Blood tests:** Since gout is caused by an excessive amount of uric acid (hyperuricemia), elevated levels of uric acid in the blood could be reflective of a gout diagnosis. Hyperuricemia is a classic feature of gout. Hyperuricemia is defined as a plasma urate level greater than 7.0 mg/dL in males and 6.0 mg/dL in females.

However, not all hyperuricemic patients have gout, so further diagnostic tests are recommended in order to proper diagnosis.

- **Synovial fluid examination:** The most accurate diagnostic test for gout is the examination of synovial fluid, the liquid that surrounds joints and provides them with protection and nutrients. It is the most reliable test for gout. In this, fluid is extracted from the affected joint and observed under the microscope. Urate crystals are found in the synovial fluid.
- **Urinalysis:** Collecting and testing urine for uric acid levels excreted gives a clue to a gout diagnosis. This test is not conclusive on its own. Gout patients tend to have higher than normal outputs of uric acid in their urine. Usually, urine is collected over a 24-hour span for a more accurate detection of uric acid output throughout the day.

Use of Biochemical Testing for the Detection of Lesch-Nyhan Syndrome

- **Overproduction of uric acid:** Overproduction of uric acid may lead to the development of uric acid crystals or stones in the kidneys, ureters, or bladder. Such crystals deposited in joints later in the disease may produce gout-like arthritis, with swelling and tenderness. The stones, or calculi, usually cause hematuria (blood in the urine) and increase the risk of urinary tract infection. Stones may be the presenting feature of the disease.
- **Activity of the HGPRTase enzyme:** Activity of the blood HGPRTase enzyme less than 1.5% of normal enzyme activity confirms the diagnosis of Lesch-Nyhan syndrome.
- **Urate to creatinine concentration ratio:** The urate to creatinine (breakdown product of creatine phosphate in muscle) concentration ratio in urine is elevated. This is a good indicator of acid overproduction. For children under 10 years of age with LNS, a urate to creatinine ratio above two is typically found.
- **Molecular genetic testing (called as diagnostic triad for LNS):** Molecular genetic studies of the *HPRT* gene mutations may confirm diagnosis of LNS, and are particularly helpful for subsequent "carrier testing" in at-risk females, such as close family relatives on the female side. Molecular genetic testing is the most effective method of testing, as **HPRT1** is the only gene known to be associated with LNS. Technique, such as PCR is used for the diagnosis of LNS.

◼ DE NOVO SYNTHESIS OF PYRIMIDINE NUCLEOTIDES

Unlike the synthesis of purine nucleotide, six-membered pyrimidine ring is made first and then attached to ribose phosphate which is donated by PRPP. The pyrimidine nucleotides are:

- Cytidine monophosphate (CMP)
- Uridine monophosphate (UMP)
- Thymidine monophosphate (TMP)

Precursors for the De novo Synthesis of Pyrimidine (Figure 18.12)

- Glutamine provides N_3
- Aspartic acid furnishes C_4, C_5, C_6, and N_1
- Carbon dioxide provides C_2.

Major Steps for De Novo Synthesis of Pyrimidine Nucleotide

- Pyrimidine biosynthesis starts with the formation of carbamoyl phosphate from glutamine, ATP, and CO_2 **(Figure 18.13)**. This reaction is catalyzed by **cytosolic carbamoyl phosphate synthetase-II (CPS-II)**, an enzyme different from mitochondrial carbamoyl phosphate synthase-l (CPS-I) required in the synthesis of urea. Differences between CPS-I and CPS-II are given in **Table 18.1**.
- Condensation of carbamoyl phosphate with aspartate forms carbamoyl aspartate in a reaction catalyzed by **aspartate transcarbamoylase and is the committed step in the biosynthesis of pyrimidine (Figure 18.13)**
- With the several subsequent reactions UMP is formed, UMP is phosphorylated to UDP. UDP is phosphorylated to UTP.
- UTP is aminated to form cytidine triphosphate (CTP).
- Deoxyuridine diphosphate (dUDP) formed from UDP by reduction is dephosphorylated to dUMP which acts as a substrate for thymidine monophosphate (TMP).
- Methylation of dUMP by N^5,N^{10}-methylenetetrahydrofolate, catalyzed by **thymidylate synthase**, forms deoxythymidine monophosphate (dTMP) (deoxythymidylate).

Regulation of De Novo Synthesis of Pyrimidine Nucleotides

The first two enzymes **carbamoyl phosphate synthetase-II** and **aspartate transcarbamoylase** are allosteric enzymes and are regulated allosterically **(Figure 18.14)**.
- Carbamoyl phosphate synthetase-II reaction 1 is feedback inhibited by UTP and activated by PRPP
- Aspartate transcarbamoylase, reaction 2, is feedback inhibited by CTP and activated by ATP.

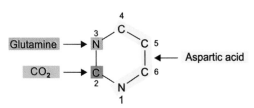

Figure 18.12: Sources of the carbon and nitrogen atoms in the pyrimidine ring.

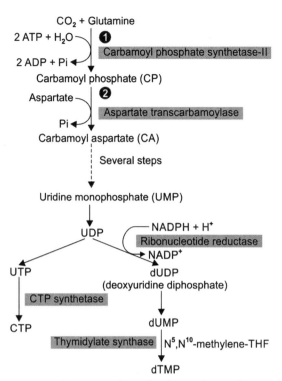

Figure 18.13: De novo pathway for the synthesis of pyrimidine nucleotide.

TABLE 18.1: Differences between CPS-I and CPS-II.

Characteristics	*CPS-I*	*CPS-II*
Cellular location	Mitochondria	Cytosol
Pathway involved	Urea cycle	Pyrimidine synthesis
Source of nitrogen	Ammonia	Glutamine
Allosteric activator	N-acetylglutamate (NAG)	NAG does not serve as an allosteric activator

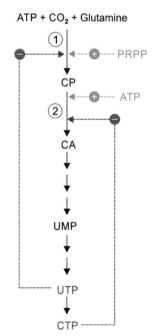

Figure 18.14: Regulation of de novo pyrimidine synthesis.

(CP: Carbamoyl phosphate; CA: Carbamoyl aspartate)

CATABOLISM OF PYRIMIDINE NUCLEOTIDES, AND ASSOCIATED DISORDERS

- Unlike the purines which degraded sparingly soluble product, uric acid, the end products of pyrimidine catabolism are highly water soluble **(Figure 18.15)**. These are:
  - CO_2
  - NH_3
  - β-alanine
  - β-aminoisobutyrate
- In humans, β-aminoisobutyrate is transaminated to methylmalonate semialdehyde which is then converted to succinyl-CoA via methylmalonyl-CoA. β-alanine can serve as precursor of acetyl-CoA.

> Since no human enzyme catalyzes hydrolysis or phosphorolysis of pseudouridine, this unusual pyrimidine nucleotide is excreted unchanged in the urine of normal subjects.

Disorders Associated with Pyrimidine Nucleotide Metabolism

Since the end products of pyrimidine catabolism are highly water soluble, overproduction of pyrimidine catabolites is rarely associated with clinically significant abnormalities.

Orotic Aciduria

- Orotic aciduria is a hereditary disorder due to defect in the enzyme **UMP synthase** that converts orotic acid to UMP in pyrimidine synthesis.
- A defect in **UMP synthase** results in the excretion of orotic acid in the urine.
- UMP synthase is a multifunctional enzyme containing both **orotate phosphoribosyltransferase** and **orotidylate decarboxylase** activity **(Figure 18.13)**. There are two types of orotic aciduria:
  1. **In type-I** there is deficiency of both enzymes, orotate phosphoribosyltransferase and orotidylate decarboxylase

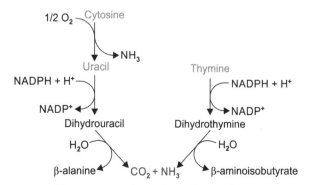

Figure 18.15: Catabolism of pyrimidines.

2. **In type-II** only orotidylate decarboxylase is deficient.

The deficiency in UMP and other pyrimidine nucleotides results in inhibition of DNA and RNA synthesis, which causes **megaloblastic anemia** and **failure to thrive** (growth retardation).

Reye's Syndrome

Reye's syndrome is a secondary orotic aciduria, which may be due to inability of severely damaged mitochondria to utilize carbamoyl phosphate in the formation of urea which then may be diverted for cytosolic over production of orotic acid.

ASSESSMENT QUESTIONS

■ STRUCTURED LONG ESSAY QUESTION (SLEQ)

1. Describe purine catabolism under the following headings:
   i. Formation of uric acid with pathway
   ii. Reference range for serum uric acid
   iii. Various hyperuricemic conditions.

■ SHORT ESSAY QUESTIONS (SEQs)

1. What is salvage pathway? Write purine salvage pathway with its significance.
2. What is gout? Give its types, causes and clinical manifestations.
3. What is Lesch-Nyhan syndrome? Write its symptoms with its biochemical basis.
4. Write regulation of de novo biosynthesis of purine nucleotide.
5. What is uric acid? How it is form in the body?

■ SHORT ANSWER QUESTIONS (SAQs)

1. Enumerate the sources of carbon and nitrogen in purine ring.
2. Explain how patients with glycogen storage disease (glucose-6-phosphatase deficiency) develop gout in early adult life.
3. Give four causes of gout.
4. What are catabolic end products of pyrimidines?
5. Write regulation of de novo biosynthesis of pyrimidine nucleotide.
6. What is the cause of severe combined immunodeficiency?
7. What is normal blood uric acid level? Mention any two conditions in which normal blood uric acid level is raised.
8. Outline the reaction by which deoxynucleotides are formed in a cell from ribonucleotides.

■ CASE VIGNETTE-BASED QUESTIONS (CVBQs)

Case Study

1. **A 50-year-old female patient complains of pain and swelling in joints and shows hyperuricemia.**
   Questions
   a. Name the probable disease.
   b. Name the enzyme defect.
   c. What is the normal value of serum uric acid?
   d. Suggest nutritional therapy.

2. **A 4-year-old boy suffered from pain in joints, showed signs of mental retardation, delayed development of milestones and had self-mutilation (self-destructive behavior of biting fingers and lips). His serum uric acid level was 10 mg/dL.**
   Questions
   a. What is the probable diagnosis?
   b. Which enzyme is defective in this disease?
   c. What is the normal level of serum uric acid in human?
   d. What is the mode of inheritance of this disease?

3. **A 50-year-old man was awakened by a severe pain in his left toe and the pain became so intense that he could not bear the weight of the bedclothes. On investigation, it is found that his serum uric acid level was high.**
   Questions
   a. Name the probable disorder.
   b. What is uric acid?
   c. Write pathway for the formation uric acid.
   d. Give normal level of serum uric acid.

4. **A 45-year-old HIV positive man was prescribed highly active retroviral medicines due to his rapidly falling CD 4 cells counts. After 2 months of beginning the therapy, the patient presented to the OPD with complaints of severe pain and swelling in the right big toe. On examination, the first metatarsophalangeal joint was red and swollen. X-ray of the right foot did not show any bony or soft tissue anomalies. Six months after the acute presentation the patient mentioned that he is an alcohol binge and consumes nonvegetarian food often.**
   Blood examination revealed:
   – Total protein   : 6.9 g/dL
   – Albumin   : 3.9 g/dL
   – Blood urea   : 37 mg/dL
   – Serum creatinine : 1 mg/dL
   – Serum uric acid   : 8.6 mg/dL
   Questions
   a. What is the probable diagnosis? Justify.
   b. What is the biochemical basis of precipitation of symptoms following alcohol binge?
   c. How glucose 6-phosphatase deficiency does affect the above diagnosis?
   d. What is the treatment and its mechanism?

5. A 2-year-old male child brought to the hospital with complains of involuntary movements of upper limb and habit of biting of lips and fingers. On examination, baby had multiple marks of biting on fingers and lips. Mother gave the history of orange discoloration of baby diaper. Laboratory studies: Sr. Uric acid : 9 mg/dL

   Questions
   a. What is the probable diagnosis? Justify.
   b. What is the cause of the above diagnosed case?
   c. Why males are mostly affected?
   d. What is the reason for orange discoloration of baby diaper?

MULTIPLE CHOICE QUESTIONS (MCQs)

1. Rate controlling step of pyrimidine biosynthesis is catalyzed by:
   a. Orotidylate decarboxylase
   b. Aspartate transcarbamoylase
   c. Carbamoyl phosphate synthase I
   d. Orotate phosphoribosyltransferase

2. Which statement for purine biosynthesis is incorrect?
   a. Requires vitamin B_{12}
   b. Assembled on ribose phosphate
   c. Requires PRPP
   d. Requires glycine

3. Purines and pyrimidines are:
   a. Dietary essential
   b. Dietary nonessential
   c. Derived from essential fatty acids
   d. Derivatives of essential amino acid

4. The two nitrogen of the pyrimidine ring are contributed by:
   a. Glutamate and ammonia
   b. Glutamine and aspartate
   c. Glutamate and glutamine
   d. Aspartate and carbamoyl phosphate

5. Nitrogen or carbon atoms are contributed to the structure of the purine ring by amino acids, *except*:
   a. Glycine
   b. Glutamine
   c. Aspartate
   d. Glutamate

6. Lesch-Nyhan syndrome may lead to:
   a. Self-destructive behavior
   b. Gout
   c. Elevated levels of PRPP
   d. All of the above

7. Hyperuricemia can result from defect in enzymes, *except*:
   a. Carbamoyl phosphate synthase II
   b. HGPRTase
   c. PRPP synthase
   d. Glucose-6-phosphatase

8. The end product of purine metabolism in human is:
   a. Creatinine
   b. Uric acid
   c. Urea
   d. Ammonia

9. The salvage pathway for purines involves enzyme:
   a. PRPP amidotransferase
   b. PRPP synthase
   c. HGPRTase
   d. Xanthine oxidase

10. Enzyme involved with immunodeficiency disease of purine metabolism is:
    a. Adenosine deaminase
    b. Xanthine oxidase
    c. PRPP synthetase
    d. HGPRTase

11. Purine salvage occurs in the tissues, *except*:
    a. RBC
    b. Brain
    c. Liver
    d. Polymorphonuclear leukocytes

12. Allopurinol is used in the treatment of:
    a. Rickets
    b. Cancer
    c. Gout
    d. Pellagra

13. Lesch-Nyhan syndrome is due to the lack of:
    a. HGPRTase
    b. APRTase
    c. Adenosine deaminase
    d. PRPP amidotransferase

14. Hereditary orotic aciduria type II is due to deficiency of the following enzyme:
    a. Dihydro-orotate dehydrogenase
    b. Orotate phosphoribosyltransferase
    c. Aspartate transcarbamoylase
    d. Orotidylate decarboxylase

15. The de novo biosynthesis of purine nucleotides differs from the de novo biosynthesis of pyrimidine nucleotides in which one of the following features?
    a. Utilizes glutamine
    b. Utilizes aspartate
    c. PRPP stimulates both
    d. Utilizes glycine

16. The source of sugar phosphate the de novo synthesis of purine nucleotides is:
    a. Ribulose-5-phosphate
    b. 5-phosphoribosyl pyrophosphate (PRPP)
    c. Glucose-6-phosphate
    d. Deoxyribose 5-phosphate

17. Which of the following statements describe pyrimidine biosynthesis in mammals?
    a. Carbamoyl phosphate synthase II (CPSII) is feedback inhibited by UTP
    b. CPS II activated by PRPP
    c. CPS II utilizes glutamine as a source of amino group
    d. a, b, and c are all correct

18. The enzyme hypoxanthine guanine phosphoribosyltransferase (HGPRTase) is involved in:
    a. Salvage of pyrimidine bases
    b. Salvage of purine bases
    c. De novo synthesis of purine nucleotides
    d. De novo synthesis of pyrimidine nucleotides

19. What is involved in formation of d-TMP from d-UMP?
    a. N^5,N^{10}-methylenetetrahydrofolate
    b. From imino folate
    c. N5 formyl folate
    d. Dihydrofolate

20. In purine biosynthesis carbon atoms at 4 and 5 position and N at 7 positions are contributed by:
    a. Glycine
    b. Glutamine
    c. Alanine
    d. Threonine

21. N^{10}-formyl and N^5N^{10}-methenyltetrahydrofolate contributes purine carbon atoms at position:
    a. 4 and 6
    b. 4 and 5
    c. 5 and 6
    d. 2 and 8

22. In purine nucleus nitrogen atom at 1 position is derived from:
    a. Aspartate
    b. Glutamate
    c. Glycine
    d. Alanine

23. Inosinic acid is biological precursor of:
    a. Uracil and thymine
    b. Purines and thymine
    c. Adenylic acid and guanylic acid
    d. Orotic acid and uridylic acid

24. Conversion of inosine monophosphate to xanthine monophosphate is catalyzed by:
    a. IMP dehydrogenase
    b. Formyl transferase
    c. Xanthine-guanine phosphoribosyltransferase
    d. Adenine phosphoribosyltransferase

25. A 10-year-old child with aggressive behavior and poor concentration is brought with presenting complains of joint pain. Mother gives history of self-mutilate his finger. Which of the following enzymes is likely to be deficient in this child?
    a. HGPRTase
    b. Adenosine deaminase
    c. APRTase
    d. Acid maltase

26. An enzyme which acts as allosteric regulator of de novo biosynthesis of purine nucleotides is:
    a. PRPP synthetase
    b. PRPP glutamyl amidotransferase
    c. HGPRTase
    d. Formyltransferase

27. Adenosine deaminase (ADA) deficiency leads to:
    a. Severe combined immunodeficiency (SCID)
    b. Orotic aciduria
    c. Gout
    d. Lesch-Nyhan syndrome

28. In the biosynthesis of purine nucleotides the AMP feedback regulates:
    a. Adenylosuccinase
    b. Adenylosuccinate synthetase
    c. IMP dehydrogenase
    d. HGPRTase

29. Pyrimidine and purine nucleoside biosynthesis share a common precursor:
    a. PRPP
    b. Glycine
    c. Fumarate
    d. Alanine

30. Pyrimidine biosynthesis begins with the formation using glutamine, ATP and CO_2, of:
    a. Carbamoyl aspartate
    b. Orotate
    c. Carbamoyl phosphate
    d. Dihydroorotate

31. The two nitrogen of the pyrimidine ring are contributed by:
    a. Ammonia and glycine
    b. Asparate and glutamine
    c. Glutamine and ammonia
    d. Aspartate and ammonia

32. A 12-year-old child presents with mental retardation and history of self-mutilation. Which of the following tests will help in determining the diagnosis?
    a. Serum lead levels
    b. Serum alkaline phosphatase levels
    c. Serum lactate dehydrogenase Levels
    d. Serum uric acid levels

33. UDP and UTP are formed by phosphorylation from:
    a. AMP
    b. ADP
    c. ATP
    d. GTP

34. The purines salvage pathway is from:
    a. Hypoxanthine and xanthine
    b. Hypoxanthine and adenine
    c. Adenine and xanthine
    d. Xanthine and guanine

35. Conversion of deoxyuridine monophosphate to thymidine monophosphate is catalyzed by the enzyme:
    a. Ribonucleotide reductase
    b. Thymidylate synthase
    c. CTP synthetase
    d. Orotidylic acid decarboxylase

36. d-UMP is converted to TMP by:
    a. Methylation
    b. Decarboxylation
    c. Reduction
    d. Deamination

37. UTP is converted to CTP by:
    a. Methylation
    b. Isomerization
    c. Amination
    d. Reduction

38. Methotrexate blocks the synthesis of thymidine monophosphate by inhibiting the activity of the enzyme:
    a. Dihydrofolate reductase
    b. Orotate phosphoribosyltransferase
    c. Ribonucleotide reductase
    d. Dihydroorotase

39. The enzyme aspartate transcarbamoylase of pyrimidine biosynthesis is inhibited by:
    a. ATP
    b. ADP
    c. AMP
    d. CTP

40. Gout is a metabolic disorder of catabolism of:
    a. Pyrimidine
    b. Purine
    c. Alanine
    d. Phenylalanine

41. Gout is characterized by increased plasma levels of:
    a. Urea
    b. Uric acid
    c. Creatine
    d. Creatinine

42. Lesch-Nyhan syndrome, the sex linked, recessive absence of HGPRTase, may lead to:
    a. Compulsive self-destructive behavior with elevated levels of urate in serum
    b. Hypouricemia due to liver damage
    c. Failure to thrive and megaloblastic anemia
    d. Protein intolerance and hepatic encephalopathy

43. The major catabolic product of pyrimidines in human is:
    a. β-alanine
    b. Urea
    c. Uric acid
    d. Guanine

44. Gout is a disorder of:
    a. Purine metabolism
    b. Pyrimidine
    c. Oxalate metabolism
    d. Protein metabolism

45. An autosomal recessive disorder, xanthinuria is due to deficiency of the enzymes:
    a. Adenosine deaminase
    b. Xanthine oxidase
    c. HGPRTase
    d. Transaminase

46. Hyperuricemia is not found in:
    a. Cancer
    b. Psoriasis
    c. Von Gierke's disease
    d. Xanthinuria

47. A child presents with hyperuricemia and delayed developmental milestones. He also has the habit of biting fingers and nails. What is the most probable enzyme deficiency?
    a. HGPRTase deficiency
    b. Phenylalanine hydroxylase
    c. Adenine deaminase
    d. Hexosaminidase A

48. A 10-year-old child presents with history of rashes self-mutilation. Which of the following investigations do you think may be suggestive of valuable for diagnosis?
    a. Lead
    b. Alkaline phosphatase
    c. LDH
    d. Uric acid

49. A 10-year-old child with aggressive behavior and poor concentration is brought with presenting complaints of joint pain and reduced urinary output. Mother gives history of self-mutilate his finger. Which of the following enzymes is likely to be deficient in this child?
    a. HGPRTase
    b. Adenine deaminase
    c. APRTase
    d. Acid maltase

50. In a patient with increased hypoxanthine and xanthine in blood with hypouricemia, which enzyme is deficient?
    a. HGPRTase
    b. Adenine deaminase
    c. APRTase
    d. Xanthine oxidase

ANSWERS FOR MCQs

1. b	2. a	3. b	4. b	5. d
6. d	7. a	8. b	9. c	10. a
11. c	12. c	13. a	14. d	15. d
16. b	17. d	18. b	19. a	20. a
21. d	22. a	23. c	24. a	25. a
26. a	27. a	28. b	29. a	30. c
31. b	32. d	33. c	34. b	35. b
36. a	37. c	38. a	39. d	40. b
41. b	42. a	43. a	44. a	45. b
46. d	47. a	48. d	49. a	50. d

DNA Replication and Repair

Competency	Learning Objectives
BI 7.2: Describe the processes involved in replication and repair of DNA and the transcription and translation mechanisms.	1. Describe replication in prokaryotes, inhibitors of replication and its clinical importance. 2. Describe replication in eukaryotes. 3. Describe telomere, telomerase and its importance. 4. Describe the DNA repair mechanisms with associated disorders. 5. Describe the cell cycle.

▐ OVERVIEW

Replication is the synthesis of deoxyribonucleic acid. Deoxyribonucleic acid is a major store of genetic information. To transfer this genetic information from a parent cell to a daughter cell during cellular reproduction, the DNA must be duplicated. **The duplication** or **synthesis of DNA is called replication**.

In this chapter, we shall study the process of replication, mechanisms used to repair different types of DNA damage and inhibitors of DNA replication.

▐ REPLICATION IN PROKARYOTES, INHIBITORS OF REPLICATION AND ITS CLINICAL IMPORTANCE

The fundamental properties of the DNA replication process are identical in all species. DNA replication is **semiconservative**. In the semiconservative replication each strand serves as a **template** for the synthesis of a new strand, producing two new DNA molecules, each with one new strand and one old strand **(Figure 19.1)**.

Replication in prokaryotes is much better understood than replication in eukaryotes. The basic requirements and components of replication are the same for prokaryotes as for eukaryotes. Therefore, an understanding of how prokaryotes

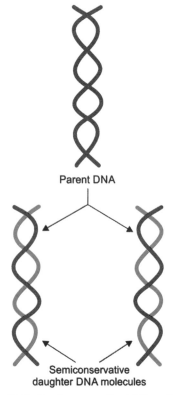

Parent DNA

Semiconservative
daughter DNA molecules

Figure 19.1: Semiconservative DNA replication.

replicate provides the understanding of how eukaryotes replicate.

Basic Requirements for Replication

Substrates

The four deoxyribonucleosides triphosphate:
1. dATP
2. dGTP
3. dCTP
4. dTTP.

Template

A template is required to direct the addition of the appropriate complementary nucleotide to the newly synthesized DNA strand. Each strand of double helix acts as a **template** for the synthesis of new strand with complementary sequences.

Primer

Primer is a **short piece of RNA** about five nucleotides in length having a free 3′ end. An RNA polymerase called **primase** synthesizes a short stretch of RNA that is complementary to one of the template DNA strands. After DNA synthesis has been initiated, the short stretch of RNA is removed by hydrolysis and replaced by DNA. DNA polymerases cannot initiate DNA synthesis without a primer.

Enzymes and Proteins

Enzymes

- **DNA polymerases** (DNA dependent DNA polymerases): The DNA synthesis is catalyzed by enzymes called **DNA dependent DNA polymerases**. They are called DNA dependent as they require DNA template. They are more commonly called **DNA polymerases**. There are three types of polymerases **(Table 19.1)**
  1. *DNA polymerase I (Pol I):* Removal of primer (has 5; to 3′ exonuclease activity)
  2. *DNA polymerase II (Pol II):* DNA proofreading and DNA repair.
  3. *DNA polymerase III (Pol III):* Leading and lagging strand synthesis.
- DNA topoisomerases (DNA gyrase)
- DNA ligase

Proteins

- DNA A protein
- DNA B protein (Helicase)

TABLE 19.1: Different types of prokaryotic DNA polymerase.

Types of polymerase	Function
DNA polymerase I	Filling of gaps (synthesis between Okazaki fragments of lagging strand); removal of primer
DNA polymerase II	DNA proofreading and DNA repair
DNA polymerase III	Leading and lagging strand synthesis

TABLE 19.2: Enzymes and proteins involved in replication.

Protein	Function
DNA A protein	Recognizes *ori* sequence; Opens duplex at specific sites in origin
DNA B protein (Helicase)	Unwinds DNA
DNA C protein	Required for DNA B binding at origin
HU (Histone like protein)	Stimulates initiation
Primase (DNA G protein)	Synthesizes RNA primer
SSB (single stranded binding protein)	Binds single stranded DNA and stabilizes the separated strand and prevents renaturation of DNA
DNA topoisomerases I	Catalyze the relaxation of supercoiled DNA by breaking just one strand of DNA
DNA topoisomerase II (DNA-gyrase)	Relieves torsional strain generated by DNA unwinding by breaking both strand of DNA
DNA polymerases	Deoxynucleotides polymerization and proofreading
DNA ligase	Seals the single strand nick between the nascent chain and Okazaki fragments on lagging strand
Tus-Ter complex	Prevents the helicase (DNA B protein) from further unwinding of DNA and facilitates the termination of replication

- DNA C protein
- Primase (DNA G protein)
- SSB (single stranded binding protein)

Enzymes and proteins involved in prokaryotic replication are given in **Table 19.2**.

Stages of Replication

The process of replication can be divided into three stages:
1. Initiation
2. Elongation
3. Termination.

Initiation

For a double stranded DNA molecule to replicate the two strands of the double helical must be separated from each other. Initiation of DNA replication involves unwinding (separation) of two complementary DNA strands and formation of **replicating fork**. This separation allows each strand to act as a **template** on which a new polynucleotide chain can be assembled.

- Prokaryotic cells, which lack nuclei, have a single **circular double stranded chromosomal DNA**. Circular DNA duplex unwinds in such a way as to form an **'eye'** or **'bubble' (Figure 19.2)**.
- Unwinding is not a random process; rather it occurs at a single, specific site at a particular DNA sequence on circular DNA. The site is called the **origin of replication, 'ori'**.

- This unwound section appears under electron microscopes as a **bubble** and is thus known as a **replicating bubble**, where active synthesis occurs. This region is called **replicating fork**.
- Replication of double stranded DNA is **bidirectional** that is, the replication forks move in both directions away from the origin **(Figure 19.2)**.
- Replication ends on the other side of DNA at a termination point. One round of synthesis involves over 4 million nucleotides in each new strand of DNA which is completed in about 40 minutes.

Formation of Prepriming Complex

- First **DNA A protein** recognizes and binds to the **origin of replication 'ori'** of the DNA and successively denatures the DNA.
- **DNA B protein** (helicase) then binds to this region and unwinds the parental DNA, and form a 'V' (fork) where active synthesis occurs. This region is called the replicating fork **(Figure 19.3)**.
- The stress produced by supercoiling (due to unwinding by helicase) is released by **topoisomerases** by cutting either one or both DNA strands. **Type I topoisomerases** cleave just one strand of DNA, whereas type II enzymes cleave both strands.

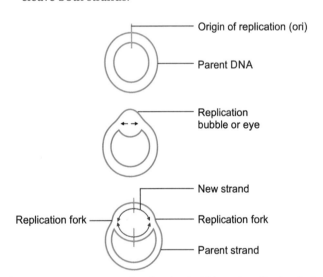

Figure 19.2: Formation of replicating bubble and replicating fork.

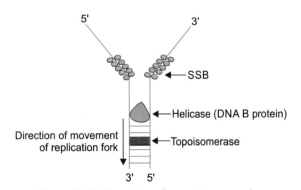

Figure 19.3: Formation of prepriming complex.

- Binding of the **single stranded binding (SSB) protein** stabilizes the separated strands and prevents their reassociation. The result of this process is the generation of structure called the **prepriming complex (Figure 19.3)**.
- Prepriming complex makes single stranded DNA accessible to other enzymes (proteins) and the primase (DNA G) is now able to insert the **RNA primer**.

Elongation

- Primase (DNA-G) synthesizes **RNA primer** complementary to template DNA strands and recruited with DNA templates
- Once **RNA primer** has been laid down on each strand, two **DNA polymerase III** complexes are assembled on each primer
- DNA polymerases synthesize DNA in **5′ to 3′ direction** but not 3′ to 5′ direction. Thus, both strands are synthesized in **5′ to 3′ direction**. DNA polymerase adds complementary nucleotides one at a time to the 3′ end of the DNA strand.
- Because of the antiparallel nature of the two strands, the direction of synthesis of DNA along the two strands is different. One strand of a DNA is made **continuously** whereas the other strand is synthesized in **fragments (Figure 19.4)**.
  - The DNA chain which runs in the **3′ to 5′ direction** is copied by polymerase III in the 5′ to 3′ direction as a continuous strand, requiring **one primer**. This new strand is known as the **leading strand**.
  - The DNA chain which runs in the **5′ to 3′ direction** is copied by polymerase III in the 5′ to 3′ direction as a discontinuous and newly synthesized DNA exists as small fragments. These fragments called **Okazaki fragments**. This new strand is known as the **lagging strand**. This requires many **RNA primers** at specified intervals after synthesis of each **Okazaki fragments**

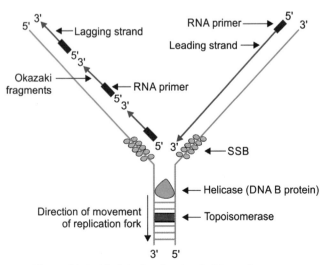

Figure 19.4: Model of replicating fork in prokaryotes.

of DNA **(Figure 19.4)**. These **Okazaki fragments** are 1000 to 2000 nucleotides long.

- Upon completion of lagging strand synthesis the RNA primers are removed from fragments by **DNA polymerase-I**.
- Polymerase-I fills the gaps that are produced by removal of the primer
- Polymerase-I cannot join two polynucleotide chains together; an additional enzyme **DNA ligase** is required to perform this function **(Figure 19.4)**.
- The **joining of Okazaki fragments** is catalyzed by **DNA ligase**. This enzyme catalyzes the formation of a **phosphodiester** bond which requires energy. In eukaryotes, ATP is the energy source. In bacteria, NAD⁺ typically plays this role.

Termination of Replication

- Replication of the circular chromosome initiates at an origin (Ori), with two replication forks proceeding in opposite directions.
- The two forks move in the opposite direction around the circular chromosome and finally meet at a **terminus region** containing specific sequences, called terminator or **'Ter'**.
- Ter sequence prevents further unwinding and replication fork motion.
- The arrest of replication fork motion at Ter sites requires the action of **Tus (terminator utilization substance)**.
- The parental and newly made circular DNA are, at this point topologically interlinked and must be separated with the help of **topoisomerase**.

Proofreading

- Deoxyribonucleic acid is copied by DNA polymerase with high fidelity (accuracy).
- **Incorrect nucleotides** are incorporated with a frequency of one in 10^8–10^{12} **bases**, which could lead to **mutation**.

- Mismatches do not lead to stable incorporations because the **all three polymerases have 3′ to 5′ exonuclease** activity (proofreading activity). Exonucleases are enzymes that cleave DNA sequences in a polynucleotide chain from either the 5′ or 3′ end one at a time.
- DNA polymerase I and II are known to remove erroneous nucleotides before the introduction of the next nucleotide. This process is known as **proofreading**. The error ratio during replication is thus kept at a very low level.

Inhibitors of Prokaryotic Replication and its Clinical Importance

Some antibacterial, and antiviral drugs and many chemotherapeutic drugs inhibit replication.

- Many antibacterial drugs inhibit the prokaryotic enzyme, **topoisomerase II** (DNA gyrase) much more than the eukaryotic one and are widely used for the treatment of urinary tract and other infections including those due to *Bacillus anthracis* (anthrax), e.g., **Novobiocin, Nalidixic acid**, and **Ciprofloxacin**, etc.
- **Camptothecin**, an antitumor drug, inhibits human **topoisomerase I**.
- Certain anticancer and antiviral drugs inhibit elongation of DNA chain, e.g., by incorporating certain nucleotide analogs, e.g.:
  - **2, 3-deoxyinosine (ddI)**
  - Adenine arabinoside (vidarabine, araA)
  - Zidovudine also known as Azidothymidine (AZT) Acyclovir
  - **Cytosine arabinoside (cytarabin, araC), etc.**

◼ EUKARYOTIC REPLICATION

Replication in eukaryotic organisms resembles that in prokaryotic cells and proceeds by a mechanism similar to that of prokaryotic replication but is not identical. Some differences are given in **Table 19.3**. Eukaryotic replication is more complex because:

TABLE 19.3: Difference between prokaryotic and eukaryotic DNA replication.

Features	Prokaryotes	Eukaryotes
Location	Cytoplasm	Nucleus
Type of DNA	Circular	Linear
RNA primer length	~50 nucleotides	9 nucleotides
DNA polymerase	Three types and designated by Roman numerals; I, II, III	Five types and designated by Greek numerals α, β, γ, δ, and ε
Number of origins	Single	Multiple
Nucleotide length of Okazaki fragments of lagging strand	1000–2000 nucleotides	~200 nucleotides
Rate of replication	~500 nucleotides per sec	50 nucleotides per sec (10 times slower than prokaryotes)
End replication problems	Does not contain ends	Involves the synthesis of special structures, called **telomeres** at the ends of each chromosome by **telomerase, a specialized polymerase that carries its own RNA template**

TABLE 19.4: Different types of eukaryotic polymerases.

Name	Function
DNA polymerase α	• Initiator polymerase • Synthesizes the RNA primer • Adds stretch of about 20 nucleotides to the primer • No exonuclease activity
DNA polymerase β	DNA repair
DNA polymerase g	Mitochondrial DNA synthesis. No exonuclease activity
DNA polymerase δ	• Lagging strand synthesis • DNA proofreading
DNA polymerase ε	• Leading strand synthesis • DNA proofreading and DNA repair

- **Size of DNA:** *E. coli* replicates 4.8 million base pairs, whereas a human diploid cell must replicate 6 billion base pairs.
- **Number of chromosome:** *E. coli* contained only **one chromosome**, the genetic information of *E. coli* is present on one chromosome only. In human beings, 23 pairs of chromosomes must be replicated
- *E. coli* chromosome is **circular**, whereas human chromosomes are **linear**. Shorting of chromosomes occur in linear chromosomes with each round of replication.
- However eukaryotic replication is regulated and coordinated with the cell cycle. The events of eukaryotic DNA replication are linked to the eukaryotic **cell cycle (discussed latter in this chapter).**

Basic Requirements for Replication

1. **Substrates:** dATP, dGTP, dCTP, dTTP
2. **Template:** Each strand of double helix acts as a template
3. **Primer:** A short piece of RNA, complementary to the template DNA strands.
4. **Proteins required for replication**
   - Origin of replication complexes (ORCs)
   - Mini chromosome maintenance (MCM) proteins (Helicase)

- Replication protein A(RPA)/Single-stranded DNA-binding protein.
- Proliferating cell nuclear antigen (PCNA)
- Replication factor-C (RFC)

5. **Enzymes:** DNA polymerases: Eukaryotes have five types of DNA polymerases **(Table 19.4)**.
   a. DNA polymerase-α
   b. DNA polymerase-β
   c. DNA polymerase-γ
   d. DNA polymerase-δ
   e. DNA polymerase-ε

Stages of Replication

The process of replication can be divided into three stages as prokaryotes:

1. Initiation
2. Elongation
3. Termination.

Initiation

- In eukaryotes replication begins at multiple sites **(Figure 19.5)** located between 30 and 300 kbp apart.
- In contrast with *E. coli* the origins of replication (Ori) in eukaryotes do not contain sharply defined **specific sequences.** Instead replication begins at sites contained exclusively of **A-T rich sequences** and is referred to as a **consensus** sequence.
- First step in eukaryotic replication is association of the **origin of replication complexes (ORC)** with the site of origin and formation replication fork **(Figure 19.5)**.
- In eukaryotes, the ORC is composed of **six different proteins** (each homologous to DNA A protein of prokaryotes) to form a **hexameric structure.**
- After the ORC has been assembled, additional proteins are recruited, including **CDC6 (cell division cycle)** and **CDT1.** These proteins in turn recruit a hexameric **helicase** having six subunits called **mini chromosome maintenance (MCM) protein (MCM2 to MCM7).**

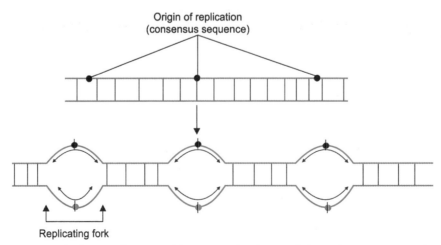

Origin of replication
(consensus sequence)

Replicating fork

Figure 19.5: Multiple sites of origin and formation of replicating fork in eukaryotic DNA replication.

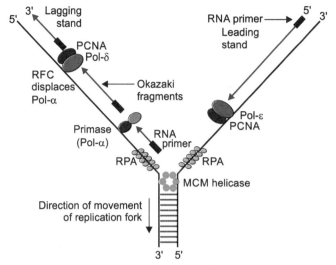

Figure 19.6: Model of replicating fork in eukaryotes.

- These proteins, including the helicase, are sometimes called **licensing factors** because they permit the formation of the initiation complex **(Figure 19.6)**.
- After the initiation complex has formed, MCM helicase separates the parental DNA strands, and single strands are stabilized by the binding of **replication protein A, (RPA),** a single-stranded DNA-binding protein.

Elongation

Eukaryotes have five types of DNA polymerases **(Table 19.4)**.
- The three types of DNA polymerases which are involved in eukaryotic DNA replication are:
  1. DNA polymerase α
  2. DNA polymerase δ
  3. DNA polymerase ε
- **DNA polymerase α** initiates the DNA replication, whereas the DNA **polymerase δ** and ε are involved in the elongation.
- Polymerase α has **primase** activity used to synthesize **RNA primers**. Polymerase α also has **DNA polymerase activity** but does not possess 3' to 5' proofreading exonuclease activity.
- After synthesis of **primer** by primase, **polymerase α** adds a stretch of about 20 deoxynucleotides to the primer.
- After **DNA polymerase α** has added a stretch of about **20 deoxynucleotides** to the primer, **replication factor-C (RFC)** replaces DNA polymerase-α, by another DNA **polymerase**. This process is called **polymerase switching** because one polymerase has replaced another.
- PCNA **(proliferating cell nuclear antigen) protein** enhances the processivity of two polymerases; **polymerase ε** and **polymerase γ**. The binding of PCNA to DNA polymerases makes the enzymes highly processive (active) and replicates long stretches of deoxyribonucleotides **(Figure 19.6)**.

- Polymerase ε and δ get recruited in place of **polymerase α.** DNA **polymerase γ** and ε is involved in the elongation.
  - The highly processive **DNA polymerase ε** synthesizes the leading strand
  - **DNA polymerase γ** synthesizes the lagging strand.
- **PCNA** holds DNA polymerase in place so that it does not slide off the DNA.
- The leading and lagging strands are formed in the same manner as in prokaryotic DNA replication.
- Both **polymerase ε** and γ enzymes have 3' to 5' proofreading exonuclease activities and can thus edit the replicated DNA.

> DNA polymerase γ occurs exclusively in the mitochondrion, where it replicates the mitochondrial genome.

Termination

- Replication continues in both directions from the origin of one replication bubble until replication of adjacent second replicon bubble meet and fuse.
- Then RNA primer is removed by **RNase H** and **FEN-1 (Flap endonuclease 1)** and the gap is filled by the freely-floating DNA polymerases.
- The nicks are joined by the DNA ligase.

> The termination of replication on linear eukaryotic chromosomes involves the synthesis of special structures, called **telomeres** at the ends of each chromosome by **telomerase (discussed latter)**.

Proofreading in Eukaryotes

- In eukaryotes **DNA polymerase δ** which is a part of replication complex, has the **3' to 5' exonuclease** activity required for this function. Enzymes that catalyze repair of mismatched bases are also present (discussed next). Consequently, eukaryotic replication occurs with high fidelity, approximately one miss pairing occurs for every 10^9 to 10^{12} nucleotides incorporated into growing DNA chains.
- Eukaryotic DNA polymerase α, β, and ε appear to be involved in DNA repair.
- Polymerase γ is located in mitochondria and, therefore, its function is related to replication of mitochondrial DNA.

> Mitochondrial DNA shows a much higher rate of mutation than nuclear DNA because polymerase-γ which copies mitochondrial DNA has no exonuclease activity.

■ TELOMERE, TELOMERASE, AND ITS IMPORTANCE

The DNA molecules in eukaryotic chromosomes are linear, i.e., have two ends. This is in contrast to bacterial chromosomes that is a closed circle, i.e., has no ends.

- The free ends of the linear chromosome are not readily replicated by cellular DNA polymerases. While replicating linear double-stranded DNA, the 5′ end of each new DNA strand will generally commence ≥100 BP short of the 5′ end of the template strand.

- Consequently, each time a cell replicates its genome in order to divide; its chromosomes become shorter **(Figure 19.7)**. This difficulty must be resolved by special mechanism which involves the synthesis of special structures, called **telomeres** (Greek: telos; end) at the ends of each chromosome by **telomerase**. Telomerase is a specialized polymerase that carries its own RNA template.

- The **telomeres** have an unusual structure. Telomeric DNA consists of hundreds of tandem (multiple) repeats of a six nucleotide G-rich sequence. In human beings, the repeating G-rich sequence is **5′-TTAGGG-3′**.

- DNA polymerase cannot synthesize the extreme 5′ end of the new strand because polymerase acts only in the 5′ → 3′ direction. The new synthesized strands would have an incomplete 5′ end after the removal of the **RNA primer (Figure 19.8)**. Consequently the new strand is always shorter than its template strand by the length of the primer. James and Watson called this **"end replication problem."**

- It is estimated that human telomeres lose about 100 base pairs from their telomeric DNA at each mitosis process. At this rate, after 125 mitotic divisions, the telomeres would be completely gone.

- Telomeric DNA is synthesized by a specialized polymerase named **telomerase**, which is a complex of protein and RNA. This internal RNA of telomerase can serve as the template for synthesizing DNA.

- Telomerase adds telomere repeat sequences to the 3′ end of DNA strands. By lengthening this strand, DNA polymerase is able to complete the synthesis of "incomplete ends of the opposite strand **(Figure 19.8)** and thus maintain the length of the telomere.

Importance of Telomeres

The telomeres have two functions:
1. To protect chromosomes from fusing with each other
2. To solve **"end replication problem"**.

Telomeres are essential for proper maintenance of chromosomes and play a major role in **aging** and **cancer**.

❖ Telomerase functions similarly to reverse transcriptase (the enzymes that copy RNA into DNA). Thus, telomerase is a specialized **reverse transcriptase** that carries its own template. Telomerase is an RNA-dependent DNA polymerase, meaning an enzyme that can make DNA using RNA as a template.

❖ Telomerase is not usually active in most somatic cells (cells of the body), but it is active in germ cells (the cells that make sperm and eggs) and some adult stem cells.

Telomerase is a Potential Target for Anticancer Therapy

❖ Telomerase is generally expressed at high levels only in rapidly growing cells. Thus, telomeres and telomerase can play important roles in cancer cell biology and in cell aging.

❖ Because cancer cells express high levels of telomerase, whereas most normal cells do not, telomerase is a potential target for **anticancer therapy**. A variety of approaches for blocking telomerase expression or blocking its activity are under investigation for cancer treatment and prevention.

❖ In contrast in absence of telomerase, the telomere will become shorter after each cell division. After reaching a certain length the cell may cease to divide and die. Thus, telomerase plays critical role in the aging process.

❖ **Progeria**, a rare disease characterized by rapid and premature aging resulting in childhood death, have short telomeres and have reduced proliferative capacity.

❖ **Cloned mammals** from adult cells have short telomeres than in normal one. Analysis of telomere length in Dolly's (cloned sheep) cells reveals that they were only 80% as long as in a normal one year old sheep. Her short telomeres do add another question to the debate about cloning mammals from adult cells.

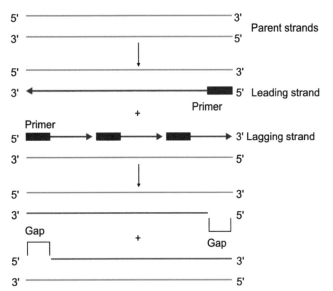

Figure 19.7: Schematic representation of end-replication problem of DNA.

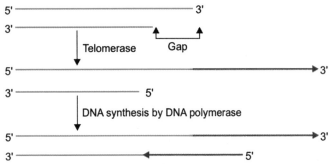

Figure 19.8: Telomere extension by telomerase.

STRIKE A NOTE

❖ Proofreading function needs 3' to 5' exonuclease activity
❖ Repair function needs 5' to 3' exonuclease activity
❖ Length of Okazaki fragments in prokaryotes is 1,000 to 2,000 base pairs
❖ Length of Okazaki fragments in eukaryotes is 100 to 250 base pairs
❖ Time taken for replication in prokaryotes is 30 minutes
❖ Time taken for replication in eukaryotes is 9 hours
❖ Telomeres assumed as a molecular countdown clock that controls aging and lifespan.

DNA REPAIR MECHANISMS WITH ASSOCIATED DISORDERS

Despite proofreading and mismatch repair during replication, some mismatched bases do persist. In addition, DNA can be damaged by mutagens produced in cells or from the environment. The environmental mutagenic agents can be either radiation or chemicals. These mutagens damage DNA, causing mutations. If the damage is not repaired, a permanent mutation may be introduced that can result in any of a number of deleterious effects leading to **cancer**.

● DNA can be damage due to the:
  ▪ Miss-incorporation of a single base
  ▪ Chemical modification of bases
  ▪ Chemical cross links between the two strands of the double helix or
  ▪ Breaks in one or both of the phosphodiester backbones.
● DNA damage may result:
  ▪ Cell death or cell transformation
  ▪ Changes in the DNA sequence that can be inherited by future generation or
  ▪ Blockage of replication process itself.
● DNA damage must be repaired to maintain the integrity of genetic information. A variety of DNA repair systems have evolved that can recognize these defects and restore the DNA molecule to its undamaged form **(Table 19.5)**.

TABLE 19.5: Types of DNA repair system.

System	Types of damage
Mismatch repair	● Mismatches ● Copying errors
Base excision repair	Base alterations or loss either spontaneously, deamination or alkylation
Nucleotide excision repair	Pyrimidine dimers may be due to chemical, radiation or spontaneous
Direct repair	Formation of O^6-methylguanine, O^4-methylthymine, and methylphosphotriesters due to alkylation
Homologous recombination (HR) and Nonhomologous end-joining (NHEJ) repair	DNA double strand breaks

● DNA repair mechanisms detect and correct damage throughout the cell cycle. The mechanisms used for the repair of DNA involve:
  1. First recognition of distorted region of the DNA.
  2. Secondly removal or excision of the damaged region of the DNA strands.
  3. Then filling of gap left by the excision of the damaged DNA by DNA polymerase.
  4. Finally sealing the nick in the strand that has undergone repair by a ligase.

Types of DNA Repair Systems

All cells have multiple DNA repair systems. The mechanisms of DNA repair include:
● Mismatch repair
● Base excision repair
● Nucleotide excision repair
● Direct repair
● Double-stranded break repair (homologous recombination and nonhomologous end-joining repair)

Mismatch Repair

Errors that occur during replication are repaired by the **mismatch repair enzyme complex**. Mismatch is repaired by **tagging template DNA** strand with **methyl groups** to distinguish it from newly synthesized strands

● Immediately after formation of replication fork, there is a short period during which the template strand is methylated but the **newly synthesized strand is not**. **Dam methylase**, (DNA adenine methyltransferase) methylates all adenine of DNA that occurs within **5'-G-A-T-C sequences**.
● Replication mismatches in the vicinity of methylated G-A-T-C sequence are then repaired according to the information in the methylated parent (template) strand. A region of the mismatched base of new unmethylated strand is removed and replaced.
● In *E. coli*, three proteins **MutS**, **MutH**, and **MutL** are required for recognition of the mutation and nicking the strand **(Figure 19.9)**.
  ▪ G-T mismatch is recognized by **MutS**.
  ▪ MutL interacts with the MutS-DNA complex, and then
  ▪ MutH endonuclease is activated by MutL.
  ▪ MutH cleaves the backbone in the vicinity of the mismatch.
● A segment of the DNA strand containing the error (erroneous **T in Figure 19.9**) is then removed by **exonuclease** and **replaced** according to the information in methylated parent (template) strand.
● New nucleotide is synthesized by DNA polymerase III and nick is sealed by **DNA ligase**.

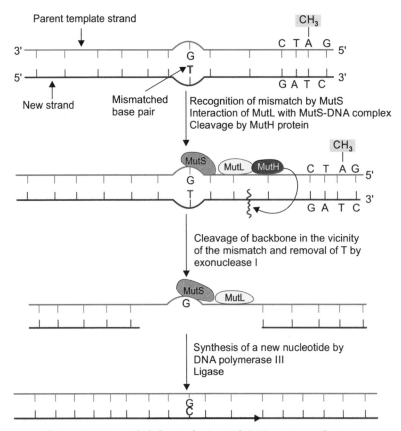

Figure 19.9: A methyl-directed mismatch DNA repair mechanism.

The increased risk for hereditary nonpolyposis colon cancer (HNPCC) or Lynch syndrome is due to inherited mutations that impair DNA mismatch repair.

Base Excision Repair

- Damage due to **base alterations** or **loss** can be corrected by **base excision repair mechanism**.
- Bases of DNA can be altered, either by:
  - Spontaneously
  - Deamination (deamination of cytosine and adenine. Deamination of adenine results in the formation of hypoxanthine and deamination of cytosine to uracil.)
  - Action of alkylating compounds.
- Every cell has a class of enzymes called **DNA glycosylases**. **DNA glycosylases** catalyze hydrolysis of the N-glycosidic bond, yielding an apurinic/apyrimidinic (AP) or abasic site in the DNA.
- DNA glycosylases
- **DNA glycosylases** recognize deaminated forms of cytosine and adenine and remove the affected base by cleaving the **N-glycosyl bond**. This creates an apurinic (devoid of A or G) or apyrimidinic (devoid of C or T) site in the DNA, both commonly referred to as an **AP sites** or **abasic site**.
- Each DNA glycosylase is generally specific for one type of lesion. **Uracil glycosylases**, for example found in most

cells, specifically remove **uracil** from DNA that results from spontaneous deamination of cytosine.
- Other DNA glycosylases recognize and remove a variety of damaged bases, including hypoxanthine (arising from adenine deamination) and alkylated bases such as 3-methyladenine and 7-methylguanine.
- Once an AP site has been formed by DNA glycosylase, another type of enzyme must repair it. Repair process begins with one of the **AP endonuclease**, enzymes that cut the DNA strand containing AP site. A segment of DNA including AP site is then removed. DNA polymerase-I in prokaryote and **DNA polymerase-β in eukaryotes** initiates repair synthesis, and DNA ligase seals the remaining nick **(Figure 19.10)**.

Nucleotide Excision Repair

- DNA lesion that caused by **pyrimidine dimers** is repaired by **nucleotide excision mechanism**. Formation of pyrimidine dimers may be due to chemical, radiation, or spontaneous.
- In nucleotide excision repair, enzyme **excinuclease** hydrolyzes two phosphodiester bonds one on either side of the distortion caused by the lesion.
  - In prokaryotes the enzyme hydrolyzes the fifth phosphodiester bond away from the damaged site on 3'-side and 8th phosphodiester bond on the 5'-side to generate a fragment of 12 to 13 nucleotides,

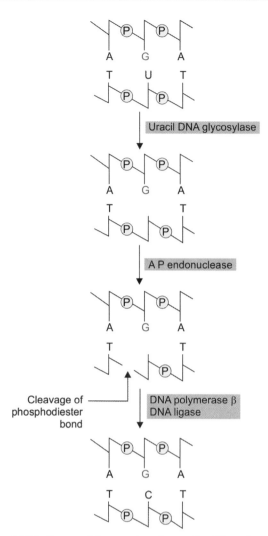

Figure 19.10: Base excision repair pathway. Uracil base formed by the deamination of cytosine is excised and replaced by cytosine.

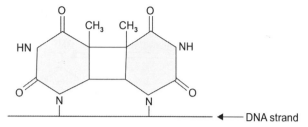

Figure 19.11: Dimer of two thymine bases.

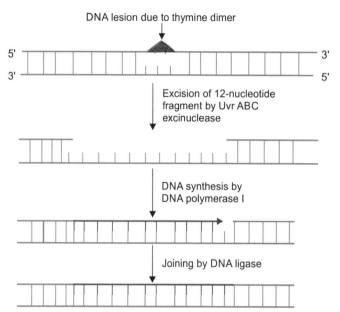

Figure 19.12: Nucleotide excision repair mechanism containing a thymine dimer.

depending on whether the lesion involves one or two bases.

- In humans and other eukaryotes, the enzyme system hydrolyzes the 6th phosphodiester bond away from the damaged site on the 3'-side and the 22nd phosphodiester bond on the 5'-side, producing a fragment of 27 to 29 nucleotides. Following the dual incision, the excised oligonucleotides are released from the duplex and the resulting gap is filled by DNA polymerase-I in prokaryotes and DNA polymerase-ε in humans. DNA ligase seals the nick.

- One of the best understood examples of nucleotide excision repair is excision of a pyrimidine dimer **(Figure 19.11)**. Three endonucleases are essential for this repair in *E. coli*, **UvrA**, **UvrB**, **UvrC**, **(UvrABC)**.
  - The **Uvr ABC** exonuclease first detects the distortion produced by the DNA damage.
  - The UvrABC enzyme then cuts the damaged DNA strand at two sites, 8 nucleotides away from the damaged site on the 5'-side and 4 nucleotides away on the 3'-side.

- The 12 residue oligonucleotide excised by this exonuclease then diffuses away.
- DNA polymerase-I enters the gap to carry out repair synthesis.
- The 3' end of the nicked strand is the primer, and the intact complementary strand is the template.
- Finally, the 3' end of the newly synthesized stretch of DNA and the original part of the DNA chain are joined by **DNA lyase (Figure 19.12)**.

Thymidine dimers are produced when adjacent thymidine residues are covalently linked by exposure to ultraviolet radiation. Covalent linkage may result in the dimer being replicated as a single base, which results in a frame shift mutation.

Direct Repair Pathway

- Several types of damage are repaired without removing a base or nucleotide. An example of direct repair is the damage caused by alkylating agents to DNA.
- Methylation of guanine bases caused by alkylating agents produces a change in the structure of DNA and is a common and highly mutagenic lesion. It tends to pair with thymine rather than cytosine during replication.

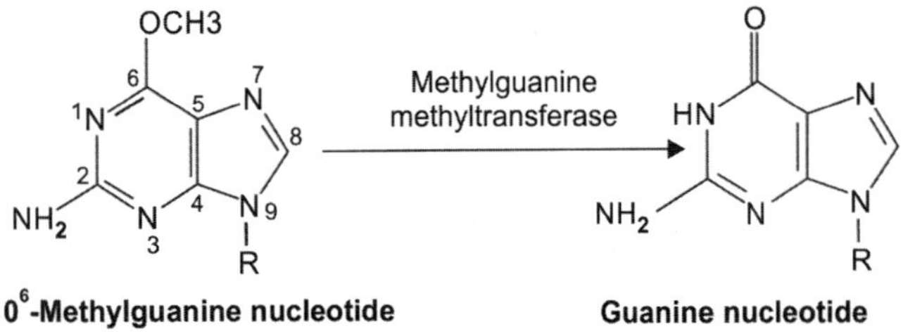

O^6-Methylguanine nucleotide → Methylguanine methyltransferase → **Guanine nucleotide**

Figure 19.13: DNA repair mechanism by O^6-Methylguanine-DNA Methyltransferase (MGMT) enzyme.

- An enzyme **methylguanine methyltransferase**, known as **MGMT**, is a DNA "suicide" repair enzyme.
- It carries out direct repair of alkylated DNA by transferring the alkyl group from the O^6 position of guanine of the DNA molecule to the **cysteine residue** of the MGMT enzyme to restore the normal base **(Figure 19.13)**. This reaction is irreversible, and thus the MGMT is said to be a "suicide" enzyme.
- The three lesions repaired by MGMT are **O^6-methylguanine**, **O^4-methylthymine**, and **methylphosphotriesters**.
- The enzyme also repairs other alkyl guanines, however, such as O^6-ethylguanine and O^6-butyl-guanine, although at a much lower efficiency.

Double-strand Break Repair

- Ionizing radiation, exposure to certain chemicals, or reactive oxygen species generated in the cell can lead to **double strand breaks (DSBs)** in **DNA**. While all the repair mechanisms discussed so far fixed damage on one strand of **DNA** using the other, undamaged strand as a **template**, these mechanisms cannot repair damage to both strands.
- Two pathways involved in the repair of double-stranded DNA breaks are:
  1. Homologous recombination (HR) and
  2. Nonhomologous end-joining (NHEJ).
- The choice between the two depends on the **phase of the cell cycle** and the exact **type of double strand breaks** to be repaired.
  - During G_0/G_1 phases of the cell cycle, DNA double strand breaks are corrected by the **nonhomologous end-joining** repair mechanism, whereas
  - During **S, G2**, and **M phases** of the cell cycle **homologous recombination** is utilized.

Homologous Recombination (HR) Repair

Homologous recombination repair commonly occurs in the late S and G2 phases of the cell, when each **chromosome** has been replicated and information from a sister chromatid can be used as a **template** to achieve error free repair.

Note that in contrast to **excision repair**, where the damaged strand was removed and the undamaged sister strand served as the template for filling in the damaged region, **HR** must use the information from another **DNA**

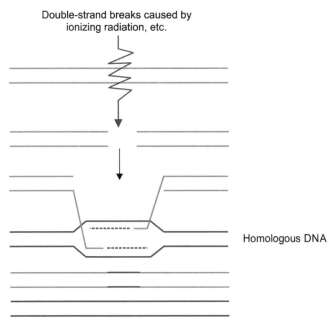

Figure 19.14: Homologous recombination DNA repair mechanism.

molecule, because both strands of the DNA are damaged in DSBs.

- This mechanism requires the presence of DNA having identical or nearly identical sequence related to the damaged DNA region for use as a template.
- Repair of a DNA double-strand break takes place by means of replication, using the homologous strand as a template to replace the damaged region of the broken DNA and no loss of genetic information normally results. **(Figure 19.14)**.
- Homologous recombination is reliable than nonhomologous end joining and does not usually cause mutations.

Nonhomologous End Joining (NHEJ)

- Nonhomologous end joining is referred to as "nonhomologous" because the break ends of the DNA are directly ligated without the need for a homologous template, in contrast to **homologous recombination** repair.
- Nonhomologous end-joining is used during G_0/G_1 **phases** of the cell cycle when sister chromatids are not available for use as HR templates.
- When these breaks occur the cell has not yet replicated the region of DNA that contains the break, so unlike the HR pathway, there is no corresponding template strand available.
- Nonhomologous end-joining rejoins the two broken ends directly. Multiple enzymes/proteins are involved in the rejoining process including:
  - Ku proteins
  - DNA ligase, and
  - DNA-dependent protein kinase (DNA-PK)

- Ku protein has ATP dependent helicase activity. It binds to both the broken ends of DNA strands.
- The DNA bound Ku protein recruits an unusual **DNA dependent protein kinase (DNA-PK)**.
- DNA-PK approximates (bring nearer) the two separated strands.
- DNA-PK phosphorylates Ku resulting in activation of the Ku helicase activity. This results in unwinding of the two ends.
- The unwound approximated DNA strands get aligned and forms base pairing. The extra nucleotide overhangs are removed by an **exonuclease** and the gaps are filled and closed by **DNA ligase (Figure 19.15)**.
- This repair mechanism involves the loss, or sometimes addition, of a few nucleotides at the cut site. So, nonhomologous end joining is likely to produce a mutation, but this is better than the loss of an entire chromosome.

Diseases Associated with DNA Repair Mechanisms

Defects in DNA repair systems increases the overall frequency of mutations and hence the probability of cancer. Genes for DNA repair proteins are often tumor suppressor gene that is they suppress tumor development.

- **Xeroderma pigmentosum** and **Cockayne syndrome** are caused by genetically defective nucleotide excision repair (NER).
  - The inherited disease xeroderma pigmentosum (XP; Greek: xeros, dry + derma, skin) is mainly characterized by the inability of skin cells to repair UV induced DNA lesions. The skin of an affected person is extremely sensitive to sunlight or UV light. The skin becomes dry and atrophy of the dermis. Skin cancer usually develops at several sites.
  - Cockayne syndrome (CS), a rare inhered disease that is also associated with defective nucleotide excision repair. Individuals with CS are hypersensitive to UV radiation and exhibit stunted growth, neurological dysfunction, premature of aging. In CS, the DNA cannot be repaired, which causes the cell to undergo apoptosis (programmed cell death).
- Defects in other repair systems can increase the frequency of other tumors. For example:
  - Hereditary nonpolyposis colorectal cancer (HNPCC), or
  - Lynch syndrome results from defective DNA mismatch repair.
- The gene for a protein called a **P53** is mutated in more than half of all tumors. P53 protein helps control the fate of damaged cells. First, it plays a central role in sensing DNA damage, then after sensing damage, it either promotes a DNA repair pathway or activates the apoptosis pathway, leading to cell death. People who inherit mutation in one of the p53 gene suffer from

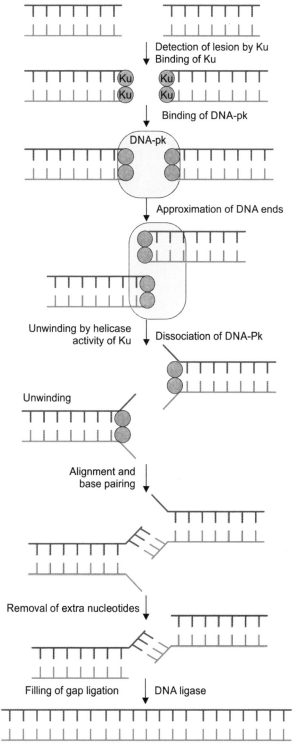

Figure 19.15: Nonhomologous end joining DNA repair mechanism.

Li-Fraumeni syndrome and leave a high probability of developing several types of cancer.

CELL CYCLE

Eukaryotic cell division occurs in four distinct phases which are collectively called the **cell cycle (Figure 19.16)**. The

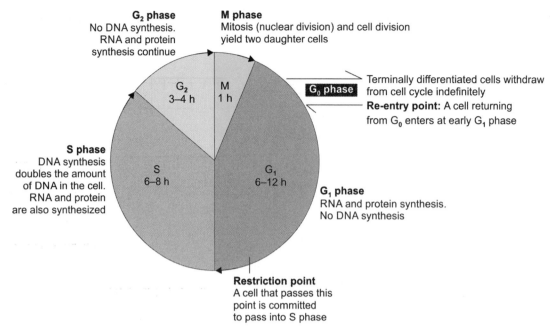

Figure 19.16: Four stages of eukaryotic cell cycle.

total duration of the cell cycle, as observed in a wide range of somatic cells ranges from 12 to 24 hours. The cell cycle of eukaryotic cells consists of four phases.

- The first **three phases** constitute **interphase**. Cells spend most of their time in these three phases, carrying out their normal metabolic activities

- The fourth phase is **mitosis**, the process of **cell division**. This phase is very brief.

Phases of Cell Cycle

- G_1 **phase** (first "gap" phase, G indicates the gap between divisions): G_1 is the first phase of the cycle. It is a preparative phase in which,
  - The enzymes necessary to replicate the genome are produced
  - Genomic DNA is checked for reliability and
  - The building materials required in mitosis begin to accumulate.
- **S phase:** S phase is the second phase, in which biosynthesis of new DNA is carried out. In the S phase, the DNA is replicated to produce copies for both daughter cells.
- G_2 **phase** (the second "gap" phase) G_2-phase is the third phase of cell cycle in which, the cell prepare to divide by synthesizing new proteins, **tubulin** for construction of the **microtubules** of the spindle apparatus and the cell approximately doubles in size.
- **M-phase:** Finally, division occurs in the brief **M-phase (mitosis)**. In the M phase, one parent cell physically divides into two daughter cells. This includes the physical separation of the duplicated genome,

termed mitosis and the subsequent separation of the cytoplasm by a process called **cytokinesis**. Although it is considered the most active phase of the cell cycle, mitosis normally accounts for the least amount of time spent in the cell cycle.

- In embryonic or rapidly proliferating tissue, each daughter cell divides again, but only after a waiting period (G_1). After passing through mitosis and into G_1, a cell either continues through another division or stops to divide, entering a **dormant phase (G_0)** that may last hours, days, or the lifetime of the cell.
- When a cell in G_0 begins to divide again, it re-enters the division cycle through the G_1 phase.
- DNA and chromosome segregation, reliability are continuously monitored throughout the cell cycle.
- Cells use special **proteins** and **checkpoint signaling** systems to ensure that the cell cycle progresses properly.
- Checkpoints at the end of G_1 and at the beginning of G_2 are designed **to assess DNA** for damage before and after S phase.
- If DNA damage or abnormalities are detected at these checkpoints, the cell is forced to undergo programmed cell death, or **apoptosis**.
- The cell cycle and its checkpoint systems can be impaired by defective proteins and can cause malignant transformation of the cell, which can lead to cancer. For example, mutations in a protein called **p**[53] which normally detects abnormalities in DNA at the G_1 checkpoint can make possible cancer-causing mutations to bypass this checkpoint and allow the cell to escape apoptosis.

In the cell cycle, the process of DNA synthesis and cell division (mitosis) are coordinated so that the replication of all DNA sequences is complete before the cell progress into the next phase of the cycle. This coordination requires several **checkpoints** that control the progression along the cycle. The timing of the cell cycle is controlled by a family of proteins, **cyclines**. Cyclines act by binding to specific cycline-dependent protein kinases (CDKs) and activating them. Mitosis takes place only after DNA synthesis.

STRIKE A NOTE

❖ Unlike the prokaryotes, where a second round of DNA synthesis can begin before cell division takes place, **eukaryotes replicate their DNA only once per cell division cycle**.

❖ Upon the appropriate signal, cells in G_0 may be stimulated to re-enter the cycle and divide.

❖ Tumor cells is that they can no longer enter G_0 phase which is the nondividing state.

ASSESSMENT QUESTIONS

STRUCTURED LONG ESSAY QUESTIONS (SLEQs)

1. Describe DNA repair systems under the following headings:
   i. Name different types of repair mechanisms
   ii. Mechanisms with diagrams of different types of repair
   iii. Clinical significance of DNA repair systems
2. Describe the replication in eukaryotes under the following headings:
   i. Process
   ii. Proofreading
   iii. Inhibitors of replication
   iv. Name DNA repair mechanisms
3. Describe the replication in eukaryotes under the following headings:
   i. Process
   ii. Proofreading
   iii. Inhibitors of replication and its clinical application
   iv. Name DNA repair mechanisms

SHORT ESSAY QUESTIONS (SEQs)

1. Name inhibitors of replication. Write its therapeutic use.
2. Write types of DNA repair mechanism. Write mechanism of any one of them.
3. What is cell cycle? Write four phases of cell cycle.
4. Difference between prokaryotic and eukaryotic replication.

SHORT ANSWER QUESTIONS (SAQs)

1. What is an Okazaki fragment? Where they are formed?
2. Enumerate component required for the process of replication.
3. Write any four differences between prokaryotic and eukaryotic replication.
4. Enumerate enzymes required for prokaryotic and eukaryotic replication
5. Write types of DNA repair mechanism.
6. What is Xeroderma pigmentosum? Write its clinical features.

7. What is telomere? Write the role of telomerase in end replication problem.
8. Write importance of telomerase in anticancer therapy and ageing.
9. What is progeria? Write its cause.

MULTIPLE CHOICE QUESTIONS (MCQs)

1. **Formation of Okazaki fragments occur in the process of:**
   a. Transcription
   b. Translation
   c. Replication
   d. Reverse transcription
2. **Which of the following enzyme joins Okazaki fragments?**
   a. DNA polymerase
   b. DNA ligase
   c. RNA polymerase
   d. Peptidyl transferase
3. **Which the following enzyme fill the gap between Okazaki fragments?**
   a. DNA polymerase
   b. RNA polymerase
   c. Translocase
   d. Helicase
4. **Which of the following eukaryotic DNA polymerases is required for mitochondrial DNA synthesis?**
   a. DNA polymerase α
   b. DNA polymerase β
   c. DNA polymerase γ
   d. DNA polymerase δ
5. **Which of the following inhibits eukaryotic protein synthesis?**
   a. Tetracycline
   b. Erythromycin
   c. Streptomycin
   d. Puromyrin
6. **All of the following enzymes are required for the synthesis of DNA, *except*:**
   a. DNA dependent DNA polymerase
   b. Helicase
   c. DNA ligase
   d. DNA dependent RNA polymerase
7. **Primer (a short piece of RNA) is required for:**
   a. DNA synthesis
   b. M-RNA synthesis
   c. t-RNA synthesis
   d. r-RNA synthesis
8. **Synthesis of DNA is also known as:**
   a. Duplication
   b. Replication
   c. Transcription
   d. Translation

9. **Replication of DNA is:**
   - a. Conservative
   - b. Semiconservative
   - c. Nonconservative
   - d. None of these

10. **Direction of new DNA strand synthesis is:**
    - a. $5' \rightarrow 3'$
    - b. $3' \rightarrow 5'$
    - c. Both (a) and (b)
    - d. None of these

11. **Formation of RNA primer:**
    - a. Leads replication
    - b. Leads translation
    - c. Leads transcription
    - d. All of the above

12. **In replication after formation of replication fork.**
    - a. Both the new strands are synthesized discontinuously
    - b. One strand is synthesized continuously and the other discontinuously
    - c. Both the new strands are synthesized continuously
    - d. RNA primer is required only for the synthesis of one new strand

13. **An Okazaki fragment contains about:**
    - a. 10 Nucleotides
    - b. 100 Nucleotides
    - c. 1,000 Nucleotides
    - d. 10,000 Nucleotides

14. **In replication RNA primer is formed by the enzyme:**
    - a. Ribonuclease
    - b. Primase
    - c. DNA polymerase I
    - d. DNA polymerase III

15. **In eukaryotes during replication, the template DNA is unwound:**
    - a. At one of the ends
    - b. At both the ends
    - c. At multiple sites
    - d. Nowhere

16. **During replication, unwinding of double helix is initiated by:**
    - a. DNA A protein
    - b. DNA B protein
    - c. Topoisomerase
    - d. Single strand binding protein

17. **In replication, the unwound strands of DNA are held apart by:**
    - a. DNA A protein
    - b. DNA B protein
    - c. Single strand binding protein
    - d. Topoisomerase

18. **In replication deoxyribonucleotides are added to RNA primer by:**
    - a. DNA polymerase I
    - b. DNA polymerase II
    - c. DNA polymerase III
    - d. All of these

19. **In replication ribonucleotides of RNA primer are replaced by deoxyribonucleotides by the enzyme:**
    - a. DNA polymerase I
    - b. DNA polymerase II
    - c. DNA polymerase III
    - d. All of these

20. **True about telomerase or telomere is/are:**
    - a. They are present at the ends of eukaryotic chromosome
    - b. Increased telomerase activity favors cancer cell
    - c. DNA dependent RNA polymerase
    - d. DNA polymerase

21. **DNA polymerase III holoenzyme possesses.**
    - a. Polymerase activity
    - b. $3' \rightarrow 5'$ Exonuclease activity
    - c. $5' \rightarrow 3'$ Exonuclease and polymerase activities
    - d. $3' \rightarrow 5'$ Exonuclease and polymerase activities

22. **Reverse transcriptase catalyses.**
    - a. Synthesis of RNA from DNA
    - b. Breakdown of RNA
    - c. Synthesis of DNA from RNA
    - d. Breakdown of DNA

23. **Consensus sequence is:**
    - a. Initiation site of replication in eukaryotes
    - b. Initiation site of replication in prokaryotes
    - c. Initiation site of transcription in eukaryotes
    - d. Initiation site of transcription in prokaryotes

24. **Eukaryotic DNA polymerase γ is located in:**
    - a. Nucleus
    - b. Nucleolus
    - c. Mitochondria
    - d. Cytosol

25. **The mammalian DNA polymerase involved in error correction is:**
    - a. DNA polymerase α
    - b. DNA polymerase β
    - c. DNA polymerase γ
    - d. DNA polymerase δ

26. **Action of 'Telomerase' is:**
    - a. DNA repair
    - b. Longevity of cell-ageing
    - c. Breakdown of telomere
    - d. None

27. **Ends of chromosomes replicated by:**
    - a. Telomerase
    - b. Centromere
    - c. Restriction endonuclease
    - d. Exonuclease

28. **Which enzymatic mutation is responsible for immortality of cancer cells?**
    - a. DNA reverse transcriptase
    - b. RNA polymerase
    - c. Telomerase
    - d. DNA polymerase

29. **All of the following cell type contains the enzyme telomerase, which protect the length of telomeres at the end of chromosomes, *except*:**
    - a. Germinal
    - b. Somatic
    - c. Hemopoietic
    - d. Tumor

30. **Telomerases are:**
    - a. DNA dependent DNA polymerase
    - b. RNA dependent DNA polymerase
    - c. DNA dependent RNA polymerase
    - d. RNA dependent RNA polymerase

31. **Which of the following mechanisms will remove uracil and incorporate the correct base?**
    - a. Direct repair
    - b. Base excision repair
    - c. Mismatch repair
    - d. Nucleotide excision repair

32. The DNA polymerase involved in base excision repair is _____.
    a. DNA polymerase α
    b. DNA polymerase β
    c. DNA polymerase σ
    d. DNA polymerase γ

33. Xeroderma pigmentosa is due to defect in:
    a. Direct repair
    b. Base excision repair
    c. Mismatch repair
    d. Nucleotide excision repair

34. Defects in mismatch repair mechanism is linked to:
    a. Xeroderma pigmentosum
    b. Cockayne syndrome (CS)
    c. Hereditary nonpolyposis colorectal cancer (HNPCC)
    d. Lesh Nyhan syndrome

35. Which of the following statements describes a difference between prokaryotic and eukaryotic DNA replication?
    a. Prokaryotic replication is discontinuous rather than semi-discontinuous
    b. Prokaryotic replication is unidirectional, rather than bidirectional
    c. DNA primers, rather than RNA primers, are used in prokaryotic replication
    d. In prokaryotic replication the same DNA polymerase synthesizes the leading and lagging strand

36. During replication of DNA, the synthesis of DNA on lagging strand takes place in segments, these segments are called:
    a. Francis Crick segments
    b. Double helix segments
    c. Kornberg segments
    d. Okazaki segments

ANSWERS FOR MCQs

1. c	2. b	3. a	4. c	5. d
6. d	7. a	8. b	9. b	10. a
11. a	12. b	13. c	14. b	15. c
16. b	17. c	18. c	19. a	20. a,b
21. d	22. c	23. a	24. c	25. b
26. b	27. a	28. c	29. b	30. b
31. b	32. b	33. d	34. c	35. d
36. d				

Transcription and RNA Processing

Competency	Learning Objectives
BI 7.2: Describe the processes involved in replication and repair of DNA and the transcription and translation mechanisms.	1. Describe processes involved in transcription, and post-transcriptional modifications in prokaryotes. 2. Describe inhibitors of prokaryotic transcription and their clinical significance. 3. Difference between prokaryotic and eukaryotic transcription. 4. Describe processes involved in transcription, and post-transcriptional modifications in eukaryotes.

■ OVERVIEW

DNA stores genetic information in a stable form that can be readily replicated. The expression of this genetic information requires its flow form DNA to RNA to protein. This flow of genetic information from DNA to RNA to protein in living cells is called the **central dogma of molecular biology**. During transcription, an enzyme system converts the genetic information in a segment of double stranded DNA into RNA strand with a base sequence complementary to one of the DNA strand.

RNA is the only macromolecule known to have a role in both the **storage** and **transmission of information** and **catalysis**. The discovery of catalytic RNAs, or **ribozymes**, has changed the actual definition of an enzyme, extending it beyond the domain of proteins.

During replication the entire chromosome is usually copied, but transcription is more selective. Only particular genes or groups of genes are transcribed at any one time and some portions of DNA genome are never transcribed. The sum of all the RNA molecules produced in a cell under a given set of conditions is called the cellular **transcriptome**.

■ PROKARYOTIC TRANSCRIPTION, AND POST-TRANSCRIPTIONAL MODIFICATIONS

Transcription is defined as the synthesis of RNA molecule using DNA as a template that results in the transfer of the information stored in double stranded DNA into a single stranded RNA; which is used by the cell to direct the synthesis of proteins. Cellular RNAs include:

- Messenger RNA (mRNA)
- Ribosomal RNA (rRNA)
- Transfer RNA (tRNA).

All are transcribed from DNA.

Similarity and Differentiation between Replication and Transcription

1. The processes of DNA and RNA synthesis are similar in that:
  ➢ They involve the general steps initiation, elongation, and termination
  ➢ Synthesis occurs in the $5' \rightarrow 3'$ direction
  ➢ Follows Watson-Crick base pairing rules.
2. These processes differ in the following respects:
  ➢ Ribonucleotides are used in RNA synthesis rather than deoxyribonucleotides
  ➢ Uracil replaces thymine as the complementary base pair for adenine in RNA synthesis
  ➢ A primer is not required in RNA synthesis
  ➢ Only a very small portion of the genome is transcribed into RNA, whereas the entire genome is copied during DNA replication
  ➢ There is no proofreading during RNA transcription (RNA polymerase lacks the nuclease activity)
  ➢ A single-strand of DNA acts as a template for synthesis of particular RNA molecules.

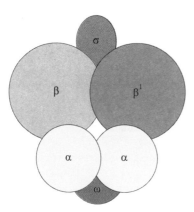

Figure 20.1: Components of prokaryotic holoenzyme RNA polymerase.

Transcription in Prokaryotes

Synthesis of RNA is best understood in prokaryotes, the description of RNA synthesis in prokaryotes is applicable to eukaryotes even though the enzyme involved and regulatory signals are different.

Basic Requirements for Transcription

Template

A single-strand of DNA acts as a template to direct the formation of complementary RNA transcript. The strand that is transcribed to RNA molecule is referred to as the **template strand** of the DNA. The other DNA strand is referred to as the **coding strand** of the gene.

Substrate

The substrates for RNA synthesis are the four ribonucleoside triphosphates:

1. ATP
2. GTP
3. CTP
4. UTP.

Enzyme

DNA dependent RNA polymerase, called **RNA polymerase (RNAP)**, is responsible for the synthesis of RNA. Prokaryotes have single RNA polymerase **(RNAP)** that transcribes all three RNAs, i.e., mRNA, rRNA and tRNA.

- RNAP contains five subunits $(2\alpha, \beta', \beta, \omega)$ which form the core enzyme.
- The active enzyme, the holoenzyme contains core enzyme and a sixth subunit called **sigma (σ) factor (Figure 20.1)**.
- The σ subunit binds transiently to the core enzyme and directs the enzyme to specific binding sites on the DNA.
- **RNA polymerase lacks a separate proofreading activity** as that of DNA polymerases. RNA polymerase requires **Mg²⁺** as well as **Zn²⁺** for its activity.

Stages of Transcription

The RNA synthesis involves:

1. Initiation
2. Elongation
3. Termination.

Initiation

- Unlike the initiation of replication, transcriptional initiation does not require a primer. **Promoter sequences** are responsible for directing RNA polymerase to initiate transcription at a particular point known as **start point** or **initiation site**.
- Promoters are characteristic sequences of DNA which are different in prokaryotes and eukaryotes. Prokaryotic genes have two promoter sequences **–10** and **–35 sites** upstream from transcription start site **(Figure 20.2)**.
- Initiation of transcription involves the binding of RNA polymerase (core enzyme + σ factor) to the template at the **promoter site (Figure 20.3)**.
- The binding of the RNA polymerase to the DNA template results in the unwinding of the DNA double helix.

Promoter Sequences in Prokaryotes

- ❖ The sequence at **–10** is called the **Pribnow box** (after David Pribnow who describe in 1975): It usually consists of the six nucleotides **T A T A A T.** It is named **–10** because it is found 10 base pairs away (upstream) from the start point. The Pribnow box is absolutely essential to start transcription in prokaryotes.
- ❖ The other **sequence at –35** (the –35 element) usually consists of the six nucleotides T T G A C A. It is named **–35** because it is found 35 base pairs upstream of the start point. Its presence allows a very high transcription rate.
- ❖ A base in the promoter region is assigned a negative number if it occurs prior, located in front (upstream) of the gene that is to be transcribed.
- ❖ Position +1 indicates the first nucleotide that will be transcribed into RNA **(Figure 20.2)**. Sequences following the first base are numbered positively and are said to be downstream of the initiation point.

Elongation

- Once the promoter region has been recognized and bound by the RNA polymerase, local unwinding of the DNA helix continues. RNA polymerase then begins to synthesize a transcript of DNA sequence and short piece of RNA is made **(Figure 20.4A)**.
- As with replication, transcription is always in the **5′ to 3′ direction**. Once a stretch of 10 nucleotides is formed, **σ factor dissociates** and RNAP moves along the template stand and continues the elongation of the transcript.
- Elongation is continued in 5′ to 3′ direction with addition of ribonucleotides ATP, GTP, CTP, and UTP complementary to template strand of DNA until termination signal is reached **(Figure 20.4B)**.

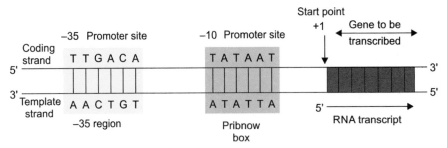

Figure 20.2: Prokaryotic promoter sites for transcription.

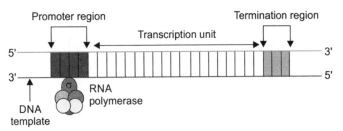

Figure 20.3: Recognition and binding of RNA polymerase to promoter of RNA in prokaryotes.

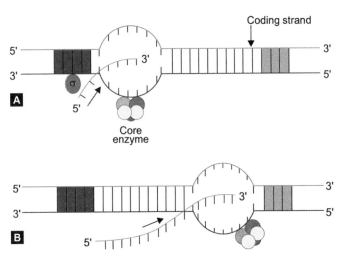

Figures 20.4A and B: Process of elongation of transcription in prokaryotes.

Termination

RNA polymerase will keep transcribing until it gets signals to stop. The process of **termination** occurs when the RNA polymerase transcribes **terminator sequence** present on template DNA. The prokaryotes have two types of termination mechanisms:

1. Rho (ρ) dependent
2. Rho (ρ) independent

Rho-dependent Termination

- In **Rho-dependent termination**, the RNA transcript contains a **binding site** for a protein called **Rho factor**.
- Rho factor binds to this sequence of a growing RNA strand and starts "climbing" up the transcript towards

RNA polymerase in 5′ 3′ direction **(Figure 20.5)** using energy released from ATP hydrolysis.

- It migrates until it reaches at **CA rich rho-utilization termination sequences (rut sequences)** on a template strand, where helicase activity of rho factor separates the RNA from DNA
- Rho (ρ)—Protein has two catalytic activities; ATPase and Helicase

Rho-independent Termination

- **Rho-independent termination** depends on specific sequences in the DNA template strand **at terminus region**, which are rich in **C and G** nucleotides.
- RNA transcribed from this region folds back on itself, and complementary C and G nucleotides pairs together to form a hairpin structure with a **stem and loop (Figure 20.6)**.
- Hairpin is followed by a sequence of four or more **uracil residues** near the **3′ end of hairpin**. RNA transcript ends within or just after them.
- RNA-DNA hybrid helix produced after hairpin, is unstable and dissociates from DNA template.

Prokaryotic Post-transcriptional Modification

- A newly synthesized RNA molecule is called **primary transcript** (pre-RNA). Primary transcript normally

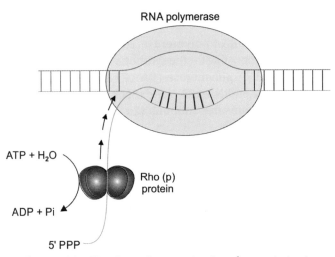

Figure 20.5: Rho-dependent termination of transcription in prokaryotes.

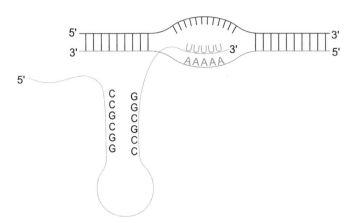

Figure 20.6: Rho-independent termination of transcription.

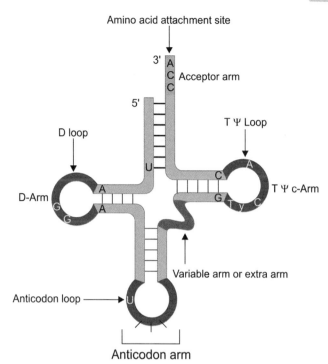

Figure 20.7: Post-transcriptional modification by addition of nucleotides and unusual bases in tRNA.

undergoes further enzymatic alteration, called **post-transcriptional modifications** to form mature functional RNAs.

- Post-transcriptional modifications give characteristics, which are needed to be functional in the cytoplasm. Post-transcriptional RNA processing is not as extensive in prokaryotes as in eukaryotes.
- In prokaryotes, **mRNA** is not post-transcriptionally processed. Prokaryotic mRNA is functional immediately upon synthesis. Indeed, its translation often begins before completion of transcript. In contrast tRNA and rRNA molecules are cleaved and chemically modified after transcription.
- Post-transcriptional modification may involve either:
  1. Cleavage of large precursor of RNA
  2. Terminal addition of nucleotides
  3. Nucleoside modification.
- Excess sequences from primary tRNA and rRNA molecules are removed by the action of **endonucleases** or **exonucleases** to smaller molecules.
- A second type of modification is the **addition of nucleotides** to the terminal of tRNA. For example, **CCA, a terminal sequence** of **acceptor arm** of tRNA required for its function is added to the 3′ ends of tRNA molecules **(Figure 20.7)**.
- A third type of processing is the modification of bases and ribose units. For example **(Figure 20.8)**:
  - Some bases of rRNA are methylated
  - Unusual bases are incorporated in tRNAs, e.g. uridylate residues are modified after transcription to form ribothymidylate and pseudouridylate. The TψC arm of tRNA contains both ribothymidine (T) and pseudouridine (ψ).

Inhibitors of Prokaryotic Transcription and their Clinical Significance

Some antibiotics prevent bacterial cell growth by inhibiting RNA synthesis. Those that inhibit RNA synthesis in

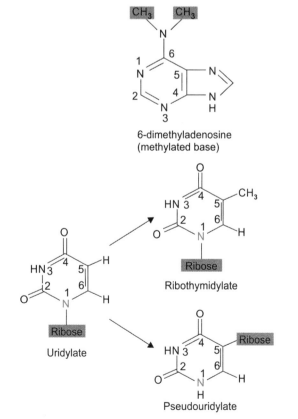

Figure 20.8: RNA processing by nucleoside modification.

prokaryotes but not in eukaryotes, serve as therapeutic drugs (antibiotics), for example,

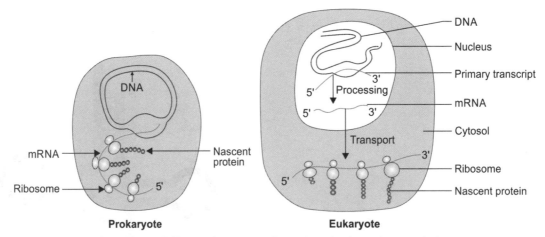

Figure 20.9: Difference between prokaryotic and eukaryotic transcription.

- **Rifampin:** It is an antituberculosis drug, which inhibits the initiation of transcription by binding β-subunit of prokaryotic RNA polymerase. Rifampin has no effect on eukaryotic nuclear RNA polymerases.
- **Dactinomycin (actinomycin D):** Dactinomycin is a therapeutic agent in the treatment of some cancer. It binds tightly and specifically to double helical DNA and thereby prevents it from being an effective template for RNA synthesis. At low concentrations, dactinomycin inhibits transcription without affecting DNA replication or translation. Its ability to inhibit the growth of rapidly dividing cells makes it an effective therapeutic agent in the treatment of cancers.
- **α-Amanitin:** α-amanitin, a compound derived from the poisonous mushroom disrupts mRNA formation in eukaryotic cells by, inhibiting RNA polymerase II and at higher concentration, RNA polymerase III. Neither RNA polymerase I nor bacterial RNA polymerase is sensitive to α-amanitin.

DIFFERENCE BETWEEN PROKARYOTIC AND EUKARYOTIC TRANSCRIPTION

1. In prokaryotes, transcription, and translation occur within the same cellular compartment. In fact, translation of bacterial mRNA begins during transcription. In eukaryotic cells, transcription, and translation occur in different cellular compartments. Transcription occurs within the nucleus and translation outside the nucleus **(Figure 20.9)**. Hence, translation can occur only after transcription has finished.
2. Another difference between prokaryotic and eukaryotic transcription is that prokaryotes translate primary transcript of mRNA without undergoing processing whereas eukaryotes extensively process mRNA primary transcripts prior to translation (discussed later).
3. In eukaryotic cells, promoter sites generally have the base sequence TATAAA centered at base –25 and CAAT

TABLE 20.1: Eukaryotic RNA polymerase.

Type of RNA polymerase	Type of RNA formed	Location
RNA polymerase I	18 S, 5.8 S, and 28 S rRNA	Nucleolus
RNA polymerase II	mRNA precursor and snRNA	Nucleoplasm
RNA polymerase III	tRNA and 5S rRNA	Nucleoplasm

centered at –75. In prokaryotic cells, promoter sites generally have the base sequence TATAAT (Pribnow box) centered at –10 and –35 region with base sequences of TTGACA (*see* **Figure 20.2**).

4. In prokaryotes, RNAs are synthesized by a single kind of polymerase. In contrast, the nucleus of a eukaryote contains three types of RNA polymerase **(Table 20.1)**.

EUKARYOTIC TRANSCRIPTION, AND POST-TRANSCRIPTIONAL MODIFICATIONS

Transcription of eukaryotic gene is a far more complicated process than transcription in prokaryotes.
- Eukaryotic transcription involves separate polymerase for the synthesis of rRNA, tRNA, and mRNA.
- Each polymerase recognizes a different type of promoter.
- In eukaryotes RNA polymerase (RNAP) does not include a removable sigma (σ) factor instead, a number of accessory proteins (transcription factors) identify promoters and recruit RNAP to the transcription start site.

Basic Requirements

- **Template:** A single-strand of DNA acts as a template to direct the formation of complementary RNA transcript. The strand that is transcribed to RNA molecule is referred to as the **template strand** of the DNA. The other DNA strand is referred to as the **coding strand** of the gene.
- **Substrate:** The four ribonucleoside triphosphates: ATP, GTP, CTP, UTP

TABLE 20.2: Proteins required for initiation of transcription of the RNAP-II promoters of eukaryotes.

Transcription protein	Functions
Initiation factors	
RNAP-II	Catalyzes RNA synthesis
TBP	Recognizes the TATA box
TFIIA	Stabilizes binding of TFIIB and TBP to the promoter
TFIIB	Binds to TBP, recruits RNAPII - TFIIF complex
TFIIE	Recruits TFIIH, has ATPase, and helicase activities
TFIIF	Binds tightly to RNAP-II, TFIIB and prevents binding of RNAP-II to nonspecific DNA sequences
TFIIH	Unwinds DNA at promoter (helicase activity) phosphorylates RNAP-II (within the CTD), recruits nucleotide excision repair proteins
Elongation factors	
• ELL • pTEFb • SII (TFIIS) • Elongin (SIII)	Phosphorylates RNAP-II (within CTD)

(RNAP-II: RNA polymerase-II; TF: transcription factor; TBP: TATA binding protein; CTD: carboxy terminal domain; ELL: eleven-nineteen lysine-rich leukemia)

- **Enzyme:** Eukaryotes have three RNA polymerases (RNAPs), which transcribe different types of genes **(Table 20.1)**. These are designated as **I, II**, and **III**. Each polymerase has a specific function. Each polymerase has a specific promoter sequences.
  1. RNA polymerase I transcribes rRNA genes,
  2. RNA polymerase II transcribes mRNA, miRNA, and snRNA. RNA polymerase II has an unusual feature, that, it consists of carboxy-terminal tail or **carboxy-terminal domain (CTD)**. The CTD has many important roles in polymerase II function, as discussed next.
  3. RNA polymerase III transcribes tRNA and 5S rRNA genes.
- **Proteins:** Proteins required for initiation of transcription are given in **Table 20.2**.

Eukaryotic Promoters

Promoter sequences of DNA are different in **prokaryotes** and **eukaryotes**. Eukaryotic promoters are complex, being composed of several different elements.

- Eukaryotic promoters placed upstream of the gene and can have regulatory elements several bases away from the transcriptional start site.
- In eukaryotic cells, promoter sites generally have the base sequence
  - TATAAA (TATA box) centered at base –25 to –30 and
  - CAAT centered at –75.
- The TATA box typically placed very close to the transcriptional start site. The **site** on the DNA from which

the first RNA nucleotide is **transcribed** is called the **+1 site**, or the initiation **site**.

Stages of Eukaryotic Transcription

Eukaryotic transcription is carried out in the nucleus of the cell by one of three RNA polymerases (RNAPs), depending on the RNA being transcribed, and proceeds in three sequential stages:
1. Initiation
2. Elongation
3. Termination.

Initiation of Transcription in Eukaryotes

- Initiation of transcription involves the binding of **RNA polymerase** to template at **promoter site**.
- **Promoter site** guides RNA polymerase to initiate transcription at a particular point known as **start point** or **initiation site**.
- RNA polymerase II (RNAP-II) is a principal enzyme to eukaryotic gene expression. For the binding of RNA polymerase to DNA template eukaryotes require many other proteins called **transcription factors (TFII)**.
- The transcription factors required for initiation of transcription are:
  - TFIIA
  - TFIIB
  - TFIIE
  - TFIIF
  - TFIIH.

Formation of Pre-initiation Complex

- First TATA binding protein, TBP associated with TFIID bind to a promoter site (TATA box).
- After binding of **TFIID-TBP** to the TATA box, five more transcription factors, **TFIIA, TFIIB, TFIIE, TFIIF,** and **TFIIH (Table 20.2)** and **RNA polymerase** link around the TATA box to form a **closed pre-initiation complex (Figure 20.10)**
- **TFIIH** has a DNA **helicase activity** that promotes the unwinding of DNA near the RNA start site or **initiator (Inr)**.
- **Opening of initiating complex** occur due to unwinding which facilitates access of RNAP to DNA template.
- TFIIH has an additional function during the initiation phase. A **kinase** activity of TFIIH **phosphorylates** the **carboxyl terminal domain (CTD)** of polymerase II at many places. Several other protein kinases also phosphorylate the CTD.
- This causes a **conformational change** in the overall complex, and the polymerase then escapes the promoter and starts transcribing RNA. Phosphorylation of CTD is also important during the subsequent elongation phase.

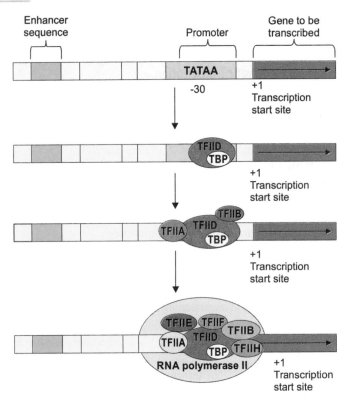

Figure 20.10: Formation of closed pre-initiation complex during eukaryotic transcription.

- After synthesis of initial 60 to 70 nucleotides of RNA, first TFIIE is released, and then TFIIH and polymerase II enter the **elongation phase of transcription**.

Elongation

- Elongation is accompanied by the release of many transcription factors.
- **TFIIF** remains associated with polymerase II throughout elongation.
- During elongation, activity of polymerase is greatly enhanced by proteins called **elongation factors**.
- Other proteins known as **activators** and **repressors** are responsible for modulating transcription rate. Activator proteins increase the transcription rate, and repressor proteins decrease the transcription rate.
- Elongation continued 5′ to 3′ direction with addition of ribonucleotide of ATP, GTP, CTP, UTP complementary to template DNA strand until **termination sequences** occur.

Termination

- The termination of transcription is different for the three different eukaryotic RNA polymerases **(Figure 20.11)**. The mechanism of termination is the least understood of the three transcription stages. RNA polymerases I and III require **termination signals**.
  - The ribosomal rRNA genes (transcribed by **RNA polymerase I**) contain a specific sequence of base

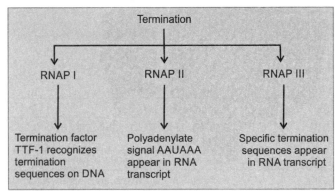

Figure 20.11: Termination of transcription for the three different eukaryotic RNA polymerases.

pairs **in DNA template** that is recognized by a termination protein called TTF-1 (Transcription Termination Factor for RNA polymerase I). This protein binds the DNA at its recognition sequence and blocks further transcription, causing the RNA polymerase I to disengage from the template DNA strand and to release its newly-synthesized RNA.

- Genes transcribed by RNA polymerase III terminate transcription in response to specific termination sequences in **the newly-synthesized RNA** which is similar to rho-independent termination of transcription in prokaryotes (formation of hairpin structure).
- RNA polymerase II lack any specific signals or sequences that direct RNA polymerase II to terminate at specific locations. RNA polymerase II terminates transcription when a **polyadenylation signal**, **AAUAAA** appears in the RNA transcript.

- RNA, thus formed is the precursor forms known as **primary transcript**. Primary transcripts undergo post-transcriptional modifications to form mature functional RNAs namely rRNA, mRNA, tRNA.

❖ When RNAP II transcription halts at site of a DNA lesion, TFIIH can interact with the lesion and recruit the entire nucleotide excision repair complex.

❖ Genetic loss of certain TFIIH subunits can produce human diseases, e.g., xeroderma pigmentosum and Cockayne syndrome, which is characterized by arrested growth, photosensitivity, and neurological disorders.

Eukaryotic Post-transcriptional RNA Processing

Virtually all RNA molecules in eukaryotes are processed to some degree after synthesis. Processing gives them the characteristics they need to be functional in the cytoplasm. A newly synthesized RNA molecule is called **primary transcript (pre-RNA)**. The most extensive processing of primary transcripts occurs in eukaryotic mRNAs and in the tRNAs of both bacteria and eukaryotes. The particular processing steps and the factors taking part vary according to the type of RNA polymerase.

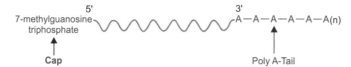

Figure 20.12: Post-transcriptional modification of a primary transcript (hnRNA). Addition of cap at near 5′ ends and a poly (A) tail at their 3′ ends.

mRNA Processing

Mature, functional mRNA is formed from extensive processing of a large precursor called **hnRNA** (heterogeneous nuclear RNA) transcript, product of RNA polymerase-II. The hnRNA (primary transcript) is extensively modified after transcription. For example:

- Primary transcripts acquire a **cap** at near 5′ ends and a **poly (A) tail** at their 3′ ends **(Figure 20.12)**
- Nearly all mRNA precursors in higher eukaryotes are **spliced** to remove **introns**.

Addition of Cap at 5′ Ends of mRNA

Capping of the primary transcript (hnRNA) is the first processing reaction. It occurs very early in transcription, after the first 20 to 30 nucleotides of transcript have been added.

- The 5′ end of eukaryotic mRNA consists of cap of **7-methylguanylate**.
  - A 7-methylguanylate cap is attached to the 5′ terminal residue of the mRNA. The addition of the guanosine triphosphate (GTP) part of the cap is catalyzed by the nuclear enzyme **guanylyl transferase**.
  - The N-7 nitrogen of the **guanine** is then methylated in the cytosol by the enzyme **guanine-7-methyltransferase**. S-adenosylmethionine is the source of the methyl group.
- Cap helps stabilize mRNAs by protecting their 5′ ends from phosphatases and ribonucleases that degrade RNAs from their 5′ end. The caps also enhance the translation of mRNA by binding of the mature mRNA to the ribosome during protein biosynthesis. Eukaryotic mRNAs lacking the cap are not translated efficiently.

> The virus needs no specialized enzymes for the synthesis of 5′ caps; instead, it borrows these structures from host-cell transcript in a process termed "cap snatching".

Addition of Poly-A Tail

- The 3′ end of most eukaryotic mRNAs is polynucleated (poly A) and called a **"tail"**. Poly A tail has a chain of 200 to 300 adenylate residues linked with phosphodiester bonds. ATP is the donor of adenylate residue. Poly A tail is not transcribed by DNA but rather is added after transcription has ended.

- Poly A tail enhances translation efficiency and involved in stabilization of mRNA. The mRNA molecule devoid of a poly-A tail is less effective template for protein synthesis than is one with poly A tail. In cytoplasm poly-A tails are slowly shortened. When the poly-A tail is completely removed, the mRNA is rapidly degraded.

Splicing of mRNA

- Most genes in higher eukaryotes are composed of **exons** and **introns**. Exons are the **coding sequence** of the gene. Introns are the **noncoding sequence** of the gene. The introns are the intervening sequences between exons.
- Introns in DNA are transcribed along with the rest of the codons of the gene by RNA polymerase. Different genes have different numbers of introns.
- The process by which introns are removed from primary transcript and exons are joined to form the mature functional mRNA is called **splicing**.
- In a RNA splicing, the introns (noncoding region) are removed from the primary transcript, and the exons (coding region) are joined to form a matured mRNA with continuous exon sequences that lay down a functional polypeptide. Some mature mRNAs are only a tenth the size of their precursors.
- This splicing must be very accurate, and very sensitive, one nucleotide slippage in a splice point would shift the reading frame and give an entirely different amino acid sequence. 15% of all genetic diseases due to mutations are due to splicing defects. Abnormal splicing causes some forms of **thalassemia**.
- Most human primary transcript (hnRNA) with multiple exons is sometimes spliced in **alternative ways** to yield different mRNAs and different proteins are called **alternative splicing**.
- Different combinations of exons from the same gene may be spliced into different mRNA, **(Figure 20.13)**, producing distinct forms of a protein for specific tissues, developmental stages, or signaling pathways.
  - Alternative splicing provides a mechanism for expanding the utility of genomic sequence through combinational control. In human beings the very different hormones are produced form a single pre-mRNA.

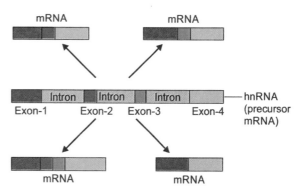

Figure 20.13: Alternative splicing.

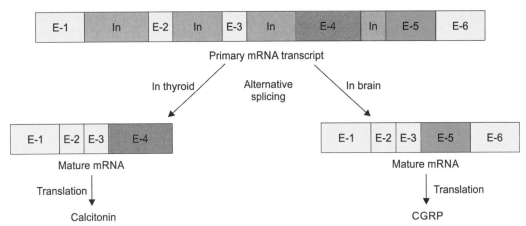

Figure 20.14: Alternative splicing of the gene encoding both calcitonin and CGRP.
(E: exon; In = intron; CGRP: calcitonin-gene-related peptide)

TABLE 20.3: Human diseases due to defects in alternative splicing.

Disorder	Affected gene or its product
Acute intermittent porphyria	Porphobilinogen deaminase
Breast and ovarian cancer	BRCA1
Cystic fibrosis	CFTR
Hemophilia A	Factor III
Lesch-Nyhan syndrome	HGPRTase
Severe combined immunodeficiency	Adenosine deaminase
Spinal muscle atrophy	SMN1 or SMN2

- For example; alternative splicing produces the gene encoding both **calcitonin** and **a neuropeptide**, **calcitonin-gene-related peptide (CGRP) (Figure 20.14)**, depending on the cell type in which the gene is expressed.
- In the thyroid gland, the **inclusion of exon 4** in one splicing pathway produces **calcitonin**; a peptide hormone that regulates calcium and phosphorus metabolism.
- In neuronal cells the **exclusion of exon 4** in another splicing pathway produces CGRP, a peptide hormone that acts as a vasodilator. In this case, only two proteins result from alternative splicing, however, in other cases, many more can be produced.
- Several human diseases that can be recognized to defects in alternative splicing are listed in **Table 20.3**.

tRNA Processing

Transfer RNA precursors are converted into mature tRNAs by following alterations **(Figure 20.15)**.

1. Cleavage of a 5′ leader sequence
2. Replacement of the 3′ terminal UU by CCA
3. Modification of several bases and sugars
4. Splicing to remove intron.

- Like those of prokaryotic tRNAs, the 5′ leader is cleaved by the endonuclease **RNase P**. RNase P is an example

of **ribozyme** as this enzyme contains both protein and RNA.

- The **3′ end of** primary transcript is processed by exonuclease, **RNase D**. CCA is then added to the 3′ end by **tRNA nucleotidyltransferase**.
- Eukaryotic tRNAs are also heavily modified on **base** and **ribose moieties**, by methylation, deamination or reduction. Unusual bases are incorporated in tRNAs, e.g., uridylate residues are modified after transcription to form **ribothymidine** and **pseudouridine**.
- In eukaryotes, introns are present in a few tRNA transcripts and must be excised by **splicing**, in which **introns** are removed by endonuclease. Introns are found in some eukaryotic tRNAs but not in prokaryotic tRNAs **(Figure 20.15)**.

rRNA Processing

Eukaryotic ribosomal RNA processing is very similar to that of prokaryotes.

- **RNA polymerase-I** transcription produces a single precursor that encodes three RNA components of the ribosome; **18S rRNA**, **28S rRNA**, and **5.8S rRNA** **(Figure 20.16)**.
- Cleavage of single precursor into three separate rRNAs; 18S rRNA, 28S rRNA, and 5.8S rRNA occur after transcription.
  - 18S rRNA is the RNA component of small ribosomal subunit (40S)
  - 28S and 5.8S rRNAs are two RNA components of large ribosomal subunits (60S).

RNA Editing

- A change in the base sequence of RNA after transcription by process other than RNA splicing is called **RNA editing**.
- Alteration of base sequence of RNA in RNA editing occurs in the cell nucleus before translation.

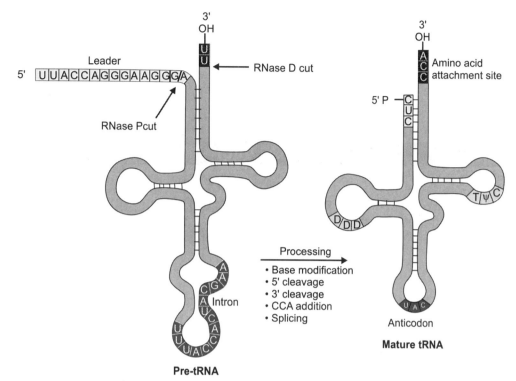

Figure 20.15: Processing of tRNA precursor to mature tRNA.

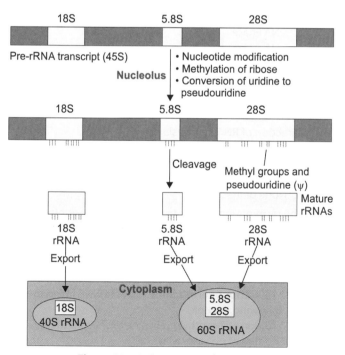

Figure 20.16: Processing of pre-rRNA transcript in eukaryotes.

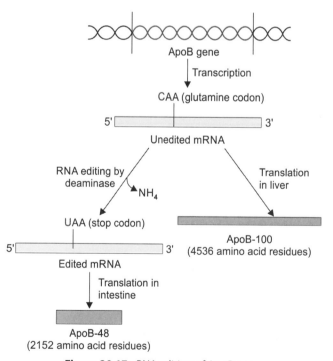

Figure 20.17: RNA editing of ApoB gene.

- The process may involve the **insertion**, **deletion**, or **substitution** of nucleotides in the RNA molecule.
- The substitution of one nucleotide for another has been observed in humans and can result in tissue specific differences in transcript, e.g., gene of apolipoprotein B, ApoB gene **(Figure 20.17)**.

- Apolipoprotein B exists in two forms:
  - ApoB-100 (4536 amino acid residues) in liver
  - ApoB-48 (2152 amino acid residues) in intestine
- ApoB gene encodes mRNA transcript in the liver which is translated into a protein called **apoB-100** with 4536 amino acid residue.

- However, in the small intestine, the same gene encodes mRNA of half the size which translated into a protein called **apoB-48** with 2152 amino acid residue.
- This happens because; in the small intestine a **cytidine** residue of mRNA is deaminated to **uridine** which changes the codon at residue 2153 from CAA (glutamine) to UAA (stop colon). The deaminase that catalyzes this reaction is present in the small intestine but not in the liver, and is expressed only at certain developmental stages.

ASSESSMENT QUESTIONS

STRUCTURED LONG ESSAY QUESTIONS (SLEQs)

1. Describe transcription mechanism in eukaryotes under the following headings:
   i. Initiation
   ii. Elongation
   iii. Termination
2. Describe transcription mechanism in prokaryotes under the following headings:
   i. Initiation
   ii. Elongation
   iii. Termination
   iv. Name inhibitors of the process
3. Describe post-transcription mechanism in eukaryotes under the following headings:
   i. mRNA processing
   ii. tRNA processing
   iii. rRNA processing

SHORT ESSAY QUESTIONS (SEQs)

1. Name the inhibitors of RNA synthesis in prokaryotes with their clinical significance.
2. Write differences between prokaryotic and eukaryotic transcription.
3. Write prokaryotic post-transcriptional RNA processing.
4. What is RNA editing? Give example.

SHORT ANSWER QUESTIONS (SAQs)

1. What is the role of RNA polymerase? Write component of prokaryotes RNA polymerase.
2. What is transcription? Name the stages of transcription.
3. Write inhibitors of prokaryotes RNA synthesis.
4. Write promoter sequences in prokaryotes and eukaryotes.
5. Write similarity and differentiation between replication and transcription.
6. Write any four factors required for initiation of transcription with their function.
7. Name any four human diseases due to defect in alternative slicing.

MULTIPLE CHOICE QUESTIONS (MCQs)

1. **A promoter site on DNA:**
   a. Transcribes repressor
   b. Codes for RNA polymerase
   c. Initiates transcription
   d. Regulates termination
2. **Which of the following true for the process of RNA synthesis?**
   a. Occurs in the 3′ to 5′ direction
   b. Require primer
   c. Does not require primer
   d. Initiated at special DNA sequences known start condos
3. **In conversion of DNA to RNA, enzyme required:**
   a. DNA-polymerase I
   b. DNA ligase
   c. DNA-polymerase III
   d. RNA polymerase
4. **Synthesis of RNA from DNA template is known as:**
   a. Replication
   b. Translation
   c. Transcription
   d. Mutation
5. **Direction of RNA synthesis is:**
   a. 5′ → 3′
   b. 3′ → 5′
   c. Both (a) and (b)
   d. None of these
6. **The termination site for transcription is recognized by:**
   a. α-subunit of DNA-dependent RNA polymerase
   b. β-subunit of DNA-dependent RNA polymerase
   c. Sigma factor
   d. Rho factor
7. **Post-transcriptional modification of hnRNA involves all of the following, *except*:**
   a. Addition of 7-methylguanosine triphosphate cap
   b. Addition of polyadenylate tail
   c. Insertion of nucleotides
   d. Deletion of introns
8. **Newly synthesized tRNA undergoes post-transcriptional modifications which include all the following, *except*:**
   a. Reduction in size
   b. Methylation of some bases
   c. Formation of pseudouridine
   d. Addition of C-C-A terminus at 5′ end

9. Post-transcriptional modification does not occur in:
   a. Eukaryotic tRNA   b. Prokaryotic tRNA
   c. Eukaryotic hnRNA   d. Prokaryotic mRNA

10. A consensus sequence on DNA, called TATA box, is the site for attachment of:
    a. RNA-dependent DNA polymerase
    b. DNA-dependent RNA polymerase
    c. DNA-dependent DNA polymerase
    d. DNA topoisomerase II

11. Introns in genes:
    a. Encode the amino acids which are removed during post-translational modification
    b. Encode signal sequences which are removed before secretion of the proteins
    c. Are the noncoding sequences which are not translated?
    d. Are the sequences that occur between two genes?

12. All of the following statements about post-transcriptional processing of tRNA are true, *except*:
    a. Introns of some tRNA precursors are removed
    b. CCA is added at 3′ end
    c. 7-methylguanosine triphosphate cap is added at 5′ end
    d. Some bases are methylated

13. Noncoding sequences in a gene are known as:
    a. Cistron   b. Nonsense codons
    c. Introns   d. Exons

14. Pribnow box is present in:
    a. Prokaryotic promoters
    b. Eukaryotic promoters
    c. Both (a) and (b)
    d. None of these

15. Hogness box is present in:
    a. Prokaryotic promoters
    b. Eukaryotic promoters
    c. Both (a) and (b)
    d. None of these

16. CAAT box is present in:
    a. Prokaryotic promoters 10 BP upstream of transcription start site
    b. Prokaryotic promoters 35 BP upstream of transcription start site
    c. Eukaryotic promoters 25 BP upstream of transcription start site
    d. Eukaryotic promoters 70–80 BP upstream of transcription start site

17. Eukaryotic promoters contain.
    a. TATA box 25 BP upstream of transcription start site
    b. CAAT box 70–80 BP upstream of transcription start site
    c. Both (a) and (b)
    d. None of these

18. Transcription is the formation of:
    a. DNA from a parent DNA
    b. RNA from a parent RNA
    c. RNA from DNA
    d. Protein from mRNA

19. Sigma and Rho factors are required for:
    a. Replication   b. Transcription
    c. Translation   d. Polymerization

20. RNA synthesis requires.
    a. RNA primer   b. RNA template
    c. DNA template   d. DNA primer

21. The site to which RNA polymerase binds on the DNA template prior to the initiation of transcription.
    a. Intron/exon junction
    b. Promoter
    c. Terminator
    d. Initiator methionine codon

22. The DNA segment from which the primary transcript is copied or transcribed is called.
    a. Coding region
    b. Initial codon
    c. Translation unit
    d. Transcriptome

23. What sequence feature of mature mRNAs listed below is thought to protect mRNAs from degradation?
    a. Special post-translational modifications
    b. 3′ poly (A)$_n$ tail
    c. 5′ methyl guanosine triphosphate cap
    d. Introns

24. The sigma subunit of prokaryotic RNA polymerase:
    a. Binds the antibiotic rifampicin
    b. Is inhibited by α-amanitin
    c. Specifically recognizes the promoter site
    d. Is part of the core enzyme

25. RNA polymerase does not require:
    a. Template (ds DNA)
    b. Activated precursors (ATP, GTP, UTP, CTP)
    c. Primer
    d. None

26. R-RNA is mainly produced in
    a. Nucleus   b. Nucleolus
    c. Ribosome   d. Endoplasmic

27. Replication and transcription are similar process in mechanistic terms because both:
    a. Use RNA primers for initiation.
    b. Use deoxyribonucleotides as precursors.
    c. Are semi conserved events
    d. Involved phosphodiester bond formation with elongation occurring in the 5′-3′ direction.

28. A segment of a eukaryotic gene that is not represented in the mature messenger RNA is known as:
    a. Intron
    b. Exon
    c. Plasmid
    d. TATA box

29. Micro RNA transcribed by:
    a. RNA polymerase I
    b. RNA polymerase II
    c. DNA polymerase
    d. None of these

30. **Normal role of micro RNA is:**
    a. Gene regulation
    b. RNA splicing
    c. Initiation of translation
    d. DNA conformational change

31. **Alternative splicing involves the removal of introns from pre-mRNA to form mRNA. When does this type of modification occur?**
    a. Before transcription
    b. After transcription
    c. During transcription
    d. During translation

32. **What is added to the 3'-end of many eukaryotic mRNAs after transcription?**
    a. Introns
    b. A poly A tail
    c. The trinucleotide 5'-CCA
    d. Exons

33. **Which of the following is not involved in the post-transcriptional processing of t-RNA?**
    a. Base modulation
    b. Attachment of CCA arm
    c. Splicing
    d. Attachment of poly-A tail

34. **Which post-transcriptional modification serves to identify the eukaryotic translation start site?**
    a. Poly(A) tail
    b. 5' cap consisting of 7-methylguanosine
    c. Intron excision
    d. Alternative splicing

◼ ANSWERS FOR MCQs

1. c	2. c	3. d	4. c	5. a
6. d	7. c	8. d	9. d	10. b
11. c	12. c	13. c	14. a	15. b
16. d	17. c	18. c	19. b	20. c
21. b	22. a	23. c	24. c	25. c
26. b	27. d	28. a	29. b	30. a
31. b	32. b	33. d	34. b	

21 CHAPTER

Genetic Code and Translation

Competency	Learning Objectives
BI 7.2: Describe the processes involved in replication and repair of DNA and the transcription and translation mechanisms. **BI 9.3:** Describe protein targeting and sorting along with its associated disorders.	1. Describe genetic code and its characteristics. 2. Describe wobble hypothesis for codon-anticodon interactions. 3. Describe eukaryotic translation, folding and processing of proteins. 4. Describe post-translational modifications. 5. Describe inhibitors of translation and their clinical importance in medicine. 6. Describe protein targeting and sorting.

OVERVIEW

Information encoded in DNA, is transcribed into RNA and then translated into protein. This path of information from DNA to ribonucleic acids RNA to protein guides the functioning of every living cell. This flow of genetic information from DNA to RNA to protein in living cells, is called the **central dogma of molecular biology (Figure 21.1)**

The chapter begins with the discussion of the genetic code then protein synthesis.

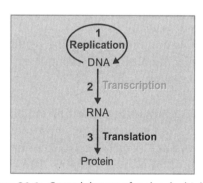

Figure 21.1: Central dogma of molecular biology.

GENETIC CODE AND ITS CHARACTERISTICS

- Information needed to direct the **synthesis of protein** is contained in **mRNA** in the form of a **genetic code. Genetic code** is the specific **sequence of nucleotides** of **mRNA** which specify particular sequence of **amino acids**.
- **Codons** are a group of **three adjacent nucleotides of mRNA** that specify amino acids of protein. Dictionary of amino acid codon in mRNA is given in **Figure 21.2**.

Characteristic Features of the Genetic Code

1. **Number of codons:** There are **64** possible codon sequences, because four nucleotide bases A, G, C and U are used to produce the three base codons, there

are therefore 4^3 or 64 (different combination of bases) possible codon sequences **(Figure 21.2)**.
2. **The code has directionality**. The code is read from the 5' end of the messenger RNA to its 3' end.
3. **Stop or termination or nonsense codons:** Three of the 64 possible nucleotide triplets (codons), **UAA, UAG** and **UGA** do not code for any amino acids, they are called **stop codons** or **nonsense codons** that normally signal termination of polypeptide chains. These **nonsense** codons are arbitrarily named **amber, ochre** and **opal**.
4. **Initiation codon:** The initiation codon AUG is the most common signal for the beginning of a polypeptide synthesis in all cells, in addition to coding for methionine residues in internal positions of polypeptides.

Second letter of codon

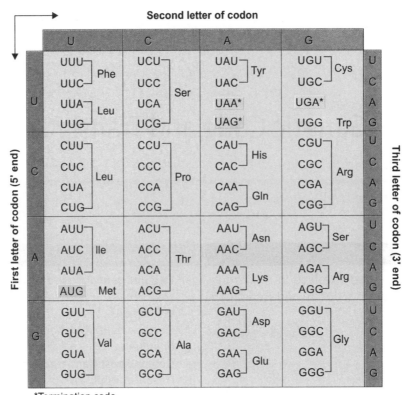

*Termination code

Figure 21.2: Dictionary of amino acid codon in mRNAs.

5. **The code is unambiguous:** For any specific codon, only a single amino acid is specified; with rare exceptions, the genetic code is unambiguous.

6. **The code is nonoverlapping:** The reading of genetic code during the process of protein synthesis does not involve any overlap of codons. Thus, the genetic code is nonoverlapping

7. **The code is without punctuation mark:** During translation, once the reading is started at a specific start codon the code is read sequentially without spacer base. The message is read in a continuing sequence of nucleotide triplets, (taken 3 at a time) until a translation stop codon is reached. For example, A U G C U A G A C U UU is read as AUG/CUA/GAC/UUU without "punctuation" between the codons.

8. **The genetic code is degenerate (multiplicity/variety):** As there are 61 codons for 20 amino acids, one amino acid has more than one codon and so the code is referred to as **degenerate** (multiplicity/diversity). This does not suggest that the code is damaged. Although, an amino acid may have more than one codon, each codon specifies only one amino acid. Codons that designate the same amino acid are called *synonyms*. The degeneracy of the code is not uniform. For example, two amino acids methionine (AUG) and tryptophan (UGG) have single codon, whereas three amino acids, arginine, leucine, and serine have six codons **(Table 21.1)**. *Degeneracy minimizes the deleterious effects of mutations.*

TABLE 21.1: Degeneracy of the genetic code.

Amino acids	Number of codons	Amino acids	Number of codons
Met	1	Tyr	2
Trp	1	Ile	3
Asn	2	Ala	4
Asp	2	Gly	4
Cys	2	Pro	4
Gln	2	Thr	4
Glu	2	Val	4
His	2	Arg	6
Lys	2	Leu	6
Phe	2	Ser	6

9. **Codon bias:** When several codons encode the same amino acid and use multiple tRNAs, not all of the codons are used with equal frequency. In a phenomenon called **codon bias**, some codons for a particular amino acid are used more frequently than others.

10. **The genetic code is almost universal:** Amino acid codons are identical in all species examined so far. This suggests that all life-forms have a common evolutionary ancestor, whose genetic code has been preserved throughout biological evolution. Exceptions to the universality of the genetic code are found in human mitochondria, where the code:

- UGA codes for tryptophan instead of serving as a stop codon
- AUA codes for methionine instead of isoleucine
- CUA codes for threonine instead of leucine.

WOBBLE HYPOTHESIS FOR CODON-ANTICODON INTERACTIONS

When several different codons specify one amino acid, the difference between them usually lies at the third base position (at the 3′ end). For example, alanine is coded by the triplets GCU, GCC, GCA and GCG. Thus, most synonyms differ only in the last base of the triplet.

Analysis of the code shows that XYC and XYU always encode the same amino acid, and XYG and XYA usually encode the same amino acid as well. For most amino acids, the first two bases of each codon are the primary determinants of specificity.

- A three base sequence on the tRNA called the **anticodon** base pair with **codons** on the mRNA.
- The first base of the codon in mRNA (read in the 5′ to 3′ direction) pairs with the third base of the anticodon **(Figure 21.3)**.
- If the anticodon triplet of a tRNA recognized only one codon triplet through Watson-Crick base pairing at all three positions, cells would have a different tRNA for each amino acid codon.
- This is not the case, however because the anticodons in some tRNAs include the nucleotide inosinate (designated 'I') which contains the uncommon base **hypoxanthine**. Inosine can form hydrogen bonds with three different nucleotides, U, C, and A **(Figure 21.4)**, although these pairings are much weaker than the hydrogen bonds of Watson-Crick base pairs G ≡ C and A = U.

	3 2 1	3 2 1	3 2 1
Anticodon (3′)	G—C—I	G—C—I	G—C—I (5′)
	≡ ≡ ≡	≡ ≡ ≡	≡ ≡ ≡
Codon (5′)	C—G—A	C—G—U	C—G—C (3′)
	1 2 3	1 2 3	1 2 3

Figure 21.4: Three different codon paring of arginine is possible when the tRNA anticodon contains inosine (I).

- For example, the anticodon (5′) ICG of yeast tRNA for arginine recognizes three arginine codons (5′) CGA, (5′) CGU, and (5′) CGC **(Figure 21.4)**. The first two bases of these codons are the same (CG) and form strong Watson-Crick base pairs with the correspond bases of the anticodon, but the third base (A, U or C) forms rather weak hydrogen bonds with the I residue at the first position of the anticodon.

Examination of these and other codon-anticodon pairing led Crick conclude that the third base of most codons pairs rather loosely with the corresponding base of its anticodon, the third base of such codons (and the first base of their corresponding anticodons) "wobbles". Crick proposed an assumption to explain these data on the basis of set of four relationships called the **"wobble hypothesis"**.

1. The first two bases of an mRNA codon always form strong Watson-Crick base pairs with the corresponding bases of the tRNA anticodon and confer most of the coding specificity.
2. The first base of the anticodon (reading in the 5′ to 3′ direction; this pairs with the third base of the codon) determines the number of codons recognized by the tRNA:
   - When the first base of the anticodon is C or A, base pairing is specific and only one codon is recognized by the tRNA.
   - When the first base is U or G, binding is less specific and two different codons may be read.
   - When inosine (I) is the first (wobble) nucleotide of an anticodon, three different codons can be recognized.
3. When an amino acid is specified by several different codons, the codons that differ in either of the first two bases require different tRNAs.
4. A minimum of 32 tRNAs are required to translate all 61 codons (31 to encode the amino acids and 1 for initiation).

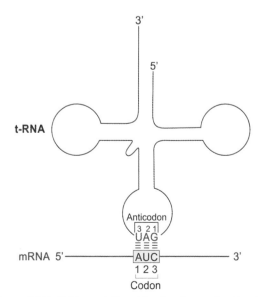

Figure 21.3: Pairing relationship of codon and anticodon.

Importance of wobble hypothesis
❖ The wobble (or third) base of codon pairs only loosely with its corresponding base in anticodon, it permits rapid dissociation of the tRNA from its codon during protein biosynthesis.
❖ If all three bases of a codon engaged in strong Watson-Crick pairing with the three bases of the anticodon, tRNAs would dissociate too slowly and this would limit the rate of protein synthesis.

Table 21.2: Differences between eukaryotic and prokaryotic protein synthesis.

Characters	Eukaryotes	Prokaryotes
Ribosome	Larger, 80S, consists of 60S and 40S subunits	Smaller, 70S, consists of 50S and 30S subunits
Initiator tRNA	Met-tRNA^{Met}	f-met-tRNA^{fmet}
Start signal	Initiating AUG closest to the 5' end of an mRNA is preceded by a cap contains methylguanosyl triphosphate	Initiating AUG of mRNA is preceded by a purine rich sequence
Initiation factors	• Contains more initiation factors than do prokaryotes • Nine are known and several consists of multiple subunits • The prefix eIF denotes a eukaryotic initiation factor	Contain three initiation factors, IF_1, IF_2 and IF_3
Termination factors	Termination is carried out by a single release factor eRF	Termination is carried by three releasing factors RF_1, RF_2 and RF_3

EUKARYOTIC TRANSLATION, FOLDING AND PROCESSING OF PROTEINS

The basics of protein synthesis are the same across all kingdoms of life. The pathway of protein synthesis is called **translation** because the language of the nucleotide sequence on the mRNA in the form of genetic code is translated into the language of an amino acid sequence.

- Translation is the process by which ribosomes convert the information carried by mRNA in the form of genetic code to the synthesis of new protein.
- Translation occurs in cytosol on ribosomes and is guided by mRNA.
- Through genetic code, the information contained in the DNA is expressed to produce a specific protein.
- There are five major stages in protein synthesis, discussed onward.

The basic plan of protein synthesis in eukaryotes is similar to that in prokaryotes. However, eukaryotic protein synthesis involves more protein components and some steps are more complicated. Some differences are listed in **Table 21.2**.

Basic Requirements for the Translation

- mRNA to be translated
- tRNAs
- Ribosomes
- Energy in the form of ATP and GTP
- Enzymes and specific factors needed for a five stage process.

Before looking at these five stages in detail in eukaryotes, we must examine three key components in protein biosynthesis the tRNA, mRNA and ribosome.

mRNA

The mRNA is a **template** for protein synthesis. The mRNA molecule is translated from **5' end to the 3' end** and resulting polypeptide chain is synthesized from the amino terminus to the carboxyl terminus. The **initiating codon AUG** is present closest to the 5' end **(Figure 21.5)**.

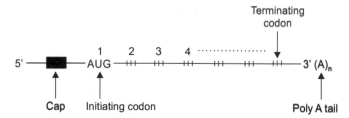

Figure 21.5: Symbolic diagram of mRNA.

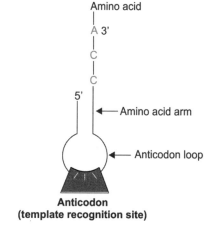

Figure 21.6: Symbolic diagram of an aminoacyl-tRNA.

- Eukaryotic mRNA is referred to as **monocistronic**, meaning that there is only one coding sequence on each mRNA molecule producing only one polypeptide chain.
- Prokaryotic mRNA is **polycistronic**, often encoding more than one polypeptide on the same mRNA.

tRNA

The tRNAs consist of a single strand of RNA folded into a precise three-dimensional structure **(Figure 21.6)**. The tRNA is the adaptor molecule in protein biosynthesis. Two arms of a tRNA are critical for its adaptor function. A tRNA molecule carries a specific amino acid in an activated form to the site of protein synthesis.

- The **amino acid arm** can carry a specific amino acid esterified by its carboxyl group to the hydroxyl group of the **A** residue at the 3' end of the tRNA.

- The anticodon arm contains the **anticodon**. The anticodon on tRNA recognizes a complementary sequence of three bases on mRNA called *codon*.

Ribosome

Ribosomes are molecular machines for making polypeptide chains. These are large complexes of **protein** and **rRNA**.

- Prokaryotic ribosomes contain about 65% rRNA and 35% protein. They composed of two unequal subunits with sedimentation coefficients of **30S** and **50S** and a combined sedimentation coefficient of **70S**.
- The ribosomes of eukaryotic cells are larger and more complex than bacterial ribosomes. They have sedimentation coefficient of about **80S**. They also have two subunits with sedimentation coefficient of **60S** and **40S (Figure 21.7)**.
- Ribosomes have three sites that bind tRNAs:
  1. Aminoacyl site (A site)
  2. Peptidyl (P) site
  3. Exit (E) site.
- The A and P sites bind to aminoacyl-tRNAs, whereas E site binds only to uncharged tRNAs that have completed their task on the ribosome.

Ribosomal subunits are identified by their **S (Svedberg unit)** values, **sedimentation coefficients** that refer to their rate of sedimentation in a centrifuge. The S values are not additive for the whole ribosome when subunits are combined, because, the sedimentation coefficient depends on the size and shape of a particle as well as molecular mass.

Stages of Translation

There are five major stages in protein synthesis, each requiring a number of components. Protein synthesis can be described in the following five phases:
1. Activation of amino acids
2. Initiation
3. Elongation
4. Termination and ribosome recycling
5. Folding and processing

Activation of Amino Acids

Amino acids are activated by attaching the amino acid to a tRNA in the first stage of protein synthesis. This reaction takes place in the cytosol, not on the ribosome.

- Each of the 20 amino acids is covalently attached to their corresponding tRNA at the expense of ATP using Mg^{2+} dependent, **aminoacyl-tRNA synthetases (AAS)**. Each enzyme is specific for one amino acid and one or more corresponding tRNAs. The carboxy group of an amino acid is esterified to the hydroxy group of the ribose unit at the 3' end of the tRNA chain **(Figure 21.8)**.
- When an amino acid is attached to the tRNA to form **aminoacyl-tRNA**, the latter can recognize a codon on mRNA by virtue of an **anticodon** triplet bases on

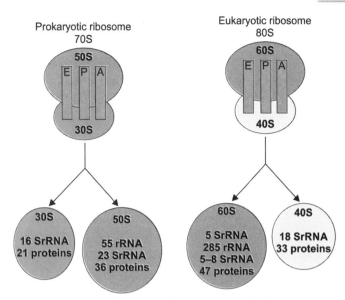

Figure 21.7: Ribosomes of prokaryotes and eukaryotes.

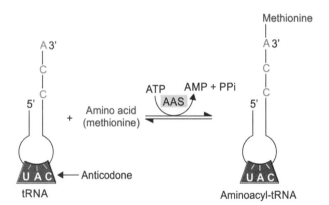

Figure 21.8: Activation of amino acid.
(AAS: aminoacyl-tRNA synthetase)

anticodon loop in the tRNA structure. When the tRNA is carrying an amino acid it is referred to as being **charged** and the amino acid as being **activated**.

Initiation

The initiation of a polypeptide chain in eukaryotes requires:
- Ribosome
- mRNA to be translated
- The initiating Met-tRNA^Met
- A set of protein factors called initiation factors.
  - In prokaryotes, three initiation factors are known **IF₁**, **IF₂** and **IF₃**,
  - In eukaryotes there are at least ten factors, designated **eIF** to indicate eukaryotic origin.

Initiation can be divided into four steps **(Figure 21.9)**:
1. Dissociation of ribosome into its 40S and 60S subunits.
2. Binding of ternary complex consisting of the **initiator methionyl-tRNA** (met-tRNA^i), GTP and **eIF-2** to the 40S ribosome to form the **43S preinitiation complex**.

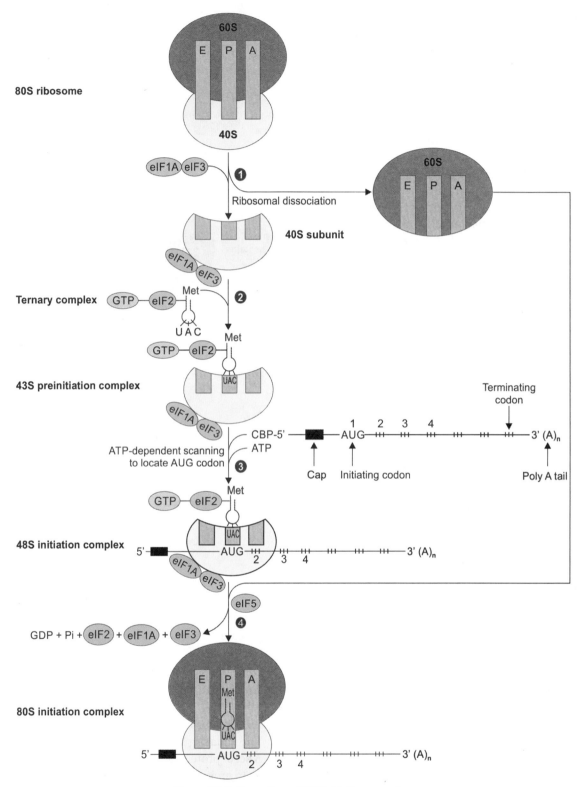

Figure 21.9: Formation of 80S initiation complex.
[CBP: cap binding protein (eIF4)]

3. Binding of mRNA to the 43S preinitiation complex to form **48S initiation complex**
4. Combination of the 48S initiation complex with the 60S ribosomal subunit to form the **80S initiation complex**.

■ **Ribosomal dissociation:** Two initiation factors eIF-3 and eIF-IA, bind to the newly dissociated 40S ribosomal subunit and prevents the reassociation with 60S subunit.

- **Formation of 43S preinitiation complex:** First it involves the binding of GTP with eIF_2. This binary complex then binds to Met-tRNA^i (a tRNA specifically involved in binding to the initiation codon AUG on mRNA. There are two tRNAs for methionine one for specifying methionine for the initiator codon, and the other for internal methionines). This **(GTP-eIF$_2$-tRNA^i)** ternary complex binds to the 40S ribosomal subunit to form **43S preinitiation complex,** which is stabilized by association with eIF$_3$ and eIF-1A.
- **Binding of mRNA to the 43S preinitiation complex to form 48S initiation complex:** The binding of mRNA to the 43S preinitiation complex forms **48S initiation complex.**
   - The 5′ terminals of most mRNA molecules in eukaryotic cells are capped by **methylguanosyl triphosphate**, which facilitates the binding of mRNA to the 43S preinitiation complex.
   - The association of mRNA with 43S initiation complex requires **cap binding protein (CBP), eIF-4F,** and **ATP.**
   - Following association of the 43S preinitiation complex with mRNA cap, the complex translocates 5′ → 3′ and scans the 43S complex to locate AUG initiator codon of mRNA forming 48S initiation complex.
- **Formation of 80S initiation complex:** Combination of the 48S initiation complex with 60S ribosomal subunit forms **80S initiation complex**. The binding of the 60S ribosomal subunit to the 48S initiation complex involves the hydrolysis of the GTP bound to eIF$_2$ by eIF$_5$ with the release of the initiation factors bound to the 48S initiation complex. These factors are then recycled. At this stage, the Met-tRNA^i is on the P site of the ribosome and is now ready for the elongation process.

Elongation

Elongation is a cyclic process on the ribosome in which one amino acid at a time is added to the nascent peptide chain. The amino acid sequence is determined by the order of the codons in the mRNA. Elongation involves following steps **(Figure 21.10):**

1. Binding of aminoacyl-tRNA specified by the next codon in the mRNA to the A site.
2. Formation of peptide bond between amino acids present in P and A site of ribosome.
3. Translocation of the ribosome along the mRNA.
4. Elimination of the deacylated-tRNA from the P and E sites.

- **Binding of aminoacyl-tRNA to the A site:** In the 80S initiation complex formed during the process of initiation, both the A site (aminoacyl or acceptor site) and E site (deacylated-tRNA exit site) are free. The binding of the appropriate aminoacyl-tRNA in the A site requires proper codon recognition.
   - The next aminoacyl-tRNA specified by the next coding triplet in the mRNA is first bound to a complex of **elongation factor eEf-1A** containing a molecule of bound **GTP.**
   - The resulting **aminoacyl-tRNA-eEf1A-GTP** complex then allows aminoacyl-tRNA to enter the A site of the ribosome with the release of eEF-1A-GDP and phosphate **(Figure 21.10).**
- **Formation of peptide bond:** In the second step of the elongation cycle, a new peptide bond is formed between the amino acids whose tRNAs are located on the A and P sites of the ribosome. This step occurs by the transfer of the **initiating methionine** from its tRNA to the amino group of the new amino acid that has just entered the A site. This step is catalyzed by **peptidyl transferase (ribozyme),** a component of 28S rRNA of the 60S subunit. As a result of this reaction, a **dipeptide tRNA** is formed on the A site and the **"empty"** initiating tRNA$_i^{Met}$ remains bound to P site **(Figure 21.11).**
- **Translocation:** In the third step of the elongation cycle the ribosome moves along the mRNA toward its 3′ end.
   - The deacylated-tRNA is attached by its anticodon to the P site at one end and by the free CCA tail to an exit (E) site of large ribosomal subunit.
   - The elongation factor EF2 binds and displaces the peptidyl-tRNA form the A site to the P site.
   - In turn, the deacylated-tRNA is in E site, from which it leaves the ribosome.
   - The hydrolysis of GTP to GDP provides energy to move mRNA forward, by a distance of one codon (three bases) and leaving the A site open for occupancy by another aminoacyl-tRNA–EFIA-GTP complex and another cycle of elongation. A eukaryotic ribosome can incorporate as many as six amino acids per seconds
   - Thus, the process of peptide synthesis occurs until a termination codon is reached.

Termination

The elongation steps are repeated until one of the three (UAA, UAG, UGA) termination or nonsense codon of mRNA appears in the A site. Once the ribosome reaches a termination codon, releasing factors are capable of recognizing the termination signal present in the A site. Prokaryotes have three release factors, **RF-1, RF-2,** and **RF-3.** Eukaryotes have only single release factor **eRF.**

- Releasing factors in conjunction with GTP and peptidyl transferase hydrolyze the peptidyl-tRNA bond (the bond between the peptide and the tRNA), when a nonsense codon occupies the A site.

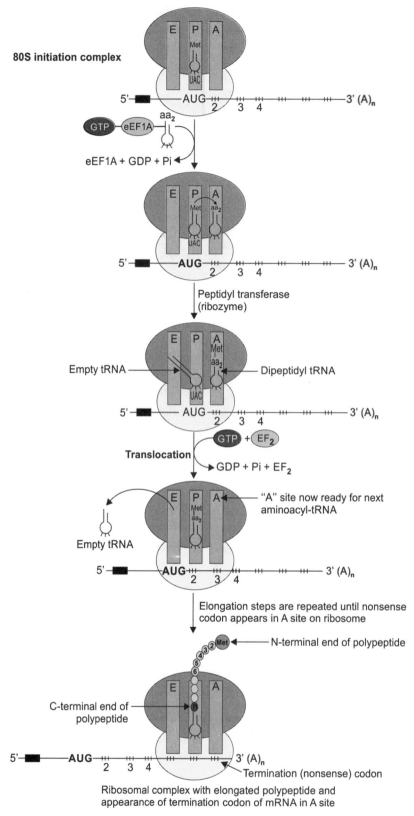

Figure 21.10: Diagrammatic representation of elongation of protein synthesis.

- This hydrolysis releases the polypeptide and tRNA from P site. Upon hydrolysis and release of the polypeptide and tRNA, the mRNA is then released from the ribosome. Ribosome then dissociates into 60S and 40S subunits, which are then recycled **(Figure 21.12)**.

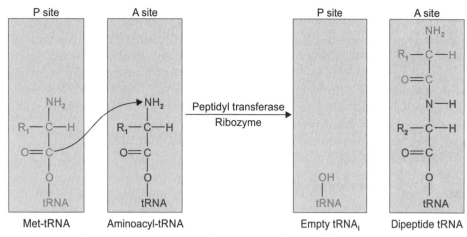

Figure 21.11: Formation of peptide bond at site of the ribosome.

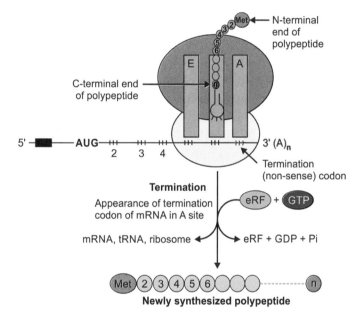

Figure 21.12: Diagrammatic representation of termination of protein synthesis.

Folding and Processing

In order to achieve its biologically active form, the new polypeptide must fold into its proper three-dimensional conformations. Before or after folding, the new polypeptide may undergo enzymatic processing, including removal of one or more amino acids (usually form the amino terminus), addition of acetyl, phosphoryl, methyl, carboxyl, or other groups to certain amino acid residues, proteolytic cleavage; and/or attachment of oligosaccharides or prosthetic groups.

Role of Molecular Chaperones in Folding of Protein

Chaperones are a group of proteins that help in protein folding. After synthesis of protein, the nascent polypeptide chain is folded and processed into its biologically active form. Not all proteins fold spontaneously as they are synthesized in the cell. Folding of many proteins requires

chaperones, proteins that interact with partially folded or improperly folded polypeptides, facilitating correct folding pathways.

Several types of molecular chaperones are found in organisms ranging from bacteria to humans. Two major families are **Hsp70** family and the **chaperonins**.

- **The Hsp70 family of proteins** with molecular weight 70,000) are more abundant in cells stressed by elevated temperatures (hence, heat shock proteins of M 70,000, or Hsp70). Hsp70 proteins bind to regions of unfolded polypeptides that are rich in hydrophobic residues. These chaperones thus protect proteins subject to denaturation by heat. Hsp70 proteins also block the folding of certain proteins that must remain unfolded until they have been translocated across a membrane. Some chaperones also facilitate the quaternary assembly of oligomeric proteins.

- **Chaperonins** are proteins that provide favorable conditions for the correct folding of other proteins, thus preventing aggregation. They prevent the misfolding of proteins. Chaperonin proteins may also tag misfolded proteins to be degraded.

Clinical Significance of Chaperones

There are many disorders associated with mutations in genes encoding chaperones that can affect muscle, bone and/or the central nervous system.

▮ POST-TRANSLATIONAL MODIFICATIONS

Before or after folding, the polypeptide may undergo processing by enzymatic action. Collectively these alterations are known as **post-translational modifications**. Post-translational modifications may include removal of part of the translated amino acid sequence or the covalent addition of one or more chemical groups required for protein activity. Some types of post-translational modifications are listed below.

Amino Terminal and Carboxyl Terminal Modifications

The first residue inserted in all polypeptides begins with a residue of N-formyl-methionine (in prokaryotes) or methionine (in eukaryotes). The formyl group, the amino terminal methionine residue and additional amino terminal and carboxyl terminal residues may be removed enzymatically. The amino group of amino terminal in most of the eukaryotic proteins is acetylated after translation.

Loss of Signal Sequence

Fifteen to thirty residues at amino terminal end of some proteins required for directing the proteins to its ultimate destination in the cell. Such signal sequences are ultimately removed by specific peptidase.

Attachment of Carbohydrate Side Chains

The carbohydrate side chains of **glycoproteins** and **proteoglycans** are attached covalently during or after the synthesis of the polypeptide chain.

Modification of Individual Amino Acids

- **Phosphorylation** of hydroxyl amino acids, e.g., serine, threonine, and tyrosine residues are phosphorylated to yield phosphoserine phosphothreonine, phosphotyrosine respectively.
- **Carboxylation** of amino acids like glutamic acid and aspartic acid, e.g., the blood clotting protein prothrombin contain a number of γ-carboxyglutamate residues.
- **Methylation**: In some proteins lysine residues are methylated enzymatically, e.g., methylated lysine residues present in muscle proteins and in cytochrome C. The calmodulin contains one trimethyllysine residue.

Addition of Isoprenyl Groups

A number of eukaryotic proteins are modified by the addition of groups derived from **isoprene**. A thioester bond (ester-bond between the COOH and –SH group) is formed between the isoprenyl group and a cysteine residue of the protein. The isoprenyl groups are derived from intermediates of the cholesterol biosynthetic pathway. Proteins modified in this way include; **Ras proteins** (products of the ras oncogenes), **G-protein, lamins** (proteins found in nuclear matrix).

The transforming (carcinogenic) activity of the ras oncogene is lost when isoprenylation of the Ras protein is blocked, this finding developed interest in identifying inhibitors of this post-translational modification pathway for use in cancer chemotherapy.

Additional Prosthetic Groups

Many prokaryotic and eukaryotic proteins require for their activity covalently bound prosthetic groups. These are attached to the polypeptide chain after it leaves the ribosome, e.g., the covalently bound **biotin** molecule in acetyl-CoA carboxylase and **heme** group of cytochrome C.

Proteolytic Processing

Insulin, some viral proteins and proteases such as trypsin and chymotrypsin are initially synthesized as larger, inactive precursor proteins. These precursors are proteolytically trimmed to produce their final, active forms.

Formation of Disulfide Cross Links

Proteins to be exported from cells, after undergoing spontaneous folding into their native conformations are often covalently cross linked by the formation of intrachain or interchain disulfide bridges between cysteine residues. The cross links formed in this way help to protect the native conformation of the protein molecule from denaturation in an extracellular environment.

INHIBITORS OF TRANSLATION AND THEIR CLINICAL IMPORTANCE IN MEDICINE

A number of commonly used pharmaceutical agents, such as variety of **antibiotics**, acts by inhibiting selectively the process of prokaryotic translation. The most useful of this class of antibiotics do not interact with component of eukaryotic ribosomal particles and thus are not toxic to eukaryotes. Such antibiotics can be used as therapeutic drugs **(Table 21.3)**.

TABLE 21.3: Inhibitors of protein synthesis.

Antibiotic	Action
Streptomycin	Inhibits initiation and causes misreading of mRNA in prokaryotes. It binds to the 30S subunit at the A site, thereby causing a cessation of chain elongation. It's binding also distorts the A site and may result in the inseration of improper amino acids
Tetracycline	Binds to the 30S subunit and inhibits binding of aminoacyl-tRNA to mRNA in prokaryotes
Chloramphenicol	Binds to the 50S ribosomal subunit and blocks the peptidyl transferase reaction in prokaryotes
Erythromycin	Binds to the 50S ribosomal subunit that inhibits the translocation reaction in prokaryotes
Lincomycin and Clindamycin	Binds to the 50S subunit and inhibits peptidyl transferase, thereby preventing peptide bond formation in prokaryotes
Puromycin	Causes premature chain termination by acting as an analog of aminoacyl-tRNA in both prokaryotes and eukaryotes
Cycloheximide	Inhibits peptidyl transferase activity of the 60S ribosomal subunit in eukaryotes

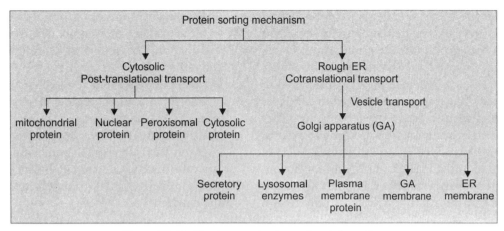

Figure 21.13: The two mechanisms of protein sorting.

- Other antibiotics inhibit protein synthesis on all ribosomes (prokaryotic and eukaryotic), e.g., **puromycin** or only on those of eukaryotic cells, e.g., **cycloheximide.** Puromycin and cycloheximide are not clinically useful but are used for research purpose.
- Toxins such as: **Diphtheria toxin** (exotoxin of *Corynebacterium diphtheriae*) inactivates an elongation factor in eukaryotes and **Ricin** of castor bean, α-**sarcin** (a fungal toxin), and **colicin** (protein secreted by some strains of *E. coli*; inhibits eukaryotic protein synthesis.

PROTEIN TARGETING AND SORTING

Protein targeting or protein sorting is the mechanism by which a cell transports proteins to the appropriate position in the cell or outside of it.

The eukaryotic cell is made up of many compartments and organelles each with specific functions that require distinct sets of proteins and enzymes. These proteins (with the exception of those produced in mitochondria) are synthesized in the cytosol. Not all newly synthesized proteins are destined to function in the cytoplasm. Eukaryotic cells can direct proteins from cytosol to internal sites such as mitochondria, the nucleus and the endoplasmic reticulum (ER). The pathways by which proteins are sorted and transported to their proper cellular location are referred to as **protein targeting** or **sorting pathways**. Proteins can be targeted to the:

- Inner space of an organelle
- Different intracellular membranes
- Plasma membrane or
- To exterior of the cell via secretion.

This delivery process is carried out based on information contained in the protein itself. Correct sorting is crucial for the cell; errors can lead to **diseases**. Protein targeting system is depending on the short sequence of amino acids called **signal sequence** at amino terminus of a newly synthesized polypeptide chain. The signal sequence directs a protein to its appropriate location in the cell and is removed during transport or when the protein reaches its final destination. There are two general mechanisms by which **sorting** take place **(Figure 21.13)**

1. In one mechanism, the protein is synthesized in the cytoplasm, and then the completed protein is delivered to its intracellular location post-translationally. Protein destined for the nucleus, chloroplast, mitochondria, and peroxisomes are delivered by this general process.

2. The other mechanism, termed as the **secretory pathway**, directs proteins into the endoplasmic reticulum (ER), cotranslationally; that is, while the protein is being synthesized. Approximately 30% of all proteins are sorted by the secretory pathway and destined for various membranes e.g., of the ER, **Golgi complex**, **plasma membrane**, as well as **lysosomal enzymes**.

Disorders Associated With Protein Targeting and Sorting

1. **Primary hyperoxaluria type-I:** Alanine/glyoxylate aminotransferase-I (AGT) deficiency can be caused by its mistargeting to mitochondria leading to primary hyperoxaluria type-I. AGT catalyzes the conversion of glyoxylate to glycine in the peroxisomes of hepatocytes. The mistargeting of AGT disrupts peroxisomal function, leading to glyoxylate being oxidized to oxalate and the deposition of calcium oxalate in the kidney and urinary tract, eventually leading to kidney failure and the deposition of calcium oxalate in almost every organ and tissue in the body.

2. **Peroxisomal biogenesis disorder (PBD):** PBD includes: **Zellweger syndrome**, the most severe; **neonatal adrenoleukodystrophy**; and **infantile Refsum's disease** the least severe. These are **autosomal recessive**

metabolic disorders that are collectively characterized by abnormal peroxisome assembly and impaired peroxisomal function. PBDs disorders often cause death in early infancy. Most PBDs are caused by defects in peroxisomal matrix protein import. Most enzymes in the peroxisomal matrix are linked to lipid metabolism and detoxification of reactive oxygen species. This results in the over-accumulation of **very long chain fatty acids and branched chain fatty acids**, such as **phytanic acid**. In addition, PBD patients show deficient levels of plasmalogens, ether-phospholipids necessary for normal brain and lung function. Collectively,

PBDs are developmental brain disorders that also result in skeletal and craniofacial dysmorphism, liver dysfunction, progressive sensorineural hearing loss, and retinopathy.

3. **Pyruvate dehydrogenase deficiency:** The first report of a defect in a mitochondrial targeting signal causing a human disease described a mutation in pyruvate dehydrogenase (PDH) that leads to PDH deficiency. The PDH complex catalyzes the oxidative decarboxylation of pyruvate to acetyl CoA, and PDH deficiency is one of the most common causes of primary lactic acidosis in infants and children.

ASSESSMENT QUESTIONS

▎STRUCTURED LONG ESSAY QUESTION (SLAQ)

1. Describe the translation process in eukaryotes under the following headings:
   - i. Basic requirements
   - ii. Different stages with diagram
   - iii. Name the drugs that inhibit translation

▎SHORT ESSAY QUESTIONS (SEQs)

1. Define genetic code. Write its characteristics.
2. Write wobble hypothesis and its importance.
3. Write difference between eukaryotic and prokaryotic protein biosynthesis.
4. What is protein targeting? Write its mechanism.
5. Write post-translational modifications
6. What are chaperones? Write role of chaperones in protein folding.
7. Name inhibitors of protein biosynthesis and write their clinical importance in medicine.

▎SHORT ANSWER QUESTIONS (SAQs)

1. What are codons? Where these are present? Name stop codons.
2. Enumerate any four inhibitors of protein biosynthesis with mode of action.
3. Write mechanism of action of chloramphenicol on translation.
4. What is protein targeting? Give two disorders of defective protein targeting.
5. Give four characteristics of genetic code.
6. Give codons of initiation and termination of protein biosynthesis.

▎MULTIPLE CHOICE QUESTIONS (MCQs)

1. **The formation of an initiation complex for polypeptide synthesis in eukaryotes requires:**
   a. A promoter
   b. Formylmethionyl-tRNA^{Met}
   c. The 60S subunit but not the 40S subunit
   d. Both 60S and 40S subunits

2. **A codon AUG is a:**
   a. Chain initiating codon
   b. Chain terminating codon
   c. Releasing factor for peptide chains
   d. Recognition site on the tRNA

3. **Release of a polypeptide chain from a ribosome is catalyzed by:**
   a. Translocase
   b. Dissociation of ribosomes
   c. Peptidyl transferase
   d. Stop codons

4. **In contrast to eukaryotic mRNA, prokaryotic mRNA:**
   a. Has a poly A tail
   b. Has 7-methylguanosine at the 5' end
   c. Can be polycistronic
   d. None of the above

5. **Erythromycin prevents synthesis of polypeptide:**
   a. By inhibiting binding of aminoacyl-tRNA to mRNA
   b. By inhibiting translocation reaction
   c. By inhibiting binding of tRNA to mRNA
   d. Blocking mRNA formation from DNA

6. **The stop codons are present on:**
   a. The coding strand of DNA
   b. The template strand of DNA
   c. The mRNA
   d. The t-RNA

7. Termination of protein biosynthesis requires presence of:
   a. Termination sequences "ter"
   b. Rho factor
   c. Nonsense codons
   d. Sigma factor

8. Which of the following drug inhibits the initiation step of translation?
   a. Cycloheximide   b. Tetracycline
   c. Streptomycin   d. Erythromycin

9. Translocase is an enzyme required in the process of:
   a. DNA replication
   b. RNA synthesis
   c. Initiation of protein synthesis
   d. Elongation of peptides in protein synthesis

10. Which of the following nucleotide base is not present in codons?
    a. Adenine   b. Guanine
    c. Thymine   d. Cytosine

11. Total number of codons are:
    a. 64   b. 61
    c. 62   d. 63

12. A gene is:
    a. A single protein molecule
    b. A group of chromosomes
    c. An instruction for making a protein molecule
    d. A bit of DNA molecule

13. Degeneracy of the genetic code means that:
    a. Codons are not ambiguous
    b. A given amino acid can be coded for by more than one base triplet
    c. A given codon can code for more than one amino acid
    d. There is no punctuation in the code sequence

14. Which of these antibiotics prevents tRNAs from attaching to the a site of the ribosome?
    a. Chloramphenicol   b. Tetracycline
    c. Streptomycin   d. Erythromycin

15. The first codon to be translated on mRNA is:
    a. AUG   b. GGU
    c. GGA   d. AAA

16. AUG, the codon for methionine is important as:
    a. A releasing factor for peptide chains
    b. A chain terminating codon
    c. Recognition site on tRNA
    d. A chain initiating codon

17. In biosynthesis of proteins, the chain terminating codons are:
    a. UAA, UAG and UGA
    b. UGG, UGU and AGU
    c. AAU, AAG and GAU
    d. GCG, GCA and GCU

18. Which of the following is not a type of post-translational modification?
    a. Proteolysis   b. Protein folding
    c. Glycosylation   d. Poly adenylation

19. Formation of initiation complex in protein biosynthesis involves:
    a. Dissociation of ribosome into its 40S and 60S subunits
    b. Formation of 48S initiation complex
    c. Formation of 80S initiation complex
    d. All of the above

20. Initiation of protein synthesis requires:
    a. ATP   b. AMP
    c. GDP   d. GTP

21. The enzyme aminoacyl-tRNA synthetase is involved in:
    a. Dissociation of discharged tRNA from 80S ribosome
    b. Charging of tRNA with specific amino acids
    c. Termination of protein synthesis
    d. Formation of peptide bond

22. Translation results in a product known as:
    a. Protein   b. tRNA
    c. mRNA   d. rRNA

23. Tetracycline prevents synthesis of polypeptide by:
    a. Blocking mRNA formation from DNA
    b. Releasing peptides from mRNA-tRNA complex
    c. Competing with mRNA for ribosomal binding sites
    d. Preventing binding of aminoacyl-tRNA

24. Which of the following is the end product of genetic information pathway?
    a. Protein   b. Lipid
    c. Carbohydrate   d. Vitamins

25. Synthesis of DNA is also known as:
    a. Duplication
    b. Replication
    c. Transcription
    d. Translation

26. Anticodons are present on:
    a. Coding strand of DNA   b. mRNA
    c. tRNA   d. rRNA

27. Codons are present on:
    a. Noncoding strand of DNA
    b. mRNA
    c. tRNA
    d. None of these

28. Nonsense codons are present on:
    a. mRNA   b. tRNA
    c. rRNA   d. None of these

29. The first aminoacyl-tRNA which initiates translation in prokaryotes is:
    a. Methionyl-tRNA
    b. Formylmethionyl-tRNA
    c. Tyrosinyl-tRNA
    d. Alanyl-tRNA

30. All the following statements about genetic code are correct, *except*:
    a. It is degenerate
    b. It is unambiguous
    c. It is nearly universal
    d. It is overlapping

31. All of the following statements about nonsense codons are true, *except*:
    a. They do not code for amino acids
    b. They act as chain termination signals
    c. They are identical in nuclear and mitochondrial DNA
    d. They have no complementary anticodons

32. A polycistronic mRNA can be seen in:
    a. Prokaryotes
    b. Eukaryotes
    c. Mitochondria
    d. All of these

33. The first aminoacyl-tRNA which initiates translation in eukaryotes is:
    a. Methionyl-tRNA
    b. Formylmethionyl-tRNA
    c. Tyrosinyl-tRNA
    d. Alanyl-tRNA

34. There are 20 amino acids with three codons in spite of the no of amino acids could be formed is 64 leading to that an amino acid is represented by more than one codon is called:
    a. Transcription
    b. Degeneracy
    c. Mutation
    d. Frame shift

35. Genetic code has triplet of nucleotides each for one amino acid. When an amino acid is specified by more than one codon, it is called:
    a. Transcription   b. Degeneracy
    c. Mutation   d. Frame shift

36. Termination process of protein synthesis is performed by all, *except*:
    a. Releasing factor   b. Stop codon
    c. Peptidyl transferase   d. UAA codon
    e. AUG codon

37. Part of eukaryotic DNA contributing to polypeptide synthesis:
    a. Exon   b. Enhancer
    c. Leader sequence   d. tRNA

ANSWERS FOR MCQs

1. d	2. a	3. c	4. c	5. b
6. c	7. c	8. c	9. d	10. c
11. a	12. d	13. b	14. b	15. a
16. d	17. a	18. d	19. d	20. d
21. b	22. a	23. d	24. a	25. b
26. c	27. b	28. a	29. b	30. d
31. c	32. a	33. a	34. b	35. b
36. e	37. a			

Regulation of Gene Expression and Gene Mutation

Competency	Learning Objectives
BI 7.3: Describe gene mutations and basic mechanism of regulation of gene expression.	1. Describe gene expression: Definition, types of gene, types of gene regulation. 2. Describe mechanism of regulation of gene expression in prokaryotes with illustration of Lac Operon. 3. Describe mechanism of regulation of gene expression in eukaryotes. 4. Describe mutations: Types, causes, consequences with examples.

OVERVIEW

Gene expression is the combined process of the transcription of a gene into mRNA, the processing of that mRNA and its translation into protein.

- The rate of expression of prokaryotic genes is controlled mainly at the level of **transcription, mRNA synthesis**.
- Eukaryotes, however, have a much larger and more complex genome than prokaryotes. Gene expression in eukaryotes is controlled by many ways. Gene regulation is more complex in eukaryotes than in prokaryotes for a number of reasons **(Table 22.1)**:
  - Eukaryotic genome is significantly larger compare to prokaryotic genome.
  - Many different cell types present in most eukaryotes.

- Eukaryotic genes are not generally organized into operons. Instead, genes that encode proteins for a given pathway are often spread widely across the genome.
- Transcription and translation are uncoupled in eukaryotes.

In this chapter, we will examine gene regulation mechanisms in prokaryotes and eukaryotes and gene mutation.

GENE EXPRESSION

Information encoded in DNA, is transcribed into RNA and then translated into protein is called the **gene expression (Figure 22.1)**. Thus, gene is expressed in the form of **protein**. The expression of the genetic information must be regulated during **adaptation**, **development**, and **differentiation**.

TABLE 22.1: Prokaryotic versus eukaryotic gene expression.

Prokaryotes	Eukaryotes
Prokaryotic mRNA is polycistronic **can encode more than one polypeptide**. A single mRNA that encodes more than one protein is referred to as a **polycistronic mRNA**	Eukaryotic mRNA is monocistronic **can encode only one polypeptide**
Prokaryotic gene expression (both transcription and translation) occurs within the **cytoplasm** of a cell due to the lack of a defined nucleus	Eukaryotic gene expression occurs in both the **nucleus** (transcription) and **cytoplasm** (translation)
In prokaryotes the processes of transcription (DNA to RNA) and translation (RNA to protein) are **coupled** occur almost simultaneously	Transcription and translation processes in eukaryotes are **uncoupled**
Prokaryotic gene expression is primarily controlled at the level of **transcription**	Eukaryotic gene expression is controlled at the many levels of **epigenetics (nongenetic influences), transcription, post-transcription, translation, and post-translation**

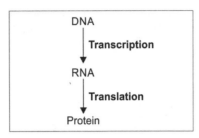

Figure 22.1: Expression of gene.

Types of Gene Regulation

There are two types of gene regulation: **Positive regulation** and **negative regulation**.

- When the expression of genetic information is quantitatively increased by the presence of a specific regulatory element, regulation is said to be **positive**.
- When the expression of genetic information is diminished by the presence of a specific regulatory element, regulation is said to be **negative**.
- The element or molecule mediating the positive regulation is said to be a **positive regulator**, an **activator** or **inducer** and element mediating negative regulation is said to be **negative regulator**, a **silencer** or **repressor**.

Types of Gene

There are two types of genes **inducible gene** and **constitutive gene**.

1. **Inducible genes** are expressed only when a specific positive regulatory substance, i.e., an inducer or activator is present. For example, the production of the enzyme β-**galactosidase** is induced by the presence of **lactose** in the prokaryotes or **glucokinase** of glycolysis is produced in response to **insulin** in human being. Insulin is an inducer of the gene glucokinase. These genes are subject to **regulated expression**.
2. **Constitutive genes:** Some genes are expressed all the time and are known as **constitutive gene** or **housekeeping genes**. Genes for ribosomes, proteins such as actin,

glyceraldehyde 3-phosphate dehydrogenase (GAPDH) and ubiquitin are an example of constitutive gene. Ribosomes are constantly being transcribed because ribosomes are constantly needed for protein synthesis. Ubiquitin functions in targeting proteins for degradation. As a result of mutation, some inducible gene products become constitutively expressed.

REGULATION OF GENE EXPRESSION IN PROKARYOTES

In prokaryotes the processes of transcription (DNA to RNA) and translation (RNA to protein) are **coupled** occur almost simultaneously. When the resulting protein is no longer needed, transcription stops. Thus, the regulation of transcription controls what type of protein and how much of each protein is expressed in a prokaryotic cell. When more protein is required, more transcription occurs. Therefore, in prokaryotic cells, the control of gene expression occurs within **cytoplasm** at the **transcriptional level**.

- In prokaryotes, the genes are often present in a linear fashion, called an **operon**.
- For example, all of the genes needed to use **lactose** as an energy source are located next to each other in the **lactose (or lac) operon**.
- Prokaryotic regulation is often dependent on the **type** and **quantity of nutrients** that surround the cell.

Lactose Operon or Lac Operon

Structure

Lac operon is a coordinated unit of gene expression to make the enzymes necessary to metabolize lactose. All genes needed to use lactose are present next **to each other** in **lactose (or lac) operon (Figure 22.2)**. The lac operon contains the following genetic elements:

- **Regulatory gene (lac i)** produces a repressor protein

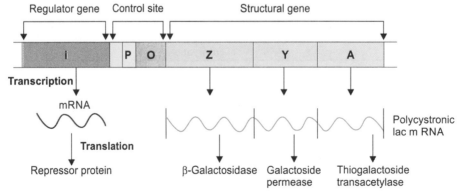

Figure 22.2: Schematic diagram of lac operon showing its protein products.

(P: promoter; O: operator; i: lac i gene; Z: lac Z gene; Y: lac Y gene; A: lac A gene)

- **A promoter site (P)** for the binding of RNA polymerase. Promoter site contains two specific regions:
  1. Catabolite activator protein binding site **(CAP site)**
  2. RNA polymerase entry site, to which RNA polymerase first becomes bound.
- **An operator site (O)**, a regulatory protein called the lac repressor binds to this site and blocks initiation of transcription.
- Three structural genes, **Z**, **Y**, and **A**, that code for β-**galactosidase**, **galactoside permease**, and **thiogalactoside transacetylase** respectively, required for lactose metabolism.
  - The β-galactosidase hydrolyzes lactose into galactose and glucose.
  - Galactoside permease is required for the transport of lactose across the bacterial cell membrane.
  - The transacetylase appears to play a role in the detoxification of compounds that also may be transported by the permease.

This arrangement of the structural genes and their regulatory genes allows for the coordinated expression of the three enzymes concerned with lactose metabolism.

Regulation of Lac Operon

- Regulation of lac operon is dependent on **type** and **quantity of nutrients** that surround the cell.
- Lac operon is regulated by following mechanism:
  - Negative regulation by **lac repressor** in absence of lactose and presence of glucose.
  - Positive regulation by **induction of expression**, in presence of lactose and absence of glucose.
  - Positive regulation by **catabolite repression** in presence of both glucose and lactose.

Negative Regulation by Lac Repressor in Absence of Lactose and Presence of Glucose

- *E. coli* bacteria usually depend on **glucose** as their source of carbon and energy. However, in absence of glucose, *E. coli* can use lactose as their carbon and energy source.
- In the absence of lactose, the cell has no need for the production of β-**galactosidase** and **galactoside permease**. Hence, regulatory molecule, the **lac repressor**, prevents expression of the lac operon in the absence of lactose.
- In presence of glucose no transcription of the *lac* operon occurs. That is because the *lac* repressor protein (a product of regulatory gene i) binds to the operator and prevents the binding of RNA polymerase and subsequent transcription of the structural genes Z, Y, and A. Under these conditions β-galactosidase and other two proteins are not made by the cells **(Figure 22.3)**.

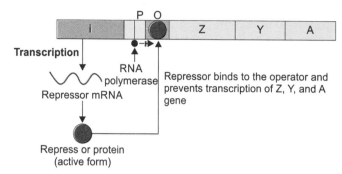

Figure 22.3: Regulation of lac operon in presence of glucose and absence of lactose.

Positive Regulation by Induction of Expression, in Presence of Lactose and Absence of Glucose

- In presence of lactose and absence of glucose in the medium, lactose acts as an **inducer**. It binds to repressor protein and inactivates it and releases the lac repressor from the operator.
- This allows RNA polymerase to bind to the promoter and move forward on the DNA and transcribe the operon. The inactive repressor no longer binds to the operator. RNA polymerase now can bind to the promoter and transcribe the three structural genes of the operon.
- RNA polymerase alone does not bind very well to the lac operon promoter. It might make a few transcripts, but it won't do much more unless it gets extra help from catabolite activator protein (CAP). CAP binds to a region of DNA just before the lac operon promoter and helps RNA polymerase to attach to the promoter, leading high levels of transcription.
- Role of catabolite activator protein (CAP):
  - CAP isn't always active (able to bind DNA). Instead, it is regulated by cyclic AMP (cAMP).
  - cAMP is made by *E. coli* when glucose levels are low or absent.
  - cAMP binds to CAP, changing its shape and making it able to bind DNA and promote transcription **(Figure 22.4)**. Without cAMP, CAP cannot bind DNA and is inactive. CAP is only active when glucose levels are low (cAMP levels are high).
  - Thus, the lac operon can only be transcribed when glucose is absent.

Positive Regulation by Catabolite Repression in Presence of Both Glucose and Lactose

When *E. coli* is exposed to both lactose and glucose, they first metabolize the glucose, although lactose is present. The cell does not induce those enzymes necessary for catabolism of lactose until the glucose has been exhausted.

- As glucose levels decrease and unavailable, cAMP levels increase.
- cAMP binds to **catabolite activator protein (CAP)** forming a complex, **cAMP-CAP**.

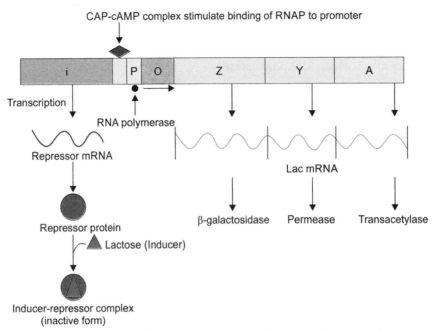

Figure 22.4: Regulation of lac operon in presence of lactose and absence of glucose.

- **cAMP-CAP** binds to the CAP binding site of promoter, stimulating the binding of the RNA polymerase to the promoter and transcription occurs **(Figure 22.4)**.
- As glucose levels increase, cAMP levels decrease and in the absence of cAMP, CAP does not bind to CAP binding site of promoter and transcription does not occur.
- Thus, the enzymes for metabolism of lactose are not produced if cells have an adequate supply of glucose even if the alternative energy source, lactose, is present at very high levels.

REGULATION OF GENE EXPRESSION IN EUKARYOTES

Eukaryotic gene expression is more complex than prokaryotic gene expression **(Table 22.1)**. Unlike prokaryotic cells, eukaryotic cells can regulate gene expression at many different levels. In eukaryotic cells, the DNA is contained inside the nucleus where it is transcribed into RNA. The newly-synthesized RNA is then transported out of the nucleus into the cytoplasm where ribosomes translate the RNA into protein **(Figure 22.5)**.

- Eukaryotic gene expression occurs in both the nucleus (transcription) and cytoplasm (translation). The regulation of gene expression can occur at all stages of the process. It is controlled at the levels of:
  1. Epigenetic (nongenetic influences)
  2. Transcription
  3. Post-transcription
  4. Translation
  5. Post-translation.

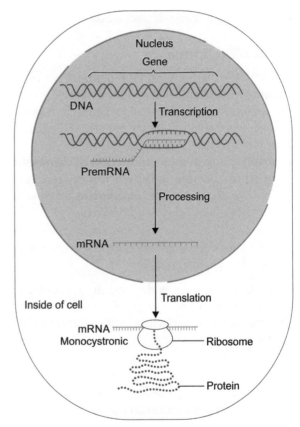

Figure 22.5: Eukaryotic expression of gene.

Epigenetic Regulation

Epigenetics means nongenetic or external influences that activate or deactivate genes without any change in DNA sequence. In eukaryotic cells, the first stage of gene expression control occurs at the epigenetic level. Epigenetic

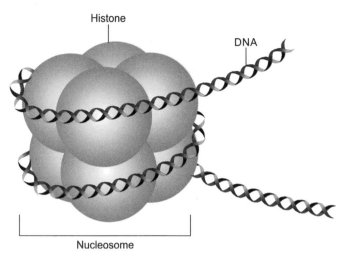

Figure 22.6: DNA is folded around histone proteins to form nucleosome which control the access of proteins to the gene.

mechanisms regulate access to the chromosomal region to allow genes to be turned on or off.

- Eukaryotic gene expression begins with control of **access to the DNA**. The DNA in the nucleus is specifically wound around **histone proteins**, folded and compacted into **chromosomes** and thus in wrapped DNA, genes are not accessible for transcription **(Figure 22.6)**.

- Nucleosome complexes can control the access of **transcription factors** to the DNA regions. In the nucleus, the process of chromatin remodeling regulates the availability of a gene for transcription.

- If a specific gene is to be transcribed into RNA, the nucleosomes surrounding that region of DNA can slide down to open that specific chromosomal region and allow for the transcriptional machinery (RNA polymerase) to initiate transcription.

- If a gene is to be transcribed, the histone proteins and DNA are modified surrounding the chromosomal region encoding that gene. This is facilitated by enzymes that modify **histones** by adding **methyl** and **acetyl** groups to their N-terminal tails of the histones **(Figure 22.7)**.

  - **Acetylation** of N-terminal tails of the histones result in loose packing of nucleosome. Acetylation reduces the net positive charge of the histones, loosening their affinity for DNA. This opens the chromosomal region to allow access for **RNA polymerase** and **other proteins**, called transcription factors, to bind to the promoter region, and initiate transcription.

  - **Methylation:** Methylation histones of DNA causes nucleosomes to pack tightly together so that transcription factors can not bind the DNA and genes are not expressed. Increased binding of methylation

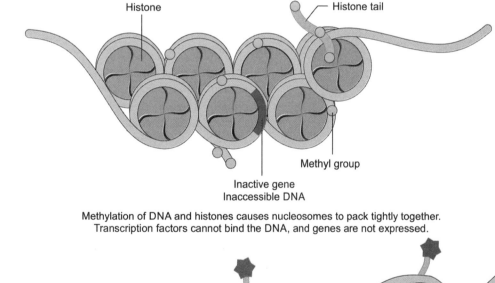

Methylation of DNA and histones causes nucleosomes to pack tightly together.
Transcription factors cannot bind the DNA, and genes are not expressed.

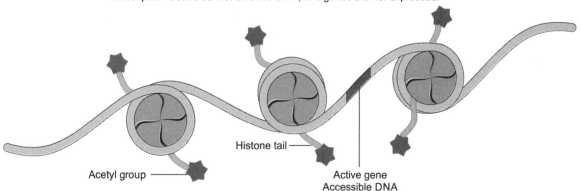

Histone acetylation results in loose packing of nucleosomes.
Transcrption factors can bind the DNA and genes are expressed.

Figure 22.7: Regulation of gene expression by acetylation and demethylation of DNA.

to histones decreases the availability of DNA for transcription.

Transcriptional Regulation

The transcriptional regulation of individual genes in eukaryotes is fundamentally similar to the transcriptional regulation of operons in prokaryotes. The major difference is that in eukaryotes the number of DNA sequence elements and regulatory factors is quite larger than in prokaryotes.

Role of Transcription Factors, Enhancers, and Repressors

Transcription Factors

- Like prokaryotic cells, the transcription of genes in eukaryotes requires the binding of an **RNA polymerase** to **promoter sequence**. **Transcription factors (TFs)** are proteins that bind to the promoter sequence and recruit RNA polymerase to the site for transcription.
- Transcription factors control the transcription of the target gene. RNA polymerase by itself cannot initiate transcription in eukaryotic cells.
- There are hundreds of transcription factors in a cell that each bind specifically to a particular DNA sequence motif.
- Transcription factors are regulated by signals produced from other molecules, e.g., hormones activate transcription factors and thus enable transcription. Hormones therefore activate certain gene and initiate transcription of the gene that is needed.

Enhancers of Transcription

- An enhancer is a DNA sequence that promotes transcription. In some eukaryotic genes, there are regions that help increase or enhance transcription called **enhancers**. They can be located upstream of a gene, within the coding region of the gene, downstream of a gene, or may be thousands of nucleotides away and called **distal control elements**. Two different genes may have the same promoter but different distal control elements, enabling differential gene expression.
- Enhancer regions are binding sites, for transcription factors. Transcription begins when the factors at the promoter region bind with the factors at the enhancer region creating a loop in the DNA **(Figure 22.8)**. This shape change allows for the interaction of the activators bound to the enhancers with the transcription factors bound to the promoter region and facilitate binding of RNA polymerase to promoter sequences.

Transcriptional Repressors

Like prokaryotic cells, eukaryotic cells also have mechanisms to prevent transcription. **Transcriptional repressors** can bind to promoter or enhancer regions and block transcription. Like the transcriptional activators, repressors

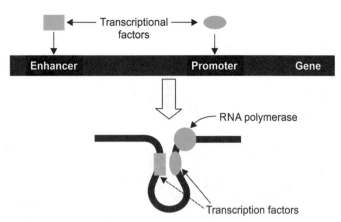

Figure 22.8 Binding of transcriptional factor to promoter and enhancer region of DNA to form a loop.

respond to external stimuli to prevent the binding of activating transcription factors.

Post-transcriptional Regulation

The processing after RNA molecule has been transcribed, but before it is translated into a protein, is called post-transcriptional modification. Post-transcriptional processing of RNA is much more extensive in eukaryotes than in prokaryotes. The two major levels at which post-transcriptional regulation taken place is:

- RNA splicing and
- RNA stability.

RNA Splicing

- RNA splicing is the first stage of post-transcriptional control. In eukaryotic cells, the RNA transcript often contains regions, called **introns** that are removed prior to translation. The regions of RNA that code for protein are called exons **(Figure 22.9)**.
- After an RNA molecule has been transcribed, but prior to its departure from the nucleus to be translated, the RNA is processed and the introns are removed by splicing.
- Differential removal of introns enables a gene to code for more than one different protein.
- Thus same gene can produce related but different proteins in different cell types.
- An example is; in thyroid gland, a **calcitonin gene** produces hormone **calcitonin**, same gene in neurons produces a neuropeptide, **calcitonin gene-related peptide** (CGRP).

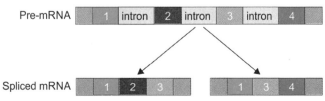

Figure 22.9: Regulation of gene expression by RNA splicing.

RNA Stability

Alterations in RNA stability may effect gene regulation in eukaryotes. Regulation of RNA stability may occur in either the **nucleus** or the **cytoplasm**.

- Before the mRNA leaves the nucleus, it is given two protective **"caps"** that prevent the end of the strand from degrading during its journey (*see* **Figure 6.17**).
  - The **5′ cap**, which is placed on the 5′ end of the mRNA, is usually composed of a **methylated guanosine triphosphate molecule (GTP)**.
  - The **poly-A tail**, which is attached to the **3′ end**, is usually composed of a **series of adenine nucleotides**.
- Once the RNA is transported to the cytoplasm, the length of time that the RNA resides there can be controlled. Each RNA molecule has a defined lifespan and decays at a specific rate. This rate of decay can influence the amount of protein in the cell.
  - If the decay rate is increased, the RNA will not exist in the cytoplasm as long, and less protein will be translated.
  - Conversely, if the rate of decay is decreased, the RNA molecule will reside in the cytoplasm longer and more protein can be translated.
- This rate of decay indicates the RNA stability. If the RNA is stable, it will be found for longer periods of time in the cytoplasm.
- The mRNA of different genes may vary considerably in their half-lives.
- Some genes that code for an **abundant product with a long duration of action**, such as the β-globin gene has long half-life (approximately 10 hours). Other genes that code for a protein with a short duration of action, e.g., **growth factors**, may produce mRNA that has a short half-life (less than 1 hour).

Role of RNA-binding Proteins (RBPs)

- Binding of **RNA-binding proteins** to the RNA can influence its stability.
- RBPs, can bind to the regions of the RNA just upstream or downstream of the protein-coding region.
- These regions in the RNA that are not translated into protein are called the **untranslated regions**, or **UTRs**. They are not introns (those have been removed in the nucleus). Rather, these are regions that regulate **mRNA localization**, **stability**, and **protein translation**.
- The region just before the protein-coding region is called the **5′ UTR**, whereas the region after the coding region is called the **3′ UTR (Figure 22.10)**.
- The binding of RBPs to these regions can increase or decrease the stability of an RNA molecule, depending on the specific RBP that binds.

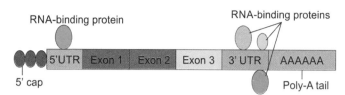

Figure 22.10: Regulation of gene expression by binding of RNA-binding proteins (RBPs) to 5′ or 3′ UTR.

Role of MicroRNAs

- In addition to RBPs that bind to and control (increase or decrease) RNA stability, other elements called **microRNAs** can bind to the RNA molecule.
- The miRNAs are made in the nucleus as longer pre-miRNAs. These pre-miRNAs are chopped into mature miRNAs by a protein called **dicer**.
- These **microRNAs**, or miRNAs, are short RNA molecules that are only 21–24 nucleotides in length.
- MicroRNAs (miRNAs) are a class of noncoding RNAs that play important roles in regulating gene expression.
- In most cases, miRNAs interact with the 3′ untranslated region (3′ UTR) of target mRNAs to induce mRNA degradation and translational repression.
- Like transcription factors and RBPs, mature miRNAs recognize a specific sequence and bind to the RNA; however, miRNAs also associate with a ribonucleoprotein complex called the **RNA-induced silencing complex (RISC)**. RISC binds along with the miRNA to degrade the target mRNA. Together, miRNAs and the RISC complex rapidly destroy the RNA molecule.

Translational Regulation

The synthesis of **proteins** is dependent on the availability of the **mRNAs encoding** them. The rate of degradation of an **mRNA** will influence how long it is around to direct the synthesis of the protein it codes for. Regulation of **translation** is used to control the production of many proteins.

- Most eukaryotic translational controls affect the initiation of protein synthesis. The initiation factors required for translation particularly **eukaryotic factor 2 (eIF$_2$)** involved in these regulatory mechanism. The action of eIF$_2$ is inhibited when it is phosphorylated by a **protein kinase**.
- For example, protein synthesis in reticulocytes is the most well described example of translational regulation. Reticulocyte (**newly produced immature red blood cells**) which contains no nuclei and therefore, no DNA for transcription, must regulate the synthesis of globin at the translational level. Globin is produced when heme levels in the cell are high. If the supply of heme is inadequate globin synthesis is inhibited. Heme acts by preventing phosphorylation of eIF$_2$. The kinase

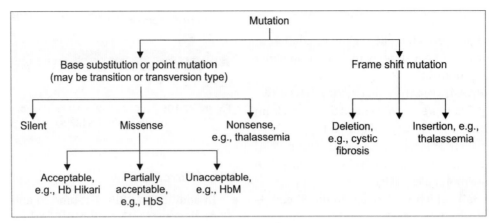

Figure 22.11: Types of mutation.

that phosphorylates eIF$_2$ is inactivated when heme is bound. Thus, when heme levels are high eIF$_2$ is not phosphorylated and, therefore, it is active in initiating the synthesis of globin. As heme levels decrease in the cell, eIF$_2$ is phosphorylated and inactivated.

Although all stages of gene expression can be regulated, the main control point for many genes is **transcription**. Later stages of regulation often refine the gene expression patterns that are "roughed out" during transcription.

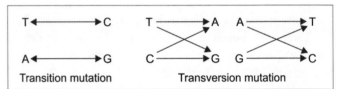

Figure 22.12: Diagrammatic representation of transition and transversion mutations.

MUTATIONS

The term mutation refers to the permanent changes in the DNA sequence due to changes in the nucleotide sequence of a DNA. Mutations in **germ cells** are transmitted to the next progeny and may give rise to inherited diseases. Mutations in **somatic cells** are not transmitted to the progeny but are important in the causation of cancers and some congenital malfunctions. Various types of mutations are given in **Figure 22.11**.

Causes of Mutations

Mutation arises by a number of different means:
- **Errors in replication**, if a mismatch base pair is not corrected during proofreading and post replication repair system
- **Error due to recombination events:** Physical crossing over of DNA during meiosis into new combinations of DNA is a normal event. In the process exchange of genetic material with each other occur, and is called recombination.
- **Spontaneous change in DNA:** For example, **deamination** or spontaneous **depurination**. Deamination is the removal of an amino group from DNA bases; e.g., deamination of cytosine to uracil. Almost all DNA bases undergo deamination in spontaneous reactions, with the exception of thymine—which does not have an amino group. **Depurination** involves the loss of purine bases (adenine and guanine) from DNA.

- **Environmental factors** like chemical mutagens and irradiations, e.g., UV light or ionizing radiation can alter the structure of DNA.

Types of Mutations

Base Substitution or Point Mutation

Point mutation occurs when only one base in DNA is altered, which may be transcribed into mRNA and therefore may result in the translation of a protein with an abnormal amino acid sequence. Single base change can be of **transition type** or **transversion type (Figure 22.12)**.
- Transition, in which one purine is replaced by another purine or one pyrimidine, is replaced by another pyrimidine.
- Transversion, in which a purine is replaced by a pyrimidine or a pyrimidine, is replaced by a purine.

Effect of Point Mutation

Single base changes in the mRNA molecules may have one of several effects when translated into protein. The effect of point mutation can be:
- Silent mutation
- Missense (wrong sense or meaning) mutation
- Nonsense mutation.

Silent Mutation

Point mutations are said to be silent when there is no detectable effect. Silent mutation leads to the formation of a codon synonym and no change in the amino acid sequence of the protein occurs due to degeneracy of the codon, e.g., a codon change from CGA to CGG does not affect the proteins because both of these codons specify arginine.

Missense Mutation

Missense mutation will occur when a different amino acid is incorporated at the corresponding site in the protein molecule. Depending upon the location of the mistaken amino acid (missense) in the specific protein, missense mutation might be:
- Acceptable
- Partially acceptable
- Unacceptable with respect to the function of that protein.

Acceptable Missense Mutations

The example of acceptable missense mutation is **Hb-Hikari.** This Hb has aspargine substituent for lysine at the 61 position in the β-chain. Hb-Hikari is a type of transversion mutation, in which either AAA or AAG changed to either AAU or AAC. The replacement of the specific *lysine with aspargine* does not alter the normal function of the β-chain in these individuals and is therefore called acceptable missense mutation.

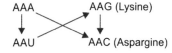

Partially Acceptable Missense Mutation

For example, HbS, *sickle hemoglobin*, in which the normal amino acid in position 6 of the β-chain, glutamic acid has been replaced by valine. The corresponding transversion might be either GAA or GAG of **glutamic acid** to GUA or GUG of **valine**.

GAA or GAG (Glutamic acid)
↓   ↓
GUA or GUG (Valine)

Unacceptable Missense Mutation

For example, *Hb M (Methemoglobin)* in which normal amino acid in position 58 of α-chain, **histidine** has been replaced by **tyrosine** and nonfunctional Hb molecule is generated which cannot transport oxygen.

CAU or CAC (Histidine)
↓   ↓
UAU or UAC (Tyrosine)

Nonsense Mutations

Nonsense mutation leads to the conversion of an amino acid codon to a stop or nonsense codon. Nonsense mutation causes the premature termination of a polypeptide chain, which is usually nonfunctional, e.g., one type of **thalassemia**, in which codon 17 of the β-chain is changed from UGG to UGA and results in the conversion of a codon tryptophan to a nonsense codon.

UGG (Tryptophan) ─────────→ UGA (Nonsense codon)

Frame Shift Mutations

Frame shift mutation **(Figure 22.13)** occurs when there is insertion or deletion of one or two nucleotides in DNA that generates altered mRNAs.

Deletion Frame Shift Mutation

- The deletion of a single nucleotide from the coding strand of a gene results in an altered reading frame in the mRNA
- Since there is no punctuation in the reading of codons, the translating machinery does not recognize that a base was missing
- Such frame shifts would result in the production of an entirely different protein after transcription and translation or indeed, no protein, at all, if a stop codon is encounter, e.g., cystic fibrosis.

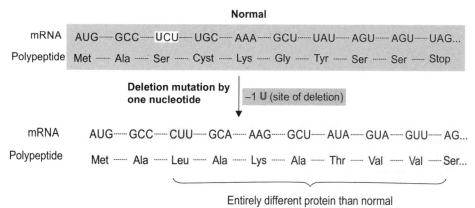

Figure 22.13: Deletion frame shift mutation by one nucleotide.

Insertion Frame Shift Mutation

Insertion may be of one or two nucleotides. As with deletions, insertions of nucleotides into genes can lead to severe frame shift mutations **(Figure 22.14)**.

If the number of nucleotides involved in deletion or insertion is three or multiples of three, frame shift does not occur. Instead, an abnormal protein, missing one or more amino acids, is synthesized. Such a mutation is likely to be less severe than a frame shift mutation.

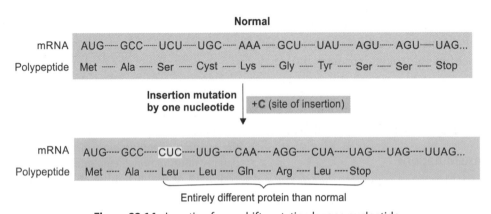

Figure 22.14: Insertion frame shift mutation by one nucleotide.

ASSESSMENT QUESTIONS

STRUCTURED LONG ESSAY QUESTIONS (SLAQs)

1. Describe mutations under the following headings:
   i. Definition
   ii. Causes
   iii. Types
   iv. Examples
2. Describe regulation of gene expression in eukaryotes under following headings:
   i. Definition of gene expression
   ii. Regulation at DNA level
   iii. Regulation at transcriptional level
3. Describe lac operon concept under the following headings:
   i. Structure
   ii. Regulation

SHORT ESSAY QUESTIONS (SEQs)

1. What is Lac operon? Give structure of Lac operon.
2. Define gene expression? Write post-transcriptional regulation.

SHORT ANSWER QUESTIONS (SAQs)

1. Write types of mutations with an example.
2. Define frame shift mutation with an example.
3. Give definition of gene expression and enumerate its levels of control in eukaryotes.
4. Draw the structure of Lac operon
5. Write role of miRNA in regulation of gene expression
6. Write role of RNA-binding proteins (RBPs) in regulation of gene expression
7. Write role of mRNA stability in regulation of gene expression

MULTIPLE CHOICE QUESTIONS (MCQs)

1. **Housekeeping genes are:**
   a. Inducible
   b. Required only when inducer is present
   c. Mutant
   d. Not regulated

2. **Lac operon transcription is inhibited by, *except*:**
   a. Glucose
   b. Glucose with inducer
   c. Inducer without glucose
   d. Both lactose and glucose

3. **All of the following statements about the repressor of lac operon of *E. coli* are true, *except*:**
   a. It is the gene product of regulatory gene
   b. It prevents the transcription of structural genes
   c. It binds to the operator region of the lac operon
   d. It requires corepressor

4. **cAMP regulates the lac operon, *except*:**
   a. By forming cAMP-CAP (catabolite activator protein) complex
   b. By binding to the promoter site
   c. By stimulating binding of RNA polymerase to promoter and by activating transcription
   d. By binding to the lac repressor to prevent transcription

5. **The portion of an operon to which a repressor binds is:**
   a. A regulatory gene   b. A promoter
   c. An initiation site   d. An operator

6. **Lac operon is a cluster of genes present in:**
   a. Human beings   b. *E. coli*
   c. Lambda phage   d. All of these

7. Lac operon is a cluster of:
   a. Three structural genes
   b. Three structural genes and their promoter
   c. A regulatory gene, an operator, and a promoter
   d. A regulatory gene, an operator, a promoter, and three structural genes

8. The regulatory i gene of lac operon:
   a. Is inhibited by lactose
   b. Is inhibited by its own product, the repressor protein
   c. Forms a repressor protein which regulates the expression of structural genes
   d. None of the above

9. RNA polymerase holoenzyme binds to lac operon at the following site:
   a. i gene
   b. z gene
   c. Operator locus
   d. Promoter region

10. Transcription of z, y, and a, genes of lac operon is prevented by:
    a. Lactose
    b. Allolactose
    c. Repressor
    d. cAMP

11. Transcription of structural genes of lac operon is prevented by binding of the repressor protein to:
    a. i gene
    b. Operator locus
    c. Promoter
    d. z gene

12. Binding of RNA polymerase holoenzyme to the promoter region of lac operon is facilitated by:
    a. Catabolite gene activator protein (CAP)
    b. cAMP
    c. CAP-cAMP complex
    d. None of these

13. Lactose or its analog act as positive regulators of lac operon by:
    a. Attaching to i gene and preventing its expression
    b. Increasing the synthesis of catabolite gene activator protein
    c. Attaching to promoter region and facilitating the binding of RNA polymerase holoenzyme
    d. Binding to repressor subunits so that the repressor cannot attach to the operator locus

14. Expression of structural genes of lac operon is affected by all the following, *except*:
    a. Lactose or its analog
    b. Repressor protein
    c. ADP
    d. CAP-cAMP complex

15. Control of gene expression in eukaryotic cells occurs at which level(s)?
    a. Only the transcriptional level
    b. Epigenetic and transcriptional levels
    c. Epigenetic, transcriptional, and translational levels
    d. Epigenetic, transcriptional, post-transcriptional, translational, and post-translational levels

16. RNA splicing occurs in the:
    a. Nucleus
    b. Cytoplasm
    c. Nuclear membrane
    d. Mitochondria

17. RNA splicing _____ removes from the RNA transcript.
    a. Exons   b. Introns
    c. Axons   d. None of these

18. The _____ of mRNA regulate localization, stability, and translation.
    a. Introns
    b. RNA binding proteins
    c. Untranslated regions
    d. Exons

19. Tightly coiled DNA is:
    a. Transcriptionally inactive
    b. Translationally regulated
    c. Known as hypermethylated
    d. Known as acetylated

20. Which of the following are involved in post-transcriptional control?
    a. Control of RNA splicing
    b. Control of RNA lifespan and decay
    c. Control of RNA stability
    d. All of the above

21. Which one of the following causes frame shift mutation?
    a. Transition
    b. Transversion
    c. Deletion
    d. Substitution of purine to pyrimidine

22. A frame shift mutation changes the reading frame because the genetic code:
    a. Is degenerate
    b. Is overlapping
    c. Has no punctuations
    d. Is universal

23. Insertion of a base in a gene can cause:
    a. Change in reading frame
    b. Garbled amino acid sequence in the encoded protein
    c. Premature termination of translation
    d. All of these

24. If the codon UAC on mRNA changes into UAG as a result of a base substitution in DNA, it will result in:
    a. Silent mutation
    b. Acceptable missense mutation
    c. Nonsense mutation
    d. Frame shift mutation

25. Hemoglobin S is an example of:
    a. Silent mutation
    b. Acceptable missense mutation
    c. Unacceptable missense mutation
    d. Partially acceptable missense mutation

26. Mutations can be caused by:
    a. Ultraviolet radiation
    b. Ionizing radiation
    c. Alkylating agents
    d. All of these

27. **Substitution of an adenine base by guanine in DNA is known as:**
    a. Transposition
    b. Transition
    c. Transversion
    d. Frame shift mutation

28. **Substitution of a thymine base by adenine in DNA is known as:**
    a. Transposition
    b. Transition
    c. Transversion
    d. Frameshift mutation

29. **A point mutation results from:**
    a. Substitution of a base
    b. Insertion of a base
    c. Deletion of a base
    d. All of these

30. **Substitution of a base can result in a:**
    a. Silent mutation
    b. Missense mutation
    c. Nonsense mutation
    d. All of these

31. **Amino acid sequence of the encoded protein is not changed in:**
    a. Silent mutation
    b. Acceptable missense mutation
    c. Both (a) and (b)
    d. None of these

32. **Sickle cell anemia is the clinical manifestation of homozygous genes for an abnormal hemoglobin molecule. The event responsible for the mutation in the B chain is:**
    a. Insertion
    b. Deletion
    c. Nondisjunction
    d. Point mutation

33. **A mutation in the codon which causes a change in the coded amino acid, is known as:**
    a. Mitogenesis
    b. Somatic mutation
    c. Missense mutation
    d. Recombination

34. **In a mutation if valine is replaced by which of the following would not result in any change in the function of protein?**
    a. Proline   b. Leucine
    c. Glycine   d. Aspartic acid

■ ANSWERS FOR MCQs

1. d	2. c	3. d	4. d	5. d
6. b	7. d	8. c	9. d	10. c
11. b	12. c	13. d	14. c	15. d
16. a	17. b	18. c	19. a	20. d
21. c	22. c	23. d	24. c	25. d
26. c	27. b	28. c	29. a	30. d
31. a	32. d	33. c	34. b	

Molecular Techniques and Applications

Competency	Learning Objectives
BI 7.4: Describe applications of molecular technologies like recombinant DNA technology, PCR in the diagnosis and treatment of diseases with genetic basis.	1. Describe recombinant DNA technique and construction of recombinant DNA. 2. Describe cloning of the DNA. 3. Describe applications of recombinant DNA technology. 4. Describe genomic and c-DNA libraries. 5. Describe DNA probes. 6. Describe Blot transfer techniques and its application. 7. Describe restriction fragment length polymorphism and its application. 8. Describe polymerase chain reaction, technique and its application in medicine.

OVERVIEW

Genetic engineering is the construction and repair of the genes of living things. Now it is possible to synthesize a gene in a laboratory and then introduce it into a living cell which will synthesize protein corresponding to that gene. Rapid progress in biotechnology is a result of following few key techniques:

- **Restriction enzyme analysis:** Restriction enzymes allow an investigator to manipulate DNA segment.
- **Blotting techniques:** Southern and Northern blots are used to separate and characterized DNA and RNA respectively. The western blot uses antibodies to characterize proteins.
- **DNA sequencing:** The precise nucleotide sequence of the molecule of DNA can be determined. Sequencing provides information concerning gene architecture, the control of gene expression and protein structure.
- **Solid-phase synthesis of nucleic acids:** Precise sequences of nucleic acids can be synthesized de novo and used to identify other nucleic acids.
- **Polymerase chain reaction (PCR):** The polymerase chain reaction leads to several fold amplification of a segment of DNA. This technique can be used to detect pathogens and genetic diseases, determine the source

of a hair left at the scene of a crime and regenerate genes from the fossils of extinct organisms.

We begin by outlining the principles of recombinant DNA, DNA cloning, and then illustrate the range of applications and potentials of many newer technologies.

RECOMBINANT DNA

Recombinant DNA is a DNA formed by the hybrid combination of two DNA fragments, derived from different sources. In vivo genes often undergo recombination.

Genes or sets of gene can also be recombined in vitro to produce new combinations that do not occur biologically.

Principle

- Recombinant DNA technology involves **isolation** and **manipulation** of DNA to make **chimeric** or **hybrid DNA** molecule. Chimeric DNA is a recombinant DNA containing genes from two different species, e.g., molecules containing both human and bacterial DNA sequences (Chimera was a mythological creature with the head of the lion, the body of goat and the tail of the snake). A number of techniques have been used to construct recombinant DNA.

- Following steps are involved in the construction of recombinant DNA:
  - Fragmentation of DNA by **restriction endonuclease** enzyme called restriction fragments.
  - Isolation of specific human DNA.
  - Insertion of isolated human DNA into vector (*a vector is a carrier DNA molecule*) to form chimeric or hybrid DNA molecule.
  - Joining of two different cut DNA fragments by DNA ligase.

Construction of Recombinant DNA

Fragmentation of DNA by Restriction Endonuclease Enzyme

Restriction endonuclease also called as **restriction enzyme**. These are found in wide variety of prokaryotes. These enzymes were originally called restriction enzymes because their presence in a given bacterium restricted the growth of foreign infective bacterial viruses (bacteriophages). The cell's own DNA is not degraded because the sequences recognized by its own restriction enzymes are methylated, thereby protected from the action of restricted endonuclease enzyme.

Restricted enzymes cut DNA of any source in a sequence specific manner in contrast to action of most other endonuclease which breaks DNA randomly. The restricted enzymes are named according to the bacteria from which they are isolated. Their name consists of a three letter abbreviation for the host organism.

- The first letter of the name is from genus of the bacteria
- The next two letters are from the name of the species
- These followed by a strain and Roman numeral indicate the order in which the enzyme was discovered in the particular organism, e.g.,
  - **EcoRI** is from *Escherichia coli*
  - **BamHI** is from *Bacillus amyloliquefaciens*
  - **Hae III** is for *Haemophilus aegyptius*

Restriction endonuclease recognizes specific base sequences of double helical DNA, usually 4–6 base pairs in length and cleaves both strands within this sequence. Most of the DNA sequences recognized by restriction endonucleases are *palindromic* (in Greek palindromic = running back again), i.e., both strands of DNA have the same sequence when read in a 5′ to 3′ direction **(Figure 23.1)**.

Action of Restriction Endonucleases

Some restriction endonucleases cleave both strands of DNA so as to leave no unpaired bases on either end. These ends are often called *blunt ends,* e.g., restriction enzyme from Hae III (*Haemophilus aegyptius*) **(Figure 23.2)**. Others, e.g., EcoRI make staggered cuts on the two strands, leaving two to four nucleotides of one strand unpaired at each resulting end. These are referred to as **cohesive ends** or *sticky ends* **(Figure 23.2)**.

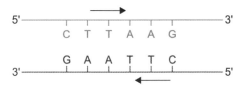

Figure 23.1: Palindromic sequence when read in 5′ to 3′ direction.

Restriction enzymes are used to cleave DNA molecules into specific fragments that are more readily analyzed and manipulated than the entire parent molecule. Different restriction fragments of DNA can base pair with each other if they have sticky ends which are complementary. Therefore, two unrelated DNA fragments can base pair with each other, if they were cleaved by the same restriction endonuclease enzyme.

Isolation of Specific Human DNA

Once DNA has been cleaved into fragments by restriction endonuclease, a particular fragment of interest can be separated by others, by **electrophoresis** or **high performance liquid chromatography (HPLC)**.

Insertion of Isolated Human DNA into Vector to form Chimeric or Hybrid DNA Molecule

A specific selected fragment of DNA of human genome is inserted into vector (carrier). *A vector is a carrier DNA molecule*, to which the fragment of DNA of interest is, attached **(Figure 23.3)**. A segment of the foreign DNA and the DNA vector are usually cleaved with the same restriction enzyme to produce complementary sticky ends in both the foreign DNA and the DNA vector. These complementary sticky ends can base pairs.

Normally, foreign DNA fragments cannot self-replicate in a cell. Therefore, they are joined together to a vector that can replicate within the host cell. Most commonly used cloning vectors are:

- **Bacterial plasmids:** Small circular duplex DNA molecule whose natural function is to confer antibiotic resistance to the host cell and replicate independently from the bacterial chromosomal DNA.
- **Bacteriophages:** Viral DNA capable of replicating in bacterial cell.
- **Cosmids:** Plasmids that contain DNA sequences from the lambda phage.

Joining of Two Different Cut DNA Fragments by DNA Ligase

After the fragments of DNA (one from human genome and another from vector DNA) have base paired, the ends are covalently joined by the action of *DNA ligase*. Restriction enzymes in conjunction with DNA ligase, therefore, can produce vector containing recombinant or **hybrid** or **chimeric DNA**.

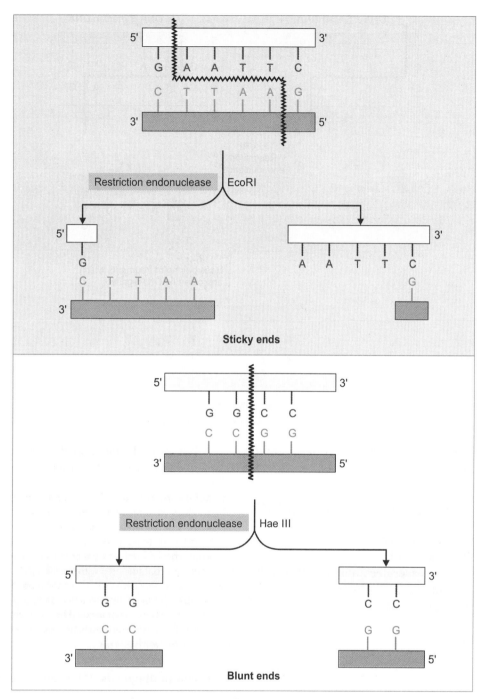

Figure 23.2: Action of restriction endonuclease:
EcoRI produces sticky ends and Hae III produces blunt ends.

CLONING OF THE DNA

Cloning is a technique developed for amplifying the quantity of DNA, in vivo using **recombinant DNA technology.** A clone is a large population of identical molecules, bacteria, or cells that arise from a common ancestor. Cloning allows for the production of a large number of identical DNA molecules, which can be produced as follows:

- **Introduction of recombinant DNA into appropriate host cell:** The recombinant DNA inserted back into bacterial cell (host cell) by the process called

transformation. Host cells that contain recombinant DNA are called transformed cells.

- **Amplification of recombinant DNA:** The host cells containing the recombinant DNA are incubated under conditions in which they replicate rapidly. As the host cell divide in addition to replicating their own DNA, they also replicate the DNA of the vector which includes the human DNA. Subsequently, relatively large quantities of human DNA can be isolated from cells.

- If the host cells are grown under conditions permitting expression of the human DNA, the human

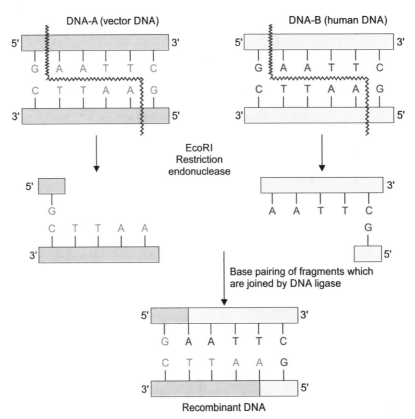

Figure 23.3: Construction of recombinant DNA molecules.

protein produced from this DNA can be isolated **(Figure 23.4)**.

APPLICATIONS OF RECOMBINANT DNA TECHNOLOGY

Let us consider how the recombinant DNA technology has been used in medicine **(Table 23.1)**.

- **Molecular basis of disease:** Recombinant DNA technology is used to understand the molecular basis of a number of diseases like:
  - Familial hypercholesterolemia
  - Sickle cell disease
  - Thalassemia
  - Cystic fibrosis
  - Muscular dystrophy, etc.
- **Diagnosis of disease:** Recombinant DNA technology is used to diagnose existing diseases.
- **Production of proteins:**
  - Using recombinant technology, human proteins can be produced in abundance for **therapy**, **research** and **diagnosis (Table 23.2)**.
  - For example, it can supply large amounts of material that could not be obtained by conventional purification methods, e.g., interferon, tissue plasminogen activating factor, etc.
  - It can provide human material, e.g., insulin and growth hormone. The primary aim of recombinant technology is to supply proteins for treatment (insulin) and diagnosis (AIDS, Ebola testing) of

human and other animal diseases and for prevention of disease (hepatitis B vaccine).

- Before the introduction of recombinant DNA technology, vaccines were made from infectious agents, which were either killed or attenuated (altered so that they can no longer multiply in an inoculated individual).
- Both types of vaccines were potentially dangerous because they could get contaminated with the live infectious agents.
- By recombinant DNA techniques, the proteins could be produced, completely free of the infectious agent, and used in the vaccines. Thus, the risk of infection could be eliminated.
- The first successful recombinant DNA vaccine to be produced was for the **hepatitis B virus**.

- **Prenatal diagnosis:** If the genetic error is understood and a specific probe (probe is a single-stranded polynucleotide of DNA or RNA that is used to identify the sequence on a target DNA) is available, prenatal diagnosis is possible. DNA from cells collected from amniotic fluid can be analyzed by **Southern blot transfer**.
- **Genetic counseling:** One means of preventing disease is avoid passing defective genes to offspring. If members of families are tested for genetic diseases, which are known to carry a defective gene, genetic counselors can inform the individuals of their risk and options. With this information people can decide in advance whether to have children.
- **Screening tests:** Tests based on the recombinant DNA techniques have been developed for many inherited

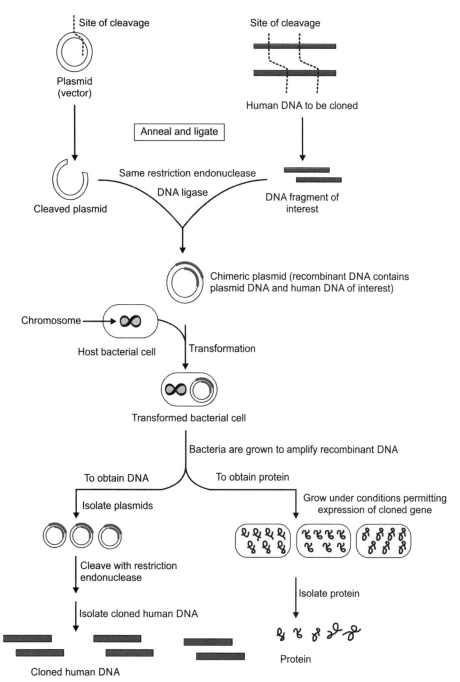

Figure 23.4: Cloning of human DNA in bacteria using recombinant DNA technology.

TABLE 23.1:	Applications of recombinant DNA technology.
1.	It offers a rational approach to understanding the molecular basis of number of diseases, e.g., familial hypercholesterolemia, sickle cell disease, thalassemia, cystic fibrosis, muscular dystrophy, vascular and heart disease, cancer and diabetes
2.	Human proteins can be produced in abundance for therapy (e.g., insulin, growth hormone, tissue plasminogen activator, etc.)
3.	Proteins for vaccine, e.g., hepatitis B and for diagnostic testing, e.g., Ebola and AIDS tests) can be obtained
4.	This technology is used both to diagnose existing diseases as well as to predict the risk of developing a given disease and individual response to pharmacological therapeutics
5.	Special techniques (DNA fingerprinting/**DNA genotyping** or **DNA profiling**) are used in forensic medicine
6.	Gene therapy for curing diseases caused by a single gene deficiency such as sickle cell disease, thalassemia, adenosine deaminase deficiency and others may be planned
7.	Genetic counseling prenatal diagnosis transgenic animal formation is possible
8.	*Commercial applications:* Agricultural applications and industrial applications

Table 23.2: Human proteins and their role produced by recombinant technology.

Protein produced	Function
Anticoagulant	Tissue plasminogen activator (TPA). It activates plasmin, an enzyme involved in dissolving clots. Used in treating heart attack victims
Human growth hormone	It is used to treat children with growth hormone deficiencies (dwarfism)
Growth factors	Stimulate differentiation and growth of various cell types
Colony-stimulating factors	Immune system growth factors. It stimulates leukocyte production used to treat immune deficiencies
Erythropoietin	Stimulates erythrocyte production used to treat anemia
Blood factors	Factor VIII promotes clotting and is used to treat hemophilic patients
Insulin	A hormone used to treat diabetes
Interferons	Used to treat cancer
Interleukins	Activates and stimulates leukocytes used in wound healing, HIV infections, cancer, immune deficiencies
Monoclonal antibodies	Used in diagnostic tests, also to transport drugs, toxins, or radioactive compounds to tumors or a cancer therapy
Superoxide dismutase	Prevent tissue damage from reactive oxygen species (ROS) when tissue is deprived of O_2 for short periods during surgery
Proteins for diagnosis	For example, for AIDS test of human and other animal diseases
Vaccines	Prevent disease

diseases. Screening can be performed on the prospective parents before conception. If they decide to conceive, the fetus can be tested for the genetic defect. In some cases if the fetus has the defect, treatment can be instituted at an early stage, even in utero. For certain diseases, early therapy leads to a more positive outcome.

- **Gene therapy:** The ultimate cure for genetic diseases is to introduce normal genes into individuals who have defective genes. The strategy is to clone a normal copy of the relevant gene into a suitable vector and incorporate into genome of a host cell. Bone marrow precursor cells are being investigated for this purpose. The introduced gene would begin to direct the expression of its protein product and this would correct the deficiency in the host cell. It is not possible at present to replace a defective gene with a normal gene at its usual location in the genome of the appropriate cells.

- Gene therapy for **sickle cell disease, thalassemia, adenosine deaminase** deficiency and other diseases may be devised. Currently gene therapy is at experimental level.

- **Transgenic animals:** Transgenic means containing genetic material into which DNA from a different organism has been artificially introduced. The introduction of normal genes into somatic cells with defective genes corrects the defect only in the treated individuals, not in their offspring. To dominate the defect for future generations the normal genes must be introduced into the germ cell line (the cells that produce sperm in males or eggs in females).

Experiments with animals indicate that gene therapy in germ cells is feasible. Genes can be introduced into fertilized eggs from which transgenic animals develop, and these transgenic animals can produce apparently normal offspring.

Transgenic approach has been used to correct a genetic deficiency in mice.

- **In forensic medicine:** Special techniques, e.g., **DNA fingerprinting** also called **DNA genotyping** or **DNA profiling** (analysis of DNA sequence differences) can be used to determine family relationships or to help identify the criminals of a crime.

- **Commercial applications:**
  - **Agricultural applications:** In agriculture, plants that are resistant to disease, insects, herbicides, and drought and temperature extremes or more efficient at fixing nitrogen are being produced using recombinant DNA technology.
  - **Industrial applications:** Industrial applications include the production of enzymes used in detergents, sugar and cheese.

GENOMIC AND c-DNA LIBRARIES

DNA library is a collection of cloned restriction fragments of DNA that represents the entire genome. The total genetic information content of an organism is represented by all the fragments in the library in the same way as human knowledge is represented by all the volumes in a book library. DNA libraries may be either:

- Genomic DNA library in which both introns (noncoding sequences) and exons (coding sequences) are represented.

- Complementary DNA (cDNA) library in which only exons are represented.

Genomic DNA Library

- In genomic DNA library both introns and exons are represented and thus, contain every sequence from the genome of a specific organism.

- The entire genomic DNA of an organism is cut into small pieces by restriction endonucleases. These cut pieces are then introduced into vectors.
- A collection of these different recombinant clones is called **genomic DNA library**.
- To produce the complete gene library about 1500 fragments are required in the case of *E. coli*, but about 10 lakh fragments for human DNA.

Complementary DNA (cDNA) Library

- In cDNA library only exons are represented. It is constructed so as to include only those genes that are expressed in a given organism or even in certain cells or tissues.
- cDNA library is a more **specialized** and **exclusive DNA library**.
- To construct cDNAs library, the mRNAs from an organism is extracted and complementary double-stranded DNAs (cDNAs) are produced from this mRNAs by **reverse transcriptase**.
- The resulting DNA fragments are then inserted into a suitable vector and cloned, creating a population of clones called a cDNA library.
- Since there will be no introns in the mRNA, the expression of the genes is easier.

■ DNA PROBES

DNA libraries contain thousands or even millions of irrelevant DNA fragments. It is difficult to pick out a specific gene (a DNA sequence of interest) from these fragments. **Probes are used to search specific gene from the DNA libraries**.

- Probe is a single-stranded polynucleotide molecule used to identify a specific fragment of DNA or RNA:
  - In a genetic library or
  - During analysis by blot transfer (Southern, or Northern) techniques.
- Probes can be composed of
  - cDNA produced from mRNA (by reverse transcriptase)
  - Fragments of genomic DNA (cleaved by restriction enzymes from the genome)
  - Chemically synthesized oligonucleotides or occasionally RNA.
- To identify the target sequence, the probe must carry a **label**. If the probe has radioactive label, it can be detected by autoradiography **(Figure 23.5)**.

■ BLOT TRANSFER TECHNIQUES AND ITS APPLICATION

Blot transfer is a technique used for visualization of specific DNA, RNA or proteins among the thousands of molecules. These are **(Figure 23.6)**:

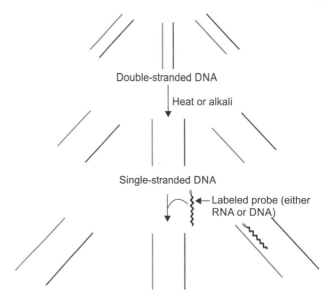

Double-stranded DNA

Heat or alkali

Single-stranded DNA

Labeled probe (either RNA or DNA)

Probe hybridize with complementary sequence of DNA

Figure 23.5: Identification of DNA sequences by using labeled probes.

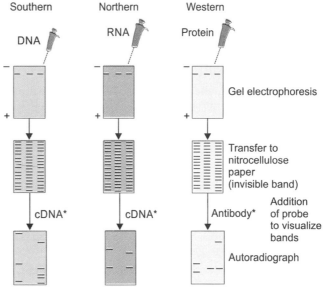

Figure 23.6: The blot transfer procedures (Asterisk signify radio-labeling).

- Southern blot (for DNA)
- Northern blot (for RNA)
- Western blot (for protein).

EM Southern developed a technique which bears his name for identifying DNA sequences on gels and the other two names Northern and Western began as laboratory jargons.

Southern Blots Transfer

- Southern blot transfer procedure is useful to detect specific DNA segment present in a given tissue and mutations in the gene.

- Steps of Southern blots transfer:
  - First DNA is extracted from cells, which is digested into many fragments with restriction enzyme.
  - The resulting fragments are separated by agarose or polyacrylamide gel electrophoresis.
  - The smaller fragments move more rapidly than larger fragments.
  - After a suitable time the DNA is denatured by mild alkali
  - Denatured DNA fragments transferred to nitrocellulose paper in an exact replica of the pattern on the gel by blotting technique, hence the name blot.
  - The paper is then exposed to the labeled cDNA probe, which hybridizes to complementary fragments on the paper.
  - The paper is exposed to X-ray film, which shows specific bands corresponding to the DNA fragment that recognized the sequence in the cDNA probe.
- Use of Southern blot:
  - Identification of specific viral or bacterial DNA in the infected sample.
  - Screening test to detect inborn errors.
  - Detect DNA mutations such as large insertion, deletion, trinucleotide repeat expansion, point mutation, and rearrangement of nucleotide.
  - In forensic medicine, to analyse DNAs from specimens at the scene of crime-blood, semen, saliva etc.

Northern or RNA Blots Transfer

- The Northern blot transfer technique is used to detect specific RNA molecules.
- In Northern blot procedures RNA is subjected to electrophoresis before blot transfer and treated similarly as that of Southern blot transfer) except that alkali is not used (alkali hydrolyzes RNA).
- The hybrids formed between RNA and cDNA can be identified by radio autography.

Western Blots Transfer

- Western blots technique is used to detect **specific protein molecules**.
- In this case, the presence of **viral proteins** in the blood is detected by **antibodies**.
- In the Western blot procedures proteins are electrophoresed and transferred to nitrocellulose paper and then probed with labeled antibodies.
- The probes are labeled to visualize the bands with which they hybridize.
- Western blot are used for:
  - Identification of specific proteins in sample
  - Detection of viral pathogens by identifying viral proteins for HIV virus or hepatitis B.

RESTRICTION FRAGMENT LENGTH POLYMORPHISM

The human genome is heterogeneous. There are normal variations of DNA sequence. Variations of DNA sequence is called polymorphism, which occurs approximately once in every 500 nucleotides or about 10^7 times per genome. In normal healthy individual, these alterations (deletion, insertion of DNA or single base substitution) occur in non-coding region of DNA or at sites that cause no change in function of encoded protein.

The differences in DNA sequences can result in variations of restriction sites and thus, in the length of restriction fragments. An inherited difference in the pattern of restriction sites is known as restriction fragment length polymorphism or restriction fragment length polymorphism (RFLP).

Application of RFLP

- Restriction fragment length polymorphism can be used to detect human genetic defects in prospective parents or in fetal tissue, for example sickle cell anemia and thalassemia.
- In forensic medicine, RFLPs is used to establish a unique pattern of DNA fragments (fingerprinting) for an individual.

POLYMERASE CHAIN REACTION: TECHNIQUE AND ITS APPLICATION IN MEDICINE

Revolutionary technique invented by **Karry B Mullis**. He got **Nobel Prize** for this in **1993.** Polymerase chain reaction (PCR) is an in vitro method for the amplification of specific segments of DNA. DNA can be amplified in vivo by cloning by recombinant DNA (discussed earlier).

Amplification of DNA by PCR is faster and technically less difficult than laborious cloning methods using recombinant DNA techniques. It is particularly used for amplifying DNA for clinical or forensic testing procedures. By PCR DNA can be amplified from a single strand of hair or single drop of blood or semen.

The Key Requirements of a PCR

- *Taq* polymerase
- Primers
- **Template DNA:** It is a DNA sample containing the segment to be amplified
- **Nucleotides (DNA building blocks):** All four deoxyribonucleotides

Taq polymerase: Like DNA replication in an organism, PCR requires a DNA polymerase enzyme that makes new strands of DNA, using template strand. The DNA polymerase typically used in PCR is called **Taq polymerase**, (this polymerase is isolated from Thermus aquatics, a bacterium that grows in hot springs). Taq polymerase is very heat-stable and is most active around 70°C, (a temperature at which a human or *E. coli* DNA polymerase would be nonfunctional). This heat-stability makes Taq polymerase ideal for PCR because high temperature is used repeatedly in PCR to denature the template DNA, or separate its strands.

PCR primers: Like other DNA polymerases, Taq polymerase requires a primer to start DNA synthesis. PCR primers are short pieces of single-stranded DNA, usually around 20 nucleotides in length. Two primers are used in each PCR reaction, and they are designed so that they flank the target region (region that should be copied). That is, they are given sequences that will make them bind to opposite strands of the template DNA, just at the edges of the region to be copied. The primers bind to the template by complementary base pairing.

When the primers are bound to the template, they can be extended by the Taq polymerase, and the region that lies between them will get copied.

The Steps of PCR

- There are three steps **(Figure 23.7):**
    1. **Strand separation (denaturation):** The two strands of the parent DNA are separated by heating the solution to **95°C for 15 seconds**. This provides single-stranded template for the next step.
    2. **Binding of primers (annealing):** The solution is then cooled to **54°C** to allow each primer to bind to a separated DNA strand. One primer binds to the 3′ end of the target on one strand, and other primer binds to the 3′ end on the complementary target strand.
    3. **DNA synthesis (extension):** The solution is then heated to 72°C (the optimal temperature for heat stable polymerases). **Deoxyribonucleotides** and heat stable **Taq polymerase** are added to the mixture to initiate the synthesis. Taq polymerase extends the primers, synthesizing new strands of DNA.
- These three steps, **strand separation, binding of primers,** and **DNA synthesis** constitute one cycle of the PCR amplification and can carried out repetitively just by changing the temperature of the reaction mixture.
- The thermostability of polymerase makes it possible to carry out PCR in a closed container.
- No reagents are added after the first cycle.
- At the completion of the second cycle, four duplexes containing the targeting sequence have been generated.
- Subsequent cycles will amplify the target sequence enormously **(Figure 23.8)**.
- Ideally, after *n* cycles, the desired sequence is amplified $2n$-fold. The amplification is million fold after 20 cycles and billion fold after 30 cycles, which can be carried out in less than 1 hour.

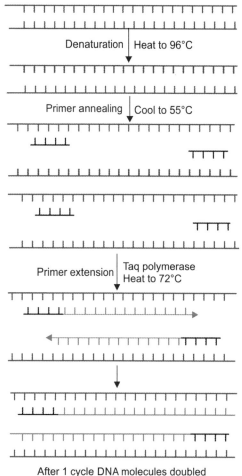

After 1 cycle DNA molecules doubled
After 20 cycles 10^6 fold amplification occur

Figure 23.7: Polymerase chain reaction (PCR).

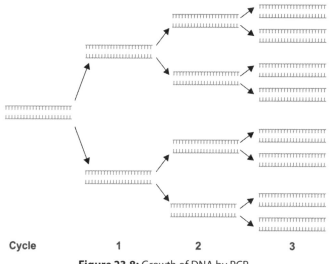

| Cycle | 1 | 2 | 3 |

Figure 23.8: Growth of DNA by PCR.

- DNA sequences amplified by PCR are analyzed using **gel electrophoresis.**

Applications of PCR

PCR is used in many research labs, and it also has practical applications in **forensics**, **genetic testing**, and **diagnostics**.

PCR can also be used to test **infectious agents**, a bacterium or DNA virus in blood or tissue sample.

Role of PCR in Detection of Infectious Agents

- PCR is extensively used in analyzing clinical specimens for the presence of infectious agents, including HIV, hepatitis, human papillomavirus, (the causative agent of genital warts and cervical cancer), Epstein-Barr virus (glandular fever), COVID-19, malaria and anthrax.
- PCR is particularly helpful in the early detection of HIV as it can identify the DNA of the virus within human cells immediately following infection, as opposed to the antibodies that are produced weeks or months after infection. PCR can also be used to determine the viral load (i.e., how much virus is circulating around the body), which is a useful measure of prognosis.
- Finding *Mycobacterium tuberculosis* bacilli in tissue specimens is slow and laborious. With PCR tubercle bacilli can be detected readily.
- Currently, PCR is used to complement microscopic examination. Malaria is traditionally diagnosed by identifying malarial parasites (*Plasmodium falciparum*) through microscopic analysis of the blood. However, PCR technology has been useful in that it can rapidly identify the species of malaria present. This is important in cases of mixed infection, and also in determining the type of drug treatment to use.
- PCR can be used to identify the bacterium **Bacillus anthracis**, the causative agent of anthrax. Because of the need to rapidly diagnose such infections, PCR has become an important tool in detecting the presence of anthrax in clinical specimens. It replaces conventional methods of using a specimen to grow the bacteria in the laboratory, which take at least 24 hours. PCR provides a rapid, sensitive and specific alternative.

Role of PCR in Cancer Diagnosis

- PCR is promising method for early detection of cancers. PCR can identify mutations of certain growth control genes, such as the **ras genes**. The capacity to greatly amplify selected regions of DNA can also be highly informative in monitoring cancer chemotherapy. Tests using PCR can detect when cancerous cells have been eliminated and treatment can be stopped; they can also detect a relapse and the need to immediately resume treatment.
- PCR is an invaluable tool as it can provide information on a patient's prognosis, and predict response or resistance to therapy. Many cancers are characterized by small

mutations in certain genes, and this is what PCR is employed to identify.

- PCR is ideal for detecting leukemia caused by chromosomal rearrangements. PCR can also be applied in monitoring leukemia patients following treatment, by counting the number of cancerous cells that are still circulating in their bodies.

Role of PCR in Analysis of Genetic Diseases and Paternity Testing

- Another important application of PCR is in the analysis of mutations that occur in many genetic diseases (e.g., cystic fibrosis, sickle cell anemia, phenylketonuria, muscular dystrophy). Because of the sensitivity of PCR, this can be done from a single cell taken from an embryo before birth.
- The paternity test is essentially carried out by PCR. A cheek swab is taken from inside the mouth of both parents and the child. The DNA is extracted from the cells obtained and is analyzed by PCR. Everyone's DNA is the same in every cell in the body. A child's DNA should have part of the mother's and father's DNA. Several locations called 'loci' on the child's DNA are examined, and the sequences of these loci are compared to the mother and father to see if there are matches from both parents.
- In clinical biochemistry and molecular biology it is used in the antenatal diagnosis of single gene mutation and in studying structural gene polymorphism.
- **Forensics and legal medicine:** PCR is also having an effect in forensics and legal medicine. It is appropriate for forensic testing procedures because only a very small sample of DNA is required as the starting material which can be obtained from a single strand of hair or a single drop of blood or semen.
  - PCR amplification of multiple genes is being used to establish biological parentage in disputed paternity and immigration cases.
  - Analysis of blood stains and semen samples by PCR have implicated blame or innocence in numerous assault and rape cases.
- **Studies of molecular evolution:**
  - PCR provides an ideal method for amplifying ancient DNA molecules so that they can be detected and characterized.
  - PCR can also be used to amplify DNA from microorganisms that have not yet been isolated and cultured. The sequences from these PCR products can be sources of significant awareness into evolutionary relationships between organisms.

ASSESSMENT QUESTIONS

STRUCTURED LONG ESSAY QUESTIONS (SLEQs)

1. Describe recombinant DNA technology under the following headings:
   i. Principle
   ii. Steps involved in construction recombinant DNA
   iii. Applications.
2. Describe cloning of DNA under the following headings:
   i. Definition
   ii. Technique
   iii. Applications
3. Describe polymerase chain reaction under the following headings:
   i. Definition
   ii. Steps involved in PCR
   iii. Applications.

SHORT ESSAY QUESTIONS (SEQs)

1. What is restriction endonuclease? Write its mode of action.
2. Write applications of recombinant DNA technology.
3. What is DNA library? Write different types of DNA library.
4. What is restriction fragment length polymorphism and its application?
5. What is cloning of DNA? Write its mechanism.
6. What is restriction endonuclease? Write its role in recombinant DNA technology.

SHORT ANSWER QUESTIONS (SAQs)

1. What is the difference between endonuclease and restriction endonuclease? Give two examples of restriction endonuclease.
2. What is the difference between genomic DNA library and c-DNA library?
3. Name the techniques used for detection of specific DNA, RNA and proteins.
4. What is blot transfer technique? Name different types with their application.
5. What is restriction fragment length polymorphism (RFLP)? Give its application.
6. What is PCR? Write its two applications.
7. What is cloning? Write its two applications.
8. Define recombinant DNA? Write its two applications.
9. What is chimeric DNA?
10. What is gene therapy? Write its applications.
11. Write different types of vectors used in recombinant DNA technology.

MULTIPLE CHOICE QUESTIONS (MCQs)

1. Restriction endonuclease has the following characteristics, *except*:
   a. Cut DNA in a sequence specific manner
   b. Named according to the bacteria from which they are isolated
   c. Most of the DNA sequences recognized by it are palindromic
   d. Cut DNA randomly
2. Most commonly used cloning vectors are:
   a. Bacterial plasmids
   b. Bacteriophages
   c. Cosmids
   d. All of the above
3. Cloning is a technique developed for:
   a. Amplifying the quantity of DNA in vivo
   b. Amplifying the quantity of DNA in vitro
   c. To search specific gene from DNA library
   d. To visualize specific DNA, RNA or proteins
4. Southern blot is a technique used for visualization of specific:
   a. RNA
   b. DNA
   c. Protein
   d. Carbohydrate
5. Polymerase chain reaction (PCR) is a technique for:
   a. Amplification of DNA in vitro
   b. Amplification of DNA in vivo
   c. Amplification of protein
   d. Amplification of RNA
6. Which one of the following enzymes is required for PCR?
   a. DNA ligase
   b. Thymidine kinase
   c. Taq polymerase
   d. Restriction endonuclease
7. Restriction endonucleases are enzymes:
   a. Used to joining DNA to cloning vector
   b. Which cleaves DNA at specific sequence?
   c. Which cleaves DNA randomly
   d. Which digest DNA molecule from ends
8. Construction of recombinant DNA requires which of the following steps.
   a. Fragmentation of DNA by restriction endonuclease enzyme
   b. Isolation of specific human DNA
   c. Insertion of isolated human DNA into vector to form hybrid DNA
   d. All of the above

9. Which of the following is correct for complementary DNA (cDNA) library?
   a. Is reverse transcribed from functional eukaryotic mRNA?
   b. Remains as a single-stranded molecule
   c. Exons as well as introns are presented
   d. All of the above.

10. Restriction endonucleases.
    a. Cut RNA chains at specific locations
    b. Excise introns from mRNA
    c. Remove Okazaki fragments
    d. Act as defensive enzymes to protect the host bacterial DNA from DNA of foreign organisms

11. Restriction endonucleases recognize and cut a certain sequence of:
    a. Single-stranded DNA   b. Double-stranded DNA
    c. RNA   d. Protein

12. Restriction endonucleases are present in:
    a. Viruses   b. Bacteria
    c. Eukaryotes   d. All of these

13. Restriction endonucleases can recognize.
    a. Palindromic sequences
    b. Chimeric DNA
    c. DNA-RNA hybrids
    d. Homopolymer sequences

14. All of the following statements about restriction endonucleases are true, *except*:
    a. They are present in bacteria
    b. They act on double-stranded DNA
    c. They recognize palindromic sequences
    d. They always produce sticky ends

15. Fragments of DNA can be identified by the technique of:
    a. Western blotting   b. Eastern blotting
    c. Northern blotting   d. Southern blotting

16. A particular RNA in a mixture can be identified by:
    a. Western blotting   b. Eastern blotting
    c. Northern blotting   d. Southern blotting

17. The first protein synthesized by recombinant DNA technology was:
    a. Streptokinase
    b. Human growth hormone
    c. Tissue plasminogen activator
    d. Human insulin

18. Trials for gene therapy in human beings were first carried out, with considerable success, in a genetic disease called.
    a. Cystic fibrosis
    b. Thalassemia
    c. Adenosine deaminase deficiency
    d. Lesch-Nyhan syndrome

19. Chimeric DNA:
    a. Is found in bacteriophages
    b. Contain unrelated genes
    c. Has no restriction sites
    d. Is palindromic

20. In addition to Taq polymerase, polymerase chain reaction requires all of the following, *except*:
    a. A template DNA
    b. Deoxyribonucleoside triphosphates
    c. Primers
    d. Primase

21. The normal function of restriction endonucleases is to:
    a. Excise introns from mRNA
    b. Polymerize nucleotides to form RNA
    c. Remove primer from Okazaki fragments
    d. Protect bacteria from foreign DNA

22. cDNA used in gene amplification in bacteria of genomic DNA because:
    a. Easy to replicate
    b. Human genome has many introns that cannot be removed by bacteria
    c. Promoter are not found
    d. Complete genome cannot be replicated

23. After digestion by restriction endonucleases DNA strands can be joined again by:
    a. DNA polymerase
    b. DNA ligase
    c. DNA topoisomerase
    d. DNA gyrase

■ ANSWERS FOR MCQs

1. d	2. d	3. a	4. b	5. a
6. c	7. b	8. d	9. a	10. d
11. b	12. b	13. a	14. d	15. d
16. c	17. d	18. c	19. b	20. d
21. d	22. a,b,d	23. b		

Nutrition in Health and Disease

Competency	Learning Objectives
BI 8.1: Discuss the importance of various dietary components and explain importance of dietary fiber. **BI 8.2:** Describe the types and causes of protein energy malnutrition and its effects. **BI 8.3:** Provide dietary advice for optimal health in childhood and adult, in disease conditions like diabetes mellitus, coronary artery disease, and in pregnancy. **BI 8.4:** Describe the causes (including dietary habits), effects and health risks associated with being overweight/ obesity. **BI 8.5:** Summarize the nutritional importance of commonly used items of food including fruits and vegetables. (Macromolecules and its importance). **BI 11.23:** Calculate energy content of different food Items, identify food items with high and low glycemic index and explain the importance of these in the diet	1. Describe various types of dietary components required for growth and the maintenance of life. 2. Describe the importance and requirement of carbohydrates, dietary fibers, fats, proteins, vitamins and minerals. 3. Describe energy requirements and factors affecting energy expenditure: BMR, SDA of food and physical activity. 4. Describe balance diet for optimal health. 5. Describe types, causes and effects of protein energy malnutrition (PEM). 6. Describe causes, effects and health risk associated with overweight/ obesity. 7. Describe dietary advice for optimal health in adult, childhood, and in pregnancy. 8. Describe dietary advice for optimal health in diabetes mellitus, and coronary artery disease. 9. Describe various groups of food items and their nutritional importance. 10. Describe energy content of different food items and its calculation. 11. Describe glycemic index and its importance in the diet.

OVERVIEW

Nutrition is the science of food and the nutrients and other substances contained in food. It is the study of their actions, interactions, and balance in relation to health and disease. Thus, nutrition is concerned with the digestion, absorption, transport, metabolism, and functions performed by the essential nutrients.

Nutrition is best defined as the composition and quantity of food intake and the utilization of the food by living organism. Study of human nutrition can be divided into three areas; **undernutrition, overnutrition,** and **ideal nutrition.** Overnutrition is a particularly serious problem in developing countries, and thus is at risk for a number of series health consequences. There is increasing interest in the concept of ideal or optimal nutrition.

DIETARY COMPONENTS REQUIRED FOR GROWTH AND THE MAINTENANCE OF LIFE

Dietary components called, **nutrients** are the necessary constituents of food required by organisms for growth and the maintenance of life. There are five classes of nutrients that contribute to an adequate diet **(Table 24.1)**. Each plays a special role. These may be divided into: **macronutrients** and **micronutrients**.

TABLE 24.1: Essential nutrients required by human beings.

Macronutrients	Micronutrients
Carbohydrates	**Vitamins**
Glucose	Fat soluble vitamins
Fiber	• Retinol (A)
Fat	• Cholecalciferol (D)
Essential fatty acids	• α-tocopherol (E)
• Linoleic acid	• Phylloquinone (K)
• Linolenic acid	Water soluble vitamins
Protein	• Thiamine (B_1)
Essential amino acids	• Riboflavin (B_2)
• Phenylalanine	• Niacin
• Valine	• Pyridoxine (B_6)
• Threonine	• Pantothenic acid
• Tryptophan	• Biotin
• Isoleucine	• Folic acid
• Methionine	• Cobalamine (B_{12})
• Histidine	**Mineral elements**
• Arginine	Macrominerals
• Leucine	Na^+, K^+, Ca^+, Mg^{++}, P, S, and Cl^-
• Lysine	Microminerals
	Cr, Co, Cu, F, I, Fe, Mn, Mo, Se, Zn

Macronutrients

These are **proteins**, **fats**, and **carbohydrates**. They form the main bulk of food. Protein, fat, and carbohydrate are sometimes referred to as **proximate principle**. They are oxidized in the body to yield energy, which the body needs. The entire energy requirement for the body is provided by these three nutrients. They supply energy at the following rates. The energy content of fat is more than twice that of carbohydrate or protein.

- **Protein:** 4 kcal/g or 17 kJ
- **Fat:** 9 kcal/g or 38 kJ
- **Carbohydrate:** 4 kcal/g or 17 kJ

In the Indian food, **proteins**, **fats**, and **carbohydrates** contribute to the total energy intake in the following proportions.

Proteins: 7–15%

Fats: 35–45%

Carbohydrates: 50–70%

- Although proteins provide energy their primary function is to provide **essential** and **nonessential amino acids** for building of body proteins. If an adequate energy supply is not provided, some protein will be burnt to provide energy.
- **Fats** particularly the vegetable oils, besides being concentrated source of energy, provide **essential fatty acids** which have a **vitamin** like function in the body.
- **Water** is the solvent of the body and transport vehicle for distributing nutrients to the tissues. Water, although not a nutrient by definition, is of course required to replace the water lost in the urine, breath, and sweat.
- **Fiber** also is not a nutrient but is being considered as a necessary food component. In plant foods, fibers (dietary fiber) which have undigestible complex molecules also contribute to the bulk and have some useful functions in the digestive tract. Role of fiber is discussed later.

Micronutrients

Vitamins and minerals are called micronutrients **(Table 24.1)**. They are called micronutrients because they are required in small amounts which may vary from a microgram to several milligrams. Vitamins and minerals do not supply energy but they play an important role in the regulation of the metabolic activity in the body and help in the utilization of **proximate principles**. Minerals are also used for the formation of body structure and skeleton.

IMPORTANCE AND REQUIREMENT OF CARBOHYDRATES, DIETARY FIBERS, FATS, PROTEINS, VITAMINS AND MINERALS

Importance and Requirement of Carbohydrates

Carbohydrates are one of three macronutrients along with proteins and fats that body requires daily. Carbohydrates are the main source of energy for brain, kidneys, heart muscles, and central nervous system. There are three main types of carbohydrates: **soluble sugars**, **starches**, and **fiber**. These dietary carbohydrates divided into two types:

1. Available or digestible carbohydrate (soluble sugars and starch)
   - Simple carbohydrates
   - Complex carbohydrates
2. Unavailable or undigestible carbohydrate (fiber).

- **The available or digestible carbohydrates** are a major source of food energy. These include:
  - **Simple carbohydrates** which comprises, soluble sugars. The term "sugars" is conventionally used to describe the mono and disaccharides. Sugar is the simplest form of carbohydrate and occurs naturally in some foods, including fruits, vegetables, milk, and milk products. Types of sugar include fruit sugar (fructose), table sugar (sucrose), and milk sugar (lactose).
  - **Complex carbohydrates** for example starch. Starch is made of many sugar units bonded together. Starch occurs naturally in vegetables, grains, beans, and peas. One of the important of carbohydrates for health is **resistant starch**. Resistant starch is defined as "starch and starch degradation products not absorbed in the small intestine of healthy humans".
- **Unavailable** or **undigestible carbohydrates** provide **dietary fiber**. Some carbohydrate is not digested and absorbed in the small intestine but rather reaches the large bowel where it is fermented. Fiber is not digested by the digestive enzymes and does not serve as a source of energy. It is however a significant component of the

diet. It occurs naturally in fruits, vegetables, whole grains, and cereals.

Importance of Carbohydrates

Carbohydrates have significant physiological effects, which is important to health, such as:

- Provision of energy carbohydrate as an energy source, yielding 4 kcal/g and provide about 50–70% of the energy requirement. Carbohydrates are the main source of energy for brain, kidneys, heart muscles, and central nervous system. Brain entirely depends on glucose for energy.
- Carbohydrates have protein sparing effect. By using carbohydrates for energy, the breakdown of proteins for energy decreases and proteins are spared to its primary function i.e., body building, synthesis of hormones, and enzymes.
- Supply of pentose sugars (ribose) for the formation of nucleic acids (RNA and DNA).
- Bowel movement:
  - It has long been known that non-starch poly-saccharides are the principal dietary component affecting **laxation**. Fermentable polysaccharides stimulate the growth of bacteria in the large gut which leads to an increase in microbial biomass in the colon. The increased biomass results in some increase in fecal weight and is one of the mechanisms whereby carbohydrate influences bowel habit. Foods which selectively stimulate the growth of gut bacteria are known as **pre-biotics**.
  - The **non-fermentable polysaccharides** are not degraded in the colon and become constituents of the stool. They have a tendency to hold water and produce a marked increase in fecal weight. Similarly, **resistant starch** can increase fecal weight.

Carbohydrate Requirement

- The minimum carbohydrate requirement for adults is 130 grams.
- This is the **minimum** amount of **carbohydrates** needed to produce enough glucose for the brain to function.
- **WHO** suggests, in balanced diet carbohydrates, should provide the energy requirements – between 50 and 70% of **daily intake** and free sugars should remain below 10% of total energy intake. Protein should make up a further 10–15% of calorie **intake**.
- Most Indian diets contain amounts more than this, providing as much as 90% of total energy intake in some cases, which make the diet **imbalanced**.

Dietary Fibers and their Importance in the Diet

Dietary fiber is the name given collectively to indigestible carbohydrates present in foods. These carbohydrates consist of **cellulose**, **pectin**, **gum**, and **mucilage**. The dietary fiber is not digested by the enzyme of the human gastrointestinal tract, where most of the other carbohydrates like starch, sugars are digested and absorbed. Plant foods are the only sources of dietary fiber. It is found in vegetables, fruits, and grains. Fiber is commonly classified as **soluble** and **insoluble**. The amount of soluble and insoluble fiber varies in different plant foods.

- **Soluble fiber:** This type of fiber dissolves in water to form a gel-like material during digestion. They increase stool bulk and may lower blood cholesterol and glucose levels. Soluble fiber can be found in fruits (such as apples, oranges and grapefruit), vegetables, legumes (such as dry beans, lentils, and peas), barley, oats and oat bran.
- **Insoluble fiber:** Insoluble fiber does not dissolve in water but can absorb and hold water. They remain unchanged during digestion. They promote the movement of intestinal contents and increases stool bulk and prevents constipation. Whole-wheat flour, wheat bran, nuts, beans and vegetables, such as cauliflower, green beans and potatoes, are good sources of insoluble fiber.

Importance of Fiber

Water holding capacity: The dietary fibers have a property of holding water and swell like sponge with a concomitant increase in viscosity. Thus, fiber adds bulk to the diet and increases transit time in the gut (gastric emptying time) due to high viscosity.

Physiological effects: Dietary fiber exerts its influence along the entire gastrointestinal tract from ingestion to excretion **(Table 24.2)**.

Adsorption of organic molecules: The organic molecules like bile acids, neutral sterols, carcinogens, and toxic compounds can be adsorbed on dietary fiber and facilitates its excretion.

It increases stool bulk: The fiber absorbs water and increases the bulk of the stool and helps to reduce the tendency towards constipation by increasing bowel movements.

Hypoglycemic effect of fiber: Recent studies have shown that gum present in fenugreek seeds (it contains 40% gum) are most effective in reducing blood sugar and cholesterol levels.

TABLE 24.2: Activities of dietary fiber along the entire GI tract.

Site	Activity
Mouth	Stimulates saliva secretion
Stomach	Delays gastric empting
Small intestine	Delays absorption
Large intestine	Traps water, binds cations
Stool	Softens, enlarges, prevents straining

Hypocholesterolemic effects of fiber: Fiber has cholesterol lowering effect. Fiber binds **bile acids** and **cholesterol**, increasing their fecal exertion, and thus, decreasing plasma and tissue cholesterol level.

Clinical Significance of Dietary Fiber

High fiber diet is associated with reduced incidence of a number of diseases like:
- Coronary heart disease (CHD)
- Colon cancer
- Diabetes
- Diverticulosis
- Hemorrhoids (piles).

Daily Recommendations for Adult

Total dietary fiber intake should be **25 to 30 grams** a day from food, not supplements.

Adverse Effect of Dietary Fiber

Dietary fiber also has some adverse effects on nutrition. Dietary fiber binds some mineral elements and prevents their proper absorption. Thus, high dietary fiber intake may lead to deficiency of mineral elements.

Importance and Requirement of Fat

Fat gets a bad rap even though it is a nutrient that we need in our diet. Dietary fats are essential to give energy and to support cell growth. Dietary fats are high energy yielding nutrients. Fat yields **9 kcal/g**. Fats are more energy-dense than carbohydrates and proteins, which provide **4 kcal/g**. Besides satisfying metabolic energy needs, there are essential functions of dietary fat, namely:
- Fats help for the absorption of the fat soluble vitamins (A, D, E, and K).
- Fat supply essential fatty acids, **linoleic acid** and **linolenic acid** to the body.
- Fat help produce important hormones like steroid hormones, prostaglandins etc.
- Dietary lipid also increases the **palatability** of food and produces a feeling of **satiety**.
- They also help protect our organs and help keep body warm.

Types of Dietary Fats

There are four major dietary fats in the foods we eat:
1. Saturated fats
2. Transfats
3. Monounsaturated fats
4. Polyunsaturated fats.

- The bad fats, **saturated** and **trans fats**, tend to be more solid at room temperature (like a butter), while monounsaturated and polyunsaturated fats tend to be more liquid (like liquid vegetable oil).

- The saturated fats and *trans* fats raise bad cholesterol (LDL) levels in blood.
- Monounsaturated fats and polyunsaturated fats can lower bad cholesterol levels and are beneficial when consumed.
- Consuming high levels of saturated or *trans* fats can also lead to heart disease and stroke.
- Replacement of saturated fats and *trans* fats with monounsaturated fats and polyunsaturated fats is recommend.

Requirement of Fat

- The daily requirement of fat is not known with certainty. As per WHO fat intake should be in balance with energy expenditure. To avoid unhealthy weight gain, total fat should not exceed 30% of the total energy intake of which at least 50% of fat intake should consist of vegetable oils rich in essential fatty acids.
- Intake of saturated fats should be less than 10% of total energy intake, and intake of trans fats less than 1% of total energy intake.

Requirement of Protein and Amino Acids

Proteins are vital to any living organism. Proteins are important constituent of tissues and cells of the body. Protein is essential for growth and repair and the maintenance of good health. They form the important component of muscle and other tissues and vital body fluids like blood. A large proportion of this will be muscle (43% on average) with significant proportions being present in skin (15%) and blood (16%).
- Protein provides the body with approximately 10 to 15% of its dietary energy and it is the second most abundant compound in the body, following water.
- The proteins in the form of enzymes and hormones are concerned with wide range of vital metabolic processes in the body.
- Protein as antibodies helps the body to defend against infections.
- Proteins supply **essential** and **nonessential amino acids** for the synthesis of protein and nitrogen for the synthesis of several key compounds such as neurotransmitter purines, pyrimidines, heme etc.

Thus, proteins are one of the most important nutrient required by the body and should be supplied in adequate amounts in the diet.

> The amino acids, which are not used for protein synthesis, are broken down to provide energy, which is a wasteful way of using proteins (this is not their primary function). Hence, diet should contain adequate carbohydrate and fat to provide energy so that the proteins in the diet are most economically used for the formation of body proteins to fulfil other functions essential to life.

TABLE 24.3: Minimum requirement of essential amino acids.

Essential amino acid	Requirement (mg/kg body weight/per day)
Phenylalanine	14
Leucine	11
Lysine	9
Valine	14
Isoleucine	10
Threonine	6
Methionine	14
Tryptophan	3

TABLE 24.4: Deficient amino acids of some important food proteins.

Protein source	Protein type	Limiting amino acid
Animal protein	Egg	Nil
	Milk	S-containing amino acid
	Meat	S-containing amino acid
	Fish	Tryptophan
Vegetable proteins	Rice	Lysine, Threonine
Cereals	Wheat	Lysine, Threonine
Pulses	Bengal gram	S-containing amino acid
	Red gram	S-containing amino acid
Oil seeds	Ground nut	Lysine, Threonine S-containing amino acid
	Soya bean	S-containing amino acid

Essential Amino Acids

Any amino acid that humans either cannot synthesize or are unable to synthesize in adequate quantity is termed "essential" and rest of the amino acids are called **nonessential** as they can synthesized in the body. An essential amino acid must be provided in the diet. An absence of an essential amino acid from the diet impairs protein synthesis and generally causes negative nitrogen balance, i.e., the total nitrogen losses in the urine, feces, and sweat exceed the dietary nitrogen intake.

Ten of the twenty amino acids found in proteins are essential for humans **(see Table 24.1)** (*Refer* **Chapter 4**). Of the 10 essential amino acids, 8 are essential at all times during life. The other two namely **histidine** and **arginine** are required in the diet during periods of rapid growth as in childhood and pregnancy and called **semi essential** or **conditional amino** acids. Each amino acid is required in differing amounts. Minimum requirements of essential amino acids are shown in **Table 24.3**.

Protein Requirement

- The requirement is dependent on the **quality** of dietary protein. The ICMR Expert Group suggested an intake of **one gram of protein per kg of body weight** for adult males and females, assuming, net protein utilization (NPU) of 65 for dietary protein. The requirement should be nearly double for growing children, pregnant, and lactating women.
- The protein requirement varies with the NPU of dietary protein. If the NPU is low, the protein requirement is high and vice versa. The NPU of the protein of Indian diets varies between 50 and 60.
- In refereeing the adequacy of dietary proteins to meet the human needs, not only the quantity but the nutritional quality of the dietary proteins also matters. Proteins present in different foods vary in their nutritional quality because of the differences in their amino acid composition. **The quality of protein depends on the pattern of essential amino acids it supplies**.
- The best quality protein is the one which provides essential amino acid pattern very close to the pattern of the tissue proteins. Egg proteins, human milk protein, satisfy these criteria and are classified as high quality proteins and serve as **reference protein** for defining the quality of other proteins. Deficient amino acids of some important food proteins are given in **Table 24.4**.

Mutual Supplementation of Proteins

It is seen that generally animal proteins are of higher biological value than proteins from plant foods. Plant proteins are of poorer quality since essential amino acids (EAAs) composition is not well balanced and a few EAAs deviate much from the optimal level present in egg. For example in comparison with egg protein, **cereal proteins** are poor in amino acid **lysine**. **Pulses** and **oil seed proteins** are rich in lysine but they are poor in **sulfur containing amino acids**. Such proteins individually are therefore **incomplete proteins**.

However, relative insufficiency of a particular amino acid of any vegetable food can be overcome by wise combination with other vegetable foods, which may have adequate level of that limiting (deficient) amino acid. The amino acid composition of these proteins **complement** each other and the resulting mixture will have an amino acid pattern better than either of the constituent proteins of the mixture.

This is the procedure normally used to improve quality of vegetable proteins. This phenomenon is called **mutual supplementation effect of amino acid**.

Thus, a protein of cereals, deficient in lysine and pulses with adequate lysine content have a mutually supplementary effect, a deficiency of an amino acid in one can be made good by an adequate level in another, if both are consumed together. Thus, the habitual diets of vegetarians in India based on cereal and pulse helps to overcome the deficiency of certain essential amino acids in one food.

Nitrogen Balance

Protein requirements can be determined by measuring **nitrogen balance**. Protein is the major dietary source of nitrogen. The output of nitrogen from the body is mainly in the form of urea and smaller quantities of other compounds in urine (like uric acid and creatinine), undigested protein (including digestive enzymes and shed intestinal mucosal cells) in feces; significant amount may also be lost in sweat and shed skin.

Nitrogen balance tells about state of protein nutrition and its loss from the body. A balance between amount of nitrogen intake in the form of dietary protein and amount of nitrogen lost or excreted in the form of urea and small amount of amino acids by an individual is known as **nitrogen balance**.

Nitrogen balance can be determined by measuring the dietary intake and output of nitrogenous compounds from the body. Measurement of total nitrogen intake gives a good estimate of protein intake by using the formula: (mg Nitrogen × 6.25 = mg protein). Protein contains approximately 16% nitrogen by weight, so 1 g of nitrogen corresponds to 6.25 g of proteins.

Catabolism of amino acids leads to a net loss of nitrogen from the body. This loss must be compensated by the diet in order to maintain a constant amount of body protein. Three states can be defined.

- **Nitrogen equilibrium: Nitrogen intake equals nitrogen excretion.**

  A normal healthy adult is in **nitrogen equilibrium** since the daily dietary intake is equal to the loss through urine, feces, and sweat. In this situation, the rate of body protein synthesis is equal to the rate of degradation and there is no change in the total body content of protein.

- **Positive nitrogen balance: Intake of nitrogen is more than excretion.**

  It shows that nitrogen is retained in the body, which means that protein is laid down. In growing **child, a pregnant woman**, or a person in recovery from protein loss, the excretion of nitrogenous compounds is less than the dietary intake and there is net retention of nitrogen in the body as protein and is called positive Nitrogen Balance.

- **Negative nitrogen balance: Nitrogen output exceeds input.**

  This occurs during **serious illness** and **major injury** and **trauma**, in **advanced cancer** or if the intake of protein is inadequate to meet requirements, there is net loss of protein nitrogen from the body e.g.,, in **kwashiorkor** and **marasmus**. If the situation is prolonged, it will ultimately lead to death.

Importance and Requirement of Vitamins and Minerals

The nutritional aspects including metabolism, biochemical functions dietary sources, requirements and associated pathological conditions for vitamins **(Chapter 9)** and for minerals **(Chapter 15)** have been discussed in much detail.

ENERGY REQUIREMENTS AND FACTORS AFFECTING ENERGY EXPENDITURE

Energy is the principal requisite for body function and growth. The energy requirement of an individual is defined as the energy intake which will balance energy expenditure in an individual, whose body size and composition and level of physical activity are consistent with long-term good health.

- For children and for pregnant and lactating women, allowances are additionally made for growth of tissue and production of milk.

- Energy intake has to be adequate to meet energy expenditure, otherwise the body's reserves will be utilized without being properly replenished, resulting in loss of body weight, impairment of various body functions and finally death.

- If, on the other hand, the energy intake is excessive, compared to the energy expenditure, the body's fuel reserves will increase, resulting in **obesity** which is also a health risk.

- Determinations of energy requirements depend, therefore, on measurements of energy expenditure. All energy in the diet is provided by three nutrients:
  - *Protein:* 4 kcal/g or 17 kJ
  - *Fat:* 9 kcal/g or 38 kJ
  - *Carbohydrate:* 4 kcal/g or 17 kJ

  The energy content of fat is more than twice that of carbohydrate or protein. If an adequate energy supply is not provided, some protein will be burnt to provide energy.

Factors Affecting Energy Expenditure

The energy expended by an individual depends on three main factors:

1. The basal metabolic rate (BMR).
2. The thermogenic effect (specific dynamic actions, SDA) of food.
3. Physical activity, and

   Besides the above four factors extra provision of energy has to be made for growth, pregnancy, and lactation.

The Basal Metabolic Rate

- The basal metabolic rate (BMR) is the energy expenditure necessary to maintain basic physiologic functions, such as:
  - The activity of the heart
  - Respiration
  - Conduction of nerve impulses
  - Ion transport across membranes
  - Reabsorption in the kidney
  - Metabolic activity such as synthesis of macromolecules.

- BMR is defined as the energy expenditure at rest, awake (but not during sleep), 8 to 12 hours after the last meal and 8 to 12 hours after any significant physical activity. The total caloric expenditure in 24 hours to complete basal state is 1,800 kcal for adult males and 1,400 kcal for adult females, assuming that the total body surface areas are 1.8 sqm and 1.6 sqm respectively.

- Basal metabolic rate can be measured by:
  - Calorimeter directly by measuring the heat dissipated under basal condition
  - Indirectly by measuring oxygen consumption.

Normal Values of BMR

- The BMR values are expressed as kcal per square meter of body surface per hour.
- In adults, BMR for:
  - Healthy males is 40 kcal/sqm/h
  - Healthy females, it is 37 kcal/sqm/h.

> ❖ Determination of BMR is useful for the diagnosis of disorders of thyroid. In hypothyroidism, BMR is low while in hyperthyroidism it is elevated.
> ❖ BMR is used in calculating caloric requirements of an individual and planning of diets.

Factors Affecting BMR

The BMR differs among different individuals. It depends on many factors as follows:

Gender or sex: The BMR of the males is slightly higher than that of females, partly due to:

- Women's lower percentage of muscle mass (lean body mass) and higher percentage of adipose tissue (that has lower rate of metabolism), when compared to men of the same body weight.
- The difference in sex hormone profile of the two genders.

Age: Decline in BMR with increasing age is probably related to loss of muscle mass (lean body mass) and replacement of muscle with adipose tissue that has lower rate of metabolism.

Nutritional state: BMR is low in starvation and under-nourishment as compared to well-fed state. Starvation leads to an adaptive decrease in BMR, which results from a decrease in lean body mass.

Body size or surface area: The BMR is directly proportional to the surface area of the subject. Larger the surface area, greater will be the heat loss and equally higher will be the heat production and BMR.

Body composition: The BMR is proportionate to lean body mass, (LBM). LBM is the body weight minus non-essential (storage triacylglycerol) weight. Adipose tissue is not as metabolically active as lean body mass. BMR is often expressed as per kilogram of lean body mass or fat-free mass. Therefore, higher the percentage of adipose tissue in the body, lower the BMR/kg body weight.

Endocrinological or hormonal state: In hyperthyroidism, the BMR is increased and in hypothyroidism it may be decreased by up to 40%, leading to weight gain.

Environmental temperature or climate: In colder climate, the BMR is higher and in tropical climates the BMR is proportionally low. Stress, anxiety and disease states, especially infections, fever, burns and cancer also increase the BMR.

Drugs: Smoking (nicotine), coffee (caffeine) and tea (theophylline) increase the BMR, whereas β-blockers tend to decrease energy expenditure.

The Thermogenic Effect of Food (TEF) or Specific Dynamic Action (SDA)

Another factor of energy expenditure is **diet induced thermogenesis**, also known as **postprandial thermogenesis** or **dietary induced thermogenesis (DIT)**. This is the energy used in the **digestion**, **absorption**, **storage** and subsequent **processing** of food. In other words, to get the energy from of the food, we must first spend some energy to digest, absorb, and transport it to the body's cells. This is called **thermogenic effect of food (TEF)** as these processes require energy and generate heat.

- Some constituents of our food have a greater effect on TEF than the others. Compared to carbohydrate and fat, protein has the highest TEF.
- In order to process a protein meal will require 30% of the calories expenditure. This means that out of every 100 g of protein consumed, the energy available for doing useful work is 30% less than the calculated value. The other two macronutrients, carbohydrate and fat, have lower thermic effect: carbohydrate digestion will cause 5–15% and fat 5% of the calories expenditure. This means most easily digested are fats.
- The thermogenic effect of food varies considerably from individual to individual. It has been suggested that in some people, a high degree of diet induced thermogenesis may be a factor which allows them to maintain their normal body weight even after overeating.
- The thermogenic effect of mixed food is 10% of overall calories.
- The thermogenic effect of food is equivalent to about 5 to 10% of total energy expenditure. This effect was originally recognized only to the metabolic processing of **protein** and was termed **specific dynamic action (SDA)**, but it is now recognized as an effect produced by the consumption of all dietary fuels.

Physical Activity

Physical activity is the largest variable affecting energy expenditure. For convenience, the activity level may be divided

TABLE 24.5: Energy expenditure during different types of activity for a 70 kg man.

Kind of activity	Calories/h
Sleeping	65
Awake lying still	77
Sitting at rest	100
Standing relaxed	105
Walking slowly (2.6 miles/h)	200
Swimming	500
Running (5.3 miles/h)	570
Walking upstairs rapidly	1100

into three groups—**sedentary**, **moderate**, and **heavy** with regard to their physical activity and requirement of energy.

- **Sedentary work people:** 2,200 to 2,400 kcal/day
- **Moderate work people:** 2,500 to 2,900 kcal/day
- **Heavy work people:** 2,900 to 3,500 kcal/day
  Table 24.5 shows energy expenditure during different types of physical activity for a 70 kg man.

▌BALANCED DIET FOR OPTIMAL HEALTH

A balanced diet is defined as one which contains a variety of foods in such quantities and proportions that the need for energy, amino acids, vitamins, minerals, fats, carbohydrate, and other nutrients is adequately met for maintaining health, vitality and general well-being and also makes a small provision for extra nutrients to withstand short duration of illness.

- In constructing balanced diet, the following principles are considered:
  - The daily requirement of protein should be met. This amounts to 10–15% of the daily energy intake.
  - The fat requirement, which should be limited to 15–30% of the daily energy intake

- Carbohydrates rich in natural fiber should constitute the remaining food energy. The requirements of micronutrients should be met.
- The dietary pattern varies widely in different parts of the world. It is generally developed according to the:
  - Kinds of food produced (which depends upon the climatic conditions of the region)
  - Economic capacity
  - Religion
  - Customs
  - Tastes and habits of the people.
- Indian Council of Medical Research (ICMR) has formulated balanced diet for different age groups, sex, and under various occupations for physical activity. These are given in **Table 24.6** and **Table 24.7**. During pregnancy and lactation, additional food is required. This is shown in **Table 24.8**. For nonvegetarians, ICMR has recommended substitution of a part of pulses by animal food **(Table 24.9)**.
- "The Food Guide Pyramid" is an outline of what to eat each day based on the dietary guidelines. The Pyramid provides information on the food types and amounts necessary to meet daily dietary requirements. The Indian adaptation of the Food Pyramid is divided into four levels of foods according to recommended consumption: **(Figure 24.1)**.
  - Cereals, legumes/beans, dairy products at the base should be eaten in sufficient quantity;
  - Vegetables and fruits on the second level should be eaten liberally;
  - Animal source foods and oils on the third level are to be eaten moderately; and
  - At the apex, highly processed foods that are high in sugar and fat are to be eaten sparingly.
- The Pyramid appeals for eating a variety of foods to get the needed nutrients by the body and at the same time the right amount of calories to maintain healthy weight.

TABLE 24.6: Balanced diet for adult suggested by ICMR.

Food item	Adult man			Adult woman		
	Sedentary work	Moderate work	Heavy work	Sedentary work	Moderate work	Heavy work
	Quantity gram per day			Quantity gram per day		
Cereals	460	520	670	410	440	575
Pulses	40	50	60	40	45	50
Leafy vegetables	40	40	40	100	100	100
Other vegetables	60	70	80	40	40	50
Roots and tubers	50	60	80	50	50	60
Milk	150	200	250	100	150	200
Oil and fat	40	45	65	20	25	40
Sugar or jaggery	30	35	55	20	20	40

TYPES, CAUSES AND EFFECTS OF PROTEIN ENERGY MALNUTRITION

When balanced diet is not consumed by a person for a sufficient length of time, it leads to nutritional deficiencies or disorders. This nutritional status is called **malnutrition**. The World Health Organization (WHO) defines malnutrition as

"the cellular imbalance between the supply of nutrients and energy and the body's demand for them to ensure growth, maintenance, and specific functions." The term protein-

TABLE 24.7: Balanced diet for children suggested by ICMR quantity gram per day.

Food items	Children		Boys	Girls
	1–3 years	4–6 years	10–12 years	10–12 years
Cereals	175	270	420	380
Pulses	35	35	45	45
Leafy vegetables	40	50	50	50
Other vegetables	20	30	50	50
Roots and tubers	10	20	30	30
Milk	300	250	250	250
Oil and fat	15	25	40	35
Sugar or jaggery	30	40	45	45

TABLE 24.8: Additional allowances during pregnancy and lactation.

Food items	During pregnancy (g/day)	Calories (kcal)	During lactation (g/day)	Calories (kcal)
Cereals	35	118	60	203
Pulses	15	118	60	203
Milk	15	83	100	83
Fat	–	–	10	90
Sugar	10	40	10	90
Total	–	293	–	521

TABLE 24.9: Suggested substitution for nonvegetarians.

Food item which can be deleted in nonvegetarian diets	Substitution that can be suggested for deleted item or items
50% of pulses (20–30 g)	One egg or 30 g of meat or fish Additional 5 g of fat or oil.
100% of pulses (40–60 g)	Two eggs or 50 g of meat or one egg +30 g meat or fish 10 g of fat or oil

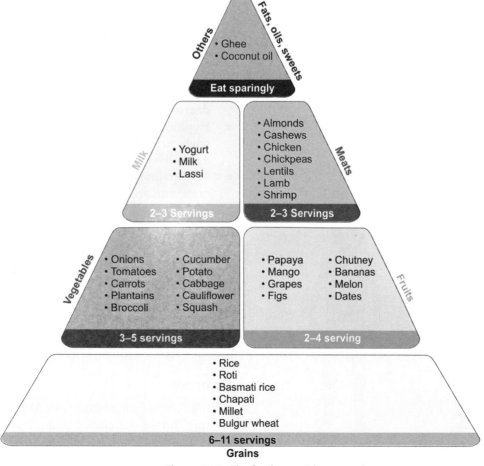

Figure 24.1: The food pyramid.

energy malnutrition (PEM) applies to a group of related disorders.

- Protein-energy malnutrition (PEM) is a common childhood disorder and is primarily caused by deficiency of **energy**, **protein**, and **micronutrients** in the diet.
- PEM manifests as underweight, stunting (poor linear growth), wasting (acute weight loss), or edematous malnutrition (kwashiorkor).
- PEM is primarily a problem in resource-limited countries. Worldwide, PEM is the leading cause of death in children under the age of 5. The highest prevalence is in Africa and south-central Asia.
- PEM is also found in developed countries under various circumstances, including fasting or anorexia nervosa (a mental health condition), cancer and severe chronic disease states.

Classification of PEM

The PEM can be classified into two form depends on the balance of nonprotein and protein sources of energy.

1. Kwashiorkor or edematous PEM.
2. Marasmus or nonedematous PEM

Kwashiorkor

- Kwashiorkor (edematous PEM) mostly occurs in children between the ages of 1 and 3 years.
- Kwashiorkor refers to conditions caused by severe **protein deficiency** in individuals with an **adequate energy intake**.
- Kwashiorkor is an African word that means **weaning disease**. When children are weaned from protein rich breast milk, they receive insufficient protein.
- **Kwashiorkor** is characterized by **(Figure 24.2)**:
  - Anorexia
  - Maintenance or gain of body fat

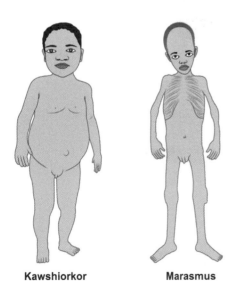

Kawshiorkor   **Marasmus**

Figure 24.2: Edematous kwashiorkor vs. emaciated marasmus.

TABLE 24.10: Features of kwashiorkor and marasmus.

Features	Kwashiorkor	Marasmus
Age of on set	1–5 years	Below 1 year
Edema	Present in lower legs, and usually in face and fare arms	None
Fatty liver	Frequent	None
Muscle wasting	Sometimes hidden by edema and fat	Severe
Fat wasting	Retained	Severe loss of subcutaneous fat
Mental changes	Irritable, moaning, apathetic	Sometimes quiet and apathetic
Appetite	Poor	Usually good
Diarrhea	Often	Often
Skin changes	Diffuse pigmentation	Usually none
Hair changes	Often sparse-straight and silky; depigmentation grayish or reddish	Texture may be modified but no depigmentation
Moon face	Often	None

- Peripheral edema due to the decrease in serum albumin
- Moon face
- Depigmented hair. The hair becomes thin, reddish brown, or gray.
- Dry, thin, wrinkled, and peeling skin
- Fatty liver
- Distended/protruded abdomen (due to enlarged liver).
- The edema is due **to low oncotic pressure** in the plasma due to **hypoalbuminemia**. Hypoalbuminemia is due to **decreased synthesis of plasma proteins** by the liver.
- Hypoalbuminemia in turn impairs the export of **triglycerides** and other lipids from the liver, resulting in a **fatty liver**.
- The major differences between kwashiorkor and marasmus are given in **Table 24.10**.

Biochemical Manifestations

- Decreased plasma albumin (<2 g/dL)
- Decreased immunity
- Decreased retinol binding protein.

Treatment

Ingestion of protein rich foods or the dietary combinations to provide about 3–4 g of protein/kg body weight/day.

Marasmus

- Marasmus (nonedematous PEM) is a chronic condition due to deficiency of both **protein** and **energy** (carbohydrate).
- Marasmus occurs in famine (extreme scarcity of food) areas when infants are weaned from breast milk and

given inadequate bottle feedings of thin watery gruels (liquid food) of native cereals or other plant foods to supplement the mother's breast milk. These watery gruels are usually deficient in both carbohydrates and proteins.

Marasmus is characterized by:

- Weight loss
- Diarrhea
- Dehydration
- Anemia
- Weakness
- Growth retardation
- Wasting of subcutaneous fat and muscle results in an **emaciated** appearance **(Figure 24.2)**
- Ribs and facial bones appear prominent
- Loose, thin skin hangs in folds

Biochemical Manifestations

- Increased serum cortisol. As the corticosteroid-binding globulin is low the free cortisol levels is high.
- Decreased fasting blood glucose
- Starvation adaptations cause serum protein and electrolyte concentrations to remain within their normal range and do not show edema.

Treatment

Not only the symptoms but the complications of disorders including infections, dehydration, and circulation disorders should be treated.

THE CAUSES, EFFECTS, AND HEALTH RISK ASSOCIATED WITH OVERWEIGHT/OBESITY

Overweight/obesity are the pathological state. Obesity is becoming a worldwide problem affecting all levels of society and is thus being described as a global epidemic.

Definition of Obesity

Overweight and obesity are defined as "abnormal or excessive fat accumulation that presents a risk to health". Childhood obesity is one of the most serious public health challenges of the 21st century. Today's lifestyle promotes the development of obesity. The lack of physical activity, sedentary lifestyle and energy-rich diet are the main causes of an excess body fat accumulation.

- Overweight and obesity in adults is classified on the basis of **Body Mass Index (BMI)**.
- BMI is defined as the weight in kilograms divided by the square of the height in meters (kg/m²).

$$BMI = \frac{Body\ weight\ (kg)}{Height\ (m^2)}$$

TABLE 24.11: Relationship between BMI and degree of obesity

Value of BMI	Degree of obesity
20–25	Normal
25–30	Overweight or obesity grade I
30–35	Over obesity or grade II
Above 35	Gross obesity or grade III

- WHO defines overweight as a BMI equal to or more than 25, and obesity as a BMI equal to or more than 30. It is same for both sexes and for all ages of adults.
- WHO classifies underweight, normal weight, overweight and obesity according to categories of BMI is given in **Table 24.11**. However, it should be considered as a rough guide because it may not correspond to the same body fat percentage in different individuals.

The Causes of Obesity

The fundamental cause of childhood overweight and obesity is an energy imbalance between calories consumed and calories expended which may be:

- Metabolic
- Hormonal
- Genetic
- Changes in lifestyle and eating habits.

Metabolic

- Obesity may result due to accumulation of **triacylglycerol**. The triacylglycerol accumulates when:
  - Caloric intake exceeds the amount needed for body function and the amount of work being done.
  - Deficiency of the enzyme **ATPase** which impairs normal energy metabolism and gain more weight.

Hormonal

- Apart from increased intake of energy rich foods and decreased exercise and physical activity, hormones also play a role in obesity and overweight.
- Several hormones including **leptin (adipokine)**, **insulin**, **sex hormones**, and **growth hormones** play a role in appetite, metabolism, body fat distribution and increased storage of excess energy in food as fats.
- Leptin is released from the adipocytes in amounts proportional to the body weight. This hormone reaches the brain and binds with its receptors and causes decrease in appetite and an increase in heat generation from energy both leading to a decrease in obesity.
- Despite of high level of leptin, obese people are not sensitive to the effects of leptin and thus do not have a reduced appetite. This could be due to **deficiency of leptin receptors** in these individuals.
- The pituitary gland in the brain produces **growth hormone**. Growth hormone also affects metabolism

of all the nutrients taken by the body. Levels of growth hormone are lower in obese people than normal individuals.

- Obesity may result from endocrine disorders like:
  - Hypothyroidism
  - Hypogonadism
  - Hypopituitarism
  - Cushing's syndrome (excess cortisol increase appetite).

Genetic

- Several genes have the potential to cause obesity in humans, e.g., mutation in **leptin gene (*ob gene*)** results in obesity.
- In normal individuals leptin leads to suppression of food intake.
- Grossly obese humans have a failure in production of leptin.

Changes in Lifestyle and Eating Habits

Unhealthy dietary habits and poor selection of food may be responsible the obesity. There has been a global shift in diet towards increased intake of **energy-dense foods** that are high in fat and sugars but low in vitamins, minerals, and other healthy micronutrients.

- Because of improper eating behaviors children consume an excess amount of energy; and their diet is deficient in elements necessary for proper development.
- The examples of such bad eating habits are: snacking highly processed and calorie-rich foods between meals eating in front of the TV screen, skipping breakfasts, drinking sugar-sweetened beverages, "eating out" frequently and "emotional eating".
- Bad eating behaviors are crucial factors for the development of obesity. Eating habits are usually formed in early childhood and parents play a very important role in their development.
- There is also a trend towards decreased **physical activity** levels due to the increasingly social and economic development and policies in the areas of transport, urban planning, the environment, food processing, distribution and marketing, as well as education.

Health Risk Associated with Obesity

Childhood obesity is associated with a higher chance of premature death and disability in adulthood. Overweight and obese children are more likely to stay obese into adulthood and to develop noncommunicable diseases (NCDs) like diabetes and cardiovascular diseases, hypertension and stroke at a younger age that reduce the overall quality of life.

The most significant health consequences of childhood overweight and obesity, which often do not become obvious until adulthood, include:

- Cardiovascular diseases (mainly heart disease and stroke);
- Diabetes;
- Musculoskeletal disorders, especially osteoarthritis; and
- Certain types of cancer at a younger age (endometrial, breast, and colon).

Prevention of Overweight and Obesity

Overweight and obesity, as well as related noncommunicable diseases, are largely preventable through changes in lifestyle, especially diet. Prevention is the most feasible option for limiting the childhood obesity epidemic. The goal in fighting the childhood obesity epidemic is to achieve an energy balance which can be maintained throughout the individual's life span. WHO recommends the following to reduce and prevent childhood overweight and obesity:

- Increase consumption of fruit and vegetables, as well as legumes, whole grains and nuts.
- Limit energy intake from total fats and shift fat consumption away from saturated fats to unsaturated fats;
- Limit the intake of sugars; and
- Be physically active and have at least 60 minutes of regular, moderate- to vigorous-intensity activity each day.

DIETARY ADVICE IN ADULT, CHILDHOOD, AND IN PREGNANCY FOR OPTIMAL HEALTH

A healthy diet helps to protect against malnutrition in all its forms, as well as noncommunicable diseases (NCDs), such as diabetes, heart disease, stroke, and cancer. However, increased production of processed foods, rapid urbanization, and changing lifestyles has led to a shift in dietary patterns. People are now consuming more foods high in energy, fats, free sugars and salt/sodium, and many people do not eat enough fruit, vegetables, and other dietary fiber such as whole grains.

The balanced and healthy diet will vary depending on individual characteristics (e.g., age, gender, lifestyle, and degree of physical activity), cultural context, locally available foods, and dietary customs. However, the basic principles of what constitutes a healthy diet remain the same.

Dietary Advice for Adults

A healthy diet includes, fruits, vegetables, legumes (e.g., lentils and beans), nuts, and whole grains (e.g., unprocessed maize, millet, oats, wheat, and brown rice).

Fruits and Vegetables

- **Fruits and vegetables:** At least 400 g (i.e. five portions) of fruit and vegetables per day, excluding potatoes, sweet potatoes, and other starchy roots is recommended. Eating at least 400 g, or five portions, of fruit and vegetables per day reduces the risk of noncommunicable diseases (NCDs) (diabetes, heart disease, stroke, and cancer) and helps to ensure an adequate daily intake of dietary fiber. Fruit and vegetable intake can be improved by:

- Always including vegetables in meals;
- Eating fresh fruit and raw vegetables as snacks;
- Eating fresh fruit and vegetables that are in season; and
- Eating a variety of fruit and vegetables.

Sugars

- Less than 10% of total energy intakes from free sugars, which is equivalent to 50 g (or about 12 level teaspoons) for a person of healthy body weight consuming about 2000 calories per day is recommended. But ideally is less than 5% of total energy intake is good for additional health benefits. Free sugars are all sugars added to foods or drinks by the manufacturer, cook or consumer, as well as sugars naturally present in honey, syrups, fruit juices, and fruit juice concentrates.
  - In both adults and children, the intake of free sugars should be reduced to less than 10% of total energy intake. A reduction to less than 5% of total energy intake would provide additional health benefits.
  - Consuming free sugars increases the risk of dental caries (tooth decay).
  - Excess calories from foods and drinks high in free sugars also contribute to unhealthy weight gain, which can lead to **overweight** and **obesity**.
  - Recent evidence also shows that free sugars influence **blood pressure** and **serum lipids**, and suggests that a reduction in free sugars intake reduces risk factors for cardiovascular diseases.
  - Sugars intake can be reduced by:
    - Limiting the consumption of foods and drinks containing high amounts of sugars, such as sugary snacks, candies, and sugar-sweetened beverages (i.e., all types of beverages containing free sugars – these include carbonated or noncarbonated soft drinks, fruit or vegetable juices and drinks, liquid and powder concentrates, flavored water, energy and sports drinks, ready-to-drink tea, ready-to-drink coffee and flavored milk drinks)
    - Eating fresh fruit and raw vegetables as snacks instead of sugary snacks.

Fats

- Less than 30% of total energy intake from fats is recommended. Unsaturated fats (found in fish, avocado and nuts, and in sunflower, soybean, canola, and olive oils) are preferable to:
  - Saturated fats, found in fatty meat, butter, palm and coconut oil, cream, cheese, ghee, and lard.

- Industrially-produced *trans*-fats, found in baked and fried foods, and pre-packaged snacks and foods, such as frozen pizza, pies, cookies, biscuits, wafers, and cooking oils, and spreads.
- Ruminant *trans*-fats, found in meat and dairy foods from ruminant animals, such as cows, sheep, goats, and camels.
- It is suggested that the intake of saturated fats be reduced to less than 10% of total energy intake and *trans*-fats to less than 1% of total energy intake. In particular, industrially-produced *trans*-fats are not part of a healthy diet and should be avoided.
- Reducing the amount of total fat intake to less than 30% of total energy intake helps to prevent unhealthy weight gain in the adult population. Also, the risk of developing NCDs is lowered by:
  - Reducing saturated fats to less than 10% of total energy intake;
  - Reducing *trans*-fats to less than 1% of total energy intake; and
  - Replacing both saturated fats and *trans*-fats with unsaturated fats in particular, with polyunsaturated fats.
- Fat intake, especially saturated fat and industrially-produced *trans*-fat intake, can be reduced by:
  - Steaming or boiling instead of frying when cooking;
  - Replacing butter, lard, and ghee with oils rich in polyunsaturated fats, such as soybean, canola (rapeseed), corn, safflower, and sunflower oils;
  - Eating reduced-fat dairy foods and lean meats, or trimming visible fat from meat; and
  - Limiting the consumption of baked and fried foods, and pre-packaged snacks and foods (e.g., Doughnuts, cakes, pies, cookies, biscuits, and wafers) that contain industrially-produced *trans*-fats.

Salt, Sodium, and Potassium

- **Salt, sodium, and potassium:** Less than 5 g of salt (equivalent to about one teaspoon) per day is recommended. Salt should be iodized.
- Most people consume too much sodium through salt (corresponding to consuming an average of 9–12 g of salt per day) and not enough potassium (less than 3.5 g). High sodium intake and insufficient potassium intake contribute to high blood pressure, which in turn increases the risk of heart disease and stroke.
- Keeping salt intake to less than 5 g per day (equivalent to sodium intake of less than 2 g per day) helps to prevent **hypertension**, and reduces the **risk of heart disease** and **stroke** in the adult population
- People are often unaware of the amount of salt they consume. In many countries, most salt comes from processed foods (e.g., ready meals; processed meats such as bacon, ham, and salami; cheese; and salty snacks) or from foods consumed frequently in large amounts (e.g.,

bread). Salt is also added to foods during cooking (e.g., bouillon, stock cubes, soy sauce, and fish sauce) or at the point of consumption (e.g., table salt).

- Salt intake can be reduced by:
  - Limiting the amount of salt and high-sodium condiments (e.g., Soy sauce, fish sauce, and bouillon) when cooking and preparing foods
  - Not having salt or high-sodium sauces on the table
  - Limiting the consumption of salty snacks
  - Choosing products with lower sodium content.
- Some food manufacturers are reformulating recipes to reduce the sodium content of their products, and people should be encouraged to check nutrition labels to see how much sodium is in a product before purchasing or consuming it.
- Potassium can mitigate the negative effects of elevated sodium consumption on blood pressure. Intake of potassium can be increased by consuming fresh fruit and vegetables.

Dietary Advice for Infants and Young Children

In the first 2 years of a child's life, optimal nutrition nurtures healthy growth and improves cognitive development. It also reduces the risk of becoming overweight or obese and developing noncommunicable diseases (such as diabetes, heart disease, stroke, and cancer) later in life. Advice on a healthy diet for infants and children is similar to that for adults, but the following elements are also important:

- Infants should be breastfed exclusively during the first 6 months of life.
- Infants should be breastfed continuously until 2 years of age and beyond.
- From 6 months of age, breast milk should be complemented with a variety of adequate, safe, and nutrient-dense foods. Salt and sugars should not be added to complementary foods.

Dietary Advice in Pregnancy

Maintaining good nutrition and a healthy diet during pregnancy is critical for the health of the mother and unborn child. A healthy balanced diet during pregnancy contains adequate energy, protein, whole grains, vitamins, and minerals, obtained through the consumption of a variety of foods, including green and orange vegetables, meat, fish, beans, nuts, pasteurized dairy products, and fruit. Sweets and fats should be kept to a minimum.

To maintain a healthy pregnancy, approximately 300 extra calories are needed each day. Mother diet should produce adequate nutrients so that maternal stores do not get depleted and produce sufficient milk to nourish her child after birth. Overall a balanced diet is obtained with an appropriate mixture of all the 5 food groups:

TABLE 24.12: Recommended dietary allowance in pregnancy.

Nutrient	Normal adult women	Pregnant women
Energy kcals		
• Sedentary	1875	+300
• Moderate	2225	+300
• Heavy	2925	+300
Protein (g)	50	+15
Fat (g)	20	30
Calcium (mg)	400	1000
Iron (mg)	30	38
Retinol (µg)	600	600
Beta carotene (µg)	2400	2400
Thiamine (mg)		
• Sedentary	0.9	+0.2
• Moderate	1.1	+0.2
• Heavy	1.2	+0.2
Riboflavin (mg)		
• Sedentary	1.1	+0.2
• Moderate	1.3	+0.2
• Heavy	1.5	+2
Niacin (µg)		
• Sedentary	12	+2
• Moderate	14	+2
• Heavy	16	+2
Pyridoxine (mg)	2.0	2.5
Ascorbic acid (mg)	40	40
Folic acid (mcg)	100	400
Vitamin B_{12} (µg)	3	+1

1. Vegetables and legumes
2. Breads and cereals
3. Milk, yoghurt, and cheese
4. Meat, poultry, fish, and alternatives
5. Fruit

Recommended dietary allowances in pregnancy is given in **Table 24.12**.

DIETARY ADVICE FOR OPTIMAL HEALTH IN DIABETES MELLITUS AND CORONARY HEART DISEASE

Dietary Advice in Diabetes Mellitus

Diabetes mellitus is a metabolic disorder characterized by **chronic hyperglycemia** associated with impaired carbohydrate, fat, and protein metabolism. These abnormalities are the consequence of either inadequate **insulin** secretion or impaired insulin action, or both.

The overall objective in the management of patients with diabetes mellitus is to reduce the risk of cardiovascular disease. Nutritional management is the basis of treatment, both for types 1 and 2, and complements the use of hypoglycemic drugs or insulin.

Dietary recommendations for people with diabetes are very similar to those given to the general population for the promotion of good health. Dietary strategies for patients with diabetes have to be considered as lifelong strategies.

The majority of patients with type 2 diabetes are overweight or obese, and this is becoming more common in patients with type 1 diabetes, especially in those, following intensive insulin therapy.

- Reduction in body weight improves outcomes in patients with both, type 1 and 2 diabetes. Blood glucose control, insulin resistance, blood pressure, and lipid abnormalities have all been shown to improve in association with weight reduction.

- Dietary contribution can also be effective in preventing the onset of type 2 diabetes in high risk individuals. Dietary involvement trials have shown that weight loss achieved in high risk individuals consuming diets with **reduced saturated fat** and **increased dietary fiber**, in conjunction with increased physical activity, can reduce risk of type 2 diabetes.

- Experts agree that patients with diabetes should consume diets in which the energy from saturated fat is less than 10% of total energy intake and cholesterol intake less than 150 mg per day.

- Foods rich in dietary fiber and/or with a **low glycemic index** make an important contribution to glucose control and can improve blood lipid profile, therefore **legumes**, **fruits**, **cereals** and other **vegetables** are recommended.

- The effectiveness of a meal in reducing blood glucose is related to the **glycemic index** of the constituent foods. The **glycemic index** is a measure of the extent to which a food raises blood glucose concentration compared with an equivalent amount of a reference carbohydrate (glucose). A diet containing mainly low glycemic index foods improves the metabolic control in diabetic patients and may have favorable effects on other cardiovascular risk factors. Therefore foods with a low glycemic index (e.g., legumes, oats, parboiled rice, and certain raw fruits) should replace, whenever possible, those with a high glycemic index.

- Additionally, in accordance with general guidelines for the promotion of good health, diabetic patients should consume less than 6 g salt per day to control blood pressure and restrict their daily alcohol intake to one or two unit alcohol (women and men respectively).

Dietary Advice in Cardiovascular Disease

The nature of dietary fat is an important determinant of coronary heart disease (CHD). It is well known that, diet governs many situations favoring the onset of "heart disease," particularly coronary heart disease. Of all the factors associated with CHD (e.g.,, plasma cholesterol, high blood pressure, cigarette smoking, and lack of physical activity) plasma cholesterol has a very high statistical significance

TABLE 24.13: Characteristics of cardio protective diets.

- Low intakes of saturated fatty acids
- Saturated and trans unsaturated fatty acids increase CHD risk; ω-6 and ω-3 polyunsaturated fatty acids are protective
- High intake of raw or appropriately prepared fruit and vegetables
- Antioxidant nutrients, flavonoids, folate and other B vitamins, nonstarch polysaccharides, whole grain cereals, nuts, soy protein, and alcohol may protect against CHD
- Lightly processed cereal foods and wholegrains are preferred
- Fat intakes are derived predominantly from unmodified vegetable oils
- Fish, nuts, seeds, and vegetable protein sources are important dietary components
- Meat, when consumed, is lean and eaten in small quantities
- Energy balance reduces rates of obesity

with the incidence of CHD. The risk of CHD appears to increase as the plasma cholesterol concentration rises. The WHO Expert Committee concludes that there is a well-established triangular relationship between habitual diet, blood cholesterol levels and CHD.

Dietary advice to reduce risk of occurrence or recurrence of cardiovascular events includes a reduction in saturated fatty acids and an increase in fruit, vegetables, and low fat dairy products. Foods to be eaten regularly include pulses, fresh fruit, vegetables and cereals, brown rice, and fish, lean meat or poultry, nuts. Foods to avoid include chips cooked in saturated fatty acids, butter or hardened margarine, sugarcoated cereals, meat fat, processed meat, cream.

A number of dietary patterns across the world have been shown to be protective against CHD is given in **Table 24.13**. For someone with heart disease, diet is a big deal. By adopting a diet that controls LDL ("bad") cholesterol, lowers blood pressure, lowers blood sugar, and helps with weight loss will help for someone with heart disease. Following nine strategies will help to plan meals for someone with heart disease:

1. Serve more vegetables, fruits, whole grains, and legumes. They're rich in fiber and other nutrients.
2. Choose fat calories wisely by:
   - Limit saturated fat (found in animal products).
   - Avoid artificial *trans* fats as much as possible.
   - When using added fats for cooking or baking, choose oils that are high in monounsaturated fat (for example, olive and peanut oil) or polyunsaturated fat (such as soybean, corn, and sunflower oils).
3. Serve a variety of protein-rich foods. Balance meals with lean meat, fish, and vegetable sources of protein.
4. Limit cholesterol. Cholesterol in foods, found in red meat and high-fat dairy products, can raise blood cholesterol levels, especially in high-risk people.
5. Serve the right kind of carbohydrates. Include foods like brown rice, oatmeal, and sweet potatoes to add fiber and help control blood sugar levels. Avoid sugary foods.

6. Eat regularly. This helps someone with heart disease control blood sugar, burn fat more efficiently, and regulates cholesterol levels.
7. Cut back on salt. Too much salt is bad for blood pressure. Instead, use herbs, spices, or condiments to flavor foods.
8. Encourage hydration. Staying hydrated makes you feel energetic and eat less.
9. Keep serving sizes in check. It can help to use smaller plates and glasses, and to check food labels to see how much is in a serving, since it's easy to eat more than you think.

GROUPS OF FOOD ITEMS AND THEIR NUTRITIONAL IMPORTANCE

Food items are categorized into **five groups by ICMR**, depending upon their type, nutritional contribution, and roles.

A balanced diet is one that includes foods from all food groups during the day. The quantities and proportions of these foods need to be such that they fulfill our daily requirements for all nutrients. Five food group plan suggested by ICMR and the nutrients supplied by each food group are given in **Table 24.14**.

Group I: Cereals and Grains

- Rice, wheat, ragi, bajra, maize, jowar, barley, rice flakes, wheat flour are the main sources of carbohydrates, which are the main energy yielding and bulk forming foods.
- They also provide variable amounts of proteins (6–12%) and vitamin B$_1$, vitamin B$_2$, folic Acid, iron, and fiber.
- Nutritive values of common cereals are given in **Table 24.15**.

Group II: Pulses and Legumes

- Commonly known as dals. Common examples are chana (Bengal gram), arhar or tuvur dal (red gram), moong dal (green gram), urad dal (black gram), peas and beans, ground-nut, soyabeans etc.
- They are sources of proteins and provide 20–25% of proteins. In fact they contain more proteins than eggs, meat, fish, etc. But they are poor in one or more essential amino acids, e.g., pulses are poor in **methionine**. Soyabean is exceptionally rich containing up to 40% of protein.
- They also provide vitamin B$_1$, vitamin B$_2$, folic acid, calcium, iron, fiber.
- Nutritive values of common pulses are given in **Table 24.16**.

TABLE 24.14: ICMR Five Food Group Plan.

Group	Food Items	Nutrients
I: Cereals and Grains	Rice, Wheat, Ragi, Bajra, Maize, Jowar, Barley, Rice flakes, Wheat Flour	Energy, protein, Vitamin B$_1$, Vitamin B$_2$, Folic Acid, Iron, Fiber.
II: Pulses and Legumes	Bengal gram, Black gram, Green gram, Red gram, Lentil (whole as well as dhals) Cowpea, Peas, Rajmah, Soyabeans, Beans	Energy, Protein, Invisible fat, Vitamin B$_1$, Vitamin B$_2$, Folic Acid, Calcium, Iron, Fiber
III: Milk and Meat Products	• *Milk:* Milk, Curd, Skimmed milk, Cheese • *Meat:* Chicken, Liver, Fish, Egg, Meat.	Protein, Fat, Vitamin B$_{12}$, Calcium. Protein, Fat, Vitamin B$_2$
IV: Fruits and Vegetables	• *Fruits:* Mango, Guava, Tomato Ripe, Papaya, Orange. Sweet Lime, Watermelon • *Vegetables (Green Leafy):* Amaranth, Spinach, Drumstick leaves, Coriander leaves, Mustard leaves, fenugreek leaves • *Other Vegetables:* Carrots, Brinjal, Ladies fingers, Capsicum, Beans, Onion, Drumstick, Cauliflower	• Carotenoids, Vitamin C and A, Fiber. • Invisible Fats, Carotenoids, Vitamin B$_2$, Folic Acid, Calcium, Iron, Fiber. • Carotenoids, Folic Acid, Calcium, Fiber
V: Fats and Sugars	• *Fats:* Butter, Ghee, Hydrogenated oils, Cooking oils like Groundnut, Mustard, Coconut. • *Sugars:* Sugar, Jaggery	• Energy, Fat, Essential Fatty Acids, and vitamin A and E • Energy

TABLE 24.15: Nutritive value of cereals and grains (values per 100 g).

	Rice	Wheat	Maize	Jowar	Bajra	Ragi
Carbohydrates (g)	78.2	71.2	66.2	72.6	67.5	72.0
Proteins (g)	6.8	11.81	11.1	10.4	11.6	7.3
Fats (g)	0.5	1.5	3.6	1.9	5.0	1.3
Energy (Kcal)	345	346	342	349	361	328
Thiamine (mg)	0.06	0.45	0.42	0.3	0.3	0.2
Niacin (mg)	1.9	5.0	0.1	3.1	2.3	2.3
Riboflavin (mg)	0.06	0.17	0.1	1.3	0.25	0.18
Calcium (mg)	33	41	26	25.0	42.0	344.0

TABLE 24.16: Nutritive value of pulses (values per 100 g).

Parameters	Bengal gram	Black gram	Red gram	Soyabean
Energy (kcal)	360	247	335	432
Proteins (g)	17	24	22	43
Fats (g)	5.3	1.4	1.7	20
Calcium (mg)	202	155	75	240
Iron (mg)	4.6	3.8	2.7	10.4
Thiamine (mg)	0.30	0.42	0.45	0.75
Niacin (mg)	2.9	2.0	2.9	3.2
Riboflavin (mg)	0.15	0.20	0.20	0.40

TABLE 24.18: Nutritive value of meat, fish and eggs (values per 100 gms).

Animal food	Proteins	Fat	Minerals (mg)
Meat, goat	21.4	3.6	1.1
Fish	19.5	2.4	1.5
Egg (hen)	13.5	13.5	1.0
Liver, goat	20.0	3.0	1.5

TABLE 24.19: Nutritive value of some common fruits (values per 100 g).

Fruits	Calories	Calcium (mg)	Iron (mg)	Carotene (mg)	Vitamin C (mg)
Banana	104	10	10.5	124	7
Grapes	71	20	1.5	0	1
Guava	54	10	0.27	0	212
Mango	74	14	1.3	2210	16
Orange	48	26	0.32	2240	68
Papaya	32	17	0.5	2740	57
Sitaphal	104	17	4.31	0	37
Amla	58	50	1.2	9	600
Dry dates	317	120	7.3	44	3
Dry raisins	308	87	7.7	24	1

Group III: Milk and Meat Products

- Examples are milk, curd, skimmed milk, cheese, chicken, liver, fish, egg, meat etc.
- Milk is the most complete food of all. It is a good source of protein (3–4%), called casein present as calcium caseinate. It is a good source of fats (3.4%), sugar (lactose), vitamins (all, except vitamin C) and minerals like calcium, sodium, potassium, magnesium, phosphorus, copper, iodine, etc. It is poor in iron. Nutritive value of milk from different sources is given in **Table 24.17**.
- **Egg:** Egg contains all the nutrients except carbohydrates and vitamins C. Eggs contain 6% protein, 6% fats and also calcium and iron. Most vitamins are also present.
- **Fish:** Fish is a good nutritive food containing 15–25% of protein with good biological value, fat soluble vitamins A and D and polyunsaturated fatty acids. Sea fish contains iodine but not fresh water fish.
- **Meat:** Meat is nothing but the flesh of animals like cattle, goat, sheep, etc. It is a good source of protein, iron, zinc, and B-group vitamins like B_{12}.
- Nutritive value of meat, fish, and eggs is given in **Table 24.18**.

Group IV: Fruits and Vegetables

- **Vegetables** are rich in vitamins and minerals and fibers. These are also called protective foods. These include:
  - **Vegetables (Green Leafy):** Amaranth, spinach, Drumstick leaves, coriander leaves, mustard leaves, fenugreek leaves

  - **Other Vegetables:** Carrots, brinjal, ladies fingers, capsicum, beans, onion, drumstick
- **Fruits** are protective foods and contain vitamins and minerals. For example:
  - Orange, guava, amla are rich in vitamin C.
  - Papaya, mangoes are rich in B-carotenes
  - Banana is rich in potassium
  - Dried raisins (kismish), dates are rich in calcium, iron and sugar.
- Nutritive values of some common fruits are shown in **Table 24.19**.

Group V: Fats and Sugars

- **Fats:** Butter, ghee, hydrogenated oils, cooking oils like Groundnut, mustard, coconut.
- Oils obtained from plants are generally liquid at room temperature. They contain unsaturated fatty acids including essential fatty acids.
- Animal fats contain vitamins A and D, which are absent in vegetable oils.
- **Sugars,** Jaggery are source of energy. Jaggery, on the other hand, also contains iron

TABLE 24.17: Nutritive value of milk (value per 100 gms).

Nutrient	Buffalo	Cow	Goat	Human
Energy (Kcal)	117	67	72	65
Fat (g)	6.5	4	4.5	3.4
Protein (g)	4.5	3.5	3.5	1.1
Lactose (g)	5	4.5	4.6	7.4
Calcium (mg)	210	120	170	28
Water (g)	81.0	87	86.8	88

Nutritional Importance of Indian Diet

❖ Yogurt for example is a source of calcium and is a low fat alternative to dips made of mayonnaise.
❖ Spinach and tomatoes are the super-foods that provide antioxidants, vitamins, and minerals to strengthen our immunity.

Contd...

Contd...

- ❖ Garlic features greatly in Indian cooking which is good for our heart, immunity, and metabolism.
- ❖ Whole grain cereals provide the necessary carbohydrate for energy and fiber for our gut health.
- ❖ Indian food is made using a variety of spices that satisfies our taste buds and giving us satiety and more so giving it vibrancy to keep it interesting.
- ❖ Turmeric used as a prime spice in Indian curries is known for its anti-inflammatory effect and prevents cancer and cardiovascular diseases.
- ❖ Indian meal uses locally available and seasonal fruits and vegetables and hence gains maximum nutritional benefits. The cooking methods like steaming, poaching, grilling or using tandoor, also helps in retaining the nutrients well.
- ❖ A traditional Indian thali will provide you a balance of carbohydrate from cereals, proteins from legumes, pulses, animal food or dairy, vitamins and minerals from vegetables and fruits that you need for a balanced diet making Indian food a healthy one around the globe.

ENERGY CONTENT OF DIFFERENT FOOD ITEMS AND ITS CALCULATION

The energy content of a food is a measure of how many calories the food contains. Determining the energy content of foods depends on the following:

- The components of food that provide energy (protein, fat, carbohydrate) should be determined by appropriate analytical methods;
- The quantity of each individual component must be converted to food energy using a generally accepted factor that expresses the amount of available energy per unit of weight; and
- The food energies of all components must be added together to represent the nutritional energy value of the food for humans.

How to Calculate the Energy Available from Foods

To calculate the energy available from a food, multiply the number of grams of:

- Carbohydrate in the food by 4 calories per gram.
- Protein in the food by 4 calories per gram
- Fat in the food by 9 calories per gram.
- Add the energy from carbohydrate, protein, and fat. The total, in calories, is the energy content of the food. This is the same information available on a nutritional label, for those foods that provide nutritional information.
- For example, 1 slice of bread with a tablespoon of peanut butter on it contains:
  - 16 grams carbohydrate = 16 g × 4 kcal/g = 64 kcal
  - 7 grams protein = 7g × 4 kcal/g = 28 kcal
  - 9 grams fat = 9 g × 9 kcal/g = 81 kcal
  - Total = 173 kcal
- Also note: 1 g alcohol = 7 kcal

GLYCEMIC INDEX AND ITS IMPORTANCE IN THE DIET

- The glycemic index (GI) is a measure of how quickly or slowly a carbohydrate food is digested and increases blood sugar levels compared with an equivalent amount of glucose
  - Higher GI carbohydrates increase blood glucose levels more quickly.
  - Lower GI carbohydrates increase blood glucose levels more slowly.
- Glycemic index ranges from **0 to 100** based on how much they raise blood glucose level.
  - **Glucose** and **galactose** have highest glycemic index (100%), as do **lactose**, **maltose**, **isomaltose**, and **trehalose**, which give rise to these monosaccharaides on hydrolysis.
  - **Fructose** and the **sugar alcohols** are absorbed less rapidly and have a lower glycemic index, as dose sucrose.
  - The glycemic index of **starch** ranges from 1 to 100. Zero for those that are not hydrolyzed at all (nonstarch polysaccharides; e.g., cellulose) and 100 for starches that are readily hydrolyzed in the small intestine.
- The extent to which starch in foods is hydrolyzed by α-amylase is determination by its structure. The amount of **amylose** and **amylopectin** basically determines the digestibility of starch and thus glycemic index. The proportion of amylose and amylopectin can vary from one variety of starch to the other.
- Starches with **lower amylose** contain will have **higher glycemic index**; inversely starches with a **higher amylose** content will have **low glycemic indexes**.
- Examples of foods with **low**, **middle** and **high GI** values include the following:
  - **High-GI foods** (with scores of 70 or higher) include white rice, white bread, potatoes, crackers, sugar-sweetened beverages, and watermelon.
  - **Medium-GI foods** (with scores of 56–69) include bananas, grapes, pineapple, ice cream, raisins, and sweet corn.
  - **Low-GI foods** (with scores of 55 and under) include green vegetables, most fruits, carrots, kidney beans, oatmeal, peanuts, peas etc.

Foods that have a low glycemic index are considered to be more beneficial since they cause less fluctuation in insulin secretion) and reduce the risk of type 2 diabetes and heart disease. The glycemic index of common foods is given in **Table 24.20**.

Importance of Glycemic Index in the Diet

- The glycemic index is used to assess how slowly or how quickly a given food cause increase in blood glucose

TABLE 24.20: The glycemic index of common foods.

Food	Examples	Glycemic index (glucose = 100)
High-carbohydrate foods	White wheat bread	75 ± 2
	Whole wheat bread	74 ± 2
	Grain bread	53 ± 2
	Wheat roti	62 ± 3
	Chapatti	52 ± 4
	White rice boiled	73 ± 4
	Brown rice boiled	68 ± 4
	Barley	28 ± 2
	Sweet corn	52 ± 5
Breakfast cereals	Cornflakes	81 ± 6
	Wheat biscuits	69 ± 2
	Oatmeal	55 ± 2
Fruits	Apple	36 ± 2
	Orange	43 ± 3
	Banana	51 ± 3
	Pineapple	59 ± 8
	Mango	51 ± 5
	Watermelon	76 ± 4
	Dates	42 ± 4
Vegetables	Potato boiled	78 ± 4
	Sweet potato boiled	63 ± 6
	Pumpkin boiled	64 ± 7
	Green banana	55 ± 6
	Vegetable soup	48 ± 5
Dairy products	Milk full fat	39 ± 3
	Milk skim	37 ± 4
	Ice cream	51 ± 3
	Yogurt	41 ± 2
	Soy milk	34 ± 4

Contd...

Contd...

Food	Examples	Glycemic index (glucose = 100)
Legumes	Peas	28 ± 9
	Kidney beans	24 ± 4
	Lentils	32 ± 5
	Soya beans	16 ± 1
Snack products	Chocolate	40 ± 3
	Popcorn	65 ± 5
	Potato crisps	56 ± 3
	Soft drink/Soda	59 ± 3
	Rice crackers/Crisps	87 ± 2
Sugars	Fructose	15 ± 4
	Sucrose	65 ± 4
	Glucose	103 ± 3
	Honey	61 ± 3

levels. Foods having low GI tend to release glucose slowly and steadily and are helpful in keeping blood glucose under control. Foods having high glycemic index release glucose rapidly.

- Eating foods with **high glycemic index** have been associated with obesity.
- For weight maintenance, low GI diet is the best for longer-term weight management
- Low GI diets can significantly reduce total and LDL cholesterol levels.
- The GI of foods has important implications for the food industry. Terms such as complex carbohydrates and simple sugars are now recognized as having little nutritional or physiological significance. The WHO/FAO recommends that these terms be removed and replaced with the total carbohydrate content of the food and its GI value.

ASSESSMENT QUESTIONS

■ SHORT ESSAY QUESTIONS (SEQs)

1. Write nutritional importance of proteins.
2. Define BMR and state the factors affecting BMR.
3. What is protein energy malnutrition (PEM)? What are the types of PEM? Write the importance features.
4. What are dietary fibers and explain their importance in human nutrition with respect to the prevention of diseases.
5. Define obesity. Write causes and health risk associated with it.
6. What is glycemic index? Give its importance.

■ SHORT ANSWER QUESTIONS (SAQs)

1. What is a complete protein?
2. What is the role of dietary fiber in the body?
3. What is biologic value of protein?
4. Name the factors affecting energy expenditure.
5. What is thermogenic effect of food?
6. What is nitrogen balance? Give its different states.
7. What are essential amino acids? Name the essential amino acids.
8. Define balanced diet. Give its importance.
9. What is meant by glycemic index of food?

10. Write parameter for the assessment of nutritive value of proteins.
11. List four differences between marasmus and kwashiorkor.
12. What is relationship between BMI and obesity?

CASE VIGNETTE-BASED QUESTIONS (CVBQs)

Case Study

1. A 4-year-old child comes with retarded growth and pedal edema. She also has discoloration of skin and hair. On enquiring by the physician, mother told the physician that child was on breast milk up to one and a half years of age and for the past two and a half years she was being given rice and dal. The laboratory data of the child showed hypoalbuminemia.

   Questions
   a. Name the probable condition.
   b. What is the cause of edema?
   c. What are the preventive measures?

2. One-year-old female child comes to OPD with retarded growth and emaciated appearance (wasting of muscles). No edema is present. The condition is diagnosed by physician as marasmus.

   Questions
   a. What is marasmus?
   b. What is the difference between marasmus and kwashiorkor?
   c. What is the cause of emaciated appearance?

MULTIPLE CHOICE QUESTIONS (MCQs)

1. Dietary fiber has following effects, *except*:
   a. Increases stool bulk
   b. Lowers cholesterol
   c. Decreases risk of cardiovascular disease
   d. Increases risk of diabetes mellitus.

2. Which of the following dietary sources has the greatest thermogenic effect?
   a. Fat   b. Protein
   c. Carbohydrate   d. Vitamins

3. Following features are seen in marasmus, *except*:
   a. Edema   b. Muscle wasting
   c. Growth retardation   d. Anemia

4. The quality of a protein is assessed by:
   a. Protein efficiency ratio (PER)
   b. Biological value (BV)
   c. Net protein utilization (NPU)
   d. All of the above

5. An obese person has the health risk of:
   a. Atherosclerosis
   b. Hypertension
   c. Coronary heart disease and stroke
   d. All of the above

6. Which of the following statements is correct for BMR?
   a. Increases in response to starvation
   b. Decreases in response to starvation

   c. Is not responsive to changes in hormone levels
   d. Increases with increasing age

7. Intake of excess protein beyond the body's need will be:
   a. Excretion of the excess protein in the urine
   b. An increase in the storage pool of protein
   c. An increased synthesis of muscle protein
   d. None of the above

8. Which of the following statement is correct for obesity?
   a. Cause metabolic changes that are usually irreversible
   b. Is caused solely by high caloric consumption
   c. Several genes have the potential to cause obesity
   d. Is associated with an increased sensitivity of insulin receptor

9. Which of the following is not correct for dietary fat?
   a. If present excess stored as triacylglycerol in adipose tissue
   b. If present excess stored as glycogen in liver
   c. Should include linoleic and linolenic acids
   d. High fat diets are associated with many health risks.

10. The caloric value for a gram of fat is:
    a. 9 kcal/g   b. 6 kcal/g
    c. 4 kcal/g   d. 5 kcal/g

11. Protein quality is assessed by:
    a. Amino acid score   b. Net protein
    c. Biological value   d. All of the above

12. Marasmus is characterized by:
    a. Growth retardation
    b. Anemia
    c. Fat and muscle wasting
    d. All of the above

13. Kwashiorkor is characterized by:
    a. Severe edema
    b. Fatty liver
    c. Depigmented hair and skin
    d. All of the above

14. The value of BMI (body index mass) of 20–25 is considered as:
    a. Normal
    b. Obesity grade I (over weight)
    c. Obesity grade II (over obesity)
    d. Obesity grade III (gross obesity)

15. Normal values of BMR for healthy male is:
    a. 80 kcal/sqm/hour   b. 40 kcal/sqm/hour
    c. 60 kcal/sqm/hour   d. 100 kcal/sqm/hour

16. Which of the following carbohydrate functions a dietary fiber?
    a. Cellulose   b. Pectin
    c. Gums   d. All of the above

17. Oxidation of which substance in the body yields the most calories:
    a. Glucose   b. Glycogen
    c. Protein   d. Lipids

18. The recommended energy intake for an adult sedentary Indian man is:
    a. 1,900 kcal/day   b. 2,400 kcal/day
    c. 2,700 kcal/day   d. 3,000 kcal/day

19. The recommended energy intake for an adult sedentary Indian woman is:
    a. 1,900 kcal/day
    b. 2,200 kcal/day
    c. 2,400 kcal/day
    d. 2,700 kcal/day

20. During pregnancy, the following should be added to the calculated energy requirement:
    a. 300 kcal/day
    b. 500 kcal/day
    c. 700 kcal/day
    d. 900 kcal/day

21. The proximate principles of diet are:
    a. Vitamins and minerals
    b. Proteins
    c. Carbohydrates and fats
    d. Carbohydrates, fats, and proteins

22. The limiting amino acid in wheat is:
    a. Leucine
    b. Lysine
    c. Cysteine
    d. Methionine

23. The limiting amino acid in pulses is:
    a. Leucine
    b. Lysine
    c. Tryptophan
    d. Methionine

24. Maize is poor in
    a. Lysine
    b. Methionine
    c. Tryptophan
    d. Lysine and tryptophan

25. Net protein utilization depends upon:
    a. Protein efficiency ratio
    b. Digestibility coefficient
    c. Digestibility coefficient and protein efficiency ratio
    d. Digestibility coefficient and biological value

26. The following is considered as reference standard for comparing the nutritional quality of proteins:
    a. Milk proteins
    b. Egg proteins
    c. Meat proteins
    d. Fish proteins

27. The amino acids present in pulses can supplement the limiting amino acids of:
    a. Cereals
    b. Milk
    c. Fish
    d. Nuts and beans

28. Kwashiorkor occurs when the diet is severely deficient in:
    a. Iron
    b. Calories
    c. Proteins
    d. Essential fatty acids

29. Clinical features of kwashiorkor include all of the following, *except:*
    a. Mental retardation
    b. Muscle wasting
    c. Oedema
    d. Anemia

30. Kwashiorkor usually occurs in:
    a. The post-weaning period
    b. Pregnancy
    c. Lactation
    d. Old age

31. Marasmus occurs from deficient intake of:
    a. Essential amino acids
    b. Essential fatty acids
    c. Calories
    d. Zinc

32. Marasmus differs from kwashiorkor in the which of these following respect:
    a. Mental retardation occurs in kwashiorkor but not in marasmus
    b. Growth is retarded in kwashiorkor but not in marasmus

c. Muscle wasting occurs in marasmus but not kwashiorkor
d. Subcutaneous fat disappears in marasmus but not in kwashiorkor

33. Obesity increases the risk of:
    a. Hypertension
    b. Diabetes mellitus
    c. Cardiovascular disease
    d. All of these

34. What is the definition of gross obesity or grade III?
    a. BMI 20–25
    b. BMI above 35
    c. BMI 25–30
    d. BMI 30–35

35. What type of diet is recommended for weight maintenance?
    a. Low protein and low GI
    b. High protein and high GI
    c. Low protein and high GI
    d. High protein and low GI

36. Pulses are a good source of _____.
    a. Carbohydrates
    b. Proteins
    c. Fats
    d. Vitamins

37. Which of the following food constituents is not digested but is still important for us?
    a. Vitamins
    b. Minerals
    c. Proteins
    d. Fiber

38. Which of the following food items is rich in iron?
    a. Rice
    b. Banana
    c. Pulses
    d. Orange

39. Among the given nutrients milk is a poor source of:
    a. Calcium
    b. Protein
    c. Carbohydrate
    d. Vitamin C

40. The energy needed to digest and absorb nutrients from food is called as:
    a. Thermic effect of food
    b. Basal metabolism
    c. Physical activity
    d. Sedentary activity

41. A 4-year-old child was born at term, with no congenital abnormalities. She is now only 70% of normal body weight. On examination she shows dependent edema of the lower extremities as well as an enlarged abdomen with palpable fluid wave. Her desquamating skin shows irregular areas of depigmentation, and hyperpigmentation. Which of the following nutritional problems is most likely present in this child?
    a. Marasmus
    b. Kwashiorkor
    c. Vitamin A toxicity
    d. Niacin deficiency

42. Marasmus and kwashiorkor are both diseases occurring in infants due to the deficiency of which nutrients?
    a. Minerals
    b. Water
    c. Vitamins
    d. Proteins

■ ANSWERS FOR MCQs

1. d	2. b	3. a	4. d	5. d
6. b	7. d	8. c	9. b	10. a
11. d	12. d	13. d	14. a	15. b
16. d	17. d	18. b	19. a	20. a
21. d	22. b	23. d	24. d	25. d
26. b	27. a	28. c	29. a	30. a
31. c	32. d	33. d	34. b	35. d
36. b	37. d	38. b	39. d	40. a
41. b	42. d			

Organ Functions, Disorders, and Function Tests

Competency	Learning Objectives
BI 6.13: Describe the functions of the kidney, liver, thyroid and adrenal glands. **BI 6.14:** Describe the tests that are commonly done in clinical practice to assess the functions of these organs (kidney, liver, thyroid and adrenal glands). **BI 6.15:** Describe the abnormalities of kidney, liver, thyroid and adrenal glands. **BI 11.17:** Explain the basis and rationale of biochemical tests done in the following conditions: • Myocardial infarction • Renal failure • Proteinuria • Nephrotic syndrome • Edema • Jaundice • Liver diseases • Thyroid disorders	1. Describe the functions, disorders and tests to assess the functions of the liver. 2. Describe the functions, disorders and tests to assess the functions of the kidney. 3. Describe the functions, disorders and tests to assess the functions of the thyroid gland. 4. Describe the functions, disorders and tests to assess the functions of the adrenal glands. 5. Describe cardiac markers and tests used to diagnose myocardial infarction (MI).

▌OVERVIEW

A large number of biochemical tests are carried out in the investigation of diseases. Tests that provide information on the functioning of particular organs are often grouped together as **organ function tests and are sometimes ordered together by a clinician**. Thus, organ function tests are the tests carried out to assess whether a particular organ is functioning normal or not. Commonly done organ function tests are briefly discussed here. For example:

- Liver function tests
- Renal function tests
- Thyroid function tests
- Adrenal function tests
- Cardiovascular disorders and cardiac markers

▌FUNCTIONS, DISORDERS AND TESTS TO ASSESS THE FUNCTIONS OF THE LIVER

The liver is one of the most versatile and important organs. The liver is the largest gland in the human body. It is situated above and to the left of the stomach and below the lungs. This vital organ carries out more than 500 roles in the human body. Alcohol abuse is one of the major causes of liver problems in the industrialized world.

Functions of the Liver

- The liver is the primary organ responsible for the metabolism of carbohydrates, lipids, proteins, porphyrins, and bile acids.

- The liver performs several roles in carbohydrate metabolism: The liver synthesizes and stores around 100 g of glycogen via glycogenesis, the formation of glycogen from glucose. When needed, the liver releases glucose into the blood by performing glycogenolysis, the breakdown of glycogen into glucose. The liver is also responsible for gluconeogenesis, which is the synthesis of glucose from certain amino acids, lactate, or glycerol.
- The liver plays several roles in lipid metabolism—it performs cholesterol synthesis, lipogenesis, and the production of triglycerides, and a bulk of the body's lipoproteins are synthesized in the liver.
- It is responsible for synthesizing most plasma proteins except the immunoglobulins, which are produced by lymphocytic plasma cell system. The liver produces albumin, the most abundant protein in blood serum. It is essential in the maintenance of **oncotic pressure**, and acts as a transport for **fatty acids** and **steroid hormones**.
- The liver plays a role in the production of clotting factors, as well as red blood cell production. Some of the proteins synthesized by the liver include coagulation factors I (fibrinogen), II (prothrombin), V, VII, VIII, IX, X, XI, XIII, as well as protein C, protein S and antithrombin.
- The liver plays a key role in digestion, as it produces and excretes **bile** required for emulsifying fats and helps the absorption of vitamin K from the diet.
- The liver is responsible for the breakdown and excretion of many waste products.
  - The liver conjugates bilirubin to bilirubin diglucuronide, facilitating its excretion into bile.
  - The liver breaks down ammonia into urea as part of the urea cycle, and the urea is excreted in the urine.
- The liver is also principle site for storage of:
  - Iron, in the form of ferritin, ready to make new red blood cells. The liver also stores and releases copper.
  - **Vitamins A**, **D**, **E**, **K**, and **B$_{12}$**. It keeps significant amounts of these vitamins stored.
- Furthermore, the liver plays an important role in the detoxification of xenobiotics and the excretion of metabolic end products such as bilirubin, ammonia, and urea. The liver produces the enzyme **catalase** in order to break down hydrogen peroxide, a very toxic substance due to it being a powerful oxidizing agent, into water and oxygen.
- The liver synthesizes **angiotensinogen**, a hormone that is responsible for raising the blood pressure when activated by renin, an enzyme that is released when the kidney senses low blood pressure.
- The liver is responsible for immunological effects—the mononuclear phagocyte system of the liver contains many immunologically active cells, acting as a 'sieve' for antigens carried to it via the portal system.

Laboratory tests for evaluation of liver disease are based, in part, on evaluation of these normal functions of the liver.

Disorders of Liver

The liver is a vital organ and supports almost every other organ in the body. Because of its multidimensional functions, the liver is also prone to many diseases. Examples of liver disease include:

Cirrhosis

Cirrhosis is a condition in which the liver does not function properly due to long-term damage. This damage is characterized by the replacement of normal liver tissue by **scar tissue** in a process known as **fibrosis**. Eventually, fibrosis can lead to liver failure as the functionality of the liver cells is destroyed.

Typically, the disease develops slowly over months or years. Initial there are often no symptoms. As the disease worsens, a person may become tired, weak, and itchy, have swelling in the lower legs, develop yellow skin, bruise easily, have fluid buildup in the abdomen, or develop spider-like blood vessels on the skin.

Cirrhosis is most commonly caused by **alcohol**, **hepatitis B**, **hepatitis C**, and nonalcoholic fatty liver disease. On-alcoholic fatty liver disease has a number of causes, including being overweight, diabetes, high blood fats, and high blood pressure.

Hepatitis

- Hepatitis is a common condition of **inflammation of the liver** caused by viruses, toxins, or an autoimmune response. Hepatomegaly refers to an enlarged liver and can be due to many causes.
- The most usual cause of this is **viral**, and the most common of these infections are **hepatitis A**, **B**, **C**, **D**, and **E**. Some of these infections are sexually transmitted. Chronic (rather than acute) infection with hepatitis B virus or hepatitis C virus is the main cause of **liver cancer**.
- Liver damage can also be caused by drugs, particularly drugs used to treat **cancer**.

Alcoholic Liver Disease

Drinking too much alcohol over long periods of time can cause liver damage and these include alcoholic hepatitis, fatty liver, and cirrhosis. It is the most common cause of cirrhosis in the world.

Jaundice

Many diseases of the liver are accompanied by jaundice caused by increased levels of bilirubin in the system. The bilirubin results from the breakup of the hemoglobin of dead red blood cells; normally, the liver removes bilirubin from the blood and excretes it through bile. For details **Refer Chapter 14.**

Primary Biliary Cholangitis (PBC)

Primary biliary cholangitis is an **autoimmune disease** of the bile ducts of liver. Due to slow progressive destruction of the small bile ducts of the liver. When these ducts are damaged, bile and other toxins cannot flow from the liver to the duodenum, called **cholestasis**. Failure to excrete waste products from the hepatocytes into the biliary tract and intestine is referred to as **cholestasis**. This can lead to fibrosis and cirrhosis.

Fatty Liver Disease

Fatty liver is the accumulation of fats within the cells of the liver to the point that more than 5–10% of the liver is fat. There are 2 types of fatty liver disease: **alcoholic liver disease** and **nonalcoholic fatty liver disease (NAFLD)**. Fatty liver disease can progress to serious complications, such as cirrhosis of the liver. For details **Refer Chapter 11**.

Liver Cancer

The most common types of liver cancer are **hepatocellular carcinoma** and **cholangiocarcinoma**. The leading causes are alcohol and hepatitis.

Tests to Assess the Functions of Liver (Liver Function Tests)

Liver diseases may be diagnosed by **liver function tests**, groups of blood tests that can readily show the extent of liver damage. Liver function tests (LFTs) are a group of tests that help in diagnosis, assessing prognosis and monitoring therapy. Different tests can give different information about hepatic dysfunction. This then allows the selection of further investigations such as ultrasound, CT scanning, magnetic resonance spectroscopy, endoscopy and liver biopsy

- As liver performs a multiple of functions like **excretion/secretion**, **metabolism**, **detoxification**, **storage**, etc., a number of tests are required to assess hepatic functions.

All the tests need not be performed in every case. The tests should be selected according to the clinical symptoms and signs.

- Several tests used earlier, e.g., **icterus index**, **thymol turbidity**, **serum cholesterol: cholesterylester ratio**, etc. have now become outdated due to lack of specificity and or sensitivity.

Liver function tests can be classified into three classes according to the function of the liver. The major commonly used liver function tests in this category are listed in **Table 25.1**.

1. **Tests based on excretory function:** It includes measurement of:
   - Serum bilirubin
   - Urine bilirubin
   - Urine bile salts
   - Urine urobilinogen
2. **Tests based on synthetic function:** It includes determination of:
   - Plasma proteins, albumins and globulins
   - Prothrombin time.
3. **Tests related to enzymes in diagnosis of liver disease**
   - Serum alanine transaminase (ALT)
   - Serum aspartate transaminase (AST)
   - Serum alkaline phosphatase (ALP).

Liver Function Tests Based on Excretory Function

An important physiologic role of the liver is the removal of toxic endogenous and exogenous substances from the blood. The tests based on excretory function of liver are related to bilirubin metabolism.

Tests Based on Bilirubin Metabolism

Bilirubin is the excretory end product of heme catabolism. It is conjugated in the liver to form bilirubin diglucuronide. Bilirubin is insoluble in water but bilirubin diglucuronide is soluble in water. The bilirubin glucuronide is excreted in

	Test	Aspect of liver function assessed	Major utility
1.	Serum bilirubin levels (total and conjugated)	Indicator of the ability of the liver to conjugate and excrete bilirubin (conjugation and excretory function)	Aids in the differential diagnosis of jaundice
2.	Total serum protein and albumin	Measure of the biosynthetic function of the liver, as the liver is the primary site of synthesis of most plasma proteins	Indicator of severity of chronic liver disease
3.	Prothrombin time	Measure of the biosynthetic function of the liver, as several coagulation factors are synthesized in the liver	Indicator of severity of acute liver disease
4.	Serum enzymes:		
	Aspartate transaminase (AST)	Serves as marker of injury to hepatocytes that contain AST in abundance	Activities of serum AST and AST are early indicator of liver damage and helps in monitoring response to treatment
	Alanine transaminase (ALT)	Serves as marker of injury to hepatocytes that contain ALT in abundance	
	Alkaline phosphatase (ALP)	Serves as marker of biliary obstruction	Aids in diagnosis of obstruction of the biliary tract

TABLE 25.1: Major liver function tests.

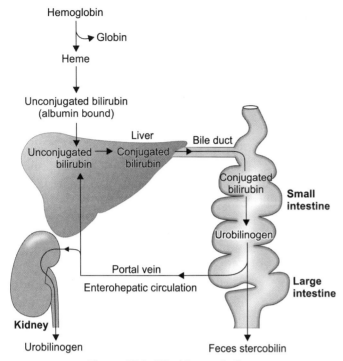

Figure 25.1: Bilirubin metabolism.

the bile and through the bile goes to the intestine. There, it is reduced by to bacterial enzymes to urobilinogen. Bilirubin metabolism is shown in **Figure 25.1**.

- Bilirubin exists in the plasma in two forms.
  1. Conjugated or direct bilirubin which is water soluble.
  2. Unconjugated or indirect bilirubin which is water insoluble.
- The normal concentration of:
  1. Total serum bilirubin is **0.1–1 mg/dL**
  2. Direct serum bilirubin ranges from **0.1 to 0.4 mg/dL**
  3. Indirect serum bilirubin is **0.2–0.7 mg/dL**.
- There are three main reasons why bilirubin levels in the body may rise.
  1. **Hemolysis:** Increased hemoglobin breakdown produces bilirubin which overwhelms a normal functioning conjugating mechanism.
  2. Failure of conjugating mechanism within the hepatocyte
  3. Obstruction in the biliary system.

Serum Bilirubin Estimation by Van den Bergh Reaction

Estimation of serum bilirubin is based on **Van den Bergh reaction**. In this reaction, when serum bilirubin is allowed to react with **Van den Bergh's diazo** reagent (sulfanilic acid and sodium nitrite in HCl) a purple colored **azobilirubin** is formed.

- **Conjugated bilirubin** being water soluble can react directly with aqueous solution of diazo reagent and so called **direct bilirubin**.
- Whereas the **unconjugated bilirubin** is water insoluble and does not react in aqueous solution. It requires addition of methyl alcohol to react with diazo reagent in the determination method and called **indirect bilirubin**.
- If both conjugated and unconjugated bilirubin is present in increased amounts, a purple color is produced immediately and the color is intensified on addition of alcohol and the reaction is called biphasic.

Clinical Interpretation

An increase in **serum bilirubin** occurs due to many causes, and results in **jaundice**. Estimation of **direct** and **indirect bilirubin** is useful for the **differential diagnosis of jaundice**. Bilirubin metabolism is deranged in three important diseases. They are:

1. **Hemolytic jaundice (prehepatic):** In **hemolytic** jaundice, **unconjugated** bilirubin is increased. Hence, Van den Bergh test is indirect positive.
2. **Hepatitis (hepatic jaundice):** In **obstructive** jaundice, **conjugated** bilirubin is elevated and Van den Bergh test is direct positive.
3. **Obstructive jaundice (posthepatic):** In **hepatic** jaundice both **conjugated** and **unconjugated** bilirubin are increased hence a biphasic reaction is observed.

Laboratory results in normal persons and patients with three different types of jaundice are shown in **Table 25.2**.

Urine Bilirubin

In normal individuals, bilirubin is not excreted in the urine. When it is present in the urine, it indicates some disease of the liver. Only conjugated bilirubin is soluble in water and is excreted in urine but not the unconjugated which is water

TABLE 25.2: Laboratory results in normal and patients with three types of jaundice.				
Condition	**Serum bilirubin**		**Urine urobilinogen**	**Urine bilirubin**
	Conjugated (direct)	*Unconjugated (indirect)*		
Normal	0.1–0.4 mg/dL	0.2–0.7 mg/dL	0.4 mg/24 h	Absent
Hemolytic or prehepatic jaundice	Normal	Increased	Increased	Absent
Hepatitis or hepatic jaundice	Increased	Increased	Normal or decreased if micro-obstruction to bile ductules is present	Present if micro-obstruction to bile ductules occurs
Obstructive or posthepatic jaundice	Increased	Normal	Absent	Present

insoluble. In urine, conjugated bilirubin can be detected by **Fouchet's test**.

Clinical Interpretation

- Conjugated bilirubin appears in urine of patients in **obstructive** and **hepatic jaundice**.
- In hemolytic jaundice, unconjugated bilirubin is increased in blood; it does not appear in urine.

Urobilinogen in Urine

The amount of urobilinogen present in urine depends on the amount of bilirubin entering the intestine. Urine urobilinogen is estimated semiquantitatively, by **Ehrlich's aldehyde reagent**.

Clinical Interpretation

- Normally, trace amounts of urobilinogen are present in urine.
- An increase in urobilinogen in urine is found in hemolytic jaundice due to excess production of bilirubin.
- In hepatitis, the urobilinogen in urine may be normal or decreased.
- In posthepatic obstructive jaundice, due to the complete or almost complete biliary obstruction, no urobilinogen is found in urine because bilirubin is unable to enter the intestine.

Liver Function Tests Based on Synthetic Function

Liver is the main source of synthesis of **plasma proteins, e.g., albumin, globulin** (except γ-globulins which are synthesized in the reticuloendothelial system), blood clotting factors, e.g., fibrinogen, prothrombin and factors V, VII, IX, X. Impaired function of liver results in decreased protein synthesis.

Determination of Serum Albumin and Globulin

The normal concentrations of serum proteins are given here:
- Total serum protein = 6–8 g/dL
- Serum albumin = 3.5–5.5 g/dL
- Serum globulin = 2–3.5 g/dL
- Albumin/globulin ratio = 1.2:1–1.6:1.

Clinical Interpretation

- Hypoalbuminemia may occur in hepatocellular disease like cirrhosis.
- Hyperglobulinemia may be present in chronic inflammatory disorders such as cirrhosis and in infectious hepatitis.
- The **albumin:globulin ratio (A:G ratio)** often provides useful clinical information. The reversal of the A:G ratio may be seen in conditions where the albumin levels are low (hypoalbuminemia) or where globulins are abnormally high, e.g., multiple myeloma. The concentration of total globulins increases due to a rise in the γ-globulins (γ-globulins synthesized by reticuloendothelial system and not by the liver) to compensate for a possible fall in the α-globulins by liver.

- Reversal of the A:G ratio is often the first investigation that raises suspicion of multiple myeloma.

Determination of Prothrombin Time

Hepatic synthetic function can be assessed by a simple coagulation test, **e.g., prothrombin time**. Various proteins that participate in blood coagulation are synthesized in the liver, e.g., fibrinogen, prothrombin (factor II) and factors V, VII, IX and X. If any one of these factors is deficient, the deficiency causes prolonged prothrombin time.

Clinical Interpretation

- An **increased prothrombin time** indicates the failure of hepatic synthesis of one or more of the above-mentioned clotting factors which is an indicator of severity of **acute liver disease**.
- As vitamin K is required for the synthesis of blood clotting factors, deficiency of vitamin K can also cause prolonged prothrombin time, which must be ruled out by estimating the prothrombin time, before and after administration of vitamin K. In case of liver disease, the prothrombin remains prolonged even after administration of vitamin K.

Tests Related to Enzymes in Diagnosis of Liver Disease

Liver cells contain several enzymes. In liver damage, these enzymes are released into blood and levels of these enzymes increase in blood. A large number of different enzymes have been used in the diagnosis of liver disease. But most commonly and routinely employed in laboratory are **(Table 25.3):**
- Serum aspartate transaminase
- Serum alanine transaminase
- Serum alkaline phosphatase.
  Other enzymes which have been found to be useful but not routinely done in the laboratory are:
- Serum 5'-nucleotidase
- Lactate dehydrogenase

TABLE 25.3: Enzyme assays in differential diagnosis of jaundice.

Enzyme assays	Hemolytic or prehepatic jaundice	Hepatic or hepatocellular jaundice	Obstructive or posthepatic jaundice
ALT or AST	Usually normal	Marked increase, goes in thousand units usually 500–1500 IU/L	Increased, usually 100–300 IU/L Do not exceed 300 IU/L
ALP	Normal	Increased slightly. Usually less than 30 KA/100 mL	Marked increase 30–100 KA/100 mL, usually more than 30 KA/100 mL

- Isocitrate dehydrogenase
- γ-glutamyl transferase.

Serum Aspartate Transaminase and Alanine Transaminase

- Liver is the richest source of:
  - **Aspartate transaminase** which is previously called **serum glutamate oxaloacetate transaminase (SGOT)**.
  - **Alanine transaminase** which is previously called **serum glutamate pyruvate transaminase (SGPT)**.
- The normal range for these enzymes is as follows:
  - AST or SGOT = 4–17 IU/L
  - ALT or SGPT = 3–15 IU/L.
- Although, both AST and ALT are commonly thought of as liver enzymes because of their high concentrations in liver, only ALT is markedly specific for liver since AST is widely present in myocardium, skeletal muscle, brain and kidney and may rise in acute necrosis of these organs besides liver cell injury.

Clinical Interpretation

- The activities of serum alanine transaminase and aspartate transaminase are significantly elevated several days before onset of jaundice in acute viral hepatitis.
- ALT is considered to be more specific for liver disease than AST, because AST is elevated in cases of cardiac or skeletal muscle injury while ALT is not.
- In hepatitis, the levels of both these enzymes (ALT and AST) are increased, which go in thousand units, usually 500–1500 IU/L.
- In obstructive jaundice also an increase occurs but usually does not exceed 200–300 IU/L.
- In hemolytic jaundice, the level of these enzymes is normal.

Alkaline Phosphatase (ALP)

The ALP is produced by many tissues, especially bone, liver, intestine and placenta and is excreted in the bile. Elevation in activity of the enzyme can thus be found in diseases of bone, liver and in pregnancy. In the absence of bone disease and pregnancy, there are elevated ALP levels generally due to hepatobiliary disease.

The normal range for ALP in the plasma is: 3–13 KA units/100 mL (King-Armstrong units).

Clinical Interpretation

- Serum alkaline phosphatase activity is elevated in **obstructive jaundice**. The enzyme ALP is normally excreted through bile. Obstruction to the flow of bile causes regurgitation of enzyme into the blood resulting in increased serum concentration.
- Slight to moderate increase is seen in hepatitis and cirrhosis.

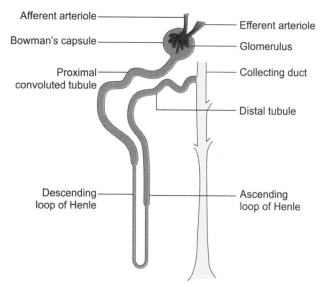

Figure 25.2: Components of nephron.

- Normal serum ALP values are found in hemolytic jaundice.
- A high activity of serum ALP is also seen in bone disease.

FUNCTIONS, DISORDERS AND TESTS TO ASSESS THE FUNCTIONS OF THE KIDNEY

The nephron is the structural and functional unit of the kidney. The component parts of the nephron are given in **Figure 25.2**.

Functions of the Kidney

The chief function of kidney is excretion of water and metabolic wastes in urine. The kidneys excrete a variety of waste products produced by metabolism and toxins into the urine. These include the nitrogenous wastes **urea** from protein catabolism, and **uric acid** from nucleic acid metabolism, **creatinine** from creatine metabolism.

1. The **glomerular filtration** and **renal tubular reabsorption** are the two major functions of kidney that are involved in the formation of urine.
   - Glomeruli provide an efficient filtration mechanism for elimination of the body waste products and toxic substances.
   - To ensure that important constituents are not lost from the body, tubular reabsorption must be equally efficient. Approximately 180 L of fluid passes into the glomerular filtrate each day, and more than 99% of this is recovered.
   - Nephron processes the blood supplied to it via **filtration**, **reabsorption**, **secretion** and **excretion**; in the formation of urine.
     - ♦ **Filtration:** Filtration takes place at the **renal corpuscle** (the glomerulus and the Bowman's

capsule). The glomerulus has a semipermeable membrane through which substances (except cells and large molecular size plasma proteins) are filtered into Bowman's capsule to make an **ultrafiltrate** that eventually becomes **urine**. The rate of filtration is approximately **120 mL/ minute**, known as **glomerular filtration rate (GFR)**. The GFR is an important parameter in clinical assessment of renal function. The kidney generates **180 liters of filtrate a day**. The process is also known as hydrostatic filtration due to the hydrostatic pressure exerted on the capillary walls.

♦ **Reabsorption:** Approximately, 80% of salt and water are reabsorbed from this glomerular ultrafiltrate in the proximal convoluted tubule. All filtered glucose and most of the amino acids are normally reabsorbed here. Low molecular weight proteins, urea, potassium, magnesium and calcium are reabsorbed to varying extent. The descending loop of Henle is highly permeable to water. Passive reabsorption of water occurs leaving the highly concentrated urine at the bottom of the loop. The ascending loop of Henle (diluting segment) is relatively impermeable to passage of water but actively reabsorbs Na$^+$ and Cl$^-$. A small fraction of filtered sodium, chloride and water is reabsorbed in the distal tubule, which responds to antidiuretic hormone (ADH), so that its water permeability is high in the presence of hormone and low in its absence.

♦ **Secretion:** Secretion is the reverse of reabsorption: molecules are transported from the peritubular capillary through the interstitial fluid, then through the renal tubular cell and into the ultrafiltrate.

♦ **Excretion:** The last step in the processing of the ultrafiltrate is excretion: the ultrafiltrate passes out of the nephron and travels through a tube called the collecting duct and then to the ureters where it is renamed urine. In addition to transporting the ultrafiltrate, the collecting duct also takes part in reabsorption. ADH controls the water permeability of the collecting tubule throughout its length.

2. The kidney participates in whole body homeostasis, regulating **acid-base balance**, **electrolyte concentrations**, **extracellular fluid volume**, and **blood pressure**. The kidney accomplishes these homeostatic functions both independently and in concert with other organs, particularly those of the endocrine system. Various endocrine hormones, for example, renin, angiotensin II, aldosterone, antidiuretic hormone, and atrial natriuretic peptide are involved in these functions.

■ **Acid-base balance:** The kidneys have two very important roles in maintaining the acid-base balance: to reabsorb and regenerate bicarbonate from urine, and to excrete hydrogen ions and fixed acids (anions of acids) into urine.

■ **Regulation of osmolality:** Osmolality is maintained by maintaining water and salt level of the body by kidney. Any significant rise in plasma osmolality is detected by the hypothalamus, which communicates directly with the posterior pituitary gland. An increase in osmolality causes the gland to secrete antidiuretic hormone (ADH), resulting in water reabsorption by the kidney and an increase in urine concentration. The two factors work together to return the plasma osmolality to its normal levels.

■ **Hormone secretion:** The kidneys secrete a variety of hormones, including erythropoietin, calcitriol, and renin. Erythropoietin is released in response to hypoxia (low levels of oxygen at tissue level) in the renal circulation. It stimulates erythropoiesis (production of red blood cells) in the bone marrow. They convert a precursor of vitamin D to its active form, calcitriol. Calcitriol, the activated form of vitamin D, promotes intestinal absorption of calcium and the renal reabsorption of phosphate. Renin synthesized by kidney is an enzyme which regulates angiotensin and aldosterone levels.

■ **Blood pressure regulation:** Although, the kidney cannot directly sense blood, long-term regulation of blood pressure predominantly depends upon the kidney. This primarily occurs through maintenance of the extracellular fluid compartment, the size of which depends on the plasma sodium concentration. The **renin-angiotensin system** (*see* **Figure 16.3)** is involved in maintenance of the extracellular fluid compartment and maintaining the blood pressure.

♦ When renin levels are elevated, the concentrations of angiotensin II and aldosterone increase, leading to increased sodium chloride reabsorption, expansion of the extracellular fluid compartment, and an increase in blood pressure.

♦ Conversely, when renin levels are low, angiotensin II and aldosterone levels decrease, contracting the extracellular fluid compartment, and decreasing blood pressure.

Disorders of the Kidney

Disorders of kidney function include **acute kidney injury (AKD)**, and **chronic kidney disease (CKD)**.

Acute Kidney Injury

Acute kidney injury (AKI) is common. In AKI, renal function deteriorates over a period of hours or days. **Chronic kidney disease** develops over months or years and leads eventually to end-stage kidney disease.

- AKI arises from a variety of problems affecting the kidneys and/or their circulation. It usually presents as a sudden deterioration of renal function.
- AKI is characterized by an increase in **serum creatinine** and urea concentrations with a **decrease in urine output** over a period of hours or days.
- AKI may be:
  - **Prerenal:** The kidney fails to receive a proper blood supply. For example, in blood loss and hypovolemia (a decreased volume of circulating blood in the body).
  - **Postrenal:** The urinary drainage of the kidneys is impaired because of a urethral obstruction. For example, in kidney stones or malignancy.
  - **Renal:** Intrinsic or intrarenal damage to kidney tissue. This may be due to variety of diseases, or renal damage. For example, in glomerulonephritis or nephrotoxicity.
- **Acute glomerulonephritis** is acute inflammation of the glomeruli that may result oliguria, hematuria, increased BUN and serum creatinine levels, decreased GFR, edema formation, and hypertension. The presence of red blood cell in the urine (hematuria) alone is insufficient evidence of acute glomerulonephritis, as blood can originate elsewhere in kidney or in the urinary tract. Other abnormalities present in acute glomerulonephritis include **proteinuria** and **anemia**.
- **The nephrotic syndrome** has been characterized by massive proteinuria, edema, hypoalbuminemia, hyperlipidemia, and lipiduria. This syndrome is characterized by increased glomerular membrane permeability that results in massive proteinuria and excretion of fat bodies. Protein excretion rates usually are greater than 2–3 g/day in the absence of a low GFR. Hematuria and oliguria may be present. As a result of the massive loss of serum proteins, primarily albumin into urine, the plasma protein concentration is decreased, with a concomitant reduction in plasma oncotic pressure. This results in fluid movement from the vascular to interstitial space with consequent edema formation.
- **Interstitial nephritis:** Inflammation of the interstitial space of the kidneys is another cause of depressed renal function. This disorder is characterized by pyuria (a condition that is characterized by an elevated number of white blood cells in the urine in the absence of infection), moderate proteinuria, and depressed GFR. Interstitial nephritis usually occurs as a reaction to medications. This reaction can be allergic, in response to any medicine, or nonallergic, in response to nonsteroidal anti-inflammatory medicines.

Chronic Kidney Disease

- CKD is a long-term condition caused by usually irreversible damage to both kidneys and associated with ill health. Patients with CKD may be without symptoms until the GFR falls to very low values (below 15 mL/minute, i.e., to 10% of normal function).
- Consequences of CKD include:
  - Disordered water and sodium metabolism
  - Acid-base imbalance:
    - Hyperkalemia
    - Abnormal calcium and phosphate metabolism
    - Anemia
- In CKD, renal tubules may lose their ability to **reabsorb** and so **concentrate urine**. Because of the impaired ability to regulate water balance, patients with renal disease may **become fluid overload** or **fluid depleted** very easily. Disorders of urine concentration and dilution occur in all renal disease as the GFR falls appreciably.
- Tubular proteinuria may occur as the result of a tubular defect in the handling of proteins. In tubular proteinuria, less than 2 g/day of protein is excreted.
- As CKD progresses, the ability of the kidneys to regenerate bicarbonate and excrete hydrogen ions in the urine becomes impaired. The retention of hydrogen ions causes **renal tubular acidosis (RTA)**. RTA is simply a **metabolic acidosis**.
- The **Fanconi syndrome** is a group of renal tubular defects that results in glucosuria, aminoaciduria, hypophosphatemia, and renal tubular acidosis.
- **Anemia** is often associated with CKD. The normochromic normocytic anemia is due to failure of erythropoietin production.
- Factors indicating increased risk of CKD include:
  - Diabetes mellitus
  - Hypertension

Kidney/Renal Function Tests

In order to assess renal function, a number of tests have been developed which give information regarding the following parameters:

- Renal blood flow
- Glomerular filtration rate
- Renal glomeruli function
- Renal tubular function
- Urinary output.

The various renal function tests have been divided into following groups **(Table 25.4)**.

1. **Urine analysis:** Urinalysis can evaluate for pH, protein, glucose, and the presence of blood in urine, which includes:
   - Physical examination
   - Chemical examination
   - Microscopic examination to identify the presence of urinary casts and crystals.
2. **Estimation of serum and urine markers of renal function**
   - Serum creatinine
   - Serum urea (or blood urea nitrogen, BUN)

TABLE 25.4: Major renal function tests.
Tests
• **Urine analysis** ➢ *Physical characteristics:* Assessment of volume, color, odor, appearance, specific gravity, and pH ➢ *Chemical characteristics:* Checking for the presence of protein, glucose, ketone bodies, blood, bile salts, bile pigments, and urobilinogen ➢ *Microscopy:* Checking for the presence of WBCs, RBCs, and casts • **Serum markers of renal function** ➢ Serum creatinine ➢ Serum urea [or blood urea nitrogen (**BUN**)] • **Estimation of glomerular filtration rate (GFR)** ➢ Creatinine clearance ➢ Inulin clearance • **Tests of renal tubular function** ➢ Osmolality in plasma and urine ➢ Water deprivation test ➢ Urine acidification test ➢ Specific proteinuria ➢ Glycosuria ➢ Aminoaciduria

- Protein in urine (proteinuria)
- Red blood cells in urine (hematuria)

3. **Estimation of glomerular filtration rate (GFR)**
   - Creatinine clearance test
   - Urea clearance test
   - Inulin clearance test
4. **Tests of renal tubular function**
   - Osmolality measurement in plasma and urine
   - Urine concentration test (water deprivation test)
   - Acid load test (urine acidification test)
   - Specific proteinuria
   - Glycosuria
   - Aminoaciduria

> ❖ Kidney biopsy and CT scan performed to evaluate for abnormal anatomy. Dialysis and kidney transplantation are used to treat kidney failure; one (or both sequentially) of these are almost always used when renal function drops below 15%.
> ❖ Nephrectomy is frequently used to cure renal cell carcinoma.

Urine Analysis

Routine urine examination is usually the first test undertaken to assess the renal function and very often it gives some important information like **proteinuria, hematuria** to do further renal investigation. Its analysis, therefore, is important in evaluating kidney function. It may reveal the disease anywhere in the urinary tract. The standard urine analysis includes:

- Physical examination
- Chemical examination
- Microscopic examination of urine.

Physical examination includes: Urine volume (this requires a timed urine sample, usually 24 hours urinary output),

appearance (clear or turbid), color, odor, pH, specific gravity and osmolality.

Volume: The daily output of urine in adult is 800–2,500 mL with an average of **1,500 mL/day**. The quantity normally depends on the water intake, the external temperature, the diet and the mental and physical state, cardiovascular and renal function.

- **Polyuria:** Volume more than 2,500 mL/day occur in:
  - Diabetes mellitus, up to 5–6 L/day
  - Diabetes insipidus, 10–20 L/day
  - Later stages of chronic glomerulonephritis, 2–3 L/day.
- **Oliguria:** Volume 500 mL/day due to:
  - Acute nephritis
  - Early stages of glomerulonephritis
- **Anuria:** Complete cessation of urine occurs in:
  - Acute tubular necrosis
  - Bilateral renal stones

Appearance: Normal urine is transparent. Turbidity in a fresh sample may indicate infection but also may be due to fat particles in an individual with nephrotic syndrome.

Color: Normal urine is pale yellow or amber color. Variation in color may be physiological or pathological. Darkening from the normal pale yellow color indicates more concentrated urine or presence of another pigment. For example, hemoglobin (hematuria) and myoglobin in urine produce a reddish coloration.

- The **presence of myoglobin** in the **urine** is due to muscle injury, rhabdomyolysis. **Myoglobin** is present in muscle cells as a reserve of oxygen.
- Hematuria (Hemoglobinuria) is due to kidney infections, kidney stones, injury or disease of urinary tract or serious kidney diseases such as pyelonephritis or cancer.

Odor: Fresh urine is normally aromatic. Foul smell indicates bacterial infection.

pH: The urine is normally acidic with a pH of about 6.0 (range 5.5–7.5). The renal tubules normally excrete hydrogen ions by mechanisms that ensure tight regulation of blood hydrogen ion concentration. Where one or more of these mechanisms fail, an acidosis results [so called renal tubular acidosis (RTA)]. Measurement of urine pH may be used to screen for RTA in unexpected metabolic acidosis. pH less than 5.3 indicates that the renal tubules are able to acidify urine and thus, is responsible for the metabolic acidosis. Alkaline urine is found in urinary tract infection.

Specific gravity: The specific gravity indicates the concentrating ability of the kidney. It normally varies from **1.016–1.025** with an average 1.02. It can vary widely depending on diet, fluid intake and renal function. If renal function is impaired, the quantity of eliminated urine will be very less. In this condition increased specific gravity may be seen.

TABLE 25.5: Some abnormal constituents of urine.

Constituent	Clinical significance	Examples of conditions in which present
Protein	• **Glomerular proteinuria** refers to the presence of albumin in urine due to a loss of integrity of the glomerular basement membrane	• Nephrotic syndrome, acute glomerulonephritis, diabetic nephropathy, etc.
	• **Overflow proteinuria** is due to the presence of abnormally high levels of low molecular weight proteins in the plasma that are filtered by the glomerulus and thus appear in the urine	• Multiple myeloma (light chains of immunoglobulins appear in urine, resulting in Bence-Jones proteinuria)
	• **Tubular proteinuria** refers to the presence of low molecular weight proteins (like β_2 microglobulin) in urine, due to impaired reabsorption of these proteins by the proximal tubule	• Fanconi's syndrome, nephrotoxicity due to amino glycoside antibiotics, heavy metals, etc.
	• **Postrenal proteinuria** refers to the presence of proteins in urine derived from the urinary tract	• Inflammation of the urinary tract associated with urinary tract infection, nephrolithiasis, and tumors of the urinary tract
Glucose	• **Hyperglycemic glucosuria:** Presence of glucose in urine is usually seen when plasma glucose rises above the renal threshold of 180 mg/dL	• Uncontrolled diabetes mellitus
	• **Renal glucosuria:** Presence of glucose in urine due to impaired reabsorption of glucose in the proximal tubule	• Fanconi's syndrome and inherited defects in the sodium glucose transporter-2 (SGLT-2)
Ketone bodies	Detectable levels in urine (ketonuria) are seen in conditions characterized by increased ketogenesis	Diabetic ketoacidosis and starvation ketoacidosis
Blood	• **Hematuria** refers to the presence of red blood cells in urine, due to bleeding into the urinary tract	• Renal stones or urinary tract infections
	• **Hemoglobinuria** refers to the presence of hemoglobin in urine, which occurs due to intravascular hemolysis	• Incompatible blood transfusions, malaria, etc.
Bile salts and bile pigments	Presence of these in urine is associated with obstruction of the biliary tract	Gallstone or carcinoma of the head of pancreas obstructing the common bile duct

Chemical Examination

• Chemical examination includes detection of the abnormal constituents of urine like: **Protein, blood, glucose, ketone bodies, bile salts** and **bile pigment, urobilinogen, nitrite** and **leukocytes (white blood cells).**

• The abnormal constituents that appear in different disease conditions are listed in **Table 25.5.**

• Most of these parameters can now be estimated semi-quantitatively at the bedside using commercially available **disposable strips (dipstick).** Dipsticks are plastic strips which is impregnated (soaked) with a number of **colored reagents 'blocks'** separated from each other by narrow bands **(Figure 25.3).**

• When the strip is manually immersed in the urine specimen, the reagents in each block react with a specific component of urine in such a way that:
  ▪ The block changes color if the component is present
  ▪ The color change produced is proportional to the concentration of the component being tested for **(Figure 25.4)**

• To test urine sample by disposable strips:
  ▪ Fresh urine is collected into a clean, dry container
  ▪ The sample is not centrifuged
  ▪ The disposable strip is briefly immersed in the urine specimen; care must be taken to ensure that all reagent blocks are covered
  ▪ The strip is then held in a horizontal position for 30 seconds to 2 minutes

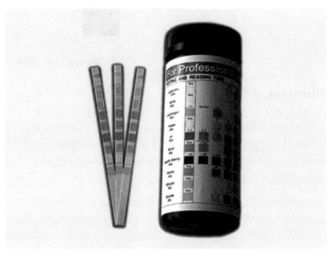

Figure 25.3: Urine multi-dipstick.

▪ The colors of the test areas are compared with those provided on a color chart **(see Figure 25.3).** The strip is held close to the color blocks on the chart, matched carefully and then discarded.

Glucose: The presence of glucose in urine (glycosuria) indicates that the filtered load of glucose exceeds the ability of the renal tubules to reabsorb all of it. This usually occurs in hyperglycemia. However, glycosuria is not always due to diabetes. The renal threshold for glucose may be lowered, e.g., in pregnancy, and glucose may enter the filtrate even at normal plasma concentrations (renal glycosuria which is unrelated to diabetes).

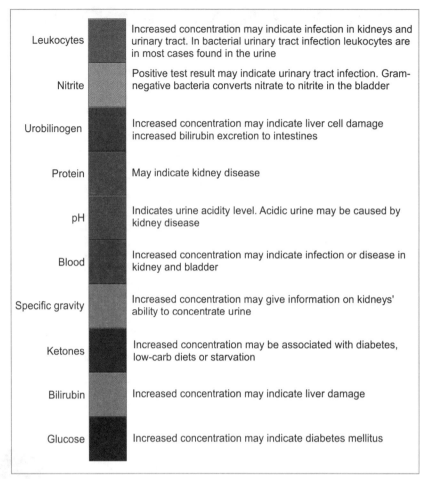

Figure 25.4: Interpretation of urine dipstick.

Bilirubin: Bilirubin exists in the blood in two forms: conjugated and unconjugated. Only the conjugated form is water-soluble, so bilirubinuria signifies the presence in urine of conjugated bilirubin. This is always pathological. Presence of bilirubin in urine is associated with obstruction of the biliary tract.

Urobilinogen: In the gut, conjugated bilirubin is broken down by bacteria to products urobilinogen or stercobilinogen. However, unlike bilirubin, urobilinogen is found in the urine of normal subjects. Thus the finding of urobilinogen in urine is of less diagnostic significance than the finding of bilirubin. High levels are found in any condition in which bilirubin turnover is increased, e.g., hemolysis.

Ketones: Ketones are products of fatty acid breakdown. Their presence usually indicates that the body is using fat to provide energy rather than storing it for later use. This can occur in uncontrolled diabetes, in which glucose is unable to enter cells (diabetic ketoacidosis), in alcoholism (alcoholic ketoacidosis) or in starvation

Protein: Proteinuria may signify abnormal excretion of protein by the kidneys due to abnormally 'leaky' glomeruli or to the inability of the tubules to reabsorb protein normally. Proteinuria and its causes are discussed in detail later.

Blood: The presence of blood in the urine (hematuria) is consistent with various possibilities ranging from malignancy through urinary tract infection to contamination from menstruation. The absence of red cells, despite a strongly positive dipstick test for blood, points towards myoglobinuria or hemoglobinuria.

Nitrite: This dipstick test depends on the conversion of nitrate (from the diet) to nitrite by the action in the urine of bacteria that contain the necessary reductase. A positive result points towards a urinary tract infection.

Leukocytes: The presence of leukocytes in the urine suggests acute inflammation and the presence of a urinary tract infection.

Microscopic Examination

- Microbiological testing of a urine specimen (usually a mid-stream specimen) is routinely performed to confirm the diagnosis of a urinary tract infection. These samples should be collected into sterile containers
- Microscopic examination of the centrifuged urinary sediment is done to detect cells like RBC, WBC, pus cells, crystals like calcium phosphate, calcium oxalate, amorphous phosphates, etc. casts, e.g., hyaline casts, granular casts, red blood casts, etc.

- Presence of crystals in the urine may be a clue to the diagnosis of a specific type of **renal calculus**. Various components are observed on microscopic examination of urine in renal disease.

Renal Stones

Renal stones (calculi) produce severe pain and discomfort and are common causes of obstruction of urinary tract. Types of renal stone include:

- ❖ **Calcium phosphate:** Associated with primary hyperparathyroidism or RTA
- ❖ **Magnesium, ammonium and phosphate:** Associated with urinary tract infection
- ❖ **Oxalate:** Associated with hyperoxaluria
- ❖ **Uric acid:** Associated with hyperuricemia
- ❖ **Cystine:** Associated with inherited metabolic disorder cystinuria.

Serum and Urine Markers of Renal Function

Serum Creatinine and Urea

Serum **urea** and **creatinine** are markers of renal function. Both these substances are primarily excreted in the urine. Deterioration of renal function is, therefore associated with increases in the serum levels of these substances:

- Creatinine is considered a better marker of renal function than urea because its blood level is not significantly affected by nonrenal factors, thus making it a specific indicator of renal function.
- A number of "prerenal" factors like dietary protein intake, renal perfusion, etc. and "postrenal" factors significantly increase blood urea levels.
- An impaired glomerular filtration results in retention of urea and creatinine, which causes in:
  - Elevation of **blood urea** (normal range 20–40 mg/dL)
  - **Creatinine** (normal range 0.5–1.5 mg/dL).
- An increase of these end products in the blood is called **azotemia**.

- ❖ BUN is the nitrogen content of urea. Urea is approximately twice that of BUN. The conversion factor is 0.357
- ❖ BUN mg/dL multiplied by 0.357 = urea (mmol/L)
- ❖ Urea (mmol/L) divided by 0.357 = BUN (mg/dL)

Proteinuria

Proteinuria refers to abnormal urinary excretion of protein. It is most often an indication of abnormal glomerular function. Detection of proteinuria is important because:

- It is associated with renal and cardiovascular disease
- It identifies diabetic patients at risk of **nephropathy** and other microvascular complications
- It predicts end-organ damage in hypertensive patients.

Types of Proteinuria

Glomerular Proteinuria

Normally, the total amount of protein excreted in urine over 24 hours is **less than 150 mg** (and less than 30 mg of albumin)

and is not detectable by routine tests. The presence of protein in urine in excess of this is referred to as **proteinuria**.

- The glomeruli of kidney are not permeable to plasma proteins and therefore do not usually allow passage of **albumin**. So plasma proteins are absent in normal urine. Protein in urine is an indicator of **leaky glomeruli** and is the first sign of **glomerular injury** before a decrease in GFR.
- Excretion of albumin in the range **30–300 mg/day** is termed **microalbuminuria**. Microalbuminuria is the earliest sign of renal damage due to **diabetes mellitus** and **hypertension**. Excretion of albumin more than 300 mg/day is indicative of significant damage to the glomerular membrane.
- When glomeruli are damaged in diseased conditions, they become more permeable and plasma proteins may appear in urine.
- The most common cause of glomerular proteinuria is due to loss of integrity of the **glomerular basement** as seen in **nephrotic syndrome** and **diabetic nephropathy**.
- When this happens, the ability of the body to replace the lost protein is exceeded, and the protein (total protein or albumin) concentration in the patient's blood falls.
- When patients become **hypoproteinemic** and **hypoalbuminemic** due to excessive proteinuria, the normal balance of **oncotic** and **hydrostatic forces** at the capillary level is disturbed, leading to loss of fluid into the interstitial space **(edema)**.

Tubular Proteinuria

- Some proteins are so small that, unlike albumin and other larger proteins; they pass through the glomerulus freely.
- The best-known examples are α_1-**microglobulin**, β_2-**microglobulin**, and **retinol-binding protein**.
- If these proteins are detected in excess in the urine, this indicates tubular rather than glomerular dysfunction, i.e., an inability of the renal tubules to reabsorb them.

Overflow Proteinuria

- Overflow proteinuria occurs when the ability of the glomeruli to retain proteins is overwhelmed by the total quantity of protein.
- The best characterized example of overflow proteinuria is seen in **multiple myeloma**.
- Multiple myeloma involves malignant proliferation of a clone of plasma cells which produce immunoglobulins.
- This results in the production of huge amounts of the immunoglobulin by the malignant clone and **light-chain fragments of immunoglobulin** are excreted in the urine. These light chain fragments of immunoglobulin called **Bence-Jones proteins**

Postrenal Proteinuria

Postrenal proteinuria refers to the presence of proteins in urine derived from the urinary tract. Postrenal proteinuria occurs with inflammation of the urinary tract associated with urinary tract infection, nephrolithiasis, and tumors of the urinary tract. Postrenal proteinuria usually resolves when the underlying condition has resolved.

Tamm-Horsfall Proteinuria
This glycoprotein gets its name from the authors of a 1952 paper describing its purification. It is one of the most abundant proteins in urine. It is not derived from the blood, but rather is produced and secreted into the filtrate by the **ascending loop of Henle**. Increased levels of it forms large aggregates that can form urinary casts that may pass into the urine.

Hematuria

Intact glomerulus does not allow the passage of RBC. But with severe glomerular damage, RBC leakage occurs. Thus, detection of microscopic hematuria or RBC casts confirms glomerular damage and is an earliest sign before the decrease in GFR.

Estimation of Glomerular Filtration Rate

These tests are performed to assess the **glomerular filtration rate**. GFR provides a useful index of the status of functioning glomeruli. Renal clearance tests are performed to determine GFR.

Clearance Test

The renal clearance test is performed to measure the glomerular filtration rate. Clearance is defined as the volume of plasma (in mL) from which a particular substance is completely cleared by the kidney per minute and is expressed as milliliters per minute. It may also be defined as that volume of plasma (in mL) containing the amount of particular substance which is excreted by kidney in urine in 1 minute. Renal clearance (C) is calculated by using following formula.

$$\text{Clearance (mL/min) } C = \frac{U \times V}{P}$$

Where,

C: Renal clearance = GFR of a substance in mL/minute
U: Concentration of substance in urine (mg/100 mL)
V: Volume of urine produced per minute (calculated by dividing the value for the volume of urine collected over 24 hours by 1440 [24 × 60])
P: Concentration of substance in plasma (mg/100 mL).

- Lower than normal GFR measurements indicate:
  - Acute tubular necrosis
  - Glomerulonephrosis
  - Acute nephrotic syndrome
  - Acute and chronic renal failure.
- In order to determine GFR, the substance should be selected in such a way that, which is:
  - Freely filtered by glomerulus
  - Should not be reabsorbed or secreted

- Should not be metabolized by the kidney
- Should not be toxic
- It should not be affected by dietary intake.
- The substances which are used for clearance tests include:
  - Endogenous creatinine and urea.
  - Exogenous inulin.

Creatinine Clearance Tests

- Even though **serum creatinine** is considered a specific marker of renal function, a significant increase in its blood level is seen only after a ~50% decline in the glomerular filtration rate has occurred. It is therefore a test of poor sensitivity.
- Measurement of **creatinine clearance**, on the other hand which gives an estimate of the GFR helps in early detection of renal failure.
- Creatinine clearance is defined as the volume of plasma (in mL) from which creatinine is completely cleared by the kidney per minute and is expressed as milliliters per minute.
- The creatinine clearance is determined by collecting urine over a 24-hour period and a sample of blood is drawn during the urine collection period. The clearance of creatinine from plasma is directly related to the GFR, which is calculated as follows:

$$\text{Creatinine clearance} = \text{GFR} = \frac{U \times V}{P}$$

Where,
U is urinary creatinine (mg/dL)
P is plasma creatinine (mg/dL)
V is volume of urine excreted (mL/minute).

- ❖ Creatinine is an excretory product derived from **creatine phosphate**.
- ❖ The excretion of creatinine is not influenced by metabolism or dietary factors.
- ❖ **Characteristics of an ideal substance to be used for Clearance Tests** are given in **Table 25.6**.
- ❖ Creatinine is freely filtered at the glomerulus and is not reabsorbed by the tubules. A small amount of creatinine is secreted by tubules. Because of these properties, the creatinine clearance can be used to estimate the GFR.

Clinical Interpretation

- The normal range for creatinine clearance is **90–120 mL/minute**.
- A decreased creatinine clearance is a very sensitive indicator of a **decreased glomerular filtration rate**.
- The reduced filtration rate may be caused by **acute** or **chronic damage** to the **glomerulus** or any of its components.
- Reduced blood flow to the glomeruli may also produce a decreased creatinine clearance.

TABLE 25.6: Characteristics of an ideal substance to be used for clearance tests.
Characteristics
• It should have a fairly constant blood level • It should be excreted from the body only in the urine • It should be freely filtered at the glomerulus • It should neither be reabsorbed nor secreted by the renal tubules

Urea Clearance Test

Urea is the end product of protein metabolism. Urea clearance may also be employed as a measure of the GFR. But urea clearance is not as sensitive as creatinine clearance because:

- Unlike creatinine, 40–60% of urea is reabsorbed by the renal tubules after being filtered at glomeruli. Hence, its clearance is less than GFR.
- Moreover, urea clearance is influenced by number of factors, e.g., dietary protein, fluid intake, infection, surgery, etc. Urea clearance is defined as the volume of plasma (in mL) that would be completely cleared off urea per minute. It is calculated by the formula as given above.

Clinical Interpretation

- The normal value of urea clearance is 75 mL/minute.
- Urea clearance between 40 and 70 mL/min indicates mild impairment, between 20 and 40 mL/min indicates moderate impairment and below 20 mL/min indicates severe impairment of renal function.

Inulin Clearance Test

Inulin is a polysaccharide of **fructose**, which is filtered by the glomerulus but not reabsorbed, secreted or metabolically altered by the renal tubule. **Inulin clearance** is considered the gold standard method for measuring GFR, as it satisfies all the criteria essential for a substance to be used in clearance test **(Table 25.6)**. The normal value of inulin clearance is **120 mL/min**.

STRIKE A NOTE

❖ Though **Inulin clearance** is considered the gold standard method for measuring GFR, however, creatinine clearance is widely used due to the **ease of estimation of creatinine** (by Jaffe's method) and the fact that it is an **endogenous substance** (as opposite to inulin, which is **exogenous** in origin and has to be injected intravenously at a constant rate).

❖ An important drawback associated with the use of clearance tests to estimate GFR is the need for an accurately timed urine sample. However, this problem can be overcome by employing formulae, which can be used to calculate an estimated value for GFR called eGFR, using serum creatinine values alone by correcting for age, sex, and body weight. One such formula is the **Cockcroft-Gault formula**, shown here.

Estimated GFR (creatinine clearance) mL/min =

$$\frac{(140 - age) \times weight~(kg) \times 0.85~(if~female)}{72 \times serum~creatinine~(mg/dL)}$$

Tests of Renal Tubular Function

- The glomeruli provide an efficient filtration mechanism for elimination of waste products and toxic substances from the body. To ensure that important constituents are not lost from the body. Tubular reabsorption must be equally efficient.
- Approximately 180 L of fluid passes into the glomerular filtrate each day, and more than 99% of this recovered.
- However, compared with glomerular filtration rate as overall assessment of glomerular function, there is no single measure of tubular function that gives overall assessment of tubular function. Urine osmolality is sometimes used to measure tubular function.
- Some disorders of tubular function are inherited, e.g., the ability of some patients to acidify urine is limited by a failure of hydrogen ion secretion.
- However, renal tubular damage is much more frequently secondary to other conditions.
- Any cause of acute kidney injury may be associated with renal tubular failure.

Osmolality in Plasma and Urine

- Urine osmolality serves as a useful general marker of tubular function. This is because of all tubular functions; the one most frequently affected by disease is the **ability to concentrate urine**.
- If the tubules and collecting ducts are working efficiently, they will be able to reabsorb water.
- Ability to concentrate urine can be assessed by measuring urine concentration (osmolality) and comparing this to the plasma (serum) osmolality.
  - If the urine osmolality is 600 mmol/kg or more, tubular function is usually regarded as intact.
  - When the urine osmolality does not differ greatly from plasma (urine/plasma osmolality ratio approximately 1), the renal tubules are not reabsorbing water.
- The urine osmolality of normal individuals varies widely depending on the state of hydration. After excessive intake of fluids, the osmotic concentration may fall as low as 50 mOsm/kg, whereas with restricted fluid intake it is up to 1,200 mOsm/kg have been observed. On average fluid intakes, 300–900 mOsm/kg are found.

Water Deprivation Test (Urine Concentration Test)

- Where measurement of urine osmolality is inconclusive, tubular concentrating and **diluting** ability test may be performed.
- Assessment of the **concentrating** and **diluting** ability of the kidney can provide the most sensitive means of detecting early impairment in renal function since the ability to concentrate or dilute urine is dependent upon:
  - Adequate GFR
  - Renal plasma flow

- Tubular mass
- Healthy tubular cells
- Presence of antidiuretic hormone.

- The urinary **specific gravity** and **osmolality** are used to measure the concentrating and diluting ability of the tubules.
- In the fluid deprivation test, fluid intake is withheld for 15 hours. The first urine sample in the morning is collected and osmolality or specific gravity is measured.
  - If osmolality exceeds **850 mOsmol/kg** or **specific gravity of 1.025**, the renal concentrating ability is considered normal.
  - Dehydration maximally stimulates ADH secretion. If kidney is normal, water is selectively reabsorbed resulting in excretion of urine of high solute concentration and urine osmolality should be at least three times that of plasma (286 mOsmol/kg).

Clinical Interpretation

In case the urine does not have specific gravity 1.025 or osmolality 850 mOsmol/kg it is sure that renal concentrating ability is impaired either due to tubular defect or decreased secretion of ADH (diabetes insipidus). So ADH test must be carried out.

- If the tubules and collecting ducts are working efficiently and if ADH is present they will be able to reabsorb water
- In polyuria of diabetes insipidus, where the hormone ADH is lacking or in nephrogenic diabetes insipidus (lack of response to ADH), the osmolality will remain constant even after fluid deprivation.

> ❖ In practice, the fluid deprivation test is extremely unpleasant for the patient. It is potentially dangerous if the patient cannot retain water. The test must be terminated if more than 3 L of urine are passed. Clinically, the loss of concentrating ability is manifested by **nocturia** (passage of urine at night) and polyuria.
> ❖ For this reason, instead of a formal water deprivation test, an alternative method is to restrict fluid overnight (8 pm–10 am) and measure urine osmolality the following morning in early morning spot urine.

Acid Load Test (Urine Acidification Test) or Ammonium Chloride Loading Test

- The acid load test is occasionally used for the diagnosis of **renal tubular acidosis** in which metabolic acidosis resulting from defective renal tubular function, specifically relating to its ability to handle hydrogen and bicarbonate.
- Ammonium chloride is administered orally in gelatine capsule (100 mg/kg body weight) to cause **metabolic acidosis** and the capacity of kidneys is assessed for the production of acidic urine. Urine samples are collected hourly for the following 8 hours.
- This test is very unpleasant for the patient and may be associated with vomiting. A more acceptable alternative

is to administer **furosemide (a synthetic diuretic compound)**, which reduces reabsorption of chloride and sodium from the loop of Henle.

Clinical Interpretation

- In normal subjects, the urine pH falls below 5.5 in at least one sample due to increase acid excretion. Normal urine pH is 5.5–7.5.
- In an individual with renal tubular acidosis this decrease does not occur, which remains between 5.7 and 7.0.

Specific Proteinuria

The appearance of abnormal amounts of protein in urine may indicate leaky glomeruli. α_1-**microglobulin** and β_2-**microglobulin** are small proteins filtered at the glomeruli, but usually they are reabsorbed by the tubular cells. An increased concentration of these proteins in urine is a sensitive indicator of renal tubular cell damage. Proteinuria is discussed in detail earlier.

Glycosuria

- The presence of glucose in urine when blood glucose is normal is usually due to the inability of the tubules to reabsorb glucose because of a specific tubular lesion. Here, the renal threshold has been exceeded. This is called renal glycosuria and is benign.
- Glycosuria also present in other disorders of tubular function, e.g., **Fanconi syndrome**. The **Fanconi syndrome** is a group of renal tubular defects that results in **glucosuria**, **aminoaciduria**, **hypophosphatemia**, and **renal tubular acidosis**.

Aminoaciduria

- Normally, amino acids in a glomerular filtrate are reabsorbed in the proximal tubules.
- They may be present in excessive amounts because either the plasma concentration exceeds the renal threshold or there is specific failure of normal tubular reabsorptive mechanisms.
- The latter may occur in the inherited disorder **cystinuria** or more commonly because of **renal tubular damage**.

▌ FUNCTIONS, DISORDERS AND TESTS TO ASSESS THE FUNCTIONS OF THE THYROID

The thyroid gland, or simply the thyroid, is an endocrine gland in the neck, consisting of two lobes. The thyroid gland secrets the hormones: **thyroxine (T_4)** and **triiodothyronine (T_3)** which primarily influence the **metabolic rate** and **protein synthesis**. The hormones also have many other effects including those on development. To understand the thyroid function tests, it is necessary to understand the following basic concepts:

- The thyroid hormones **triiodothyronine (T_3)** and **thyroxine (T_4)** are produced from **tyrosine** and **iodine.**
- The function of the thyroid gland is to take iodine from the circulating blood, combine it with the amino acid **tyrosine** of thyroglobulin and convert it to the thyroid hormones **thyroxine (T_4)** and **triiodothyronine (T_3).**
- T_4 has four iodine atoms, whereas T_3 has three.
- The thyroid gland secretes mostly **T_4**, the concentration of which in plasma is around **100 nmol/L.**
- Peripheral tissues, especially **liver** and **kidney**, deiodinate T_4 to produce approximately two-thirds of the circulating **T_3**, present at a concentration of around **2 nmol/L.**
- T_3 is more biologically active; it binds to receptors and triggers the effects of the thyroid hormones.
- After secretion, only a very small proportion of the thyroid hormones travel freely in the blood. Most are bound to:
  - Thyroxine-binding globulin, TBG (about 70%)
  - Transthyretin (10%)
  - Albumin (15%).
- Only small amount of the hormone (0.03% of T_4 and 0.3% of T_3) is free which is not bound to protein have hormonal activity.
- However, it is the free portion of the thyroid hormones that is the true determinant of the thyroid status of the patient.
- Hormone production by the thyroid gland is tightly regulated through **hypothalamic-pituitary-thyroid axis (HPTA) (Figure 25.5).** The components of the HPTA axis are:
  - Thyrotropin-releasing hormone (TRH)
  - Thyroid-stimulating hormone (TSH)
  - Thyroid hormones
- Formation of triiodothyronine (T_3) and thyroxine (T_4) by thyroid is regulated by **thyroid-stimulating hormone** secreted from the anterior pituitary gland, which itself is regulated by **thyrotropin-releasing hormone** produced by the hypothalamus.
- Thyroid hormones provide negative feedback to the TSH and TRH:
  - If the thyroid is producing too much thyroid hormone, this will suppress the circulating TSH.
  - If the thyroid is not secreting enough thyroid hormone, TSH will be very high-attempting to stimulate the gland to secret more.
- This negative feedback also occurs when levels of TSH are high, causing TRH production to be suppressed.

Functions of Thyroid

The thyroid hormones T_3 and T_4 have a number of **metabolic, cardiovascular** and **developmental effects** on the body. The primary function of the thyroid is the production of hormones, **triiodothyronine (T_3)** and **thyroxine (T_4)** and the peptide hormone **calcitonin.** The thyroid hormones have a wide range of effects on the human body. These include:

- **Metabolic:** The thyroid hormones increase the **basal metabolic rate** and have effects on almost all body tissues. Appetite, the absorption of substances, and gut motility are all influenced by thyroid hormones. They increase the absorption in the gut, uptake by cells, and breakdown of glucose. They stimulate the breakdown of fats, and increase the number of free fatty acids. Despite increasing free fatty acids, thyroid hormones decrease cholesterol levels, perhaps by increasing the rate of secretion of cholesterol in bile.
- **Cardiovascular:** The hormones increase the rate and strength of the heartbeat. They increase the rate of breathing, intake and consumption of oxygen, and increase the activity of mitochondria. Overall, these factors increase blood flow and the body's temperature.
- **Developmental:** Thyroid hormones are important for normal development. They increase the growth rate of young people, and cells of the developing brain are a major target for the thyroid hormones T_3 and T_4. Thyroid hormones play a particularly crucial role in brain maturation during fetal development and first few years of postnatal life.
- The thyroid gland also produces the hormone **calcitonin**, which helps regulate blood calcium levels. Parafollicular cells produce calcitonin in response to high blood calcium. Calcitonin decreases the release of calcium from bone, by decreasing the activity of osteoclasts, cells which break down bone. Bone is constantly resorbed by osteoclasts, and is deposited by osteoblasts in a process called ossification. Calcitonin effectively stimulates deposition of calcium into bone. The effects of calcitonin are opposite those of the

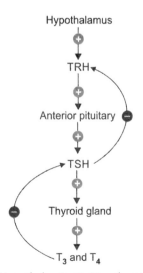

Figure 25.5: Hypothalamic pituitary thyroid axis (HPTA).
(TRH: thyrotropin-releasing hormone; TSH: thyroid-stimulating hormone)

parathyroid hormone (PTH) produced in the parathyroid glands.

Disorders of Thyroid Gland

Hyperthyroidism

- Excessive production of the thyroid hormones is called hyperthyroidism, which is most commonly a result from:
  - Graves' disease
  - Toxic multinodular goiter
  - Solitary thyroid adenoma
  - Thyroiditis
- Hyperthyroidism often causes a variety of nonspecific symptoms. The clinical features of hyperthyroidism may include:
  - Weight loss inspite normal or increased appetite
  - Sweating and decreased tolerance of heat
  - Tremor, palpitations, anxiety and nervousness
  - In some cases, it can cause chest pain, diarrhea, and hair loss and muscle weakness.

Hypothyroidism

- Hypothyroidism usually develops slowly. An underactive thyroid gland results in hypothyroidism.
- The clinical features of hypothyroidism may include:
  - Weight gain
  - Lethargy and tiredness
  - Constipation
  - Heavy menstrual bleeding
  - Hair loss
  - Cold intolerance
  - Slow heart rate.
  - Many other associated signs including, anemia, dementia, muscle stiffness.
- Hypothyroidism is most commonly occur in:
  - **Hashimoto's thyroiditis:** The autoimmune disease due to destruction of thyroid gland
  - Iodine deficiency is the most common cause of hypothyroidism worldwide
  - Radioiodine or surgical treatment of hyperthyroidism
  - Congenital defects such as blocks in the biosynthesis of T_4 and T_3
  - Myxedema

Goiter

An enlarged thyroid gland is called a goiter **(Figure 25.6)**. Goiter may be due to iodine deficiency, autoimmune disease (both Grave's disease and Hashimoto's thyroiditis), infection, and inflammation. Globally, iodine deficiency is the common cause of goiter:

- Some forms of goiter are associated with pain, whereas many do not cause any symptoms.

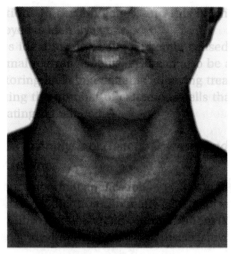

Figure 25.6: A patient with goiter

- Enlarged goiters may extend beyond the normal position of the thyroid gland to below the sternum, around the airway or esophagus.
- Goiters may be associated with hyperthyroidism or hypothyroidism, relating to the underlying cause of the goiter. Thyroid function tests may be done to investigate the cause and effects of the goiter.

Graves' Disease

Graves' disease is an **autoimmune disorder** that is the most common cause of **hyperthyroidism**. In Graves' disease, for unknown reason autoantibodies develop against the thyroid-stimulating hormone receptor.

- These antibodies activate the receptor, leading to development of a goiter and symptoms of **hyperthyroidism**, such as heat intolerance, weight loss, diarrhea and palpitations.
- Occasionally such antibodies block but do not activate the receptor, leading to symptoms associated with **hypothyroidism**.
- In addition, gradual protrusion of the eyes may occur, called Graves' ophthalmopathy **(Figure 25.7)**.

Thyroiditis

Inflammation of the thyroid is called thyroiditis. Inflamed thyroids may cause symptoms of hyperthyroidism or hypothyroidism.

Thyroid Function Tests

- A number of tests can be used to assess the function of the thyroid, the presence of diseases, and the success or failure of treatment. Blood tests in general aim to measure thyroid function or to determine the cause of thyroid dysfunction. They may reveal:
  - Hyperthyroidism (high T_3 and T_4)
  - Hypothyroidism (low T_3, T_4), or

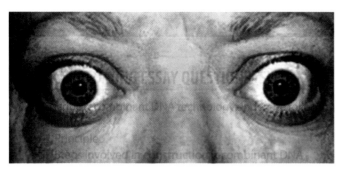

Figure 25.7: Protrusion of the eyes (Graves' ophthalmopathy) in a patient with Graves' disease.

- ■ Subclinical hyperthyroidism (normal T_3 and T_4 with a low TSH).
- The evaluation of the thyroid status is not a simple procedure because it does not depend solely on the measurement of circulating thyroid hormone. One or more of the following factors may be abnormal and these have to be sorted out and evaluated.
  - ■ The concentration of **thyroid-binding protein (TBG)** and its degree of saturation with T_3 and T_4
  - ■ Concentration of **free T_3 and T_4.** T_4 is preferred, because in hypothyroidism T_3 levels may be normal.
  - ■ The status of **hypothalamus** and **anterior pituitary** with their respective outputs of TRH and TSH. TSH levels are considered the most sensitive marker of thyroid dysfunction.
  - ■ The response of the pituitary to TRH and response of the thyroid to TSH.
- Lastly, antibodies against components of the thyroid, particularly **antithyroid peroxidase (anti-TPO)** and **antithyroglobulin antibodies** can be measured. These may be present in normal individuals but are highly sensitive for autoimmune-related disease.
- Ultrasound of the thyroid may be used to reveal whether structures are solid or filled with fluid, helping to differentiate between nodules and goiters and cysts. It may also help differentiate between malignant and benign lesions.
- A fine needle aspiration biopsy may be taken simultaneously of thyroid tissue to determine the nature of a lesion.
- Computed tomography of the thyroid plays an important role in the evaluation of thyroid cancer. CT scans often incidentally find thyroid abnormalities, and thereby practically becomes the first investigation modality.
- The main thyroid function tests commonly done in clinical practice are **(Table 25.7).**
  1. Serum thyroid-stimulating hormone (TSH)
  2. Serum free thyroxin (T_4) and triiodothyronine (T3)
  3. Tests for autoimmune thyroid diseases include tests for:
     - ♦ TSH receptor antibodies
     - ♦ Thyroglobulin antibodies
     - ♦ Thyroid peroxidase antibodies.

TABLE 25.7: Major thyroid function tests.
Tests
• Serum thyroid-stimulating hormone (TSH)
• Serum free thyroxin (T_4) and triiodothyronine (T_3)
• TSH receptor antibodies
• Thyroglobulin antibodies
• Thyroid peroxidase antibodies

Serum Thyroid-stimulating Hormone

The measurement of plasma thyroid-stimulating hormone in a basal blood sample provides the single most sensitive, specific and reliable test of thyroid status. Stimulation of the thyroid gland by the TSH, which is produced by the anterior pituitary gland, will cause the release of stored thyroid hormones.

- When T_4 and T_3 are too high, TSH secretion decreases.
- When T_4 and T_3 are too low, TSH secretion increases.
  This measurement is used in the diagnosis of **primary hypothyroidism** (thyroid gland failure).

Normal values of serum TSH: 2–6 µU/mL.

Clinical Interpretation

- Increased levels of serum TSH are seen in primary **hypothyroidism** due to absence of negative feedback control on the pituitary (*see* **Figure 25.5**).
- Decreased levels of serum TSH are associated with:
  - ■ Primary hyperthyroidism (thyroid gland failure)
  - ■ Secondary hypothyroidism (anterior pituitary failure)
  - ■ Tertiary hypothyroidism (hypothalamic failure)

Serum Free T_3 and T_4

This is a measure of that fraction of circulatory T_4 and T_3 that exists in the free state in the blood, unbound to protein. Measurement of free thyroxine levels will help establish the diagnosis in most cases where an abnormal value is obtained **(Table 25.8).** Free thyroid hormone concentrations provide more reliable means of diagnosing thyroid dysfunction than measurement of total serum T_4 and T_3.

Normal values of free serum T_4 and T_3
- Free T_4 = 10–27 pmol/L
- Free T_3 = 3–9 pmol/L.

Clinical Interpretation

- Increased values are associated with hyperthyroidism and thyrotoxicosis.

TABLE 25.8: Laboratory diagnosis of thyroid disorders.

Free thyroxin	TSH levels	
	High	**Low**
High	Secondary hyperthyroidism	Primary hyperthyroidism
Low	Primary hypothyroidism	Secondary hypothyroidism

- **Primary hyperthyroidism:** Increased levels of T_3 and T_4 with decreased levels of TSH
- **Secondary hyperthyroidism:** Increased levels of T_3 and T_4 with increased levels of TSH
- Decreased values are associated with hypothyroidism.
  - **Primary hypothyroidism:** Decreased levels of T_3 and T_4 with increased levels of TSH
  - **Secondary hypothyroidism:** Decreased levels of T_3 and T_4 with decreased levels of TSH

Serum Total T_4 and T_3

Changes in total thyroid hormone concentration are far less sensitive indices of thyroid function than is TSH; for this reason, they should not be measured alone. The concentration of total serum thyroxine can be affected by changes in the concentration of **thyroid-binding globulin**, in the absence of thyroid disease. Because more than 99.9% of thyroid hormone is protein bound. Serum total T_4 and T_3 are clinically meaningful only if the functional levels of thyroid-binding proteins in blood are known. This test is a good index of thyroid function when TBG is normal.

The normal values of total T_4 and T_3

- T_4 = 5–12.5 μg/dL.
- T_3 = 70–200 ng/dL.

Clinical Interpretation

- Values can be increased in:
  - Hyperthyroidism
  - Increased concentration of TBG (as in pregnancy and with estrogen therapy).
  Thyroid-binding globulin levels rise during pregnancy in response to elevated estrogen levels. Because the majority of T_4 and T_3 circulates bound to TBG the total T_4 and total T_3 measurements will also rise, but the levels of free T_4 and free T_3 will not be affected.
- Values can be decreased in:
  - Hypothyroidism
  - Decreased concentration of TBG (as in nephrosis due to loss of TBG in urine and in liver disease in which there is a decreased synthesis of TBG).

Thyroid Autoantibodies

Autoimmune thyroid diseases produce **antibodies** against components of thyroid. Several types of antibody against thyroid tissue have been detected in serum of patients with thyroid disease. Measuring these antibodies helps demonstrate the presence of the autoimmune disorders. For example:

- **Graves' disease** is commonly associated with the presence of antibodies against the **TSH receptor**.
- **Hashimoto's thyroiditis** (autoimmune thyroiditis) is associated with the presence of antibodies against

thyroid peroxidase (**TPO antibodies**, previously called **antimicrosomal antibodies**).

- Measurement of **Thyroglobulin (Tg) antibody** is of particular use in assessing the presence of any **remnant thyroid tissue** after thyroidectomy, performed for malignancy

> ❖ **Thyroid peroxidase (TPO)** is an enzyme normally found in the thyroid gland. TPO plays an important role in the production of thyroid hormones.
> ❖ **Thyroglobulin (Tg)** is a glycoprotein made by the thyroid gland that serves as the source for thyroxine (T_4) and triiodothyronine (T_3) production within the lumen of thyroid follicles.

Clinical Interpretation

- **Thyroid peroxidase** and **thyroglobulin** antibodies are present in the serum of patients with immunological mediated thyroid disease, e.g., Hashimoto's thyroiditis and Graves' disease.
- They may also be found in a small proportion of healthy individuals, the incidence being higher in relations of patients with hyperthyroidism.
- After successful thyroidectomy for thyroid malignancy Tg antibody concentration in blood will fall to undetectable levels. The reappearance of Tg in blood is strongly suggestive of tumor recurrence.

FUNCTIONS, DISORDERS AND TESTS TO ASSESS THE FUNCTIONS OF THE ADRENAL GLANDS

The adrenal glands are endocrine glands. They are found above the kidneys. Each gland has an outer cortex and an inner medulla.

Functions of Adrenal Gland

The adrenal gland secretes a number of different hormones, these hormones are involved in a number of essential biological function.

- The adrenal cortex produces three main types of steroid hormones:
  1. **Mineralocorticoids**—such as **aldosterone**
  2. **Glucocorticoids**—such as **cortisol**
  3. **Androgens—sex hormones**
- The medulla produces the **catecholamines; adrenaline** and **noradrenaline**.

Mineralocorticoids

- In the kidneys, aldosterone acts on the distal convoluted tubules and the collecting ducts by increasing the reabsorption of **sodium** and the excretion of both **potassium** and **hydrogen ions**.
- The amount of sodium present in the body affects the extracellular volume, which in turn influences blood

pressure. Therefore, the effects of aldosterone in sodium retention are important for the regulation of blood pressure.

- Mineralocorticoid secretion is regulated mainly by the renin angiotensin-aldosterone system (RAAS).

Glucocorticoids

Glucocorticoids are under the regulatory influence of **the hypothalamus-pituitary-adrenal (HPA) axis (Figure 25.8)**. Glucocorticoid synthesis is stimulated by adrenocorticotropic hormone (ACTH), a hormone released by the anterior pituitary. In turn, production of ACTH is stimulated by the presence of corticotropin-releasing hormone (CRH), which is released by the hypothalamus. Excess glucocorticoid acts as an inhibitor of both CRH and ACTH synthesis. Glucocorticoids have many effects on metabolism.

- As their name suggests, they increase the blood glucose level by increasing the mobilization of amino acids from protein and the stimulation of synthesis of glucose from these amino acids in the liver by gluconeogenesis.
- In addition, they increase the levels of free fatty acids, which cells can use as an alternative to glucose to obtain energy.
- Glucocorticoids also have effects unrelated to the regulation of blood sugar levels, including the suppression of the immune system and a potent anti-inflammatory effect.

Androgens

The adrenal glands produce **male sex hormones,** or **androgens,** the most important of which is **dehydroepiandrosterone (DHEA)**. These hormones are converted to more potent androgens such as testosterone and dihydrotestosterone (DHT) or to estrogens (female sex hormones) in the gonads.

Catecholamines

The adrenal medulla produces the **catecholamines; epinephrine (adrenaline)** and **norepinephrine (noradrena-** line**),** which function to produce a rapid response throughout the body in stress situations. Release of catecholamine is stimulated by the activation of the sympathetic nervous system.

Adrenaline and noradrenaline increase blood pressure and heart rate. Actions of adrenaline and noradrenaline are responsible for the **fight or flight response,** characterized by a quickening of breathing and heart rate, an increase in blood pressure, and constriction of blood vessels in many parts of the body.

Disorders of Adrenal Gland

The normal function of the adrenal gland may be impaired by conditions such as infections, tumors, genetic disorders and autoimmune diseases, or as a side effect of medical therapy. These disorders affect the gland either directly (as with infections or autoimmune diseases) or as a result of the dysregulation of hormone production (as in some types of Cushing's syndrome) leading to an excess or insufficiency of adrenal hormones and the related symptoms.

Cushing's Syndrome

Cushing's syndrome is the manifestation of **glucocorticoid excess**. It can be the result of a prolonged treatment with glucocorticoids or due to alterations in the HPA (hypothalamic-pituitary-adrenal axis) axis or the production of cortisol.

- Causes can be further classified into **ACTH-dependent** or **ACTH-independent**. The most common cause of endogenous Cushing's syndrome is a **pituitary adenoma** which causes an excessive production of **ACTH**.
- The disease produces a wide variety of signs and symptoms which include obesity, diabetes, increased blood pressure, excessive body hair (hirsutism), osteoporosis, depression, and most distinctively, stretch marks in the skin, caused by its progressive thinning.

Primary Aldosteronism

When the adrenal gland produces excess aldosterone, the result is primary aldosteronism. Causes for this condition are bilateral hyperplasia (excessive tissue growth) of the glands, or aldosterone-producing adenomas (a condition called Conn's syndrome).

Primary aldosteronism produces hypertension and electrolyte imbalance, increasing potassium depletion and sodium retention.

Adrenal Insufficiency

Adrenal insufficiency (the deficiency of glucocorticoids) occurs in about 5 in 10,000 in the general population. Diseases classified as **primary adrenal insufficiency** (including Addison's disease and genetic causes) directly affect the adrenal cortex. If a problem that affects the

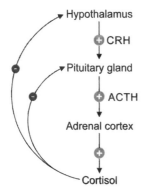

Figure 25.8: Hypothalamic pituitary adrenal axis (HPAA).
(CRH: corticotropin-releasing hormone; ACTH: adrenocorticotropic hormone)

hypothalamic-pituitary-adrenal axis arises outside the gland, it is a **secondary adrenal insufficiency**.

Addison's Disease

Addison's disease refers to **primary hypoadrenalism**, which is a deficiency in **glucocorticoid** and **mineralocorticoid** production by the adrenal gland:

- Addison's disease is most commonly an autoimmune condition, in which the body produces antibodies against cells of the adrenal cortex.
- Worldwide, the disease is more frequently caused by infection, especially from tuberculosis.
- A distinctive feature of Addison's disease is **hyperpigmentation of the skin**, which presents with other nonspecific symptoms such as fatigue.

Secondary Adrenal Insufficiency

In secondary adrenal insufficiency, a dysfunction of the hypothalamic-pituitary-adrenal axis leads to decreased stimulation of the adrenal cortex due to:

- Suppression of the axis by glucocorticoid therapy is the most common cause of secondary adrenal insufficiency.
- **Tumors** that affect the production of adrenocorticotropic hormone by the pituitary gland.
- This type of adrenal insufficiency usually does not affect the production of mineralocorticoids, which are under regulation of the renin-angiotensin system instead.

Congenital Adrenal Hyperplasia

Congenital adrenal hyperplasia (CAH) is a group of **autosomal recessive** disease in which mutations of **enzymes** that are responsible for synthesis of **steroid hormones** (cortisol, aldosterone, and, in very rare cases, androgen) occur. All forms of CAH are characterized by **low levels of cortisol**, **high levels of ACTH**, and **adrenal hyperplasia (overgrowth)**.

- The most common form of congenital adrenal hyperplasia is due to deficiency of **21β-hydroxylase**. 21β-hydroxylase is necessary for production of both mineralocorticoids and glucocorticoids, but not androgens. Therefore, ACTH stimulation of the adrenal cortex induces the release of excessive amounts of adrenal androgens, which can lead to the development of ambiguous genitalia and secondary sex characteristics.
- It is further characterized by **hypotension**, **hyponatremia**, **hyperkalemia**, and **metabolic acidosis**. Complications of CAH include **severe hypoglycemia**, **adrenal insufficiency**, and/or a failure to thrive.
- Treatment of CAH involves lifelong glucocorticoid replacement therapy. Patients with a 21β-hydroxylase deficiency also require mineralocorticoid replacement with fludrocortisone.

Adrenal Function Tests

The adrenal gland makes many different hormones and is divided into two distinct zones: The medulla and the cortex. The medulla makes hormones called **catecholamines**, such as **adrenaline**. The cortex primarily makes the hormones **cortisol** and **aldosterone**. Diseases of the adrenal gland can often be diagnosed with blood tests that measure the levels of these different hormones, although most adrenal gland disorders affect only the adrenal cortex.

A clinical diagnosis of adrenal hyperfunction (Cushing's syndrome) or hypofunction (Addison's disease) is confirmed by adrenal function tests.

Purpose of the Adrenal Hormone Tests

- To evaluate patients with suspected dysfunction of the adrenal glands.
- To aid in the diagnosis and evaluation of adrenal abnormalities, such as Cushing's syndrome, Addison's disease, adrenal adenoma, or adrenal hyperplasia.
- DHEA-S (dehydroepiandrosterone-sulfate—a sex hormone (androgen) synthesized by the adrenal gland—is a precursor to testosterone) may be measured to determine the cause of hirsutism (abnormal growth of hair on a woman's face and body), amenorrhea (an abnormal absence of menstruation), or infertility in women and to evaluate precocious puberty in children.

Blood Cortisol

Blood cortisol is one of the basic tests used to assess adrenal gland function. Secretion of cortisol from adrenal gland shows diurnal variation; serum cortisol is highest during the early morning hours and lowest around midnight. Loss of this diurnal variation is one of the earliest signs of **adrenal hyperfunction**.

- Cortisol levels rise and fall throughout the day, so a single blood sample may not be effective at diagnosing a deficiency or overproduction.
- Measurement of serum cortisol in blood samples drawn at midnight and 8 AM is, therefore, useful as test. A diagnosis of adrenal hyperfunction is confirmed by **dexamethasone suppression test** which demonstrate failure of suppression of the early morning concentration of cortisol following the administration of **1 mg dexamethasone** (a synthetic glucocorticoid) at midnight.

Adrenocorticotropin Hormone

Adrenocorticotropin hormone, or ACTH, is a hormone made by the pituitary gland that stimulates the adrenal glands to make cortisol. As a result, it can be measured to assess adrenal function. If the adrenal glands are not working effectively, the pituitary secretes more ACTH to stimulate them to make more cortisol. As a result, people with poorly functioning adrenal glands typically have elevated ACTH levels.

Adrenal Stimulation Test

Another way to more accurately measure adrenal gland function is to measure cortisol levels before and after stimulation of the adrenal glands. For this test, the cortisol level is measured and then the patient is injected with a synthetic form of ACTH called cosyntropin. After 45 minutes, the blood cortisol level is measured again to see if the adrenal glands produced more cortisol in response to the cosyntropin. Failure of the blood cortisol levels to rise suggests adrenal gland malfunction.

Corticotropin-releasing Hormone

The corticotropin-releasing hormone test can also be used to test adrenal gland function. First, baseline levels of ACTH and cortisol are measured. Then, corticotropin-releasing hormone, a chemical that stimulates the release of ACTH is injected. Cortisol and ACTH levels are measured every 15 minutes. Typically, ACTH levels peak after 15–30 minutes, and cortisol levels peak 30–40 minutes after the injection of corticotropin-releasing hormone. Failure of cortisol levels to rise after an increase in ACTH suggests adrenal failure.

Blood 18-Hydroxycortisol

18-hydroxycortisol, a product of cortisol metabolism, is an unusual steroid produced in excessive amounts in patients with primary hyperaldosteronism.

Measuring blood levels of this hormone can help to determine whether primary hyperaldosteronism is caused by a tumor called adrenal adenoma, or by overgrowth (hyperplasia) of adrenal tissue; levels are significantly higher in people with an adenoma.

DHEA-S (dehydroepiandrosterone-sulfate)

DHEA-S, or dehydroepiandrosterone-sulfate, a sex hormone (androgen) synthesized by the adrenal gland is a precursor to **testosterone**. In women, the adrenal glands are the major, and sometimes only, source of androgens.
- Elevated DHEA-S levels are associated with virilism (male body characteristics), hirsutism (excessive hair growth), amenorrhea (absence of menstruation), and infertility.
- Adrenal abnormalities such as tumors may lead to abnormally high DHEA-S levels.

CARDIAC MARKERS AND TESTS USED TO DIAGNOSE MYOCARDIAL INFARCTION

Myocardial Infarction

Myocardial infarction (MI) occurs when there is a sudden block in blood flow in one or more of the coronary arteries and this cuts off blood supply to a part of the heart muscle,

causing necrosis (massive cell death a permanent damage). If the block is severe, the heart can stop beating (cardiac arrest).

The major causes of acute myocardial infarction (AMI) are **atherosclerotic plaque rupture** and **thrombus formation**. Myocardial ischemia and subsequent infarction usually begin in the endocardium and spread toward the epicardium. When the necrosis occurs through the full thickness of the myocardium, the infarct is termed **transmural**.

Irreversible cardiac injury occurs if occlusion is complete for at least 15–20 minutes. Irreversible injury occurs maximally when occlusion is sustained 4–6 hours, but most of the damage occurs within the first 2–3 hours. Restoration of flow within the first 4–6 hours is associated with salvage of myocardium, but the salvage is greater if restoration occurs in 1 or 2 hours. Coronary thrombosis undergoes spontaneous lysis within 10 days.

Diagnosis of Acute Myocardial Infarction

- The diagnosis of AMI established by the **World Health Organization (WHO)** requires at least two of the following criteria:
  - A history of chest pain
  - Evolutionary changes on the ECG
  - Elevation of cardiac enzymes and proteins (cardiac markers).
- AMI is usually diagnosed by the history of crushing chest pain and characteristic ECG changes. When the ECG fails to demonstrate an AMI, **cardiac markers** are used. Biochemical tests complement the ECG findings.

Cardiac Markers

After myocardial infarction, a number of intracellular **enzymes** and **proteins** are released from the damaged cells. They have diagnostic importance and are called **cardiac markers**. Cardiac markers are useful in the detection of acute myocardial infarction or minor myocardial injury.

- The cardiac markers of major diagnostic interest include enzymes such as:
  - Creatine kinase (CK)
  - Lactate dehydrogenase (LD)
  - Serum aspartate aminotransferase also called serum glutamate transaminase.
- Nonenzyme proteins such as:
  - Cardiac troponin T and I (cTnT and cTnI).

Although, the cardiac markers are all myocardial proteins they differ in their location within myocyte, release after damage and clearance from the serum. Plasma **creatine kinase**, (possibly with CK-MB isoenzyme) measurements are requested most often, less often total LD or LD_1 (heart specific) may be requested, particularly if more than 36 hours have elapsed since the episode of chest pain. In

Marker	Abnormal activity detectable (hours)	Peak value of abnormality (hours)	Duration of abnormality (days)
CK	3–8	10–24	3–4
CK-2 (MB)	3–8	10–24	2–3
LDH (Total) and LDH$_1$	8–12	72–144	8–14
AST/SGOT	6–12	24–48	4–6
Troponin I (cTnI)	3–8	24–48	3–5
Troponin T (cTnT)	3–8	72–100	5–10

TABLE 25.9: Cardiac markers and time course after onset of acute myocardial infarction.

(CK: creatine kinase; LDH: lactate dehydrogenase; SGOT: serum glutamate transaminase; AST: aspartate transaminase

Table 25.9 various cardiac markers with time course after onset of acute myocardial infarction is listed.

Enzyme Cardiac Markers

Creatine Kinase

Creatine kinase (CK) has three isoenzymes (**Refer Chapter 5**) CK-2 or CK-MB isoenzyme is specific for the heart.

Reference values

- Normal values for total CK ranges from 10 to 100 U/L.
- The upper limit for CK-MB activity = 6 U/L.

Clinical interpretation
Increased activity:

- There is a rise in total CK activity following a myocardial infarction. The degree of increase varies with the extent of the tissue damage. CK is the first enzyme to appear in serum in higher concentration after myocardial infarction and is probably the first to return to normal levels if there is no further coronary damage.
- The serum total CK activity may be increased in some cases of coronary insufficiency without myocardial infarction. So, the simultaneous determination of CK-MB isoenzyme and LDH$_1$ isoenzyme help to make the diagnosis.
- The CK-MB isoenzyme starts to increase within 4 hours after an acute myocardial infarction and reaches a maximum within 24 hours.
- CK-MB is a more sensitive and specific test for AMI than total CK.

Lactate Dehydrogenase

Lactate dehydrogenase (LDH) is distributed widely in liver, cardiac muscle, kidney, skeletal muscle, erythrocytes and other tissues. Because LDH is not tissue-specific enzyme, serum total LDH is increased in a wide variety of disease including heart disease. LDH has five isoenzymes (**Refer Chapter 5**). LDH$_1$ is specific for the heart.

Reference values
Total   LDH = 125–290 U/L
         LDH$_1$ = 100 U/L

LDH$_2$ = 115 U/L
LDH$_3$ = 65 U/L
LDH$_4$ = 40 U/L
LDH$_5$ = 35 U/L

The use of LDH and LDH isoenzymes for detection of AMI is declining rapidly. The troponin tests are much more useful, as will be explained later in the chapter.

Clinical interpretation

- For patients having an AMI, serum total LDH values become elevated at 12–18 hours after onset of symptoms, peak at 48–72 hours and returns to normal after 6–10 days **(Figure 25.9)**.
- Significant elevation of LDH$_1$ and LDH$_2$ (LDH$_1$ >LDH$_2$) occurs within **24–48 hours** after **myocardial infarction** (MI). The LDH$_1$ increase over LDH$_2$ in serum after AMI. Normally LDH$_2$ is present in higher concentration than LDH$_1$. But this pattern is reversed in MI and called **flipped pattern** of LDH.
- The combination of an elevated CK-MB and a flipped pattern of LDH isoenzyme in a patient suspected of having a myocardial infarct makes the diagnosis certain. The combination never occurs in coronary insufficiency without a myocardial infarction.

Serum Aspartate Aminotransferase/Serum Glutamate Oxaloacetate Transaminase

Aspartate aminotransferase is also known as **aspartate transaminase, (AST)**. It was known formerly as **serum glutamate oxaloacetate transaminase**.

Reference values
The normal concentration of serum AST is 6 U/L–25 U/L.

Clinical interpretation

- The plasma AST level starts increasing **after 6–8 hours** after the onset of chest pain with **peak values 18–24 hours** proportional to the extent of cardiac damage and the values fall to normal level by the fourth or fifth day, provided no new infarct has occurred.

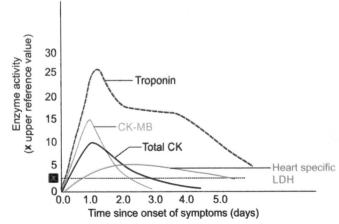

Figure 25.9: Enzyme activity after myocardial infarction (troponin which is not an enzyme is also shown).

- The increase in activity is not as great as for CK, nor does it rises as early after the infarct.
- It is much less specific indication of myocardial infarction than the rise in CK, because so many other conditions, e.g., liver, muscle or hemolytic disease, can cause a rise in serum AST. Prolonged myocardial ischemia, congestive heart failure is also associated with an increased AST level.

Nonenzyme Cardiac Markers

Cardiac Troponin

- The contractile proteins include the regulatory protein **troponin**. Troponin is a complex of three protein subunits:
  1. Troponin C (TnC), the calcium-binding component
  2. Troponin I (TnI), the inhibitory component
  3. Troponin T (TnT), tropomyosin-binding component
- The troponin subunits exist in a number of isoforms. However, cardiac-specific **troponin T (cTnT)** and **troponin I (cTnI)** forms are the most useful cardiac markers of myocardial infarction. Cardiac-specific troponin forms are currently the most sensitive and specific cardiac markers of MI available.

Clinical interpretation

The initial rise in cardiac troponins (cTnI and cTnT) after myocardial infarction occurs at about the same time as CK and CK–MB, but this rise continues for longer than for most of the enzyme (possibly because of later release of insoluble troponin from the infarcted muscle). Following general clinical impressions can be made regarding cTnT and cTnI.

- For patients having MI serum **cTnT** and **cTnI** values become elevated above the normal level at **4–8 hours** after the onset of the symptoms. Thus, the initial rise of both cTnT and cTnI are similar to those of CK-2 after MI.
- Secondly, cTnT and cTnI also can remain elevated up to 5–10 days respectively, after an MI occurs. The long time interval of cardiac troponin increase means it can replace the LDH isoenzyme assay in the detection of late presenting MI individuals.
- Thirdly, the very low to undetectable, cardiac troponin values in serum from individuals without cardiac disease permits the use of cTnT and cTnI to offer better risk assessment than use of CK-2.
- Cardiac specificity of troponin T and I eliminates a false diagnosis of MI in patients with increase CK-2 concentrations after skeletal muscle injuries.
- cTnT has been shown to differentiate individuals with increased CK-2 due to skeletal muscle injury from those individuals with concomitant MIs.
- Furthermore cTnT has been an excellent marker of myocardial injury in the presence of sepsis, drug-induced toxicities, chronic diseases, malignancies hematological disorders and noncardiac surgery.
- When cTnI and total CK in serum were compared in individuals with extreme skeletal muscle injury but without cardiac muscle injury, cTnI remained undetectable even when peak values of CK-2 were greater than, 200 U/L and total CK reached more than 50,000 U/L. cTnI was not elevated unless myocardial injury was detected concomitantly.

Thus, measurement of cTnI has been shown as a sensitive and specific cardiac marker for diagnosis of AMI, preventing the increased incidence of false diagnosis associated with elevated CK-2 concentrations. Thus, clinical evidence has been shown that either cTnT or cTnI can be replaced CK-2 as the test of choice to rule in or rule out MI.

ASSESSMENT QUESTIONS

▌STRUCTURED LONG ESSAY QUESTIONS (SLEQs)

1. Describe liver function tests under following headings:
   i. Any four disorders of liver
   ii. Tests based on bilirubin metabolism
   iii. Enzymes assay
   iv. Tests based on synthetic functions
2. Describe kidney function tests under following headings:
   i. Serum and urine markers of renal function
   ii. Tests based on glomerular filtration rate
   iii. Urine analysis (physical and chemical)
3. Describe adrenal function tests under following headings:
   i. Functions of adrenal
   ii. Disorders of adrenal
   iii. Tests that are commonly done in clinical practice to assess the functions of the adrenal
4. Describe thyroid function tests under following headings:
   i. Functions of thyroid
   ii. Disorders of thyroid
   iii. Tests that are commonly done in clinical practice to assess the functions of the thyroid
5. Describe biochemical tests perform to diagnose myocardial infarction under following headings:
   i. Enzymes
   ii. Nonenzymes

SHORT ESSAY QUESTIONS (SEQs)

1. Name the enzymes in liver function tests with clinical significance.
2. Enumerate the liver function tests and how Van den Bergh test distinguishes different types of jaundice.
3. What is a clearance test? Write creatinine clearance test.
4. What is polyuria? Give different types of polyuria.
5. Write any two kidney function tests based on tubular function.
6. What is hypothalamic pituitary thyroid axis (HPTA)?

SHORT ANSWER QUESTIONS (SAQs)

1. Enumerate thyroid function tests and give normal values of T_3 and T_4.
2. Write clinical interpretation of estimation of serum thyroid-stimulating hormone (TSH) in TFT.
3. What is renal clearance? Why creatinine clearance is superior to urea clearance?
4. Enumerate different kidney function tests.
5. Give four kidney diseases.
6. Write four functions of thyroid.
7. Name two disorders of thyroid gland.
8. Write clinical interpretation of alkaline phosphatase with respect to liver function.
9. Write clinical interpretation of a alanine transaminase with respect to liver function.
10. What is nephrotic syndrome?
11. What is hypothalamic pituitary adrenal axis (HPAA)?

CASE VIGNETTE-BASED QUESTIONS (CVBQs)

Case Study

1. **A man aged 38 years presenting with a serum creatinine of 1.7 mg/dL. 24 hours urine of 2160 mL is collected and found to have creatinine concentration in urine of 0.85 g/dL.**

   Questions
   a. Calculate the creatinine clearance and comment on the results.
   b. Write normal creatinine clearance value.
   c. Define creatinine clearance.
   d. Which are the other clearance tests?

2. **A 4-year-old male child is admitted with the history of recurrent episode of puffiness of the face, generalized weakness and loss of appetite. Following were the results of urine and blood investigations.**
   Blood:
   – **Total protein: 4.9 g/dL**
   – **Albumin: 2.5 g/dL**
   – **Globulin: 2.4 g/dL**
   – **Total cholesterol: 450 mg/dL**
   – **Blood urea: 97 mg/dL**
   – **Serum creatinine: 1.8 mg/dL**
   Urine: Total protein in 24-hour urine collection: 4.5 g/day.

Questions
a. What is the probable diagnosis?
b. Justify your diagnosis.
c. Why are his albumin levels low?
d. What is the reason of facial puffiness in this child?
e. Mention the normal ranges of all parameters tested.

3. **A 50-year-old housewife complains of progressive weight gain of 9 kg in 1 year, fatigue, postural dizziness, loss of memory, slow speech, deepening of her voice, dry skin, constipation, and cold intolerance. Her menstrual cycles had stopped 3–4 years back. On physical examination, the vital signs include a temperature 96.8°F, pulse 58/minute and regular, BP 110/60. She is moderately obese and speaks slowly and has a puffy face, with pale, cool, dry, and thick skin. The thyroid gland is not palpable. Laboratory studies:**

   – **CBC and differential WBC are normal.**
   – **Serum T_4 concentration   : 3.8 µg/dL**
   – **Serum TSH   : 20 µU/mL**
   – **Anti-TPO   : ++++**
   – **FT4   : 4.0 pmol/L**
   – **Serum cholesterol   : 255 mg/dL**

   Questions
   a. What is the probable diagnosis? Justify.
   b. How T_4 and T_3 synthesis is regulated?
   c. What are the common causes of the above diagnosed case?
   d. What are the reasons behind the above said symptoms?
   e. What is the importance of FT_3 and FT_4 over total T_4 and T_3?

MULTIPLE CHOICE QUESTIONS (MCQs)

1. **Conjugated hyperbilirubinemia with raised alkaline phosphatase levels are found in:**
   a. Viral hepatitis
   b. Obstructive jaundice
   c. Hemolytic jaundice
   d. Neonatal physiological jaundice

2. **Inulin clearance is used to assess:**
   a. Renal threshold
   b. Concentrating ability of tubules
   c. GFR
   d. Diluting ability of tubules

3. **In hemolytic jaundice:**
   a. Urinary urobilinogen excretion is increased
   b. Serum conjugated bilirubin is increased
   c. Serum alkaline phosphatase is increased
   d. Bilirubin is excreted in urine

4. **Prothrombin time in obstructive jaundice:**
   a. Decreases
   b. Increases after parenteral injection of vitamin K
   c. Normal
   d. Normalizes after parenteral injection of vitamin K

5. Positive direct Van den Bergh's reaction indicates presence of:
   a. Conjugated bilirubin   b. Unconjugated bilirubin
   c. Urobilinogen   d. Bile salts

6. Failure of concentrating capacity of urine is assessed by measurement of:
   a. Inulin clearance test
   b. Fluid deprivation test
   c. Acid load test
   d. Creatinine clearance test

7. Which of the following tests measures GFR accurately?
   a. Creatinine clearance   b. Urea clearance
   c. Inulin clearance   d. None of the above

8. Which of the following is not a feature of obstructive jaundice?
   a. Increased level of serum unconjugated bilirubin
   b. Increased level of serum conjugated bilirubin
   c. Absence of urobilinogen in stool
   d. Increased level of alkaline phosphatase

9. Absence of urobilinogen in urine occurs in:
   a. Obstructive jaundice   b. Hemolytic jaundice
   c. Hepatic jaundice   d. All of the above

10. In obstructive jaundice which of the following enzymes is diagnostically important?
    a. Alkaline phosphatase
    b. Acid phosphatase
    c. Lactate dehydrogenase
    d. Creatine phosphokinase

11. The normal value of urea clearance is:
    a. 54 mL/min   b. 75 mL/min
    c. 110 mL/min   d. 130 mL/min

12. Average creatinine clearance in an adult man is about:
    a. 54 mL/min   b. 75 mL/min
    c. 110 mL/min   d. 130 mL/min

13. Inulin clearance in an average adult man is about:
    a. 54 mL/min   b. 75 mL/min
    c. 110 mL/min   d. 120 mL/min

14. A simple way to assess tubular function is to withhold food and water for 12 hours and then measure:
    a. Serum urea   b. Serum creatinine
    c. Urine output in 1 hour d. Specific gravity of urine

15. Among the following, the most sensitive indicator of glomerular function is:
    a. Serum urea   b. Serum creatinine
    c. Urea clearance d. Creatinine clearance

16. All the following statements about inulin are correct, *except*:
    a. It is completely nontoxic
    b. It is completely filtered by glomeruli
    c. It is not reabsorbed by tubular cells
    d. It is secreted by tubular cells

17. Excretion of albumin in microalbuminuria occurs in the range of:
    a. 30–300 mg/day   b. 30–800 mg/day
    c. 0.3–3 gm/day   d. None of the above

18. Azotemia is:
    a. An increase of blood urea and creatinine
    b. An increase of blood glucose and ketone bodies
    c. An increase of blood T_3 and T_4
    d. An increase of urine urea and creatinine

19. Serum urea and creatinine are markers of:
    a. Liver function   b. Renal function
    c. Pancreatic function d. Gastric function

20. Tests of renal tubular function is:
    a. Urine concentration test (Water deprivation test)
    b. Urine dilution test (Excess water intake test)
    c. Acid load test (Urine acidification test)
    d. All of the above

21. The adrenal cortex produces which of the following hormone:
    a. Adrenaline   b. Calcitonin
    c. Epinephrine   d. Aldosterone

22. What is the signs and symptoms of aldosteronism? (Hypersecretion of aldosterone) *except*:
    a. Hypotension   b. Hypernatremia
    c. Hypokalemia   d. Alkalosis

23. What is Cushing's syndrome?
    a. High aldosterone   b. High cortisol
    c. High corticosteroid d. Low cortisol

24. What will happen to the adrenal cortex if there is hypersecretion of ACTH from the pituitary?
    a. Unilateral cortical hyperplasia
    b. Cortical adenoma
    c. Bilateral cortical hyperplasia
    d. Cortical inflammation

25. Primary hyperaldosteronism, also known as Conn's Syndrome, is associated with which of these?
    a. High K^+ level   b. Low K^+ level
    c. High renin level   d. Low renin level

26. In secondary hyperaldosteronism, which is the most important feature?
    a. High renin level   b. Low renin level
    c. High K^+ level   d. High Na^+ level

27. Which of these are the clinical features of hyperaldosteronism?
    a. Retention of Na^+
    b. Edema from retention of water
    c. Hyperkalemia
    d. Hypertension

28. For the ACTH-dependent Cushing's syndrome, which of these are the prominent features, *except*:
    a. Hyperkalemia   b. Hypokalemia
    c. Hypoglycemia   d. Muscle wasting

29. Dexamethasone suppression test is a function test of which of the following:
    a. Liver   b. Kidney
    c. Thyroid   d. Adrenal

30. Following are the cardiac markers, *except*:
    a. Troponin
    b. Myoglobin
    c. CK-MB
    d. Alkaline phosphatase

31. **Increased plasma level of which of the following is a risk factor of CHD, *except*:**
    a. LDL-cholesterol
    b. HDL-cholesterol
    c. Triglyceride
    d. Homocysteine

32. **Overproduction of cortisol leads to:**
    a. Cushing's syndrome
    b. Addison's disease
    c. Congenital adrenal hyperplasia
    d. None of these

33. **Anti-TSH receptor antibodies are most specific to which disease?**
    a. Graves' disease
    b. Hashimotos thyroiditis
    c. Postviral thyroiditis
    d. Atrophic thyroiditis

34. **Which antibodies are characteristics of Graves' disease?**
    a. Anti-TPO
    b. Anti-TRH receptor
    c. Anti-TSH receptor
    d. Anti-thyroglobulin

35. **TPO antibodies are most specific to which disease?**
    a. Graves' disease
    b. Hashimotos thyroiditis
    c. Postviral thyroiditis
    d. Atrophic thyroiditis

36. **Which of the following amino acid is the precursor for the synthesis of thyroid hormones?**
    a. Tryptophan   b. Tyrosine
    c. Alanine   d. Proline

37. **Which of the following proteins is the precursor for the thyroid hormone, and also a marker of thyroidal cancer?**
    a. Thyroalbumin
    b. Thyroglobulin
    c. Thyroid binding globulin
    d. All of the above

38. **The majority of the thyroid hormones in the blood are bound to proteins. Which of the following is not the thyroid hormone-binding proteins in the plasma?**
    a. Albumin
    b. Thyroglobulin
    c. Thyroid binding globulin
    d. None of the above

ANSWERS FOR MCQs

1. b	2. c	3. a	4. d	5. a
6. b	7. c	8. a	9. a	10. a
11. b	12. c	13. d	14. d	15. d
16. d	17. a	18. a	19. b	20. d
21. d	22. a	23. b	24. c	25. a,d
26. a	27. a,b,d	28. a	29. d	30. d
31. b	32. a	33. a	34. b	35. b
36. b	37. b	38. b		

Extracellular Matrix

Competency	Learning Objectives
BI 9.1: List the functions and components of the extracellular matrix (ECM). **BI 9.2:** Discuss the involvement of ECM components in health and disease.	1. Describe types, functions, and components of the extracellular matrix (ECM). 2. Describe the structure and functions of proteins of ECM: Collagen, elastin, fibrillin, fibronectin, laminin. 3. Describe the structure and functions of proteoglycans and glycoproteins of ECM. 4. Describe the disorders associated with components of ECM.

OVERVIEW

The extracellular space in the tissues of multicellular animals is filled with gel like material, called **extracellular matrix (ECM)**. ECM is also called **ground substance**. ECM often referred to as **"connective tissue,"** that provide structural and biochemical support for surrounding cells.

This chapter describes the basic biochemistry of the major classes of biomolecules found in the ECM and illustrates their biomedical significance as well as diseases relating the components of ECM are also briefly discussed.

TYPES, FUNCTIONS, AND COMPONENTS OF THE EXTRACELLULAR MATRIX

The extracellular matrix (ECM) is secreted by cells. It is a three-dimensional network of extracellular macromolecules, such as **collagen**, **enzymes**, and **glycoproteins**. ECM holds the cells together and provides a porous pathway for diffusion of **nutrients** and **oxygen** to individual cells. The composition of ECM varies between multicellular structures; however, **cell adhesion**, **cell-to-cell communication**, and **differentiation** are common functions of the ECM.

Types of the Extracellular Matrix

The ECM has two basic forms:

1. **Basement membrane:** The basement membrane is a thin layer of ECM that forms between the epithelial and endothelial cells. It surrounds muscle, fat, and nerve cells. It provides **mechanical structure**, **separates different cell types**, and **signals for cell differentiation**, **migration**, and **survival**.

2. **Interstitial matrix:** Interstitial matrix is present between various animal cells (i.e., in the intercellular spaces). Gels of polysaccharides and fibrous proteins fill the interstitial space and act as a **compression buffer** against the stress placed on the ECM.

Functions of the Extracellular Matrix

- ECM holds the cells together and provides a porous pathway for diffusion of nutrients and oxygen to individual cells.
- ECM protects the organs and also provides elasticity where required, for example, in blood vessels, lungs, and skin.
- Due to the sturdiness of fibrous proteins, collagen, and elastin of ECM, it can act as a compression buffer against the stress and can resist the mechanical pressures without collapsing.
- ECM regulates cell processes such as **growth**, **migration**, and **differentiation**. The extracellular matrix directs the **morphology** of a tissue by interacting with cell-surface receptors and by binding to the surrounding growth factors which then stimulate signaling pathways.

- The proteins and glycosaminoglycans of ECM form a gel like structure which provides a flexible mechanical support and functions as a cushion and lubricant against mechanical shocks.
- More direct applications of the extracellular matrix include its role in supporting growth and wound healing. For instance, bone growth depends on the extracellular matrix since it contains the minerals needed to harden the bone tissue.
- Moreover, the extracellular matrix has an important role in tissue repair which can be utilized as a therapeutic target.

Components of the Extracellular Matrix

Components of the ECM are produced intracellularly by cells and secreted into the ECM via exocytosis. Once secreted, they then aggregate with the existing matrix. The extracellular matrix contains:

1. Water
2. Fibrous proteins: The main fibrous proteins that build the extracellular matrix are **collagen** and **elastin**
3. Glycoproteins: The main glycoproteins are **fibrilin**, **fibronectin**, and **laminins**
4. Proteoglycans: Glycosaminoglycans (GAGs) attached to extracellular matrix proteins.

- **Collagens** are the major structural component of the ECM. In the matrix, collagen will give the cell **tensile strength** and facilitate **cell-to-cell adhesion** and **migration**. Collagens provide scaffolding for the attachment of laminin, proteoglycans and cell surface receptors.
- **Elastins** in contrast to collagens, give elasticity to tissues, allowing them to stretch when needed and then return to their original state. This is useful in blood vessels, the lungs, in skin, and the ligamentum nuchae. These tissues contain high amounts of elastins.
- **Fibrillin** is a glycoprotein, which is essential for the formation of elastic fibers found in connective tissue. Fibrillin is secreted into the extracellular matrix by fibroblasts and becomes incorporated into the insoluble microfibrils, which appear to provide a scaffold for deposition of elastin.
- **Fibronectins** are glycoproteins that connect cells with collagen fibers in the ECM, allowing cells to move through the ECM. Fibronectins also help at the site of tissue injury by binding to platelets during blood clotting and facilitating cell movement to the affected area during wound healing.
- The **laminin** is a glycoprotein. They are secreted and incorporated into cell-associated extracellular matrix. Laminin is vital for the maintenance and survival of tissues. Defective laminins can cause improper formation of muscles, leading to muscular dystrophy,

lethal skin blistering disease (junctional epidermolysis bullosa) and defects of the kidney filtration (nephrotic syndrome).

- **Proteoglycans:** Glycosaminoglycans (GAGs), attached to extracellular matrix proteins known as proteoglycans. Proteoglycans have a net negative charge that attracts positively charged sodium ions (Na^+), which attracts water molecules via osmosis, keeping the ECM and resident cells hydrated. Proteoglycans may also help to trap and store growth factors within the ECM.

Clinical Significance of ECM

- ❖ Biologic scaffold materials composed of extracellular matrix (ECM) have been used in a variety of surgical and tissue engineering/regenerative medicine applications. Extracellular matrix has been found to cause regrowth and healing of tissue. ECM is associated with remodeling properties including **angiogenesis**, and **stem cell recruitment**.
- ❖ In human fetuses, for example, the extracellular matrix works with stem cells to grow and regrow all parts of the human body, and fetuses can regrow anything that gets damaged in the womb. The matrix stops functioning after full development. It has been used in the past to help horses heal torn ligaments, but it is being researched further as a device for tissue regeneration in humans.
- ❖ In terms of injury repair and tissue engineering, the extracellular matrix serves two main purposes.
  - ➤ First, it prevents the immune system from triggering from the injury and responding with inflammation and scar tissue.
  - ➤ Next, it facilitates the surrounding cells to repair the tissue instead of forming scar tissue.
- ❖ Extracellular matrix proteins are commonly used in cell culture systems to maintain stem and precursor cells in an undifferentiated state during cell culture and function to induce differentiation of epithelial, endothelial, and smooth muscle cells in vitro.

STRUCTURE AND FUNCTIONS OF MAJOR PROTEINS OF ECM

Several types of **fibrous proteins**, including **collagen**, **elastin**, **fibronectin**, and **laminin**, are found in varying amounts within the extracellular matrix of different tissues. These proteins are produced by **fibroblasts**, but they aren't secreted in their active form. Rather, they are released as 'precursor' molecules; their subsequent incorporation into the extracellular matrix is guided by the fibroblasts in accordance with the functional needs of a particular tissue.

Structure and Function of Collagen

Collagen is derived from Greek words meaning to produce **glue**. When collagen fibers are warmed slightly in dilute acid; they dissociate and go into solution. If the solution is cooled, fibers will reform but if it is boiled, gelatine results, and denaturation is irreversible.

Collagen is the main protein of connective tissue and the most abundant protein in mammals. It has great **tensile strength** and is present to some extent in nearly all organs and serves to hold cells together.

Structure of Collagen

All collagen types have **triple helical** structure. The basic structural unit of collagen is **tropocollagen**, which consists of **three polypeptide** chains called α-**chains**. These three polypeptide chains twisted around each other in a **triple helix** forming a rope like structure **(Figure 26.1)**.

The three helically interwind polypeptides are of equal length, each having about 1000 amino acids residues. The three polypeptide chains are held together by **hydrogen bonds** between chains. Multiple types of collagen in human tissues arise from different triple helical combinations of polypeptides. In human tissues, 19 distinct types of collagen have been identified. **Table 26.1** summarizes the most abundant types of collagen found in human tissues.

Structure of α-chain of Collagen

Collagen has an unusual amino acid composition with 33% of the total residues being **glycine (Gly)**, 10% **proline (Pro)**, 10% **hydroxyproline (Hyp)** and 1% **hydroxylysine (Hyl)**. Two amino acids that are found in collagen, 4-**hydroxyproline** and 5-**hydroxylysine (Figure 26.2)** are not present in most proteins. In collagen, **tyrosine**

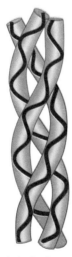

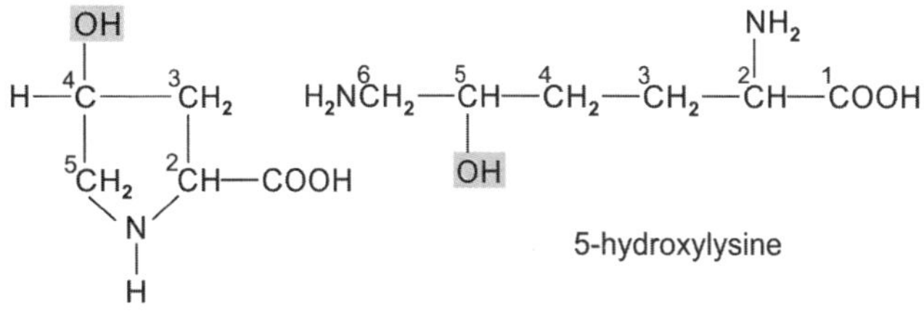

Figure 26.2: Two special amino acids found in collagen.

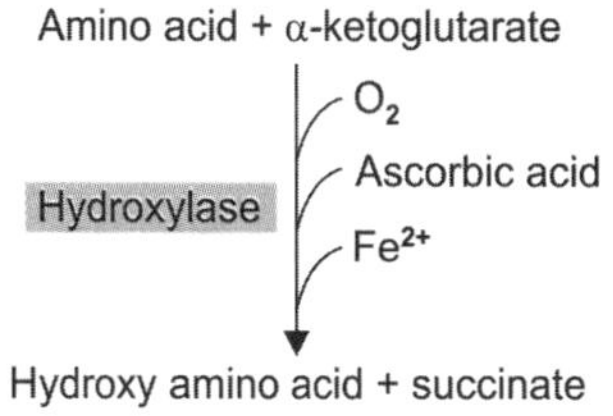

Amino acid + α-ketoglutarate

Hydroxylase → O_2, Ascorbic acid, Fe^{2+}

Hydroxy amino acid + succinate

Figure 26.3: Hydroxylation of amino acid to hydroxy amino acid.

is present in low amounts and the essential amino acid **tryptophan** is absent. **Cysteine** also is absent and, thus, no disulfide cross-links are present.

- **Hydroxyproline** and **hydroxylysine** are derived from **proline** and **lysine** in enzymatic process of post-translational modification. Tropocollagen is an example of a protein that undergoes extensive post-translational modification.

- Hydroxyproline is formed by the hydroxylation of proline residues catalyzed by the enzyme **prolyl hydroxylase**. **Hydroxyproline is involved in stabilizing the triple helical structure of collagen**.

- Lysine may also be modified to hydroxylysine through the action of **lysyl hydroxylase**. These hydroxylation reactions require **Fe²⁺**, **ascorbic acid (vitamin C)**, **oxygen** and α-**ketoglutarate (Figure 26.3)**. Ascorbic acid, reducing agent maintains prolyl hydroxylase in an active form by keeping its iron atom in the reduced ferrous state.

- In addition to hydroxylation reactions, the formation of stable triple helices requires **glycosylation**. A few hydroxylysine residues of collagen are covalently bound to carbohydrate units, mostly a **disaccharide of glucose and galactose (Figure 26.4)**. The number of carbohydrate units per tropocollagen depends on the tissue. For example, tendon tropocollagen (type-I) contains 6 units, whereas those in the lens capsule (type-II) have 110 units of carbohydrate.

- The primary structure of collagen is unusual in that, collagen has regular arrangement of amino acids in each of the α-chains of the tropocollagen. The sequence generally follows the pattern **(Gly-X-Y)**, where Gly for glycine and X and Y, for any amino acid residues. Most of the time X is for proline and Y is for hydroxyproline **(Figure 26.5)**. Thus, glycine, the smallest amino acid is

Figure 26.1: Triple helical structure of collagen.

TABLE 26.1: Most abundant types of collagen found in human tissues and their distribution.

Types of collagen	Distribution
I	Skin, tendon, bone, cornea
II	Articular cartilage, intervertebral disk, vitreous body
III	Fetal skin, cardiovascular system, reticular fibers
IV	Basement membrane
V	Placenta, skin

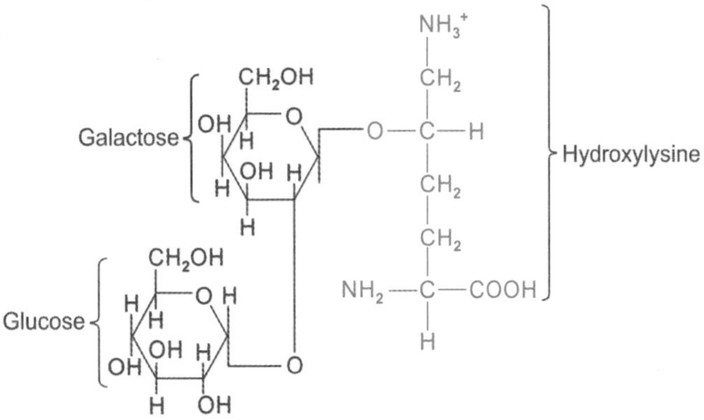

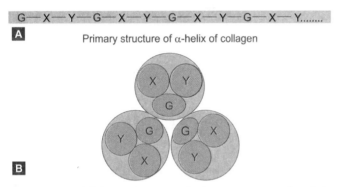

Figure 26.4: Glycosylated hydroxylysine.

G—X—Y—G—X—Y—G—X—Y—G—X—Y........

A

Primary structure of α-helix of collagen

B

Figures 26.5: (A) Representation of primary structure of α-chain of collagen; (B) Cross-section of triple helical structure showing position of glycine in the central core of the helix of collagen, where, G = Glycine, X and Y = any other amino acid mostly proline and hydroxyproline.

found in every third position of the polypeptide chain. This is necessary because **glycine** is the only amino acid small enough to be accommodated in the limited space available in the central core of the helix **(Figure 26.5)**.

- Each α-chain forms a **left-handed helix**. This helix is unlike the typical α-helix in that there is no intrachain peptide hydrogen bonding, because they contain high proportion of proline and hydroxyproline residues. Since nitrogen atom of proline and hydroxyproline residues in a peptide linkage has no substituted hydrogen (as it has imino NH group instead of amino NH$_2$ group) for the formation of hydrogen bond with other residue.

- The three α-chains are then wound around each other to form a tight, **right-handed triple helix** or super coil. Interchain hydrogen bonding between glycine's NH group in the peptide bond and the carbonyl (C = O) groups of amino acids in adjacent peptides stabilizes the triple helical structure. This triple helix is extremely strong. The triple helix resists unwinding because it and its three α-chains are coiled in opposite directions, a principle used also in the steel cables of suspension bridges.

- Individual tropocollagen molecules spontaneously laterally aggregate to form fibril. These fibrils of tropocollagen molecules become connected and

stabilized by intra- and intercovalent cross-links through copper requiring enzyme **lysyl oxidase**. These cross-links are important for the tensile strength of the fibers. Because of its cross-linkages, it has no capacity to stretch.

- The **intramolecular cross-links** are formed between lysine residues within the same tropocollagen molecule.

- The **intermolecular cross-links** are formed by joining of two hydroxylysine residues and one unmodified lysine residue of different tropocollagen molecules.

STRIKE A NOTE

- ❖ Collagen synthesized in absence of ascorbic acid (vitamin C) is insufficiently hydroxylated and because proline and lysine residues are not hydroxylated hydrogen bonding with triple helices and cross-linking between triple helices cannot occur and collagen molecules cannot stabilized. This abnormal collagen cannot properly form fibers and thus, causes the skin lesions, blood vessel fragility, loose teeth, bleeding gums in scurvy.
- ❖ Mutation of a single glycine residue in collagen leads to connective tissue disorder which can be lethal, e.g., **osteogenesis imperfecta**.
- ❖ Collagen is unique in its high content of helix destabilizing amino acids, **proline**, **hydroxyproline**, and **glycine**. These prevent the formation of the usual α-helical and β-pleated structure. Instead, it forms a **triple helical** secondary structure.
- ❖ Destruction of elastin by **elastase** is normally inhibited by α-trypsin, the genetic deficiency of which can result in **emphysema**.

Structure and Function of Elastin

Elastin occurs with collagen in connective tissues. Elastin is a **rubber-like protein**, which can stretch to several times their length and then rapidly return to their original size and shape when the tension is released. Elastin is present in large amounts, particularly in tissues that require these physical properties, e.g., lung, blood vessels, and ligaments. Smaller quantities of elastin are also found in skin, ear cartilage, and several other tissues.

Elastin differs from collagen in several properties. **Table 26.2** summarizes the main differences between collagen and elastin. In contrast to collagen, there is only one genetic type of elastin.

- The basic subunit of elastin fibrils is **tropoelastin**, which contains about 800 amino acid residues.

- Unlike collagen, elastin does not contain repeat (Gly-X-Y) sequences.

- Although elastin and collagen contain similarly high amounts of glycine and proline and both lack cysteine and tryptophan elastin contains less hydroxyproline and no hydroxylysine and glycosylated hydroxylysine.

- Elastin has very high content of **alanine** and other nonpolar aliphatic residue, i.e., **valine**, **leucine** and **isoleucine**.

TABLE 26.2: Differences between collagen and elastin.

Collagen	Elastin
Many different genetic types	One genetic type
It has no capacity to stretch	It has capacity to stretch and subsequently to recoil
Primary structure has repeating (Gly -X-Y) sequences	Primary structure has no repeating (Gly-X-Y) sequences
Formation of triple helical secondary structure	No formation of triple helix
Presence of hydroxylysine	No hydroxylysine present
Glycosylated hydroxylysine is present	No glycosylated hydroxylysine present
Formation of intramolecular aldol cross-links	Formation of intramolecular desmosine cross-links

- The major cross-links formed in elastin are the **desmosines**, which is derived from the condensation of three allysine (oxidized form of lysine) residues with lysine. These cross-links permit the elastin to stretch in two dimensions and subsequently recoil during the performance of its physiologic functions.

STRUCTURE AND FUNCTION OF PROTEOGLYCANS AND GLYCOPROTEINS

Proteoglycans

Proteoglycans are important in the structural organization of the extracellular matrix. Proteoglycans are found in every tissue of the body, mainly in the ECM intracellular **ground substance**. They are associated with each other and also with the other major structural components of the matrix, collagen and elastin, in specific ways. Some proteoglycans bind to collagen and others to elastin. **Table 26.3** list several proteoglycans along with their GAG chains, and tissue localization.

Some proteoglycans (e.g.,, decorin) can also bind **growth factors** such as TGF-β, modulating their effects on cells. Some of the proteoglycans interact with certain **adhesive proteins** such as fibronectin and lamin, also found in the matrix.

- The GAGs present in the proteoglycans are **negatively charged (anion)** and hence bind positively charged cations such as Na$^+$ and K$^+$. This Na$^+$ attracts water by osmotic pressure into extracellular matrix keeping the ECM and resident cells hydrated. Because of the long extended nature of the polysaccharide chains of GAGs and their ability to gel, the proteoglycans can act as **sieves**, restricting the passage of large macromolecules into the ECM but allowing relatively diffusion of small molecules.
- As well as due to their extended structures and the huge macromolecular aggregation, they occupy a **large volume** of the matrix relative to proteins.

TABLE 26.3: Some important proteoglycans present in the ECM.

Type	Proteoglycans	GAG type	Tissue
Small interstitial proteoglycans	Decori	CS	Connective tissue
	Biglyca	CS	Connective tissue
Aggrecan family of matrix proteoglycans	Aggrecan	CS, HA, KSII	Cartilage
	Brevican	CS	Brain
	Neurocan	CS	Brain
HS proteoglycans	Periecan	HS	Basement membrane
	Agrin	HS	Basement membrane
	Syndecans	HS, CS	Epithelial cells
	Glypicans	HS	Epithelial cells
	Serglycin	CS	Mast cells
KS proteoglycans	Lumican	KS 1	Broad
	Keratocan	KS 1	Broad
	Fibromodulin	KS 1	Broad
	Mimecan	KS 1	Broad
	Claustrin	KS 2	CNS
HS proteoglycans	Periecan	HS	Basement membrane
	Agrin	HS	Basement membrane
	Syndecans	HS, CS	Epithelial cells

- The major glycosaminoglycans are:
  - Hyaluronic acid (HA)
  - Chondroitin sulfate (CS)
  - Keratan sulfate (KS) I and II
  - Heparan sulfate (HS)
  - Heparin
- Various glycosaminoglycans exhibit differences in structure and have characteristic distributions and different functions **(For details Refer Chapter 2)**.

Glycoproteins

Glycoproteins are proteins to which oligosaccharides are covalently attached. The main function of glycoprotein is to facilitate adhesion between various elements of connective tissue. Some glycoproteins present in ECM are:

- **Fibrillins:** Structural components of microfibrils
- **Fibronectin:** An important glycoprotein involved in cell adhesion and migration
- **Lamin:** Major protein component of **basal lamins**. Basal lamins are specialized areas of the ECM that surround epithelial and other cells, for example muscle cells.

DISORDERS ASSOCIATED WITH COMPONENTS OF ECM

The extracellular matrix (ECM) of connective tissues is essential for normal development and tissue function. Mutations in ECM genes result in a wide range of serious inherited disorders.

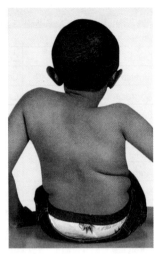

Figure 26.6: A patient with osteogenesis imperfecta.

- Mutations in genes that are responsible for production of collagen can lead to number of disorders. For example:
  - Osteogenesis imperfect
  - Number of types of Ehlers-Danlos syndrome
  - Epidermolysis bullosa
- Marfan's syndrome is due to mutations in genes coding for **fibrilin**, a glycoprotein.
- **Mucopolysaccharidoses** a group of genetic disorders is due to deficiencies of enzymes that degrade proteoglycans (the glycosaminoglycans; GAGs), a specific component of ECM.

Osteogenesis Imperfecta

Osteogenesis imperfecta (OI) is a group of genetic disorders that mainly affect the **bones**. The term "Osteogenesis imperfecta" means imperfect bone formation **(Figure 26.6)**. People with this condition have bones that break (fracture) easily, so also called **brittle bone syndrome**.

- Osteogenesis imperfecta is caused by multiple genetic defects in the **synthesis of type-I collagen**.

- The disorder is characterized by fragile bones, thin skin, abnormal teeth, and weak tendons. The sclera is often abnormally thin and translucent and may appear blue owing to a deficiency of connective tissue.
- Many of these mutations are single base substitutions that replace glycine in the (Gly-X-Y) repeat sequence by another bulkier amino acid **cysteine**, preventing the correct folding of the collagen chains into a triple helix and their assembly to form collagen fibrils.
- Treatments include bone-strengthening medications, physical therapy, and orthopaedic surgery.

Ehlers-Danlos Syndrome

Ehlers-Danlos syndrome (formerly called Cutis hyperelastica) is a group of inherited disorder of **connective tissue**, that mostly affect the skin, joints, and blood vessel walls.

- A number of forms of Ehlers-Danlos syndrome is caused by genetic defects in proteins involved in synthesis of collagens type I, III, and V.
- This is characterized by translucent, elastic and hyperextensibility of the skin, excessively flexible joints that can dislocate, and abnormal tissue fragility **(Figure 26.7)**.

Epidermolysis Bullosa

Epidermolysis bullosa is a rare heritable disorder due to mutation in gene encoding collagen. It is characterized by skin breaks and blistering of the skin and epithelial tissue **(Figure 26.8)**. Three kinds of epidermolysis bullosa are known:

1. **Dystrophic form:** This is due to mutations in gene encoding type VII collagen. This collagen forms fibrils that anchor the basal lamina to collagen fibrils in the dermis. Reduction in these anchoring fibrils result in the blistering in the dermis.

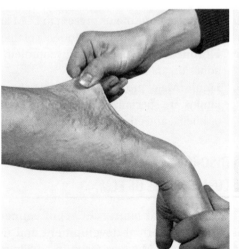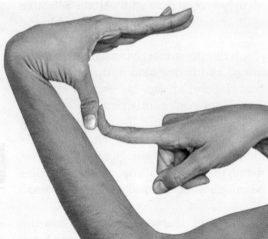

Figure 26.7: Ehlers-Danlos syndrome: Fragile stretchy skin and joint hypermobility.

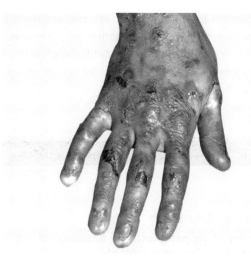

Figure 26.8: Epidermolysis bullosa skin blisters.

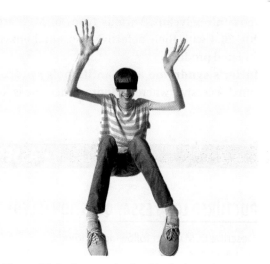

Figure 26.9: A person having Marfan's syndrome.

2. **Junctional form:** Junctional form is due to defects in the laminin which leads to blistering in dermal-epidermal junction.

3. **Simplex form:** Simplex form is due to mutations in keratin filaments which results in blistering in the epidermis.

Marfan's Syndrome

Marfan's syndrome is an inherited disease of connective tissue. Abraham Lincoln may have had this condition. Marfan's syndrome is relatively rare genetic disorder caused by mutations in genes coding for **fibrillin**, a glycoprotein, which gives stability to the elastic fibers.

Mutations in fibrillin affect the eyes, the skeletal system and cardiovascular system. Marfan's syndrome is characterized by:

- Ectopia lentis, i.e., dislocation of the lens (due to weakness of the suspensory ligaments).
- Tall structure, long arms and legs, hyper extensibility of the joints **(Figure 26.9)**.

Mucopolysaccharidoses

The mucopolysaccharidoses are genetic hereditary disorders (1:30,000 birth) characterized by excessive **accumulation of glycosaminoglycans** in various tissues causing symptoms such as skeletal and extracellular matrix deformities and mental retardation.

Mucopolysaccharidoses result from deficiency of one or more **lysosomal hydrolases** that are required for the degradation of **dermatan sulfate** and for **heparan sulfate**. This results in the presence of oligosaccharides in the urine, because of incomplete lysosomal degradation

TABLE 26.4: Types of mucopolysaccharidoses and their enzyme detects.

Mucopolysaccharidoses	Alternative designation	Enzyme defect	Accumulated products
Hurler	MPS I H	L-Iduronidase	Dermatan Sulfate Heparan Sulfate
Scheie	MPS I S	L-Iduronidase	Dermatan Sulfate
Hunter	MPS II	Iduronate Sulfatase	Dermatan Sulfate Heparan Sulfate
Sanfilippo A	MPS IIIA	Heparan Sulfate N Sulfatase	Heparan Sulfate
Sanfilippo B	MPS IIIB	N-Acetyl Glucosaminidase	Heparan Sulfate
Sanfilippo C	MPS IIIC	Glucosaminide N-acetyltransferase	Heparan Sulfate
Sanfilippo D	MPS IIID	N Acetylgucosamine Sulfatase	Heparan Sulfate
Morquio A	MPS IVA	Galactosamine 6 Sulfatase	Keratan Sulfate Chondroitin 6-Sulfate
Morquio B	MPS IVB	Beta Galactosidase	Keratan Sulfate
Maroteaux Lamy	MPS VI	N Acetyl Galactosamine 4 Sulfatase (Aryl Sulfatase B)	Dermatan Sulfate
Sly	MPS VII	Beta Galactosidase	Dermatan Sulfate Heparan Sulfate

of glycosaminocans. Various types of MPS are given in **Table 26.4** with their defective lysosomal enzyme and accumulated product.

Hurler's syndrome and **Sanfilippo's syndrome** are autosomal recessive, whereas **Hunter's disease** is X-linked.

Both Hurler's and Hunter's syndrome are characterized by skeletal deformities and mental retardation, which in severe cases may result in death. In contrast Sanfilippo's syndrome the physical defects are relatively mild while mental retardation is severe.

ASSESSMENT QUESTIONS

STRUCTURED LONG ESSAY QUESTION (SLEQ)

1. Describe ECM under following headings:
   i. Functions
   ii. Components
   iii. Disorders

SHORT ESSAY QUESTIONS (SEQs)

1. Write components and functions of extracellular matrix.
2. Write structure and functions of collagen.
3. Write structure and functions of elastin.
4. Give difference between collagen and elastin.
5. What is proteoglycan? Write role of proteoglycans in extracellular matrix.
6. Write disorders associated with components of ECM.

SHORT ANSWER QUESTIONS (SAQs)

1. What is Marfan's syndrome? Write its clinical features.
2. What is osteogenesis imperfecta? Write its clinical features.
3. Collagen has triple helical structure. Why?

MULTIPLE CHOICE QUESTIONS (MCQs)

1. **Basic components of ECM are, *except*:**
   a. Collagen
   b. Elastin
   c. Proteoglycans
   d. Cholesterol
2. **Hydroxylation of proline requires which of the following?**
   a. Vitamin C
   b. Fe^{2+}
   c. Zinc
   d. All of the above
3. **Collagen contents of helix destabilizing amino acid is:**
   a. Glycine
   b. Serine
   c. Alanine
   d. Threonine
4. **Cross-links present in collagen are, *except*:**
   a. Aldol condensation
   b. Schiff base
   c. Lysinonorleucine
   d. Desmosine
5. **The basic subunit of elastic fibrils is:**
   a. Troponin
   b. Tropoelastin
   c. Tensin
   d. Laminin
6. **Which of the following is not a genetic disorder of collagen?**
   a. Marfan's syndrome
   b. Osteogenesis imperfecta
   c. Scurvy
   d. Epidermolysis bullosa
7. **A deficiency of copper affects the formation of normal collagen by reducing the activity of:**
   a. Propyl hydroxylase
   b. Lysyl oxidase
   c. Lysyl hydroxylase
   d. Glucosyl transferase
8. **Which of the following is the odd one out?**
   a. Elastins
   b. Collagens
   c. Spectrins
   d. Proteoglycan
9. **Which of the following is not a fibrous protein type?**
   a. Elastin
   b. Proteoglycan
   c. Collagen
   d. Laminin
10. **Which of the following diseases are linked with genetic defects in collagen-encoding genes?**
    a. Osteogenesis imperfecta
    b. Marfan's syndrome
    c. Mucopolysaccharidoses
    d. Menkes disease
11. **The most abundant protein in the human body is:**
    a. Elastin
    b. Laminin
    c. Casein
    d. Collagen
12. **Which of the following is not a component of the extracellular matrix?**
    a. Laminin
    b. Fibrilin
    c. Fibronectin
    d. All of the above
13. **The fibrous proteins of the extracellular matrix are embedded in polysaccharides known as:**
    a. Glycosaminoglycans
    b. Pectins
    c. Hemicelluloses
    d. Procollagen
14. **Connective tissue fibers are produced by**
    a. Macrophages
    b. Mast cells
    c. Fibroblasts
    d. All of the above
15. **Mucopolysaccharidoses a group of genetic disorders is due to deficiencies of enzymes that degrade:**
    a. Proteoglycans
    b. Collagen
    c. Fibronectin
    d. Elastin

ANSWERS FOR MCQs

1. d	2. d	3. a	4. d	5. b
6. c	7. b	8. c	9. b	10. a
11. d	12. d	13. a	14. c	15. a

Immune System

Competency	Learning Objectives
BI 10.3: Describe the cellular and humoral components of the immune system and describe the types and structure of antibody. **BI 10.4:** Describe and discuss innate and adaptive immune responses, self/nonself-recognition and the central role of T-helper cells in immune responses. **BI 10.5:** Describe antigens and concepts involved in vaccine development.	1. Describe various organs and cells involved in the immune system. 2. Describe innate and adaptive immune systems with their components. 3. Describe antibody/immunoglobulins: Structure, types, and functions. 4. Describe self/nonself-recognition. 5. Describe innate immune responses. 6. Describe adaptive immune responses and role of helper T cells in immune responses. 7. Describe immunological memory. 8. Describe antigens: Definition, structure and types. 9. Describe various types of vaccine. 10. Describe disorders of human immunity.

OVERVIEW

The environment consists of numerous **pathogens**, which include bacteria, protists, fungi and other infectious organisms. Many of these infectious agents cause diseases. We are constantly exposed to pathogens in food and water, on surfaces, and in the air. The human body has the ability to resist almost all types of infectious organisms or toxins that tend to damage the tissue or organs. This defense system consists of **specialized cells** and **soluble molecules** which are capable of providing protection from a majority of this disease agents. This protective system is called the **immune system**. Immune system:

● Provides defenses against pathogens
● Removes dead or worn out cells like RBCs
● Identifies and destroys abnormal cancer cells
● Protects from autoimmune diseases
● Rejects tissues cells of foreign antigens.

THE ORGANS AND CELLS INVOLVED IN THE IMMUNE SYSTEM

The immune system is found throughout the body and is made up of many different **cells**, **organs**, and **tissues** that collectively protect the body from bacterial, parasitic, fungal, viral infections and from the growth of the tumor cells. The cells of the immune system can engulf bacteria, kill parasites or tumor cells or kill viral infected cells. The organs and tissues of the system can be classified into two main groups **(Figure 27.1)**:

1. **Primary lymphoid organs:** The **bone marrow** and the **thymus** constitute the **primary lymphoid** organs.
2. **Secondary lymphoid organs:** The **secondary lymphoid organs** include the **spleen** and **lymph nodes**, as well as **lymphoid tissues**. Lymphoid tissues are clumps of lymphoid tissue that are found in many parts of the body, especially in the linings of the digestive tract and the

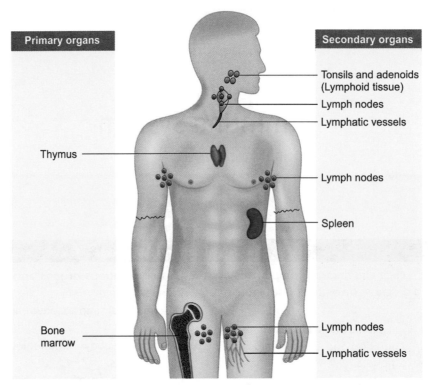

Figure 27.1: Primary and secondary organs of the immune system.

airways and lungs-regions that serve as gateways to the body. These tissues include the **tonsils**, **adenoids**, and **appendix**.

Primary Lymphoid Organs

The **bone marrow** and the **thymus** constitute the primary lymphoid organs.

Bone Marrow

Bone marrow is the soft, highly vascular and flexible **connective tissue** within bone cavities. The major function of bone marrow is to generate **blood cells**. All these cells originate from **stem cells**. This cell is called a **"stem"** cell because all the other specialized cells arise from it. Bone marrow is a central organ where all the immune cells are born. **Hematopoietic (blood-forming) stem cells (HSCs)** give rise to **two** other types of stem cells **(Figure 27.2)**:
1. **Myeloid progenitor cells** and
2. **Lymphoid progenitor cells**.

Myeloid Progenitor Cells

These give rise to **red blood cells, platelets**, and the **cells of the innate immune** system. The cells of the immune system are:
- **Granulocytes** include **neutrophils, eosinophils**, and **basophils**. These immune cells defend the body against foreign invaders (bacteria, viruses, and other pathogens) and become active during allergic reactions.

- **Monocytes:** These large white blood cells migrate from blood to tissues and develop into **macrophages** and **dendritic cells**. Macrophages and dendritic cells are the most important cells in hand over the antigen to immune system cells for initiating primary immune responses against antigen. They are often referred to as **antigen presenting cells (APCs)**.

Lymphoid Progenitor Cells

These give rise to cells essential to adaptive immunity:
- **T-lymphocytes** and **B-lymphocytes**. B-lymphocytes remain in the marrow to mature, while T-lymphocytes travel to the thymus.
- **Natural killer NK cells**, like B and T cells, are derived from the lymphoid progenitor cell. However, NK cells have been classified as components of the **innate immune system (Figure 27.2)**.

Thymus

T cells, formed from hematopoietic stem cells (HSCs) in the bone marrow are called **prothymocytes** (immature thymocytes). Prothymocytes leave the bone marrow and migrate into the **thymus** for the maturation and become **mature T cells**. While in the thymus, the developing T cells start to express **T cell receptors (TCRs)** and other receptors called **CD4** and **CD8** receptors. All T cells express TCRs, and either CD4 or CD8, not both. So, some T cells will express CD4, and others will express CD8.

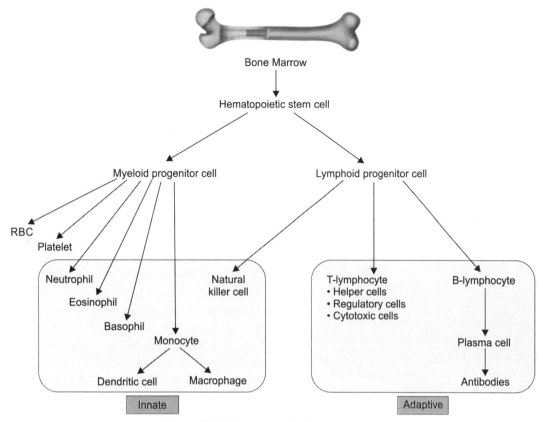

Figure 27.2: The cells of the immune system.

- Three types of mature T cells produced by thymus are:
  1. **Helper T (CD4⁺ T) cells**
  2. **Cytotoxic (CD8⁺ T) T cells**
  3. **Regulatory T cells**
- After maturation process, T cells that are beneficial to the immune system are spread, while those T cells that might evoke a harmful autoimmune response are eliminated.
- The maturation of thymocytes within the thymus can be divided into three steps, collectively referred to as **thymic selection** which includes:
  1. Development of a functional **T-cell receptor (TCR)**
  2. Positive selection
  3. Negative selection
  - **The first step** of thymic selection involves the development of **T-cell receptor (TCR)** through which these cells are activated by antigen presenting cells (APCs).
  - **The second step** of thymic selection involves the **positive selection of thymocytes**. Thymocytes that can interact appropriately with **major histocompatibility complex (MHC)** molecules are stimulated for further process of maturation, whereas thymocytes that do not interact appropriately are not stimulated and are eliminated by apoptosis.
  - **The third** and final step of thymic selection involves **negative selection** to remove **self-reacting thymocytes** (those that react to self-antigens) by **apoptosis**. Thymocytes with defective TCRs

are removed by negative selection through the stimulation of apoptosis. This final step is referred to as **central tolerance** because it prevents self-reacting T cells from reaching the bloodstream and potentially causing autoimmune disease, which occurs when the immune system attacks healthy "self" cells.

> It has been estimated that the three steps of thymic selection eliminate 98% of thymocytes. The remaining 2% that exit the thymus migrate through the bloodstream and lymphatic system to sites of secondary lymphoid organs/tissues, such as the **lymph nodes**, **spleen**, and **tonsils** where they await activation through the presentation of specific antigens by APCs. Until they are activated, they are known as mature **naïve T cells**.

Secondary Lymphoid Organ

The secondary lymphoid organs include the **spleen** and **lymph nodes**, as well as **lymphoid tissues**.

Spleen

The spleen is the largest **secondary lymphoid** organ in the body. It is an **immunologic filter** of the blood. The most important functions of the spleen are:
- Clearance of microorganisms and antigens from the blood stream.
- Synthesis of **immunoglobulins** and **properdin** (required for the complement activation).
- Removal of abnormal red blood cells (RBCs)

- In the spleen, B cells become activated through APCs and differentiate into antibody-secreting **plasma cells** that produce large amounts of **antibodies**.

Lymph Nodes

A lymph node is a **secondary organ of the lymphatic system**. Lymph nodes are found throughout the body and are linked by the **lymphatic vessels (Figure 27.1)**. Lymph nodes contain **lymphocytes** that include **B** and **T cells**. The entire lymph node is enclosed by a tough fibrous capsule.

Lymph nodes are important for the proper functioning of the immune system. Lymph nodes work like **filters**. It filters bacteria, viruses, parasites, other foreign materials (even cancer cells) that are brought to the nodes via lymphatic vessels. Antigens are filtered out of the lymph in the lymph node before returning the lymph to the circulation.

Lymphoid Tissues

They are clumps of lymphoid tissue that are found in many parts of the body, especially in the linings of the digestive tract and the airways and lungs-territories that serve as gateways to the body. These tissues include the **tonsils**, **adenoids**, and **appendix**.

INNATE AND ADAPTIVE IMMUNE SYSTEMS AND THEIR COMPONENTS

The immune system protects from infection with **layered defenses** of increasing specificity. The two main classes of the immune system are the **innate immune (natural) system** and the **adaptive** or **acquired immune system**.

1. The **innate (natural) immune system** is the **first line of defense** which provides an immediate, but nonspecific response.
2. The **adaptive immune system** is the **second line of defense**. If pathogens successfully bypass the innate response a second line of defense, the adaptive immune system is activated by the innate response.

Innate Immunity and Its Components

Innate immunity refers to **defense mechanisms** that are present even before infection (pre-existing) and hence provides immediate protection against exposure to a new pathogen. Such innate responses are **not specific** to a particular pathogen.

The innate immune system is always general, or **nonspecific**, meaning anything that is identified as **foreign** or **nonself** is a target for the innate immune response. The innate immune system is activated by the presence of antigens and their chemical properties. There is two types of innate system:

- The innate **humoral immune** system and
- The innate **cellular** or **cell mediated immune** system.

Innate Humoral Immune System and Its Components

The **humoral innate** immune system is essentially made up of **physical** and **chemical barriers** that aim to keep viruses, bacteria, parasites, and other foreign particles out of our body or limit their ability to spread and move throughout the body. It involves a variety of substances found in the humor (the body fluid used to be called humorous) which protects against **extracellular microbes** and their **toxins** **(Table 27.1)**. These are:

1. **Physical and chemical barriers:** This system does not confer long lasting immunity against a pathogen. These defense mechanisms include:
   - **Skin:** Before any immune factors are triggered, the skin functions as a continuous, impenetrable barrier to potentially infectious pathogens. Pathogens are killed or inactivated on the skin by desiccation (drying out) and by the skin's acidity.
   - Regions of the body that are not protected by skin such as the eyes and mucus membranes have alternative methods of defense:
     - **Tears** consisting of antibacterial enzyme **lysozyme**
     - **Mucus** secretions that trap and rinse away pathogens

TABLE 27.1: Components of the innate and adaptive immune system.

Innate immunity		Adaptive immunity	
Humoral components	**Cellular components**	**Humoral components**	**Cellular components**
1. **Physical and chemical barriers:** ➤ Skin; by desiccation (drying out) and by the skin's acidity ➤ Tears; antibacterial enzyme lysozyme ➤ Mucus secretions ➤ Cilia in the nasal passages and respiratory tract ➤ Gastric acid in stomach ➤ Antimicrobial peptides, e.g., β-defensins ➤ Process of urination; flushes pathogens from the urinary tract 2. **Plasma proteins:** Proteins of the complement system 3. **Other circulating proteins:** ➤ Mannose binding lectin ➤ C-reactive protein	1. **White blood cells (leukocytes):** ➤ Neutrophils ➤ Eosinophils ➤ Basophils ➤ Monocytes ◆ Macrophages ◆ Dendritic cells 2. **Natural killer cells (NK)**	1. **Antibody:** Immunoglobulin, e.g., IgA, IgG, IgD, IgM, and IgE	1. **Activated T cells**, e.g., ➤ Helper T cell ➤ Cytotoxic T cell ➤ Regulatory T cell

- ♦ **Cilia** in the nasal passages and respiratory tract that push the mucus with the pathogens out of the body.
- Throughout the body are other defenses, such as the:
  - ♦ **Low pH** of the stomach, which inhibits the growth of pathogens
  - ♦ Blood small **antimicrobial peptides** like **defensins** that bind and disrupt bacterial cell membranes
  - ♦ Process of **urination**, which flushes pathogens from the urinary tract.
2. **Plasma proteins (proteins of the complement system): Complement proteins** are some of the most important plasma proteins of the innate humoral immune system. It contains about 20 different proteins and is named for its ability to "complement" the killing of pathogens by **antibodies**. Complement proteins are divided into the following five groups by function.
   i. Proteins **C1**, **C4**, **C2**, and **C3** (in order of activation) require for the activation of the complement system by **classic pathway**.
   ii. Proteins **C3**, **factor B** and **D**, and **properdin** require for the activation of the complement system by the **alternative pathway**.
   iii. Proteins **C5** through **C9** of the membrane which **attack complex**.
   iv. Proteins as **inhibitors** and **inactivators** of the classic and alternative pathways, include **C1**, inhibitor factors **H** and **I** and **C4 binding protein** (C4 bp)
   v. Proteins as **cellular receptors** for activated or cell bound components.
3. **Other circulating proteins:** Mannose-binding lectin and **C-reactive protein**, both of which coat microbes for phagocytosis and complement activation.

Innate Cellular Immune System and its Components

Innate cellular immune system is carried out by **cells**, **neutrophils**, **eosinophils**, and **basophils (Figure 27.2)** and is responsible for defense against **intracellular microbes**. Despite the **physical** and **chemical barriers**, pathogens may enter the body through skin abrasions or punctures, or by collecting on mucosal surfaces in large numbers that overcome the mucus or cilia. Some pathogens have developed specific mechanisms that allow them to overcome physical and chemical barriers.

When pathogens do enter the body, the cellular innate immune system responds with **inflammation, pathogen engulfment**, and **secretion** of **immune factors** and **proteins**. The inflammatory response actively brings immune cells to the site of an infection by increasing blood flow to the area.

The cellular innate immune system has **specific cells** with **receptors** that recognize **pathogen-associated molecular patterns (PAMPs)** present on the pathogen's surface. Many bacteria, viruses, and protozoa have **glycoproteins** and **glycolipids** on their surface that have distinctive shapes (referred to as **"pathogen-associated molecular patterns"** or **PAMPS**) that enable them to recognize in a nonspecific way as "nonself" by the innate cellular immune system.

There are many types of **white blood cells** or **leukocytes** of the cellular innate immune system that work to defend and protect the human body **(Table 27.1)**. The following cells are leukocytes of the innate immune system:

1. **Monocytes:** These large white blood cells migrate from blood to tissues and develop into **macrophages** and **dendritic cells (Figure 27.2)**.
2. **Macrophages:** When there is tissue damage or infection, the monocytes leave the bloodstream and enter the affected tissue or organ and start cleanup task by engulfing unwanted particles and 'eating' them and begin to swell, increasing their diameter these cells are now called **macrophages**.

   They are often referred to as **scavengers** or **antigen presenting cell (APC)**. They play important role in the initiation of cell-mediated immune responses. Most invading organisms are first phagocytized and partially digested by the macrophages. Macrophages then present these antigens by cell-to-cell contact directly to the T and B-lymphocytes, thus leading to activation of the specified lymphocytes.

   The macrophages in addition secrete **interleukin**, which promotes still further growth and reproduction of the specific lymphocytes.
3. **Dendritic cells:** In addition to function as macrophage precursors, monocytes have the capacity to differentiate into **dendritic cells (*see* Figure 27.2)**. Dendritic cells are **antigen-presenting cells**. These are more efficient APCs than macrophages. Dendritic cells are phagocytes in tissues that are in contact with the external environment; therefore they are located mainly in the skin, nose, lungs, stomach, and intestine.

   Dendritic cells have **Toll-like receptors (TLRs)** that bind to PAMPs (pathogen-associated molecular patterns) of pathogens, triggering rapid **cellular responses** directed against the pathogens. Dendritic cells also act as bridge between the innate immune system and the adaptive immune system.
4. **Neutrophils:** Neutrophils are **phagocytic cells** that are also classified as **granulocytes** because they contain granules in their cytoplasm. These granules are very toxic to bacteria and fungi, and cause them to stop proliferating or die on contact. Neutrophils are typically the first cells to arrive at the site of an infection.
5. **Eosinophils:** Eosinophils are granulocytes and target multicellular parasites. Eosinophils secrete a range of highly **toxic proteins** and **free radicals** that kill bacteria and parasites. The toxic proteins and free radicals also cause tissue damage, so activation and release of toxins by eosinophils is highly regulated to prevent any unnecessary tissue damage.

TABLE 27.2: Distinguishing factors between natural killer (NK) cells and cytotoxic T cells.

Characteristic	NK cells	Cytotoxic cells
Surface markers	**CD16** and **CD56**	**CD3** and **CD8**
Immunity	Innate	Acquired
MHC restriction	No	MHC-I restricted
Target cells	Virus infected cells and tumor cells	Virus infected cells and tumor cells
Mechanism of cytotoxicity	By perforins and granzymes	By perforins and granzymes
Memory	No	Yes

6. **Basophils:** Basophils are also granulocytes that attack multicellular parasites. Basophils release **histamine**. Histamine increases the permeability of the capillaries to white blood cells and some proteins, to allow them to come across pathogens in the infected tissues.

7. **Natural killer cells (NK):** Natural killer cells are third category of lymphocytes that are neither B nor T cells. They do not mature in thymus. They are large granular lymphocytes. They are present in the spleen, lymph nodes, bone marrow, and blood. They work more effectively against viruses and tumor cells. NK cells differ from **cytotoxic T** cells in many aspects **(Table 27.2)** such as:

   - NK cells lack the T cell markers such as CD3, CD4, or CD8 molecules (hence are called null cells), instead possess specific surface markers as **CD16** and **CD56**.
   - They do not require prior sensitization and involvement of **major histocompatibility complex (MHC) antigen** to kill microbes.
   - NK cells are part of **innate immunity**; they do not require the prior exposure to microbial antigen.
   - NK cells do not differentiate into **memory cells**.

Adaptive Immune System and Its Components

Adaptive immunity is an immunity that occurs after exposure to an antigen either from a pathogen or a vaccination. The adaptive, or acquired, immune response takes days or even weeks to become established. This is much longer than the innate response. However, adaptive immunity is more **specific** to pathogens and has **memory**. By convention the term "immune response," refers to adaptive immunity.

Adaptive immune system is activated when the innate immune response is insufficient to control an infection. In fact, without information from the innate immune system, the adaptive response could not be prepared. There are two types of adaptive immune system:

- Adaptive **humoral immune system**, which is controlled by activated **B cells** and **antibodies**.
- Adaptive **cell-mediated immune system** which is carried out by **T cells**.

Components of the Adaptive Humoral Immune System

The humoral immune system is controlled by activated **B cells** and **antibodies**. **Antibody (Ab)** also known as **Immunoglobulin (Ig)**, is the protein produced by B cells in response to the presence of a foreign substance, called an **antigen**. (The types, structure and functions of antibody are discussed onwards).

Components of the Adaptive Cellular Immune System

The adaptive cellular immune system depends on **T-lymphocytes** to carry out its tasks.

T-lymphocytes are derived from **hematopoietic stem cells**, in the bone marrow. After they are made in the bone marrow, they need to mature and become activated. Maturation of **T cells** occurred in the **thymus**. T cells contain a various types of cells with extremely different functions. Three types of mature T cells are:

1. Helper T cells (CD4+ T cells)
2. Cytotoxic T cells (CD8+ T cells)
3. Regulatory T cells

All T cells produce a cell surface **glycoproteins called, cluster of differentiation (CD)** molecules. **CD4** and **CD8** are the two most important CD molecules, used for differentiation of the cells and is a **coreceptor** on the T cell. **Helper T cells** and **regulatory T cells** are characterized by the expression of **CD4** on their surface, whereas **cytotoxic T cells** are characterized by the expression of **CD8**. The different classes of T cells play different functional roles in the immune system:

- **Helper T cells (CD4+ T cells):** Helper T cells express **CD4** on their surface and help in the activation of cytotoxic T and B cells, and other immune cells. The helper T cells function indirectly to identify pathogens for other cells of the immune system. These cells are important for extracellular infections, such as those caused by certain bacteria, helminths, and protozoa.
- **Cytotoxic T cells (CD8+ T cells):** Cytotoxic T cells express **CD8** on their surface, and are responsible for removing virus infected host cells and tumor cells. Cytotoxic T cells are the principal effector cells of **cell mediated immune response**. Naive cytotoxic T cells respond to viral or tumor peptide antigens which are processed by the target host cells and presented along with **MHC class I** molecules. Activated cytotoxic T cells in turn secrete cytotoxic enzymes that lyse the target cells.
- **Regulatory T cells:** Regulatory T cells express **CD4** and help distinguish between **self** and **nonself** molecules, and by doing so, reduce the risk of autoimmune diseases. Regulatory T cells deactivate T cells and B cells when needed, and thus prevent the immune response from becoming too intense.

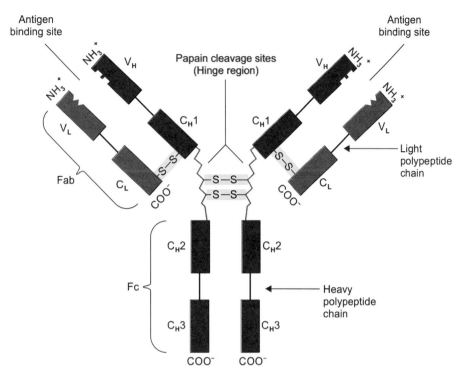

Figure 27.3: Schematic structure of immunoglobulin G (IgG).

ANTIBODY/IMMUNOGLOBULINS: STRUCTURE, TYPES, AND FUNCTIONS

Antibody is a protective protein produced by the immune system in response to the presence of a **foreign substance, called an antigen**. Each type of antibody is unique and defends the body against one specific type of antigen.

Structure of Antibody/Immunoglobulin

B cells are responsible for the synthesis of **antibodies**. **Antibodies are** also known as **immunoglobulins (Ig)**. Immunoglobulins are **glycoproteins** made up of **four polypeptide** chains:

1. Two identical **heavy chains (H)** and
2. Two identical **light chains (L)**.

- The term **"light"** and **"heavy"** refer to **molecular weight**. Light chains have a molecular weight of 25,000 whereas heavy chains have a molecular weight of 50,000 to 70,000.
- The four chains are linked by **disulfide bonds**. Pairs of heavy and light chains combine to form **Y-shaped** molecule. All antibodies have the same basic structure **(Figure 27.3)**.
- An individual antibody molecule always consists of identical H chains and identical L chains.
- L chain may be either of two types, **Kappa (κ)** or **Lambda (λ)** but not both.
- The heavy chains may be of five types and are designated by Greek letter: **alpha (α)**, **gamma (γ)**, **delta (δ)**, **mu (μ)**, **epsilon (ε)**.

TABLE 27.3: Different types of antibodies (immunoglobulins, Ig) corresponding to the type of heavy chains.

Antibody types	Types of H chains
IgG	γ (gamma)
IgA	α (alpha)
IgM	μ (mu)
IgD	δ (delta)
IgE	ε (epsilon)

- Immunoglobulins are named as per their heavy chain type as **IgA, IgG, IgD, IgM, and IgE (Table 27.3)**.
- The L and H chains are subdivided into **variable** and **constant** regions. The region that changes to various structures depending on antigens is called the variable region, and the region that has a constant structure is called the constant region.
- L chain consists of one **variable (V_L)** and one **constant (C_L)** region. Most H-chains consist of one **variable (V_H)** and **three constant (C_H1, C_H2, and C_H3)** regions.
- The amino acid sequence of variable region varies greatly among different antibodies. These variable regions give the antibody its specificity for binding antigen.
- The constant region determines the mechanism used to destroy antigen.
- IgG and IgA have three C_H regions whereas IgM and IgE have four.
- Each immunoglobulin molecule has **hinge region** between C_H1 and C_H2, which allows a better fit with the antigen surface.

- The variable regions of both the light and heavy chains form two **antigen-binding sites**, whereas the constant region of heavy chain is responsible for various biologic functions, e.g., complement activation and binding to cell surface receptors. Complement binding site is in the C_H2 region.
- The constant region of the light chain has no known biological function.
- The variable regions of both L and H chains have three extremely variable amino acid sequences at the amino terminal end called **hypervariable region**. Hypervariable region form the **antigen binding site**.
- The specificity of antibodies is due to these hypervariable regions.
- Enzyme papain splits the immunoglobulin molecule in the hinge region into two fragments named as:
  - **Fab** (Fragment for antigen binding) and
  - **Fc** (crystallizable fragment or fragment for complement binding (*see* **Figure 27.3**).
- **Fc** is the constant part of the molecule and does not participate in antigen binding. However, the Fc fragment is associated with secondary effects after binding of complement.
- **Fab** is the variable parts of the molecule and is the site of antigen binding. The variation in amino acid content allows a wide range of specific activity.

Types of Antibodies

Human antibodies are classified into five types (IgG, IgA, IgM, IgD, and IgE) according to their H chains, which provide each type with distinct characteristics and roles **(Table 27.4)**.

IgG (Heavy Chain γ)

- IgG is a smaller **monomeric** molecule with **two antigen binding sites**. There are four subclasses, IgG_1 to IgG_4 based on antigenic differences in the H-chains and on the number and location of disulfide bonds.
- It is produced mainly in the **secondary response** and constitutes an important **defense against bacteria** and **viruses**. Secondary immune response is the reaction of the immune system when it contacts an antigen for the second and subsequent times.
- IgG is the major class of immunoglobulin found in the serum which accounts for 70% of the total.

- IgG is the only antibody that **crosses the placenta** and therefore is the class of **maternal antibody** that protects the fetus. The important functions of IgG are given in **Table 27.4**.

IgA (Heavy Chain a)

- IgA is the **second most abundant class** constituting about 20% of serum immunoglobulins.
- IgA occurs in two forms:
  - Secretory IgA and
  - Serum IgA.
  - **Secretory IgA** is a **dimeric molecule (Table 27.4)** formed by two monomer units, joined together at their carboxy terminals by a protein termed **J-chains** (J for joining). Additionally secretory IgA has a **secretory component** attached to dimer. Secretory component is a polypeptide that provides for IgA passage to the mucosal surface and also protects IgA from being degraded in the intestinal tract. Secretory IgA found in external secretions such as **colostrum**, **saliva**, **tears** and **respiratory**, **intestinal** and **genital tract secretions**. It prevents attachment of microorganisms like bacteria and viruses to mucous surfaces from antigenic attack and prevents access of foreign substances to the circulation.
  - Some **serum IgA** exists as **monomeric** form. IgA found in internal secretions such as **synovial**, **amniotic**, and **pleural** and **CSF** is of the serum type IgA.

IgM (Heavy Chain μ)

- It is a **pentamer** consisting of five identical immunoglobulin molecules, joined together by disulfide bridges **(Table 27.4)**. This pentamer is closed in a ring structure by J-chain **(Figure 27.4)**.
- IgM is the main immunoglobulin **produced early in the primary response**. IgM can be produced by fetus in certain infections.
- IgM accounts for some 10% of normal serum immunoglobulin.
- As IgM is a pentamer it has 10 antigen binding sites and is the most efficient immunoglobulin in **agglutination**, **complement activation** and other antibody reactions and is important in defense against bacteria and viruses.

TABLE 27.4: Structure and characteristics of different types of antibodies.			
Types	Structure	Characteristics	Functions
IgG	**Monomer**	• Main antibody in the secondary response • It is only antibody which crosses the placenta and is the only maternal antibody which protects the fetus • Classified into four classes IgG_1, IgG_2, IgG_3, and IgG_4	• Neutralizes bacterial toxins and viruses • Opsonizes bacteria, making them easier to phagocytize • Activates complements which enhances bacterial killing

Contd...

Contd...

Types	Structure	Characteristics	Functions
IgA	**Monomer or dimer** Or **Dimer** J-chain	• Major component of colostrum • Also occurs in saliva, tears and respiratory, intestinal and genital tract secretions	• Secretory IgA prevents attachment of bacteria and viruses to mucous membranes and helps protect mucous surface from antigenic attack • Prevents access of foreign substances to the circulation
IgM	**Monomer or pentamer** J-chain	• Main antibody in the primary response to an antigen • Produced by fetus	• Activates complement, promotes phagocytosis, and causes lysis of antigenic cells (bacteria) • Antigen receptor on the surface of B-lymphocytes
IgD	**Monomer**	Labile molecules. These facts have made the study of IgD function difficult	May function as an antigen receptor. No known antibody function
IgE	**Monomer**	Binds mast cells and basophils, leads to rupture of the cell membrane, degranulation and release of histamine	• Antiallergic and antiparasitic • Mediates immediate hypersensitivity by causing release of histamine from mast cells and basophils upon exposure to antigen • Defends against worm infections by causing release of enzymes from eosinophils

- IgM present on the surface of **B-lymphocytes** are **monomer**, where it functions as an antigen binding **receptor** for antigen recognition.
- The natural blood group antibodies, anti-A and anti-B are IgM.

IgD (Heavy Chain δ)

It is a **monomer** and resembles IgG structurally. IgD has no known antibody function but may function as an **antigen receptor**. Like IgM, it is present on the surface of many **B-lymphocytes**. The circulating concentration of IgD in blood is very low. **IgD is labile** which made the study of IgD function difficult.

IgE (Heavy Chain ε)

- IgE is a **monomeric** molecule similar to IgG.

- Although IgE is present in **trace amounts**, in normal (approximately 0.004%) persons with allergic activity have greatly increased amounts.
- IgE is responsible for **anaphylactic** (shortness of breath coupled with lowered blood pressure) type of **hypersensitivity** and **allergy**.
- Its main activity is mediated by **mast cells** or **basophils** which release **histamine**.
- In the allergic response, the plasma cell produces IgE-antibodies. Binding of IgE to mast cells and basophils leads to rupture of the cell membrane and release of **histamine** present in granules of mast cells and basophils. Histamine is responsible for anaphylactic hypersensitivity reaction.
- IgE also functions in immunity to certain **parasites** such as helminths like Schistosoma mansoni, Trichinella

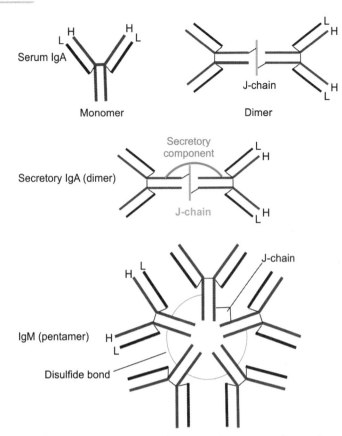

Figure 27.4: Monomeric, dimeric, and pentameric forms of immunoglobulins.

spiralis, and fasciola hepatica. It defends against these worm infections by causing release of worm destroying enzymes from eosinophils.

Functions of Antibody

- IgG provides long-term protection because it persists for months and years after the presence of the antigen that has triggered their production.
- IgG protect against bacteria, viruses, neutralize bacterial toxins, trigger compliment protein systems, and bind antigens to enhance the effectiveness of phagocytosis.
- Main function of IgA is to bind antigens on microbes before they invade tissues. It aggregates the antigens and keeps them in the secretions so when the secretion is expelled is along with the antigen.
- IgA are also first defense for mucosal surfaces such as the intestines, nose, and lungs.
- IgM is involved in the ABO blood group antigens on the surface of RBCs.
- IgM enhance ingestions of cells by phagocytosis.
- IgE bind to mast cells and basophils which participate in the immune response.
- IgD is present on the surface of B cells as a B cell receptor, BCR and plays a role in the induction of antibody production.

▮ SELF/NONSELF-RECOGNITION

An immune response is a reaction, which occurs for the purpose of defending against foreign invaders. In an immune response, the immune system recognizes the **antigens** on the surface of substances or microorganisms, such as bacteria or viruses, and attacks and destroys, or tries to destroy, them. Cancer cells also have antigens on their surface. The immune system realizes these antigens as foreign and mounts an immune response against them.

In order to be effective, the immune system needs to be able to recognize which particles are **foreign** or **nonself**, and which are a part of our body or **self**. Let's understand first what is self and nonself and how does the body recognize?

- **Self** refers to particles, such as **proteins** and other molecules that are a part of, or made by our body. Something that is self should not be targeted and destroyed by the immune system. The non-reactivity of the immune system to self-particles is called **tolerance**.
- **Nonself** refers to particles that are not made by our body, and are recognized as potentially harmful. These are sometimes called **foreign bodies**. Nonself-particles or bodies can be bacteria, viruses, parasites, pollen, dust, and toxic chemicals. The nonself-particles and foreign bodies that are infectious or pathogenic, like bacteria, viruses, and parasites, make proteins called **antigens** that allow the human body to know that they intend to cause damage. An **antigen** is a foreign or "nonself" macromolecule that on entry into the body stimulates an immune response against that substance.

Basis for Self-recognition

The immune system has the capacity to distinguish between **body cells (self)** and **foreign materials (nonself)**. The immune system can make this distinction because all nucleated cells of the body possess identification molecules on its surface. The self-identification molecules are called **major histocompatibility complex molecules (MHC)**. They are also called **HLA antigens (human leukocyte antigens)** which help in identification of body cells (self) and foreign materials (nonself).

Body's immune system normally recognizes MHC as self. The immune system will not normally react to cells bearing **MHC**. This is due to the mechanism of **immunological tolerance**. **Immunological tolerance** is an unresponsiveness of the immune system to an antigen to produce an immune response. Immunological tolerance to self-antigen provides the basis for self-recognition. The T cells recognize MHC- self antigen complex as the self-antigens and do not react against them.

A cell with molecules on its surface that are not identical to those on the body's own cells is identified as being foreign. The immune system then attacks that cell. Such a cell may be a cell from transplanted tissue or one of the body's cells that has been infected by an invading microorganism or altered by cancer. (HLA molecules are what doctors try to match when a person needs an organ transplant).

> ❖ A self-marker (MHC) labels the body's cells as a 'friend' and is tolerated by the immune system.
> ❖ An antigen is a molecule that the immune system recognizes as foreign (nonself) and treats as a foe (enemy).

INNATE IMMUNE RESPONSES

The innate immune responses are the **first line of defense** against invading pathogens. They are also required to initiate specific adaptive immune responses.

Innate Humoral Response

1. **Role of physical and chemical barriers:** Most simply **physical and chemical barriers** of the body prevent the entry of pathogens such as bacteria and viruses into the body are as follows:
   - Before any immune factors are triggered, the skin functions as a continuous, impermeable barrier to potentially infectious pathogens. Pathogens are killed or inactivated on the skin by desiccation (drying out) and by the skin's acidity. Skin and respiratory tract secrete **antimicrobial peptides** such as the **β-defensins**. In addition, beneficial microorganisms that coexist on the skin compete with invading pathogens, preventing infection.
   - Regions of the body that are not protected by skin (such as the eyes and mucus membranes) have alternative methods of defense, such as **tears** and **mucus secretions** that trap and rinse away pathogens. **Cilia** in the nasal passages and respiratory tract that push the mucus with the pathogens out of the body. Enzymes such as **lysozyme** and **phospholipase A$_2$** in saliva, tears, and breast milk are also **antibacterial**.
   - In the stomach, **gastric acid** and **proteases** serve as powerful chemical defense against pathogens. The **low pH of the stomach** inhibits the growth of pathogens.
   - **Lung surfactant** is also a component of innate humoral immunity, providing protection against inhaled microbes.
2. **Role of complement system:** A group of approximately 20 types of soluble proteins many of which are **enzyme precursors**, called a **complement system** (also called the **complement cascade**). It functions to destroy **extracellular pathogens**. The complement proteins primarily synthesized by **liver** and small amounts are synthesized by **monocytes** and other cell types. All these complement proteins are present normally in the plasma and are capable of responding immediately

to infecting microorganisms. The complement system is so named because of their ability to assist or complement the activity of the **antibody** in fighting infection. The enzyme precursors of complement protein are normally inactive. When activated, these proteins come together to initiate the immune response by the following ways:

- **Opsonization:** Opsonization is a process in which foreign particles are marked for phagocytosis.
- **Chemotaxis:** Chemotaxis is the phenomenon in which the direction of a cell's locomotion is determined by extracellular chemicals. Chemotaxis uses **cytokines** and **chemokines** to attract **macrophages** and **neutrophils** to the site of infection, to destroy the pathogens in that area. Chemokines are a type of cytokines that are released by **infected cells** to initiate an immune response.
- **Cell lysis:** Lysis is the breaking down or destruction of the membrane of a cell. The proteins of the complement system puncture the membranes of foreign cells, destroying the integrity of the cell membrane of the pathogen. Destroying the membrane of foreign cells or pathogens weakens their ability to proliferate and helps to stop the spread of infection.
- **Agglutination:** Agglutination is the clumping of cells aided by **antibodies** and **lectins**. Agglutination binds pathogens together to prevent them from interfering with the normal physiological processes of the body.

Innate Cellular Response

Cellular innate immune responses depend on the body's ability to recognize specific features of pathogens that are not present in the normal uninfected host cells. These include **pathogen-associated molecular patterns (PAMPs)** on the pathogen's surface. PAMPs are the **molecular tags** of carbohydrate, polypeptide, and nucleic acid that are expressed by viruses, bacteria, and parasites which are not present in the uninfected host cells. PAMPs also activate **complement**, a group of blood proteins that act together to disrupt the membrane of the microorganism, to target micro-organisms for **phagocytosis** by **macrophages** and **neutrophils**, and to produce an **inflammatory response**.

- The phagocytic cells use a combination of degradative enzymes, antimicrobial peptides, and reactive oxygen species to kill the invading microorganisms.
- In addition, they release signaling molecules that trigger an inflammatory response which induce adaptive immune response.
- Cells infected with viruses produce **interferons (cytokine)**, which induce a series of cell responses to inhibit viral replication and activate the killing activities of natural killer (NK) cells and cytotoxic T cells **(Figure 27.5)**.

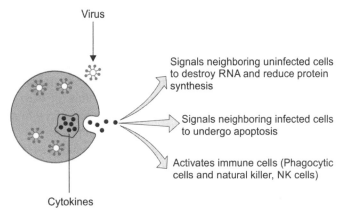

Figure 27.5: Immune response of interferon released by an infected cell to stop the infection.

Recognition of PAMP and Release of Cytokines

When a pathogen enters the body, the specific cells of the innate immune system (*see* **Figure 27.2**) in the blood and lymph detect the specific **pathogen-associated molecular patterns (PAMPs)** on the pathogen's surface. The specific cells of the innate immune system have receptors through which they recognize these PAMPs.

- **Macrophages** recognize PAMPs via complementary **pattern recognition receptors (PRRs)**. The binding of PRRs with PAMPs triggers the release of **cytokines**, which signal that a pathogen is present and needs to be destroyed along with any infected cells.
- A **cytokine** is a **chemical messenger** that regulates cell differentiation, proliferation and gene expression to affect immune responses. At least 40 types of cytokines exist in humans that differ in terms of the cell type. Cytokines are released by the infected cells which bind to nearby uninfected cells and induce those cells to release cytokines, which results in a **cytokine burst**.
- One type cytokine, **interferon** which is released by infected cells work by signaling neighboring uninfected cells to **destroy RNA** and **reduce protein synthesis**, signaling neighboring infected cells to **undergo apoptosis** (programmed cell death), and **activating immune cells (Figure 27.5)**.
- In response to interferons, uninfected cells alter their gene expression, which increases the cells' resistance to infection. One of the functions of an interferon is to **inhibit viral replication**. They also have other important functions, such as **tumor surveillance**.
- Cytokines also send feedback to cells of the nervous system to bring about the overall symptoms of feeling sick, which include lethargy, muscle pain, and nausea. These effects may have developed because the symptoms encourage the individual to rest and prevent them from spreading the infection to others. Cytokines also increase the core body temperature, causing a fever, which causes the liver to withhold iron from the blood.

Without iron, certain pathogens, such as some bacteria, are unable to replicate; this is called **nutritional immunity**.

- ❖ The term **cytokines** refer to different set of small proteins that include the **interleukins (IL)**, **interferons (IFN)**, and **chemokines**.
- ❖ The interleukin derived their name from cells in which they are synthesized and from which they are secreted. Many of these proteins are produced by **leukocytes** and act on leukocytes. The human genome encodes more than 50 interleukins.
- ❖ **Interferon was the first described member of the class of protein molecules now known as cytokines. Interferons (IFN)** on the other hand, derive their name from their ability to inhibit, or interfere, with the replication of infecting viruses.
- ❖ **Chemokines** are small proteins secreted by activated white blood cells. They are known for their role in controlling the migration (chemotaxis) of leukocytes and other cells to a site of infection or injury.

Phagocytosis and Inflammation

The **cytokines** enhance **inflammation**, the **localized redness**, **swelling**, **heat**, and **pain** that result from the movement of leukocytes and fluid through increasingly permeable capillaries to a site of infection. The population of leukocytes that arrives at an infection site depends on the nature of the infecting pathogen.

- Both **macrophages** and **dendritic cells** engulf pathogens and cellular debris through phagocytosis.
- **Neutrophils** are also phagocytic leukocytes that engulf and digest pathogens. Neutrophils contain **lysosomes** that digest engulfed pathogens.
- **Eosinophils** are involved in the allergic response and in protection against helminthes (parasitic worms). Neutrophils and eosinophils are particularly important leukocytes that engulf large pathogens, such as bacteria and fungi.
- **Mast cells** produce inflammatory molecules, such as **histamine**, in response to large pathogens. Histamines cause nearby capillaries to dilate and neutrophils and monocytes leave the capillaries.
- Monocytes become macrophages when they move from the circulation into the tissues. When they enter the tissues they begin to swell, increasing their diameter, these cells are now called macrophages. Neutrophils, dendritic cells and macrophages release chemicals to stimulate the inflammatory response.
- A hypersensitive immune response to harmless antigens, such as in pollen, often involves the release of histamine by basophils and mast cells.

Role of Natural Killer (NK) Cells

NK cells are constantly patrolling the body and works more effectively against viruses, controlling potential infections and tumor cells, preventing cancer progression. Natural killer cells kill microbes by following mechanisms:

Receptor Interaction

NK cells are not MHC restricted. They directly recognize certain ligands (e.g., glycoproteins) present on the surface of altered host cells like virus-infected cells or tumor cells. However, such ligands are also present on normal cells. NK cells are capable of distinguishing normal host cells from the altered cells with the help of two types of receptors present on NK cell surface.

1. When **CD16 receptors** (activation receptors) are engaged with ligands (antigen) present on the target cells; NK cells become activated.

2. **C-type lectin receptors** (inhibitory receptors) recognize a part of MHC I molecule which is present on the surface of all normal nucleated cells. Binding of inhibitory receptors to MHC-I molecules of normal cells generates an inhibitory signal that suppresses the NK cells. However, an infected cell or a tumor cell is usually incapable of synthesizing MHC I molecules. In such cases, there would not be any inhibitory signal. Hence, binding of activation receptor to its ligand leads to activation of NK cells.

   ■ NK cells release **cytotoxic granules** when they come in close contact with the target cell. The **perforin** molecules from the granules form pores in the target cell membrane through which the **granzymes** enter the target cell and kill the target cells by inducing **apoptosis**.

   ■ This mechanism of lysis of target cell by NK cells is similar to that of cytotoxic T cells. The only difference is that, the enzymes are **constitutively** expressed in NK cell cytoplasm (i.e., they are cytotoxic all the time, even without exposure to the antigen) while in cytotoxic T cells the enzymes are **inducible**, expressed only after stimulation.

Antibody-dependent Cell-mediated Cytotoxicity (ADCC)

NK cells possess **Fc receptors** on their surface that can bind to the Fc region of the **antibody-coated viruses** and subsequently cause lysis of the antibody-coated viruses by releasing cytotoxic granules like **perforins** and **granzymes**. This phenomenon is known as **antibody-dependent cell-mediated cytotoxicity (ADCC)**.

▌ADAPTIVE IMMUNE RESPONSES AND THE ROLE OF HELPER T CELLS

Adaptive immune response is activated when the innate immune response is insufficient to control an infection. In fact, without information from the innate immune system, the adaptive response could not be able. The **adaptive** immune response takes much longer days or even weeks to become established than the innate response. However, adaptive immunity is more **specific** to pathogens and has **memory**.

Adaptive Humoral Immune Responses

Antibodies provide **adaptive humoral** immunity. The **B-cells** are responsible for formation of antibodies. **B cells**, which are derived from the **bone marrow**, differentiate into antibody-secreting **plasma cells** that produce **antibodies** (*see* **Figure 27.2**).

Mechanism of Production of Antibodies

● B cell is triggered when the **antigen** binds to a B cell. Then the B cell engulfs the antigen by endocytosis and digests it into fragments of peptides. These degraded pieces of antigen bound to its unique class II MHC molecules are displayed on the cell surface which activates B cells for the production of plasma cell **(Figure 27.6)**.

● When a helper T (CD4+ T) cell detects that a B cell is bound to a relevant antigen, it binds to B cells. When this happens helper T cell secretes specific **cytokines** that induce the B cell to proliferate rapidly. B cells then make thousands of identical (clonal) copies of **antibody producing plasma cells (Figure 27.7)**.

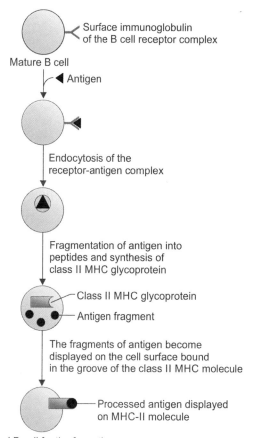

Surface immunoglobulin of the B cell receptor complex

Mature B cell

◀ Antigen

Endocytosis of the receptor-antigen complex

Fragmentation of antigen into peptides and synthesis of class II MHC glycoprotein

Class II MHC glycoprotein

Antigen fragment

The fragments of antigen become displayed on the cell surface bound in the groove of the class II MHC molecule

Processed antigen displayed on MHC-II molecule

Activated B cell for the formation antibody producing plasma cell

Figure 27.6: Activation of B cells for the production of plasma cells.

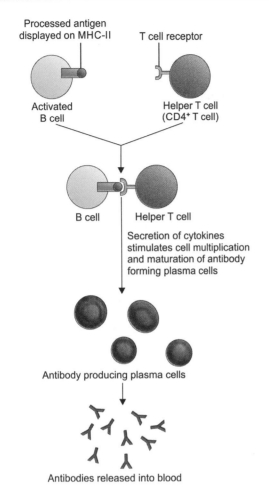

Processed antigen
displayed on MHC-II

T cell receptor

Activated
B cell

Helper T cell
(CD4⁺ T cell)

B cell

Helper T cell

Secretion of cytokines
stimulates cell multiplication
and maturation of antibody
forming plasma cells

Antibody producing plasma cells

Antibodies released into blood

Figure 27.7: Production of antibodies from activated B cell.

- Different cytokines stimulate B cells to produce different antibody producing plasma cells.
- Plasma cell then secretes the antibody corresponding to the **surface immunoglobulin** found on the stimulated parent cell. Secreted antibodies enter the blood and are able to find, neutralize and eliminate antigens.
- If antibodies bind to antigens (bacteria or parasites) it acts as a signal for **polymorphonuclear (PMN) leukocytes (neutrophils, eosinophils, and basophils)** or **macrophages** to engulf and kill them.
- Another important function of antibodies is to initiate the **"complement system."** When antibodies bind to antigen (cells or bacteria), plasma complement proteins bind to the antibodies and destroy the bacteria by creating holes in them.
- Antibodies can also signal **natural killer cells** to kill viral or bacterial infected cells.

❖ Surface immunoglobulins (IgM and IgD), present on the surface of B cells, constitute the **B cell receptor (BCR)**. B cells recognize antigen via the BCR.
❖ In addition to membrane immunoglobulin, the B cells also express several other molecules that are essential for B cell function. These include: **complement receptors (CD21), Fc receptors** and **CD40**.

Contd...

Contd...

❖ Complement receptor-21 (CD21) is also the receptor for the **Epstein-Barr virus (EBV)** and hence EBV readily infects B cells.
❖ The formation of antibodies that occurs on first exposure to a specific antigen is called **primary response**. The formation of antibodies that occurs after second exposure to the same antigen is **secondary response**.
❖ The potency of primary response is weak and short life (only few weeks). The secondary response by contrast, begins rapidly after exposure to the antigen (often within hours), is far more potent and forms antibodies for many months rather than for only a few weeks

Mechanism of Action of Antibodies

Each antibody is specific for a particular antigen because of its unique structural organization of amino acids in the variable portions of both the light and heavy chains. There are two variable sites on the monomer antibody for attachment of antigens, making antibody **bivalent (Figure 27.8)**. IgM which consists of 10 light and 10 heavy chains has as many as 10 binding sites.

The antibodies can inactivate the invading agent in one of several following mechanisms (**mnemonic: PANIC**), by binding antigen via antigen binding region (Fab) of antibody.

- **Precipitation:** Precipitation makes soluble antigens insoluble aiding elimination by opsonization and phagocytosis.
- **Agglutination:** The antibody binds multiple antigenic particles by cross-linking together into a clump for easier removal
- **Neutralization:** Antibodies may block the attachment of viruses or bacterial toxins to membrane receptor by covering the toxic sites of the antigenic agent by antibodies.

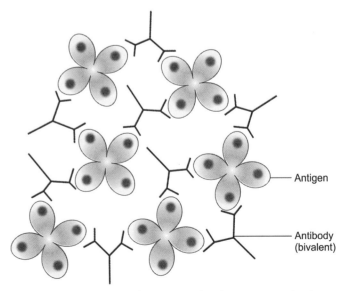

Antigen

Antibody
(bivalent)

Figure 27.8: Binding of antigen molecules to one another by bivalent antibody.

- **Inflammation:** Antibodies may trigger an inflammatory response by releasing histamine. Inflammation raises the blood flow to the area of injury or infection cause redness, swelling, heat, and pain.
- **Complement activation:** The activation of the complement system is initiated by the binding of one of the complement molecules to the Fc portion of the antibody. Complement proteins perforate a membrane which leads to cell lysis.

Adaptive Cellular Immune Response and Role of Helper T Cells, Cytotoxic T Cells, and Regulatory T Cells

T-lymphocytes are responsible for acquired cellular immune response. T cells can only recognize antigens that are bound to receptor molecules of **antigen-presenting cells** (APCs), dendritic cells and macrophages.

The receptor molecules are called, **Major histocompatibility complex class I (MHC-I)** and **class II (MHC-II)**. These MHC molecules are **membrane-bound surface receptors** on antigen-presenting cells, dendritic cells, and macrophages.

If the antigen presenting cells present antigen to T cells, the T cells become activated. Activated T cells proliferate to form **helper T (CD4$^+$T) cells** and **cytotoxic T (CD8$^+$T) cells**. The activated T cells in turn react specifically against the antigen presented by the APCs.

Role of Helper T (CD4$^+$T) Cells

As their name implies they help in the functions of the immune response by several ways. Helper T cells express **T cell receptors (TCR)** that recognize antigen bound to **class II MHC molecules**. Helper T cells have no cytotoxic activity and do not kill infected cells or clear pathogens directly. They instead control the immune response through **cytokines**, by directing other cells to perform these tasks.

- The activation of helper T cells causes it to release number of proteins called **cytokines** and other stimulatory signals that stimulate the activity of **macrophages, cytotoxic (killer) T cells** and **B cells**.
- Cytokines act as the regulator of immune functions by acting on other cells of the immune system and bone marrow and help determine which type of immune responses the body will make to particular pathogens.
- In absence of the cytokines the immune system is almost paralyzed.
- The helper T cells can differentiate into several distinct subtypes; each of these subtypes secretes a different panel of cytokines that initiate the immune response in a specific direction. Helper T cells play a key role in various immunologic processes **(Figure 27.9)**, such as:
  - Activation of cytotoxic T cells and macrophages
  - Maturation of B cells into plasma cells and memory B cells
  - Antibody production by B cells
  - Recruitment of eosinophils and basophils to the loci of infection/inflammation
  - Amplification of microbicidal activity of macrophages
  - Development of tolerance or suppression of inflammatory responses
  - Stimulation of suppressor cells.

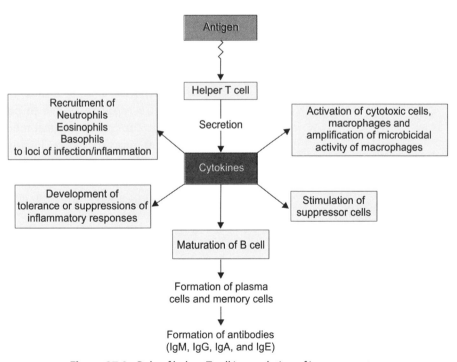

Figure 27.9: Role of helper T cell in regulation of immune system.

Helper T cells are destroyed by the acquired immunodeficiency syndrome (AIDS) virus and body becomes unprotected against infectious disease.

Role of Cytotoxic T (CD8+) Cells

Cytotoxic T cells are also called **killer cells** because these cells are capable of killing directly certain tumor cells, and infected host cells. Cytotoxic T cells directly attack cells carrying certain foreign or abnormal molecules on their surfaces. Cytotoxic T cells recognize small fragments of the viral proteins carried on the surface of an infected cell by body's own **class I MHC** protein molecules.

- The protein of the infecting virus is processed into fragments which combine with **class I MHC** protein molecule and brought to the surface of the infected cell. There the complex is recognized by a cytotoxic T cell **(Figure 27.10)**. Cytotoxic T cells are activated when their T cell receptor (TCR) binds to this specific **antigen-MHC-I** complex molecule.

- Recognition of this **antigen MHC-I** complex is assisted by CD8 receptor of the cytotoxic T cell. The cytotoxic T cell then travels throughout the body in search of cells where the MHC-I receptor bear this antigen.

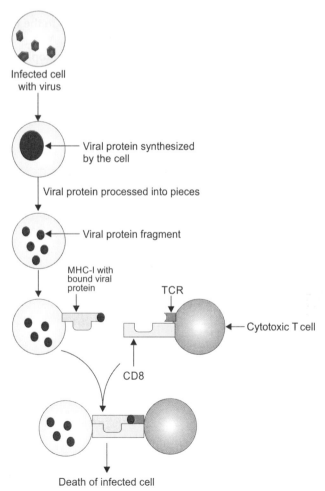

Figure 27.10: Role of cytotoxic T cell.

- After binding, the cytotoxic T cell secretes hole forming proteins called **perforins**. Perforins make hole in the plasma membrane of the attacked cell through which fluid from interstitial space flows rapidly into the attacked cell. The attacked cells then become swollen and it dissolves shortly thereafter. Cytotoxic T cell activation is tightly controlled and requires activation signals provided by **helper T cells**.

Role of Regulatory (Suppressor) T Cells

Regulatory T cells express **CD4** and another receptor, called **CD25** are capable of regulating the function of both cytotoxic T cells and helper T cells and prevent the excessive immune reactions that may cause damage to the body's own tissue. The regulatory T cells help distinguish between **self** and **nonself** molecules, and by doing so, reduce the risk of **autoimmune diseases**.

IMMUNOLOGICAL MEMORY

Immunological memory is the ability of the body to "remember" foreign substance previously encountered and react again promptly if the same pathogen is detected again. This response is called **secondary immune response**, which is quicker and stronger than the **primary response**. It occurs even after many years since the first exposure.

When B cells and T cells are activated and begin to reproduce duplicate cells, some of their offspring will become long **lived memory cells**. Throughout the lifetime these memory cells will remember each specific pathogen encountered and can mount a strong response if the pathogen is detected again. This is **"adaptive"** because it occurs during the lifetime of an individual as an adaptation to infection with that pathogen and prepares the immune system for future challenges.

A host organism needs time, often days, to mount an immune response against a new antigen, but memory cells permit a rapid response to pathogens previously encountered. The immunological memory may be **passive** (short-term memory) or **active** (long-term memory).

- In **passive immunity**, antibodies come from outside the person's body. Passive immunity is usually short-term, lasting from a few days up to several months. Several layers of passive protection are provided by the mother.
  - During pregnancy, antibody IgG, is transported from mother to baby directly across the placenta so human babies have high levels of antibodies even at birth, with the same range of antigen specifies as their mother.
  - Breast milk also contains antibodies that are transferred to the gut of the infant and protect against bacterial infections until the newborn can synthesize its own antibodies.

In medicine, protective passive immunity can also be transferred artificially from one individual to another via antibody rich serum.

TABLE 27.5: Cellular distribution of MHC-molecules.

MHC molecules	Cellular distributions
Class I proteins	All nucleated cells and platelets
Class II proteins	B cells
	Activated T cells
	APCs: Macrophages, Dendritic cells
	Epithelial cells

- **Long-term active memory** is developed after infections by activation of B and T cells. When a clone of T cells is activated by an antigen, many of the newly formed T cells are preserved in the lymphoid tissue to become additional T cells of that specific clone which are called **memory cells**. These memory cells even spread throughout the lymphoid tissue of the entire body. On subsequent exposure to the same antigen anywhere in the body, release of activated T cells occurs far more rapidly and much more powerfully than had first exposure.

- Similarly a few of the activated B lymphocytes do not go on to form plasma cells but instead form some new B-lymphocytes similar to those of the original clone. They also circulate throughout the body to all the lymphoid tissue. However, they remain dormant until activated once again by the same antigen. These lymphocytes are called **memory cells**. Subsequent exposure to the same antigen will cause a much rapid, and much more potent antibody response this second time.

ANTIGEN: DEFINITION, STRUCTURE AND TYPES

Definition

A substance that is capable of stimulating an immune response is known as **antigen**. An **antigen** that induces an immune response is called an **immunogen**.

Structure

The antigens are mostly the **conjugated proteins** like **lipoproteins**, **glycoproteins**, and **nucleoproteins**. On the surface of antigens are regions, called **antigenic determinants** or **epitope** (in Greek; epi – upon, topos - place) that fit and bind to T cell receptor (TCR) molecules present on the surface of the lymphocytes. Each antigen carries many epitopes.

Types

Antigens are categorized in to five types based on their source/**origin** and **immune response**.

1. Exogenous antigens
2. Endogenous antigens
3. Auto antigens
4. Complete antigens/immunogens
5. Haptens/incomplete antigens

- **Exogenous antigens:** These are antigens which are foreign to host body hence are also called **foreign antigens**, e.g., bacteria, fungi, viruses etc. These are antigens that enters the body from the outside, e.g., through inhalation, ingestion, or injection. These antigens enters the body or system and start circulating in the body fluids and trapped by the APCs (Antigen presenting cells such as macrophages, dendritic cells etc.). The uptakes of these exogenous antigens by APCs are mainly mediated by the phagocytosis.

- **Endogenous antigens:** These are antigens which originate from own host body (self-antigens). **Major histocompatibility complex (MHC)** antigens are self-antigens that help in identifying and rejecting the foreign antigens. These are **cell surface glycoproteins**.

  They are also called **HLA antigens (human leukocyte antigens)**, as they were first identified on the membrane of leucocytes. However, afterward they were found to be present on the surface of all body cells except red cells. On the basis of their chemical structure, tissue distribution, and function, the MHC antigens are classified into two major groups **(Table 27.5)**:
  1. Class I: MHC I antigen
  2. Class II: MHC II antigen

  - **MHC I antigen:** MHC I antigens are present on the cell membranes of all nucleated cells and platelets except red cells (red cells contain blood group antigens). MHC I molecules hand over antigens to **cytotoxic T cells**.

  - **MHC II antigen:** MHC II antigens are present on the surface of B-cells, activated T-cells, monocytes, antigen presenting cells (APCs), and on some epithelial cells. MHC-II molecules hand over antigens to **helper T cells** to trigger the appropriate immune response.

- **Auto antigens:** Auto antigens are normal "self" protein or complex of proteins or nucleic acid that is attacked by the host's immune system, causing an **autoimmune disease**. These are not immunogenic under normal condition however due to genetic and environmental factors immunological tolerance is lost and immune response is generated leading to the generation of autoantibodies.

- **Complete antigens/immunogens:** A substance that induces specific immune response can be called as **immunogen**. Antigens which are able to generate immune response by themselves are known as **complete antigens**. These are generally molecules with high molecular weight. They possess antigenic properties denovo and are usually protein in nature. Some of them can be polysaccharide in chemical nature.

- **Haptens/Incomplete antigens:** Antigens which are unable to generate the immune response themselves are termed as incomplete antigens however on coupling with carrier proteins they can be immunogenic. They are also called **haptens** (Greek: hapten- to grasp). When a molecule of haptens is coupled to carrier proteins they become able to generate immune response and function as an immunogen.

They generally have low molecular weight and are usually nonprotein substances, e.g., capsular polysaccharide of pneumococcus, polysaccharide C of streptococci, cardiolipin antigens, etc. Carrier molecule is a nonantigenic component and helps in provoking the immune response, e.g., serum protein such as albumin or globulin.

VACCINE

The administration of vaccines is called **vaccination** (also called **immunization**). Vaccination is a method of active immunization. Vaccination is one of the most effective ways to prevent diseases. Vaccines protect against more than 25 life-threatening diseases, including measles, polio, tetanus, diphtheria, meningitis, influenza, tetanus, typhoid, and cervical cancer.

The principle behind **vaccination** is to introduce an antigen from a pathogen in order to stimulate the immune system and develop specific immunity against that particular pathogen without causing disease associated with that organism.

Vaccinations induce long-term immunity to specific pathogenic infections by initiating a primary immune response, which results in production of **memory cells**. When exposed to the actual pathogen, the memory cells trigger a more potent secondary immune response. As a consequence of this more potent immune response, disease symptoms do not develop. Individual becomes immune to pathogen.

The immunity to infection following a vaccination depends on how long the memory cells survive. Memory cells may not survive a lifetime and individuals may subsequently require a booster shot to maintain immunity.

Types of Vaccine

A vaccine is a biological preparation that provides active acquired immunity to a particular infectious disease. The word "vaccine" was created by **Edward Jenner**. The word actually comes from the name for a cowpox (smallpox of the cow) virus, *vaccinia*. In Latin word **vacca** means cow.

The discovery and utilization of vaccines represents a significant milestone in modern medical history. The pioneering work of **Edward Jenner** and **Louis Pasteur** in the eighteenth and nineteenth centuries reveled that inoculation with inactivated forms of a pathogen could protect against subsequent infection with the active pathogen.

A vaccine typically contains a weakened or attenuated form of the disease causing pathogen, its toxins, or one of its surface proteins (antigens) but is incapable of triggering disease. The active component of a vaccine that is responsible to protect against a particular viral/bacterial infection can often consists of many forms as:

1. Whole pathogen vaccines
2. Killed or inactivated vaccines
3. Live attenuated (weakened) vaccines
4. Subunit vaccines
5. Toxoid vaccines
6. Nucleic acid vaccine: (RNA vaccine, DNA vaccine)

- **Whole pathogen vaccines:** The oldest and most well-known method of vaccination is to use the whole disease-causing pathogen in a vaccine to produce an immune response similar to that seen during natural infection. Using the pathogen in its natural state would cause active disease and could potentially be dangerous to the individual receiving it and risk the disease spreading to others. To avoid this, modern vaccines use pathogens that have been altered.

- **Live attenuated vaccines:** Live attenuated vaccines contain whole bacteria or viruses which have been "weakened"(attenuated) so that they generate a protective immune response but do not cause disease in healthy people.

For most modern vaccines this "weakening" is achieved through genetic modification of the pathogen either as a naturally occurring phenomenon or as a modification specifically introduced by scientists.

Live vaccines tend to create a strong and lasting immune response. However, live vaccines may not suitable for people whose immune system doesn't work, either due to drug treatment or underlying illness. This is because the weakened viruses or bacteria could in some cases multiply too much and might cause disease in these people.

Live vaccines are:

- Measles, mumps, rubella (MMR combined vaccine) vaccine
- Rotavirus vaccine
- Smallpox vaccine
- Chickenpox vaccine

- **Inactivated or killed vaccines:** Inactivated vaccines contain whole bacteria or viruses, which have been killed or have been altered, so that they cannot replicate. Because inactivated vaccines do not contain any live bacteria or viruses, they cannot cause the diseases against which they protect, even in people with severely weakened immune systems. However, inactivated vaccines do not always create such a strong or long-lasting immune response as live attenuated vaccines.

Inactivated vaccines are:

- Hepatitis A vaccine
- Flu vaccine
- Polio vaccine
- Rabies vaccine

- **Subunit vaccines:** Subunit vaccines do not contain any whole bacteria or viruses at all. Instead, these vaccines typically contain a purified protein component from the surface of the pathogen. Such proteins can be either isolated from infected material (such as blood from chronically infected patients) or generated by **recombinant methods**. The first recombinant antigen vaccine approved for human use is **hepatitis B vaccine**. The advantage of subunit vaccines over whole pathogen vaccines is that the immune response can focus on recognizing a small number of antigen targets. Subunit vaccines do not always create such a strong or long-lasting immune response as live attenuated vaccines. They usually require repeated doses initially and subsequent booster doses in subsequent years. Subunit vaccines are:
  - Hepatitis B vaccine
  - HPV (Human papillomavirus) vaccine
  - Pneumococcal disease vaccine
- **Toxoid vaccines:** Some bacteria release toxins (poisonous proteins) when they attack the body, and it is the toxins rather than the bacteria itself that we want to be protected against. The immune system recognizes these toxins in the same way that it recognizes other antigens on the surface of the bacteria, and is able to mount an immune response to them.

  Toxoid vaccines are made from a toxin (produced by certain bacteria, e.g., tetanus or diphtheria) that has been made harmless but that produces an immune response against the toxin. They trigger a strong immune response. Toxoid vaccines are safe because they cannot cause the disease they prevent and there is no possibility of reversion to virulence. They are stable, as they are less susceptible to changes in temperature, humidity, and light.

  Toxoid vaccines are:
  - Diphtheria vaccine
  - Tetanus vaccine
  - Pertussis (whooping cough) vaccine
- **Nucleic acid vaccines:** Nucleic acid vaccines work in a different way to other vaccines in that they do not supply the protein antigen to the body. Instead, they provide the genetic instructions of the antigen to cells in the body and in turn the cells produce the antigen, which stimulates an immune response. Nucleic acid vaccines are quick and easy to develop.
  - **RNA vaccines:** RNA vaccines use mRNA (messenger RNA) covered with a lipid (fat) membrane. This fatty cover both protects the mRNA when it first enters the body, and also helps it to get inside cells by fusing with the cell membrane.
    - When this is injected into body, cells start to synthesize the relevant viral protein for example Covid-19's 'spike' protein.
    - This mRNA typically persists a few days, but in that time sufficient antigen is made to stimulate an immune response.
    - It is then naturally broken down and removed by the body.
    - RNA vaccines are not capable of combining with the human genetic code (DNA).
    - Two RNA Covid-19 vaccines have been approved for use: Pfizer-BioNTech and Moderna.
  - **DNA vaccines:** DNA is more stable than mRNA. DNA vaccines are typically administered along with a technique called **electroporation**.
    - This uses low level electronic waves to allow the bodies' cells to take up the DNA vaccine.
    - DNA must be transcribed to mRNA within the cell nucleus which subsequently translated to protein antigens, which stimulate an immune response. There are currently no licenced DNA vaccines, but there are many in development.

> However, despite the success of vaccines in the prevention of many devastating diseases, several pathogens have posed a significant challenge to vaccine development. For example, development of an effective HIV vaccine is difficult or impossible. Because the mechanism for replication of HIV is prone to error, a population of HIV presents an ever-changing group of coat proteins. Indeed, the mutation rate of HIV is more than 65 times higher than that of influenza virus.

DISORDERS OF HUMAN IMMUNITY

Inappropriate responses of immune cells and molecules themselves can disrupt the proper functioning of the entire system, leading to host-cell damage that can become fatal. Failures of host defense causes:

- Immunodeficiency
- Autoimmunity
- Hypersensitivity

Immunodeficiency

Immunodeficiency is a failure, insufficiency, or delay in the response of the immune system, which may be **acquired** or **inherited**. Immunodeficiencies occur when one or more of the component of the immune system is inactive. Immunodeficiency can allow pathogens or tumor cells to gain a base and replicate or proliferate to high enough levels so that the immune system becomes overwhelmed.

- **AIDS (acquired immunodeficiency syndrome)** and some types of **cancer** cause **acquired** immunodeficiency.

- AIDS is due to of **human immunodeficiency virus (HIV)** infection with certain pathogens that attack the T cells of the immune system itself.
- **Chemical exposure**, including certain medical treatments such as **chemotherapy**, for instance, radiation exposure can destroy populations of lymphocytes and elevate an individual's susceptibility to infections and cancer.
- **Malnutrition** is the most common cause of immunodeficiency. Diets lacking sufficient protein are associated with impaired **cell-mediated immunity**, **complement activity**, **phagocytic function**, **IgA antibody concentrations**, and **cytokine production**. Deficiency of single nutrients such as **iron**, **copper**, **zinc**, **selenium**; vitamins A, C, E, B_6, and folic acid (vitamin B_9) also reduces immune responses.
- Immunodeficiencies can also be **inherited**.
  - **Chronic granulomatous** disease where phagocytes have a reduced ability to destroy pathogens is an example of an inherited or congenital immunodeficiency.
  - Rarely, primary immunodeficiencies that are present from birth may also occur. For example, **severe combined immunodeficiency disease (SCID)** is a condition in which children are born without functioning B or T cells.
  - The loss of the thymus at an early age through genetic mutation or surgical removal results in **severe immunodeficiency** and a high susceptibility to infection.

Autoimmunity

Failure to differentiate host cells from a foreign invader can trigger an autoimmune response in which the body's immune system attacks its own tissues and organs. The resulting damage may be cumulative, such as occurs in rheumatoid arthritis and multiple sclerosis, or acute, such as the complete destruction of pancreatic islets cells that

TABLE 27.6: Autoimmune diseases.

Organ specific	Systemic
• Autoimmune atrophic gastritis of pernicious anemia • Autoimmune hemolytic anemia • Autoimmune thrombocytopenia • Autoimmune hepatitis • Hashimoto thyroiditis • Grave's disease • Insulin dependent diabetes mellitus • Multiple sclerosis	• Systemic lupus erythematosis • Rheumatoid arthritis • Reiter's syndrome • Inflammatory myopathies

occurs in type 1 dibetes. **Table 27.6** lists several of the more commonly encountered autoimmune disorders.

Hypersensitivity

Hypersensitivity is an immune response that damages the body's own tissues. Types of hypersensitivities include **immediate**, and delayed, based on the mechanisms involved and the time course of the hypersensitive reaction.

Immediate hypersensitivity: Immediate or anaphylactic reaction often associated with **allergy**. On first exposure to an allergen, an antibody (IgE) is synthesized by plasma cells. The antibodies bind to mast cells which release histamines and other modulators that cause the symptoms of allergy.

The effects of an allergic reaction range from mild symptoms like sneezing and itchy, watery eyes to more severe or even life-threatening reactions involving intensely itchy marks or rashes, airway constriction with severe respiratory distress, and reducing blood pressure caused by dilating blood vessels and fluid loss from the circulatory system.

Delayed hypersensitivity: Delayed hypersensitivity is a **cell-mediated immune response** that takes approximately one to two days to develop. This type of hypersensitivity involves the helper T cell cytokine-mediated inflammatory response and may cause local tissue lesions or contact dermatitis (rash or skin irritation). Delayed hypersensitivity occurs in some individuals in response to contact with certain types of jewelry or cosmetics.

ASSESSMENT QUESTIONS

STRUCTURED LONG ESSAY QUESTIONS (SLEQs)

1. Describe innate immune system under following headings:
   i. Definition
   ii. Types
   iii. Components
   iv. Response
2. Describe adaptive immune system under following headings:
   i. Definition
   ii. Types
   iii. Components
   iv. Response
3. Describe antibodies (Immunoglobulins) under following headings:
   i. Definition
   ii. Types
   iii. Structure
   iv. Formation
   v. Mechanism of action

SHORT ESSAY QUESTIONS (SEQs)

1. Write role of helper T cell in regulation of immune system.
2. List and write nonspecific barrier mechanisms for defense against microorganisms.
3. Write the difference between innate (natural) and adaptive (acquired) immunity
4. What is "complement system" and how it contributes to our body's immune defenses?
5. Write the role of antibodies in an immune response.
6. What is vaccine? Write different types.
7. Give disorders due to failure of defense mechanism.
8. Write cells and organs involved in immune system.

SHORT ANSWER QUESTIONS (SAQs)

1. What is primary and secondary immune response?
2. Define immunologic tolerance.
3. What is meant by antigen and epitope?
4. Enumerate two antigen presenting cells. And their formation.
5. Write the difference between passive and active immunity.
6. Write the difference between a primary and secondary immune response.
7. List the causes of immunodeficiency.
8. What is meant by immunological memory.
9. Write the role of the macrophages and dendritic cells.
10. Write the role of the neutrophils in immune system.
11. Write the role of the eosinophils and basophils in immune system.
12. Write the role of the natural killer cells.
13. Write the role of the helper T-cells.
14. Write the role of the cytotoxic T-cells.
15. Write the role of the regulatory T-cells.
16. What is the role of the B-lymphocytes?
17. Write the role of the plasma cells in immune system.
18. What is histocompatibility molecules.

MULTIPLE CHOICE QUESTIONS (MCQs)

1. **A helper T-lymphocyte is known to recognize which of the following on a presenting cell?**
   a. HLA class I antigen
   b. HLA class II antigen
   c. CD8 antigen
   d. Surface immunoglobulin
2. **Which of the following cells are phagocytic?**
   a. Macrophages
   b. Monocytes
   c. Neutrophil polymorphonuclear leukocytes
   d. All of the above
3. **Which of the following is known to be involved in the initial presentation of antigen to T-lymphocytes?**
   a. Dendritic cells
   b. Plasma cells
   c. Platelets
   d. Erythrocytes
4. **Which of the following control the immune response?**
   a. Cytotoxic T cell
   b. Helper T cell
   c. Supressor cell
   d. Natural killer cell

5. **Performin a protein secreted by:**
   a. Helper T cell
   b. Cytotoxic cell
   c. Natural killer cell
   d. Supressor cell
6. **Following are the antigen presenting cells (APCs), except:**
   a. Macrophages
   b. B-lymphocytes
   c. Dendritic cells
   d. Helper T cell
7. **Antibodies are secreted by:**
   a. Stem cells
   b. Tissue cells
   c. Plasma cells
   d. Membranous cells
8. **Immunological destruction of body tissue or product due to antibodies reacting with it as antigen is called:**
   a. Anaphylaxis
   b. Autoimmune diseases
   c. Prophylaxis
   d. Immunodeficiency disease
9. **Innate immunity is:**
   a. Active acquired immunity
   b. Passive acquired immunity
   c. Inborn immunity
   d. Both B and C
10. **Innate immunity is provided by:**
    a. Phagocytes
    b. Antibodies
    c. T-lymphocytes
    d. B-lymphocytes
11. **Which one engulfs foreign materials:**
    a. Macrophages
    b. Plasma cells
    c. Mast cells
    d. Lymphocytes
12. **Macrophages are derived from:**
    a. Neutrophils
    b. Lymphocytes
    c. Monocytes
    d. Basophils
13. **Memory cells are formed from:**
    a. Erythropoietic stem cells
    b. Monocytes
    c. T-lymphocytes
    d. B-lymphocytes
14. **Segments of antigen that are recognized by antibody are:**
    a. Memory regions
    b. Epitopes
    c. Nondeterminants
    d. Self limitation
15. **Passive immunity is:**
    a. Acquired through natural overt or latent infection
    b. Acquired through vaccination
    c. Acquired through readymade antibodies
    d. Acquired by activating immune system of the body
16. **Passive immunity is obtained through injecting:**
    a. Antibiotics
    b. Vaccines
    c. Antibodies
    d. Antigens
17. **Resistance developed in an individual as a result of antigenic stimulus is:**
    a. Natural immunity
    b. Active acquired immunity
    c. Passive acquired immunity
    d. Artificial immunity
18. **The two types of immunity in humans are:**
    a. Intrinsic and extrinsic
    b. Innate and the acquired
    c. Internal and external
    d. Overt and covert

19. **Another name for innate immunity is:**
    a. Nonspecific immunity
    b. Is immunity
    c. Is specific immunity
    d. None of the above

20. **The two types of lymphocytes are:**
    a. Platelets and erythrocytes
    b. B cells and the T cells
    c. Platelets and the T cells
    d. T cells and erythrocytes

21. **The physical barriers that form part of the immune system are:**
    a. The skin and the mucosal membranes
    b. The bones and the mucosal membranes
    c. The skin and bones
    d. The skin, body temperature, and the mucosal membranes

22. **Chemical barriers that form part of the immune system are:**
    a. Tears and urine
    b. Hair, breast milk, sweat, saliva, stomach acid
    c. Tears, breast milk, sweat, saliva, stomach acid, and faeces
    d. Tears, breast milk, sweat, saliva, stomach acid

23. **Neutrophils, eosinophils and basophils are known as:**
    a. Granulocytes
    b. Astrocytoma
    c. Platelets
    d. Buffers

24. **With acquired immunity the body fails to achieve specific immunity to a specific threat.**
    a. True
    b. False

25. **The acquired immune system is based upon the lymphocytes.**
    a. True
    b. False

26. **Where do precursor T-lymphocytes develop into fully competent but not yet activated T-cells?**
    a. The thymus gland
    b. The bone marrow
    c. The lymph nodes
    d. The spleen

27. **Which of the following is not a feature of a secondary immune response to an antigen, when compared to the first response to the same antigen?**
    a. The antibody is generated faster
    b. More antibodies are produced
    c. The antibody produced has greater affinity for the antigen
    d. Antibody is generated without T cell help

28. **What is the normal immunological role of the CD8+ T cell?**
    a. Helps B-lymphocytes to develop into plasma cells
    b. Kills virus infected cells
    c. Secretes antibodies
    d. Rejects transplanted tissue

29. **In order to initiate an adaptive immune response, antigenic peptide must be presented to antigen-specific T cells. Which one type of cell presents this antigen to T cells?**
    a. Dendritic cell   b. Epithelial cell
    c. Neutrophil   d. Plasma cell

30. **Which of the following cell types or systems is not part of an innate immune response to a pathogen?**
    a. Phagocytes
    b. Natural killer cells
    c. The inflammatory response
    d. Cytotoxic T-lymphocytes

31. **The concept of vaccination was first developed by:**
    a. Louis Pasteur
    b. Edward Jenner
    c. Carl Landsteiner
    d. Joseph Miester

32. **The first vaccine was developed by:**
    a. Louis Pasteur
    b. Edward Jenner
    c. Carl Landsteiner
    d. Joseph Miester

33. **A vaccine can be:**
    a. An antigenic protein
    b. Weakened pathogen
    c. Live attenuated pathogen
    d. All of these

34. **Which of the following statement is true regarding vaccination?**
    a. Vaccination is a method of active immunization
    b. Vaccination is a method of passive immunization
    c. Vaccination is a method of artificial passive immunization
    d. Vaccination is a method of natural passive immunization

35. **Active immunity may be gained by:**
    a. Natural infection   b. Vaccines
    c. Toxoids   d. All of these

36. **The first recombinant antigen vaccine approved for human use is:**
    a. Hepatitis B vaccine
    b. Hepatitis A vaccine
    c. Pneumococcal disease vaccine
    d. DPT vaccine

ANSWERS FOR MCQs

1. b	2. d	3. a	4. b	5. b
6. d	7. c	8. b	9. c	10. a
11. a	12. c	13. d	14. b	15. c
16. c	17. b	18. b	19. a	20. d
21. d	22. d	23. a	24. b	25. a
26. a	27. d	28. b	29. d	30. d
31. b	32. a	33. d	34. a	35. d
36. a				

28 CHAPTER

Biochemistry of Cancer

Competency	Learning Objectives
BI 10.1: Describe the cancer initiation, promotion oncogenes, and oncogene activation. Also focus on p53 and apoptosis. **BI 10.2:** Describe various biochemical tumor markers and the biochemical basis of cancer therapy.	1. Describe characteristics of cancer cell and biochemical changes occur in cancer cell. 2. Describe molecular basis of cancer (carcinogenesis). 3. Describe various carcinogens. 4. Describe oncogenes and proto-oncogenes. 5. Describe tumor suppressor genes, retinoblastoma (RB) gene and P53 gene. 6. Describe apoptosis in physiologic and pathologic conditions. 7. Describe various biochemical tumor markers. 8. Describe the biochemical basis of cancer therapy.

OVERVIEW

A neoplasm refers to any abnormal new growth of tissue. It may be **benign** or **malignant** in nature. A mass of tissue formed as a result of abnormal excessive, uncoordinated, autonomous, and purposeless proliferation of cells is called **tumor**. Tumors may be **"benign"** (i.e., it does not invade or spread to distant sites in the body and does not destroy the tissue in which it originates, i.e., a noncancerous tumor) or **"malignant"** (i.e., it invades and destroys the tissue in which it originates and can spread to other sites in the body via the blood stream and lymphatic systems).

The term cancer is usually associated with malignant tumors. It may be defined as **"malignant neoplasm."**

The branch of science dealing with the study of neoplasm or tumor is called **oncology** (oncos = tumor, logos = study).

CHARACTERISTICS OF CANCER CELL AND BIOCHEMICAL CHANGES OCCUR IN CANCER CELL

Cancer cells are characterized by certain main properties **(Figure 28.1)**:
1. They proliferate rapidly.
2. Show diminished growth control.

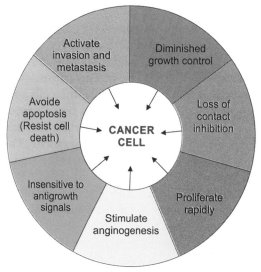

Figure 28.1: Major characteristics of cancer cells.

3. Show loss of contact inhibition. Malignant tumors show faster rate of growth due to loss of contact inhibition and form multilayers instead of a monolayer. Contact inhibition is a process of arresting cell growth when cells come in contact with each other. As a result, normal cells stop proliferating when they form a monolayer. Contact

inhibition is a powerful anticancer mechanism that is lost in cancer cells.

4. They invade (attack) local tissues and spread, or metastasize, (distant spread) to other parts of the body. (Benign tumors do not invade or metastasize). Invasion and metastasize is the hallmark of malignant tumors. **Metastasis is the spread of cancer cells from the place where they first formed to another part of the body**. In metastasis, cancer cells escape from the original (primary) tumor, travel through the blood or lymph system, and form a new tumor in other organs or tissues of the body.

5. They are self-sufficient in growth signals and are insensitive to antigrowth signals.

6. They stimulate local angiogenesis (stimulation of blood vessel growth).

7. They are often able to avoid apoptosis.

Biochemical Changes which Occur in Cancer Cell

❖ Increased synthesis of RNA and DNA.
❖ Increased activity of ribonucleotide reductase required for the formation of deoxyribonucleotides from ribonucleotides.
❖ Increased rates of aerobic and anaerobic glycolysis. Thus, more pyruvate is produced than can be metabolized. This in turn results in excessive production of lactate and lactic acidosis results.
❖ Synthesis of certain fetal proteins, e.g., carcino embryonic antigen.
❖ Inappropriate synthesis of certain growth factors and hormones.
❖ Alterations of the cell surface due to changes in the composition of glycoproteins or glycosphingolipids.

MOLECULAR BASIS OF CANCER (CARCINOGENESIS)

Carcinogenesis means mechanism of induction of cancer. Agents, which can induce cancer, are called **carcinogens**. Carcinogenesis is a gradual multi step process involving many generations of cells. The various causes may act on the cell one after another. Ultimately, the cells so formed are **genetically** and **phenotypically transformed cells** having phenotypic features of malignancy, like **excessive growth**, **invasiveness** and distinct **metastasis**. The main principles of the molecular basis of cancer are summarized in **Figure 28.2**.

● In cancer there are either genetic abnormalities in the cell, or there are normal genes with abnormal expression.
● The genetic abnormalities may be inherited or induced by carcinogenic agents, namely chemicals, viruses, and radiation. The mutated cells transmit their characters to the next progeny of cells and result in cancer. In normal cell growth, there are four regulatory genes.
  1. DNA repair genes regulate the repair of DNA damage that has occurred during mitosis.
  2. Proto-oncogenes are growth promoting genes.
  3. Antioncogenes are growth inhibiting or growth suppressor genes.
  4. Apoptosis regulatory genes control the programed cell death.

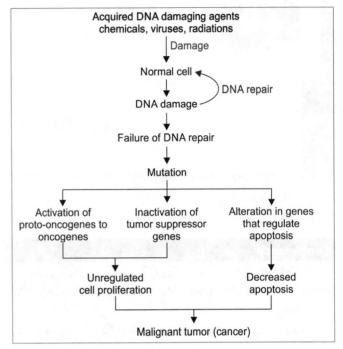

Figure 28.2: Molecular basis of cancer (carcinogenesis).

● In cancer the **transformed cells** are produced due to genetic damage to these normal controlling genes. The corresponding abnormalities in these four genes are as under:
  1. Failures of **DNA repair genes** and thus inability to repair the DNA damage resulting in **mutation**.
  2. Activation of proto-oncogene to **oncogenes** causing transformation of cell (mutant form of normal proto-oncogene is termed oncogene). Gene products of oncogenes are called **oncoproteins**.
  3. Inactivation of cancer **suppressor genes** (i.e., inactivation of antioncogenes) permitting the cellular proliferation of transformed cells.
  4. Alteration in genes that regulate apoptosis.

CARCINOGENS

There are three classes of carcinogens, exposure to which result in tumor formation. These are:
  1. Chemicals
  2. Radiant energy
  3. Certain oncogene viruses.

Chemical Carcinogens

A wide variety of chemical compounds are carcinogenic. It is estimated that 80% of human cancers are caused by environmental factors, principally chemicals. A variety of mutations in DNA can result from exposure of human to chemical carcinogens, some of which contribute to the development of cancer.

TABLE 28.1: Important chemical carcinogens.

Carcinogen	Class	Examples
Initiators of carcinogenesis		
Direct carcinogens	• Alkylating agents (anticancer drugs) • Acylating agent	Cyclophosphamide, chlorambucil, nitrosourea
Indirect carcinogens (Procarcinogens)	Polycyclic aromatic hydrocarbons	Benzo(a)pyrene, dimethylbenzanthracene. Tobacco, smoke, fossil fuel, e.g., coal, tar, mineral oil, smoked animal foods, industrial, and atmospheric pollutants
	Aromatic amines	β-Naphthylamine, benzidine, acetylaminofluorene, Azo dyes used for coloring foods
	• Naturally occurring compounds (derived from plant and microbial sources) • Miscellaneous compounds	• Aflatoxin B1, dactinomycin, betel nuts (compounds in betel nuts are unknown) • Nitrosamines, vinyl chloride, asbestos, arsenical compounds, metals like nickel, lead, chromium, cobalt, etc.
Promoters of carcinogenesis		Phenols, hormones (estrogen), phenobarbital, artificial sweetners like saccharine and cyclamates

Basic mechanism of chemical carcinogenesis is by induction of mutation in the **proto-oncogenes** and **antioncogenes**. Depending upon the mode of action of carcinogenic chemicals they are divided into two groups:

1. Initiators of carcinogenesis: Direct and Indirect
2. Promoters of carcinogenesis.

Initiators of Carcinogenesis

These are the chemical carcinogens which can initiate the process of abnormal new growth of cells. Initiation is the first stage in carcinogenesis. Chemicals acting as initiators of carcinogenesis can be grouped into two categories **(Table 28.1)**.

1. **Direct carcinogens:** Some chemicals interact directly with DNA and can induce cellular transformation without undergoing any prior metabolic activation, e.g., anticancer drugs like cyclophosphamide, chlorambucil, and nitrosourea
2. **Procarcinogens or indirect carcinogens:** These require metabolic activation to become carcinogenic. One or more enzyme catalyzed reactions convert procarcinogens to active carcinogens **(ultimate carcinogens) (Figure 28.3)**. Examples of procarcinogens are:
   - Aromatic hydrocarbons, e.g., Benzo[a]pyrene, Tobacco smoke, industrial and atmospheric pollutants.
   - Aromatic amine, e.g., Benzidine, β-naphthylamine, azo dyes, used in rubber industries.
   - Naturally occurring products, e.g., Aflatoxin B1.
   - Inorganic compounds, e.g., Vinyl chloride, asbestos, metals like nickel, lead, chromium, etc.
   - Nitrosamine compounds, e.g., Dimethylnitrosamine, diethylnitrosamine found in whisky, new car interiors, tobacco smoke.

Promoters of Carcinogenesis

Certain chemical substances are not carcinogenic but they help the initiated cell to proliferate further are called **promoters** of **carcinogenesis**. For example, phenols, phenobarbital, artificial sweeteners like saccharine and cyclamates **(Table 28.1)**.

Action of Chemical Carcinogens

Direct or indirect acting carcinogens are usually **electrophiles**, i.e., they are deficient in electrons (free radicals). These free radical carcinogens can covalently bind to **purines, pyrimidines**, and **phosphodiester bonds of DNA** causing unrepairable damage. This unrepaired damage generates **mutations in DNA** and mutation in DNA may lead to **cancer**.

In either case following steps are involved in transforming the target cell into the initiated cell.

- **Metabolic activation:** Majority of chemical carcinogens is indirect or procarcinogens requires metabolic activation, while direct carcinogens which are electrophilic (electron deficient) do not require this activation.
- The indirect carcinogens are activated in the liver by the **cytochrome P$_{450}$** located in the endoplasmic reticulum (ER). Indirect acting substances become electrophilic (electron deficient) after metabolic activation.
- Following this step, both types of chemical carcinogens behave alike, and these electrophiles interact with **DNA, RNA**, and other **proteins** producing mutagenesis **(Figure 28.3)**.
- The change in DNA may lead to the initiated cell. Most of the time the damaged DNA is repaired or detoxified by enzyme like **glutathione transferase**. The unrepaired damage produced in the DNA of the cell becomes permanent and irreversible, which are the characteristics of the initiated cell.

Radiant Energy

Radiant energy can be carcinogenic. **Ultraviolet rays** and **ionizing radiation**, i.e., **x-rays, α-, β- and γ-rays** are mutagenic and carcinogenic. These rays damage DNA which

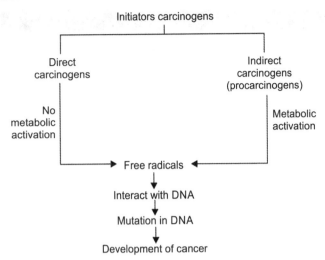

Figure 28.3: Action of chemical carcinogens.

TABLE 28.2: Some important oncogenic viruses that cause human cancer.

Virus	Genome	Type of cancer
Human papilloma virus (HPV)	DNA	Cancer of cervix
Human herpes viruses type I	DNA	Kaposi sarcoma
Hepatitis B virus (HBV)	DNA	Hepatocellular carcinoma
Human papilloma virus (HPV)	DNA	B-cell lymphoma, nasopharyngeal cancer, Burkitt lymphoma
Human T-cell leukemia virus type I	RNA	Adult T-cell leukemia
Hepatitis C	RNA	Hepatocellular carcinoma

is the basic mechanism of carcinogenicity with radiant energy. These agents can damage DNA in a number of ways as given below:

- Formation of pyrimidine dimers in DNA
- Formation of apurinic or apyrimidine sites by elimination of corresponding bases
- Formation of single or double strands breaks or cross linking of DNA.
- Additionally, x-rays, and γ-rays can induce formation of reactive oxygen species (ROS), **free radicals**. Formation of highly reactive *free radicals* can interact with DNA and other macromolecules leading to molecular damage. Damage to the DNA results in mutagenesis and thereby probably contributes to carcinogenic effects of radiant energy.

The main source of UV radiation is the sunlight; others are UV lamps, welder's arcs. In humans excessive exposure of UV rays can cause various forms of skin cancers. The risk of developing a skin cancer due to ultraviolet radiation increases with increasing frequency and intensity of exposure and decreasing melanin content of skin.

Oncogenic Viruses

Both DNA and RNA viruses have been identified as being able to cause cancer in humans **(Table 28.2)**. RNA oncogenic viruses are **retroviruses**, i.e., they contain the enzyme **reverse transcriptase**. RNA oncogenic viruses use RNA as the genome. All retroviruses are not oncogenic.

Mechanism of Viral Oncogenesis

The genetic material of viruses is incorporated into the genome of the host cell.

- The DNA virus infects the host cell. Then DNA virus binds tightly to host cell DNA and causes alterations in gene expression and thus causes cell transformation by altering the types of protein made in cell. Viral oncoproteins are thought to bind to tumor suppressors and inactivate them. DNA viruses often act by down regulating the expression and/or function of **tumor suppressor genes P53** and **RB** and their protein products.
- The RNA viruses use RNA as the genome. The RNA gets copied by **reverse transcriptase** to produce single strand of viral DNA. Single strand of viral DNA is then copied to form another strand of complementary DNA, resulting in double stranded viral DNA called the **provirus**. The provirus is then integrated into the DNA of the host cell DNA and results in various activities such as:
  - Deregulation of the cell cycle
  - Inhibition of apoptosis
  - Abnormalities of cell signaling pathways.

ONCOGENES AND PROTO-ONCOGENES

An **oncogene** is an altered gene derived by "activation" of normal cellular **proto-oncogenes**. When proto-oncogenes get mutated they become oncogenes. Cellular proto-oncogenes code for a number of proteins, e.g., **growth factors, receptors, transcription factors**, and other proteins involved in cell growth. Oncogenes encode a wide variety of altered proteins that accelerate cell growth or cell division. **(Table 28.3)**.

Oncogenes are genes capable of causing cancer. In the cancer cell their normal proto-oncogenes are permanently changed to oncogenes and the balance between factors stimulating and the factors inhibiting cell growth is permanently lost resulting in increased proliferation of cells. The effect of oncogenes on cell growth has been compared **to putting one's foot on the accelerator of an automobile**, whereas the action of tumor suppressor genes resembles **putting one's foot on the break**.

- Proto-oncogenes are activated to oncogenes by various mechanisms:
  - Promoter and enhancer insertion
  - Chromosomal translocation
  - Gene amplification
  - Point mutation.

TABLE 28.3: Some oncogenes and their mutated protein product.

Oncogenes	Location	Mutated protein product related to
jun	Nucleus	Transcription factor
fos	Nucleus	Transcription factor
myc	Nucleus	DNA-binding protein
ras	Cytoplasm	GTP-binding protein
rat	Cytoplasm	Protein kinase (serine)
abl	Cytoplasm	Protein kinase (tyrosine)
src	Cytoplasm	Protein kinase (tyrosine)
trk	Cell membrane	Growth factor receptor
erbB	Cell membrane	Growth factor receptor
fms	Cell membrane	Growth factor receptor
sis	Cell membrane	Growth factor

- When oncogenes are expressed, they produce mutated versions of:
  - Growth factors
  - Receptors for growth factors
  - Proteins involved in signaling gene expression in the nucleus.

Thus, various factors that cause cancer may all act through their effects on proto-oncogene. Radiation and chemical carcinogens may cause mutations in the proto-oncogene; viruses may introduce promoters into the host cells, which regulate proto-oncogene expression causing the genes to lose their normal controls.

TUMOR SUPPRESSOR GENES

A **tumor suppressor gene** produces a protein product that normally suppresses cell growth or cell division. It regulates **cell cycle** and **apoptosis**. These tumor suppressor genes, sometimes called **recessive** *oncogenes* or **antioncogenes**.

When such a gene is altered by mutation, the inhibitory effect of its product is lost or diminished, leading to increased cell growth or cell division. Inactivation by mutation of tumor suppressor gene removes certain mechanisms of growth control and can cause some types of tumor. Two of the most widely studied tumor suppressor genes are **retinoblastoma (RB) gene** and **P53 gene**.

- The **retinoblastoma (RB) tumor suppressor gene** was the first tumor suppressor gene discovered. The RB gene lies on chromosome 13. RB gene codes for a **nuclear transcription protein**, **pRB**. Mutation of RB gene leads to several human tumors, most commonly **retinoblastoma**.
- **P53 tumor suppressor gene (P53 gene)** is located on chromosome 17. P53 gene codes for **tumor suppressor protein p53 (p53)**. This protein acts as a tumor suppressor. It prevents multiplication of genetically

damaged cells and acts as **"molecular policeman."** Thus, it is also called a **Gatekeeper gene**, or **Guardian of the genome**. When the DNA of a normal cell is damaged by any carcinogenic agent, it causes activation of p53 protein. The two major functions of p53 in the normal cell cycle are as under:

- **Inhibition of mitotic activity:** p53 prevents the cell to enter G_1 phase transiently. This breathing time in the cell cycle is utilized by the cell to repair the DNA damage.
- **Promotion of apoptosis:** p53 acts together with another antioncogene, RB gene, and identifies the genes that have damaged DNA, which cannot be repaired by inbuilt system. P53 directs such cells to apoptosis by activating apoptosis and bringing the defective cells to an end by apoptosis.

A mutation in the *p53 gene* affects a cell's ability to undergo apoptosis; thus a cell with this mutation may continue to divide and develop into a tumor. Germline mutation in *p53*, influence individuals to a wide range of tumor types at an early age; this is known **as Li-Fromeni syndrome**. Infection with the human **papillomavirus** interferes with the action of p53, potentially leading to the development of **cervical cancer**.

APOPTOSIS

Apoptosis is an **enzymatic process** in which cells destined to die. The fundamental event in apoptosis is the activation of enzymes called *caspases* (so named because they are *cysteine proteases* that cleave proteins after *asp*artic residues).

In the process of apoptosis the cells' own nuclear DNA and nucleoproteins are broken down by the enzyme and then the cell is fragmented. Fragments of the apoptotic cells then break off; giving the appearance that is responsible for the name (apoptosis, Greek "dropping off" or falling off). These fragments are quickly extruded and phagocytosed without causing an inflammatory response.

The plasma membrane of the apoptotic cell remains intact, but the membrane is altered in such a way that the cell and its fragments become targets for phagocytes. In normal cells, **phosphatidylserine** is present on the inner leaflet of the plasma membrane, but in apoptotic cells this phospholipid "flips" out and is present on the **outer layer** of the membrane, where it is recognized by **macrophages**.

This facilitates prompt clearance of the dead cells before their cellular contents leaked out and which can result in inflammation. Therefore, cell death by this pathway does not produce an inflammatory reaction in the host. Thus, **apoptosis** differs from **necrosis**, which is characterized by loss of membrane integrity, enzymatic digestion of cells, leakage of cellular contents, and frequently a host reaction.

Causes of Apoptosis

- Apoptosis occurs normally in many situations, and serves to eliminate potentially harmful cells and cells that have undergone their usefulness.
- It is also a pathologic event when cells are damaged beyond repair, especially when the damage affects the cell's DNA or proteins; in these situations, the irreparably damaged cell is eliminated.

Apoptosis in Physiologic Situations

Death by apoptosis is a normal phenomenon that serves to eliminate cells that are no longer needed and to maintain a steady number of various cell populations in tissues. The programed destruction of cells is important during **embryogenesis**, including **implantation, organogenesis, developmental involution, and metamorphosis**.

Apoptosis in Pathologic Conditions

Apoptosis eliminates cells that are genetically altered or injured beyond repair without causing a severe host reaction, thus keeping the damage as limited as possible. Exposure of cells to radiation or chemotherapeutic agents induces DNA damage, and if this is too severe to be repaired it triggers apoptotic death. In these situations, elimination of the cell may be a better alternative than risking mutations in the damaged DNA, which may progress to malignant transformation.

When DNA is damaged, the **p53 protein** accumulates in cells. It first arrests the cell cycle (at the G_1 phase) to allow time for repair. However, if the damage is too extreme to be repaired successfully, p53 triggers apoptosis by stimulating synthesis of **pro-apoptotic proteins**.

When p53 is mutated or absent (as it is in certain cancers), it is incapable of inducing apoptosis, so that cells with damaged DNA are allowed to survive. In such cells, the DNA damage may result in **mutations** that lead to **neoplastic transformation**.

■ TUMOR BIOMARKERS

Many cancers are associated with abnormal production of **enzymes**, **proteins**, and **hormones** that can be measured in plasma or serum. These molecules are known as **tumor biomarkers**, which may suggest the presence of a type of cancer. Some of them are listed in **Table 28.4**.

- Tumor biomarkers can be used in a number of ways including:
  - Screening in general population
  - Differential diagnosis in symptomatic individuals
  - Clinical staging of cancer
  - Prognosis of disease
  - Evaluation of success of treatment
  - Detection of recurrence of cancer
  - Monitoring of response to therapy.
- Among these monitoring, treatments and detecting recurrence of the disease and the determination of

TABLE 28.4: Tumor markers commonly used in clinical practice.

Malignancy	Tumor marker (s)	Suggested roles
Adrenal carcinoma	• Steroids, catecholamines	• Diagnosis
Breast	• CA 15-3, CA 27.29 • ER/PR/Her-2neu	• Monitoring, recurrence • Response to therapy
Carcinoid	• 5-HIAA	• Diagnosis
Colorectal, stomach, pancreas	• CEA, CA 19-9	• Monitoring, prognosis
Chorio-carcinoma	• β-hCG	• Monitoring, prognosis, diagnosis
Germ cell tumors	• AFP, β-hCG • LDH, PLAP (Seminoma)	• Monitoring, prognosis, diagnosis • Monitoring, prognosis
Hepatoma	• AFP	• Screening, monitoring, prognosis, diagnosis
Lymphomas	• LDH • Cytogenetic alterations	• Diagnosis, prognosis • Diagnosis
Melanoma	• Tyrosinase	• Diagnosis
Myeloma	• Immunoglobulins	• Diagnosis, prognosis
Ovarian	• CA 125	• Monitoring, diagnosis, recurrence
Prostate	• PSA	• Screening, monitoring, prognosis, diagnosis
Sarcomas	• Cytogenetic alterations	• Diagnosis
Thyroid	• Thyroglobulin • Calcitonin	• Screening, monitoring • Screening, monitoring, prognosis

(AFP: alfa fetoprotein; β-hCG: beta human chorionic gonadotropin; CA: carbohydrate antigen; CEA: carcinoembryonic antigen; ER: estrogen receptor; HIAA: hydroxy indole acetic acid; LDH: lactate dehydrogenase; PLAP: placental alkaline phosphatase; PR: progesterone receptor; PSA: prostate-specific antigen)

TABLE 28.5: Some benign conditions associated with rise in tumor markers.

Marker	Associated nonmalignant conditions
Alfa fetoprotein (AFP)	Viral hepatitis, liver injury, IBD, pregnancy
β-human chorionic gonadotropin (β-hCG)	Testicular failure, marijuana smokers, pregnancy
Carcinoembryonic antigen (CEA)	Smokers, Inflammatory bowel disease, hepatitis, cirrhosis, pancreatitis, gastritis
Carbohydrate antigen (CA 125)	Peritoneal irritation, endometriosis, pelvic inflammatory disease, hepatitis, pregnancy
Prostatic acid phosphatase (PAP) Prostate-specific antigen (PSA)	Prostatitis, benign prostatic hyperplasia

the progression of disease status after the completion of initial therapy are the most useful roles for tumor markers.

- Tumor markers provide an aid to diagnosis, but only when used in conjunction with clinical and radiological evidence, often tumor biomarker concentrations may be increased in clinical conditions not associated with malignancy. Many tumor markers may be elevated in benign conditions **(Table 28.5)**. For example, carcinoembryonic antigen (CEA) is elevated in a variety of noncancerous gastrointestinal disorders, and prostate specific antigen (PSA) synthesized by prostate is elevated in prostatitis and benign prostatic hyperplasia.
- Tumor markers are of little value in screening for asymptomatic disease.
- No single marker is useful for all types of cancer or for all patients with a given type of cancer. Markers are most

often detected in advanced stages of cancer rather than early stages, when they would be more helpful.

Types of Tumor Markers

Oncofetal Oncogenes

Oncofetal antigens are proteins produced during fetal life. These proteins are present in high concentrations in the sera of fetuses and decreases to low level or disappear after birth. These proteins reappear in cancer patients because certain genes are reactivated as the result of the malignant transformation of cells, e.g., α-fetoprotein (AFP) and carcinoembryonic antigen (CEA).

Alpha-fetoproteins (AFP), carcinoembryonic antigen (CEA) have been widely used for the diagnosis of different types of cancers such as liver cancer, colorectal cancer, and pancreatic cancer. A high level of CEA can be a sign of certain types of cancers. These include cancers of the colon and rectum, prostate, ovary, lung, thyroid, or liver.

Hormones

In cancer hormones are produced by two separate routes. First, the endocrine tissue that normally produces the hormone can produce excess amounts. Second, a hormone may be produced at a distant site by a nonendocrine tissue that normally does not produce the hormone (ectopic syndrome).

Elevation of a given hormone is not diagnostic of specific tumor because a particular hormone may be produced by a variety of cancers. Several hormones that are used as tumor biomarkers are listed in **Table 28.6**.

Carbohydrate Markers

Carbohydrate tumor markers either are antigens on the tumor cell surface or secreted by tumor cells. Carbohydrate

TABLE 28.6: Hormones that are used as tumor biomarkers.

Hormone	Type of Cancer
Adrenocorticotropic hormone (ACTH): Normally produced by the corticotropic cells of the anterior pituitary	Lung (small cell)
Antidiuretic hormone (ADH): ADH helps to regulate water balance in the blood. Normally ADH is elevated in response to high blood osmolality	Lung, adrenal cortex, pancreatic, intestine
Calcitonin: Normally secreted in response to increased serum calcium to inhibit release of calcium from bone	Thyroid, lung, breast, renal, liver
Gastrin: Considered diagnostic as a tumor marker when elevated 10 times the upper limit of normal	Gastrinoma
Glucagon: Highly metastatic. Continued elevated glucose levels as glucagon produced is not under control of feedback mechanisms	Glucagonoma (islet-cell pancreatic tumor)
Human chorionic gonadotropin (hCG): Normally elevated during pregnancy	Embryonal, placenta, testicular, choriocarcinoma
Insulin: Persistent increased insulin levels even in fasting state	Insulinoma
Parathyroid hormone (PTH)	Liver, renal, breast, lung
Prolactin	Pituitary, renal, lung

TABLE 28.7: Carbohydrate tumor biomarkers.

Tumor marker	Type of cancer
CA 15-3 CA 27-29 CA 549	Breast
CA 19-9	• Colorectal • Stomach • Pancreas
CA 125	Ovarian

TABLE 28.8: Enzymes as a tumor biomarker.

Tumor marker	Type of cancer
Prostatic acid phosphatase (PAP)	Prostate
Prostate-specific antigen (PSA)	Prostate
Alkaline phosphatase	Bone metastasis.
Neuron-specific enolase	Small-cell lung carcinoma
Lactate dehydrogenase (LDH)	Germ cell tumors Lymphomas
Tyrosinase	Melanoma

markers are high molecular weight **glycoproteins**. They usually are abbreviated CA for carbohydrate antigen **(Table 28.7)**.

Enzymes

Elevated enzyme levels may signal the presence of malignance. Enzymes were used historically as tumor biomarkers before the discovery of oncofetal antigens and the introduction of monoclonal antibodies. The elevated levels of enzymes are either due to the expression of the fetal form of the enzyme or the ectopic production of enzymes.

Enzymes are present in much higher concentrations inside cells and are released into the systemic circulation as the result of tumor necrosis or a change in the membrane permeability of the cancer cells. By the time enzymes are released into the systemic circulation, the metastasis of tumors may have occurred. Most enzymes are not unique for a specific organ; therefore enzymes are most suitable as nonspecific tumor markers **(Table 28.8)**.

■ BIOCHEMICAL BASIS OF CANCER THERAPY

Many cancer treatments are available. Cancer can be treated by **surgery, chemotherapy, radiation therapy, hormonal therapy**, and **targeted therapy (including immunotherapy)**. The choice of therapy depends upon the location and grade of the tumor and the stage of the disease, as well as the general state of the patient.

Surgery and **radiation therapy** are the principal methods of treating the **primary tumor**. For many early stage cancers surgery alone has a good chance of cure. Unfortunately, many patients cannot be cured surgically.

Radiotherapy in combination cytotoxic chemotherapy has meant in such conditions.

The options of cancer therapies
❖ **Surgery:** The goal of surgery is to remove the cancer or as much of the cancer as possible.
❖ **Chemotherapy:** Chemotherapy uses drugs to kill cancer cells.
❖ **Radiation therapy:** Radiation therapy uses high-powered energy beams, such as X-rays or protons, to kill cancer cells.
❖ **Hormone therapy:** Some types of cancer are operated by body's hormones. Examples include breast cancer and prostate cancer. Removing those hormones from the body or blocking their effects may cause the cancer cells to stop growing.
❖ **Targeted drug therapy:** Targeted drug treatment focuses on specific abnormalities within cancer cells that allow them to survive.
❖ **Immunotherapy:** Immunotherapy, also known as biological therapy, uses body's immune system to fight cancer.

Biochemical Basis of Chemotherapy

Cytotoxic chemotherapy has been the main mode of **drug treatment** of cancer. Chemotherapeutic drugs are not cancer specific. These drugs not only act against specific cancer cells, but also act on the normal cells, such as bone marrow, skin, and GI tract mucosa. This action on normal cells produces undesired side effects. It kills cells by promoting apoptosis and sometimes necrosis. Different cytotoxic drugs work at different stages in the cell cycle. Chemotherapeutic drugs are classified according to their mode of action as discussed below:

1. **DNA damaging drugs**
   i. **Alkylating agents:** They act by covalently binding to DNA forming **cross-link DNA strands**, interfering with DNA synthesis and causing strand breaks. For example cyclophosphamide, busulfan, chlorambucil etc.
   ii. **Platinum compounds:** They cause interstrand cross links of DNA and are nonalkylating agents. For example, cisplatin, carboplatin, and oxaliplatin.
2. **Antimetabolites:** Antimetabolites are usually **structural analogues** of naturally occurring metabolites that interfere with normal synthesis of nucleic acids by falsely substituting purines and pyrimidines in metabolic pathways. Antimetabolites can be divided into:
   i. **Folic acid analogues**, e.g., methotrexate. This is structurally similar to folic acid and binds preferentially to **dihydrofolate reductase**, the enzyme responsible for the conversion of folic acid to tetrahydrofolate (folinic acid) active form of folic acid.
   ii. **Pyrimidine analogues**, e.g., **5-Fluorouracil**, consist of a uracil molecule with substituted fluorine atom. It acts by blocking the enzyme **thymidylate synthase**, which is essential for pyrimidine synthesis.
   iii. **Arabinosides** inhibit DNA synthesis by inhibiting **DNA polymerase**.

iv. **Purine analogues**, e.g., 6- mercaptopurine and 6-thioguanine. Purine analogues are potent inhibitors of DNA synthesis due to their direct inhibitory effect on **ribonucleotide reductase**.

3. **DNA repair inhibitor**
   i. **Epipodophyllotoxins:** These are semisynthetic derivatives of podophyllotoxin which inhibit **topoisomerase**. Topoisomerase enzymes allow unwinding and uncoiling of supercoiled DNA. **Etoposide** inhibits enzyme **topoisomerase II**. **Irinotecan** inhibits **topoisomerase I**.
   ii. **Cytotoxic antibiotics:** A group of medicines that contain chemicals which are toxic to cells, preventing their replication or growth, and so are used to treat cancer. Examples are doxorubicin, daunorubicin, dactinomycin, epirubicin, and idarubicin.

4. **Antitubulin agents**
   i. **Vinca alkaloids:** Drugs such as vincristine, vinblastine, and vinorelbine act by binding to tubulin and inhibiting microtubules formation during mitosis.
   ii. **Taxanes:** Paclitaxel and docetaxel bind to tubulin dimers and prevent their assembly into microtubules.

Biochemical Basis of Radiotherapy

Radiation delivers energy to tissues, causing **ionization** and **excitation** of atoms and molecules. The biological effect is exerted thorough the generation of single- and double-strand DNA breaks. This in turn induces apoptosis of cells through the production of short lived **free radicals** (oxygen derived free radicals) which damage proteins and membranes.

Biochemical Basis of Hormonal Therapy

The growth of some cancers can be inhibited by providing or blocking certain hormones. Common examples of hormone-sensitive tumors include certain types of **breast** and **prostate cancers**. **Estrogen** is capable of stimulating the growth of breast and endometrial cancers and **androgen** is capable of stimulating the growth of prostate cancer.

Removal of these hormones (growth factors) from the body or blocking their effects may result in **apoptosis** and that slows or stops the growth of breast and prostate cancers that use hormones to grow. In certain cancers, administration of hormone such as progestogens may be therapeutically beneficial.

Biochemical Basis of Targeted Drug Therapy

Cancer cells have changes in their genes (DNA) that make them different from normal cells. Cancer cells can grow faster than normal cells and sometimes spread. Targeted drugs target those differences that help a cancer to grow. There are many different targets on cancer cells and different drugs that target them. Some targeted drugs called **biological therapies**. Targeted drugs might:

- Stop cancer cells from dividing and growing
- Seek out cancer cells and kill them
- Encourage the immune system to attack cancer cells
- Stop cancers from growing blood vessels
- Help carry other treatments such as chemotherapy, directly to the cancer cells.

There are many different types of targeted drugs that can be grouped according to the effect they have. For example,

- **Cancer growth blockers** stop the proteins that trigger the cancer cell to divide and grow.
- **Antiangiogenic drugs** (drugs that block cancer blood vessel growth) can slow the growth of the cancer and sometimes shrink it. They stop cancers from growing blood vessels. A cancer needs a good blood supply to provide itself with food and oxygen and to remove waste products. The process of growing new blood vessels is called **angiogenesis**.
- Other groups include a particular type of drug, such as a **monoclonal antibody**. These target specific proteins on cancer cells (monoclonal antibodies are also a type of immunotherapy, discussed later).

Biochemical Basis of Immunotherapy

Immunotherapy uses our immune system to fight cancer. It works by helping the immune system to recognize and attack cancer cells. Some types of immunotherapy are also called **targeted treatments** or **biological therapies**. There are different types of immunotherapy:

- **Monoclonal antibodies (MABs):** Trigger the immune system by attaching themselves to proteins on cancer cells. This makes it easier for the cells of the immune system to find and attack the cancer cells. This process is called **antibody dependent cell mediated cytotoxicity (ADCC)**. Antibodies are found naturally in our blood and help us to fight infection. MAB therapies mimic natural antibodies, but are made in a laboratory. Monoclonal means all one type. So each MAB therapy is a lot of copies of one type of antibody.
- **Cytokines:** Cytokines are a group of proteins in the body that play an important part in enhancing the immune system. **Interferon** and **interleukin** are types of cytokines found in the body. Scientists have developed man made (recombinant proteins) versions of these to treat some types of cancer.

ASSESSMENT QUESTIONS

■ STRUCTURED LONG ESSAY QUESTIONS (SLEQs)

1. Describe carcinogens under following headings:
   i. Types
   ii. Mechanism of each type
2. Describe tumor marker under following headings:
   i. Types with examples
   ii. Clinical application

■ SHORT ESSAY QUESTIONS (SEQs)

1. What is tumor marker? Write its clinical application and give examples.
2. Write biochemical basis of chemotherapy.
3. What is meant by tumor suppressor genes? Give examples of tumor suppressor genes.
4. Define apoptosis. Write apoptosis in physiologic and pathologic conditions.
5. Describe molecular basis of cancer (carcinogenesis).

■ SHORT ANSWER QUESTIONS (SAQs)

1. Mention four tumor markers with their specific diagnostic application.
2. Enumerate carcinogens with examples.
3. Give characteristic features of cancer cells.
4. What is tumor suppressor gene? Name two examples.
5. What is Oncogenes? Name two examples with their mutated protein product.
6. What are proto-oncogenes? Enumerate mechanisms of its activation.
7. What is the antineoplastic (anticancer) effect of methotrexate.

■ MULTIPLE CHOICE QUESTIONS (MCQs)

1. **Activation of proto-oncogenes to oncogenes occurs by following mechanisms, *except*:**
   a. Promoter insertion
   b. Chromosomal translocation
   c. Gene amplification
   d. Post-translational modification
2. **All of the following statements regarding proto-oncogene are true, *except*:**
   a. They are present in normal cells
   b. They are present only in cancer cells
   c. They code for growth factors, receptors and other proteins involved in cell proliferation
   d. When they get mutated, they become oncogenes
3. **Which of the following statements regarding tumor suppressor genes are true?**
   a. Normal genes
   b. Antioncogenes

   c. Mutation of this gene causes tumor formation
   d. All of the above
4. **Regarding oncogenes which of the following are true:**
   a. When proto-oncogene get mutated they become oncogene
   b. Oncogenes are genes capable of causing cancer
   c. When oncogenes are exposed they produce mutated version of growth factors
   d. All a, b, and c are true
5. **Retinoblastoma (RB) gene is a:**
   a. Proto-oncogene
   b. Oncogene
   c. Carcinogen
   d. Antioncogene
6. **Genes capable of causing cancer are, *except*:**
   a. Mutagens
   b. Oncogenes
   c. Carcinogens
   d. Antioncogenes
7. **Which one of the following is not a tumor marker?**
   a. Alpha-fetoprotein
   b. Carcino embryonic antigen
   c. Prostatic acid phosphatase
   d. Parathormone
8. **Tumor suppressor genes are sometimes called:**
   a. Antioncogenes
   b. Proto-oncogenes
   c. Oncogenes
   d. Proximate carcinogens
9. **A normal cell can be transformed into a cancer cell by which of the following:**
   a. Ionizing radiation
   b. Mutagenic chemicals
   c. Oncogenic bacteria
   d. All of the above
10. **Proto-oncogenes are present in:**
    a. Oncoviruses
    b. Cancer cells
    c. Healthy human cells
    d. Prokaryotes
11. **Retinoblastoma can result from a mutation in:**
    a. ras proto-oncogene
    b. erbB proto-oncogene
    c. p53 gene
    d. RB1 gene
12. **RB1 gene is:**
    a. A tumor suppressor gene
    b. Oncogene
    c. Proto-oncogene
    d. Activated proto-oncogene
13. **Which of the following is an active cell death process?**
    a. Apoptosis   b. Necrosis
    c. Lysis   d. None of the above

14. **Apoptotic bodies can be recognized with the presence of these on the surface**
    a. Phosphatidyl tyrosine
    b. Phosphatidylinositol
    c. Phosphatidylcholine
    d. Phosphatidylserine

15. **Which of the following cell cannot be killed by apoptosis**
    a. Immune cells
    b. Cells with DNA damage
    c. Cancer cells
    d. Cell infected with viruses

16. **PSA is mainly used to detect**
    a. Colorectal cancer
    b. Breast cancer
    c. Liver cancer
    d. Prostate cancer

17. **p53 is *except*:**
    a. Oncogene
    b. Tumor suppressor protein
    c. Prevents the cell to enter G1 phase transiently
    d. Promote apoptosis

ANSWERS FOR MCQs

1. d	2. b	3. d	4. d	5. d
6. d	7. d	8. a	9. d	10. c
11. d	12. a	13. a	14. d	15. c
16. d	17. a			

Xenobiotics and Detoxification

Competency	Learning Objectives
BI 7.5: Describe the role of xenobiotics in disease.	1. Define biotransformation and detoxification. 2. Describe phase-I reactions of detoxification of xenobiotics. 3. Describe phase-II reactions of detoxification of xenobiotics. 4. Describe biological effects of xenobiotics and its role in disease.

OVERVIEW

We are exposed to a wide variety of foreign chemicals (*xenobiotic*); both naturally occurring compounds in plant foods, and synthetic compounds in medicine, food additives, preservatives, and environmental pollutants. These foreign compounds are known as *xenobiotic* (Greek, *xenos* "stranger"). These harmful chemical agents may enter the human body through various routes such as inhalation, ingestion, skin contact, etc. Knowledge of the metabolism of xenobiotic is essential for an understanding of pharmacology and therapeutics, toxicology, and management of disease. Many of the **xenobiotics in plant foods** have potentially beneficial effects, for example acting as **antioxidants**.

BIOTRANSFORMATION AND DETOXIFICATION

We encounter many xenobiotic that must be metabolized before being excreted. Xenobiotic can produce a variety of biological effects, including, toxicity, immunologic reactions, and cancer. In the past the metabolic processes that lead to the disposal of foreign compounds have been referred to as *detoxification* mechanisms. However, the term is not always appropriate, because the detoxified products are sometimes more toxic than the original substance. *Biotransformation* has been suggested as a preferable term.

- **Biotransformation** refers to the process by which xenobiotic (foreign) or endogenous chemicals are enzymatically modified (metabolized) to chemicals that differ in their **excretability**, **biological activity**, and **toxicity**. Normally, the biological activity of a chemical decreases during biotransformation, called **detoxication** but this is not always the case.

- The major purpose of biotransformation is to chemically modify (metabolize) poorly excretable **lipophilic** compounds to more **hydrophilic** chemicals. Biotransformation is normally not required for xenobiotics with high water solubility because of rapid excretion in urine.

- Biotransformation either produces inactive metabolites from the parent compound (detoxification, e.g., toluene metabolized to inactive hydroxyl and carboxyl metabolites), or produces active metabolites (bioactivation, e.g., benzene is oxidized to toxic quinone metabolites or methanol to formic acid).

Source of Xenobiotics

- Foreign chemicals (xenobiotics): drugs, food additives, insecticides, pollutants, etc.
- Compounds produced in the body which are to be eliminated: bilirubin, steroids, ammonia, etc.
- Compounds produced in the intestine by bacterial putrefaction and fermentation: Indole and skatole (from tryptophan), histamine (from histidine), tyramine (from tyrosine), etc.

Site of Detoxification

- Liver is the major site of detoxification. The liver plays the most important role in the biotransformation reactions. Many xenobiotics are poorly soluble in water (lipophilic), biotransformation converts them to relatively water-soluble (hydrophilic) derivatives, which may be more readily eliminated in the aqueous urine and/or bile.
- Kidney and intestines are involved to a lesser extent.
- The overall mechanism of detoxification is to increase the water solubility (polarity) of toxic products and thus facilitate their excretion from the body. For convenience the metabolism of xenobiotics is grouped into two phases:
  1. Phase-I reactions
  2. Phase-II reactions

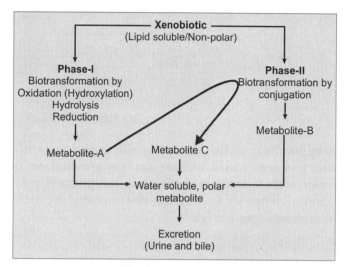

Figure 29.1: Metabolic reactions of xenobiotics.

PHASE-I: REACTIONS OF DETOXIFICATION OF XENOBIOTICS

- Phase-I reactions transform hydrophobic chemicals to more polar products. Most of the reactions of phase-I are either:
  - Oxidation (largely hydroxylation)
  - Reduction or
  - Hydrolysis
- Metabolites of phase-I reactions may be excreted without further reactions or is subsequently conjugated with conjugating agent (phase-II reaction) for excretion **(Figure 29.1)**.
- Minor reactions like **deamination, desulfuration, dealkylation, epoxidation**, etc. are also included under phase-I. However, in phase-I, the main reaction involved is **hydroxylation**.

Oxidation

A large number of foreign substances which include alcohols, aldehydes, amines, aromatic hydrocarbons, and certain drugs are destroyed in the body by oxidation.

- In phase-I the major reaction involved is **hydroxylation**, catalyzed by **cytochrome P$_{450}$** enzymes. Cytochrome P$_{450}$ enzyme absorbs light at 450 nm, when exposed to light. P stands for pigment. Cytochromes P$_{450}$ are heme containing enzymes present in microsomes (fragment of endoplasmic reticulum) of the liver.
- There are at least 57 cytochrome P$_{450}$ genes in the human genome. There are about 100 different cytochrome P$_{450}$ isoenzymes with varying degrees of specificity for different substrates.
- It catalyzes an oxidation reaction in which carbon–hydrogen (C–H) bond oxidizes into carbon–hydroxyl (C–OH) bond.
- Cytochrome P$_{450}$ needs a **molecule of oxygen (O$_2$)**, and one of the oxygen atoms is incorporated into the

xenobiotic which becomes a **hydroxyl group** and other is reduced to **water**. Hence, Cytochrome P$_{450}$ is also called **monooxygenase** or **mixed function oxidases (MFOs)**. They also called hydroxylases.

- General reaction of cytochrome P$_{450}$ is shown in **Figure 29.2** which requires coenzyme **NADPH**.
  - XH represents a wide variety of xenobiotics including drugs, carcinogens, pesticides, petroleum products, and pollutants.
  - One oxygen atom is introduced to the xenobiotic substrate (XH) to convert xenobiotic to water soluble hydroxylated xenobiotic form (X-OH). The other oxygen atom is reduced to water (H$_2$O).
  - Approximately, 50% of the drugs that are ingested in humans are metabolized by cytochrome P$_{450}$ enzyme. The **cytochrome P$_{450}$** enzymes are present in mitochondria and in microsomes.
- **Microsomal cytochrome P$_{450}$** enzymes are important for the hydroxylation of many xenobiotics such as drugs, carcinogens, and environmental agents (pollutants). Their hydroxylated products are more water soluble than their lipophilic substrates, facilitating their excretion.
- **Mitochondrial cytochrome P$_{450}$** enzymes catalyze **steroidal hydroxylation** and play important role in hormone synthesis and breakdown, cholesterol synthesis, and vitamin D metabolism.
- In addition to hydroxylation, cytochrome P$_{450}$ enzymes catalyze a wide range of reactions, for example those involving **deamination, dehalogenation, desulfuration, epoxidation, peroxygenation**, and **reduction**.

In some cases, phase-I metabolic reactions convert xenobiotics from inactive to biologically active compounds. For example, oxidation of **methanol** in phase-I metabolism, results in the production of **formic acid** a more toxic compound than methanol. Compounds which become

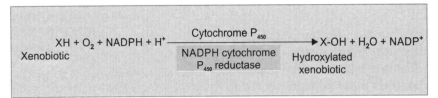

Figure 29.2: Mode of action of cytochrome P$_{450}$

more reactive in phase-I metabolism that can be conjugated with **glucuronic acid**, **sulfate**, **acetate**, **glutathione**, or **amino acids** in **phase-II metabolism**. This produces polar compounds that are water soluble and can therefore readily be excreted in urine or bile.

Various nutrients are required in order for the Phase I detoxification system to be carried out efficiently. Cytochrome P$_{450}$ reactions generate free radicals and this can cause secondary damage to cells. An adequate supply of key antioxidants is therefore essential to prevent tissue damage. Reduced glutathione, superoxide dismutase and additional nutrients such as beta carotene, vitamin E, and selenium will act as antioxidants. Other nutrient co-factors required for cytochrome P$_{450}$ reactions include riboflavin, niacin, magnesium, and iron have been shown to support Phase I of liver detoxification.

Reduction

Reduction is less common than oxidation. The major groups of compounds which are reduced and detoxified by the liver are **azo compounds** and **nitro compounds**. Some important reactions are:

- Aldehydes may be reduced to alcohol, e.g.

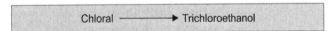

- Aromatic nitro compounds are reduced to amines, e.g.

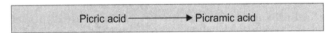

- Compounds with S-S bonds reduced to -SH, e.g.

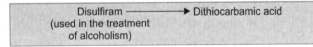

Hydrolysis

Foreign compounds that are esters, amides or glycosides are subject to hydrolysis by esterases, amidases, and glycosidases, e.g.

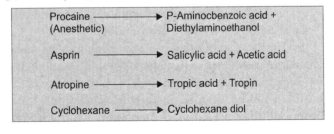

PHASE-II: REACTIONS OF DETOXIFICATION OF XENOBIOTICS

Phase II reactions involve conjugation reactions that add polar functional groups, such as glucose or sulfate to produce more polar metabolites which become more water soluble and can be readily excreted in the aqueous urine and/or bile.

In phase-II, the hydroxylated or other compounds produced in phase-I (known as intermediates) are altered further by conjugation reactions **(Figure 29.1)**. Some substances enter phase-II reactions directly without prior metabolism (phase-I reaction) but conjugation (phase II reaction) occurs more frequently subsequent to preliminary modification of the molecule by phase-I reactions (hydroxylation, reduction, and hydrolysis). There are six major **conjugation** reactions occur in phase-II:

1. Sulfate conjugation (sulfation)
2. Glucuronidation (conjugation with glucuronic acid).
3. Glutathione conjugation
4. Acetylation
5. Amino acid conjugation
6. Methylation

Each of these reactions works on specific types of intermediates. These reactions work by adding a molecule to the intermediate from phase I, making it less toxic and soluble in water. Then the final product can be flushed out of the body through the urine or the bile.

Sulfate Conjugation (Sulfation)

This is the pathway where toxins attach with sulfur-containing compounds. The sulfur donor for conjugation reactions is **phosphoadenosyl phosphosulfate (PAPS)**. This compound is called active sulfate. Sources of **PAPS** include the sulfur-bearing amino acids such as **methionine** and **cysteine**.

- **Sulfotransferase** transfers sulfate from PAPS to the alcoholic OH of the phenol, cresol, indole, skatole, steroids or to the NH$_2$ of aliphatic and aromatic amines to form various etheral sulfates. The general reaction can be represented as follows:

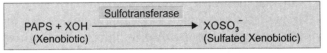

- This is the main liver detoxification reaction that neutralizes some commonly prescribed drugs such as acetaminophen (also known as Paracetamol or Tylenol), food additives, aspartame, toxins produced by intestinal bacteria, neurotransmitters, steroid hormones, certain environmental toxins, and phenolic compounds.

- Sulfation is also used to detoxify some normal body chemicals and is the main pathway for the elimination of steroid (glucocorticoids, mineralocorticoids, androgens, estrogens, and progestogens) and thyroid hormones.
- **Adrenal androgen dehydroepiandrosterone** is an endogenous example of such conjugation reaction.

- ❖ A diet low in methionine and cysteine has been shown to reduce sulfation. In some cases, sulfation can be increased by supplemental sulfate, extra amounts of sulfur-containing foods in the diet.
- ❖ Large doses of N-acetyl-cysteine (NAC) are a standard treatment for Tylenol (paracetamol or acetaminophen) overdose.
- ❖ Since sulfation is also the primary route for the elimination of neurotransmitters, dysfunction in this system may contribute to the development of some nervous system disorders.
- ❖ Many sufferers from Parkinsonism, motor neuron disease and Alzheimer's disease as well as environmental illness, tend to have a reduced ability to produce sulfate from the amino acid cysteine in their body, and instead accumulate cysteine.
- ❖ Sulfate is produced by the action of the enzyme **cysteine dioxygenase** on cysteine. This process is known as sulphoxidation.

Glucuronidation (Conjugation with Glucuronic Acid)

Glucuronidation is the combining of glucuronic acid with toxins, which requires the enzyme **UDP-glucuronyl transferase (UDPGT)**. Glucuronic acid is a metabolite of glucose formed in glucuronic acid pathway. Glucuronic acid participates in detoxification reactions as its UDP-derivative, **UDP-glucuronic acid**.

- Glucuronidation is a major inactivating pathway for a huge variety of exogenous and endogenous molecules such as pollutants, fatty acid derivatives, retinoids, bile acids, and bilirubin **(Figure 29.3)**.
- Many of the commonly prescribed drugs or medications are detoxified through this pathway. Some of them are:
  - 2-acetylaminofluorene (a carcinogen)
  - Morphine
  - Chloramphenicol
  - Salicylic acid
  - Indomethacin

- Mercaptobenzothiazole
- Dapsone
- Sulfathiazole etc.
- This pathway also helps to detoxify food additives (such as benzoates), aspartame, menthol, vanillin (synthetic vanilla), and preservatives.

Glutathione Conjugation

Glutathione (γ-glutamyl-cysteinyl-glycine) is a tripeptide composed of three amino acids, cysteine, glutamic acid, and glycine. Glutathione is available through two routes: diet and synthesis. Dietary glutathione (found in fresh fruits and vegetables, cooked fish, and meat) is absorbed well by the intestine.

- Glutathione conjugation helps to detoxify and eliminate poisons in the liver, lungs, intestines, and kidneys.
- The attachment of glutathione to toxins helps to detoxify and eliminate fat soluble toxins, especially heavy metals like mercury, cadmium, and lead. The general reaction can be represented as follows:

$$X + G\text{–}SH \xrightarrow{\text{Glutathione S-transferase}} X\text{–}S\text{–}G$$

Where,   X = Xenobiotic
         GSH = Reduced glutathione
         X–S–G = Glutathione conjugate

- Glutathione-S-transferase (GST) also detoxifies other fat soluble environmental toxins such as many solvents, herbicides, fungicides, polycyclic aromatic hydrocarbons, and lipid peroxides.
- Decreased glutathione conjugation capacity may increase toxic burden and increase **oxidative stress**.
- Glutathione-S-transferase gives protection against oxidative stress (especially by reducing hydrogen peroxide and by regenerating oxidized vitamins C and E).
- Glutathione is a very important antioxidant and anti-cancer agent in the body. Its production requires the presence of amino acids such as cysteine, glutamic acid, and glycine.
- Smoking increases the rate of utilization of glutathione, both in the detoxification of nicotine and in the neutralization of free radicals produced by the toxins in the smoke.

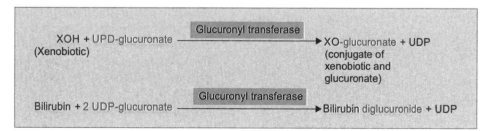

Figure 29.3: General reaction for conjugation with glucuronic acid. Conjugation reaction with bilirubin.

Acetylation

In this pathway, **acetyl Co-A** is attached to toxins to make them less harmful and easy to excrete. These reactions are catalyzed by **N-acetyltransferase** acetylation is represented by:

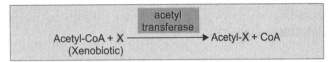

- Conjugation of toxins with acetyl-CoA is the primary method by which the body eliminates sulfa drugs. Acetylation is the chief detoxification reactions for the compounds containing aromatic amines such as histamine, serotonin, PABA, P-amino salicylic acid, aniline, isoniazid (antituberculosis drug) and procaine amide.
- N-acetyl transferase detoxifies many environmental toxins, including tobacco smoke, and exhaust fumes.

> Acetylation system appears to be especially sensitive to genetic variation, with those having a poor acetylation system being far more susceptible to sulfa drugs and other antibiotics.

Amino Acid Conjugation

The conjugation of toxins with amino acids occurs in this pathway. The amino acids commonly used in this pathway include **glycine**, **glutamine**, and **cysteine**. These amino acids help to excrete many toxic chemicals, xenobiotics from the environment.

- Many aromatic carboxylic acids are conjugated with glycine, e.g.,

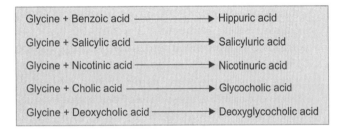

- Salicylates and benzoate are detoxified primarily through glycination. Benzoate is present in many food substances and is widely used as a food preservative.
- Toluene, the most popular industrial organic solvent, is converted by the liver into benzoate, which, like aspirin and other salicylates, must then be detoxified by conjugation with the amino acid glycine.
- A large dose of glycine is used in treating aspirin overdose.
- In normal metabolic pathway phenylacetate is conjugated with glutamine to phenylacetylglutamine.

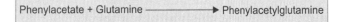

Methylation

A few xenobiotics are subjected to methylation for their excretion. Most of the methyl groups used for detoxification comes from S-adenosylmethionine (SAM). SAM is synthesized from the amino acid methionine, a process which requires the nutrients choline, vitamin B_{12}, and folic acid. The reaction is catalyzed by methyltransferase. This pathway is used to detoxify;

- Pyridine, nicotinic acid, nicotinamide, thyroxine is N-methylated
- Estrogens
- Epinephrine and norepinephrine.

STRIKE A NOTE

- ❖ Formation of bilirubin diglucuronide is a normal metabolic reaction for detoxification of bilirubin.
- ❖ Cholic acids and deoxycholic acid are conjugated with glycine to form glycocholic acid and deoxyglycocholic acid respectively are the examples of normal metabolic detoxification reactions.
- ❖ In normal metabolic pathway phenylacetate is conjugate with glutamine to phenylacetylglutamine
- ❖ In normal metabolic pathway, potentially toxic hydrogen peroxide is reduced to water by glutathione peroxidase.
- ❖ Adrenal androgen dihydro-epiandrosterone is an endogenous example of conjugation reaction by sulfation
- ❖ In cyanide poisoning sodium nitrite as nitroglycerine is given which forms methemoglobin, which has higher affinity for cyanide, pulls cyanide from cytochrome oxidase.

ROLE OF XENOBIOTICS IN DISEASE

Xenobiotics can produce a variety of biological effects, including **toxicity**, **immunological reactions** and **cancer (Figure 29.4)**.

People are exposed to xenobiotics in the environment they live. Xenobiotics disrupt **mitochondrial function** and cause **free oxygen radical** and **free nitrogen radical** formation. As ATP production decreases in mitochondrial dysfunction, free oxygen radicals, and free nitrogen radicals also increase. Decreased production of ATP causes complaints of **fatigue** and **weakness**.

- Increased production of free oxygen radicals and free nitrogen radicals damages **lipid**, **protein**, and **DNA** structure in the cell and causes **apoptosis**, **inflammation**, and **cancer**.
- Mitochondrial dysfunction plays an important role in the pathophysiology of age related chronic diseases such as metabolic syndrome; **diabetes**, **coronary artery disease**, **acute coronary syndrome**, **stroke**, **Alzheimer's disease**, **Parkinson's**, **depression** and **cancer**.
  1. Exposure to high levels of toxins depletes glutathione faster than it can be produced or absorbed from the diet. This results in increased susceptibility to

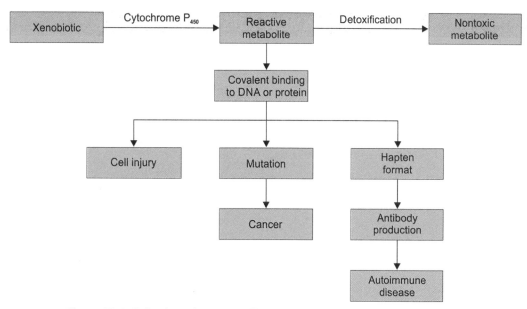

Figure 29.4: Role of xenobiotics in cell toxicity, cancer, and autoimmune diseases.

toxin-induced diseases, such as cancer, especially if phase I detoxification system is highly active.

2. Exposure to high levels of xenobiotics increases the level of **cytochrome P_{450}**. Cytochrome P_{450} could protect against certain carcinogens but enhance the **metabolic activation** of others. For example:
   - Activation of anticarcinogen, such as **indole-3-carbinol** also could act as promoters or tumor-enhancing agents.
   - Some chemicals, e.g., benzo[α]pyrene become carcinogenic after activation by cytochrome P_{450} in the endoplasmic reticulum.

3. Covalent binding of metabolites of xenobiotic to **DNA, RNA**, and **protein** can lead to **cell injury (cytotoxicity), mutation** or **autoimmune diseases**. For example:
   - In response to damage to DNA, the **DNA repair mechanisms** of the cell are activated. Activation of DNA repair mechanisms stimulates the **ADP-ribosylation** of the DNA binding protein.
   - **ADP-ribosylation** is a reversible post-translational modification process in which multiple ADP-ribose units are covalently attached to DNA binding proteins by **Poly-ADP-ribose polymerase (PARP)** enzymes.

   - The PARP transfers ADP-ribose units to proteins associated with cell signaling, DNA repair, gene regulation, and apoptosis.
   - The source of ADP-ribose is **NAD$^+$**. In this transfer reaction, the N-glycosidic bond of NAD$^+$ that links the ADP-ribose molecule and the nicotinamide group is cleaved.
   - During DNA damage or cellular stress PARPs are activated, leading to an increase **ADP-ribosylation** and a decrease in the amount of NAD$^+$ cofactor. In turn, this leads to severely impaired ATP formation and cell death.

4. The reactive metabolite of a xenobiotic may bind to a **protein**, and alters its **antigenicity**. Altered antigenicity of a protein stimulates **antibody production**. The resultant antibodies react not only with the modified protein but also with unmodified normal protein, so potentially initiating **autoimmune disease**.
   - Metabolites of a xenobiotic on its own will not stimulate antibody production, but does so when bound to a modified protein which acts as a **hapten**.
   - Hapten (a small molecule) which, when combined with a protein, can stimulate the production of antibodies.

ASSESSMENT QUESTIONS

SHORT ESSAY QUESTIONS (SEQs)

1. What is biotransformation? Describe phase II reactions.
2. Write various conjugating agents involved in biotransformation with examples.
3. Write the mechanism of oxidation of xenobiotics by cytochrome P_{450}.
4. Write the effect of xenobiotics on various diseases.

SHORT ANSWER QUESTIONS (SAQs)

1. What is biotransformation? Name different reactions for biotransformation.
2. Give four examples of detoxification by conjugation.
3. Role of cytochrome P_{450} in detoxification reactions.
4. Write detoxification reaction by conjugation with glucuronic acid.

MULTIPLE CHOICE QUESTIONS (MCQs)

1. **Toxic cyanides are conjugated with:**
   a. Cysteine
   b. Active sulfate
   c. Glucuronic acid
   d. Thiosulfate
2. **All of the following are detoxifying agents, *except*:**
   a. Glycine
   b. Glutathione
   c. Glucuronic acid
   d. Glycogen
3. **All of the following are true for cytochrome P_{450}, *except*:**
   a. Is also called mixed function oxidase
   b. Uses NADPH
   c. Associated with smooth endoplasmic reticulum
   d. Is an allosteric enzyme
4. **Biotransformation by oxidation is catalyzed by:**
   a. Cytochrome c
   b. Cytochrome aa_3
   c. Cytochrome b
   d. Cytochrome P_{450}

5. **All of the following compounds are detoxified by sulphation, *except*:**
   a. Indole
   b. Phenol
   c. Cresol
   d. Benzoic acid
6. **Phase II xenobiotic reactions include all the following, *except*:**
   a. Glucuronidation
   b. Sulfation
   c. Hydroxylation
   d. Methylation
7. **Which of the following statement is correct for glutathione, *except*:**
   a. Glutathione (GSH) can be conjugated with toxic molecules and detoxify them.
   b. Glutathione is a dipeptide derived from glutamic acid and cysteine.
   c. Glutathione helps to maintain the SH groups of certain proteins in reduced state.
   d. Glutathione involved in the transport of certain amino acids.
8. **Phase I reactions includes:**
   a. Oxidation
   b. Reduction
   c. Hydrolysis
   d. All of the above
9. **Phase I xenobiotic reactions include all the following, *except*:**
   a. Oxidation
   b. Reduction
   c. Hydroxylation
   d. Methylation
10. **Hippuric acid is:**
    a. Benzoyl glutamine
    b. Benzoyl acetate
    c. Benzoyl lactate
    d. Benzoyl glycine

ANSWERS FOR MCQs

1. d	2. d	3. d	4. d	5. d
6. c	7. b	8. d	9. d	10. d

Free Radicals and Antioxidants

Competency	Learning Objectives
BI 7.6: Describe the antioxidant defense systems in the body. **BI 7.7:** Describe the role of oxidative stress in the pathogenesis of conditions such as cancer, complications of diabetes mellitus and atherosclerosis.	1. Describe free radical, reactive oxygen species (ROS) and reactive nitrogen species (RNS). 2. Describe biological and external sources of free radical and reactive oxygen species. 3. Describe oxidative damage. 4. Describe different types of antioxidant defense systems against free radicals in the body. 5. Describe oxidative stress and effect of oxidative stress in cancer, diabetes mellitus and atherosclerosis.

OVERVIEW

Several types of reactive species are generated in the body as a result of metabolic reactions in the form of **free radicals**. These species may be either oxygen derived or nitrogen derived and called **pro-oxidants**. They attack macromolecules including protein, DNA and lipid etc., causing cellular/tissue damage. To counter their effect, the body is gifted with another category of compounds called **antioxidants**. These antioxidants are produced either endogenously or received from exogenous sources and include **enzymes, minerals** and **vitamins**.

In a healthy body, pro-oxidants and antioxidants maintain a ratio and a shift in this ratio towards pro-oxidants gives rise to **oxidative stress**. In human, antioxidant defense mechanism has developed to protect biological systems against oxidative stress. The following chapter focuses on causes, role and control of oxidative stress in the development and progression of various human diseases.

FREE RADICAL, REACTIVE OXYGEN SPECIES AND REACTIVE NITROGEN SPECIES (RNS)

Free radicals are oxygen-containing molecules that has one or more unpaired electrons, making it highly reactive with other molecules. They react quickly with nearest stable molecule to capture electron, in need to gain stability. Thus, they can initiate chain reactions by extracting an electron from a neighboring molecule to complete its own orbit.

The most important radicals are derived from **molecular oxygen** and certain oxides of nitrogen especially **nitric oxide**. These free radicals may act as signaling molecules in physiological and biochemical activities or may provide defense against invading microorganisms. Failure of these protective mechanisms may lead to pathological conditions.

- **Oxygen-derived free radicals** and related nonradical compound (H_2O_2) is referred to as **reactive oxygen species (ROS)**. Not all reactive oxygen species are free radicals, e.g., singlet oxygen and hydrogen peroxide. When 2 free radicals share their unpaired electrons, nonradical forms are created **(Figure 30.1)**. Reactive oxygen species are produced by living organisms as a result of normal cellular metabolism which are summarized in **Table 30.1**. At low-to-moderate concentrations, they function in physiological cell processes, but at high concentrations, they produce adverse changes to cell components, such as lipids, proteins, and DNA.

- **Reactive nitrogen species (RNS)** are a family of antimicrobial molecules derived from **nitric oxide ($^{\bullet}NO$)** and **superoxide ($O_2^{\bullet-}$)** produced via the enzymatic activity of inducible **nitric oxide synthase 2 (NOS2)** and **NADPH oxidase** respectively. NOS2 is expressed

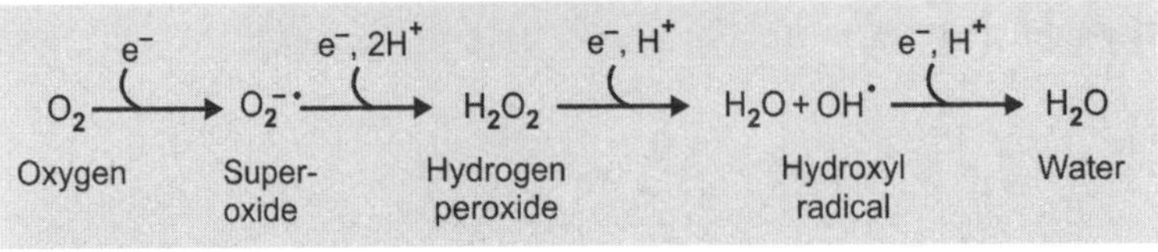

Figure 30.1: Formation of reactive intermediates from molecular oxygen.

TABLE 30.1: Major reactive oxygen species (ROS) formed during normal cellular activities.

Oxidant	Formula
Superoxide anion	$O_2^{-\bullet}$
Hydrogen peroxide	H_2O_2
Hydroxyl radical	$OH^\bullet$
Hypochlorous acid	$HOCl$
Peroxyl radicals	$ROO^\bullet$
Hydroperoxyl radical	$HOO^\bullet$

primarily in macrophages after induction by cytokines and microbial products. Reactive nitrogen species act together with reactive oxygen species to damage cells, causing nitrosative stress. Therefore, these two species are often collectively referred to as ROS/RNS.

BIOLOGICAL SOURCES AND EXTERNAL SOURCES OF FREE RADICALS AND REACTIVE OXYGEN SPECIES

Biological Sources of Free Radicals and Reactive Oxygen Species

ROS are produced from molecular oxygen as a result of normal cellular metabolism. ROS are produced during normal cellular activities, during pathological events, and during disease state. Free radical species persist for only a very short time (19^{-9}–10^{-12} seconds). The 4 major ROS that are of physiological significance are:

1. Superoxide anion ($O_2^{-\bullet}$)
2. Hydroxyl radical ($OH^\bullet$)
3. Hydrogen peroxide (H_2O_2)
4. Nitric oxide (NO)

- Various enzymatic reactions occurring in cells require oxygen. In such type of reactions free radicals are generated as byproducts. For example:
  - **Xanthine oxidase**, which catalyzes hypoxanthine to uric acid in the catabolism of purine nucleotide, generates **superoxide** during reduction of molecular oxygen (dioxygen).
  - **Cytochrome P$_{450}$ enzyme complex** found in endoplasmic reticulum and responsible for the **hydroxylation** of a wide range of endogenous and exogenous (xenobiotics) molecules, generates **superoxide** as an intermediate.

- The reactions catalyzed by **cyclooxygenase** and **lipooxygenase** (in the synthesis of prostaglandins from arachidonic acid) both lead to the formation of **hydroxyl** and **peroxyl radicals**.
- The free radical **nitric oxide** is produced in various cells in mammalian system. Nitric oxide radical is produced from **L-arginine** by **nitric oxide synthase (NOS)**.
- Nitric oxide is itself a radical, and can react with superoxide to yield **peroxynitrite**, which decomposes to form the highly reactive **hydroxyl (OH$^\bullet$) radicals**.
- Phagocytic cells, such as monocytes, macrophages, neutrophils and eosinophils form large quantities of free radical **superoxide ($^\bullet O_2^-$)** for the destruction and removal of foreign cells.

Physiological and Biochemical Significance of Free Radicals Formed by Normal Cellular Metabolism

- Nitrous oxide acts as an **intracellular signaling molecule** and performs many biological functions. It acts as a **vasodilator**, increases blood flow and lowers blood pressure.
- ROS provides **defense** against invading microorganisms:
  - Phagocytic cells, (monocytes, macrophages, neutrophils and eosinophils) form large quantities of free radical, **superoxide ($^\bullet O_2^-$)** for destruction and removal of foreign cells.
  - During the process of phagocytosis of foreign particles (such as bacteria), the phagocytic cells are activated and they rapidly increase consumption of oxygen from surrounding tissues.
  - Oxygen from surrounding tissues is consumed for the production of **superoxide** and **hydrogen peroxide**. **NADPH oxidase** located in plasma membrane, converts molecular oxygen into **superoxide**. NADPH oxidase is inactive in resting phagocytic cells, and is activated upon contact with various ligands with receptors in the plasma membrane.
  - Next superoxide is converted into **hydrogen peroxide** by **superoxide dismutase (SOD)**. In the presence of **myeloperoxidase (MPO)**, a lysosomal enzyme present within the phagolysosome, peroxide plus chloride ions are converted into **hypochlorous acid (HOCl)** that kills the bacteria. Excess H_2O_2 is either neutralized by **catalase** or by **glutathione peroxidase**
  - **Respiratory burst (oxidative burst)** is generated due to rapid release of reactive oxygen species from tissues **(Figure 30.2)**.

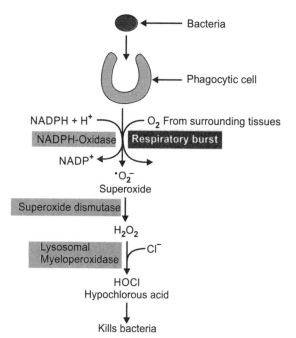

Figure 30.2: The respiratory burst during phagocytosis by neutrophil.

■ This is accompanied by metabolisms of large quantity of glucose through the **hexose monophosphate shunt** to regenerate the NADPH required for the reduction of molecular oxygen to generate superoxide.

> Genetic deficiencies of **NADPH oxidase** system cause **chronic granulomatosis**, a disease characterized by persistent and multiple infections of the skin, lungs, bone, liver and lymphocytes.

External Sources of Free Radicals and Reactive Oxygen Species

Environmental factors responsible for the generation of **harmful free radicals** are:

● **Ionizing radiation (X-rays and UV rays)** can lyse water, leading to the formation of hydroxyl radicals. These hydroperoxide species react with redox active metal ions, such as Fe and Cu, and induce oxidative stress.

● Transition **metal ions like, Cu^+, CO^+, Ni^{2+}, and Fe^{2+}** can react nonenzymatically with oxygen or hydrogen peroxide, again leading to the formation of **hydroxyl radicals**.

● **Cigarette smoke** contains many oxidants and free radicals and organic compounds, such as superoxide and nitric oxide.

● **Ozone exposure** can cause lipid peroxidation and induce influx of neutrophils into the airway epithelium. Particulate matter (mixture of solid particles and liquid droplets suspended in the air) catalyzes the reduction of oxygen.

● **Hyperoxia** refers to conditions of higher oxygen levels than normal partial pressure of oxygen in the lungs

or other body tissues. It leads to greater production of reactive oxygen and nitrogen species.

OXIDATIVE DAMAGE

Tissue damage caused by oxygen radicals is often called **oxidative damage**. Though, reactive oxygen species that is essential for normal physiology, but is also believed to accelerate the process of **aging** and to mediate **cellular degeneration in disease states**. These agents together produce highly active singlet oxygen (excited state of molecular oxygen), hydroxyl radicals (•OH), and peroxynitrite that can attack **proteins, lipids**, and **DNA**.

● The reactive intermediates which are formed during its physiological or biochemical functions usually remain tightly bound in the active sites of the enzymes, until the reaction is finished. These free radicals usually have only a transient existence in the catalytic process. But occasionally, they may escape from the active site of the enzyme and lead to a destructive effect.

● They collide another molecule and either gain or donate an electron in order to achieve stability. While doing this they generate a new radical from the molecule with which they collided, thus they can initiate a chain reactions.

Effect of Free Radicals on DNA, Proteins and Lipids

Oxygen radicals can damage to **DNA, proteins** and **lipids** in cell membranes and plasma lipoproteins and may cause **mutations, cancer, autoimmune disease, atherosclerosis** and **coronary artery disease**.

● Interaction of free radicals with bases in **DNA** can lead to chemical changes that, if not repaired, may be inherited in daughter cells. Chemical changes in DNA may leads to **mutation** and **cancer**.

● Oxidative damage to **unsaturated fatty acids** in cell membranes and **plasma lipoproteins** leads to the formation of **lipid peroxides** that can chemically modify plasma low density lipoprotein (LDL). This leads to the development of **atherosclerosis** and **coronary artery disease**.

● Chemical modification of amino acids in proteins, leads to proteins that are recognized as nonself by the immune system. The resultant antibodies will also cross react with normal tissue proteins, and thus initiating **autoimmune disease**.

ANTIOXIDANT DEFENSE SYSTEMS

Every cell that utilizes enzymes and oxygen to perform functions is exposed to oxygen free radical reactions that have the potential to cause serious damage to the cell. There are various mechanisms of protection against radical

TABLE 30.2: ROS and their antioxidants.

Reactive species	Antioxidant
Superoxide free radical ($^\bullet O_2^-$) Hydroxyl free radical (OH$^\bullet$)	Superoxide dismutase Vitamin E, β-Carotene
Hydrogen peroxide (H_2O_2)	Catalase, glutathione peroxidase
Lipid peroxides (LOO$^\bullet$)	Glutathione peroxidase
Peroxy free radical (ROO$^\bullet$)	Vitamin E and C

damage. **Antioxidants** are molecules present in cells that prevent free radical formation by donating an electron to the free radicals without becoming destabilized themselves. Antioxidants are able to trap free radicals generated by cellular metabolism or exogenous sources at different levels:

- They may prevent the initiation of chain reactions by removing free radicals
- They may scavenge free radicals generated in chain reactions, thereby interrupting the chain reaction, which prevents attack on lipids, amino acids in proteins, double bond of the polyunsaturated fatty acids, and DNA bases, avoiding formation of lesions and loss of cell integrity.
- They may remove peroxides, thereby preventing further generation of ROS.

Table 30.2 shows ROS and their antioxidants.

Types of Antioxidant Defense Systems

There are two main lines of defense against ROS **(Figure 30.3)**.
1. Enzymatic antioxidant systems also called scavenger enzymes
2. Nonenzymatic antioxidant systems.

Enzymatic Antioxidant System or Scavenger Enzymes

The major enzymes of these systems include:
- Superoxide dismutase (SOD)
- Catalase

- Glutathione peroxidase.
- Glutathione reductase

> **Superoxide Dismutase** has two isomers:
> 1. **SOD-1** is a cytosolic copper and zinc-containing enzymes
> 2. **SOD-2** is a mitochondrial manganese-containing enzyme.

- Superoxide is the primary ROS produced in a number of enzyme catalyzed reactions. A family of **superoxide dismutase** catalyze the reaction between superoxide and protons to yield oxygen and hydrogen peroxide. The hydrogen peroxide is then removed by **catalase** and various **peroxidases (Figure 30.4)**. Most enzymes that produce and require superoxide are contained in the peroxisomes, together with superoxide dismutase, catalase, and peroxidases.

- **Glutathione peroxidase** is a **selenium**-containing enzyme and can act on lipid hydroperoxides as well as H_2O_2 using glutathione (GSH) as the reducing agents. The peroxides that are formed by radical damage to lipids in membranes and plasma lipoproteins are reduced to hydroxy fatty acids by glutathione peroxidase, and the oxidised glutathione is reduced by NADPH-dependent glutathione reductase **(Figure 30.5)**.

Nonenzymatic Antioxidant System

Nonenzymatic antioxidants system includes:
1. **Vitamins:** Vitamin E, C, and A (carotenoids)
2. **Minerals:** Manganese, copper, zinc and selenium.

Vitamin Antioxidant System

- Few vitamins have antioxidant activity and help in detoxification of free radical. These vitamins are:
  - Tocopherol (vitamin E)
  - β-carotenes (vitamin A)
  - Ascorbic acid (vitamin C)

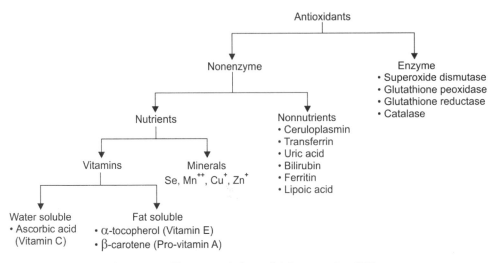

Figure 30.3: The two main lines of defense against ROS .

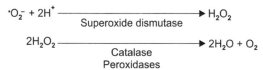

Figure 30.4: Role of enzymes as an antioxidant.

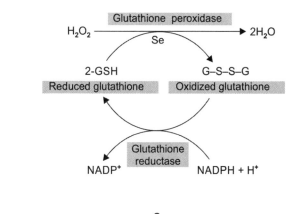

Figure 30.5: Role of glutathione as an antioxidant.

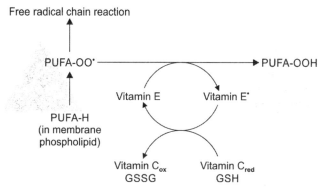

Figure 30.6: Role of vitamin E as an antioxidant.
(PUFA: polyunsaturated fatty acid in membrane phospholipid; PUFA-OO$^•$: peroxy radical of polyunsaturated fatty acid; PUFA-OOH: hydroxyperoxy radical of polyunsaturated fatty acid; vitamin E$^•$: tocopheroxyl radical; GSH: reduced glutathione; GSSG: oxidized glutathione)

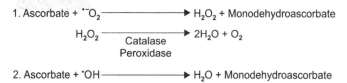

Figure 30.7: Antioxidant role of vitamin C.

- Vitamin E is as a **chain-breaking, free radical trapping** antioxidant in cell membranes and plasma membranes. It reacts with **lipid peroxide radicals** formed by peroxidation of polyunsaturated fatty acids.
- Reduced form of vitamin E (EH) can break the chain process by reacting with lipid peroxide radical and itself forming a free radical **tocopheroxy radical (E$^•$)**. The resulting vitamin E$^•$ radical is stable and relatively unreactive, as it is able to delocalize the unpaired electron within its structure and does not propagate the chain reaction. The tocopheroxyl radical persists long enough to undergo reduction back to tocopherol:

$$\underset{\substack{\text{Lipid peroxide} \\ \text{radical}}}{\text{LOO}^•} + \underset{\substack{\text{reduced} \\ \text{vitamin E}}}{\text{EH}} \longrightarrow \text{LOOH} + \underset{\substack{\text{Tocopheroxyl} \\ \text{radical}}}{\text{E}^•}$$

- The tocopheroxyl radical is reduced back to tocopherol by reaction with **vitamin C** and **carotenoids** permitting the vitamin E once more to act as an antioxidant **(Figure 30.6)**.
- Vitamin C is also able to reduce and detoxify oxygen intermediates in cells. The resultant, stable, monodehydroascorbate radical then undergoes enzymic or nonenzymic reaction to yield ascorbate and dehydroascorbate, neither of which is a radical **(Figure 30.7)**.

Minerals Antioxidant System

- The activity of the antioxidant enzymes depends on supply of minerals:
  - Manganese
  - Copper
  - Zinc
  - Selenium
- Manganese, copper and zinc are required for the activity of **superoxide dismutase**
- Selenium is required for the activity of **glutathione peroxidase**.

  Table 30.2 shows ROS and their antioxidants.

Other Antioxidants

In addition to enzymes, vitamins, and minerals, there appear to be many other compounds that have antioxidant properties. For example:
- Nonenzymatic compounds such as **ferritin, transferrin, bilirubin, ceruloplasmin**, and **uric acid, bilirubin** and **lipoic acid**.
- **Coenzyme Q10 (CoQ10, or ubiquinone)**, which is essential to energy production and can also protect the body from destructive free radicals.
- Substances in plants called **phytochemicals** are being investigated for their antioxidant activity and health-promoting potential.

OXIDATIVE STRESS AND ITS ROLE IN PATHOGENESIS

The cells produce free radicals during normal metabolic processes. However, cells also produce antioxidants that neutralize these free radicals. In general, the body is able to maintain a balance between antioxidants and free radicals.
- Chemical compounds and reactions capable of generating potential toxic reactive oxygen radicals (free radicals) can be referred to as **pro-oxidants**.

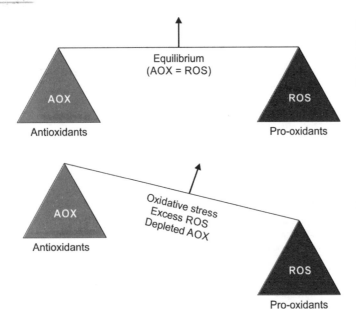

Figure 30.8: Balance between pro-oxidants and antioxidants define oxidative stress.

- On the other hand, substances and reactions those neutralize or remove free radicals by donating an electron, scavenging them, suppressing their formation or opposing their actions are **antioxidants**.

  In a normal cell, there is an appropriate **pro-oxidant (ROS): antioxidant** balance occurs **(Figure 30.8)**. This balance between antioxidants and ROS can be disturbed because of either depletion of antioxidants or accumulation of ROS due to ingestion of certain chemicals or drugs, or exposure to ionizing radiation.

Oxidative Stress

An imbalance between **oxidants** and **antioxidants** is the fundamental cause of **oxidative stress**. **Oxidative stress** is an imbalance of free radicals and antioxidants **(Figure 30.8)**, which can lead to cell and tissue damage. Several factors contribute to oxidative stress and excess free radical production. These factors can include:

- **Diet:** A person's diet is an important source of **antioxidants**. Foods such as fruits and vegetables provide many essential antioxidants in the form of vitamins and minerals that the body cannot create on its own. Cells naturally produce antioxidants is **glutathione**.
- **Lifestyle:** Healthy lifestyle and intake of generous amounts of antioxidant-rich fruits and vegetables are strongly recommended to combat oxidative stress. The neutralizing effect of antioxidants helps protect the body from oxidative stress
- **Environmental factors** such as pollution and radiation: External substances, such as cigarette smoke, pesticides, and ozone, can also cause the formation of free radicals in the body.

Effect of Oxidative Stress

The effects of oxidative stress vary and are not always harmful. For example:

- Oxidative stress that results from **physical activity** may have beneficial, regulatory effects on the body. Exercise increases free radical formation, which can cause temporary oxidative stress in the muscles. However, the free radicals formed during physical activity regulate tissue growth and stimulate the production of antioxidants.
- The body's natural **immune response** can also trigger oxidative stress temporarily. Infections and injuries trigger the body's immune response. Immune cells called macrophages produce free radicals while fighting off invading germs. These free radicals can damage healthy cells, leading to inflammation. Under normal circumstances, inflammation goes away after the immune system eliminates the infection or repairs the damaged tissue.
- However, long-term oxidative stress damages **DNA**, **proteins**, and **lipids** in cell membranes and plasma lipoproteins and leads to many **pathophysiological conditions** in the body.
- Continued oxidative stress can lead to **chronic inflammation**, which in turn could mediate most chronic diseases including **cancer**, **diabetes mellitus**, **cardiovascular disorders**, **atherosclerosis**, **neurological disorders**, and **autoimmune diseases**. Uncontrolled oxidative stress can accelerate the **aging** process. We discuss some of these conditions below:
- Free radicals can lead to DNA modifications in several ways, which involves **degradation of bases**, **single** or **double-stranded DNA breaks**, **purine, pyrimidine modifications**, and **cross-linking with proteins**. Free radical damage to DNA in germline cells in ovaries and testes can lead to heritable mutations. Free radical damage to DNA in somatic cells may lead to **cancer**.
- Chemical modification of amino acids in proteins, leads to proteins that are recognized as nonself by the immune system. The resultant antibodies will also cross-react with normal tissue proteins, and thus initiating **autoimmune disease**.
- Chemical modification in proteins or lipids in plasma low-density lipoprotein (LDL) leads to formation of abnormal LDL that is not recognized by the liver LDL receptors, and so is not cleared by the liver. The modified LDL is taken up by macrophage scavenger receptors. Lipid-engorged macrophages penetrate and accumulate under endothelium. This leads to the development of **atherosclerotic plaques**, which can block blood vessel.
- Oxidative stress causes **hypertension**. An imbalance in superoxide and nitric oxide production may account

for reduced vasodilation, which in turn can develop **hypertension**. Hypertension is often associated with metabolic abnormalities such as **dyslipidemia**, **atherosclerosis, diabetes mellitus (impaired glucose tolerance), insulin resistance**, and **obesity**.

- The effects of oxidative stress may contribute to several **neurodegenerative conditions**, such as **Alzheimer's disease** and **Parkinson's disease**. The brain is particularly vulnerable to oxidative stress because brain cells require a substantial amount of oxygen. The brain consumes 20% of the total amount of oxygen the body needs to fuel itself. Brain cells use oxygen to perform intense metabolic activities that generate free radicals.

These free radicals help support brain cell growth, neuroplasticity, and cognitive functioning.
- During oxidative stress, excess free radicals can damage brain cells and even cause cell death, which may increase the risk of **Parkinson's disease**.
- Oxidative stress also alters essential proteins, such as **amyloid-beta peptides** (a membrane protein that normally plays an essential role in neural growth and repair). Oxidative stress may modify these peptides in way that influences the accumulation of amyloid plaques in the brain and destroy nerve cells, leading to the loss of thought and memory in Alzheimer's disease. This is a key marker of Alzheimer's disease.

ASSESSMENT QUESTIONS

SHORT ESSAY QUESTIONS (SEQs)

1. Define free radicals. Write biological sources of reactive oxygen species (ROS).
2. What is oxidative damage? Describe damaging effect of ROS on biomolecules.
3. Describe the mechanism and dietary antioxidants that protect against radical damage.
4. What is oxidative stress? Write role of oxidative stress in pathogenesis.
5. Describe the mechanism enzymatic antioxidants that protect against radical damage.
6. Describe inter-relationship between antioxidant systems.
7. Write physiological and biochemical significance of free radicals

SHORT ANSWER QUESTIONS (SAQs)

1. Define antioxidant. Name any two vitamins with antioxidant property.
2. Name antioxidant enzymes, vitamins and minerals.
3. What is reactive oxygen species (ROS)? How are they formed?
4. Name enzyme reactions in which free radicals are functional products.
5. Which are the biological targets for attack by free radicals?
6. What is oxidative stress?
7. Name nutrients as antioxidants.
8. Give different ROS and their antioxidants.
9. Basic mechanism of action of antioxidant.
10. Write causes of production of external reactive oxygen species.
11. Give different ROS and their antioxidants.

MULTIPLE CHOICE QUESTIONS (MCQs)

1. **The following enzymes act as antioxidants, *except*:**
   a. Superoxide dismutase
   b. Lactate dehydrogenase
   c. Catalase
   d. Glutathione peroxidase

2. **All of the following are antioxidant nutrients, *except*:**
   a. Vitamin E
   b. Vitamin C
   c. Carotenoid and flavonoids
   d. Phylloquinone

3. **Free radicals are:**
   a. Chemical species with unpaired electron
   b. Ion having both positive and negative charge
   c. Positively charged ion
   d. Negatively charged ion

4. **The minerals function as antioxidants, *except*:**
   a. Manganese
   b. Copper
   c. Zinc
   d. Iron

5. **α-tocopherol prevents rancidity by virtue of this property:**
   a. Antioxidant
   b. Oxidant
   c. Hydrogenation
   d. Phosphorylation

6. **During respiratory burst, all the following ROS are formed, *except*:**
   a. Superoxide
   b. Hydrogen peroxide
   c. Hydroxy radical
   d. Nitric oxide

7. **The main biological target for attack by free radicals are,** *except*:
   a. PUFA   b. Protein
   c. DNA   d. Glycosaminoglycans

8. **Enzyme responsible for respiratory burst is:**
   a. NADPH-oxidase
   b. Nitric oxide synthase
   c. Glutathione peroxidase
   d. Catalase

9. **Which of the following is not generating oxygen radicals?**
   a. Action of xanthine oxidase
   b. Action of superoxide dismutase
   c. Reactions catalyzed by cyclooxygenase
   d. Ultraviolet radiation

10. **Which of the following is not the result of oxygen radical action?**
    a. Peroxidation of unsaturated fatty acids in membranes
    b. Damage to DNA

c. Oxidations of amino acids in proteins which leads to impaired transport function
d. Activation of macrophages

11. **Regarding respiratory burst, which the following is correct?**
    a. During phagocytosis NADPH oxidase leads to the production of superoxide
    b. Genetic deficiency of NADPH oxidase cause chronic granulomatosis disease
    c. Rapid consumption of the oxygen
    d. All of the above

▌ANSWERS FOR MCQs

1. b	2. d	3. a	4. d	5. a
6. d	7. d	8. a	9. b	10. d
11. d				

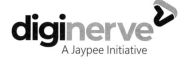
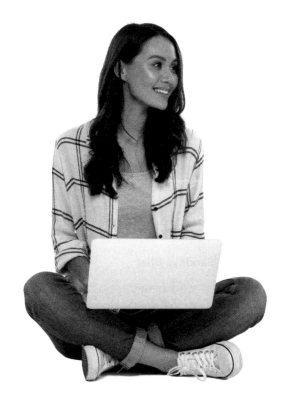

YOUR GUIDE AT EVERY STEP

Expert Knowledge Anytime, Anywhere

**SCAN QR CODE
FOR MORE DETAILS**

WHY CHOOSE US

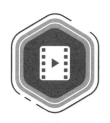

**Video
Lectures**

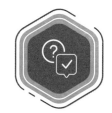

**Self-Assessment
Questions**

**Top
Faculty**

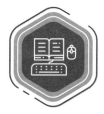

**New CBME
Curriculum**

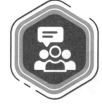

**Clinical Case
Based Approach**

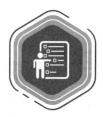

**NEET
Preparation**

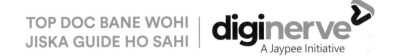
Video Lectures | Notes | Self-Assessment

UnderGrad Courses Available

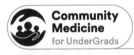

Community Medicine for UnderGrads	by Dr. Bratati Banerjee
Forensic Medicine & Toxicology for UnderGrads	by Dr. Gautam Biswas
Medicine for UnderGrads	by Dr. Archith Boloor
Microbiology for UnderGrads	by Dr. Apurba S Sastry, Dr. Sandhya Bhat & Dr. Deepashree R
OBGYN for UnderGrads	by Dr. K. Srinivas
Ophthalmology for UnderGrads	by Dr. Parul Ichhpujani & Dr. Talvir Sidhu
Orthopaedics for UnderGrads	by Dr. Vivek Pandey
Pathology for UnderGrads	by Prof. Harsh Mohan, Prof. Ramadas Nayak & Dr. Debasis Gochhait
Pediatrics for UnderGrads	by Dr. Santosh Soans & Dr. Soundarya M
Pharmacology for UnderGrads	by Dr. Sandeep Kaushal & Dr. Nirmal George
Surgery for UnderGrads	by Dr. Sriram Bhat M (SRB)

Index

Page numbers followed by *f* refer to figure and *t* refer to table